Equine Diagnostic Ultrasonography

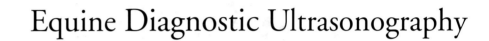

Equine
Diagnostic
Ultrasonography

EDITED BY:

NORMAN W. RANTANEN, DVM, MS

Diplomate, ACVR
Consultant in Diagnostic Ultrasound
Fallbrook, California

ANGUS O. McKINNON, BVSc, MSc

Diplomate, ACT and ABVP
Private Practice
Goulburn Valley Equine Hospital
Shepparton, Australia

Senior Research Fellow
Monash University
Victoria, Australia

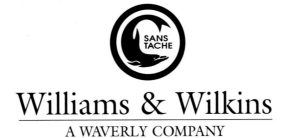

Williams & Wilkins
A WAVERLY COMPANY

BALTIMORE • PHILADELPHIA • LONDON • PARIS • BANGKOK
BUENOS AIRES • HONG KONG • MUNICH • SYDNEY • TOKYO • WROCLAW

Editor: Carroll C. Cann
Managing Editor: Paula Brown
Marketing Manager: Diane M. Harnish
Production Coordinator: Danielle Hagan
Project Editor: Kathy Gilbert
Text/Cover Designer: Dan Pfisterer
Typesetter: Maryland Composition Co., Inc.
Printer/Binder: Edwards Brothers, Inc.

Copyright © 1998 Williams & Wilkins

351 West Camden Street
Baltimore, Maryland 21201-2436 USA

Rose Tree Corporate Center
1400 North Providence Road
Building II, Suite 5025
Media, Pennsylvania 19063-2043 USA

Accurate indications, adverse reactions and dosage schedules for drugs are provided
in this book, but it is possible that they may change. The reader is urged to review the
package information data of the manufacturers of the medications mentioned.

Printed in the United States of America

First Edition,

Library of Congress Cataloging-in-Publication Data

Equine diagnostic ultrasound / edited by Norman W. Rantanen, Angus O. McKinnon.
   — 1st ed.
      p.   cm.
     Includes bibliographical references.
     ISBN 0-683-07123-8
     1. Horses—Diseases—Diagnosis.   2. Veterinary ultrasonography.
  I. Rantanen, Norman W.   II. McKinnon, A. O.
  SF951.E545   1998
  636.1'089607543—dc21
                                         97-33085
                                           CIP

*The publishers have made every effort to trace the copyright holders for borrowed mate-
rial. If they have inadvertently overlooked any, they will be pleased to make the necessary
arrangements at the first opportunity.*

To purchase additional copies of this book, call our customer service department at
(800) 638-0672 or fax orders to **(800) 447-8438.** For other book services, including
chapter reprints and large quantity sales, ask for the Special Sales department.

Canadian customers should call **(800) 665-1148,** or fax **(800) 665-0103.** For all other
calls originating outside of the United States, please call **(410) 528-4223** or fax us at
(410) 528-8550.

Visit Williams & Wilkins on the Internet: **http://www.wwilkins.com** or contact our
customer service department at **custserv@wwilkins.com**. Williams & Wilkins customer service representatives are available from 8:30 am to 6:00 pm, EST, Monday
through Friday, for telephone access.

                                        98 99 00 01 02
                        1 2 3 4 5 6 7 8 9 10

This book is dedicated to three very important people in my life: My late father, Onni M. Rantanen, self taught son of Finnish immigrants who through his hard work made it easy for me; the kindest person I've ever known. My late father-in law, Roy W. Jacobson, also self taught, and an important mentor in my life. And my wife, Marlene, partner in life, who continues as my advisor and main ally without whom I would be lost.

—NORMAN W. RANTANEN

Dedicated to those people whose untiring efforts in the field of ultrasonography have resulted in our vast body of knowledge and current equipment. Diagnostic ultrasonography has revolutionized my approach to veterinary medicine, so much so that I would not wish to practice again without it.

—ANGUS O. McKINNON

Preface

Ultrasound diagnosis has become an integral part of virtually every facet of equine medicine and surgery. This integration has preceded a complete reference text. Our aim has been to cater to that need with a text that was designed to be useful, regardless of the level of expertise. In this text the novice can begin with a discussion of the physical principles necessary to understand the technology and then rapidly advance to the chapters on normal anatomy and scanning techniques. The accomplished sonographer can use the text as a reference for the many disease conditions presented.

The material is aimed at both private and academic equine veterinarians, however in some instances, special techniques (e.g. color flow Doppler) are included to further clarify investigation of certain problems; realizing that this technology, with few exceptions, is relegated to large referral centers because of cost.

All aspects of equine sonography are covered in detail including physics, mare and stallion reproduction; abdominal and thoracic evaluation; tendon, ligament and joint examination; and ocular, endocrine and neonatal investigation. A generous use of color illustrations enhances the book. A list of ultrasound machines that are available for animal applications is provided in the appendix. Readers should realize that equipment changes from year to year, but basic types of instrument design and function are standard and are not likely to change in the near future.

This book has a special emphasis on the musculoskeletal system with comprehensive chapters on tendon and ligament injuries in performance horses. These chapters are rich in high quality figures and include numerous long term follow-up examinations. Diagnosis and technique are stressed throughout the text, however, because of the significance of tendon and ligament injuries, a multiauthored chapter on treatment methods has been included.

We are excited and also hopeful that equine sonographers will utilize this book as a reference for the many applications in horses.

The authors wish to acknowledge Carroll Cann and Susan Hunsberger, Williams and Wilkins, for their infinite patience and careful guidance throughout this lengthy process. AOM wishes to thank Aloka for their generosity in providing equipment for his use in preparing material for his chapters.

Contributor Affiliations

Gregg P. Adams, DVM, MS, PhD
Professor of Veterinary Anatomy
Department of Veterinary Anatomy
Western College of Veterinary Medicine
University of Saskatchewan
Saskatoon, Saskatchewan, Canada

Fairfield T. Bain, DVM
Diplomate, ACVIM
Diplomate, ACVP
Diplomate, ACVECC
Hagyard-Davidson-McGee
Lexington, Kentucky

Don R. Bergfelt, MS, PhD
Research Associate
Department of Animal Health and Biomedical Science
University of Wisconsin-Madison
Madison, Wisconsin

William V. Bernard, DVM
Diplomate, ACVIM
Rood and Riddle Equine Hospital
Lexington, Kentucky

David S. Biller, DVM
Diplomate, ACVR
Associate Professor, Head of Radiology
Department of Clinical Sciences
Kansas State University College of Veterinary Medicine
Manhattan, Kansas

T. L. Blanchard, DVM, MS
Diplomate, ACT
Professor of Theriogenology
Department of Large Animal Medicine and Surgery
Texas A&M College of Veterinary Medicine
College Station, Texas

Larry C. Booth, DVM, MS
Diplomate, ACVS
College of Veterinary Medicine
Iowa State University
Ames, Iowa

Larry R. Bramlage, DVM, MS
Diplomate, ACVS
Rood and Riddle Equine Hospital
Lexington, Kentucky

T. Douglas Byars, DVM
Diplomate, ACVIM
Director, Equine Medicine Hospital
Hagyard-Davidson-McGee
Lexington, Kentucky

Elaine M. Carnevale, DVM, MS, PhD
Assistant Professor
Department of Animal Science, Food and Nutrition
Southern Illinois University
Carbondale, Illinois

Nancy L. Cook, DVM
S Equine
Buellton, California

Sandra Curran, DVM, MS
Animal Health and Biomedical Sciences
University of Wisconsin
Madison, Wisconsin

Richard M. DeBowes, DVM, MS
Diplomate, ACVS
Professor of Surgery and Head
Department of Clinical Sciences
College of Veterinary Medicine
Kansas State University VMTH
Manhattan, Kansas

Jean-Marie Denoix, DVM, PhD
Maisons-Alfort
France

Sue Dyson, MA, VMB, PhD, DEO, FRCVS
Head, Equine Clinical Services
Animal Health Trust
Suffolk, England

Earl M. Gaughan, DVM
Diplomate, ACVS
Associate Professor of Surgery
Department of Clinical Sciences
Kansas State University VMTH
Manhattan, Kansas

Ronald L. Genovese, VMD
Randall Veterinary Hospital
Warrensville Heights, Ohio

Lisa J. Gift, DVM, MS
Diplomate, ACVS
Staff Surgeon
Pilchuck Veterinary Hospital
Snohomish, Washington

Brian C. Gilger, DVM, MS
Diplomate, ACVO
Assistant Professor
Department of Companion Animal
*   and Special Species Medicine*
North Carolina State University
Raleigh, North Carolina

Karon L. Hoffmann, MVSc, MRCVS, DVCS
Department of Veterinary Clinical Sciences
The University of Sydney
NSW, Australia

Gary R. Johnston, DVM, MS
Diplomate, ACVR
Department of Clinical Science
College of Veterinary Medicine
Washington State University
Pullman, Washington

Renée Léveillé, DVM
Diplomate, ACVR
College of Veterinary Medicine
The Ohio State University
Columbus, Ohio

Thomas V. Little, DVM, PhD
Diplomate, ACT
Equine Medical Associates
Lexington, Kentucky

Charles C. Love, DVM, PhD
Gainesway Farm
Lexington, Kentucky

Andrew McGladdery, BVMS, Cert. ESM, MRCVS
Beaufort Cottage Stables
High Street
Newmarket, Suffolk
United Kingdom

Angus O. McKinnon, BVSc, MSc
Diplomate, ACT
Diplomate, ABVP
Private Practice
Goulburn Valley Equine Hospital
Shepparton, Australia
Senior Research Fellow
Monash University
Victoria, Australia

Roger A. Pierson, MS, PhD
Professor of Obstetrics and Gynecology
Department of Obstetrics and Gynecology
University of Saskatchewan
Royal University Hospital
Saskatoon, Saskatchewan, Canada

Roy R. Pool, DVM, PhD
Consolidated Veterinary Diagnostic, Inc.
Sacramento, California

Raymond L. Powis, PhD
Fellow AIUM
Ultrasound Consultant
Redmond, Washington

Norman W. Rantanen, DVM, MS
Diplomate, ACVR
Consultant in Diagnostic Ultrasound
Fallbrook, California

W. Rich Redding, DVM, MS
Diplomate, ACVS
Equine Surgery and Ultrasound Diagnostic
*   Consultant*
North Carolina State University
College of Veterinary Medicine
Raleigh, North Carolina

Johanna M. Reimer, VMD
Diplomate, ACVIM
Rood & Riddle Equine Hospital
Lexington, Kentucky

Ronald D. Sande, DVM, MS, PhD
Diplomate, ACVR
Professor of Radiology
Department of Clinical Sciences
Veterinary Teaching Hospital
Washington State University
Pullman, Washington

David. G. Schmitz, DVM, MS
Diplomate, ACVIM
Associate Professor of Medicine
Department of Large Animal Medicine and Surgery
College of Veterinary Medicine
Texas A&M University
College Station, Texas

Edward L. Squires, MS, PhD
Department of Physiology
Colorado State University
Fort Collins, Colorado

Josie L. Traub-Dargatz, DVM, MS
Diplomate, ACVIM
Professor of Equine Internal Medicine
Department of Clinical Science
College of Veterinary Medicine and Biomedical Sciences
Colorado State University
Fort Collins, Colorado

Russell L. Tucker, DVM

Diplomate, ACVR
Assistant Professor of Radiology
Department of Clinical Sciences
Veterinary Teaching Hospital
Washington State University
Pullman, Washington

Dickson D. Varner, DVM, MS

Diplomate, ACT
Department of Large Animal Medicine and Surgery
Texas A&M University
College Station, Texas

David A. Wilkie, DVM, MS

Diplomate, ACVO
Associate Professor and Head Ophthalmology
Department of Veterinary Clinical Sciences
The Ohio State University
Columbus, Ohio

Robert H. Wrigley, BVSc, MS, DVR, MRCVS

Diplomate, ACVR
Associate Professor
Department of Radiological Health Sciences
College of Veterinary Medicine and Biomedical Sciences
Colorado State University
Fort Collins, Colorado

Equine Diagnostic Ultrasonography

Edited by:
Norman W. Rantanen
Angus O. McKinnon

Part I: Principles

Part II: Examination Procedures and Normal Anatomy

Part III: Reproductive Ultrasonography —The Mare

Part IV: Reproductive Ultrasonography— The Stallion

Part V: Musculoskeletal Ultrasonography

1. Ultrasound Science for the Veterinarian

RAYMOND L. POWIS

Diagnostic ultrasound no longer sits at the cutting edge of veterinary medicine. It is, in fact, well integrated into the day-to-day decisions of many practicing clinicians. These individuals are still few in number, however, and therein lies the purpose of this chapter, which is to provide a foundation of ultrasound science and instrumentation so that more interested people can embark on the road to imaging success. Fortunately, today's veterinarian does not have to rediscover most of the important ultrasonic relationships. Diagnostic ultrasound has already developed and matured in its human applications, and we can tap into this medical experience to gain an understanding of how this form of imaging can help or hinder veterinary clinical decisions.

The evolution of human diagnostic ultrasound provides three benefits for the veterinarian new to these imaging systems: (1) the large number of current manufacturers means that several machines are available with an ever-growing technology, (2) the wealth of experience in this field is all well documented in journals and books, and (3) we have a good idea about how much instrumentation an individual should know to be able to scan, produce, and, finally, interpret ultrasonic images. As it turns out, an overdose of ultrasound science seems to produce as many problems as an underdose.

Although modern ultrasonography equipment is automated to a great extent, a skilled, knowledgeable operator is still key to getting good images. Even with good image-making, interpretation requires a solid knowledge of instrumentation to determine whether a machine is telling the truth or lying. In the end, all ultrasound machines both tell the truth and lie. Success comes from separating one from the other.

The operator sits at the strategic focus of three independent forces: living tissue, ultrasound as a wave and beam, and the electronics that finally manipulate the echo signals into an image. Importantly, operators themselves can introduce variabilities as large as any resulting from these three forces.

The purpose of this discussion, then, is to provide some understanding of the interactions among the first three independent variables to make life a little easier for the fourth. The science and instrumentation that compose this chapter are not ends in themselves but only the start of a journey, a continuing process of learning as information, technology, and the full expression of animals in health and disease contribute to the body of information we call clinical ultrasound.

The first step on the road is a look at the basic nature of ultrasound.

EVENTS WITHIN THE TISSUES

Forming Waves

Ultrasound is sound, but at very high frequencies. The fact that it is sound means that the wave is mechanical and not electromagnetic. In turn, its mechanical nature means that it must have a medium to carry the waves. Wave frequencies range from 1,000,000 Hz (1 megahertz, or Mhz) to 25 Mhz. Most of the imaging systems operate in a frequency range of 2.25 Mhz to 10 Mhz, which falls into a portion of the frequency spectrum called radio frequencies (rf).

Mechanical waves appear in two forms: transverse and longitudinal. Waves traveling down a vibrating string are called *transverse waves*, because the motion of the string is transverse to the direction in which the wave energy is traveling. In contrast, sound traveling through air or water forms longitudinal waves, as the medium particles move in the same direction as the traveling energy (Fig. 1.1).

The traveling longitudinal waves form regions of compression and rarefaction. Within these regions are rapid changes in temperature and pressure, which occur so fast that the events remain localized. If we could look directly at the waves, they would form a series of repeated events. The distance from one region of compression or rarefaction to the next identical event is called a *wave length*. As the frequency of the sound increases, the wave length decreases. This relationship appears as a simple equation:

$$c = f\lambda \qquad \text{(Eq. 1.1)}$$

where c is the propagation speed of ultrasound in meters per second, f is the ultrasound frequency in Hertz, and λ is the wavelength in meters.

Because many ultrasonic properties are a function of wavelength, we are interested in a means of rapidly getting to the wavelength of any ultrasound frequency. One of the important constants in ultrasound is the average propagating velocity in soft tissue, which is 1540 meters per second. Using this value and transposing the equation to calculate λ, equation 1 becomes:

$$\lambda(mm) = \frac{1.54}{f(MHz)} \qquad \text{(Eq. 1.2)}$$

1

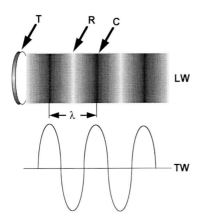

Figure 1.1. Transverse and longitudinal waves. Longitudinal waves (LW) are formed by particles moving in the same direction as the energy is moving. A transverse wave (TW) has particle motion transverse to the direction of wave propagation. C = compression; R = rarefaction; T = transducer; λ = wavelength.

where λ is in mm and the frequency is in Mhz. For example, a 3-Mhz ultrasonic wave produces a wavelength of 0.5 mm, calculated as follows using equation 1.2:

$$0.5 mm = \frac{1.54}{3.0}$$

In like manner, a 5.0-Mhz wave has a wavelength of 0.3 mm.

All waves have a common property called *superposition*; that is, waves add simply to one another to form new waves. An important property of waves is their *phase*. *Phase* really means timing, so waves in phase go through their cycles at the same time; waves out of phase go through their cycles at different times. Adding together waves that are in phase produces larger waves, sometimes with new frequencies. Adding together waves out of phase produces smaller waves. If the phase difference is exactly 180°, the two waves added together produce no wave motion, yet wave energy is still present in the space occupied by the waves (Fig. 1.2).

An important characteristic of wave superposition is that the primary waves are not lost when they form a new wave. Applying the right tool (either mathematical or electronic) to the combined wave permits us to separate out the primary waves that made the combined wave.

As noted earlier, mechanical waves need a propagating medium, but their relationship is not simple. The waves and the medium interact.

Wave and Medium Interactions

The propagating medium determines how fast the ultrasound moves, how easily the waves can be formed, and how well the traveling waves can remain moving together. The speed of energy coupling in the medium determines the propagating speed. At the same time, a measure of how easily the waves can be formed is called *acoustic impedance*.

Although diagnostic ultrasound operates within the elastic limits of the tissues, formation of compressions and rar-

efactions in tissues is not perfect. As the waves move through the tissues, they begin as organized motion with all portions of the wave moving in unison. Then, small local imperfections cause the motion to become more random. In this manner, the tissue converts the ultrasonic energy into heat (random motion). This heat production takes energy away from the waves, which is a process called *absorption*. Ultimately, tissue absorption limits how far the ultrasound can effectively penetrate into the tissues, and finally, the diagnostic effectiveness of the image.

In general, absorption increases as the distance the wave travels increases and as the frequency increases. Higher frequencies are absorbed faster than lower frequencies, producing a basic ultrasound doctrine that lower frequencies are necessary to see deeper into the tissues. But soft tissue has even more to offer.

Tissues are composed of small clusters of cells that interact with the traveling waves to produce wave *scattering*. Scattering is a process in which a small particle (or group of cells) that is smaller than a wavelength captures and re-radiates a small amount of the traveling wave energy. The re-radiated energy moves out in all directions. Scattering both removes wave energy and supplies echoes that make up a large portion of an ultrasonic image. This is the same scattering process that prevents the headlights on a car from illuminating normal distances in a fog (Fig. 1.3).

Attenuating Ultrasound

The combination of absorption and scattering accounts for most of the energy lost in a traveling ultrasonic wave. The combined effect is called *attenuation*, and because it is a function of frequency and depth, it appears in units of dB/cm per Mhz. Table 1.1 shows some typical attenuation rates.

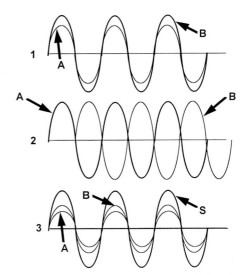

Figure 1.2. Superposition properties of waves. 1, Waves in phase (A and B) have the same events occurring at the same time. 2, Waves 180° out of phase have the same events occurring exactly opposite to one another. 3, Wave A and wave B added together simply (superposition) form the new wave S.

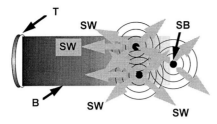

Figure 1.3. Scattering as part of absorption. As ultrasound travels through tissue, scattering bodies (SB) reflect the ultrasound in all directions (SW), reducing the energy in the ultrasound beam (B). T = transducer.

The dB is a form of comparison of quantities and also a source of some confusion. At the same time, this unit of measure is used so widely in ultrasound that knowing its meaning opens the door to understanding many of the electronic events inside the sonograph. It is also useful in reading what the ultrasound machine is doing with gain and output power levels. The dB equation comes in two delicious flavors:

$$dB = 10 Log_{10}(P_1/P_0) \qquad \text{(Eq. 1.3)}$$

where P_1 is a measured power, P_0 is a reference power, and Log_{10} is the logarithm to the base 10. The second equation appears as:

$$dB = 20 Log_{10}(V_1/V_0) \qquad \text{(Eq. 1.4)}$$

which is the same equation for a measured voltage V_1 and a reference voltage V_0. The real difference between the two is the scaling factors 10 and 20.

A logarithm is an exponent of the base number. For example, the log_{10} of 1000 (which is 10^3) is 3. Because changes in power and voltages in ultrasound are so large, the dB is a very handy way of expressing these changes.

Table 1.1.

Typical Tissue Propagation Velocities and Attenuation Rates

Tissue	Velocity (m/s)	dB/cm/Mhz
Blood	1540–1565	0.18
Fat	1476	0.63
Fat (eye)	1582	
Liver		
Normal	1585	0.94
Diseased	1570	
Kidney	1558–1572	1.0
Spleen	1570–1578	
Connective tissue	1545	
Skeletal muscle		
Longitudinal	1592	1.30
Cross-sectional	1545	3.30
Heart muscle	1568–1580	1.80
Neural tissue	1524–1540	
Bone	3406–4030	20.0
Skull	3360	
Lung	ND	41.0

ND = No data available.

Central to the dB is its role as a ratio of numbers. When someone expresses a dB value, the first question should be "Relative to what?" The reference could be an input or output voltage, current, or power. If it is a power or energy value, use equation 1.3; if it is a voltage or current value, use equation 1.4.

Despite these complex-looking equations, some uncomplicated numerical relationships can be used to keep things in perspective. For example, a 3-dB change in power is a 50% change; a 10-dB change in power is a 10-dB change.

Reflections within the Tissues

As any text on histology can attest, tissues are not uniform, and this applies as well to the local density (ρ) and the ultrasonic propagation velocity (c). As a result, ultrasonic waves are constantly encountering changes in soft tissue, changes that affect the ability of the tissue to form the sonic waves.

The impedance of the tissue in forming ultrasonic waves is expressed through the arithmetic product of these two parameters and is called the acoustic impedance.

$$Z = \rho c \qquad \text{(Eq. 1.5)}$$

When the waves encounter a change in acoustic impedance (Z), a portion of the incident wave energy reflects back. Just how much reflection occurs depends on the relative reflectivity, which in turn depends upon the change in acoustic impedance. At a reflecting interface, then, either one or both of these characteristics can change. The equation that expresses the interface reflectivity (R) is as follows:

$$R = \frac{(Z_1 - Z_2)}{(Z_1 + Z_2)} \qquad \text{(Eq. 1.6)}$$

where Z_1 and Z_2 are the two acoustic impedances on either side of the interface and R is the wave pressure reflectivity. The reflectivity increases with the difference in acoustic impedance across the interface. The greater the difference, the greater the reflection. For example, a 90% difference in impedance produces a 99% (almost total) reflection, whereas a 10% difference produces only a 5% reflection.

Although a reflection depends upon a difference in acoustical impedance, the reflected wave undergoes another change that depends on whether it sees an impedance change from low to high or high to low. A change from high to low impedance, for example, produces a reflection *in phase* with the incident wave. In contrast, an impedance change from low to high shifts the phase of the reflected wave 180°. Figure 1.4 illustrates these changes in reflection. This phase change in the reflected wave coupled with the addition of waves has important consequences that will be considered later in this discussion.

The lateral size of an interface has an effect on the reflection process as well. If an interface width is larger than a wave length, the reflection is very mirror-like; that is, the

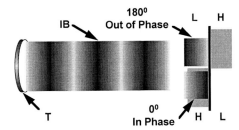

Figure 1.4. Changing phase in reflections. Changes in acoustic impedance not only cause reflections but also change the phase of the reflection. An interface changing from low impedance (L) to a high impedance (H) causes a 180° change in phase for the reflection, whereas a high (H) to low (L) impedance change does not shift the phase relative to the incident beam (IB). T = transducer.

angle of reflection is equal to the angle of incidence (Fig. 1.5). This form of reflection is called *specular reflection.* The immediate consequence of this form of reflection is that an ultrasound beam must be perpendicular to the interface for the echo to return to the transducer.

On the other hand, if the width of the interface is smaller than a wave length, the reflection follows a different set of rules called *scattering.* The scattering process requires an interaction between the reflecting particle and the ultrasonic waves. The particle simply captures a bit of the incident ultrasound and re-radiates that energy in all directions. Consequently, although the reflected energy from a scattering body is quite small, it radiates in all directions. As a result, a small portion of the scattered energy can reach the transducer, regardless of its position.

Scattering also occurs off small irregularities in a specular reflecting interface. Reflections at these tissue boundaries contain both specular and scattering reflections. In general, the best definition of boundaries comes from specular reflection, that is, when the ultrasound beam is perpendicular to the interface, but scattering defines the boundary at other times. Meanwhile, the best tissue information comes from scattering, which is largely independent of the direction in which the waves are traveling.

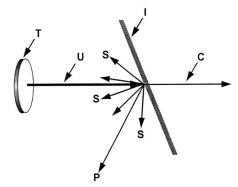

Figure 1.5. Specular and scattering reflections. Incident ultrasound (U) experiences a mirror-like principle (P) reflection at a large, specular interface (I). If the reflectivity coefficient is not 100%, a portion of the incident ultrasound continues on (C). At the same time, small surface irregularities scatter some of incident the ultrasound (S). T = transducer.

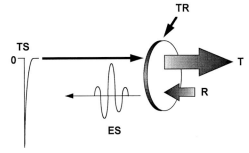

Figure 1.6. The transducer as an interface. The transducer is the point of exchange between the electrical events in the machine and the mechanical events in the tissues. ES = electronic echo signal; R = returning mechanical echo signal; T = transmitted ultrasound burst; TR = transducer; TS = transmit signal.

TRANSDUCERS AND SCANHEADS

In general, mechanical waves come from vibrating objects. In this case, the ultrasound comes from the vibration of a mechanical device called a *transducer.* As the name implies, a transducer carries pure transformation properties, changing one form of energy into another. In this case, the transformation is from electrical to mechanical energy, and mechanical back to electrical energy. These transformation capabilities of an ultrasound transducer depend on its *piezoelectric* or "pressure electric" characteristics. These include the fact that pressing on the transducer makes a voltage, and applying a voltage changes the shape of the transducer.

The transducer is an interface between two worlds (Fig. 1.6): the mechanical world of ultrasonic waves, tissues, ultrasound-tissue interactions, and energy loss; and the electronic world that represents the internal organization and signal processing of a sonograph that transforms the arriving echoes into electrical echo signals.

Producing and Receiving Ultrasound

Making ultrasound means a transducer must vibrate at an ultrasonic frequency. If a transducer is visualized as a thin material wafer (Fig. 1.7), vibration occurs along the thickness of the wafer. In turn, the thickness of the wafer determines the natural resonant frequency of the transducer. It also follows that the thinner the transducer, the higher its natural vibrating frequency.

Producing this sort of oscillation requires changing the shape of the transducer very rapidly and letting it vibrate naturally. Traditionally, a sonograph used a sharp electrical

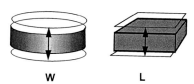

Figure 1.7. Transducer vibrational modes. Both wafer-shaped (W) and linear-shaped (L) transducers vibrate in the thickness mode. If the linear transducer is small enough laterally, it can vibrate in these directions as well, introducing additional frequencies.

pulse to excite the transducer into vibration. The voltage caused the transducer to change shape. The quick release of the stressing voltage lets the transducer vibrate at its natural resonant frequency.

The exciting voltage comes from a circuit called a *transmitter*, which sets up an automatic interdependence between the transmitter and the transducer. Many of the current machine designs have moved away from the voltage spike to one or two cycles of an alternating voltage at the natural transducer frequency. Regardless of whether the system uses a spike or an oscillating voltage, the transmitter and the system transducers have to be electronically matched to optimize the transfer of electrical energy to the transducer and to control the character of the mechanical vibration.

On the other side of events, when an ultrasonic wave travels through a transducer, an electrical voltage appears across the transducer that mimics the oscillation and character of the mechanical echo signal. This is the electrical signal the system amplifies and processes to produce an image. The transducer, however, typically receives not one wave but many waves from many different targets that add in the transducer to produce the final form of the electrical output signal. Here the simple wave summing process has an important outcome. The transducer is *phase-sensitive*, that is, it produces an electrical signal according to the sum of all the waves passing through it at any instant in time. As mentioned earlier, the phase of an echo signal depends on the change in acoustical impedance at the reflector. It is not unlikely, then, that under the right conditions, a transducer might receive waves of the same amplitude but exactly 180° out of phase, producing no electrical output. Despite the zero output, wave energy is still passing through the transducer.

This phase sensitivity of a transducer produces an image effect called *speckle* that represents the same sort of constructive and destructive interference patterns seen in a laser light. The speckle, in turn, comes from the addition of all the signals, both specular and scattering, that arrive at a transducer at any time. The separation of the returning echoes that creates the speckle depends on tissue organization. Speckle, therefore, is also a function of the scattering site organization in the tissues, contributing significantly to the textural pattern seen in the final image.

Although a transducer may be producing all sorts of ultrasound, placing the device in contact with the skin does not guarantee that ultrasound will reach the inside of the body. Any air between the transducer face and the skin surface reduces the amount of ultrasound reaching the interior of the body. As it turns out, air molecules are much farther apart than body fluids and soft tissues. In fact, they are too far apart to support an adequate transmission of ultrasound, and the space between the transducer and the body must be filled with a coupling material. The coupling works both ways, transferring sound into the body and coupling the

returning echoes back into the transducer to form the echo signals.

In human scanning, this interface is not difficult to establish. With animals, it becomes a major problem because body hair can trap air and dirt so well that ultrasound cannot penetrate. Squirting some ultrasonic gel on the hair is not good enough. Along with all the basic scanning axioms of ultrasound, none is more important for veterinary work than making sure the coupling between the transducer and an animal's skin supports an efficient transfer of ultrasound both into and out of the body.

Forming and Focusing the Ultrasound Beam

If a transducer is excited continuously, it forms an *ultrasonic beam* that extends from the transducer face into the tissue. Alternatively, when a transmitter excites a transducer into vibration for only a moment, the resulting short burst of ultrasound acts as if it were part of a beam similar to the one produced by a continuous vibration. Thus, although a pulsed ultrasound system does not strictly have a beam, it is convenient to think of it as a beam to better understand the needs and methods used to form and shape the transducer output.

To improve the ability of an imaging system to separate small adjacent structures within the tissues, the ultrasound beam requires as much focusing as possible. This focusing follows rules similar to those for focusing light with a lens. In general terms, ultrasound leaves the face of a focused transducer and advances toward a focal point, forming a focal spot, with a surrounding region of narrowness called the *focal zone* (Fig. 1.8). Outside the focal zone, the focusing is poorer, and the ability to separate structures laterally is also poorer. Clearly, the goal for any scanning problem is to place a focal zone (narrowest portion of the beam) over the anatomic region of interest. This is actually electronically possible in some of the new imaging systems.

Forming a Scanhead

Because of their small size and thinness, transducers are fragile devices. They may also receive large voltages from a transmitter, which should not be experienced by either the operator or the patient. Finally, a transducer may need to be aggressively manipulated to produce necessary images.

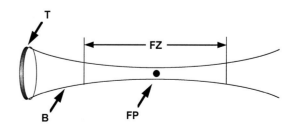

Figure 1.8. Focused beam formation. A focused beam forms a region of narrowness called a focal zone (FZ), with a central focal point (FP). B = ultrasound beam; T = transducer.

These are all good reasons for placing the transducer inside some sort of housing. This combination of housing and transducer(s) is called a *scanhead*.

A single, focused transducer has just one focal point. It may handle a moderate range of scanning problems, but it cannot handle them all. Its inflexibility limits its useful range of clinical applications. One solution to this problem is to change the transducer frequency, focal point, and range of focus by switching among several different transducers within a single scanhead. The operator simply uses a front panel switch to choose the transducer frequency and focusing needed for a particular scanning problem.

These changes can also be carried out electronically. In this case, the scanhead is made of many small, unfocused transducers that are manipulated in concert to produce, focus, and steer an ultrasound beam. Ironically, the individual elements of the scanhead are unfocused even though their collective behavior produces a focused beam. The most common forms of these multielement transducers are the linear phased array, the linear array, the curved linear array, and the annular array.

This is a good point to end this discussion on transducers temporarily and look at how to build an image, which will link transducer motion and beam production with making one-dimensional and two-dimensional images. We will return to the transducer on a more practical basis later.

FORMING A DISPLAY

Echo-Ranging Process

The fundamental events that make an image in ultrasound depend on the echo-ranging process. In turn, an echo-ranging system rests on a number of assumptions about how ultrasound behaves in tissues and an internal ability to count time after sending out a burst of ultrasonic energy. Within any echo-ranging system is an even more basic event called the *pulse-listen cycle*. Image-building and internal timing revolve around the pulse-listen cycle.

Everything begins with a relationship among distance, velocity, and time, expressed in the following simple equation:

$$d = vt \qquad \text{(Eq. 1.7)}$$

where distance is d, velocity is v, and time is t. If the velocity is constant, we can measure distance by counting time between events. In this case, the time interval starts when the system sends out a burst of ultrasonic energy that ends with the arrival of an echo. Thus, the system sends out a "pulse" and "listens" for the returning echo.

The total distance traveled by the incident ultrasound and returning echo is the sum of the distance to the target and the distance from the target back to the transducer (Fig. 1.9). The target range or distance from the transducer is the total waiting time divided by two times the velocity of propagation for ultrasound, or

$$r = \frac{vt_i}{2} \qquad \text{(Eq. 1.8)}$$

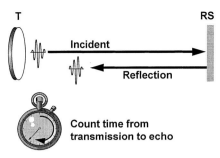

Figure 1.9. The echo-ranging process. The echo-ranging system sends out a burst of ultrasound that travels to the reflecting surface (RS). The system counts time until the reflection reaches the transducer. With a constant and known propagation velocity, the reflector range is a simple calculation from the measured time interval. T = transducer.

where r is the target range, v is the transmission velocity, and t_i is the total interval time between transmission and echo reception.

Underlying these equations are some assumptions about how the ultrasound and tissue are behaving. The first assumption is that the tissue has a uniform propagation velocity regardless of the direction in which the ultrasound is traveling. The second assumption is that ultrasound paths in and out of the tissue are straight and the same.

In essence, echo ranges are a calculation, and we could simply display them as a set of numbers representing various echo ranges for all the targets. This may be an accurate display, but it is hardly a useful format. A better way is to use a display device that shows position from the start of events and still functions like a clock. We could then position the echoes on the display according to each echo arrival time. Currently, the best technology for this sort of display is the *cathode ray tube* (CRT).

A CRT comprises an electron source, an electron beam, along with a variety of ways of moving and controlling the shape of the electron beam (Fig. 1.10). When the electron beam strikes a phosphorous surface, the phosphor emits visible light. As a result, we can see the position of the beam as a display spot, with a size proportional to the amount of

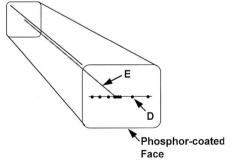

Figure 1.10. The cathode ray tube (CRT) display. The fundamental tool for displaying image information is the CRT, which moves a focused electron beam (E) over a glass phosphor-coated surface. The electron beam forms a set of dots (D) with a brightness proportional to the current in the electron beam. The electron beam has nearly zero inertia, and a controlled beam movement can be used to clock and position the returning echoes.

focus in the beam and a brightness proportional to the current in the beam. We can change or modulate the position, size, and intensity of the beam to obtain information. In this manner, the CRT can express the range and strength of the returning echo signal. Let's put things together now to form a primary display.

A-mode Display

A basic echo-ranging device (Fig. 1.11) consists of an ultrasound source and receiver (the transducer), a transmitter to excite the transducer into vibration, an internal receiver to amplify and shape the echo signals, a display to show the echoes, and a central timer to coordinate the events within the system.

The central timer coordinates two initial events: the transmitter exciting the transducer into vibration, and starting the electron beam movement at a constant rate across the CRT display. The starting point of this sweep represents the skin–transducer interface along the x-axis. To make the distances in the tissue exactly match the distances on the display, the electron beam moves at half the tissue propagation velocity. When the echo signal returns from a target, we use that signal amplitude to move the electron beam along the y-axis. The stronger the echo signal, the further the electron beam moves. This display pattern is called an *amplitude modulation,* or *A-mode,* display (Fig. 1.12).

A single pulse-listen cycle can give us the range information, but the CRT display quickly fades after a single event. In order to keep things visible, we can set up a pattern of pulse-listen cycles, with a listening time defined by how far we want to look into the tissues. If we are looking close to the skin, the listening time can be very short. Looking further into the tissues requires a longer listening time. The result is a *pulse repetition frequency* or *pulse repetition rate,* expressed as PRF or PRR. This rate can vary from as slow as 60 Hz to as fast as 16,000 Hz, or 16 kHz.

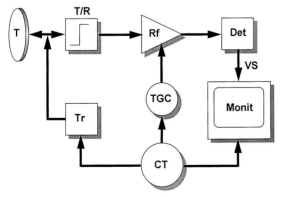

Figure 1.11. The basic echo-ranging device. An ultrasonic echo-ranging device requires a transducer (T) to make and receive ultrasound and a transmitter (Tr) to excite the transducer. The echo signals pass through the transmit-receive switch (T/R) to a receiver (Rf), then to a detector (Det), and finally to a monitor (Monit). The central timer (CT) coordinates events at the transmitter, the time gain compensation curve (TGC), and the monitor. VS = postdetection video signal.

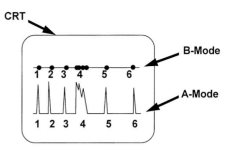

Figure 1.12. Formation and relationship of the A-mode and B-mode traces. The system forms an A-mode display by sweeping the electron beam over the cathode ray tube (CRT) face and moving the beam laterally proportionally to echo-signal amplitude. The B-mode trace has the same timed movement, but the beam forms spot with a brightness proportional to the echo-signal amplitude.

An A-mode display shows two essential qualities of the returning echoes: the echo source range and the amplitude of the echo signal, which form an A-mode trace.

B-mode Trace

Unfortunately, an A-mode display alone does not give a good picture of internal anatomy. If, however, we change the form of echo strength modulation from a y-axis movement to a beam spot intensity, we can encode the same information as before but in a new format. This change forms a brightness-modulation, or *B-mode,* display. The resulting line of dots is called a *B-mode trace* (Fig. 1.12). By forming and combining a large number of these B-mode traces, we can compose a two-dimensional picture of the internal anatomy.

So far, the display organization matches distances in the tissues to distances on the display. Although this is useful for our discussion, it lacks some reality. It would be better to scale the image down to a more efficient size. This still requires showing accurate distances into the tissues, but distances are scaled to fit the size of a smaller CRT face. Since the ultrasound average soft tissue propagation velocity is 1540 m/s, we can scale the information on the display according to time. For example, it takes 6.5×10^{-6} seconds or 6.5 microseconds to travel 1 cm into the tissue. Thus, traveling 1 cm out and back takes 13 microseconds. If we place a clock in the display circuitry that is coordinated with the CRT trace and puts up a marker every 13 microseconds, we have a way of showing 1-cm intervals on the display. With such a marker system, we can measure electronically the depth and location of structures in the tissues.

Displaying Echo Signals

We have discussed the making of both A-mode and B-mode traces. They provide information on echo-source depth and the amplitude of the returning echo, but by themselves, they offer little anatomy or information about how echo-sources may be moving over time.

An early and effective form of display based on the B-mode trace is the *time-motion* (or *motion-modulation)* display, known also as *TM* (or *M-mode)* display.

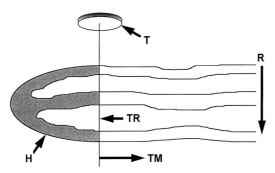

Figure 1.13. Forming an M-mode display. An M-mode display shows reflector motion along the beam axis. A B-mode trace (TR) sweeps across the display (TM) showing the reflector (R) motion. It is commonly used to show heart (H) motion. T = transducer.

Forming an M-mode display requires producing a B-mode trace in the y-axis and moving it along the x-axis as a function of time (Fig. 1.13). As the trace moves, echosource movements become easy to identify and even quantitate. This display form is an accurate means of measuring heart dimensions and detailing heart valve motion and other structures. It remains a central part of all echocardiograms.

Making a two-dimensional image requires using the B-mode trace and moving it again, but this time, the motion is linked to the position of the ultrasound beam in space (Fig. 1.14). If the ultrasound beam motion follows a sector pattern, the B-mode trace mimics this motion on the display. If the motion is linear, the B-mode trace is also linear. The image that appears on a typical scanning display, then, is the composite of many B-mode traces collected together on the CRT at the same time.

Each line of sight in the image comes from a single pulse-listen cycle. One complete image with all the lines of sight on display is called an *image frame*. The number of lines of sight that make the image frame varies greatly, depending on design and diagnostic endpoints. The number of lines can range from 100 to 512 per frame. The number of frames formed each second (fps) is called the system *frame rate*, which can vary from less than one per second to as high as 30 fps. The slow rates are used for soft tissue imaging, whereas high rates are used for echocardiography.

DISPLAY PATTERNS AND TRANSDUCER MOVEMENT

In general, the movement pattern of an ultrasound beam defines the shape of the display: linear motion makes a linear display; sector motion makes sector displays.

In turn, the means of moving ultrasound beams comes in two forms: mechanical and electronic. Mechanical systems rely either on wobbling a single transducer in a sector pattern (called a wobbler) or moving several different transducers mounted in a common rotating cylinder (called a rotating scanhead) (Fig. 1.15).

In contrast, electronic scanners move the beam electronically, employing no mechanical parts. These devices include linear phased arrays, linear arrays, and curved linear arrays (Fig. 1.16). A hybrid system that combines both electronic and mechanical components is the annular array, which uses an electronic means to focus the ultrasound beam but a mechanical system to move the resulting ultrasound beam.

In general, mechanical systems usually form a sector scanning pattern, except for some unusual scanners that move the transducer on a linear track. Linear phased arrays can also form a sector scanning pattern, whereas curved arrays form a truncated sector (Fig. 1.16). Finally, linear arrays focus the beam using the same techniques as linear phased arrays, but the beams remain perpendicular to the arrays to form a rectangular scanning pattern.

SIGNAL PROCESSING ORGANIZATION

All of the current imaging devices are based on an echo-ranging process that places restrictions on the internal design of the sonograph. The fundamental echo-ranger we

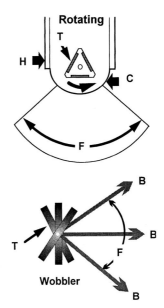

Figure 1.15. Mechanical beam motion. Mechanical scanning uses two basic techniques. The rotating system depends on mounting several transducers (T) in a moving cylinder, inside a casing (C). A wobbler rocks a single transducer (T) to form a sector scanning field (F). H = handle.

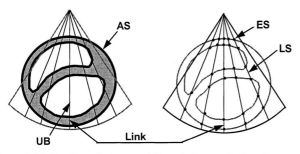

Figure 1.14. The B-mode trace and B-mode image. As the ultrasound beams (UB) move over the anatomic surface (AS), a matching B-mode trace appears on the display with the same position and angle as the beam, locating the echo signals (ES) along each line of sight (LS).

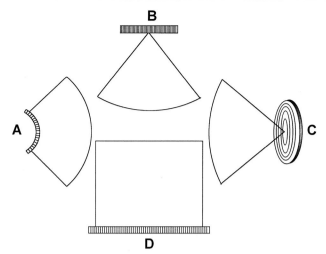

Figure 1.16. Electronic beam motion. Electronic transducers use many separate elements phased together to form and sometimes steer the ultrasound beam. The curved linear array (A) uses a mechanical curve to produce a truncated sector field. The linear phased array (B) electronically focuses and steers the beams to form a sector field. The annular array (C) uses its elements to focus the beam but uses a wobble to form the scanning field. The linear array (D) uses phasing to focus the beam and switches this control down the linear array to form the rectangular scanning field.

examined earlier divides further into specific signal processing steps (Fig. 1.17). Some of these steps may involve the use of digital techniques or local computer control, but the descriptive function remains the same.

Transmitter

The transmitter delivers the excitation voltage to the transducer, which causes a mechanical transducer vibration. The

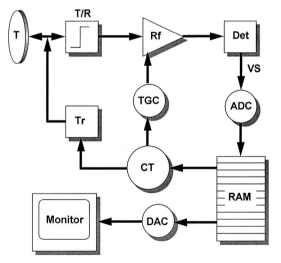

Figure 1.17. The digital echo-ranging sonogram. The timing arrangements for this organization are the same as those shown in Figure 1.11. The digital segments are expanded to show the role of the digital scan converter. After conversion and processing, the video signals (VS) go to the monitor. ADC = analog-to-digital converter; CT = central timer; DAC = the digital-to-analog converter; Det = detector; RAM = random access memory; Rf = receiver; T = transducer; TGC = time gain compensation control; T/R = transmit-receive switch; Tr = transmitter.

voltages can vary from 10 or 20 volts to several hundred, delivered as a spike or as a short oscillating voltage, typically lasting 1 to 2 μseconds. The transducer functions as both a mechanical vibrator and an electrical circuit element that must match the transmitter electronically. Each manufacturer uses a different set of parameters to match the transmitter to the transducer, ensuring problems for a user unwise enough to mix transducers from one manufacturer with the machine of another. When many of the transducers had similar connectors, this confusion could happen. Scanhead connectors are now so unique for each manufacturer that a transducer-machine crossover has little chance of happening.

Once the burst of transmitted ultrasound leaves the transducer, the system listens for the returning echoes on the same transducer. The transmit-receive switch makes dual use of the same transducer possible.

Transmit-Receive Switch

Most systems operate with a single transducer assembly to make and receive ultrasound. This arrangement requires placing a high voltage on the transducer during transmission while still being able to handle the much smaller voltages coming from the transducer during the receive portion of the cycle. Significantly, the system receiver is designed to accept only the small voltages that represent the echo signals, ranging from 1 volt to a few microvolts. The transmit-receive (TR) switch protects the receiver during transmission then passes the much smaller echo signals on to the receiver during the receiving portion of the pulse-listen cycle.

In the end, the TR switch does more than just protect the receiver. It also imposes a window on the echo signals (Fig. 1.18) that can reach the receiver, defining both the largest and smallest electrical signal the receiver can see. This window sets the *input signal dynamic range*, which determines how far the system can see into the tissues. The

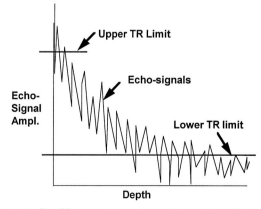

Figure 1.18. The TR (transmit-receive) switch window. Echo signals from the transducer fall off at an exponential rate from near the transducer to the distant portions of the image. The TR switch sets the upper and lower limit of the echo signals that can reach the receiver, and as a consequence, sets the penetration limit of the sonogram.

output power control on the front panel controls the range of echo signals that enter the input dynamic range window, which sets up the relationship between the system output power and how far the system can see into the tissues. From the TR switch, echo signals go to the radio frequency (rf) receiver.

RF Receiver

The system receiver is a radio frequency (rf) amplifier, capable of amplifying electrical signals within the rf spectrum. It accepts and amplifies the signals that pass through the TR switch. If an ultrasound system operates between 2.25 and 10 Mhz, the receiver must be able to handle more than just these frequencies. A typical ultrasound receiver provides 40 to 90 dB of amplification or *gain*, representing an increase in voltage of 100 to 30,000 times the input signal amplitude, respectively. Usually the front panel *gain* or *system gain* control sets the amount of receiver amplification in this portion of the system.

In addition, the amplifying behavior of the receiver is not constant. It is modified by another controlling voltage that changes the gain of the amplifier as a function of time. The operator uses this controlling voltage to shape the way the receiver gain changes over time to match the tissue imaging conditions. This process is called *time gain compensation* (TGC) or *depth gain compensation* (DGC). It provides two important signal processes: first, it decreases the range of echo signals that go on to the next signal processing stage; second, it compensates for the tissue-based attenuation.

Applying Time Gain Compensation

As we found earlier, the tissue attenuation process changes the echo signal strength as a function of depth. This means that a reflector close to the transducer has a larger echo signal than the same reflector deeper in the tissues. Clearly, to portray a segment of soft tissue as having uniform reflectivity, the same reflectors need to have the same echo signal amplitudes regardless of depth. We can achieve this by changing the receiver gain, decreasing it for close signals and steadily increasing its gain as echo signals arrive from the deeper tissues. If the system produces a gain increase that just matches the rate at which the echo signals decrease (Fig. 1.19), like reflectors will not only look alike, but unlike reflectors will look different.

Setting the TGC function is the "art" part of the imaging process. An incorrectly set TGC can either introduce noise into an image, which can mask information, or remove important clinical information from the image. Setting up the TGC curve requires having some landmarks, namely, the initial gain, TGC slope, TGC knee, and final gain.

The TGC function is set to ensure the delivery of both large and small signals to the display, all of which convey image information. This requires setting the initial gain to

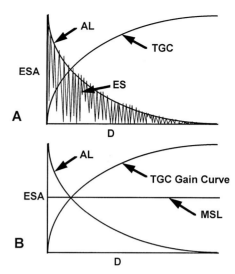

Figure 1.19. Application of time gain compensation control (TGC). A, The uncompensated echo signals (ES) follow an exponential attenuation line (AL). Balancing things out requires applying a TGC with a curve that mirrors the attenuation line. B, The result of a correct TGC is that all the like signals (maximum signal line, or MSL) appear at the same amplitude. D = image depth; ESA = echo signal amplitude.

handle the strong echoes in the near portions of the image and the TGC slope to match the tissue attenuation rate. This also means that often the compensation (slope) does not extend over the full image depth. When the TGC is correctly set, like reflectors can be expected to look alike over the TGC slope but not beyond the TGC knee.

TGC adjustments come in two primary forms: segmented and curve-adjusted (Fig. 1.20). Segmented TGC divides the image depth into segments and provides a separate con-

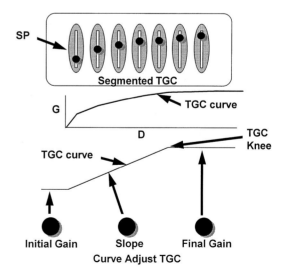

Figure 1.20. Time gain compensation control (TGC) can be adjusted using either a segmented system or curve adjust technique. The segmented system uses sliding potentiometers (SP) to control a portion of the TGC. The resulting curve is shown below the segments; G = gain; D = depth. The curve adjust technique controls the initial gain, the slope of the TGC, and the final gain. The slope should closely match the attenuation rate, and the region of compensation extends from the start of the slope to the TGC knee.

trol for each segment. Typically, sliding potentiometers provide the individual controls. In contrast, a curve-adjusted TGC usually has three controls: an initial gain, a slope, and an overall gain control. Some of the simpler systems have a fixed curve that is adjustable as near-field and far-field gain. Regardless of the control style, however, the imaging goal is to make like reflectors look alike so unlike reflectors look different. From the rf amplifier, the compensated echo signals go to the detector.

Detecting Echo Signals

After echo signals are compressed and compensated by TGC, they are *demodulated* or *detected*. This process removes the rf information and leaves just the shape of the original echo signal envelope (Fig. 1.21). This extraction occurs first through *rectification* and then through *filtering* of the rf signals. The detector not only removes the rf but also shapes the echo signals to provide a desired image quality. Some sonographs have a "sharpening" control that makes the leading edge of the echo signals steeper to help improve image sharpness.

The signals emerging from the detection process are called *video signals* not because they go to a video display but because of the range of frequencies they cover. These signals represent the reflecting interfaces within the tissues, from the largest to the smallest. These signals span what is called the *video dynamic range*, which can take on values from 30 to 60 dB (amplitude ratios of 31:1 to 1000:1), depending upon the system and dynamic range control settings. Importantly, the dynamic range control on most sonographs changes only the video dynamic range. From here, the echo signals move on to the digital scan converter.

DIGITAL SCAN CONVERTER

The digital scan converter (DSC) was the seat of a major technologic revolution in ultrasound. When ultrasound went "digital," this was where it began. Scan converters, as the name implies, change one form of scanning into another. In this case, it converts the scanning rate (movement and sampling) of the transducer or scanhead into a standard

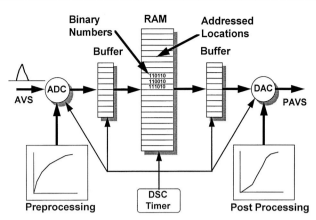

Figure 1.22. Detailed digital scan converter. The digital scan converter (DSC) first converts the analog video signal (AVS) into binary numbers at the analog-to-digital converter (ADC). It is temporarily stored in a buffer, then moves to the random access memory (RAM). Preprocessing controls the conversion rules from analog-to-digital signals. Coming out of the RAM, the signals go again through a buffer and finally into a digital to analog converter (DAC) to produce the processed analog video signal (PAVS). The final conversion rules are expressed in the postprocessing curves. The DSC timer coordinates all events, including the system pulse repetition frequency (PRF).

video format suitable for existing video technologies. It does this by accepting information at the transducer scanning rate and storing it in a digital memory, then scanning out of that memory at a conventional television format. Because the detected echo signals are analog, they must first be converted into a digital format (Fig. 1.22), then stored digitally, recovered digitally, and finally converted back into analog signals suitable for the monitor electronics.

Because the timing requirements in the scan converter are so rigid, the coordination of all timing within the sonograph for the PRF comes from the DSC.

Analog-to-Digital Conversion

The scan converter's memory accepts only digital signals, so an analog-to-digital (ADC) converter makes the first signal change. Unlike analog signals, digital signals take on discrete, specific values. For example, an analog video signal can take on any value within the operating limits of the video dynamic range. Digital signals, however, take on discrete numerical values over a range equivalent to the video dynamic range.

The digital numerical code is binary, that is, based on the number 2. The available digital values are expressed in terms of bits, where each bit can take on values of 0 or 1. Thus, an ADC with 4 bits available, can take on 2^4 or 16 values. In like manner, a 6-bit or an 8-bit system can have 2^6 or 64 values and 2^8 or 256 values, respectively. Each digital value can be a separate gray scale intensity; thus a 16-value system has 16 grays, a 64 value system 64 grays, and so on. As it turns out, the number of grays in an image influences its perceived smoothness, its ability to separate one gray level from another, and the overall image texture.

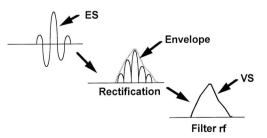

Figure 1.21. Echo signal detection. The envelope of the echo signal (ES) forms the final signal for display. First the ES is rectified then the receiver (rf) is filtered out to leave just the envelope to express the video signal (VS).

Preprocessing

As noted earlier, analog signals have an indefinite set of values and digital signals have a finite set. Converting one to the other requires some rules, and these rules are called *preprocessing*. The "pre" comes from its position, before the memory. All digital systems have preprocessing, but the rules within that preprocessing can vary greatly from one system to another. Some sonographs have fixed preprocessing curves, and others permit changes to be made in the preprocessing curves with a front panel control.

As the number of available gray levels decreases, the preprocessing curve plays an increasingly important role in overall image quality. Nonlinear preprocessing curves (Fig. 1.23) permit enhancing of the differences among gray levels for low, medium, and high amplitude signals. Many of the sonographs with large video dynamic ranges and high quality displays simply make the conversion log-linear, that is, dividing the dynamic range of the echo signals expressed in dB into digital intervals of equal size. Clearly, preprocessing works only on images entering the memory (and therefore in the real time format); it does not work on images already stored in the memory.

Storing Data in the Digital Scan Converter

The digital memory is a random access memory (RAM); that is, we can store and retrieve information in a random manner. That means a system can store information in one format and retrieve it using another. RAM is a set of addressed memory locations that can accept data in any sequence. The number of bits stored in each memory location usually matches the ADC; that is, a 6-bit RAM matches a 6-bit ADC. Each of these memory locations is mapped to a fixed location on the CRT display called a *picture element* or *pixel* (Fig. 1.24). Each pixel can take on only one gray value at a time, according to the number stored at the corresponding memory locations.

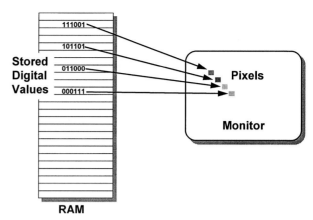

Figure 1.24. Memory mapping to the display. Each addressed memory location in the random access memory (RAM) represents a fixed pixel on the display screen, with a gray scale value that corresponds to the stored digital value in the RAM.

The digital format provides a stable, reproducible gray scale display. It permits not only real time imaging with a constantly renewing image but also a stable frozen image suitable for photography, which were the key reasons for moving to the DSC in the first place.

Converting Digital Signals to Analog Signals

Coming out of the RAM, digital signals are in the right sequence to produce the image but need to be converted back to analog voltages for the monitor. The digital-to-analog converter (DAC) provides this conversion. The conversion changes the format of the signals but not the content of the signals. Although the analog signals can assume any value between limits, their digital origin limits the analog signals to discrete values, producing a digital appearing display. Similar to the first conversion, this one has a set of rules also.

Postprocessing

Postprocessing is another set of rules that connect the digital values in the RAM to the voltages that drive the CRT display. The "post" comes from its location after the RAM storage. Because it is after the RAM, it works on both real time and static frozen images. If the monitor has a color capability, the assignments can produce pseudo-color images, also called color B-mode images.

The assignments can be linear or nonlinear, enhancing the presentation of echo signals in the low, medium, or high amplitude ranges (Fig. 1.25). The assignments can also affect the smoothness of the image.

Delivering Data to the Display

The CRT has its own influence on the appearance of the final image. Color monitors, for example, use three different electron beams and three different phosphors to produce the three primary colors (red, green, and blue, hence the RGB monitor). Combining the three colors produces

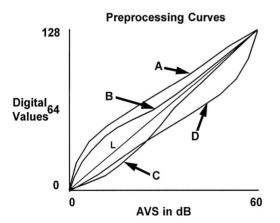

Figure 1.23. Preprocessing curves. The preprocessing curves set the rules for converting analog signals into binary numbers. The log-linear conversion (L) is a simple division of the analog video signal (AVS) into equal decibel steps. Curve A elevates all values, B emphasizes the low-range signals, C depresses the low-range signals, and D depresses over nearly the whole signal range.

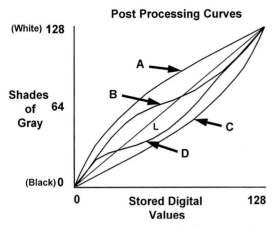

Figure 1.25. Postprocessing curves. The digital system produces discrete analog values at the digital scan converter output. Mapping the stored values into shades of gray is the postprocessing function. A enhances all signals toward white; B enhances just the lower signals; C depresses all signals; and D elevates the smaller signals and depresses the larger signals. L = log-linear relationship.

the many colors that are possible on the contemporary color display. In general, color monitors do not produce the same crispness in an image that single phosphor, monochromatic monitors produce. This technology is changing, however, and even by the time this manuscript is printed, color monitors may be comparable to single phosphor monitors.

DOPPLER AND DUPLEX TECHNOLOGY

One of the major improvements beyond the basic diagnostic imaging is the addition of Doppler signal processing. This technology comes in a variety of forms, from the basic hand-held continuous wave system to the latest in color flow imaging, all of which are dedicated to looking at blood flow events. All of these technologies are based on the Doppler effect, with its basic rules expressed through the Doppler equation.

The combining of continuous wave or pulsed Doppler with basic gray scale imaging is called *duplex imaging*, which is used for examining both vascular and cardiac blood flow events.

The targets for a Doppler system are the moving red blood cells (RBCs) within the cardiovascular system. In fact, the echo sources are not individual RBCs but clusters of RBCs functioning as scattering units, and within the ultrasound beam are many scattering units returning many echoes at any time that sum together to form a composite signal.

Doppler Effect

Echoes arising from stationary reflectors produce echoes with the same frequency as the incident waves. When the reflectors are in motion, however, the echo wave frequency changes. The amount of change depends on the amount of motion and the direction of this motion relative to the receiving transducer. This is the same effect that produces

the changing tone of a car horn as the car passes by. Locked within this change in frequency is information about the direction and character of the motion.

Doppler Equation

The Doppler equation expresses the relationship among the various factors that influence the changes in frequency. The Doppler equation appears as follows:

$$\Delta f = \frac{2F_o V Cos\theta}{c} \qquad \text{(Eq. 1.9)}$$

where Δf is the Doppler shift frequency, F_o is the unaltered carrier frequency, V is the speed of the target, θ is the Doppler angle, and c is the propagation velocity of ultrasound within the tissues.

The typical combination of events with biologic tissues places the Doppler shift frequencies within the human audio range. As a result, the first Doppler analysis tool was simply listening to the Doppler sounds. Even with the more sophisticated analytical tools now available, listening to the sequence of Doppler sounds is still valuable.

Continuous Wave Doppler

The basic Doppler device is the continuous wave (CW) Doppler. These are widely used clinical tools in human medicine and are valuable here to give a perspective on Doppler instrumentation. Figure 1.26 shows the basic CW Doppler organization.

A CW system transmits and receives continuously using two separate transducers next to one another in a common housing. A transmitter sends a continuous sine wave at frequency F_o to the transmitting transducer. The receiving transducer continuously receives the echoes, transforming them into a continuous electrical signal. The system then

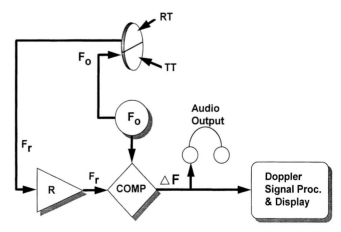

Figure 1.26. Basic continuous wave (CW) Doppler system. The CW Doppler is on continuously and compares the transmitted signal (F_o) with the received signal (F_r). The difference (ΔF) reveals the Doppler shift frequencies. The Doppler shift frequencies can be listened to or processed electronically for frequency components. RT = receive transducer; TT = transmit transducer; COMP = frequency comparator.

compares the two signals, the received signal F_r and transmitted signal F_o, producing Δf, which is the difference between the two. Common to all Doppler systems, then, is a comparison between transmitted and received signals.

The output audio frequencies can go either to an audio output such as headphone or to a speaker. The audio could also go to an analysis system that examines the frequency content of the Doppler shift frequencies and displays the various frequency components.

Spectral Display

The most widely used form of audio analysis is the fast Fourier transform (FFT) device. It takes the complex audio signals that contain signals from the many scattering targets in the blood and separates them into the basic signal frequencies and amplitudes. The FFT system samples a small portion of the analog Doppler signals, converts them into digital numbers, and extracts the frequency components digitally (Fig. 1.27). The output of the FFT is a set of discrete component frequencies and the component amplitudes. These components are then depicted on a spectral display.

The spectrum has three basic axes: frequency on the y-axis, time on the x-axis, and signal amplitude in gray scale on the z-axis (Fig. 1.28). The FFT takes a small but finite amount of time to extract frequency information, which divides the x-axis into small time intervals. These intervals can vary from 1 millisecond (ms) to 100 ms long. The FFT also divides its range of detectable frequencies into intervals called *frequency bins*. Each bin contains a small range of indistinguishable frequencies. An FFT can have from 32 to 256 bins. Typical values are 64 or 128 bins. A general rule abides here: the greater the number of frequency bins, the longer the extraction time. Bin numbers such as 64 and 128 optimize the sampling time interval.

The display divides motion events into movement

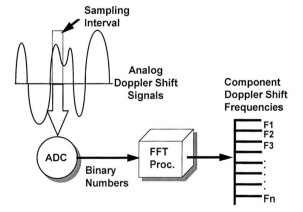

Figure 1.27. The fast Fourier transformation (FFT) system. FFT permits rapid, on-line analysis of frequency components contained in Doppler shift signals. The system first samples a portion of the analog signals and through an analog-to-digital converter (ADC) converts the amplitudes to binary numbers, which are then processed by the FFT program, producing the Doppler frequency components and amplitudes.

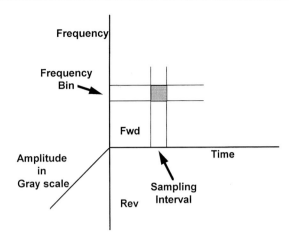

Figure 1.28. The spectral display. A Doppler display needs to show the frequency components, their amplitudes, and how they change with time. A spectral display shows the frequency components from the fast Fourier transformation (FFT) y-axis as frequency bins, with both forward (Fwd) and reversed (Rev) motion, representing motion towards and away from the transducer. The sampling interval for the FFT and the bins form pixels with a gray scale proportional to the frequency component amplitude.

towards the transducer (upward) and movement away from the transducer (reverse).

Pulsed Doppler

CW Doppler systems carry with them a standard range problem. Because the transmitting beam is on continuously, the system cannot spatially separate one vessel or flow event from another within the beam. Everything within the beam is summed together.

An alternative approach is to send out a burst of ultrasound and wait for echoes from a specific region, then process these echoes for Doppler information. This technique is called *pulsed Doppler*. The bursts of ultrasound are coherent; that is, they are sent at a specific time (PRF) and carrier frequency. This permits internal signal processing much like the simple frequency comparison in the CW system. The operator sets the Doppler sampling position using a range-gate control (Fig. 1.29) anywhere over the displayed depth. Movement within the range-gate becomes Doppler signals in the output.

Pulsed Doppler systems have one major drawback, however. They cannot handle Doppler shift frequencies above a fixed sampling limit set by the system PRF. If Doppler frequencies occur that are above this limit, the signals alias; that is, they take on the appearance of lower frequencies, representing movement in the opposite direction, and wrap around the spectral display (Fig. 1.30). In contrast, CW systems do not have a PRF and therefore do not alias. For this reason, CW Doppler capabilities are often part of Doppler systems used for echocardiography.

Basic Duplex System

The range-gate gives a pulsed Doppler a means of isolating the Doppler interrogation to specific regions, but knowing

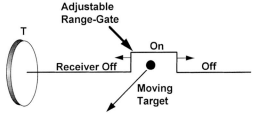

Figure 1.29. The essential range-gate Doppler system. Using pulsed Doppler, a system can send out a burst of ultrasound and wait for echoes from a specific range to arrive at the transducer (T). At the proper time, the system gates the receiver on and processes the echo signals for the Doppler shift frequencies. The sampling time appears on the display as a range-gate that is adjustable for both size and position by machine controls.

Table 1.2.
Doppler Angles and Error Rates

Angle (Degrees)	% Error/degree
0	0.015
5	0.167
15	0.482
20	0.65
55	2.5
60	3.0
65	3.8
75	6.5
80	9.9
85	20.0
88	50.0
89	100.0

the actual location of the range-gate with certainty requires an image. Within the image should be anatomic information from the soft tissues and an electronic marker that indicates the location of the Doppler sampling site as well as the position of the Doppler ultrasound beam relative to the flow pattern.

The early Duplex systems simply added a pulsed or CW Doppler to a basic imaging system. The integration is more complete now, producing sophisticated duplex scanners with advanced Doppler technology.

With directional information about flow, the user can estimate the blood velocities and relate the values to the physiology of the heart or vessels.

Velocity Calculations

The velocity calculation uses the transposed Doppler equation and a solution for the absolute target velocity. This velocity equation is as follows:

$$V = \frac{\Delta F_c}{2 F_o Cos\theta}$$ (Eq. 1.10)

The most important part of this equation is the $1/Cos\ \theta$ term, which is very nonlinear. The nonlinear aspects of this term mean that at the correct angle, small changes in the angle caused by errors in estimating the Doppler angle can produce large errors in the velocity calculations (Table 1.2).

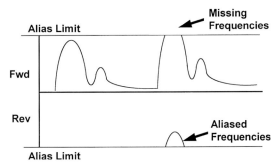

Figure 1.30. Doppler high frequency aliasing. If the higher Doppler shift frequencies exceed the aliasing limit, the high frequency information appears as lower frequencies in the opposite direction. Fwd = forward motion towards the transducer; Rev = motion away from the transducer. Aliasing limits exist in both directions.

When the Doppler angle is close to 0°, the error is small. For example, an angle of 0 ± 20 degrees still produces acceptable accuracies of less than 6%. As the Doppler angle approaches 70°, however, the error jumps to 15% per degree.

These errors can creep into any calculation in which the major flow events are not parallel to the vessel or heart wall and the user is unable to detect or correct for the flow deviation.

Although this section on Doppler is very small, the topic is not. Indeed, Doppler is a complicated technology requiring additional knowledge and skills well beyond basic imaging. The additional reading list at the end of this chapter provides good sources for detailed Doppler information.

SOME PRACTICAL CONSEQUENCES OF ULTRASOUND SCIENCE

Making Sure the Imaging System Works

A fundamental problem with all ultrasound imaging systems is determining whether or not they are working correctly. Subtle changes can occur within the sonograph that can remove important information without producing a major change in the image. Often, the machine goes through a series of small changes that are hard to discern, except for a growing problem of getting good images in a clinical setting. In this situation, it is hard to separate the possibility of a difficult animal from an improperly working sonograph.

The best way to solve this sort of problem is to regularly scan a standard set of known targets under known conditions and retain copies of the images for comparison. The central testing tool for this sort of quality assurance is the *tissue equivalent phantom*. This device is made of plastic and gel with a set of internal targets (nylon pins) that provide a standard source of echoes for the sonograph. The gel ensures a constant velocity of propagation at 1540 m/s and a fixed attenuation rate. Most manufacturers use the tissue equivalent phantom for part of the final machine inspection and may include an image of the phantom in the machine's paperwork.

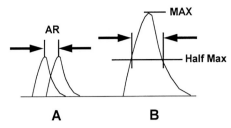

Figure 1.31. System axial resolution. System specifications can express axial resolution (AR) as the ability to separate two echo signals (A) or as the −6 dB or half maximum (MAX) width of a single echo signal (B).

Measurement protocols can be found in many of the current ultrasound physics texts and articles on quality assurance. In addition, the American Institute of Ultrasound in Medicine (AIUM) has publications on quality assurance testing protocols.

Some of the central measurements that are possible on the phantom include axial resolution, lateral resolution, and contrast resolution.

Axial Resolution

Axial resolution is a measure of the ability to show two separate targets positioned along the beam axis as two (Fig. 1.31). Because the display presentation comes from the envelope of the echo signal, the length and shape of the echo signals affect axial resolution. In general, the longer the echo signal vibration, the poorer the axial resolution.

Improving axial resolution requires shortening the effective echo pulse length. We can shorten the echo signal two ways: first, we could increase the transducer damping to shorten the total time of the transducer vibration; second, we could increase the operating ultrasound frequency. Because vibrations are a mechanical process, damping a low frequency or a high frequency transducer produces the same number of vibrations. A higher frequency, however, has shorter, faster cycles, which effectively shortens the overall pulse length.

Manufacturers often express the axial resolution as a pulse length at a specific amplitude below the peak value (Fig. 1.31). A common value is the −6 dB pulse width, which is the pulse width at half the signal maximum amplitude. A basic rule here is that a measured axial resolution on a tissue equivalent phantom should be less than 3 λ of the transducer center operating frequency. For example, one wavelength at 5.0 Mhz is 0.3 mm, and three wavelengths is 0.9 mm.

Lateral Resolution

As the name suggests, lateral resolution is a measure of a system's ability to separate two echo sources placed transverse to the beam axis as two. The closer the echo sources can be and still be separated, the better the resolution. Clearly, this form of resolution depends upon the width of the ultrasound beam (Fig. 1.32). In general, the narrower the beam,

the better the resolution. Considering a typical beam formation, it means that lateral resolution is best at the focal point, better in the focal zone, and becomes geometrically poorer outside the focal zone.

As mentioned earlier, the ability to focus a beam depends on the relationship between the ultrasound wavelength and the effective transducer aperture. Indeed, the half maximum beam width (HMBW) for a focused transducer is expressed as follows:

$$HMBW = 1.22\frac{\lambda}{D}f_z \qquad \text{(Eq. 1.11)}$$

where $HMBW$ is the half maximum beam width, λ is the operating wavelength, D is the effective aperture diameter, and f_z is the focal point range along the beam axis. This equation provides (1) clues about the rules of focusing and the way focusing changes with transducer size, (2) the center operating transducer frequency (wavelength), and (3) how far out the focusing is intended to be. Clearly, at any range, improving transducer focusing can come from increasing the frequency (decreasing the wavelength) or increasing the transducer aperture.

At the same time, as we increase transducer frequency, tissue attenuation increases, taking away the deeper fields of view. In addition, frequency-dependent tissue attenuation also decreases the focusing and moves the focal point closer to the transducer. One solution for this loss in penetration and focusing could be to increase the size of the transducer and lower frequency to focus deeper into the tissues.

Contrast Resolution

Contrast resolution is a measure of the ability of a system to show adjacent differences in echo signal amplitude in gray scale. The closer the echo signals are in amplitude and still are detected as two different amplitudes is a measure of this ability. A good contrast resolution means that echo signals

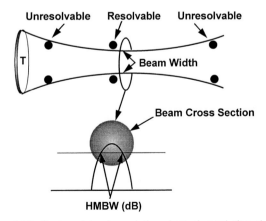

Figure 1.32. System lateral resolution. Lateral resolution depends upon the beam width. If the beam is smaller than the separation, a system can show the two targets as two. If the beam is larger, however, the two echoes blur into one. The half maximum beam width (HMBW) is a measure of the effective beam width and expresses the lateral resolution. T = transducer.

with nearly the same amplitude, representing echo sources with nearly the same reflectance, can be visually separated.

Contrast resolution depends on both the characteristics of the machine-display system and the processing properties of the human visual system. Despite claims to the contrary, the human eye can see more than 100 shades of gray on a typical monitor and will process visualized boundaries for increased contrast (Mach bands). Sonographs with gray scale tagging in pseudocolors provide an opportunity for an objective interrogation of the image for specific echo signal amplitudes.

Temporal Resolution and Frame Rates

The finite transmission velocity for ultrasound sets an upper limit on how quickly an ultrasound system can acquire information. This, in turn, limits the rate at which the ultrasound forms images. As the frame rate of a real time image decreases, its ability to depict motion accurately decreases. In addition, the system fails to sample the motion often enough to track position changes. If the frame rate becomes too slow, a form of motion aliasing occurs as moving structures seem to move in a paradoxical fashion or slower than reality. This aliasing follows the same rules as Doppler high frequency aliasing. Figure 1.33 shows some basic relationships between theoretical frame rates, lines of sight, and display depths.

Balancing Resolution and Penetration

We learned earlier than lower frequencies penetrate deeper into the tissues; however, lower frequencies do not focus as well because their apertures are limited in size. These limitations produce a need to balance the requirements for penetration against the ability to focus the ultrasound beam.

Complicating things further, the ultrasound beam is made of not just one frequency but many. The sharper the ultrasound pulse, the wider the range of frequencies that appear in the beam. At the same time, the tissues function like a low pass filter, removing the higher frequencies and

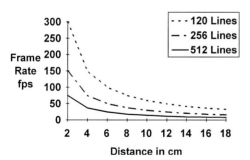

Figure 1.33. Real time frame rate variables. A real time system must wait for the ultrasound to return to the transducer from the deepest portions of the image, which limits frame rates (frames per second, fps) with increasing depth and increasing lines of sight. These theoretical values decrease markedly as processing time goes for internal housekeeping in the digital scan converter or other digital parts of the sonograph.

leaving the lower frequencies. As a result, imaging through tissues always pulls the focal point closer to the transducer and makes it larger in reality than it is in theory.

As a general rule, as the transducer frequency decreases, both lateral and axial resolution become poorer than they are when transducers with higher frequencies and relatively larger apertures are used.

Choosing the Right Field of View

Current real time systems offer a wide range of transducer arrays to handle a variety of human scanning problems. The image format can be sector shaped or rectangular. Some of the linear arrays can form trapezoidal fields of view. In general, linear arrays have larger contact areas with the skin.

Phased arrays and mechanical sector scanners, on the other hand, offer a relatively small contact area. Regions close to the skin have a limited image width, but deeper parts can be quite large (Fig. 1.16). The sector format means that the lines that form the scanning field are closer together near the transducer than deeper in the field. This is a simple consequence of the geometry of the scan. The curved linear array can modify this relationship somewhat, with a larger field of view closer to the transducer.

Linear arrays offer a rectangular field of view, with a similar line-resolution close and far from the transducer. Clearly, the linear array is a preferred pattern for looking at structures close to the skin surface.

Linear arrays also often carry the focusing deeper into the field because they can form larger apertures than linear phased arrays. On the other hand, they do not have the wide field presentation of the sector scanner at depth.

Differences between Doppler Imaging and Conventional Imaging

Because of the reflection differences between soft tissue and blood, a Doppler system and a conventional imaging system may have the same output power but present different levels of performance. It is not uncommon in a duplex system to have a clear image of vessel walls at depth, for example, but the Doppler ultrasound may not have signals strong enough from the blood to get any signals above the system noise.

This imbalance in performance often forces the manufacturer to increase the output power of the Doppler portion of the duplex system to provide similar performance for both parts of the duplex system. As a result, the imaging portion of a machine may have output power intensities of 400 to 500 milliwatts (mW)/cm^2 while the Doppler portion may be operating at intensity of 2500 mW/cm^2 or more.

Calculating Accurate Blood Velocities

The transposed Doppler equation (equation 1.10) provides a handy means of calculating blood velocities. An accurate calculation, however, requires an equally accurate determination of the angle between the ultrasound beam and the blood flow. The accuracy requirements become more critical as the Doppler angle increases (Table 1.2). The error is nonlinear, in that small changes in angle produce large changes in value with angles of more than 70°.

Velocity calculations are the normalizing means of handling Doppler information. That is, if only the Doppler equation is being used, the maximum Doppler shift frequency increases with an increasing carrier frequency. How then can you compare your work at 3.0 Mhz with published data at 5.0 Mhz? Even more disconcerting, the two measurements may be at entirely different Doppler angles, which also modulates the Doppler shift frequencies. Clearly, a calculated velocity appears to be independent of the carrier frequency and Doppler angle, but as we have seen, the calculation may not be accurate if too much error exists in the sampling location and the Doppler angle determination. The rule here is to make velocity calculations at fixed angles and approach all of these calculations with care.

Output Power and Its Effects

In the beginning of this discussion, we noted the interaction between ultrasound and the tissue carrying it. A lot of research has examined this interaction to determine if any deleterious effect on tissue may be occurring. It is clear that ultrasound does not produce tumors or mutations, but it has an ability to cause other mechanical events, including tissue heating.

Thermal effects certainly are a potential problem as the mechanical energy of ultrasound becomes transformed into local heat. Indeed, many of the early bioeffects of high levels of ultrasound to animal fetuses could be mimicked by simply overheating the fetus. It is clear, from both measurements and theoretical calculations, that localized heat-ing can occur in the proximity of a soft tissue–bone interface, precisely the situation for in utero scanning of a fetus and scanning of neonatal heads. A close watch on the human bioeffects literature will provide good guidelines to understand any possible effects that might occur from long-term fetal scanning in animals.

SUMMARY

We have looked at the formation of waves and how ultrasonography shapes and uses them to make images. The real discussion of instrumentation is not finished; it has only begun. As more engineering effort goes into improving the quality of ultrasonic images, changes can be expected in the fundamental signal processing at the heart of today's sonographs. Some suggested reading can fill in the many empty spaces in this discussion. Nevertheless, the information in this chapter is a more than adequate step into these publications.

SUGGESTED READING

Godshalk C, ed. Third Animal Ultrasound Seminar and Wet-Lab Course Syllabus (AIUM #AS92). Rockville, MD: American Institute of Ultrasound in Medicine, 1992.

Hatle L, Angelsen B. Doppler Ultrasound in Cardiology, Physical Principles and Clinical Applications. Philadelphia: Lea & Febiger, 1982.

McDicken WN. Diagnostic Ultrasonics, Principles and Use of Instruments. 2nd ed. New York: John Wiley & Sons, 1981.

Powis RL, Powis WJ. A Thinker's Guide to Ultrasonic Imaging. Munich: Urban & Schwarzenberg, 1984.

Powis RL, Schwartz RA. Practical Doppler Ultrasound for the Clinician. Balitmore: Williams & Wilkins, 1991.

Rantanen NW, ed. Veterinary Clinics of North America, Equine Practice 1986; 2.

2. Echocardiography

KARON L. HOFFMANN

Two-dimensional B-mode, M-mode, and Doppler echocardiography methods are internationally accepted as valuable diagnostic aids used for the assessment of cardiac structure and function. Echocardiography should be performed after the clinical history has been taken and a thorough examination has been performed. By following a protocol for the examination of the equine heart and by becoming familiar with normal echocardiographic findings, the sonographer will ensure that the heart has been fully examined for evidence of a pathologic process. This chapter describes the equipment required for two-dimensional B-mode, M-mode, and Doppler echocardiography; gives suggested imaging protocols that permit images and measurements to be made in standard anatomic planes; and presents a review of the normal dimensions of the equine heart.

TWO-DIMENSIONAL B-MODE AND M-MODE ECHOCARDIOGRAPHY

Equipment Requirements

Real-time echocardiography requires an ultrasound system that has a wide sector field of view (90°), a frame rate of at least 30 frames/second, minimal or adjustable frame averaging, simultaneous electrocardiogram, and, if possible, cine loop recall.

A wide sector or "pie-shaped" field of view enables the relationship of the cardiac structures to be viewed in each plane, without requiring frequent repositioning of the transducers on the body wall. Frame averaging by the superimposition of images from other stages of the cardiac cycle should not be used in echocardiography so that the stages of the cardiac cycle may be accurately measured. A simultaneous electrocardiogram is essential for precise timing of cardiac events. Cine loop recall allows the sonographer to review some of the preceding frames. Cine recall not only is useful for selecting the appropriate frame for cardiac measurements but also is invaluable in veterinary sonography to recall a previous frame after an animal has moved unexpectedly.

Sonographic Transducers

The transducer selected for echocardiography should have the highest frequency that permits acoustic penetration of the heart. The following frequencies may be used: 2.0 or 2.5 Mhz for adult racing Thoroughbreds and heavy horses, 2.5

or 3.5 Mhz for lighter adult horses and obese ponies, 3.5 or 5.0 Mhz for ponies and older foals, and 5.0 or 7.5 Mhz for newborn foals and miniature horses. The transducer should have a small contact surface or "footprint" that can be placed and rotated at an intercostal space. The transducer needs to remain in contact with the skin as it is angled and rotated; thus, a transducer with a small curved face is an advantage.

Imaging Variables

Before an echocardiograpic examination is begun, certain imaging variables should be selected.

Because of the constant movement of the heart, the frame rate selected should be higher than that used for imaging other organs. The dynamic range determines the range of echo amplitudes to be displayed. To produce an image of high contrast, a lower dynamic range should be selected for cardiac imaging. The gray scale of the image may also be modified by selecting various postprocessing curves. Edge enhancement may be used to accentuate tissue interfaces within the heart. Low-level echoes can be removed from the image by changing the reject level. In M-mode, reject levels of 5% or more may be selected, but as a general rule, a minimum reject level should be selected to help define the cardiac structures without eliminating low-amplitude echo information. If a cardiac calculation package is available, this may be selected from the control panel menu, and an integrated electrocardiogram should be selected for accurate timing of the cardiac events.

To image the entire heart of the adult athletic horse, a depth of 25 or 30 cm is used. If the maximum depth available on the sonographic system is less than 25 cm, the measurements of the left side of the heart must be made from images from the left hemithorax. Power settings are used to increase or decrease the intensity of the entire image and may be preset at 60 to 80% of maximum power. The power level may need to be increased during echocardiography to ensure ultrasound penetration to the deepest structures.

Overall gain levels are used to change the intensity of the entire image by decreasing or increasing the amplification of the received echoes. Moreover, the amplification of echoes may be adjusted in relation to depth using the time gain compensation (TGC). After the initial TGC adjustments, in which the amplification of the echoes from the near field is decreased and echoes in the far field are increased, few adjustments are usually necessary during the remainder of the echocardiographic examination.

Preparation of the Horse

The hair coat should be clipped or shaved from both sides of the thorax at the second to fourth intercostal spaces from just below the level of the elbow to approximately 10 cm above the elbow. The skin should be washed to remove debris and scurf, and coupling gel should be applied.

If an integrated electrocardiogram is available, electrode conduction paste or alcohol is applied to the skin at the site of attachment of each electrocardiogram electrode. The "left arm" electrode should be attached to the skin at the left sixth intercostal space at the level of the point of the elbow, the "right arm" electrode should be attached to the skin at the level of the dorsal margin of the right scapula, and the "right leg" electrode should be attached to the skin on the right side of the neck.

Table 2.1
Two-Dimensional Echocardiographic Examination

Image Planes	Structures Imaged
Images from the right hemithorax	
Parasternal long axis views	
Left ventricular inlet view (four-chamber image)	LA, LV, CT, MV, LVPW, RA, RV, SW, TV
Left ventricular outflow view (five-chamber image)	AO, AV, CT of MV, LA, LV, LVOT, RV, SW
Parasternal short axis views	
Left ventricle at the level of the papillary muscle	LV, PMs, LVPW, RV, SW
Left ventricle at the level of the chordae tendineae	CT, LV, LVPW, RV, SW
Left ventricle at the level of the mitral valve	LV, LVOT, MV, RV, SW
Heart base at the level of the aortic root	AO, AV, LA, PA, PV, RA, RVOT, TV
Parasternal cranial short axis angled views	AO, R coronary artery, PA, PV, RA, RVOT, SVC, TV
Right ventricular outflow view	
Images from the left hemithorax	
Parasternal caudal long axis views	
Left ventricular inlet view (two- or four-chamber image)	LA, LV, MV, RA, RV, SW, TV
Apical view (four- or five-chamber image)	AO, LA, LV, LVOT, MV, RA, RV, SW, TV
Parasternal cranial long axis view	
Left ventricular outflow view	AO, AV, LVOT, SW, RA, RV, TV
Parasternal cranial angled views	
Pulmonary artery and pulmonary valve view	AO, PA, PV, RVOT
Right atrium and cranial venous return view	AO, CrVC, RA

AO = aorta, AV = aortic valve, CrCV = cranial vena cava, CT = chordae tendineae, LA = left atrium, LV = left ventricle, LVOT = left ventricular outflow tract, LVPW = left ventricular posterior wall, MV = mitral valve (left atrioventricular valve), PA = pulmonary artery, PM = papillary muscle, PV = pulmonary valve, RA = right atrium, RV = right ventricle, RVOT = right ventricular outflow tract, SVC = superventricular crest, SW = interventricular septal wall, TV = tricuspid valve (right atrioventricular valve).

Adapted with permission from Long KJ, Bonagura JD, Darke PGG. Standardised imaging technique for guided M-mode and Doppler echocardiology in the horse. Equine Vet J 1992;24:226–235.

Examination

Routine two-dimensional B-mode echocardiography involves imaging the heart from both the left and right sides of the thorax in standard anatomic planes (Table 2.1) (1). Multiple views are provided of the ascending aorta, aortic valve leaflets, cranial vena cava, mitral valve, chordae tendineae, left atrium, left ventricle, left ventricular outflow tract, mitral valve, pulmonary artery, pulmonary muscles, pulmonary valve, left ventricular posterior wall, right atrium, right ventricle, right ventricular outflow tract, superventricular crest, interventricular septum, and tricuspid valve (see Table 2.1).

M-mode imaging is used to measure the excursions of the chamber walls and valves, as well as the thickness of septum and the ventricular walls during systole and diastole. Standard measurements and calculations are made principally from M-mode images made in the right parasternal short axis planes. An echocardiographic protocol, using standard anatomic planes, ensures that the heart is examined systematically and thoroughly for evidence of a pathologic process.

Descriptions of the placement and angulation of the sonographic transducer for equine echocardiography have been given by Carlsten (2), Reef (3), and Long, Bonagura, and Darke (1). Although these authors have described similar echocardiographic planes, the approach to transducer placement varies. Long, Bonagura, and Darke (1) used the location of the apex beat and the elbow to describe the position of the transducer on the thorax, combined with descriptions of transducer rotation and angulation, whereas Carlsten (2) aligned the transducer to surface anatomic features, and Reef (3) used a combination of anatomic placement with descriptions of transducer angulation. The following descriptions of the echocardiographic planes summarize the different approaches described by the various authors.

Images from the Right Hemithorax (see Table 2.1) (1)
Right Parasternal Long Axis Planes

LEFT VENTRICULAR INLET VIEW: FOUR-CHAMBER IMAGE (Fig. 2.1) (4). The transducer is placed at the right fourth or fifth intercostal space (Fig. 2.1A) just dorsal to the olecranon. The sector shaped sonographic beam is aligned vertically (0°), and the center of the sector image is then adjusted to image the left ventricular inlet and the interventricular septum. Long, Bonagura, and Darke (1) used this view as a reference point from which other views were obtained (Fig. 2.1B,C). The transducer can be located on the body wall so the left ventricle at the level of the chordae tendineae is in the center of the image and the interventricular septal wall is almost horizontal on the image. The transducer can also be directed dorsally or ventrally, to image the four chambers (Fig. 2.1B,C).

Carlsten (2) placed the transducer on the right thoracic wall at the fourth or fifth intercostal space, 20 to 25 cm lateral to the right sternal border. The sonographic beam was parallel to a line drawn from the dorsocaudal edge of the right scapula to the xiphoid cartilage of the sternum. Small

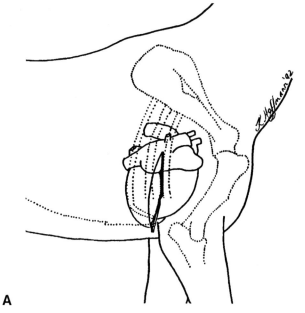

A

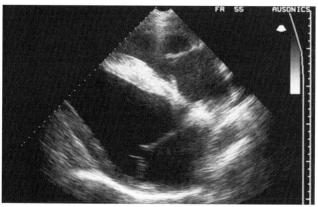

B

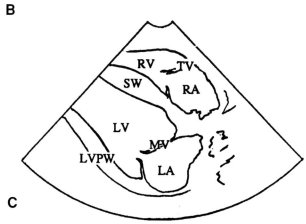

C

Figure 2.1. Right parasternal long axis, left ventricular inlet view (four chamber). A centimeter scale, time gain compensation curve, and gray-scale bar are displayed to the right of the image. Similar scales were present in all other figures in this chapter. **A,** Schematic drawing of transducer placement and rotation. **B,** Sonogram of a normal equine heart. **C,** Schematic drawing of the sonogram in **B.** LA = left atrium; LV = left ventricle; LVPW = left ventricular posterior wall; MV = mitral valve; RA = right atrium; RV = right ventricle; SW = septal wall; TV = tricuspid valve. Reprinted with permission from Hoffmann KL. Echocardiography of the horse. Veterinary Applications Module. Lane Cove, Australia: The University of Sydney/Ausonics International Proprietary, Ltd, 1993.

dorsal and caudal adjustments of the beam plane were made until the long axis image was obtained. Reef (3) obtained similar images when the transducer was placed at the right fourth intercostal space and was directed caudally from the right cardiac window toward the opposite left fifth intercostal space at approximately the level of the mitral valve.

The cardiac structures imaged in this plane include the left atrium, left ventricle, mitral valve, chordae tendineae of the mitral valve, left ventricular posterior wall, right atrium, right ventricle, septal wall, and tricuspid valve (Fig. 2.1B,C).

LEFT VENTRICULAR OUTFLOW VIEW: FIVE-CHAMBER IMAGE (Fig. 2.2) (4). The transducer is again placed at the right fourth or fifth intercostal space, and the previous reference view (left ventricular inlet view, four-chamber image) is obtained. The edge of the sector beam plane is then rotated approximately 30° clockwise, and the center of the sonographic sector is directed (Fig. 2.2A) slightly cranially and or slightly dorsally (1), to provide a long axis view of the aorta (Fig. 2.2B,C).

A similar view was described by Carlsten (2). In this report, the transducer was placed at the right second or third intercostal space, with the sonographic beam parallel to a line drawn from the dorsocaudal edge of the right scapula to the xiphoid cartilage of the sternum (Fig. 2.2A). Small adjustments were then made to the beam plane, and the beam was directed dorsally to demonstrate outflow from the left ventricle (Fig. 2.2B,C).

The cardiac structures imaged in this plane include the aorta, aortic valve, left atrium, left ventricle, mitral valve, chordae tendineae of the mitral valve, left ventricular outflow tract, right atrium, right ventricle, and septal wall (Fig. 2.2B,C).

Right Parasternal Short Axis Planes (Fig. 2.3A) (4). For the right parasternal short axis planes, the transducer was again placed in the reference position (left ventricular inlet view, four-chamber image, see Fig. 2.1) or just ventral to it.

LEFT VENTRICLE AT THE LEVEL OF THE PAPILLARY MUSCLES (Fig. 2.3B,C). The edge of the sonographic sector is then rotated 80° to 90° counterclockwise, and the center of the sector is directed slightly caudally, dorsally, or ventrally to obtain a true short axis view at the level of the papillary muscles. The cardiac structures imaged in this plane include the left ventricle, papillary muscles, left ventricular posterior wall, right ventricle, and septal wall (Fig. 2.3B,C).

LEFT VENTRICLE AT THE LEVEL OF THE CHORDAE TENDINEAE (Fig. 2.3D,E). The center of the sector beam is then directed slightly caudally and dorsally to obtain a view at the level of the chordae tendineae (1). For M-mode studies, the M-mode cursor may be placed across the ventricles between the papillary muscles and chordae tendineae. The ventricular dimensions should be measured just below the level of the mitral valve (Figs. 2.4A,B and 2.5A) (4). The cardiac structures imaged in this plane include the left ventricle, chordae tendineae of the mitral valve, left ventricular posterior wall, right ventricle, and septal wall (see Fig. 2.3D,E).

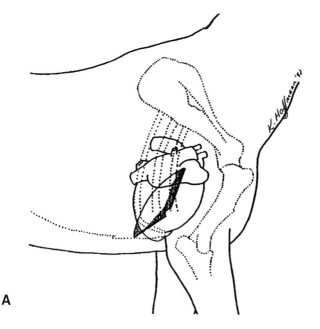

A

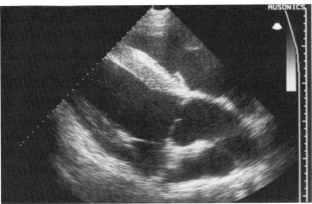

B

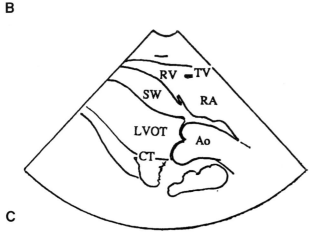

C

Figure 2.2. Right parasternal long axis, left ventricular outlet view. **A,** Schematic drawing of transducer placement and rotation. **B,** Sonogram of a normal equine heart. **C,** Schematic drawing of the sonogram in **B.** Ao = aorta, CT = chordae tendineae; LVOT = left ventricular outflow tract; RA = right atrium; RV = right ventricle; SW = septal wall; TV = tricuspid valve. Reprinted with permission from Hoffmann KL. Echocardiography of the horse. Veterinary Applications Module. Lane Cove, Australia: The University of Sydney /Ausonics International Proprietary, Ltd, 1993.

LEFT VENTRICLE AT THE MITRAL VALVE LEVEL (see Fig. 2.3F,G). The short axis image at the level of the mitral valve is obtained by placing the transducer in the reference position and then rotating the transducer 60° to 80° counterclockwise while directing the center of the sonographic sector dorsally and either slightly cranially or caudally (1). The M-mode cursor is placed across the mitral valve at this level (Figs. 2.4C,D and 2.5B). The cardiac structures imaged in this plane include the left ventricle, mitral valve, left ventricular outflow tract, right ventricle, and septal wall (see Fig. 2.3F,G).

HEART BASE AT THE LEVEL OF THE AORTIC ROOT (see Fig. 2.3H,I). The aortic valve is shown in the short axis view when the transducer is placed in the reference position and rotated 30° counterclockwise (−30°); the rotation is varied between −20° and −60° to optimize the short axis view (1). The center of the sonographic beam is directed cranially and dorsally. For M-mode observations and measurements, the M-mode cursor is placed across the aortic valve (Figs. 2.4D,E and 2.5C) (4).

Carlsten described the same views by placement of the transducer at the fourth or fifth intercostal space, 20 to 25 cm lateral to the right sternal border. The beam plane was roughly parallel to a line drawn from the right coxofemoral joint to the right olecranon. The beam plane was then swept from the apex to the base of the heart. During the sweep (see Fig. 2.3A), the transducer position was moved 5 to 8 cm dorsally to maintain a short axis view (2).

The right parasternal short axis planes are traditionally imaged for M-mode examination and measurements. Routine M-mode cursor placements within the two-dimensional images are presented in Figure 2.4. The cardiac structures images in this plane include the aorta, aortic valve leaflets, left atrium, pulmonary artery, pulmonary valve, right atrium, right ventricular outflow tract, and tricuspid valve (see Fig. 2.3 H,I)

Right Parasternal Cranial Short Axis Angled Planes: Right Ventricular Outflow View (Fig. 2.6) (4). To view image the pulmonary artery and right ventricular outflow tract, the sonographic beam can be directed further cranially from the previous view of the aorta or by placing the transducer cranially at the right second or third intercostal space (Fig. 2.6A) rotating the sonographic beam 30° counterclockwise and directing the beam cranially and dorsally (1).

Carlsten (2) described the same view by positioning the transducer over the second or third intercostal space, with the right thoracic limb of the horse pulled forward. The sonographic beam was directed parallel to a line drawn from the right coxofemoral joint to the right olecranon.

The cardiac structures imaged in this plane include the aorta, right coronary artery, pulmonary artery, pulmonary valve, right atrium, right ventricular outflow tract, superventricular crest, and tricuspid valve (Fig. 2.6B,C).

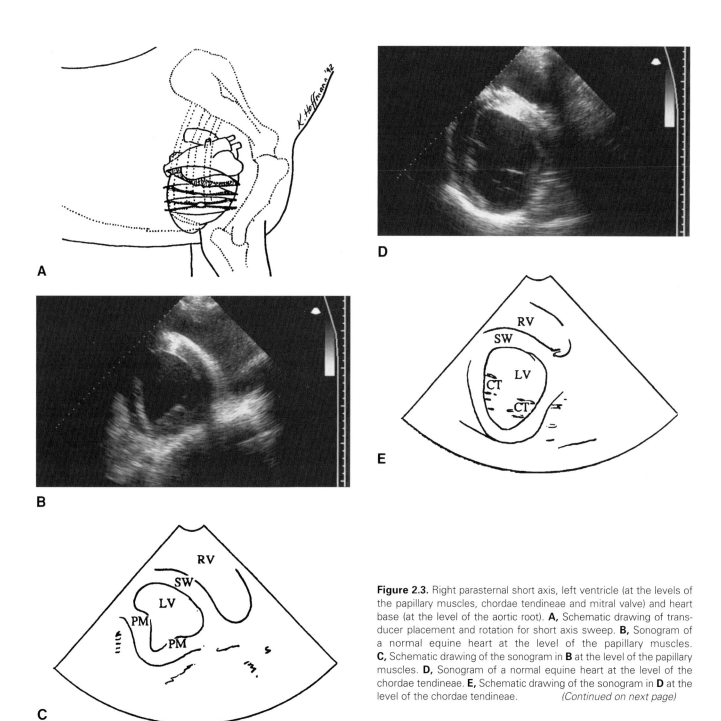

Figure 2.3. Right parasternal short axis, left ventricle (at the levels of the papillary muscles, chordae tendineae and mitral valve) and heart base (at the level of the aortic root). **A,** Schematic drawing of transducer placement and rotation for short axis sweep. **B,** Sonogram of a normal equine heart at the level of the papillary muscles. **C,** Schematic drawing of the sonogram in **B** at the level of the papillary muscles. **D,** Sonogram of a normal equine heart at the level of the chordae tendineae. **E,** Schematic drawing of the sonogram in **D** at the level of the chordae tendineae. *(Continued on next page)*

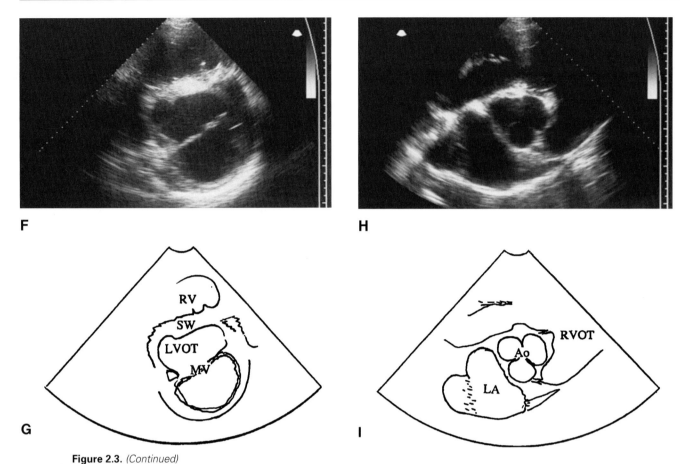

Figure 2.3. *(Continued)*
F, Sonogram of a normal equine heart at the level of the mitral valve. **G,** Schematic drawing of the sonogram in **F** at the level of the mitral valve. **H,** Sonogram of a normal equine heart at the heart base, at the level of the aortic root. **I,** Schematic drawing of the sonogram in **H** at the heart base, at the level of the aortic root. Ao = aorta; CT = chordae tendineae; LA = left atrium; LV = left ventricle; LVOT = left ventricular outflow tract; MV = mitral valve; PM = papillary muscle; RV = right ventricle; RVOT = right ventricular outflow tract; SW = septal wall. Reprinted with permission from Hoffmann KL. Echocardiography of the horse. Veterinary Applications Module. Lane Cove, Australia: The University of Sydney /Ausonics International Proprietary, Ltd, 1993.

Images from the Left Hemithorax

Left Parasternal Caudal Long Axis Planes

LEFT VENTRICULAR INLET VIEW: TWO- OR FOUR-CHAMBER VIEW (Fig. 2.7) (4). Long, Bonagura, and Darke (1) described the left ventricular inlet view as the standard reference image for the left hemithorax. From this reference image, other left thoracic views are oriented. The transducer is placed caudal to the left olecranon and dorsal to the left apical impulse (Fig. 2.7A), with the edge of the sector directed vertically (0°). This provides a long axis view of the left atrium and left ventricle; the mitral valve and left ventricular inlet are also shown. The center of the sonographic beam is then adjusted to cross the left ventricle at the level of the chordae tendineae, and the interventricular septum is oriented almost horizontally across the sector sonographic image (Fig. 2.7**B,C**). The image is a four-chamber view if the depth of view incorporates all four chambers and a two-chamber view if only the left ventricle, mitral valve, and left atrium are imaged.

Reef (3) also obtained this image by placing the transducer in the fourth or fifth intercostal space at a level midway between the point of the shoulder and the point of the elbow.

The cardiac structures imaged in this plane include the left atrium, left ventricle, mitral valve, chordae tendineae of the mitral valve, right atrium, right ventricle, septal wall, and tricuspid valve (Fig. 2.7B,C).

APICAL FOUR- OR FIVE-CHAMBER VIEW (Fig. 2.8) (4) The left apical view displays the long axis of the heart as vertically as possible. Initially, the transducer is placed in the left reference position (left ventricular inlet view, see Fig. 2.7) or caudal and ventral to it. The edge of the sonographic sector is then rotated between 0° to 40° counterclockwise and the center of the sonographic beam is directed dorsally (Fig. 2.8A) with a slight cranial or caudal angulation (1).

The left apical view is also obtained by placing the transducer in the left fourth or fifth intercostal space over the apex beat; the edge of the sonographic beam is directed vertically (0°). The transducer is then angled cranially and dorsally. This view optimally images the left ventricular inflow

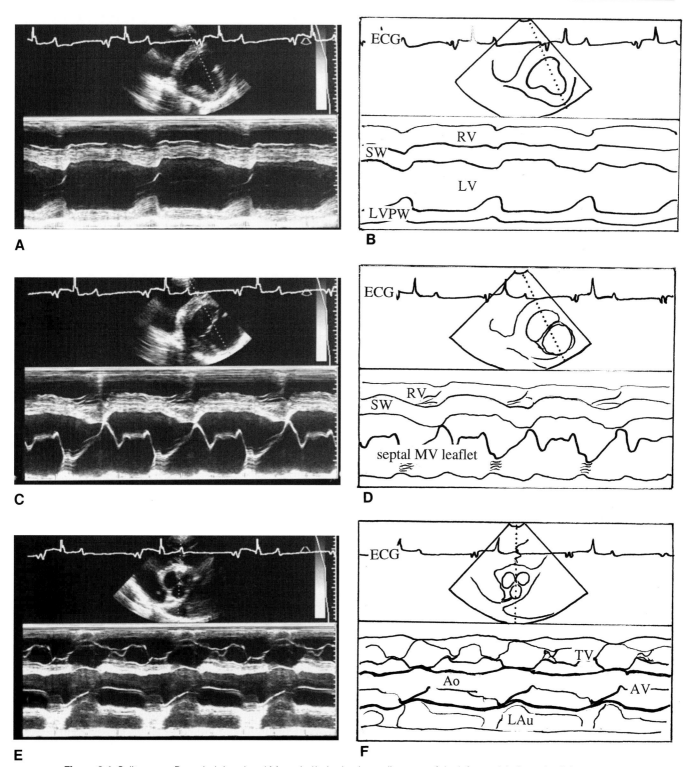

Figure 2.4. Split screen B-mode (*above*) and M-mode (*below*) echocardiograms of the left ventricle from the right parasternal short axis view. **A,** Sonogram of M-mode cursor placement between the two papillary muscles for M-mode echocardiogram of the left ventricle. **B,** Schematic drawing of the sonogram in **A. C,** Sonogram of M-mode cursor placement at the mitral valve level for M-mode echocardiogram. **D,** Schematic drawing of the sonogram in **C. E,** Sonogram of M-mode cursor placement at the aortic valve level for M-mode echocardiogram of the aortic root. **F,** Schematic drawing of the sonogram in **E.** Ao = aorta; AV = aortic valve leaflet; ECG = electrocardiogram; Lau = left auricle; LV = left ventricle; LVPW = left ventricular posterior wall; MV = mitral valve; RV = right ventricle; SW = septal wall; TV = tricuspid valve. Reprinted with permission from Hoffmann KL. Echocardiography of the horse. Veterinary Applications Module. Lane Cove, Australia: The University of Sydney/Ausonics International Proprietary, Ltd, 1993.

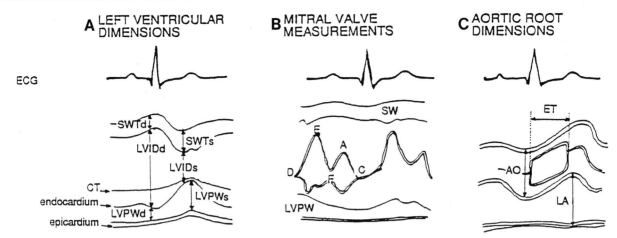

Figure 2.5. Schematic drawing of M-mode measurements. **A,** Left ventricular dimensions. **B,** Mitral valve motion. *A* = cranial motion of the septal mitral leaflet, *C* = closure of the septal mitral valve, *D* = position of mitral valve at onset of diastole, *E* = fully opened position of the septal mitral leaflet, *F* = caudal opened position of the septal mitral leaflet. **C,** Aortic root measurements. AO = aortic diameter; CT= chordae tendineae; ECG = electrocardiogram; ET = ejection time; LA = left atrium/auricle; LVIDd = left ventricular internal diameter in diastole; LVIDs = left ventricular internal diameter in systole; LVPW = left ventricular posterior wall; LVPWd = left ventricular posterior wall in diastole; LVPWs = left ventricular posterior wall in systole; SW = septal wall; SWTd = septal wall thickness in diastole; SWTs = septal wall thickness in systole. Reprinted with permission from Hoffmann KL. Echocardiography of the horse. Veterinary Applications Module. Lane Cove, Australia: The University of Sydney /Ausonics International Proprietary, Ltd, 1993.

(four chambers). To include left ventricular outflow and the aorta (five chambers, Fig. 2.8**B,C**), the sector remains vertical or is rotated as much as 30° counterclockwise; the transducer is then angled, even more cranially than in the four-chamber view (Bonagura, personal communication).

The cardiac structures imaged in this plane include the aorta, left atrium, left ventricle, left ventricular outflow tract, mitral valve, right atrium, right ventricle, septal wall, and tricuspid valve (Fig. 2.8**B,C**).

Left Parasternal Cranial Long Axis Plane: Left Ventricular Outflow View (Fig. 2.9) (4). The transducer is placed in the second to fourth intercostal space. The edge of the sonographic beam is rotated 90° to 120° clockwise, and the center of the sonographic beam is directed slightly cranially and dorsally (Fig. 2.9**A**) to bring the ascending aorta into the long axis. The cardiac structures imaged in this plane include the aorta, aortic valve, left ventricular outflow tract, right atrium, right ventricle, septal wall, and tricuspid valve (Fig. 2.9**B,C**).

Left Parasternal Cranial Angled Planes

PULMONARY ARTERY AND PULMONARY VALVE VIEW (Fig. 2.10) (4) For the cranial angled planes, the transducer is placed ventrally at the left second or third intercostal space. The edge of the sonographic beam is rotated 45° counterclockwise, and the transducer is angled caudally and steeply dorsally (1). The cardiac structures imaged in this plane include the aorta, pulmonary artery, pulmonary valve, right ventricular outflow tract, and right coronary artery (Fig. 2.10**B,C**).

RIGHT ATRIUM AND CRANIAL VENOUS RETURN VIEW (Fig. 2.11) (4) Again, the transducer is placed at the left second or third intercostal space. The edge of the sonographic beam is rotated 90° to 120° clockwise from vertical (Fig. 2.11**A**) The transducer is then angled moderately dorsally and slightly cranially or caudally (Bonagura, personal communication). The cardiac structures imaged in this plane include the aorta, cranial vena cava, and the right atrium (Fig. 2.11**B,C**).

Normal Findings

The standard imaging planes provide multiple views of cardiac ultrasonographic anatomy including the ascending aorta, aortic valve leaflets, cranial vena cava, mitral valve, chordae tendineae, left atrium, left ventricle, left ventricular outflow tract, mitral valve, pulmonary artery, pulmonary muscles, pulmonary valve, left ventricular posterior wall, right atrium, right ventricle, right ventricular outflow tract, superventricular crest, interventricular septum, and tricuspid valve (see Figs. 2.1 through 2.3 and 2.6 through 2.11) (4). To interpret echocardiographs, the sonographer must be familiar with the normal sonographic anatomy demonstrated in the previously described standard planes.

M-mode measurements made of normal horses and foals have been reported (Tables 2.2 [1, 5–8], 2.3 [9], and 2.4 [10]). The mean fractional shortening values reported for the Thoroughbred foal are lower than those reported for the pony foal and approximately half the mean values reported for the adult horse. The reason for this difference is unknown.

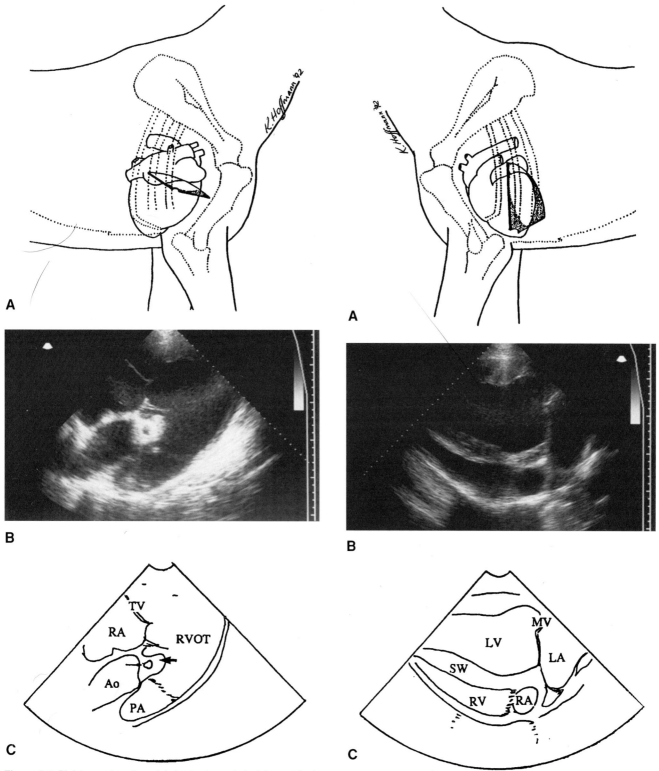

Figure 2.6. Right parasternal cranial short axis angled, right ventricular outflow view. **A,** Schematic drawing of transducer placement and rotation. **B,** Sonogram of a normal equine heart. **C,** Schematic drawing of the sonogram in **B.** *Small arrow* = right coronary artery; *large arrow* = superventricular crest. Ao = aorta; PA = pulmonary artery; RA = right atrium; RVOT = right ventricular outflow tract; TV = tricuspid valve. Reprinted with permission from Hoffmann KL. Echocardiography of the horse. Veterinary Applications Module. Lane Cove, Australia: The University of Sydney/Ausonics International Proprietary, Ltd, 1993.

Figure 2.7. Left parasternal caudal long axis, left ventricular inlet view. **A,** Schematic line drawing of transducer placement and rotation. **B,** Sonogram of a normal equine heart. **C,** Schematic line drawing of the sonogram in **B.** LA = left atrium; LV = left ventricle; MV = mitral valve; RA = right atrium; RV = right ventricle; SW = septal wall. Reprinted with permission from Hoffmann KL. Echocardiography of the horse. Veterinary Applications Module. Lane Cove, Australia: The University of Sydney/Ausonics International Proprietary, Ltd, 1993.

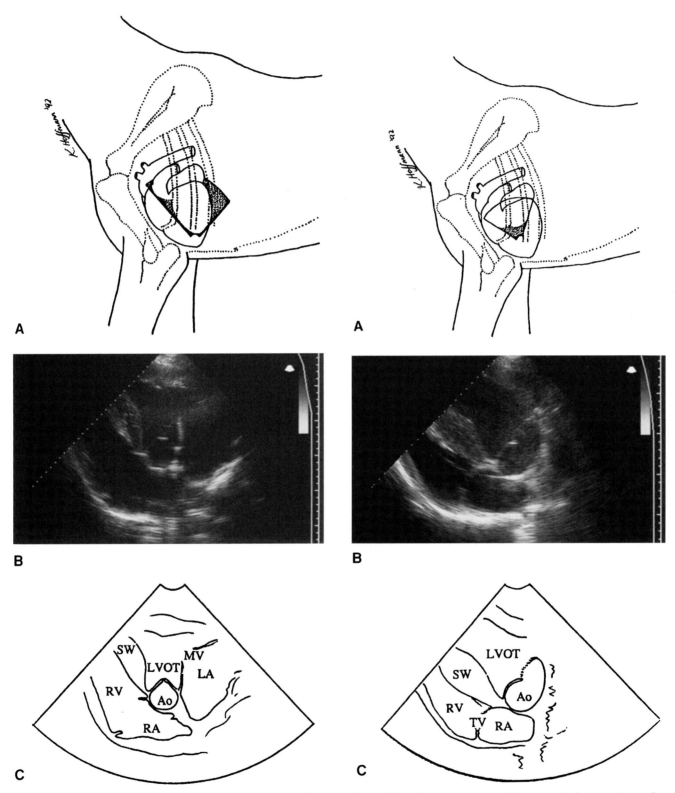

Figure 2.8. Left parasternal caudal long axis, left apical view (four-chamber or five-chamber image). **A,** Schematic line drawing of transducer placement and rotation. **B,** Sonogram of a normal equine heart. **C,** Schematic drawing of the sonogram in **B.** Ao = aorta; LA = left atrium; LVOT = left ventricular outflow tract; MV = mitral valve; RA = right atrium; RV = right ventricle; SW = septal wall; TV = tricuspid valve. Reprinted with permission from Hoffmann KL. Echocardiography of the horse. Veterinary Applications Module. Lane Cove, Australia: The University of Sydney/Ausonics International Proprietary, Ltd, 1993.

Figure 2.9. Left parasternal cranial long axis, left ventricular outflow view. **A,** Schematic drawing of transducer placement and rotation. **B,** Sonogram of a normal equine heart. **C,** Schematic drawing of the sonogram in **B.** Ao = aorta; LVOT = left ventricular outflow tract; RA = right atrium; RV = right ventricle; SW = septal wall; TV = tricuspid valve. Reprinted with permission from Hoffmann KL. Echocardiography of the horse. Veterinary Applications Module. Lane Cove, Australia: The University of Sydney/Ausonics International Proprietary, Ltd, 1993.

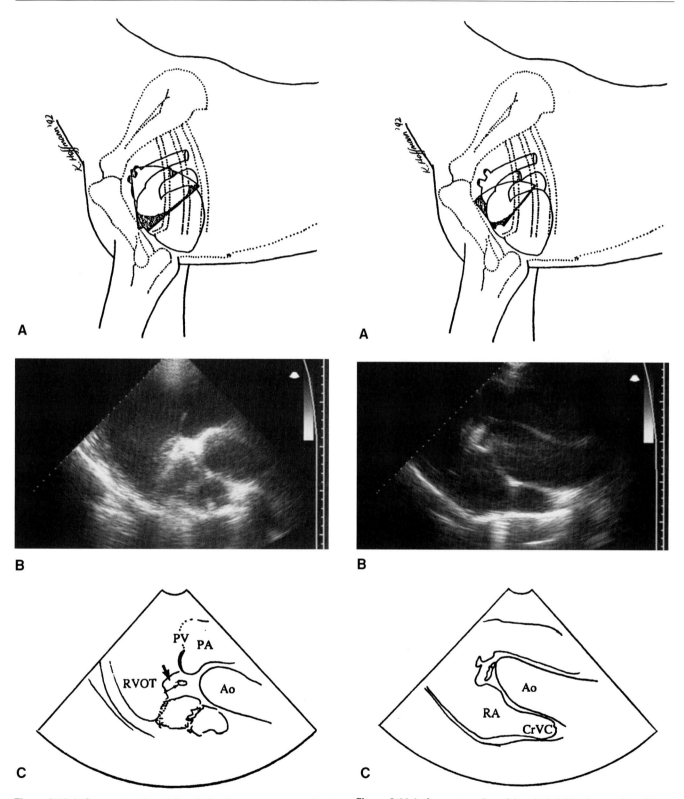

Figure 2.10. Left parasternal cranial angled, pulmonary artery and pulmonary valve view. **A,** Schematic drawing of transducer placement and rotation. **B,** Sonogram of a normal equine heart. **C,** Schematic drawing of the sonogram in **B.** Ao = aorta; PA = pulmonary artery; PV = pulmonary valve; RVOT = right ventricular outflow tract. Reprinted with permission from Hoffmann KL. Echocardiography of the horse. Veterinary Applications Module. Lane Cove, Australia: The University of Sydney/Ausonics International Proprietary, Ltd, 1993.

Figure 2.11. Left parasternal cranial angled, right atrium and cranial venous return. **A,** Schematic line drawing of the transducer placement and rotation. **B,** Sonogram of a normal equine heart. **C,** Schematic drawing of the sonogram in **B.** Ao = aorta; CrVC = cranial vena cava; RA = right atrium. Reprinted with permission from Hoffmann KL. Echocardiography of the horse. Veterinary Applications Module. Lane Cove, Australia: The University of Sydney/Ausonics International Proprietary, Ltd, 1993.

The M-mode images of the mitral valve (see Fig. 2.4C,D) can be made from the right or left parasternal short axis planes. The normal motion of the mitral valve, as studied by M-mode echocardiography, has been described by Wingfield, Miller, Voss, Bennett, and Breukels (11). After atrial systole, the septal (cranial) mitral valve leaflet makes a cranial motion (see Fig. 2.5B, peak A). The septal mitral valve leaflet then makes a rapid caudal motion that leads to the closure of the mitral valve (point C) at the onset of ventricular systole. As the ventricles empty during systole, the mitral annulus and therefore the closed septal mitral valve leaflet move cranially. Point D corresponds to the onset of diastole; the septal mitral valve leaflet then moves cranially to its fully opened position (peak E). As the ventricles fill, the septal mitral valve leaflet remains open but moves caudally (see Fig. 2.5B, point F). The slope from E to F reflects the rate of ventricular filling. With rapid heart rates, the E-F slope decreases with diminishing ventricular filling. The caudal mitral valve demonstrates a reciprocal pattern of motion with a lower amplitude than that of the septal mitral valve leaflet. The values for E-F slope in the normal adult horse and foals are presented in Tables 2.2, 2.3, and 2.4.

From the M-mode images made in the right (see Fig. 2.4E,F) or left parasternal short axis view of the aortic valve, measurements of the ejection time, aortic root dimensions, and left atrial (or auricle, depending on the angulation) dimensions are made (see Fig. 2.5C). The ejection time is the time that the aortic valve leaflets are open during systole. Measurements of the ejection time for normal adult horses

(see Table 2.2) and measurements of the aortic dimensions, left atrial/auricular dimensions, and the ratio of the left atrium to aortic diameter for the normal adult horse, Thoroughbred foal, and pony foal are given (see Tables 2.2, 2.3, and 2.4).

These normal M-mode measurements may be used in combination with two-dimensional B-mode images in the assessment of cardiac structures in the horse.

DOPPLER ECHOCARDIOGRAPHY

Doppler echocardiography is used for the investigation of murmurs created by turbulent flow of blood within the heart and the great vessels. Doppler technology enables the sonographer to determine blood velocity as well as the direction of blood flow. In the horse, Doppler echocardiography should be performed when investigating holosystolic, pansystolic murmurs (grade 3/6 or greater) and holodiastolic murmurs (12). In the horse, systolic ejection murmurs and protodiastolic and late diastolic murmurs are usually physiologic flow murmurs. After auscultation of the heart during physical examination, much information will have already been obtained about the cardiac structures that are likely to be involved and the areas and direction of the turbulent flow. This clinical information should then be used in the selection of imaging planes and the alignment of the Doppler signal to the direction of turbulent flow.

The horse is considered a poor subject for quantitative

Table 2.2
Normal Values for M-Mode Echocardiography in Mature Horses

Reference Parameter	5 Mean (cm)	6 Mean (cm)	1 Mean (cm)	7 Mean (cm)	8 Mean (cm)
Body weight sd	445 kg ± 87	482 kg ± 45	517 kg	—	300 kg
RVID (d) sd	—	5.9 ± 0.6	3.8 ± 0.9	—	—
RVID (s) sd	3.9 ± 0.6	4.7 ± 0.6	2.7 ± 1.0	—	—
SWT (d) sd	3.1 ± 0.6	3.8 ± 0.3	3.0 ± 0.4	2.4 ± 0.1	1.9–4.4
SWT (s) sd	4.8 ± 0.7	4.7 ± 0.5	4.6 ± 0.6	3.6 ± 0.1	3.3–6.2
LVID (d) sd	11.1 ± 1.3	11.3 ± 1.4	11.9 ± 0.7	9.8 ± 0.3	9.3 ± 0.3
LVID (s) sd	6.1 ± 0.9	7.3 ± 0.8	7.4 ± 0.7	6.8 ± 0.2	5.7 ± 0.2
FS sd	44.1% ± 6.4	35.3% ± 3.9	38.8% ± 4.6	—	38.6% ± 1.6
LVPWT (d) sd	2.9 ± 0.5	—	2.4 ± 0.3	1.9 ± 0.7	—
LVPWT (s) sd	4.5 ± 0.6	—	—	2.8 ± 0.1	3.2 ± 0.2
AoD (d) sd	7.3 ± 0.8	7.8 ± 0.4	8.5 ± 0.5	—	7.7 ± 0.16
AoD (s) sd	8.8 ± 0.6	—	—	—	7.3–8.6
LAD from RPLA sd	5.6 ± 0.1	—	—	—	—
LAD (d) from the LPLA sd	—	11.0 ± 0.8	—	—	—
LAD (s) from the LPLA sd	—	12.6 ± 1.3	—	—	—
LA: AO from LPLA sd	0.8 (RPLA) ± 0.2	1.4 (s) ± 0.1	—	—	—
E–F slope (cm/s) sd	22.8 ± 6.9	—	—	—	17.7 ± 0.87
ET (s) sd	0.43 ± 0.04	—	—	—	—

Ao = aorta, AoD = aortic root dimension, cm = centimeter, d = diastole, E–F = E point and F point of the mitral valve in M-mode, ET = ejection time, FS = left ventricular fractional shortening, kg = kilograms, LA = left atrium, LAD = left atrial diameter, LPLA = left parasternal long axis, LVID = left ventricular internal diameter, LVPWT = left ventricular posterior wall thickness, RPLA = right parasternal long axis, RVID = right ventricular internal diameter, s = systole, sd = standard deviation, SWT = interventricular septal wall thickness, — = not measured.

Table 2.3
Normal Values for M-Mode Echocardiography for Thoroughbred Foals (n = 16)

Age	Birth	1 hr	2 hr	4 hr	12 hr	24 hr	48 hr	4 dy	7 dy	14 dy	1 mth	2 mth	3 mth
HR (bpm)	99	87	80	82	102	96	91	89	93	91	76	55	54
	± 17	± 17	± 12	± 16	± 13	± 11	± 15	± 10	± 22	± 17	± 17	± 12	± 14
Body Wt	45.1	45.1	45.1	45.1	45.5	47.0	48.1	51.2	56.9	64.7	80.6	96.5	111.8
(kg)	± 8.6	± 8.6	± 8.6	± 8.6	± 8.9	± 9.0	± 8.7	± 9.0	± 10.1	± 12.5	± 13.6	± 12.9	± 16.1
RVTDd	2.2	2.4	2.3	2.1	2.2	2.4	2.8	2.5	2.6	2.5	2.6	2.9	2.7
(cm)	± 0.6	± 0.3	± 0.5	± 0.6	± 0.5	± 0.4	± 0.5	± 0.9	± 0.3	± 0.9	± 0.3	± 0.1	± 0.2
SWT	1.1	1.1	1.1	1.1	1.3	1.3	1.3	1.3	1.4	1.3	1.4	1.4	1.5
(cm)	± 0.3	± 0.2	± 0.1	± 0.4	± 0.2	± 0.3	± 0.2	± 0.2	± 0.2	± 0.2	± 0.2	± 0.3	± 0.1
LVIDd	6.0	6.2	6.0	5.9	5.7	5.8	5.9	6.2	6.5	6.9	7.4	7.5	7.8
(cm)	± 0.4	± 0.6	± 0.7	± 0.4	± 0.6	± 0.5	± 0.6	± 0.7	± 0.5	± 0.5	± 0.7	± 0.7	± 0.7
LVIDs	4.6	4.9	4.9	4.8	4.8	4.7	5.0	5.4	5.5	6.0	6.5	6.9	6.9
(cm)	± 0.4	± 0.5	± 0.6	± 0.4	± 0.6	± 0.6	± 0.4	± 0.8	± 0.4	± 0.1	± 0.1	± 0.2	± 0.9
FS%	24.31	22.62	22.46	17.10	19.54	21.33	22.77	18.61	20.08	20.17	16.25	18.18	21.06
	± 6.47	± 6.6	± 6.0	± 0.17	± 3.59	± 2.93	± 4.82	± 3.72	± 5.01	± 3.76	± 1.77	± 4.51	± 1.37
LVPWT	0.5	0.5	0.6	0.6	0.5	0.6	0.6	0.6	0.7	0.8	1.3	1.5	1.6
(cm)	± 0.1	± 0.04	± 0.1	± 0.03	± 0.1	± 0.04	± 0.1	± 0.04	± 0.1	± 0.1	± 0.1	± 0.2	± 0.2
AoD	3.09	2.86	2.84	3.02	3.39	3.70	3.60	3.57	3.61	3.75	4.19	3.95	4.34
(cm)	± 0.20	± 0.30	± 0.31	± 0.30	± 0.28	± 0.25	± 0.28	± 0.31	± 0.29	± 0.26	± 0.21	± 0.16	± 0.32
LAD	3.33	3.23	3.02	3.01	3.22	3.01	2.99	3.07	3.23	3.27	3.52	3.48	3.82
(cm)	± 0.98	± 0.75	± 0.54	± 0.48	± 0.73	± 0.70	± 0.56	± 0.67	± 0.50	± 0.84	± 0.92	± 0.75	± 0.60
LA/AO	1.08	1.13	1.06	1.00	0.95	0.81	0.83	0.86	0.90	0.87	0.84	0.88	0.88
	± 0.34	± 0.30	± 0.21	± 0.16	± 0.28	± 0.15	± 0.15	± 0.17	± 0.15	± 0.26	± 0.14	± 0.14	± 0.33
E–F slope	24.05	15.15	16.76	11.76	14.98	13.61	14.75	13.70	15.13	15.89	16.32	19.51	26.50
(cm/s)sd	± 13.57	± 4.40	± 9.77	± 2.44	± 3.43	± 2.38	± 2.57	± 3.00	± 3.14	± 2.09	± 3.67	± 2.40	± 5.07

Ao = aorta, AoD = aortic root dimension, bpm = beats per minute, d = diastole, ET = ejection time, E–F = E point and F point of the mitral valve in M-mode, FS = left ventricular fractional shortening, LA = left atrium, LAD = left atrial dimension, LVID = left ventricular internal dimension LVPWT = left ventricular posterior wall thickness, RVID = right ventricular internal diameter, s = systole, sd = standard deviation, SWT = interventricular septal wall thickness, Wt = weight
Adapted with permission from Stewart JH, Rose RJ, Barko A. Echocardiography in foals from birth to three months old. Equine Vet J 1984;16:332–341.

analysis of normal intracardiac flow because of the limited number of cardiac windows that allow Doppler alignment with normal flow (13). However, much useful information can be gathered from the evaluation of flow profiles and flow direction and from quantitative analysis. Doppler pulsed wave values have been reported in normal Standardbreds (13), Warmbloods (14), Thoroughbreds, and Thoroughbred crosses (15).

Equipment Requirements

Color flow, pulsed wave, and continuous wave Doppler systems are currently used in the evaluation of blood flow. Color flow Doppler may evaluate the magnitude and direction of flow and indicate turbulence by the spectral variance. Pulsed wave Doppler provides information on the direction, velocity, and characteristics of flow at a given

Table 2.4
Normal Values for M-Mode Echocardiography for Pony Foals

	Mean ± sd	Range	Linear Regression (x = weight in kg)	Correlation Coefficient
Body Wt (kg)	27 ± 10	14–57	—	—
RVTDd (cm)	—	0.8–2.0	0.016x + 0.9	r = 0.55
SWTd (cm)	1.1 ± 0.2	0.7–1.4	—	—
LVTDd (cm)	—	2.6–6.3	0.047x + 2.6	r = 0.74
LVIDs (cm)	—	1.5–4.7	0.038x + 1.5	r = 0.65
	34% ± 8%	24–50%	—	—
LVPWTd (cm)	0.9 ± 0.2	0.6–1.3	—	—
AoDd (cm)	—	2.1–3.8	0.021x + 2.2	r = 0.63
LADs from RPLA (cm)	—	1.6–3.4	0.023x + 1.6	r = 0.62
LA/AO from RPLA	0.82 ± 0.1	0.55–1.08	—	—
E–F slope (cm/s)	15 ± 4.9	8–30	—	—

Ao = aorta, AoD = aortic root dimension, d = diastole, E–F = E point and F point of the mitral valve M-mode, FS = left ventricular fractional shortening, LA = left atrium, LAD = left atrial dimension, LVID = left ventricular internal diameter, LVPWT = left ventricular posterior wall thickness, RVID = right ventricular internal diameter, s = systole, sd = standard deviation, SWT = interventricular septal wall thickness, Wt = weight, — = not measured.
Adapted with permission from Lombard CW, Evans E, Martin L, et al. Blood pressure, electrocardiogram and echocardiogram measurements in the growing pony foal. Equine Vet J 1984;16:342–347.

depth. Continuous wave Doppler may provide further quantitative information on the high velocity flows. All three Doppler modalities may be used in one examination.

Transducer Selection

Unlike the optimal B-mode images created when the ultrasound beam is perpendicular to the structures, the optimal Doppler signal is created when the ultrasound beam is parallel to flow. Moreover, measurements of high-velocity flow require a lower-frequency transducer than that required for B-mode imaging. Therefore, although simultaneous B-mode and Doppler imaging are advantageous for Doppler alignment, less than optimal B-Mode images are demonstrated during the examination.

Alignment of Doppler Beam to Blood Flow

Because maximum velocity can only be calculated if the Doppler beam is spatially aligned to blood flow, failure to align the beam reduces the amplitude of the signal of the frequency shift that is equal to the product of the true amplitude and the cosine of the angle of intercept. This reduction is not linear. At a 20° angle of incidence, the estimated velocity of the signal is decreased by 6%, and the pressure difference is underestimated by 12%, however, at angles greater than 20°, the error rapidly increases. That is, at 30° the velocity is underestimated by 13% and the pressure difference by 25%, at 40° the velocity is underestimated by 24% and the pressure difference by 41%, and at 60° the velocity is underestimated by 50% and the pressure difference by 75%. Even in the normal heart, the direction of flow can only be assumed from the two-dimensional image. Multiple Doppler transducer positions should be used to search for the best possible alignment to flow and therefore the best Doppler signal.

Angle correction computations are available for use with most Doppler equipment. Both overestimation and underestimation of velocities and pressure differences are possible when the true angle of intercept is unknown from the two-dimensional image. One of the applications of color flow may be to help to determine the direction of blood flow, thus enabling the angle of intercept of the Doppler beam to be minimized. Angle correction, if used at all, must be applied with care.

Wall Filter (Low-Frequency Filter)

A filter is used to eliminate low-frequency and high-intensity noise that is usually generated by the relatively slow-moving and strongly reflecting cardiac chamber walls. The degree of wall filtering required varies, but it is usually in the range of 100 to 400 hz. When the low-frequency signals are removed from the audio signal, the accompanying high-frequency signals become easier to hear. A wall filter setting that is too high eliminates useful lower-frequency information.

Sample Volume Size for Pulsed Wave Doppler

When using pulsed wave Doppler, the sample volume size may be increased up to 10 or 15 mm or decreased to 1 mm. A larger sample volume is useful when searching for a small jet in a large chamber. Once the flow has been located, the sample volume may then be reduced to interrogate and evaluate the flow more accurately.

Color M-Mode

Color M-mode is used to analyze the timing of flow events precisely. The cursor is not only an M-mode cursor but a Doppler cursor as well. The color M-mode is a combination of the standard M-mode of structures encountered by the cursor and a color M-mode display of flow along the path of the cursor.

Preparation of the Horse

The horse must stand quietly with little body sway or movement to enable a complete Doppler echocardiographic examination to be performed. If necessary, sedation may be required to facilitate the examination. The haircoat is clipped or shaved, and the electrocardiographic electrodes are placed as previously described for two-dimensional B-mode and M-mode examination.

Examination

Before commencing the Doppler examination, it is advisable to turn down the volume control, so the horse will not be frightened by the sudden loud noise of the Doppler signal. The volume can be increased once the horse is comfortable with the noise.

Multiple transducer positions should be used to examine velocities for each cardiac chamber and vessel (Table 2.5) (1). After the flow to be interrogated is located, the transducer direction is altered to bring in the loudest audible signal and to record the highest velocity and least velocity spread (18). Qualitative assessment of flow with color Doppler may be made in an almost infinite number of imaging views and may help to locate flows through anatomic defects or eccentric jet flows. As previously stated, optimal Doppler waveforms are obtained when the Doppler sample volume or cursor is aligned parallel to flow.

The image planes described in the following sections are those that best approximate alignment to expected blood flow given the anatomic limitations of the horse's thorax. Color flow Doppler can be used to locate areas of highest velocity for spectral Doppler analyses.

Images from the Right Hemithorax
Right Parasternal Long Axis Views

Dorsal Location Right Ventricular Inlet View (Fig. 2.12) (4). The transducer is placed in the fourth or fifth intercostal space, dorsal to the level of the olecranon process. The sector edge is directed vertically toward the dorsum of

Table 2.5
Image Planes for Doppler Echocardiographic Examination

Image Planes	Flow Examined
Images from the right hemithorax	
Parasternal long axis views	
Dorsal location right ventricular inlet	RV inflow, TI, VSD, ASD, *MI, *AI
Apical ventricular inlets	RV inflow, TI, VSD, *MI, *AI
Parasternal short axis view	
Left ventricle at the level of the mitral valve	VSD, *MI
Heart base at the level of the pulmonary artery	RV inflow, PI, TI
Parasternal angled view	
Dorsal location RVOT	RV inflow, PI, TI, pulmonary outflow, subpulmonic VSD (TS, PS)
Images from the left hemithorax	
Parasternal long axis views	
Left ventricular inlet view	LV inflow, MI, *VSD
Apical five-chamber view	Aortic outflow, AI, VSD
Parasternal cranial angled views	
Left ventricular outflow tract/aorta	Aortic outflow, AI
Right ventricular inlet/outlet	RV inflow, TI, PI

* Eccentric flow may be detected although the Doppler signal may not be optimally placed for maximum velocities.
ASD = atrial septal defect, MI = mitral insufficiency, PI = pulmonary insufficiency, PS = pulmonary stenosis, TI = tricuspid insufficiency, TS = tricuspid stenosis, VSD = ventricular septal defect, ( ) = less common.
Adapted with permission from Long KJ, Bonagura JD, Darke PGG. Standardised imaging technique for guided M-mode and Doppler echocardiology in the horse. Equine Vet J 1992;24:226–235.

the horse (0°). The sector is then rotated up to 90° clockwise (Fig. 2.12A), and the axial beam is then adjusted through a complete range cranially and dorsally to image the right ventricular inflow (1). Reef and colleagues (13) also used the foregoing view to obtain right ventricular inlet (atrial outflow) Doppler recordings and left ventricular outflow and recordings of flow in the ascending aorta. Although this view, in the normal horse, is used primarily for the right ventricular inflow, in horses with abnormal flow it may be used for the investigation of tricuspid insufficiency (Fig. 2.12B,C), ventricular septal defects, atrial septal defects, and mitral insufficiency and aortic insufficiency with eccentric flow. For routine measurements of right ventricular inflow, the sample volume or cursor is placed in the right ventricle at the point of maximal tricuspid opening, just distal to the tricuspid annulus for tricuspid valve flow and in the distal 25% of the right atrium, just above the valve leaflets. For descriptions of the sample volume or cursor placement in patients with abnormal flow, see the section of this chapter on specific investigations.

APICAL VENTRICULAR INLETS VIEW (Fig. 2.13) (4). The transducer is placed in the fourth or fifth intercostal space at, or just dorsal to, the level of the olecranon process. The edge of the sonographic sector is rotated from 0° up to 45° clockwise, and center of the sector beam is then directed dorsally

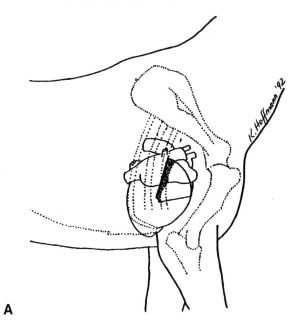

A

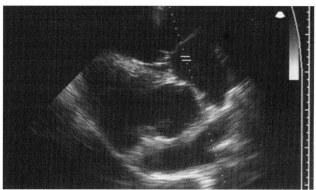

B

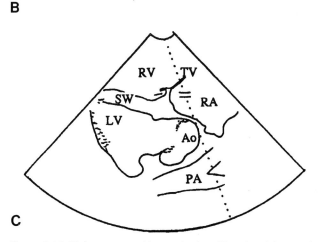

C

Figure 2.12. Right parasternal long axis, dorsal location right ventricular inlet. **A,** Schematic drawing of transducer placement and rotation. **B,** Sonogram of a pulsed wave sample volume placed in the right atrium for tricuspid insufficiency. **C,** Schematic drawing of the sonogram in **B.** Ao = aorta; LV = left ventricle; PA = pulmonary artery; RA = right atrium; RV = right ventricle; SW = septal wall; TV = tricuspid valve. Reprinted with permission from Hoffmann KL. Echocardiography of the horse. Veterinary Applications Module. Lane Cove, Australia: The University of Sydney/Ausonics International Proprietary, Ltd, 1993.

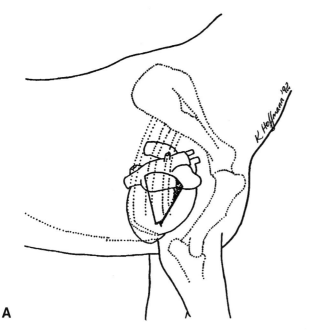

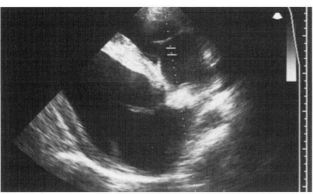

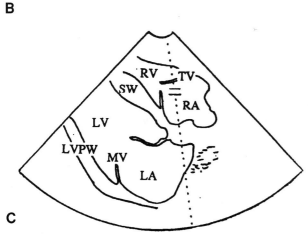

Figure 2.13. Right parasternal long axis, apical ventricular inlets. **A,** Schematic drawing of transducer placement and rotation. **B,** Sonogram of a pulsed wave sample volume placed in the right atrium for tricuspid insufficiency. **C,** Schematic drawing of the sonogram in **B.** LA = left atrium; LV = left ventricle; LVPW = left ventricular posterior wall; MV = mitral valve; RA = right atrium; RV = right ventricle; SW = septal wall; TV = tricuspid valve. Reprinted with permission from Hoffmann KL. Echocardiography of the horse. Veterinary Applications Module. Lane Cove, Australia: The University of Sydney/Ausonics International Proprietary, Ltd, 1993.

and slightly cranially (Fig. 2.13A) to image the right ventricular inflow (1). This view (Fig. 2.13B,C) should also be used in conjunction with the dorsal location right ventricular inlet view (see Fig. 2.12B,C) to investigate right ventricular inflow (15), tricuspid insufficiency, ventricular septal defects, atrial septal defects, and mitral insufficiency and aortic insufficiency with eccentric flow.

Right Parasternal Short Axis Views

LEVEL OF THE MITRAL VALVE. As previously described for two-dimensional echocardiography, short axis images at the level of the mitral valve (see Fig. 2.3F,G) are obtained by placing the transducer in the reference position and then rotating the sector between 60° to 80° counterclockwise while directing the center of the sector slightly cranially or caudally and dorsally (1). Eccentric mitral regurgitant flow may be located in this view, as well as flow through an interventricular septal defect.

LEVEL OF THE PULMONARY ARTERY (Fig. 2.14) (4). The transducer is placed in the fourth intercostal space at or just dorsal to the level of the olecranon process (Fig. 2.14A). The sector edge is then rotated 20° to 60° counterclockwise, and the center of the sonographic sector is angled dorsally and strongly cranially (1). This view may be used in the interrogation of the right ventricular inflow and outflow as well as the investigation of suspected tricuspid or pulmonary insufficiency (Fig. 2.14B,C). For right ventricular outflow measurements, the sample volume or cursor is placed just above the valve in the pulmonary artery (15). Care should be taken to keep the sample volume in the center of the vessel.

Right Parasternal Angled View: Dorsal Location Right Ventricular Outflow View (Fig. 2.15) (4). Reef and associates (13) obtained this view by placing the transducer in the third intercostal space and directing the transducer cranially (Fig. 2.15A) to obtain a sagittal view of the right atrium, tricuspid valve, right ventricular outflow tract, pulmonary valve, and pulmonary artery (Fig. 2.15 B,C). Long, Bonagura, and Darke (1) also obtained this view by placing the transducer in the third intercostal space, dorsal to the level of the olecranon process. The sector edge was then rotated 30° counterclockwise, and the center of the sonographic sector was adjusted cranially and dorsally (Fig. 2.15A) to view right ventricular inflow and outflow (Fig. 2.15B,C). This view is used for the investigation of tricuspid inflow (15), tricuspid insufficiency, pulmonary insufficiency, subpulmonary ventricular septal defects, and, less commonly, tricuspid or pulmonary stenosis.

Images from the Left Hemithorax

Left Parasternal Caudal Long Axis Views

LEFT VENTRICULAR INLET VIEW (Fig. 2.16) (4). The transducer is placed caudal to the left olecranon process and ventral or caudal to the left apical impulse. The sector edge is rotated 0o to 40o counterclockwise, and the center of the

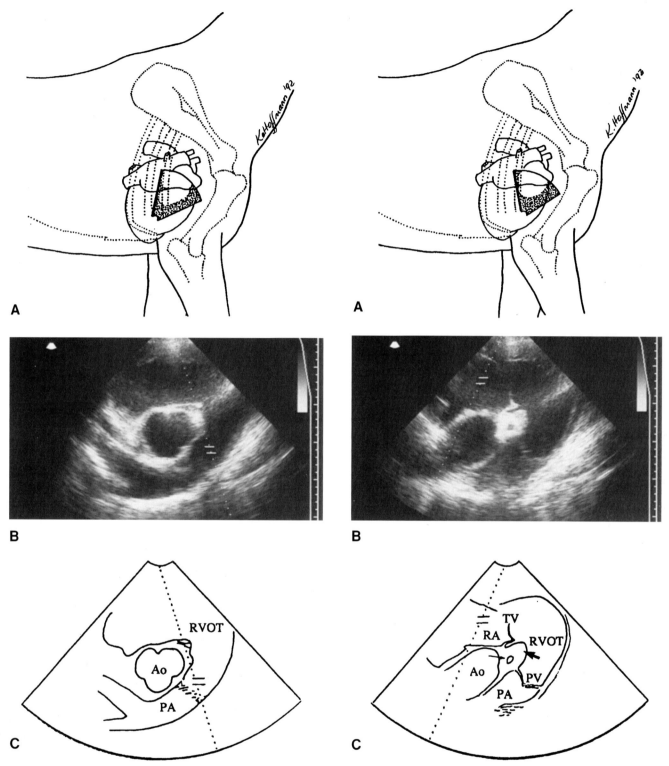

Figure 2.14. Right parasternal short axis view, heart base at the level of the pulmonary artery. **A,** Schematic drawing of transducer placement and rotation. **B,** Sonogram of a pulsed wave sample volume placed in the right ventricular outflow tract for pulmonary insufficiency. **C,** Schematic drawing of the sonogram in **B.** Ao = aorta; PA = pulmonary artery; RVOT = right ventricular outflow tract. Reprinted with permission from Hoffmann KL. Echocardiography of the horse. Veterinary Applications Module. Lane Cove, Australia: The University of Sydney/Ausonics International Proprietary, Ltd, 1993.

Figure 2.15. Right parasternal angled, dorsal location right ventricular outflow view. **A,** Schematic drawing of transducer placement and rotation. **B,** Sonogram of a pulsed wave sample volume placed in the right atrium for tricuspid insufficiency. **C,** Schematic drawing of the sonogram in **B.** Ao = aorta; PA = pulmonary artery; PV = pulmonary valve; RA = right atrium; RVOT = right ventricular outflow tract; TV = tricuspid valve; large arrow = superventricular crest; small arrow = right coronary artery. Reprinted with permission from Hoffmann KL. Echocardiography of the horse. Veterinary Applications Module. Lane Cove, Australia: The University of Sydney/Ausonics International Proprietary, Ltd, 1993.

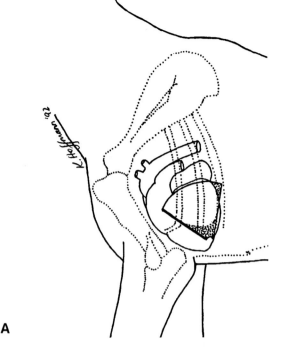

A

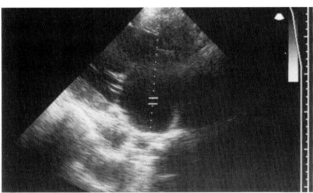

B

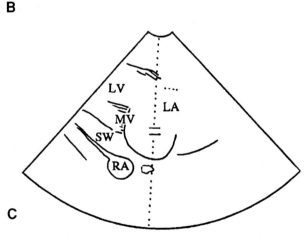

C

Figure 2.16. Left parasternal long axis, left ventricular inlet view. **A,** Schematic drawing of transducer placement and rotation. **B,** Sonogram of a pulsed wave sample volume placed in the left atrium for mitral insufficiency. **C,** Schematic drawing of the sonogram in **B.** LA = left atrium; LV = left ventricle; MV = mitral valve; RA = right atrium; SW = septal wall. Reprinted with permission from Hoffmann KL. Echocardiography of the horse. Veterinary Applications Module. Lane Cove, Australia: The University of Sydney/Ausonics International Proprietary, Ltd, 1993.

sonographic sector is directed dorsally and either slightly cranially or caudally (Fig. 2.16A) to image the left atrium (1). Reef and colleagues (13) obtained a similar image by positioning the transducer in the fifth left intercostal space, just ventral to the point of the shoulder. From this position, a long axis view was made. These images (Fig. 2.16B,C) may be used to investigate left ventricular inflow, mitral insufficiency, and flow through an interventricular septal defect. For left mitral valve flow, the sample volume or cursor is positioned in the left ventricle just below the mitral annulus at the point of maximal opening of the mitral valve. For routine left atrial flow measurements, the sample volume or cursor is placed on the atrial side of the mitral valve (Fig. 2.16B,C).

APICAL FIVE-CHAMBER VIEW (Fig. 2.17) (4). The transducer is placed caudal to the left olecranon process and ventral to the left apical impulse. The sector edge is rotated 0° to 30° counterclockwise, and the center of the sonographic sector is directed both cranially and dorsally (Fig. 2.17A) from the caudal edge of the intercostal space (1). This view may be used to investigate aortic outflow, aortic insufficiency (Fig. 2.17B,C), and flow through an interventricular septal defect. The sample volume or cursor may be positioned in the outflow tract between the septal wall and the opened septal mitral valve leaflet or, for aortic outflow measurements, the sample volume or cursor may be positioned in the ascending aorta just above the sinus of Valsalva.

Left Parasternal Cranial Angled Views

LEFT VENTRICULAR OUTLET AND AORTA VIEW. The transducer is placed caudal to the left olecranon process and ventral to the left apical impulse. The edge of the sonographic sector is rotated 30° clockwise, and the center of the sector plane is directed dorsally and either cranially or slightly caudally to obtain the left ventricular outflow tract and aorta in long axis (1). This view may be difficult to obtain in some horses, but, when possible, it is used in the investigation of aortic outflow and aortic insufficiency.

RIGHT VENTRICULAR INLET AND OUTLET VIEWS (Fig. 2.18) (4). The transducer is placed as cranially as possible in the ventral part of the left second or third intercostal space (Fig. 2.18A). The edge of the sonographic sector is rotated to 30° clockwise and angled dorsally and slightly caudally (1). The image obtained is used in the investigation of right ventricular inflow and tricuspid and pulmonary insufficiency (Fig. 2.18B,C). To obtain a view of the pulmonary artery, Reef and associates (13) placed the transducer further dorsally, just below the level of the point of the shoulder.

Specific Investigations
Ventricular Function

Aspects of ventricular function may be studied during the inflow (atrioventricular valves) and outflow (aortic and pulmonary) of blood in the heart. In the tricuspid and mitral valves, when the sample volume is placed on the ventricular

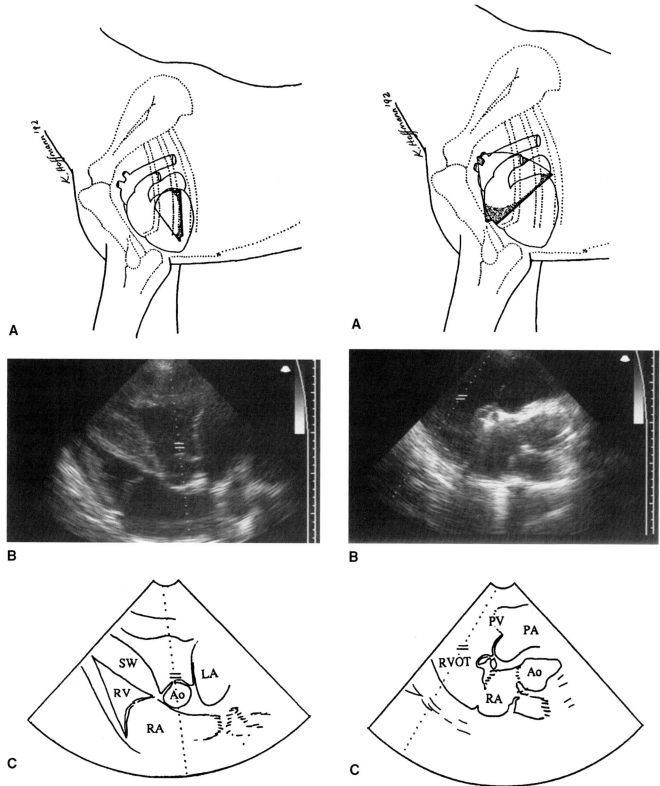

Figure 2.17. Left parasternal long axis, apical five-chamber image. **A,** Schematic drawing of transducer placement and rotation. **B,** Sonogram of a pulsed wave sample volume placed in the left ventricular outflow tract for aortic insufficiency. **C,** Schematic drawing of the sonogram in **B.** Ao = aorta; LA = left atrium; RA = right atrium; RV = right ventricle; SW = septal wall. Reprinted with permission from Hoffmann KL. Echocardiography of the horse. Veterinary Applications Module. Lane Cove, Australia: The University of Sydney/Ausonics International Proprietary, Ltd, 1993.

Figure 2.18. Left parasternal angled, right ventricular inlet and outlet view. **A,** Schematic drawing of transducer placement and rotation. **B,** Sonogram of a pulsed wave sample volume placed in the right ventricular outflow tract for pulmonary insufficiency. **C,** Schematic drawing of the sonogram in **B.** Ao = aorta; PA = pulmonary artery; PV = pulmonary valve; RA = right atrium; RVOT = right ventricular outflow tract. Reprinted with permission from Hoffmann KL. Echocardiography of the horse. Veterinary Applications Module. Lane Cove, Australia: The University of Sydney/Ausonics International Proprietary, Ltd, 1993.

side of the leaflets so that it remains between the leaflets during diastole (Blissett and Bonagura), the peak E (peak velocity during the phase of rapid ventricular filling), peak A (peak velocity during atrial contraction), and deceleration time (measured from peak E to the point where the slope of the slowing flow would intercept the base line) can be measured (Table 2.6).

In the aortic and pulmonary arteries, the peak velocity, peak acceleration (from the onset of the spectral waveform to the start of the peak velocity plateau), velocity time integral (tracing the modal velocity of the Doppler signal), preejection period (time from the onset of the QRS to the start of the spectral waveform), and ejection time can be measured (Table 2.7). Horses must be as calm as possible during the study because subtle changes in autonomic tone may influence heart rate and therefore affect Doppler values.

Tricuspid inflow measurements are the least variable when measured in the right parasternal angled view dorsal location compared with the right parasternal long axis view. The tricuspid E and A peaks are significantly greater in the angled view than they are when measured in the long axis view (15). E and A velocities are higher and the deceleration time of the E signal is shorter in the mitral valve compared with the tricuspid valve. Also, aortic blood flow velocity recorded from the right hemithorax is lower than that recorded from the left hemithorax (14, 15).

There is no difference in horses with or without ejection murmurs in the maximum recorded velocity in either the pulmonary or aortic outflow. However, the peak acceleration time of the aortic waveforms is lower and the time to peak acceleration is longer in horses with ejection murmurs (15). Also, horses with left-sided early diastolic flow murmurs have a higher peak E velocity in the mitral inflow than do horses that do not have the murmur.

Ventricular Septal Defects. Ventricular septal defects may be demonstrated in the right parasternal long and short axis views (see Figs. 2.1, 2.2, and 2.3) and in the left parasternal long and short axis views (see Figs. 2.5, 2.6, and 2.7). Sub-pulmonary ventricular septal defects are best investigated in the cranial and dorsal right parasternal angled view (see Fig. 2.15) of the right ventricular outflow tract (1). When investigating ventricular septal defects, if the defect is not visible, the entire septum should be interrogated to identify the

Table 2.6
Pulsed Wave Doppler Measurements of Tricuspid and Mitral Inflow in Normal Adult Horses (Mean ± SD)

Variable	TV (angled)	TV (long)	MV
E peak velocity (m/s)	0.90 ± 0.10	0.65 ± 0.10	0.70 ± 0.14
E decel (s)	—	0.24 ± 0.04	0.22 ± 0.03
A peak velocity (m/s)	0.69 ± 0.14	0.53 ± 0.12	0.42 ± 0.10

Angled = angled view in dorsal location, decel = deceleration, long = long axis view, MV = mitral valve, SD = standard deviation, TV = tricuspid valve.
Adapted with permission from Blissett KJ, Bonagura JD. Pulsed wave Doppler echocardiography in normal horses. Equine Vet J 1995(Suppl 19); 38–46.

Table 2.7
Pulsed Wave Doppler Measurements of Pulmonary and Aortic Outflow in Normal Adult Horses (Mean ± SD)

	PA Outflow	AO Outflow
Peak velocity (m/s)	0.91 ± 0.08	0.94 ± 0.09
Accel time (s)	0.21 ± 0.03	0.12 ± 0.02
VTI (cm)	25.74 ± 3.07	25.37 ± 3.21
PEP (s)	0.06 ± 0.02	0.08 ± 0.02
ET (s)	0.50 ± 0.03	0.47 ± 0.03

Accel = acceleration, AO = aortic, ET = ejection time, PA = pulmonary artery, PEF = preejection period, SD = standard deviation, VTI = velocity time integral.
Adapted with permission from Blissett KJ, Bonagura JD. Pulsed wave Doppler echocardiography in normal horses. Equine Vet J 1995(Suppl 19); 38–46.

shunt. Once located, the area of abnormal flow in the right ventricle and/or right ventricular outflow tract is mapped with pulsed wave Doppler or color flow Doppler echocardiography. The maximum flow velocity through the defect may be measured by continuous wave Doppler (12), or if the defect is unrestricted, the lower velocity may be measured by pulsed wave Doppler.

Tricuspid Insufficiency. Most tricuspid regurgitation jets are detected in the dorsal and the apical right parasternal long axis views (see Figs. 2.12 and 2.13) of the right ventricular inlet (12). Regurgitant flow may also be found in the right parasternal short axis view at the level of the pulmonary artery (see Fig. 2.14) and the right parasternal angled view (see Fig. 2.15) of the right ventricular outflow tract (1). The sample volume or cursor may be placed in the right atrium just above the tricuspid leaflets. Multiple transducer positions should be used. Once a regurgitant jet is identified, pulsed wave or color flow Doppler may be used to map the direction and extent of the abnormal flow, and continuous wave Doppler echocardiography may be used to document the maximum velocity of flow.

Pulmonary Insufficiency. The right parasternal short axis view at the level of the pulmonary artery (see Fig. 2.14) and the right parasternal angled view of the dorsal location of the right ventricular outflow (see Fig. 2.15) are the suggested views for the Doppler interrogation of the pulmonary valve (1). The sample volume or cursor may be placed in the right ventricular outflow tract just below the pulmonary valve. Once regurgitant flow is found, the direction and extent of the flow should be mapped and the maximum velocity measured.

Mitral Insufficiency. The left parasternal caudal long axis view of the apical left ventricular inlet (see Fig. 2.16) is the preferred view for the investigation of the mitral valve (1). The sample volume is placed on the atrial side of the mitral valve, and the regurgitant jet is located. The left atrium is examined by pulsed wave Doppler or color flow Doppler to map the extent of the regurgitant flow in the atrium (12). Because flow occurs from a chamber of high pressure to one of low pressure, the pressure drop is high, and as such continuous wave Doppler is usually necessary to measure the high-velocity regurgitant flows. If the animal has congestive heart failure, the associated higher diastolic pressures and lower ventricular pressures may result in a regurgitant flow of lower velocity.

Aortic Insufficiency. The left ventricular outflow tract is investigated for a regurgitant jet from the aortic valve into the left ventricular outflow tract (12). This investigation is best performed from the left parasternal caudal long axis five-chamber view (see Fig. 2.17) or the left parasternal cranial angled view (see Fig. 2.9) of left ventricular outflow tract and the aortic valve (1). The sample volume or cursor may be placed in the left ventricular outflow tract, below the aortic valve and between the septal leaflet of the mitral valve and the septal wall. Again, the extent and direction of the regurgitant flow should be interrogated, and maximum velocity should be measured.

Other Conditions. Other shunts or jets can be investigated in a similar fashion. The sonographer should obtain a view that aligns the suspected abnormal flow parallel to the Doppler cursor, use pulsed wave or color flow Doppler (or both) to map the direction and extent of the abnormal flow, and document the maximum flow velocity with continuous wave Doppler echocardiography.

Normal Findings

When the Doppler sample volume or cursor is aligned to flow, most normal flow is laminar. Laminar flow is present when most red blood cells are moving in the same direction at approximately the same velocity. Moreover, laminar flow has a high, clean, audible signal, whereas disturbed or nonlaminar flow contains mixed-frequency sounds and has a rough quality. In animals with anatomic defects, nonlaminar flow is frequently found and is characterized by red blood cells moving at different velocities or in different directions. Although laminar flow usually indicates the absence of disease, it may be present in abnormal jets from discrete anatomic lesions, for example, valvular stenoses (18). The normal ventricular inflow aligns to the septum in the right ventricle and the lateral left ventricular wall (18).

The initial report on normal intracardiac blood flow in the horse (13) demonstrated the difficulties of alignment of the Doppler cursor to flow when standard two-dimensional imaging planes were used. The flow velocities reported by Reef and associates (13) were angle corrected from 20° up to 70°.

Regurgitant flow patterns of normal valves have been described in dogs (19) and in people (18, 19). These regurgitant flows were considered mild, and in human patients, they did not extend 1cm beyond the closed valve. These mild regurgitant flows in patients with structurally normal hearts by two-dimensional echography are considered to be physiologic valvular regurgitations. Similar mild valvular regurgitations have been observed in the horse (Bonagura, personal communication) and in human patients (18).

The use of standard protocols for the examination of the equine heart, as described in this chapter, combined with the knowledge of the normal two-dimensional anatomy, M-mode measurements, and Doppler investigative skills will ensure that the heart is fully examined for evidence of structural disorders and flow abnormalities.

REFERENCES

1. Long KJ, Bonagura JD, Darke PGG. Standardized imaging technique for guided M-mode and Doppler echocardiography in the horse. Equine Vet J 1992;24:226–235.
2. Carslten JC. Two-dimensional, real-time echocardiology in the horse. Vet Radiol 1987;28:76–87.
3. Reef VB. Echocardiographic examination in the horse: the basics. Compend Contin Educ Pract Vet 1990;12:1312–1319.
4. Hoffmann KL. Doppler echocardiography of the horse and Echocardiography of the horse. Veterinary applications module. Lane Cove, Australia: University of Sydney/Ausonics International Proprietary, Ltd, 1993.
5. Lescure F, Tamzali J. Valeurs de reference en echocardiographie TM chez le cheval de sport. Rev Med Vet 1984;135:405–418.
6. Voros K, Holmes JR, Gibbs C. Measurement of cardiac dimensions with two-dimensional echocardiography in the living horse. Equine Vet J 1991;23:461–465.
7. O'Callaghan MW. Comparison of echocardiographic and autopsy measurements of cardiac dimensions in the horse. Equine Vet J 1985;17:61–368.
8. Pipers FS, Hamlin RL. Echocardiography in the horse. J Am Vet Med Assoc 1977;170:815–822.
9. Stewart JH, Rose RJ, Barko A. Echocardiography in foals from birth to three months old. Equine Vet J 1984;16:332–341.
10. Lombard CW, Evans E, Martin L, et al. Blood pressure, electrocardiogram and echocardiogram measurements in the growing pony foal. Equine Vet J 1984;16:342–347.
11. Wingfield WE, Miller CW, Voss JL, et al. Echocardiography in assessing mitral valve motion in 3 horses with atrial fibrillation. Equine Vet J 1980;12:181–184.
12. Reef VB. Large animal diagnostic procedures guide. Lane Cove, Australia: Ausonics International Proprietary, Ltd, 1990.
13. Reef VB, Lalezari K, De Boo J, et al. Pulsed-wave Doppler evaluation of intracardiac blood flow in 30 clinically normal Standardbred horses. Am J Vet Res 1989;50:75–83.
14. Weinberger T. Doppler-echocardiographue beim Pfred. PhD thesis, 1991, University of Hanover, Germany.
15. Blisset KJ, Bonagura JD. Pulsed wave Doppler echocardiography in normal horses. Equine Vet J 1995;(Suppl 19):38–46.
16. Goldberg SJ, Allen HD, Marx GR, et al. Doppler echocardiography. 2nd ed. Philadelphia: Lea & Febiger, 1988.
17. Kirberger RM, Bland-Van der Berg P, Darazs B. Doppler echocardiography in the normal dog. Part 1: velocity findings and flow patterns. Vet Radiol Ultrasound, 1992;33:370–379.
18. Sahn DJ, Marciel BC. Physiological valvular regurgitation: Doppler echocardiography and the potential for iatrogenic heart disease. Circulation 1988;78:1075–1977.
19. Choong CY, Abascal VM, Weyman J, et al. Prevalence of valvular regurgitation by Doppler echocardiography in patients with structurally normal hearts by two-dimensional echocardiography. Am Heart J 1989;117:636–642.

3. Thoracic Ultrasound

NORMAN W. RANTANEN

The clinician may question the rationale of using diagnostic ultrasound to examine lungs, which are usually filled with air, with a modality that does not penetrate air; however, ultrasound has become the preferred method of characterizing equine thoracic disease. When ultrasound is combined with radiology, both aerated and nonaerated lungs as well as the thoracic space can be thoroughly evaluated. Since the first reports of thoracic ultrasonographic examination of horses appeared in the literature (1–3), several authors have stressed the diagnostic and prognostic importance of this modality in evaluating thoracic disease (4–9).

Horses have a high incidence of low-grade pneumonia, as evidenced by the frequency of pleuropneumonia occurring after shipping and after administration of general anesthesia. I surveyed 168 horses of all ages and of various breeds (predominantly thoroughbreds) presented for elective surgical procedures and found that 29% had ultrasonographic evidence of pneumonia (unpublished data). Presence of lung surface consolidation or pleural effusion was considered ultrasonographic evidence of pneumonia. Many of these horses had pneumonia confirmed with transtracheal wash, culture, and cytologic examination. In one study, a large percentage of racehorses tested positive for lung inflammation based on transtracheal wash examination (10). The high percentage of thoroughbred racehorses with exercise-induced pulmonary hemorrhage suggests a high incidence of lung disease (11).

The purpose of this chapter is threefold: (a) to review cross-sectional thoracic and surrounding cranial abdominal anatomy; (b) to discuss scanning techniques and pertinent ultrasonographic physical principles peculiar to the highly reflective air-filled lung; and (c) to describe the normal ultrasonographic appearance of the lungs and thoracic space. Although reference must be made to the heart during a discussion of thoracic ultrasound, the reader is referred to Chapters 2 and 28 for definitive cardiac ultrasound. The abnormal thorax is covered in Chapter 29.

NORMAL ANATOMY

Figures 3.1 through 3.6 were made from an equine cadaver frozen in an upright position before sectioning. They are viewed from the caudal aspect with the dorsal at the top. The cranial thorax contains the cranial lung lobes, trachea, esophagus, cranial vascular segment, fat, and, depending on the horse's age, remnants of the thymus. The cranial thorax is deep to the triceps muscles and muscles of the lateral thoracic wall (see Fig. 3.1). The heart is normally covered by air-filled lung except at the cardiac notches. The right cardiac notch extends from approximately the third rib to the

fourth intercostal space. The left cardiac notch extends from the third rib to about the sixth rib (see Fig. 3.2). The cupula of the diaphragm apposes the caudal cardiac border. The lungs caudal to the cardiac notches, cranial and lateral to the diaphragm occupy the deepest part of the thorax. Fluid effusion accumulates in this area, and consolidation secondary to pneumonia is usually found because of gravity (see Fig. 3.3).

The liver is the predominant structure ventral to the right lung border. It may appose the diaphragm on the right side, or the diaphragmatic flexure of the colon may be seen deep to the diaphragm. The diaphragm is usually parallel to the body wall when it is seen ventral to the lung borders (see Fig. 3.4). Its obvious importance is that it divides the abdomen and the thorax. When the diaphragm cannot be found, diaphragmatic hernia should be suspected. The duodenum is seen at about the level of the twelfth thoracic vertebra medial to the right liver lobe and lateral to the right dorsal colon (see Fig. 3.5). It extends to the ventral aspect of the right kidney. A variable amount of lung covers the right liver lobe during normal respiration.

The spleen is the predominant parenchymal organ on the left side. The liver usually occupies the space deep to the diaphragm in the left cranial abdomen. The spleen is usually medial, but occasionally lateral, to the left liver lobe and rarely is found in the right cranial abdomen. The spleen extends from its cranial position to a position lateral to the left kidney in the lumbar fossa.

The lungs extend caudally to the level of the right kidney (see Fig. 3.6). During scanning, the lung partially covers the right kidney and a considerable portion of the spleen during inspiration. The right lung is thicker than the left because of the position of the heart in the left side of the thorax. The right accessory lung lobe that surrounds the caudal vena cava is normally not accessible to ultrasound. The cranial vascular segment, esophagus, and trachea are normally not imaged with ultrasound. The caudal vena cava is normally not imaged unless significant pleural effusion displaces the lung dorsally enough to allow the sound beam to penetrate the mediastinum caudal to the heart. Occasionally, in animals with massive lung consolidation, the caudal vena cava can be imaged through the lung.

SCANNING TECHNIQUES AND PHYSICAL PRINCIPLES

Because the lung surfaces are within 3 to 4 cm of the skin in most horses, they can be scanned with frequencies as high as 7.5 Mhz, which penetrate about 5 to 7 cm. Frequencies of 2.0 to 7.5 Mhz can be used because significant findings are straightforward and parenchymal detail is

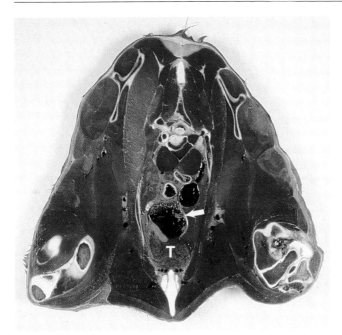

Figure 3.1. Cross-section of the cranial thorax made through the third and fourth thoracic vertebral junction at about the third intercostal space. The section is through the cranial wall of the right auricle (*arrow*). A remnant of the thymus (T) can be seen ventral to the right auricle in the ventral most aspect of the thoracic cavity. Dorsal is at the top and the section is viewed from the caudal aspect.

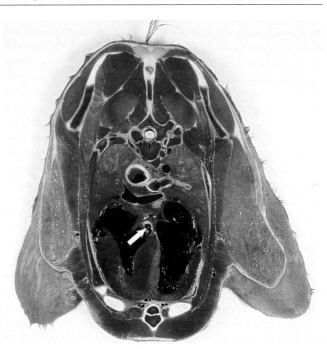

Figure 3.2. Cross-section of the thorax made through the central body of the sixth thoracic vertebra at about the fifth and sixth ribs through the heart at the level of the aortic origin (*arrow*). The relation of the triceps muscles can be seen. Dorsal is at the top and the section is viewed from the caudal aspect.

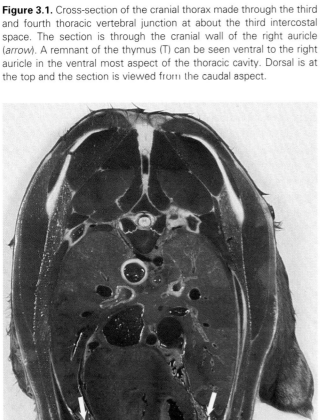

Figure 3.3. Cross-section made through the caudal end of the seventh thoracic vertebra through the caudal aspect of the heart just cranial to the diaphragm. The section cut through the head of the seventh rib dorsally and through the distal end of the sixth ventrally. Note the fat in the ventral thorax (*arrows*). Dorsal is at the top and the section is viewed from the caudal aspect.

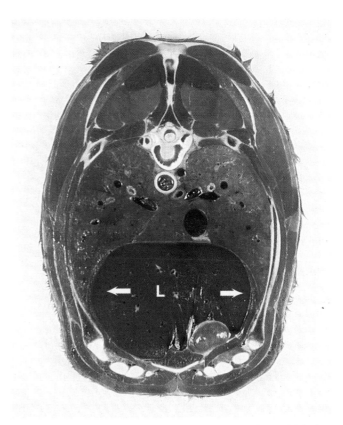

Figure 3.4. Cross-section through the caudal end of the eighth thoracic vertebra and the seventh ribs. The liver (L) is adjacent to the diaphragm (*arrows*).

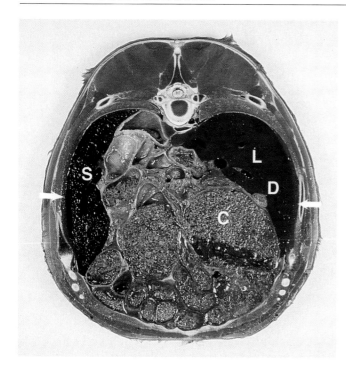

Figure 3.5. Cross-section through the thirteenth and fourteenth thoracic vertebral junction showing the spatial relationship of the right liver lobe (L), duodenum at the level of the major papilla (D), right dorsal colon (C), and spleen (S) ventral to the lung borders. The lungs were not expanded in this postmortem section, but when the lungs are aerated, a considerable amount of lung is superimposed over the liver and spleen, especially during inspiration. The diaphragm (*arrows*) is normally seen parallel to the body surface. Dorsal is at the top and the section is viewed from the caudal aspect.

not as important to make pertinent findings. Lateral resolution is not as great a factor as it is for other tissues. Lower frequencies, however, allow penetration to the deeper landmarks ventral and medial to the lung margins and extend further into large lung consolidations and massive effusions.

Clipping the animal's hair is usually not necessary to image lung surfaces successfully. This is especially true of well-groomed performance horses, many of which have already had a whole body clip. Some owners and trainers are reluctant to allow close clipping of hair for various reasons, such as when horses are to be sold and when horses are racing and showing. Aqueous gel should be spread on the horse's skin in the direction of the hair to eliminate trapped air. Wetting the hair with water or alcohol before applying aqueous gel helps to eliminate trapped air. Scans can be made with just alcohol application in most horses, but the

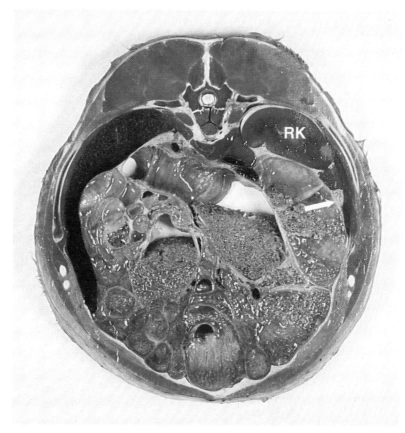

Figure 3.6. Cross-section made through the mid-body of the sixteenth thoracic vertebra at the level of the right kidney (RK). The duodenum (*arrow*) can be seen ventral to the kidney. A small portion of liver was between the kidney and duodenum on this section, showing the close association of these structures. The section was made cranial to the left kidney through the spleen. During inspiration, the caudal lung can extend over the cranial aspect of the right kidney and spleen. Dorsal is at the top and the section is viewed from the caudal aspect.

alcohol may have to be replenished because of evaporation. (Remember, alcohol is flammable.) Mineral oil is not recommended because it may damage the scanhead cables. The skin should be adequately prepared, however, whenever image quality is suboptimal or when invasive techniques such as thoracentesis or biopsy are performed.

The *entire lung surfaces* should be scanned bilaterally. Significant pneumonia and small effusions are usually found ventrally because of gravity; however, significant lung disease can be found anywhere on the lung surface. The scanhead should pass between all the costal margins from the dorsal limit to the ventral lung margins. Extra time should be allotted for examination of the ventral margins of the lungs in the deepest portion of the thorax caudal to the heart and along the margins of the cardiac notches including the cranial lung lobes. If the horse has a history of exercise-induced pulmonary hemorrhage, the caudodorsal and dorsal lung surfaces should be examined carefully. Pleural roughening and surface consolidation can be found in these sites. At some time during the examination, the cranial lung lobes and the cranial thoracic space should be imaged to rule out pneumonia or cranial thoracic abscess. The horse's forelimbs need to be extended forward to facilitate examining the cranial thorax. The cranial lung lobes should have smooth echogenic appearances; however, it is difficult to direct the beam perpendicular to the surface of the lung to create the characteristic parallel artifact.

ULTRASONOGRAPHIC APPEARANCE OF THE NORMAL LUNG AND THORACIC SPACE

The parietal and visceral pleural interface appears as a thin, echolucent black line immediately superficial to the white echogenic line corresponding to the air in the lung. Air is a near-perfect reflector because of its low density and its slow propagation velocity of sound compared with soft tissue (see Chap. 1). Therefore, when the sound beam encounters the normal air-filled lung, it reverberates between the transducer and the lung surface. This reverberation creates a characteristic parallel concentric artifact forming parallel lines in the image corresponding to the lung surface and intercostal muscle fascial planes (Fig. 3.7). Each time the sound reflects back to the transducer, another line is recorded deeper in the image because of the time delay. The echoes forming the reverberation lines deep to the pleural surface are artifacts. When the parallel concentric artifact is seen, the lung surface is flat, highly reflective, and normal.

When the lung surface (or sound–air interface) is irregular and not flat, the shape of the artifact changes dramatically. Small pleural irregularities cause a different-shaped gas reverberation artifact sometimes referred to as a "comet tail." It appears as a white artifactual streak arising from the lung surface (Fig. 3.8). These artifacts are more obvious on scans made with divergent beams such as sector, convex, and annular-array scanheads than with linear-array images. The divergent beam accentuates the "comet tails." The same artifacts on the linear-array image are vertical and are

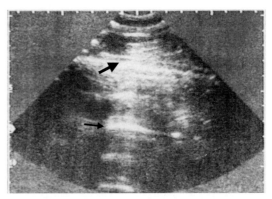

Figure 3.7. Reverberation artifact caused by the highly reflective air-filled lung. Scans were made with a 3.5-Mhz annular-array scanhead. Reflection arises from the lung surface (*large arrow*) as well as from the fascial planes of the intercostal muscles. The first major reverberation line is a mirror image reflection of the skin surface (*small arrow*); the line may have an upward "curve" corresponding to indentation of the skin if the scanhead has a convex shape.

more difficult to see (Fig. 3.9). These so-called comet tails indicate that the pleura (or sound–air interface) has small irregularities. In other words, the air–sound interface is not flat. The visceral pleural surface may appear as an irregular line. Anatomically normal horses of any age may have a few of these irregularities along the ventral margins of both lungs. A few of these small artifacts *do not* allow a diagnosis of lung disease to be made. The comet tails are artifacts and provide no anatomic information about the lung deep to their origins. Their significance is as indicators that the sound beam's encounter with the subpleural air is no longer flat at those sites.

The thoracic cavity is usually filled to capacity with lungs, heart, fat, and vessels. A small amount of fluid, the *liquor pleurae,* is present in the thorax. This fluid helps to create the thin echolucency of the parietal and visceral pleural interface seen on the scans. This fluid can measure up to a few centimeters. It should only be seen in the ventral thorax, and no fibrin tags or echogenic particles should be vis-

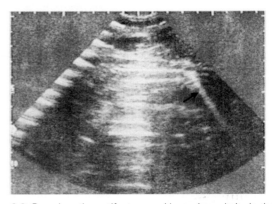

Figure 3.8. Reverberation artifact caused by an irregularity in the visceral pleura commonly referred to in the literature as a "comet tail" (*arrow*). Note the persistence of the parallel concentric artifact from the more normal lung surface.

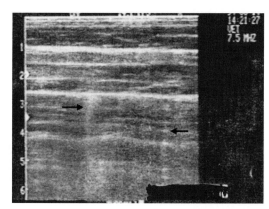

Figure 3.9. Comet tail artifacts produced with a linear array scanhead. Because of the rectangular shape of the image, the artifacts are not as obvious (*arrows*) as those produced by divergent beams.

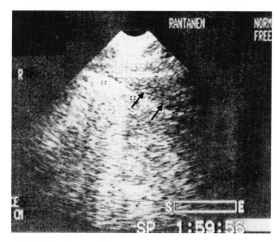

Figure 3.11. The lung margin is displaced from the parietal thoracic wall by a normal accumulation of fat (*arrows*). This should not be misinterpreted as exudate (see Fig. 3.3).

ible. When a small amount of fluid is seen in the thorax, it is most often on the right side (Fig. 3.10).

Fat deposits can displace the ventral lung margin from the thoracic wall. The clinician must not misinterpret fat deposition as displacement of the lung by fluid. This phenomenon is most prominently seen on the right side (Fig. 3.11). Fat is echogenic, has a parenchymal texture, and "jiggles" as the heart beats. Fluid surrounding the lung tip is usually more echolucent, and the lung tip waves or flutters with the heart's motion. Fluid around the ventral lung margin is usually evident because of the echolucent space and the bizarre motion caused by the hydraulic waves from the heart.

Normal pericardial fluid is not obvious in the healthy horse, but it can be seen if the heart is scanned in long axis transverse to the coronary groove during systole. As the heart shortens during systole, the pericardial sac is displaced from the heart, and the space fills with the normal *liquor pericardii* (Fig. 3.12). Pericardial effusion is usually apparent and appears as a homogeneous space separating the epicardium from the pericardial sac.

The thymus in younger foals can be seen cranial to the heart. The thymus has a parenchymal appearance, and blood vessels may be seen coursing through it (see Chap. 5,

Fig. 5.1). This structure should not be mistaken for exudate. Most foals with pneumonia do not develop significant pleural effusion.

LIMITATIONS OF THORACIC RADIOGRAPHY

The value of thoracic radiography cannot be disputed; however, certain problems are peculiar to the horse (12, 13). Pulmonary radiographic examination of the horse is usually limited to lateral views unless a recumbent or sedated foal can be positioned in a dorsoventral or ventrodorsal position for apposing views. Therefore, the radiographs cannot be interpreted as accurately as they can in smaller species because structures in both lungs must be evaluated on the same two-dimensional image. Coupled with the summation artifact is magnification of the ribs, vessels, and airways nearest the x-ray tube. This problem necessitates the taking of standing right and left lateral views so magnification does not obscure lesions.

Because apposing views cannot be taken, the entire lung cannot be assessed radiographically. The cross-sections in Figures 3.1 through 3.6 readily show that lung is superim-

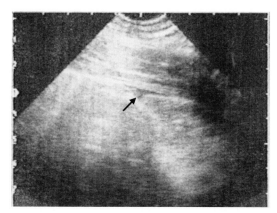

Figure 3.10. A small amount of normal echolucent fluid is often found, especially when the right ventral thorax is scanned (*arrow*).

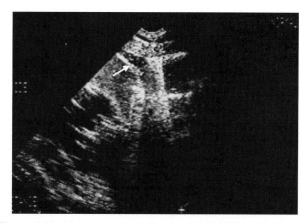

Figure 3.12. Normal amount of pericardial fluid (liquor pericardii) encountered when the heart is scanned (*arrow*). M = cardiac muscle.

posed over liver, spleen, and gut deep to the diaphragm. On lateral radiographs, lung caudal to the leading edge of the diaphragm cannot be assessed radiographically because of the high density of the superimposed tissues.

Most horses that undergo radiography are tranquilized before the procedure to reduce movement and to ensure safety. Tranquilization of the horse decreases the amount of inspired air, thereby increasing the interstitial density of the lungs and effectively eliminating any difference between mild interstitial pneumonia and normal lung. These two populations blend radiographically. Equine thoracic radiographs usually include observation of an "increase in interstitial density."

In horses with significant lung disease, radiographs can be within normal limits, or they can show an acceptable degree of interstitial density increase. In other words, significant pleural irregularities, small consolidations, and significant small effusions can be present and not seen radiographically. Diagnostic ultrasound is sensitive in detecting these small but significant indicators of lung disease.

REFERENCES

1. Rantanen NW. Pleural effusion in horses. Proceedings 25th Annual Meeting. American Institute of Ultrasound in Medicine, 1980. New Orleans, LA.
2. Rantanen NW. Ultrasound appearance of normal lung borders and adjacent viscera in the horse. Vet Radiol 1981;22:217–219.
3. Rantanen NW, Gage L, Paradis MR. Ultrasonography as a diagnostic aid in pleural effusion in horses. Vet Radiol 1981;22:211–216.
4. Rantanen NW. Diseases of the thorax. Vet Clin North Am Equine Pract 1986;2:49–66.
5. Reef VB. Ultrasonographic evaluation. In: Beech J, ed. Equine respiratory disorders. Philadelphia: Lea & Febiger, 1991.
6. Reimer JM, Reef VB, Spencer PA. Ultrasonography as a diagnostic aid in horses with anaerobic bacterial pleuropneumonia and/or pulmonary abscessation: 27 cases (1984–6). J Am Vet Med Assoc 1989;194:278–282.
7. Reimer JM. Diagnostic ultrasonography of the equine thorax. Compend Contin Educ Pract Vet 1990;12:1321–1327.
8. Byars TD, Dainis CM, Seltzer KL, et al. Cranial thoracic masses in the horse: a sequel to pleuropneumonia. Equine Vet Jour, No Amer Ed 1991;23:22–24.
9. Byars TD, Halley J. Uses of ultrasound in equine internal medicine. Vet Clin North Am Equine Pract 1986;2:253–258.
10. Sweeny CR, Humber KA, Roby KAW. Cytologic findings of tracheobronchial aspirates from 66 thoroughbred racehorses. Amer Journ of Vet Res 1991;53:1172–1175.
11. Pascoe JR, O'Brien TR, Wheat JD, et al. Radiographic aspects of exercise-induced pulmonary hemorrhage in racing horses. Vet Radiol 1983;24:85–92.
12. Farrow CS. Equine thoracic radiology. J Am Vet Med Assoc 1981;179:776–781.
13. Farrow CS. Radiographic aspects of inflammatory lung disease in the horse. Vet Radiol 1981;22:107–114.

4. Abdominal Ultrasonography

DAVID G. SCHMITZ

The advent of diagnostic ultrasonography has empowered the veterinary clinician with a noninvasive means of evaluating the equine abdominal cavity and its various organs, tissues, and contents. The technique is simple, the procedure is painless, and the portability of equipment makes it possible to perform a sonographic examination almost anywhere that electricity is available. Minimal preparation of the patient is required before examination, and results of examination procedures are available almost instantaneously. For these and other reasons, abdominal ultrasonography has become an important and increasingly used diagnostic modality in equine practice (1).

Several factors need to be kept in mind when attempting to obtain diagnostic images of abdominal structures. A standardized examination protocol for the various abdominal organs is helpful in performing a complete examination of the area of interest. As with any other diagnostic technique, a standardized method of evaluation helps to ensure a complete examination and reduces the incidence of misdiagnosis or nondiagnosis. When an area of interest is evaluated in the same way in all patients, the sonographer also acquires the ability to make certain subjective assessments about the tissue examined.

Scanning the area of interest in at least two planes is mandatory to a complete examination. Many artifacts in the ultrasound image are generated during the course of an examination, and these can make interpretation and subsequent diagnosis more difficult. When an area of interest is scanned in at least two planes, the sonographer is much better equipped to differentiate between artifact and structural change within a tissue. Lesions are repeatable findings and should be evident in more than one scan plane, whereas artifactual change may be evident in only one scan plane. Scanning a tissue in two planes gives added information about the size and configuration of the area of interest, as well as providing information about the spatial relationship of the area of interest to other organs or tissue landmarks.

The sonographer must scan as much of an organ or tissue as possible. This frequently necessitates scanning a region of the abdominal cavity and may require that both sides of the abdomen be examined, such as in renal or hepatic sonograms. Focal areas of involvement within an organ or tissue may become apparent only when the tissue is examined as completely as possible. These focal changes could be missed if only selected portions of an organ were examined. A good example is a focal abscess or neoplastic lesion, which could be missed if the organ were not examined in its entirety.

When evaluating structures within the abdomen, the sonographer should assess the structures or tissues adjacent to the area of interest as well. This gives added information about the area of interest and helps one to make judgments about the size, shape, location within the abdomen, and spatial relationship of the area of interest to other known landmarks. These findings are helpful in determining whether a questionable sonographic finding is abnormal or a variation of normal, rather than the result of disease or malfunction.

The sonographer must be familiar with the cross-sectional anatomy of the abdomen. Diagnostic ultrasound essentially represents a reflection of the various tissues or structures encountered when a thin slice is taken through the abdomen, starting at the skin edge and penetrating in a straight line into the internal depths of the abdominal cavity (1). The image portrayed on the screen of the ultrasound machine is a two-dimensional representation of a three-dimensional object, namely, the organ or tissue evaluated. It is imperative to be familiar with the spatial arrangement of the abdominal organs and to know their anatomic location before an accurate sonographic examination can be performed.

Scanning of the equine abdomen has certain limitations. The large size of the horse's abdomen tends to degrade the image quality of the sonogram. The large body size and distance of the organ from the skin edge necessitates the use of a lower-frequency transducer. As a result, the resolution of the image is compromised to some extent, and a certain amount of detailed information about the structure is lost. Subtle changes or detail may be missed until the disease process has progressed to a point where changes in echotexture can be observed with the lower-frequency transducers.

Another drawback to abdominal scanning is the presence of variable amounts of gas within the intestine. The intestinal tract occupies a significant amount of the available space in the equine abdomen. Because air or gas acts as a barrier to the sound beam, the presence of excessive bowel gas makes an imaging window difficult to find (2). As a result, many structures or organs cannot be evaluated by ultrasound unless the gas is removed or displaced.

TECHNIQUES OF ABDOMINAL SCANNING

Transcutaneous Approach

The equine abdomen lends itself to being scanned either transcutaneously or transrectally (in appropriate circumstances). Transcutaneous imaging has the benefits of requiring minimal restraint and being performed on the standing animal. It is helpful to examine the animal in a quiet environment and with the horse at rest. Motion makes scanning more difficult, so if the horse is moving or is excited, the examination is prolonged and more difficult to accomplish. Moreover, much of the abdominal content must be examined by scanning through the intercostal spaces. An elevated respiratory rate makes scanning more difficult because the aerated lung acts as a sound barrier to the deeper structures. If the horse is resting quietly, a greater portion of the abdomen can be examined when the horse has exhaled and the lung border has retracted dorsally and cranially.

When a transcutaneous examination is performed, the transducer is applied directly on the animal over the area of interest (see Patient Preparation). As noted previously, this examination requires knowledge of the topographic and cross-sectional anatomy of the equine abdomen. The sonographer must know where the desired tissue or organ is located within the abdomen before beginning the examination. Many of the abdominal organs can be scanned (either partially or in their entirety) by transcutaneous placement of the transducer. The diaphragm, the ventral portion of the right and left liver lobes, the large colon, the cecal and stomach mucosal margins, the duodenum, both kidneys, the spleen, and occasionally the distended urinary bladder can all be evaluated in this manner. Figure 4.1 is a schematic drawing of the abdominal viscera.

Transrectal Approach

In horses of appropriate size, the abdomen can be scanned by transrectal placement of the transducer. The same precautions employed when doing a routine rectal examination should be adhered to when performing a sonographic evaluation transrectally. The horse should be suitably restrained and sedated if necessary. Caudal epidural anesthesia may be helpful, particularly if the horse has excessive rectal contractions or if the sonographer is attempting to examine a structure deep within the abdomen. All feces and air should

be removed from the rectum before the examination. A coupling agent should be applied to the transducer before insertion into the rectum. Suitable coupling agents for transrectal use include most of the commercially available obstetric lubricants, mineral oil, and water-soluble lubricating jellies. After the couplant has been applied, the transducer is held within the sonographer's hand and is slowly advanced into the horse's rectum. The transducer is manipulated by the sonographer's hand until contact is made with the desired structure. If an air interface has been acquired during this procedure, gently moving the transducer slowly back and forth may displace the air or gas and may thus allow contact of the transducer with the rectal wall so a suitable image may be obtained. Structures that can be evaluated by transrectal ultrasonography include portions of the gastrointestinal tract, the urinary bladder, the urethra, the left kidney and occasionally the right kidney, the spleen, the caudal portion of the abdominal aorta, the iliac arteries, the cranial mesenteric artery in some horses, and the accessory sex glands in the male and the reproductive tract of mares (3). Additionally, the ventral back muscles, some lymph nodes, and the peritoneal surfaces of the body wall and abdominal organs can be evaluated sonographically (3). Abnormal masses palpated within the abdomen are also candidates for sonographic evaluation.

Transducer Selection

Both linear-array and sector scanners can be used to examine the abdomen. Linear-array transducers may be a little more user-friendly when performing a transrectal examination, but sector scanners can also be used for transrectal scanning. The sector scanners alternatively may offer the advantage of a small "footprint" or surface contact area when scanning transabdominally and are particularly useful

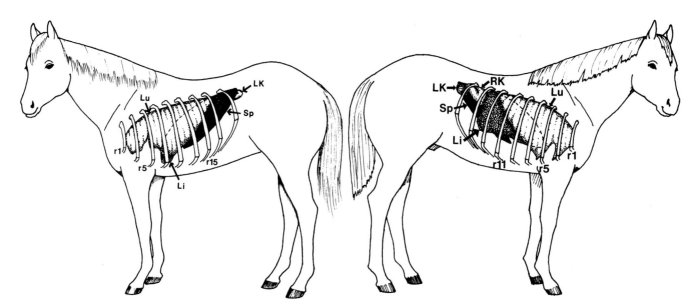

Figure 4.1. Schematic drawing of the abdominal viscera as viewed from both sides. Li = liver; LK = left kidney; Lu = lung; r = rib; RK = right kidney; Sp = spleen.

when scanning in the intercostal spaces. Their small footprint allows evaluation of deeper structures in two planes with minimal acoustic shadowing from the ribs. Linear-array transducer footprints are typically much larger than are those of sector scanners, and although they may be useful when evaluating the abdomen ventral to costal margins, they are not well suited for evaluation of structures deep to the intercostal spaces. When they are used in the intercostal spaces, a transverse (dorsoventral) view may be obtained, but it is almost impossible to obtain a diagnostic image when the linear transducer is oriented longitudinally or perpendicular to the ribs.

Ultrasound machines with convex-array or annular-array technology have become available. These machines are suitable for abdominal imaging, and each offers certain technical advantages that may improve image quality over that obtained from less sophisticated machines. In general, the foregoing comments regarding linear-array transducers apply to convex-array transducers, and the statements regarding sector scanners likewise apply, in general, to annular-array transducers.

Because of the size of the equine abdomen and the distance of the internal structures from the skin edge, a 2.5- to 5.0-Mhz transducer is typically required. The lower-frequency transducers are useful for identifying deeper structures and for performing a cursory scan of the abdomen, but a 5-Mhz transducer should be used, when possible, to obtain greater resolution and definition of the desired structures. A 7.5-Mhz transducer is useful only for evaluating superficial structures such as the body wall and adjacent peritoneal surfaces. A 7.5-Mhz transducer is also valuable for transrectal evaluation of the distal aorta and iliac arteries, for small structures close to the rectal wall or within the pelvis, and for detection of very early pregnancy or evaluation of the reproductive tracts of male and female horses.

Factors Affecting Image Quality

Various factors during the examination can affect the quality of the ultrasound image. The greatest impediment to obtaining a diagnostic image on a transcutaneous scan is poor contact between the skin and the transducer (likewise, between the rectal mucosa and the transducer when performing a transrectal examination). The transducer should be manipulated on the skin surface until suitable contact is made between the skin and the transducer. In addition, trapped air between the skin and the transducer reduces image quality, as does the presence of dirt, oils, and debris on the skin or hair surface. Removal of these substances before scanning allows the best possible image to be obtained. If a suitable image is not obtained, cleansing the skin with soap and water and applying copious amounts of couplant should greatly improve the image (see Patient Preparation).

Fat causes attenuation of the sound wave and makes imaging tissues difficult in an obese animal. The presence of fat around any tissue results in poor resolution of the tissue and imparts a hazy appearance to the image. The sound wave does not penetrate as deeply into tissue in an obese horse, and a higher power setting on the ultrasound machine is required when scanning an obese horse compared with the setting required for a thin animal. In extremely obese horses, obtaining a diagnostic image of structures within the abdomen from a transcutaneous approach can be almost impossible.

The angle with which the ultrasound beam strikes a tissue influences the echo returning from the tissue. The greatest echo return occurs when the sound wave strikes a tissue interface at a 90° angle. If the sound wave strikes the tissue at an oblique angle, a hypoechoic artifact is usually generated. Therefore, the best resolution of a desired structure occurs when the transducer is held perpendicular to the surface of the underlying tissue of interest. This technique favors recording echoes that would otherwise be lost by reflection of the sound wave in a direction away from the transducer (1, 4).

The machine settings also greatly influence the ultrasound image (see Chapter 1). Suitable power adjustment must be made to image the desired structure adequately. The time gain compensation curve should be adjusted, when possible, to yield a uniform representation of the desired tissue from the near field through the far field of the image. In general, this requires some reduction in the near-field gain setting and enhancement (or increase) of the far-field gain setting. The object of adjusting the gain settings is to provide an equal, uniform echo return from all depths of the tissue of interest.

PATIENT PREPARATION

For most examination procedures, minimal preparation of the horse is required. The horse should be adequately restrained to minimize motion and to protect the equipment. This is particularly true if a transrectal examination is to be performed, because adequate restraint is necessary under these circumstances for the horse's safety as well. Most horses can be examined while they are standing with minimal restraint. Occasionally, a mild sedative or tranquilizer may be indicated.

It is imperative to remove any air in the space between the transducer and the skin when performing an examination. This is accomplished by thoroughly wetting the skin in the desired area with copious amounts of coupling gel, alcohol, mineral oil, or, in some cases, water and scanning gel. Clipping the hair and thoroughly cleansing the underlying skin to remove dirt, oil, and debris before applying the coupling gel result in the best possible image. However, when clipping the hair is not possible or is undesirable, the use of copious amounts of coupling gel or other suitable material such as alcohol may allow an adequate image to be obtained. A cursory examination of the abdomen may be performed without clipping the hair, but when detailed information about an abdominal structure is desired, hair removal is necessary.

Before a transrectal examination, every effort should be made to remove all air and feces from the horse's rectum. A coupling agent should also be used in this procedure. Suitable materials include mineral oil, obstetric lubricants, and water-soluble lubricating jellies.

BODY WALL

The body wall itself is often overlooked when the abdomen is examined, probably because few abnormalities of the abdominal wall are presented for veterinary evaluation. The desire or need to evaluate the abdominal wall of horses is increasing, however, particularly with the advancement of other veterinary procedures and with the increased number of abdominal surgical procedures performed. As with any diagnostic modality, increased awareness of the technique frequently leads to increased use of the modality, particularly if useful information is generated.

Technique

The body wall itself is best examined with a 7.5-Mhz transducer. Even then, if the area of interest is in the superficial layers of the body wall, a stand-off pad may be required for optimal resolution. A 5.0-Mhz transducer with a stand-off pad can be used, but the resolution obtained with this transducer may be less than optimal. If fine detail is required, the higher-frequency transducer should be used. If the operator is interested only in the structural integrity of the body wall or if there are large defects in the muscle or linea alba, the lower-frequency transducer may provide that information.

Both sector and linear-array transducers can be used to examine the abdominal wall, and both provide diagnostic information. For the most part, preference of one transducer over the other is largely a matter of personal choice. However, linear-array transducers may provide better resolution in the near-field image, and they are generally easier to manipulate in the inguinal area of most horses. Sector transducers can be difficult to maneuver to obtain a diagnostic image in the inguinal area, and hence, they can be bothersome to the horse. The region of interest should be examined in two planes at right angles to each other, and the best image is obtained when the transducer is held perpendicular to the skin edge in the area of interest.

Normal Anatomy

The abdominal wall of the horse can be essentially divided into two parts, the linea alba and the lateral abdominal wall muscles. The linea alba is a fibrous raphe extending from the xiphoid cartilage to the prepubic tendon. It is found on the ventral midline and is composed chiefly of the aponeuroses of the internal and external abdominal oblique and transverse abdominal muscles and partly by fibers of the rectus abdominis muscle. Its width is variable, but is generally less than 1 cm in the adult horse. Separating the linea alba from the peritoneum is a layer of fascia, the fascia

transversalis, which can contain significant amounts of fat in the well-conditioned horse. In extremely thin horses, this fascia is thin and contains little fat (5). In the cranial abdominal floor, the falciform ligament attaches the middle liver lobe to the sternal part of the diaphragm and to the abdominal floor for a variable distance (5). In the well-conditioned horse, this structure can also contain significant amounts of fat.

The abdominal muscles essentially comprise the lateral walls of the abdominal cavity. The most superficial muscle, the external abdominal oblique, is the most extensive abdominal muscle. Superficial to the external abdominal oblique muscle, however, is the sheet of elastic tissue termed the abdominal tunic. This fibroelastic structure assists the abdominal muscles in supporting the abdominal contents and is practically coextensive with the external oblique muscle. Ventrally, the abdominal tunic becomes thickened and intimately adherent to the aponeurosis of the external oblique muscle. Laterally, it becomes gradually thinner. Deep to the external oblique is the internal abdominal oblique muscle. The third and innermost muscle group on the lateral abdominal wall is the transverse abdominal muscle. The aponeuroses of these muscles, along with the abdominal tunic, are the primary components of the linea alba.

The rectus abdominis muscle is confined to the ventral part of the abdomen, extending from the sternum to the pubis. It does not contribute to the musculature of the lateral abdominal wall. Superficially, this muscle is bounded by the aponeuroses of the oblique muscles, which constitute the external rectus sheath.

Sonographic Appearance

The skin surface is represented sonographically by a bright echogenic line. When one uses a 7.5-Mhz transducer, the layers of the skin and subcutaneous tissues are not well delineated but are represented by a hypoechoic space that typically ranges from 7 to 10 mm in thickness. Because the linea alba is composed almost exclusively of fibrous connective tissue, its sonographic appearance is usually echogenic and homogeneous. The thickness of the body wall at the ventral midline generally ranges from 2 to 4 cm, and the distance between the adjacent rectus abdominis muscles is about 2 to 3 cm (6) (Fig.4.2).

The lateral abdominal wall contains much more muscle tissue than does the linea alba, so its sonographic appearance differs from that of the linea alba. The skin and subcutaneous tissue are again represented by a 7- to 10-mm thick hypoechoic space. The fascial sheaths of the abdominal muscles are echogenic when compared with the muscle bellies themselves, and they travel in a linear, parallel direction. They tend to separate the various muscles from one another. The muscle bellies are relatively hypoechoic, but fascial planes within the muscle bellies impart some internal echo pattern to the body of the muscle. The total thickness of the lateral abdominal wall is several centimeters, but it

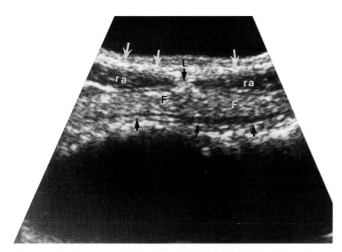

Figure 4.2. Sonogram of the ventral abdominal midline. Skin edge is at the top of the sonogram. *Large arrows* point to the abdominal tunic and aponeuroses of the abdominal oblique muscles; *small arrows* point to the peritoneal interface. F = fat in the fascia transversalis; L = linea alba; ra = rectus abdominis muscles.

varies with the size, body condition, and muscular development of the individual horse. The peritoneum is typically seen as a bright, smooth echogenic line on the deep surface of the body wall. With a 5.0-Mhz transducer, however, the interface between the peritoneum and the bowel wall may not be clearly discernable (Fig. 4.3).

Indications for Scanning

Any abnormal lumps, bumps, or swellings or other clinically palpable abnormalities involving the body wall are indications for an ultrasonographic evaluation of the area. Evaluation of the abdominal wall is particularly useful in the assessment of known or suspected body wall defects, such as those occurring with abdominal, umbilical, scrotal, inguinal, and postsurgical incisional hernias, as well as in

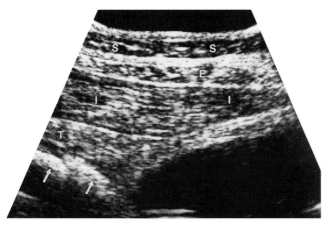

Figure 4.3. Sonogram of the lateral body wall. Skin edge is at the top of the sonogram and dorsal is to the left. *Arrow* points to bowel wall interface. E = external abdominal oblique muscle; I = internal abdominal oblique muscle; S = subcutaneous tissue; T = transverse abdominal muscle.

the assessment of postoperative sites for complications. In one report, ultrasonographic evaluation of postsurgical ventral midline celiotomies was an easy, reliable, and objective method for detecting and monitoring the progression of incisional complications such as edema formation, suture sinus, and abscess formation and dehiscence in a group of ponies (6).

LIVER

The liver is the largest parenchymal organ in the horse's abdomen, and it is commonly associated either primarily or secondarily with various disease processes. Ultrasonic evaluation of the liver can give information regarding the size, shape, position, and texture of the organ, thus providing the clinician with additional valuable diagnostic information. Hepatic ultrasonography is also extremely useful clinically to locate an area of liver suitable for biopsy procurement.

Technique

A lower-frequency transducer (2.5 to 3.5 Mhz) is often necessary to examine the liver in a 500-kg horse. Because the liver is such a large organ, the ultrasound beam should be able to penetrate to a depth of 20 to 25 cm to evaluate as much of the organ as possible. Once a cursory examination of the liver has been made, however, it is often advantageous to examine the more superficial areas of the liver with a 5.0-Mhz transducer. This provides better resolution and greater detail of the image. The liver should be examined in its entirety on both right and left sides of the horse for completeness. Linear-array and sector scanners can be used, but the smaller footprint of the sector scanners makes them more effective when imaging through the intercostal spaces. Because much of the liver is located deep to the ribs, it is easier to direct the beam in more than one plane when scanning with a sector transducer in the intercostal spaces.

Normal Anatomy

The liver is found in the cranial ventral abdomen, adjacent to the abdominal surface of the diaphragm. The greater part of the liver lies to the right of the median plane, except when the right lobe is atrophied. The liver is roughly divided into three lobes: right, middle, and left (5) (Fig. 4.4A).

The right lobe is the largest, except in older horses, in which it becomes atrophied to a variable extent. Its cranial margin is adjacent to the diaphragm, opposite approximately the sixth intercostal space. The right lobe extends caudally and dorsally. The dorsal part of the right lobe is termed the caudate lobe, which ends in a pointed caudate process that contacts, and forms a cavity for, the right kidney (Fig. 4.4B).

The middle lobe is the smallest, but differentiation of the right from the middle lobe in the adult horse is usually not possible. The anatomic arrangement of the liver within the abdomen and the lack of a suitable sonographic window make it almost impossible to evaluate the middle lobe. The

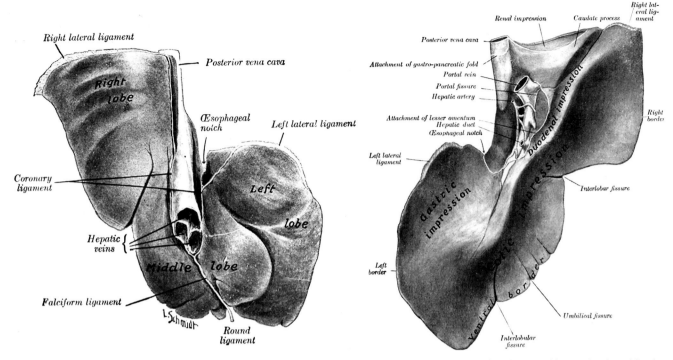

Figure 4.4. A, Parietal surface of liver of young horse, hardened in situ. **B**, Visceral surface of liver of middle-aged horse, hardened in situ. Reprinted with permission from Sisson S. The anatomy of the domestic animals. 4th ed. Philadelphia: WB Saunders, 1953.

left liver lobe generally is found in the left cranial ventral abdomen in the seventh through ninth intercostal spaces.

The porta hepatis (portal fissure) is a depression on the visceral surface of the liver to the right of the median plane. At this point, the portal vein, hepatic artery, and the hepatic plexus of nerves enter the liver, and the hepatic duct and lymph vessels exit the liver parenchyma. Although this fissure serves as an anatomic landmark in humans and some other animal species, it is not visible sonographically in the normal horse because of its location in the abdomen.

Sonographically, the liver is imaged on the right side, generally from the sixth through the fifteenth intercostal spaces. It is found ventral to the lung margin, and it extends from the cranial ventral abdomen caudodorsally to the level of the right kidney. A variable amount of liver parenchyma visibly extends ventrally from the lung border. The thickness of the right lobe varies, but to date, no parameters for normal size have been reported. However, in young to middle-aged horses, the thickest part of the liver (measured from the lateral to the medial surface of the right lobe just caudal to the ventral lung margin) is expected to measure 6 to 9 cm (7).

The amount of liver imaged from the right side can vary. In older horses, the right lobe may have atrophied such that little or no liver parenchyma can be found. Other factors that influence the extent of liver seen are the amount of material in the large colon, the volume of the thorax, the degree of lung excursion during respiration, the presence of pleural or peritoneal effusion, and the presence of disease or other conditions that may induce visceral displacement, such as ascites and late-term pregnancy (7, 8). The ventral

edge of the liver is expected to end in a "sharp," well-defined angular border.

On the left side, the liver is evaluated sonographically in the cranial ventral abdomen, generally in the seventh through ninth intercostal spaces. When seen, it is usually just caudal and adjacent to the diaphragm. The spleen usually lies medial to the liver, but it may be found between the body wall and the liver. The liver–spleen interface is frequently seen (Fig. 4.5).

On both sides of the abdomen, the ventral lung margin defines the dorsal boundary of liver parenchyma observed sonographically, and the lateral boundaries of the liver are usually adjacent to the body wall or the diaphragm. On the right side, the medial border of the liver is adjacent to the large colon and is readily discernable. The medial boundary of the left liver lobe is adjacent to the stomach wall dorsally and the large colon ventrally, but this boundary is seldom visualized sonographically.

Sonographic Appearance

Sonographically, the normal liver resembles a gross cross-section of liver (Fig. 4.6). The portal veins have echogenic walls and anechoic centers of varying size. They are diffusely scattered throughout the liver parenchyma and tend to run at roughly right angles to the hepatic veins; that is, when the portal vessels are scanned in a longitudinal plane, the hepatic veins are usually evident in cross-section. In the normal liver, minimal branching of the portal veins is evident. The main portal vein exiting the liver is rarely seen in the adult, owing to its depth and location in the abdomen.

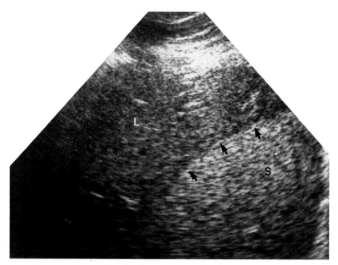

Figure 4.5. Sonogram of the liver and spleen taken in the left cranioventral abdomen. Skin edge is at the top and dorsal is to the left. *Arrows* point to liver-spleen interface. L = liver; S = spleen.

The hepatic veins generally appear as anechoic vascular structures of varying size also scattered throughout the liver parenchyma. Their walls generally do not produce an echo, but if seen, they are not nearly as well defined as those of the portal veins. Occasionally, blood can be seen flowing in the hepatic veins, but for the most part, they appear as anechoic structures within the liver. Likewise, the posterior vena cava is rarely seen in the adult horse, also because of its depth and location within the abdomen. The hepatic arteries are not visualized sonographically, and the biliary system is usually not discernable.

The margin of the liver should appear smooth and linear to curvilinear, depending on its location. The border may

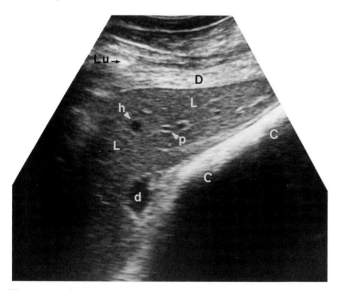

Figure 4.6. Sonogram of the liver in the right eleventh intercostal space at about the level of the point of the shoulder. Skin edge is at the top and dorsal is to the left. C = large colon; D = diaphragm; d = duodenum; h = hepatic vein; L = liver parenchyma; Lu = ventral lung margin; p = portal vein.

be represented by a weak echo suggestive of a capsule. The overall echogenicity of the liver is generally greater than that of the kidney, but less than that of the spleen. The normal liver, however, may be isoechoic with kidney. The right kidney–liver interface in approximately the dorsal fifteenth intercostal space is the region of choice for comparing the relative echogenicities of these two organs.

Indications for Scanning

A liver scan is indicated whenever clinical signs or laboratory findings suggest liver disease or dysfunction. Because the technique is noninvasive, it causes no harm to the horse and potentially generates valuable diagnostic information regarding the size, shape, location, and texture of the liver parenchyma. It is valuable in differentiating focal disease states, such as abscess or neoplasia, from generalized hepatic diseases, and it also aids procurement of suitable biopsy or aspiration samples. Hepatic ultrasonography is helpful in monitoring disease processes involving the liver, because many changes suggestive of resolution or progression of a lesion can be observed. Prognostic information is often gained when the liver is scanned multiple times during the course of a hepatic disease process.

KIDNEYS

The evaluation of horses with renal disease can present the veterinary practitioner with several unique problems. It is often difficult to differentiate between acute and chronic renal failure when the horse is first presented for evaluation, because the acute onset of chronic renal failure is clinically similar to the onset of acute renal failure. The size of many adult horses makes them unlikely or unsuitable candidates for certain radiographic diagnostic procedures such as intravenous pyelography, contrast cystography, and excretory urography. Other more sophisticated renal diagnostic modalities, such as scintigraphy, are available at few referral facilities. Renal ultrasonography offers the advantages of being noninvasive and nonpainful, and it is usually accessible. Valuable diagnostic information can be gained immediately on scanning the horse, and appropriate treatment can be initiated in a timely manner.

Technique

The kidneys in the adult horse are usually scanned transcutaneously, but transrectal sonographic evaluation can be performed in suitable horses in certain circumstances. Both linear and sector scanners can be used. However, when the kidneys are being scanned transcutaneously, sector scanners offer the advantages of having a smaller footprint and they provide better resolution of structures in the far field of the image. Transrectal sonographic evaluation of the kidneys can also be accomplished by using either type of transducer (9).

A 15-cm field of view is usually necessary to evaluate the right kidney, and at least a 20-cm field of view is necessary for scanning the left kidney. In extremely large horses, the renal parenchyma may extend beyond the depth of penetration of the transducer. Because of the depth of the kidneys, a 2.5- to 3.5-Mhz transducer is necessary, particularly when imaging the left kidney. In many cases, the right kidney can be suitably imaged using a 5.0-Mhz transducer (10–12).

When examining either kidney, multiple scanning planes are necessary to evaluate the entire organ. Seldom is the whole kidney seen on one view. This necessitates rocking the transducer cranially, caudally, dorsally, and ventrally from any one position on the horse's body, and it also requires that the kidney be examined in more than one intercostal space and at different regions of the same intercostal space (5).

Certain limitations are encountered when scanning the kidneys in horses. Because of the anatomic location of these organs, only a lateral approach is possible when scanning transcutaneously. This interferes with obtaining accurate measurements of the dimensions of the kidney, because the entire organ is not visible in a single view. Moreover, certain organs and structures medial and ventral to the kidneys cannot be evaluated when the kidneys are scanned from the lateral side.

Another limitation to transcutaneous scanning of the kidneys is that, occasionally, gas-filled bowel is situated in such a manner in the abdominal cavity that it interferes with visualization of either kidney (11). This can happen in the normal horse in the absence of gastrointestinal tract disease or bowel displacement. When this situation arises, the sonographer may repeat the examination at a later point, in the hope that the gas-filled viscus has moved, or the horse may be subjected to a transrectal sonographic examination of the kidneys. Finally, lower-frequency transducers are required to image the kidneys, and the limitations of the

resolving power of these transducers may preclude detection of small changes in architecture and texture (12)

Normal Anatomy

The right kidney grossly resembles an equilateral triangle with the angles rounded off. In the middle portion of its medial border, a deep notch, termed the renal hilus, serves as the entry for the vessels and nerves supplying the kidney. At this same area, the ureter exits the kidney (5) (Figs. 4.7**A** and 4.8). The right kidney is found in the fifteenth to seventeenth intercostal spaces, at the level of the tuber coxae. It is bounded dorsally by the transverse process of the first lumbar vertebra and by the last two to three ribs. The cranial pole is rounded and lies in the renal impression of the liver. The caudal pole is thinner and narrower than the cranial region (5, 11, 12). The lateral surface of the kidney contacts the abdominal wall and the caudal extremity of the diaphragm. The duodenum curves around its ventrolateral border, and the cecum is located ventromedially to the kidney (11, 12).

The left kidney is bean shaped and is longer and narrower than the right kidney (5). The renal hilus of the left kidney also is found at about the mid-point of the kidney, along its medial border (see Fig. 4.7). The left kidney is located in the last few intercostal spaces on the left side and caudal to the eighteenth rib in the paralumbar fossa (11, 12). It is situated below the transverse processes of the lumbar vertebrae and is often found slightly ventral to the level of the tuber coxae. This places it slightly more ventrally in the abdominal cavity than the right kidney.

The lateral border of the left kidney contacts the medial surface of the spleen. The medial border lies adjacent to the aorta and adrenal gland. Ventromedially, various parts of the gastrointestinal tract may contact the left kidney, and its dorsal surface is related to the left crus of the diaphragm,

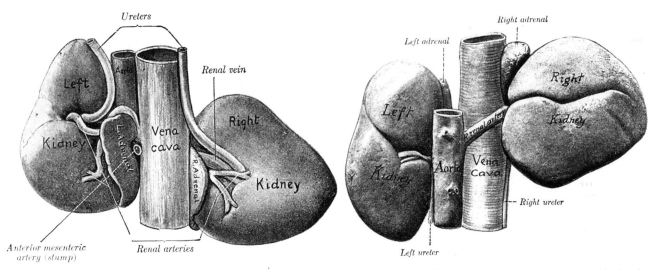

Figure 4.7. A, Ventral view of kidneys and adrenal glands, hardened in situ. **B**, Dorsal view of kidneys and adrenal glands, hardened in situ. L = left; R = right. Reprinted with permission from Sisson S. The anatomy of the domestic animals. 4th ed. Philadelphia: WB Saunders, 1953.

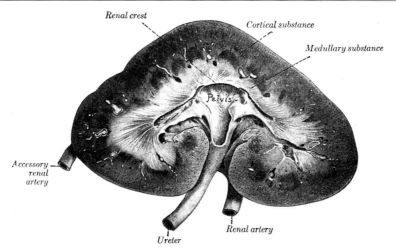

Figure 4.8. Horizontal section of kidney. The renal vein has been removed. Sections of interlobar arteries found between the cortical and medullary regions appear white in this figure. Reprinted with permission from Sisson S. The anatomy of the domestic animals. 4th ed. Philadelphia: WB Saunders, 1953.

the iliac fascia, and the psoas muscles (5). The caudal pole is usually larger than the cranial pole.

Sonographic Appearance

In the normal horse, both kidneys have a smooth capsular surface represented sonographically as a thin, linear to curvilinear echogenic line that outlines the margins of the organ. The capsule is best seen on the lateral and medial surface of the kidney. The cranial and caudal poles of the kidney are usually less well defined because of the artifact generated by refraction of sound waves from those regions (10).The capsule is best visualized with a 5.0-Mhz transducer. The renal cortex appears as a homogeneous area of fine echoes that is hypoechoic to the surrounding tissue. The renal cortex is hypoechoic to isoechoic with the liver,

hypoechoic relative to the spleen, and more echogenic than the medullary portion of the kidneys. The renal cortex resembles a series of Roman arches surrounding the medullary regions and is approximately 1 to 2 cm in thickness when measured from the renal capsule to the corticomedullary junction (11, 12). The corticomedullary junction is usually distinct, particularly when a 5.0-Mhz transducer is used. Normally, the medullary regions are hypoechoic to the cortex or anechoic and are surrounded by the cortex.

The renal pelvis is usually seen as an echogenic line or band in the central portion of the kidney (11). The increased echogenicity of this region is due to intrapelvic fat and fibrous tissue. The pelvic recesses are virtually anechoic and usually measure less than 1 cm in diameter (10, 12) (Fig. 4.9).

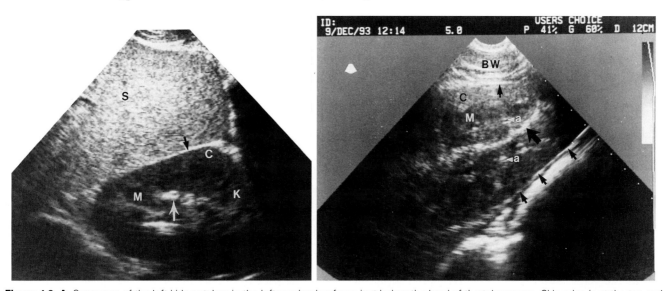

Figure 4.9. A, Sonogram of the left kidney taken in the left paralumbar fossa just below the level of the tuber coxae. Skin edge is at the top and dorsal is to the right. *Small arrow* points to renal capsule; *large arrow* points to intrapelvic fat and fibrous tissue. C = cortical region; K = left kidney; M = medullary region; S = spleen. **B**, Sonogram of the right kidney taken in the fifteenth to sixteenth intercostal space at the level of the tuber coxae. Skin edge is at the top and dorsal is to the left. *Small arrows* point to renal capsule; *large arrow* points to intrapelvic fat and fibrous tissue. a = interlobar arteries; BW = body wall musculature; C = cortical regions; M = medullary regions.

The interlobar arteries form an arciform network of vessels that may be apparent as small (2- to 3-mm diameter) circular structures evenly spaced within the medulla and pelvic area. They have echogenic margins and anechoic centers (3, 11). The abdominal aorta and the caudal vena cava are only rarely seen in some horses. The renal artery and vein may occasionally be seen, but differentiation between these vessels and a dilated ureter is almost impossible when using real-time B-mode ultrasonography. Doppler sonography is used when it is necessary to evaluate these structures.

The normal ureter is not recognized transcutaneously in most horses unless it is dilated. The ureter is even difficult to recognize on transrectal images. Distended ureters are probably best evaluated transrectally using a 5.0-, or preferably, a 7.5-Mhz transducer. They appear as circular to oval structures with a moderately echogenic rim and an anechoic to hypoechoic center. They vary in size, according to the degree of distention.

The kidneys usually measure 10 to 14 cm medially to laterally. Their length is often difficult to determine because of the inability to image the entire organ in a single view. The left kidney is deeper than the right kidney and usually requires a lower-frequency transducer to obtain an image. As a result, the resolution and detail observed in the left kidney are frequently inferior to those seen in the right kidney. However, by no means should the left kidney be excluded when a sonographic examination of the urinary system is performed.

When performing an ultrasound examination of the kidneys, the far-field image of the kidney frequently appears hypoechoic or may even become anechoic relative to the near-field or more superficial part of the kidney. This is particularly true when scanning the right kidney. If this occurs, the machine should be adjusted in an attempt to even out the image such that both near-field and far-field regions have a more uniform sonographic appearance.

Other factors that affect the sonographic image are that the caudal aspect of the left kidney may be "shadowed" by gas-filled bowel in the normal horse (12), and the cranial margin of the right kidney may be obscured by aerated lung during inspiration. The image obtained when the kidneys are scanned transrectally may be superior to that obtained from a transcutaneous examination, because the kidney is closer to the focal zone of the transducer. A higher-frequency transducer improves the resolution of the image.

Indications for Scanning

The kidneys should be evaluated ultrasonographically whenever clinical signs or laboratory abnormalities suggest renal disease or dysfunction. Additional indications for ultrasonographic examination of the kidneys include the identification of palpable masses or abnormalities in the region of the kidneys on rectal palpation and further definition of renal abnormalities discovered on rectal examination.

Ultrasonography can be useful to differentiate acute from chronic renal disease and to differentiate focal from diffuse renal involvement. Horses with acute renal disease or failure may not have abnormal sonographic findings, but ultrasonographic abnormalities are almost always observed in horses with chronic renal failure (11, 12). In addition, diffuse renal parenchymal disease can be sonographically differentiated from focal diseases such as renal cysts, tumors, abscesses, and hematomas. Ultrasonography is helpful in identifying sites for biopsy or aspiration of renal tissue, and it can also be used to monitor the progression of renal disease in an individual animal. Prognostic information may be gained after an initial examination, such as in a horse with severe renal fibrosis, or by repeat examinations during the course of disease in a particular horse.

Renal ultrasonography is reported to be superior to radiography for diagnosis of nephrolithiasis (12). Ultrasound has the ability to detect much smaller calculi than those observed by radiography. Conventional radiography enables one to detect only large calculi, and high-energy x-ray equipment is required. As a result, the radiation exposure to personnel makes it less than ideal and potentially dangerous (12).

Certain problems may be encountered when scanning the kidneys by the transcutaneous approach. The presence of bowel gas may preclude imaging part or all of the kidney, or the resolution of the renal image may be less than desirable. The state of hydration of the horse, the amount of body fat, and the depth of the kidney from the skin surface can all adversely affect image quality. These factors may prevent adequate visualization of the kidneys and may dictate a transrectal approach (11, 12). A transrectal examination is also indicated if specific information regarding the ureters is desired.

In many horses, a transrectal examination allows the transducer to be placed directly on the left kidney. This permits use of a higher-frequency transducer so maximal resolution of the image is obtained. This technique is particularly useful in visualizing small lesions (such as mineralization or calculi formation) involving the left kidney (12).

SPLEEN

The spleen is one of the largest organs in the abdominal cavity, yet it is seldom the primary site of disease in the horse. However, many systemic disease processes can secondarily affect the spleen, so it should not be overlooked when evaluating the abdominal cavity. The spleen can vary in size in a normal animal within a short period of time (minutes to hours), a feature that makes it difficult to establish normal size dimensions in the adult horse. For the most part, diseases of the spleen that cause changes in its sonographic appearance are those that induce focal changes within the organ or those that cause a gross constant enlargement of the spleen.

Technique

The spleen is usually imaged transcutaneously from the left side of the horse. In certain instances, transrectal examination of the caudal portion of the spleen may be indicated. Both linear-array and sector scanners can be used, but again, sector scanners offer certain advantages over linear-array transducers that may make them more desirable for imaging splenic tissue.

Because of the size of the spleen in the adult horse and because the dimensions of the spleen can vary so dramatically, a 20-cm field of view is the minimal requirement for examining the spleen in most adult horses. Therefore, a 3.0-Mhz or lower-frequency transducer is usually necessary. The more superficial portions of the spleen can be examined with a 5.0-Mhz transducer, and in horses of smaller stature, the entire spleen may also be observed with this transducer. The higher-frequency transducer allows better resolution of splenic tissue and is particularly valuable in evaluating small lesions.

Normal Anatomy

The spleen is situated on the left side of the abdomen, in close relation to the left part of the greater curvature of the stomach. Dorsally, the spleen contacts the diaphragm and sublumbar muscles, the dorsal part of the stomach, and the left kidney. The long axis of the spleen courses cranioventrally, with the lateral border contacting the diaphragm and lateral body wall. The more cranial portion of the spleen often becomes situated on the medial border of the liver, but in some horses, it is found on the lateral side of the liver, between the liver and the lateral body wall. The ventral margin of the spleen becomes a tapered apex and may reach the ventral midline. In some normal horses, the splenic apex may even cross the abdominal floor at the ventral midline to extend into the right half of the abdomen. The medial surface of the spleen contacts the greater curvature of the stomach and other portions of the gastrointestinal tract, including portions of the small colon, the left parts of the large colon, and the small intestine. The medial surface of the spleen is divided into two unequal parts by a longitudinal ridge; on this ridge is a groove, the hilus, in which the vessels and nerves supplying the spleen are located. The caudal splenic margin extends to the last few intercostal spaces, frequently reaching the paralumbar fossa. Cranially, the spleen can often be located in the ninth or tenth intercostal space (5).

When scanning a horse, the spleen is usually located along the entire left ventral lung border. Caudodorsally, the spleen is found lateral to the left kidney and serves as the sonographic window for scanning the left kidney. From the caudal dorsal flank area, the spleen can usually be seen coursing cranioventrally under the lung margin, often extending to or beyond the ventral abdominal midline. In the more cranial abdomen, the spleen is usually found medial to the left liver lobe, but occasionally it is observed

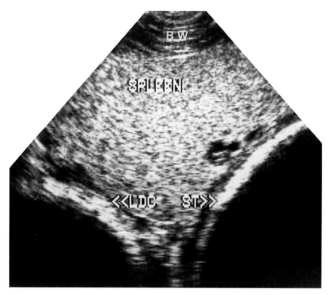

Figure 4.10. Sonogram of the spleen taken in the left tenth to twelfth intercostal space just ventral to ventral lung margin. Skin edge is at top and dorsal is to the right. The hypoechoic rim separating the spleen from the stomach mucosal/gas interface represents the musculature of the stomach wall. BW = body wall musculature; LDC = left dorsal colon; ST = stomach mucosal/gas interface.

lateral to the liver (2, 13). The cranial region of the spleen is bounded medially by the greater curvature of the stomach dorsally and by the large colon ventrally. This relationship is most readily seen in the left tenth to twelfth intercostal spaces just ventral to the ventral lung margin. It is not evident in all horses (Fig. 4.10).

Sonographic Appearance

The spleen is the most echogenic of the abdominal organs in the horse. The capsule is identified as an echogenic linear to curvilinear thin line surrounding the spleen. The splenic parenchyma has a finely mottled homogeneous pattern throughout and is of moderate echogenicity (Fig. 4.11). Infrequent small blood vessels may be seen in longitudinal and cross-sectional views, but the spleen has few visible vascular structures (3). A large central vein can usually be identified in the longitudinal plane and frequently can be seen exiting at the hilus (Fig. 4.12). The brighter echotexture, coupled with the relative lack of parenchymal vessels and the presence of the large central vein, helps to differentiate spleen from liver on the sonographic image.

The thickness of the spleen varies in adult horses, but measurements of 5 to 20 cm have been reported (3, 13). Chemical restraint may result in splenic enlargement, a fact that must be considered when assessing the size of the spleen (13).

Indications for Scanning

Because the spleen is rarely the primary site of disease in the horse, it may be overlooked when examining the abdominal cavity during the course of a diagnostic workup. However,

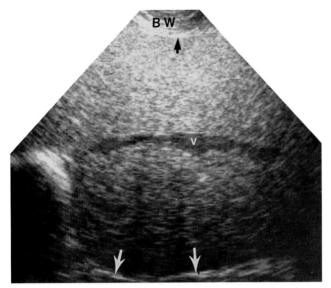

Figure 4.11. Sonogram of the spleen taken in the left mid-abdomen ventral to the ventral lung margin. Skin edge is at top and dorsal is to the left. *Arrows* point to the splenic capsule. BW = body wall musculature; v = central vein.

the spleen is frequently affected secondarily by systemic disease processes. The spleen should be examined sonographically in the course of a thorough abdominal examination. Abnormal findings in laboratory parameters or clinical findings suggestive of disease involving the abdominal cavity are indications for a thorough examination of the entire abdomen, including the spleen.

Rectal examination findings of palpable masses or abnormal structures in the left lateral abdomen indicate the need for sonographic evaluation. Abdominal abscesses, metastat-

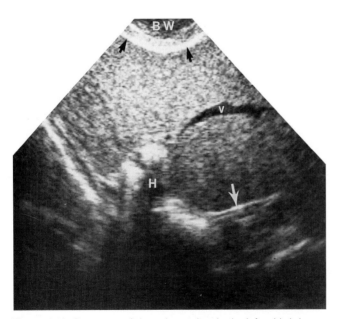

Figure 4.12. Sonogram of the spleen taken in the left mid-abdomen ventral to the ventral lung margin. Skin edge is at top and dorsal is to the left. *Arrows* point to splenic capsule. BW = body wall musculature; v = central vein shown exiting at hilar region (H).

ic tumors, hematomas, and other disease processes can affect the spleen and may be identified with sonographic evaluation. Likewise, the identification of such lesions indicates the possibility of ultrasound-guided biopsy or aspiration of the suspect lesion.

Other indications for sonographic evaluation of the spleen include hemoabdomen associated with trauma and evaluation of the abdomen for dorsal displacement of the left large colon over the nephrosplenic ligament. In the former instance, splenic fracture or rupture may be the cause of the hemoabdomen, and sonographic evaluation of the spleen may be helpful in evaluating the integrity of the spleen. Sonographic evaluation of the left paralumbar space may be particularly valuable in aiding the diagnosis of dorsal displacement of the left colon. In horses of suitable size, this diagnosis is frequently based on rectal palpation findings. However, young horses, small individuals, or other circumstances may preclude the use of rectal examination, and sonographic evaluation of the area can be extremely helpful in diagnosing the condition.

URINARY BLADDER

The urinary bladder of the horse is readily examined by traditional modalities such as rectal palpation and endoscopic visualization. Both these techniques have certain limitations, however, and circumstances occur when neither of these modalities can be used to evaluate a horse with suspected urinary bladder disease or dysfunction. Ultrasonographic examination of the bladder is an additional diagnostic tool that can provide information about the urinary bladder (14). This technique provides more information than rectal palpation alone and provides information in addition to that gained from endoscopic visualization of the bladder lumen. The bladder wall is best evaluated by ultrasound, as is the orientation of the bladder to other structures within the abdominal cavity. Moreover, transcutaneous sonographic evaluation of the bladder can be performed when rectal examination is not possible.

Technique

The urinary bladder can generally be evaluated both transcutaneously and rectally in most adult horses. Individual circumstances may dictate the approach, but transrectal evaluation is generally preferable because the entire bladder is more readily evaluated, and the transducer can usually be placed in close proximity to the bladder. This allows use of a higher-frequency transducer, which provides greater resolution of the examined structures. Both linear-array and sector transducers can be used. A 5-Mhz transducer is appropriate for most examinations, particularly if the transrectal approach is used.

When evaluating the bladder transrectally, all feces should first be removed from the horse's rectum and distal small colon, and any air in the rectum should be expelled. A water-soluble lubricant/couplant should be applied to the transducer to maintain good contact with the rectal wall. Most commercially available lubricants used for rectal palpation are suitable couplants for transrectal sonographic examinations. For transcutaneous examination of the bladder, the skin in the caudal ventral abdomen should be prepared by clipping the hair and cleaning extraneous dirt and debris from the area. A suitable couplant should then be applied to the skin. In larger horses, a 3.5-Mhz or lower-frequency transducer may be necessary to evaluate the bladder if this approach is used.

The urinary bladder is best evaluated when it is filled with fluid (15). The bladder is more readily identified if it is full, and the bladder wall is better identified and evaluated in this manner. Additionally, bladder contents are usually best seen and evaluated when they are suspended in a fluid medium. Administration of oral fluids, the appropriate use of diuretics, or retrograde infusion of a suitable sterile solution can accomplish this task.

Ballottement or manipulation of the bladder can also be performed from a transrectal approach. This may aid visualization and improve resolution of luminal contents, and it can help to differentiate free-floating material in the lumen from tissue or objects that may be attached to the bladder wall. Ballottement may also facilitate identification and evaluation of the bladder wall itself.

Normal Anatomy

The urinary bladder in the normal horse differs in form, size, and position relative to its contents. It is found at the floor of the pelvic inlet or slightly beyond, and, when distended, it extends forward along the ventral abdominal floor. The dorsal surface is related to the rectum and secondary sex glands in the male and to the body of the uterus and vagina in the female. The anterior end or vertex of the bladder is typically rounded. As filling occurs, the body of the bladder takes on a symmetric ovoid shape that changes with the degree of filling. The caudal portion of the bladder narrows to form the neck, which subsequently joins the urethra (5).

Sonographic Appearance

The bladder wall is sonographically represented by a uniformly thin, smooth echogenic interface (3, 15) (Fig. 4.13). When distended, the bladder wall appears thinner than when empty (3). In humans, mean bladder wall thickness varies from approximately 2.7 mm when almost empty to about 1.5 mm when distended. The upper limit for a normal distended bladder is about 3 mm, and for a normal empty bladder it is approximately 6 mm (15). Values for bladder wall thickness in horses have not been reported. When determining wall thickness, measurements should be taken at the bladder floor because axial resolution is better than lateral resolution, and more accurate measurements can be obtained (15). In horses, the rectal wall or vaginal wall thickness may be difficult to differentiate from that of

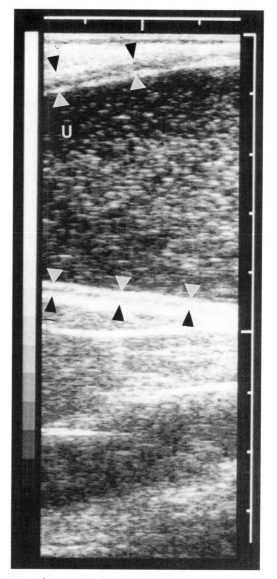

Figure 4.13. Sonogram of urinary bladder obtained transrectally. Dorsal is at the top. *Arrowheads* demarcate the bladder wall. U = urine within urinary bladder.

the bladder wall, particularly when a transrectal approach is used. These structures are all within the near-field image, and ring-down artifact may make their identification nearly impossible. Wall thickness and outline should be evaluated, because irregularities in the bladder wall appear as an abnormal density or discontinuity of the wall echo.

The sonographic appearance of urine in normal horses varies from anechoic to that of varying degrees of echogenicity (Fig. 4.14). Small echogenic particles (one to several millimeters in size) are frequently seen in bladder contents and represent calcium carbonate crystals or mucoid material (3, 14). The amount of crystalluria present depends on diet; horses fed alfalfa or calcium supplements may have increased amounts of calcium carbonate crystals in urine. An increased amount of crystals consequently augments the amount of echogenic material seen sonographically. Increased amounts of mucous or mucoid material in

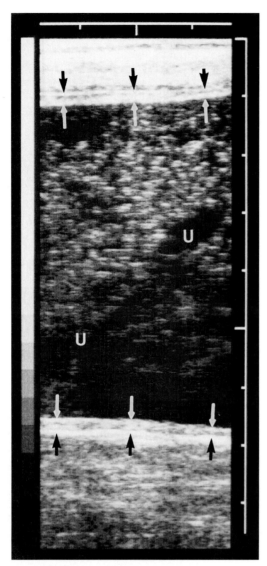

Figure 4.14. Sonogram of urinary bladder obtained transrectally. Dorsal is at the top. *Arrows* delineate the bladder wall. U = urine within the urinary bladder.

urine also enhances the echogenicity of that urine. Large amounts of both crystals and mucoid material in urine may impart a more homogeneous hyperechoic appearance to the urine such that it appears similar to that of the spleen (3). Precipitation or sedimentation of bladder contents appears as an amorphous area of echogenicity in the bladder floor. Manipulation of the bladder should cause re-suspension of this sediment. The varying degrees of echogenicity imparted by urine in normal horses can make sonographic identification of abnormal urine tedious.

Indications For Scanning

The most obvious indication for sonographic evaluation of the urinary bladder is the presence of clinical signs of cystitis or production of abnormal urine. Other indications include suspicion of cystic calculi or tumors or masses associated with the bladder wall (2, 3, 14). Bladder atony may

be assessed from the standpoint that failure to void urine usually results in excessive sludging of urine contents. Additionally, the integrity of the bladder wall may need to be evaluated after an episode of severe trauma or subsequent to pelvic fractures.

GASTROINTESTINAL TRACT

Disturbances involving the gastrointestinal tract frequently occur in the horse. Diagnostic tests are available to aid the diagnosis of these diseases, but imaging the gastrointestinal tract in horses generally has had unsatisfactory results. The abdomen of the adult horse is generally too thick to obtain good-quality radiographs, but diagnostic ultrasound can provide valuable information about the digestive tract and has become a useful tool in diagnosis of certain diseases of the bowel. Although gas in the bowel lumen makes sonographic visualization of many of the abdominal structures impossible, much information can be gained by attempting to scan various portions of the gastrointestinal tract. Information regarding bowel motility and the spatial arrangement of many parts of the gastrointestinal tract to surrounding structures is readily obtainable if the surface of the bowel is accessible to the sound beam. The presence or absence of fluid or ingesta within the bowel lumen may be discernable, and the relative size and shape of certain parts of the tract can be determined sonographically.

Technique

Scanning of the various portions of the gastrointestinal tract is routinely done with the horse standing. Both transcutaneous and transrectal approaches can be used, depending on which portion of the bowel is to be examined. Preparation of the region of interest is similar to that for other transcutaneous abdominal or transrectal examinations. A 5-Mhz or lower-frequency transducer is usually necessary, and selection of transducer frequency depends on the desirable depth of the field to be examined. Both linear-array and sector transducers can be used. A 7.5-Mhz transducer may be selected if transrectal examination of the readily palpable structures is desired.

Normal Anatomy

Stomach

The stomach is a sharply curved, J-shaped structure situated in the craniodorsal part of the abdominal cavity. It is located behind the diaphragm and liver and is situated mainly to the left of the median plane (Fig. 4.15). The convex parietal surface is directed forward, upward, and toward the left, where it lies adjacent to the diaphragm and liver. The greater curvature is extensive, and its left part lies adjacent to the medial border of the spleen. The ventral portion of the greater curvature rests on the left parts of the large colon. The left extremity of the stomach forms a rounded cul-de-sac (saccus caecus), which lies ventral to the left crus

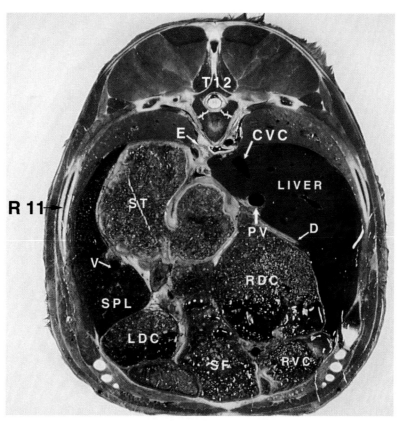

Figure 4.15. A frozen cross-section made at the level of the twelfth thoracic vertebra (T12). The section is viewed from posterior, with the left side on the reader's left. The fairly constant relationship of the spleen (SPL), splenic vein (V), and the stomach fundus (ST) is an important landmark. CVC = caudal vena cava; D = duodenum (thin slice); E = esophagus; LDC = left dorsal colon; PV = portal vein; RDC = right dorsal colon; RVC = right ventral colon; R11 = 11th rib; SF = sternal flexure. Reprinted with permission from Rantanen NW. Diseases of the abdomen. Vet Clin North Am Equine Pract. WB Saunders, 1986; 2.

of the diaphragm and medial to the base of the spleen. The right extremity is much smaller than the left and is continuous with the duodenum. This portion of the stomach lies to the right of the median plane and comes in contact with the visceral surface of the liver (5). The right portion of the stomach is positioned such that it is inaccessible to the ultrasound beam and is therefore not available for sonographic evaluation. Of the peritoneal folds (ligaments) that help to hold the stomach in place, only the gastrosplenic ligament is sonographically visible. This fold of omentum passes from the left part of the greater curvature of the stomach to the hilus of the spleen (5).

Duodenum and Small Intestine

The duodenum comprises the fixed part of the small intestine and is about 3 to 4 feet in length in the adult horse. Immediately distal to the pylorus, the duodenum is directed to the right and forms an S-shaped curve. The convex portion of the second part of this curve is directed ventrally, where it comes in contact with the medial surface of the middle and right lobes of the liver. It then passes dorsally and caudally along the right dorsal part of the colon. On reaching the level of the right kidney and base of the cecum, the duodenum curves medially to join the jejunum medial to the base of the cecum (Fig. 4.16). The remaining portions of the small intestine vary in location but lie chiefly in the dorsal part of the left half of the abdomen (5).

Cecum

The cecum is positioned to the right of the median plane, extending from the right paralumbar area ventrally, anteriorly, and medially to end on the abdominal floor behind the xiphoid cartilage (Fig. 4.17). The base extends as far cranially as the right fourteenth or fifteenth rib, and caudally to the tuber coxae. The apex generally lies on the ventral abdominal floor, on or to the right of the medial plane, and ends several inches behind the xiphoid cartilage. The right (lateral) side of the organ lies adjacent to the right abdominal wall, the diaphragm, the duodenum, and the liver. The left side of the cecum lies against the left and terminal parts of the large colon, the mesenteric root, and the small intestine (5).

Large Colon

The large colon in situ is positioned such that it consists of four parts (Fig. 4.18). The right ventral colon begins at the medial surface of the cecal base and passes downward and forward along the right costal arch and floor of the abdomen. At the region of the xiphoid cartilage, it bends sharply backward to the left (sternal flexure) to continue as

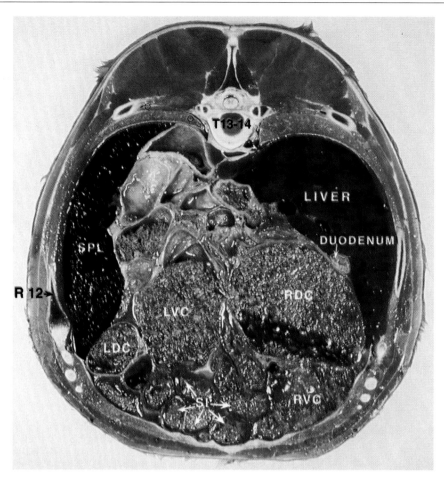

Figure 4.16. A frozen cross-section made at the junction of the thirteenth and fourteenth thoracic vertebrae (T13-14). The section is viewed from posterior, with the left side on the reader's left. The liver is the predominant parenchymal organ ventral to the right lung. LDC = left dorsal colon; LVC = left ventral colon; RDC = right dorsal colon; RVC = right ventral colon; R12 = twelfth rib; SI = small intestine; SPL = spleen. Reprinted with permission from Rantanen NW. Diseases of the abdomen. Vet Clin North Am Equine Pract 1986; 2.

the left ventral colon. The left ventral colon passes caudally along the abdominal floor to the left of the cecum and, on reaching the pelvic inlet, bends sharply dorsally and anteriorly (pelvic flexure) to form the left dorsal colon. The left dorsal colon then passes forward dorsal or lateral to the left ventral colon to reach the diaphragm and left liver lobe, where it turns backward and to the right (diaphragmatic flexure) to end in the right dorsal colon. The right dorsal colon then passes backward dorsal to the right ventral colon to reach the medial surface of the base of the cecum, where it becomes constricted and continues as the small colon (5).

The ventral parts of the large colon are mainly in contact with the abdominal wall laterally and ventrally. On the right side, the colon is usually separated from the abdominal wall by the cecum, but exceptions can occur. On the left side, the left dorsal and ventral colons are generally in contact with the left lateral ventral abdominal wall, and more cranially, they are usually positioned medial to the spleen (5).

The coils of the small colon lie chiefly dorsal to the left large colon in the space between the stomach and the pelvic inlet. The small colon is mingled with the small intestine in this space (5).

Sonographic Appearance

Certain sonographic findings are typical of all portions of the gastrointestinal tract and should be kept in mind when examining the various portions of this system. Intraluminal gas is echogenic and is usually associated with complete or partial distal acoustic shadowing. Fluid in the lumen, on the other hand, allows propagation of sound waves, and no acoustic shadowing is evident. Motion of tiny particles is typically seen within the fluid. These particles represent trapped intraluminal "micro" gas bubbles or ingesta. The hypoechoic rim frequently seen surrounding the luminal contents represents the bowel wall. The outer echogenic border of the bowel wall is produced by periserosal fat.

With higher resolution, five distinct layers of the bowel wall may be identified: first, the luminal surface is echogenic; second, the mucosa is hypoechoic; third, the submucosa has increased echogenicity; fourth, it is followed by a hypoechoic muscular layer; and fifth, the outer layer represents the echogenic serosa and periserosal fat (15). With less resolution, however, only three layers may be identified. These are the echogenic luminal surface and serosal layers that lie on either side of the hypoechoic bowel wall.

Even though intraluminal gas produces partial or complete distal acoustic shadowing, information can be gained from sonographic evaluation of various portions of the gastrointestinal tract. Real-time evaluation of the intestinal tract displays the characteristic changes in configuration of the bowel produced by peristaltic contractions or motion of the intraluminal contents. These findings can aid in the identification of certain regions of the tract and can assess size, shape, motility, and location of these segments.

Stomach

The stomach is examined transcutaneously from the left side of the horse in approximately the tenth through thirteenth intercostal spaces, in the region immediately ventral to the ventral lung margin. The transducer may be angled dorsally up under the lung margin to gain visualization of a greater portion of the organ. The stomach is medial to the spleen and typically is represented by a hypoechoic wall with an echogenic luminal surface (Fig. 4.19). The splenic vessels found along the hilus of the spleen are situated between the spleen and the stomach wall and can serve as an anatomic landmark when examining this region. The stomach echo can be found extending ventrally from the

ventral lung margin for a variable distance in the intercostal spaces named previously. Frequently, the stomach–left dorsal colon interface can be seen medial to the spleen in the middle to lower regions of the left abdominal wall (Fig. 4.20).

The stomach wall itself is typically hypoechoic to the adjacent tissues and is represented by a uniformly smooth, curvilinear space adjacent to the high-amplitude gas echo of the luminal surface. Peristaltic activity is rarely seen when real-time evaluation of the stomach is performed. No values are available for normal wall thickness in the horse, but values of 4 to 5 mm are considered upper limits for wall thickness in humans (16).

Duodenum and Small Intestine

The duodenum is scanned transcutaneously from the right side of the horse. It may be located in the tenth to twelfth intercostal spaces at about the level of the mid-abdomen to slightly lower. It is immediately adjacent to the medial border of the liver and can usually be traced to the region just ventral to the right kidney in the fifteenth to sixteenth intercostal space (Fig. 4.21). The size and configuration of the duodenum vary with degree of filling and the state of

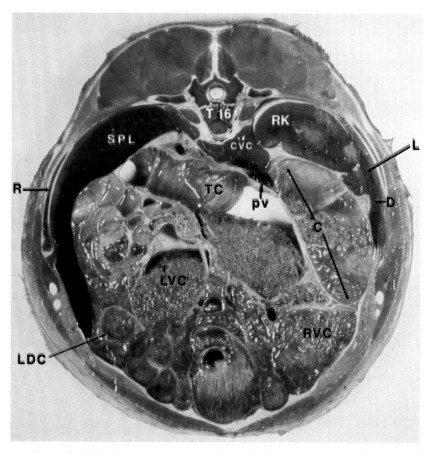

Figure 4.17. A frozen cross-section made at the sixteenth thoracic vertebra (T16). The section is viewed from posterior, with the left side on the reader's left. The right kidney (RK) lies medial-ventral to the last few ribs. The liver (L) apposes the cranial pole of the right kidney. C = cecum; cvc = caudal vena cava; D = descending duodenum; LDC = left dorsal colon; LVC = left ventral colon; pv = portal vein; RVC = right ventral colon; R = fifteenth rib; SPL = spleen; TC = transverse colon. Reprinted with permission from Rantanen NW. Diseases of the kidney. Vet Clin North Am Equine Pract 1986; 2.

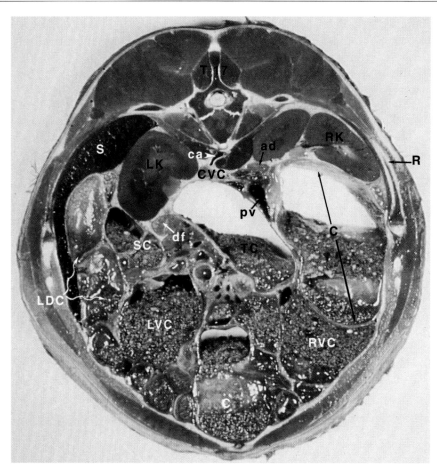

Figure 4.I8. A frozen cross-section made at the seventeenth thoracic vertebra (T17). The section is viewed from posterior, with the left side on the reader's left. The cranial pole of the left kidney (LK) is visualized. ad = right adrenal gland; ca = celiac artery; C = cecum; CVC = caudal vena cava; df = duodenal-jejunal flexure; LDC = left dorsal colon; LK = left kidney; LVC = left ventral colon; pv = portal vein; R = sixteenth rib; RK = right kidney; RVC = right ventral colon; S = spleen; SC = small colon; TC = transverse colon. Reprinted with permission from Rantanen NW. Diseases of the kidney. Vet Clin North Am Equine Pract 1986; 2.

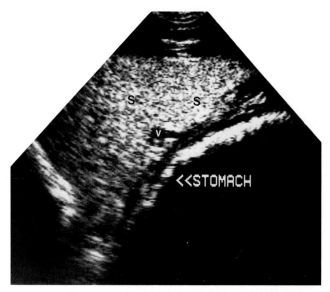

Figure 4.19. Sonogram of the spleen and stomach wall taken from the left mid-abdomen just ventral to the ventral lung margin. Skin edge is at top and dorsal is to the right. The hypoechoic rim separating the spleen (S) from the luminal surface of the stomach represents the muscular portion of the stomach wall. A splenic vessel (v) is seen exiting at the hilar region of the spleen.

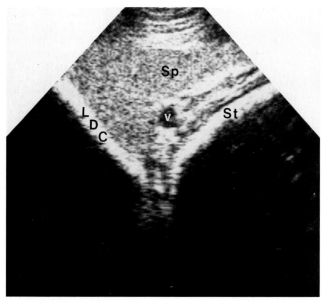

Figure 4.20. Sonogram taken in the left mid to lower abdomen at approximately the eleventh to twelfth intercostal space. Skin edge is at top and dorsal is to the right. A splenic vessel (v) is visible at the hilar region of the spleen. LDC = gas interface of the left dorsal colon; Sp = spleen; St = gastric mucosal/luminal interface.

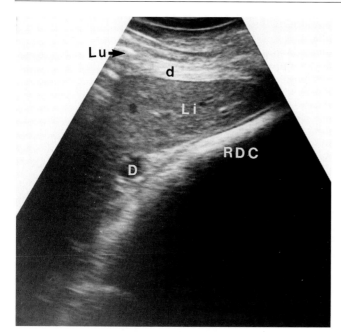

Figure 4.21. Sonogram taken in right twelfth intercostal space at the level of the mid-abdomen. Skin edge is at top and dorsal is to the left. The duodenum (D) is found on the medial border of the liver in approximately the tenth to twelfth intercostal space. Peristaltic activity during real-time imaging aids identification of this structure. d = diaphragm; Li = liver; Lu = ventral lung margin; RDC = right dorsal colon.

contraction. It assumes a generally rounded appearance in cross-section and has a tubular configuration when seen in long axis. The wall is thin and is hypoechoic relative to the lumen contents (3). Again, normal values for wall thickness are not available for horses, but 3 mm is considered the upper limit for small intestinal wall thickness in humans (16).

The duodenum typically exhibits a rapid rate of contraction and normally does not stay dilated with fluid or gas for any prolonged period (2). The duodenum should always contain some fluid, and the absence of this finding should be cause for concern. The persistence of a gas echo and the absence of fluid within the lumen should be considered abnormal findings and necessitate further evaluation of the patient.

Other portions of the small intestine are seen as rounded structures in transverse section and assume a tubular configuration in long axis. They can be identified by their lack of haustra or sacculations and can contain both fluid and gas echoes. Peristalsis may be evident during real-time evaluation of these structures. Because of the location of most of the small intestine, failure to identify portions of this part of the gastrointestinal tract during evaluation of the abdomen in the horse should not be considered abnormal.

Cecum

The cecal base is found in the right paralumbar fossa and last few intercostal spaces below the level of the tuber coxae and ventral and medial to the right kidney. The cecum

extends a variable distance down the right flank and lateral abdomen. Sonographically, it is usually represented by a high-amplitude gas echo that generally has a smooth curvilinear appearance (Fig. 4.22). On occasion, some evidence of sacculation maybe evident. The cecal wall is usually not specifically identified as an echolucent rim adjacent to the luminal gas echo. Peristaltic activity or motion of the cecal base is occasionally observed during real-time examination.

Large Colon

The right and left parts of the large colon can be examined in the middle to lower parts of their respective sides of the abdomen. The large colon is usually found adjacent to the body wall in the most ventrolateral aspects of the abdomen, except where noted previously. The sonographic appearance of the large colon is similar to that of the cecum in that it is characterized by a high-amplitude gas echo representing the luminal surface. The wall itself is infrequently identified. Specific to the large colon, however, are the haustral markings, which are readily evident sonographically. These markings are specific to the large bowel and can be used for identification as well as to assess peristaltic activity (Fig. 4.23).

Indications For Scanning

The primary indication for sonographic evaluation of the stomach is to evaluate the stomach wall for the presence of neoplastic disease. Squamous cell carcinoma is one of the most frequent neoplasms involving the stomach, and it has been documented sonographically (13). Other tumors can involve the stomach, and when primary or metastatic neoplastic disease is suspected, the stomach wall should be included in the evaluation of the patient.

Real-time ultrasound is an excellent method of assessing the presence or absence of gross motility of the intestinal

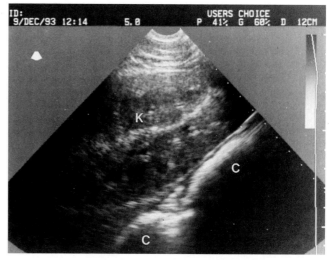

Figure 4.22. Sonogram taken in the right sixteenth intercostal space at the level of the tuber coxae. Skin edge is at top and dorsal is to the left. The high amplitude gas echo outlining the base of the cecum (C) is ventral and medial to the right kidney (K).

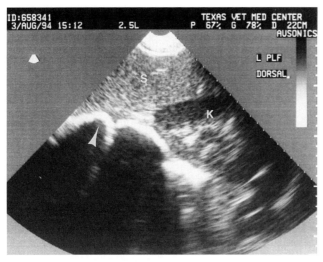

Figure 4.23. Sonogram taken in the left paralumbar fossa. Skin edge is at top and dorsal is to the right. The haustral markings (*arrowhead*) that identify the large colon are medial to the spleen (S) and ventro-medial to the left kidney (K) in this image. The sacculations of the large colon are usually readily apparent on real-time examination.

tract. The effectiveness of bowel wall motion in producing aboral transit of ingesta may not be determined sonographically, but gross wall motion can be detected. Because normal bowel always exhibits some degree of motility, lack of motility or ileus can be determined as well, and persistent ileus is abnormal and should be further investigated. Persistent ileus coupled with distention of the intestinal tract should warrant evaluation of the patient for some type of intestinal obstruction. Some of the causes for intestinal obstruction include volvulus or torsion of some portion of the gastrointestinal tract, bowel displacement, intraluminal foreign bodies such as fecaliths or enteroliths, intussusception, strangulating lipoma, and various other conditions. Many of these primary causes of obstruction can be specifically identified with ultrasound.

Ultrasound is also useful in diagnosing certain displacements of the intestinal tract. Because the location and sonographic appearance of various parts of the intestinal tract are known, alterations from normal are useful in determining which structures may be displaced and the possible location of the displacement. A good example is renosplenic entrapment (dorsal displacement) of the left colon, which is readily identifiable sonographically (17).

Other conditions in which ultrasound may provide useful information are in the assessment of horses with duodenitis–proximal jejunitis (anterior enteritis); evaluation of intestinal serosal surfaces for the presence of adhesions or metastatic neoplastic disease; evaluation of the mesentery for masses (abscesses, tumors, or lymph node enlargement); and evaluation of the abdominal cavity for the presence of excess fluid (ascites) or evidence of peritonitis.

ABDOMINAL AORTA AND GREAT VESSELS

The sonographic evaluation of the vasculature system has made great strides in recent years, and much information

has been generated regarding vascular diseases with the aid of this technique. Real-time B-mode ultrasonography provides information regarding the relative size, shape, and location of various vascular structures. It can be a crude means of assessing blood flow, in that movement of blood components is often seen in medium-sized and larger vessels with the aid of a 5-Mhz or higher-frequency transducer. It is also useful to document the presence of intravascular thrombosis.

More critical evaluation of blood flow, however, necessitates the use of Doppler ultrasound. This specialized application of sound waves interacting with a flowing medium (such as blood in the vascular system) complements two-dimensional ultrasonographic findings, but it is a science in itself and beyond the scope of this discussion. For purposes of this chapter, only B-mode real-time ultrasound evaluation of the great vessels is discussed.

Technique

The major vessels in the abdomen of the horse, such as the aorta and its associated branches, the vena cava, and other major venous structures in the abdomen, are occasionally identified during transcutaneous evaluation of the abdomen. However, only isolated segments of these vessels are typically seen in this manner, and a thorough systematic evaluation of the abdominal vasculature is not possible from a transcutaneous approach. Additionally, the presence of gas in the bowel lumen obscures many areas and structures within the abdominal cavity and makes the sonographic evaluation of many of these vascular structures difficult or impossible.

In spite of these limitations, the terminal aorta, several of its branches, and their corresponding venous structures can be evaluated from a transrectal approach in many horses (3). The length of the aorta examined depends on the size of the horse, its disposition or suitability for transrectal scanning, and the presence of bowel gas or other factors that may interfere with a satisfactory examination.

The horse is prepared by evacuating as much feces from the rectum and distal small colon as possible. Sedation may be required in some horses before initiating the procedure. Caudal epidural anesthesia is also often helpful in reducing or eliminating rectal straining during the procedure and often allows greater relaxation of the rectum. This allows better and safer maneuverability of the transducer within the rectum. Another procedure has been described whereby 20 mg propantheline bromide is given intravenously before the examination to aid in rectal dilation and to inhibit rectal straining (18). However, this product is not currently approved for use in equine species. A 7.5-Mhz transducer is preferred for vascular examination, although a 5-Mhz transducer can be used. Both sector and linear-array transducers are satisfactory if their size is small enough to use in rectal examinations.

The terminal aorta and its branches are identified at or just cranial to the pelvic inlet on the dorsal midline of the abdomen. Pulsation within the aorta helps to identify it and aids in placement of the transducer on its ventral surface, with the scan surface of the transducer directed dorsally. Once the distal aorta has been identified, the internal and external iliac arteries and associated veins can be located by moving the transducer caudally to the origin of these structures, then tracing them distally as far as possible by appropriate manipulation of the transducer within the rectum. The iliac arteries are usually best visualized with the transducer positioned obliquely to the long axis of the colon (3).

The cranial mesenteric artery is not accessible for examination in some horses (3), most commonly because of the size of the horse and for the reasons discussed previously. A technique has been described for evaluation of this artery in appropriate horses (18).

Initially, the aorta is identified and traced cranially to the origin of the cranial mesenteric artery. At this point, the transducer is moved to the left of the aorta with the scan surface directed dorsally and to the right. After the artery has been identified, it can be imaged distally by positioning the transducer such that the scan surface of the transducer

is directed cranially and to the right. By moving the transducer ventrally in this position, transverse scans of the artery can be obtained (18). Again, bowel gas may preclude visualization of the structures on any given exam, and repeated attempts may be necessary to image this artery satisfactorily.

Normal Anatomy

The aorta is positioned along the dorsal midline surface of the abdominal cavity and terminates at about the level of the fifth or sixth lumbar vertebra (5). The paired external iliac arteries originate from the aorta under the fifth lumbar vertebra, usually just cranial to the origin of the internal iliac arteries (Fig. 4.24). They descend along the side of the pelvic inlet adjacent to the tendons of the psoas minor muscles to the level of the anterior border of the pubis. Beyond this point, they continue as the femoral arteries (5). The external iliac arteries lie adjacent and anterior to their corresponding veins.

The internal iliac arteries result from the terminal bifur-

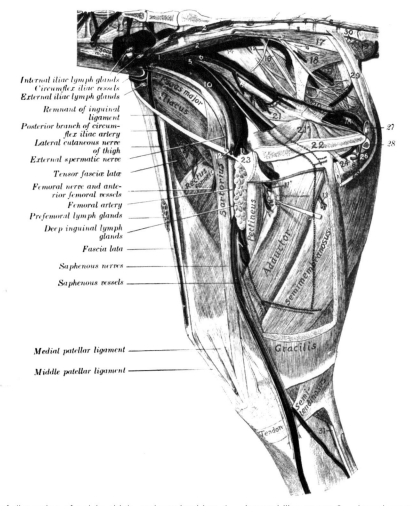

Figure 4.24. Medial view of dissection of pelvis, thigh, and proximal leg. 1 = internal iliac artery; 2 = lateral sacral artery; 6 = internal pudic artery; 10 = external iliac artery. Reprinted with permission from Sisson S. The anatomy of the domestic animals. 4th ed. Philadelphia: WB Saunders, 1953.

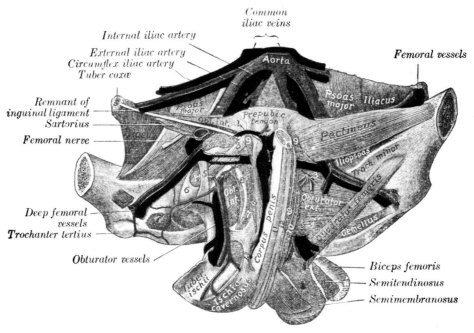

Figure 4.25. Deep dissection of ventral wall of pelvis of male horse. Reprinted with permission from Sisson S. The anatomy of the domestic animals. 4th ed. Philadelphia: WB Saunders, 1953.

cation of the aorta at about the fifth or sixth lumbar vertebra (Fig. 4.25). They diverge from the aorta at approximately a 60° angle, passing backward under the wing of the sacrum, then course downward along the pelvic surface of the shaft of the ilium (5).

The venous structures can vary in their anatomic arrangement. Generally, the internal and external iliac veins join at the level of the sacroiliac articulation to form the respective right and left common iliac veins. These two large but short trunks join at about the fifth lumbar vertebra above the terminal part of the aorta and to the right of the median plane. The confluence of these two veins forms the posterior vena cava, which courses cranially along the right hand side of the abdominal aorta.

Sonographic Appearance

The sonographic appearance of the major elastic arteries in the equine abdomen is similar with the exception of the variability in size of the different vessels. The elastic arteries should maintain their shape, even under moderate pressure, and the vessel walls exhibit pulsatile movement. Blood within the lumen is typically anechoic, although occasional swirling movement is noted within the vessel. Stagnant blood flow or slow-moving blood has an increased echogenic appearance. Higher gain settings can also create an increased echogenic appearance to moving blood.

The luminal surface of the larger arteries should have a smooth sonographic appearance, and the wall of the vessel should have a uniform thickness and echogenic pattern (19, 20). In vitro studies, however, have demonstrated a thin hyperechoic luminal layer in approximately 45% of normal arterial specimens (19). The arterial wall is usually

indistinguishable from the surrounding connective tissue (20) (Fig. 4.26).

The sonographic appearance of the venous structures of the abdomen may differ slightly form that of the arteries. Blood flow within the veins is generally slower, and therefore the blood within the veins may take on a slightly increased echogenic appearance. Venous walls are thinner than arterial walls and frequently are not specifically identified sonographically. Veins are also collapsible when pressure is applied to them, and they should distend distally if constant pressure is applied to a focal area. If pressure is applied to a vein such that blood flow is drastically reduced, the stagnated blood takes on an echogenic character. Release of the pressure allows blood flow to return to normal, and the blood again takes on an anechoic appearance.

Sonographic evaluation of the abdominal vasculature is best accomplished by transrectal examination. Even so, gas within the lumen of the various segments of the intestinal tract prevents visualization of any vascular structure deep to the gas. Manipulation of the transducer within the rectum is often necessary to evaluate as much of a vascular structure as possible.

Indications For Scanning

Probably the most common reason for sonographic evaluation of the abdominal vasculature is suspicion of aortic–iliac thrombosis. Horses affected with this disease typically exhibit exercise-associated lameness or pain involving one or both rear limbs. Sonographic evaluation of the terminal aorta and iliac arteries can provide a definitive diagnosis of this condition (21–23). Aortic–iliac thrombosis has also

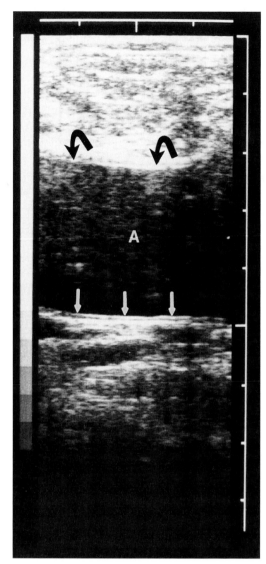

Figure 4.26. Sonogram of the distal abdominal aorta obtained transrectally, with the scanhead directed towards the lumbar spine. The ventral wall of the aorta (*curved arrows*) is often difficult to distinguish from the surrounding connective tissue. The dorsal wall (*small arrows*) of the aorta (A) is readily identified in this image.

been diagnosed sonographically in two stallions that exhibited ejaculatory failure (24).

Other disease conditions that may warrant sonographic evaluation of the abdominal vasculature include verminous arteritis (19, 20) and the presence of unilateral or bilateral rear limb edema. In the latter instance, the caudal vessels of the abdomen may be evaluated for the presence of intraluminal or extraluminal masses causing obstruction of venous return from the leg.

DIAPHRAGM

Technique

The diaphragm lies adjacent or close to the chest wall in almost all scan planes in which it is observed. Therefore, a higher-frequency transducer is required for positive identification and assessment of this structure. The diaphragm may be identified with a 3-Mhz or lower-frequency transducer, but a 5- or 7.5-Mhz transducer is preferable, particularly if the diaphragm itself is to be evaluated. Both linear-array and sector transducers can be used, but the small footprint of the sector transducer typically allows better visualization of the diaphragm through the intercostal spaces. Regardless of which transducer is employed, the gain settings should be set to enhance the near-field image, because the diaphragm lies so close to the skin surface. Before examination, the skin is prepared as for other transcutaneous sonographic evaluations.

Normal Anatomy

The diaphragm is a large, singular dome-shaped muscle that separates the thoracic and abdominal cavities. The thoracic side is strongly convex, and the corresponding abdominal surface is concave. This muscle is composed of a muscular rim and a tendinous central portion. The outer muscular rim can be subdivided into three areas. The costal muscular portion originates from its attachments to the cartilages of the ribs, beginning at about the eighth rib and extending caudally to include the last rib. From the tenth rib backward, the attachments to the ribs occur at an increasing distance above the costochondral junctions, such that at the last rib, the upper limit of attachment is only 4 to 5 inches from the ventral limit of attachment. Anteriorly, the origin extends from the ninth costal cartilage to insert on the xiphoid cartilage. The muscle fibers of the diaphragm curve dorsomedially and forward from these points of origin to join the tendinous central portion. The sternal part attaches to the upper surface of the xiphoid cartilage, and the lumbar part attaches to the ventral longitudinal ligament and thus to the first four or five lumbar vertebrae (5). Of the three different parts of the muscular diaphragm, only portions of the costal part ventral to the lung margin are accessible for sonographic evaluation.

The thoracic surface of the diaphragm is adjacent to the visceral pleura of the lung, the pericardium, and the parietal pleura of the thoracic wall in the ventral parts of the thorax. The abdominal surface is largely covered by peritoneum and is related to the liver, the right colon and intestines, and the right kidney on the right side. On the left side, the abdominal surface is related to the liver, the spleen, the stomach, and portions of the left colon and intestines.

Sonographic Appearance

The diaphragm is visualized in the intercostal spaces ventral to the lung margin on both sides of the thorax. It lies adjacent and parallel to the body wall in the ventral most part of the thorax, then gradually diverges dorsally and medially to disappear behind the echogenic lung interface.

The sonographic appearance of the diaphragm may change slightly, depending on the varying amounts of mus-

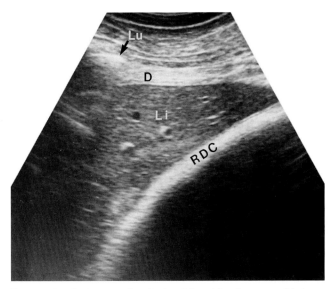

Figure 4.27. Sonogram taken in the right mid to lower twelfth intercostal space. Skin edge is at top and dorsal is to the left. The diaphragm (D) is an important landmark separating the thoracic and abdominal cavities. Li = liver; Lu = ventral lung margin; RDC = luminal surface of right dorsal colon.

cle and fibrous tissue present, but it is characteristically identified by its curvilinear parallel echogenic fascial planes with a hypoechoic muscular portion sandwiched between the more echogenic outer fascial rims (25) (Fig. 4.27). Only a small linear portion is identified in any one plane, however, because structures are best visualized when their surfaces are perpendicular to the ultrasound beam. The curved shape of the diaphragm thus precludes complete visualization of the structure, even when large amounts of pleural fluid are present (26). Little if any change is noted in the sonographic appearance of the diaphragm when comparing inspiratory with expiratory movements.

Indications For Scanning

The diaphragm is an extremely important landmark in the sonographic evaluation of the abdomen or thorax of the horse, because it serves to separate and partially define the boundaries of these two large body cavities and their respective contents. Other specific indications for evaluating the diaphragm include the suspicion of a diaphragmatic hernia or rupture (26, 27) and evaluation of the diaphragm as a possible implantation site for metastatic neoplastic disease (13). The diaphragm may also be examined for possible sites of fibrous adhesion between it and other abdominal organs, particularly when horses exhibit clinical signs referable to abdominal discomfort, chronic intermittent colic, or peritonitis.

EFFECT OF PREGNANCY ON ABDOMINAL IMAGING

Early pregnancy in the mare has no significant effect on the location of various organs within the abdominal cavity. However, in mid-term and late-term pregnancy, the developing fetus and associated uterine structures begin to occu-

py an increasing amount of space within the abdomen. Subsequently, the abdominal organs that are not rigidly fixed can be displaced from their more normal or anticipated location (13). Organs that can be variably displaced include the colon, cecum, liver, spleen and urinary bladder. Failure to identify these organs in their expected location or visualization of decreased amounts of these structures in late-term pregnancy should not be regarded as specific signs of disease. Because the late-term fetus typically occupies the ventral cranial abdomen, the cecum, colon, liver and spleen may all be displaced dorsally. Likewise, the diaphragm may have a more cranial excursion, and the urinary bladder may be displaced to either side of the midline in these mares.

Another factor to consider in middle to late pregnancy is differentiation of uterine fluid from peritoneal fluid. When attempting to differentiate these two fluid compartments, every effort should be made to identify the uterine wall. This is best accomplished by first identifying the fetus, then subsequently finding the uterine wall. Because the heavy gravid uterus typically occupies the ventral part of the abdomen, this area should be initially examined to attempt to identify the fetus or uterus. Alternatively, the sonographer may have greater success in identifying the fetus by beginning the examination in the caudal ventral portion of the abdomen, then progressing anteriorly until the gravid uterus is identified.

To differentiate peritoneal fluid from uterine fluid, the abdominal cavity should initially be evaluated in the lower sixth or seventh intercostal space immediately caudal to the diaphragm. Usually, any significant amount of peritoneal fluid initially accumulates in the cranioventralmost part of the abdomen and can be seen immediately adjacent to the abdominal surface of the diaphragm. Larger amounts of peritoneal fluid may actually displace the liver from its close apposition to the diaphragm, and the other abdominal organs may be identified within the fluid echo. The various abdominal organs may actually appear to be floating within a fluid medium when large quantities of peritoneal fluid are present. A significant aspect of differentiating peritoneal fluid from uterine fluid is that various abdominal organs or structures can be identified within the fluid medium in the case of ascites, whereas these same structures *cannot* be identified within the fluid echo of uterine fluid.

REFERENCES

1. Schmitz DG. Understanding the principles of equine ultrasonography. Vet Med 1991;86:748.
2. Rantanen NW. Abdominal ultrasonography. Equine Vet Data 1985;6:331.
3. Schmidt AR. Transrectal ultrasonography of the caudal portion of abdominal and pelvic cavities in horses. J Am Vet Med Assoc 1989;194:365.
4. Rantanen NW, Ewing RL III. Principles of ultrasound application in animals. Vet Radiol 1981;22:196.
5. Sisson S. The anatomy of the domestic animals. 4th ed. Philadelphia: WB Saunders, 1953.

6. Wilson DA, et al. Ultrasonographic evaluation of the healing of ventral midline abdominal incisions in the horse. Equine Vet J 1989;7 (Suppl):107.

7. Rantanen NW. Diseases of the liver. Vet Clin North Am Equine Pract 1986;2:105.

8. Reef VB, Johnston JK, Divers TJ, et al. Ultrasonographic findings in horses with cholelithiasis: eight cases (1985–1987). J Am Vet Med Assoc 1990;196:1836.

9. Rantanen NW: Diseases of the kidneys. Vet Clin North Am Equine Pract 1986;2:89.

10. Penninck DC, Eisenberg HM, Teuscher EE, et al. Equine renal ultrasonography: normal and abnormal. Vet Radiol 1986; 27:81.

11. Kiper ML, Traub-Dargatz JL, Wrigley RH. Renal ultrasonography in horses. Compend Contin Educ Pract Vet 1990;12:993.

12. Rantanen NW. Renal ultrasound in the horse. Equine Vet Educ 1990; 2:135.

13. Rantanen NW: Diseases of the abdomen. Vet Clin North Am Equine Pract 1986;2:67.

14. Traub-Dargatz JL, McKinnon AQ. Adjunctive methods of examination of the urogenital tract. Vet Clin North Am Equine Pract 1988; 4.

15. Mittelstaedt CA. Lower urinary tract. In: Mittelstaedt CA, ed. General ultrasound. New York: Churchill Livingstone, 1992.

16. Mittelstaedt CA. Gastrointestinal tract. In: Mittelstaedt CA, ed. General ultrasound. New York: Churchill Livingstone, 1992.

17. Santschi EM, Slone DE Jr, Frank WM II. Use of ultrasound in horses for diagnosis of left dorsal displacement of the large colon and monitoring its nonsurgical correction. Vet Surg 1993;22:281.

18. Wallace KD, Selcer BA, Becht JL. Technique for transrectal ultrasonography of the cranial mesenteric artery of the horse. Am J Vet Res 1989;50:1695.

19. Wallace KD, Selcer BA, Tyler DE, et al. In vitro ultrasonographic appearance of the normal and verminous equine aorta cranial mesenteric artery and its branches. Am J Vet Res 1989; 50:1774.

20. Wallace KD, Selcer BA, Tyler DE, et al. Transrectal ultrasonography of the cranial mesenteric artery of the horse. Am J Vet Res 1989; 50:1699.

21. Tithof PK, Rebhun WC, Dietze AE. Ultrasonographic diagnosis of aorto-iliac thrombosis. Cornell Vet 1985;75:540.

22. Reef VB, Roby KA, Richardson DW, et al. Use of ultrasonography for the detection of aortic-iliac thrombosis in horses. J Am Vet Med Assoc 1987;190:286.

23. Edwards GB, Allen WE. Aorto-iliac thrombosis in two horses: clinical course of the disease and use of real-time ultrasonography to confirm diagnosis. Equine Vet J 1988;20:384.

24. McDonnell SM, Love CC, Martin BB, et al. Ejaculatory failure associated with aortic-iliac thrombosis in two stallions. J Am Vet Med Assoc 1992;200:954.

25. Rantanen NW. Diseases of the thorax. Vet Clin North Am Equine Pract 1986;2:49.

26. Hartzband LE, Kerr DV, Morris EA. Ultrasonographic diagnosis of diaphragmatic rupture in a horse. Vet Radiol 1990;31:42.

27. Everett KA, Chaffin MK, Brinsko SP. Diaphragmatic herniation as a cause of lethargy and exercise intolerance in a mare. Cornell Vet 1992;82:217.

5. Neonatal Sonography

JOHANNA M. REIMER

Many disorders in the equine neonate can be evaluated readily with diagnostic ultrasound. The heart, lungs, liver, spleen, and kidneys of the foal can be examined with ultrasound, as in the adult horse. Gastrointestinal sonography is often more rewarding in the foal than it is in the adult, because less gas-filled large colon is present, and small intestinal disorders are more prevalent. Ruptured bladders and internal umbilical remnant infections lend themselves readily to sonographic evaluation. Sonography can also be useful for evaluating several musculoskeletal disorders in the foal, such as synovial effusions, fractures, osteomyelitis, and tendon and ligament injuries.

THORACIC SONOGRAPHY

Lungs and Pleural Cavity

Pneumonia in the neonate is most frequently interstitial, and it rarely produces pleural effusion or cranioventral consolidation. Radiography often provides a better indication of the type and severity of disease in foals with pneumonia, although in some cases sonography adds complementary information (1). Thoracic sonography should be strongly considered in foals with suspected hemothorax, as a result of rib fractures, for example, and diaphragmatic hernias.

A 7.5-Mhz transducer generally provides optimal image quality of the neonatal lung surface. In foals with large pleural effusions or extensive regions of lung consolidation, a 5.0-Mhz transducer may be adequate, and sometimes even necessary. The sonogram must be performed with the foal standing or in sternal recumbency (2). Any fluid or intestinal contents within the pleural cavity will lie beneath air-filled lung and will therefore be hidden by the lung if the foal is in lateral recumbency. The procedure for thoracic sonography is otherwise the same as that described for the adult (see Chapter 3). The sonographic appearance of the lung surface is identical to that of the adult; the lung surface is represented by a bright linear echo, with equidistant reverberation artifacts below this line. Minimal, if any, pleural fluid should be present.

The cranial mediastinum is also accessible for sonographic evaluation in the foal. The thymus is easily visualized in some foals up to several months of age and should not be confused with a mass or abscess. The thymus appears as a homogenous parenchymatous structure, just beneath and medial to the lung in the cranial mediastinum (Fig 5.1) (2).

Heart

Congenital and acquired cardiac defects are best investigated with echocardiography. Pericardial diseases and endo-carditis, which are generally seen in older foals, and congenital cardiac defects are, with few exceptions, easily documented with echocardiography (1). The clinician should be aware that severe congenital cardiac defects, typically those with right-to-left shunts (cyanotic congenital cardiac disease), may not be associated with a murmur. Contrast (bubble) studies are easy to perform and are useful in determining whether right-to-left intracardiac shunting exists, either in the setting of a congenital cardiac defect or when reversion to fetal circulation is suspected. Pulmonary hypertension may occur secondary to profound septicemia, endotoxemia, hypoxemia, or pneumonia. If the foramen ovale or ductus arteriosus has not yet fibrosed, the increase in pulmonary pressure can result in a reversion to fetal circulation. This potential cause of hypoxemia unresponsive to oxygen administration in the critically ill neonate can be investigated with echocardiographic techniques. Doppler echocardiography, a method used to evaluate blood flow, is most commonly used to investigate the source and significance of pathologic murmurs. Information regarding the presence and degree of valvular regurgitation or cardiac shunts may be obtained with Doppler echocardiography. Patent ductus arteriosus is actually difficult to demonstrate with two-dimensional echocardiography; however, Doppler echocardiography enables documentation of left-to-right patent ductus arteriosus.

A 5.0-Mhz transducer and depth of field of 15 to 20 cm provide optimum image quality of the heart in the neonatal foal (3). The transducer is positioned at the right cardiac window, which is generally located at the fourth intercostal space, halfway between the point of the shoulder and the elbow. The standard imaging views (both B-mode and M-mode) employed in the adult are also used in the neonate (see Chapter 2). An additional view that can be performed in the recumbent neonate is the subxiphoid view (1). This view is of greatest application in Doppler flow studies in which the aortic flow velocity can be determined and cardiac output can be subsequently estimated. Critical attention must be paid to cardiac anatomy, including the venous and arterial communications in the neonate, if congenital defects are suspected.

Contrast studies are performed by the rapid intravenous injection of agitated saline, with simultaneous echocardiography. The right atrium and ventricle are opacified with microbubbles. Appearance of bubbles in the left atrium, left ventricle, or aorta is indicative of right-to-left shunting. In foals with left-to-right shunting, as in a foal with a left-to-right ventricular septal defect, for example, negative contrast (a lack of bubbles within a chamber otherwise opacified with bubbles) at the level of the shunt may be identified (3).

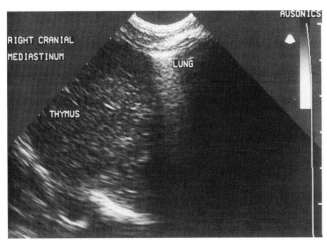

Figure 5.1. Cranial mediastinum of a 1-day-old Thoroughbred foal. The image was obtained from the right third intercostal space. Notice the parenchyma-like architecture of the thymic tissue. Dorsal is to the right, ventral is to the left.

ABDOMEN

Gastrointestinal Tract

Sonographic evaluation of the intestinal tract should be considered in foals with abdominal pain, abdominal distention, or suspected ruptured viscus. Sonography enables the evaluation and characterization of intestinal distention, lumen contents, motility, wall thickness, and peritoneal fluid. In some cases, the results of sonography can be of greater diagnostic value than those of radiography, such as in the case of small intestinal intussusception. Abdominal sonography should be performed before abdominocentesis or radiography, because these procedures may be found to be unnecessary or too risky based on the results of the sonogram (4).

A 7.5-Mhz transducer generally provides optimal image quality of the intestinal tract of the foal. A built-in fluid bath or handheld stand-off pad may be necessary for adequate visualization of structures close to the abdominal wall (such as small quantities of peritoneal fluid or detailed images of adjacent small intestine), whereas a 5.0-Mhz transducer may be necessary to penetrate deeply within the abdomen (as in foals with many loops of fluid filled intestine, which provide a larger window for penetration of the ultrasound beam). The abdomen should be thoroughly clipped, as for surgery, to ensure that as much intestine as possible is evaluated. The sonogram should be performed with the foal standing, because fluid-filled or edematous intestine is located at the most dependent portion of the abdomen (5). A segment of the duodenum may also be seen in the region ventral to the right kidney coursing from the cranial–mid-dorsal abdomen near the liver dorsally towards the caudal pole of the right kidney; therefore, the region of the right kidney should also be clipped if evaluation of this area is desired (6).

Normal small intestine in the foal often appears as amorphous motile tissue, and little fluid is seen within the lumen of the small intestine (Fig 5.2) (4). Little or no peritoneal fluid should be seen. The sonographic appearance of various intestinal disorders is described in Chapter 35.

The large and small colons generally contain little gas as compared with the adult. The contents of the colon can appear fluid-like, or echogenicity may resemble that of soft tissue. Meconium may be visualized if there is minimal gas in the surrounding intestine. The stomach may also be identified and may be filled with material of variable echogenicity or gas.

Urinary Tract

Sonography of the bladder is of value in the diagnostic workup of foals with uroperitoneum or dysuria and in monitoring bladder distention of recumbent foals to assist in determining the need for catheterization. The bladder is best imaged with a 7.5- to 5.0-Mhz transducer. The neonatal bladder is easily visualized from the caudoventral abdomen. The bladder appears as a round or oval structure containing anechoic fluid. In foals that have undergone repeated catheterizations, or in those with an indwelling urinary catheter, large amounts of mucous and sediment may be seen within the bladder.

The urachus can be identified coursing from the umbilical stump to the apex of the bladder. The urachal lumen should not be visible. The lumen is infrequently discernible in foals with patent urachus without concurrent infection, and any fluid within the lumen of the urachus most often represents purulent material. The urachus should be examined carefully for any evidence of disruption in foals with uroperitoneum or subcutaneous edema, which may be due to subcutaneous urine dissection.

Sonography of the kidneys in the neonate is of value in differentiating whether renal azotemia is due to a congenital anomaly, a rare situation, or to acute renal disease. In older animals, in which renal disease may be in a chronic stage, ultrasonography is also valuable. The kidneys can be

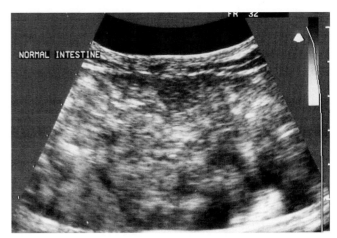

Figure 5.2. Ventral abdominal view of a 1-week-old Thoroughbred foal shows normal small intestine. The intestine has an amorphous appearance, and no peritoneal fluid is grossly visible. This image was obtained with a 7.5-Mhz transducer with a built-in fluid off-set.

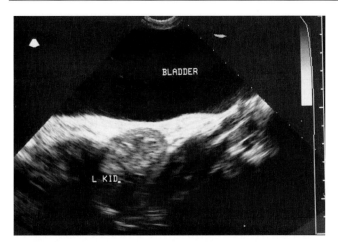

Figure 5.3. Sonogram of the normal left kidney of a neonatal foal visualized through the bladder from the ventral abdomen.

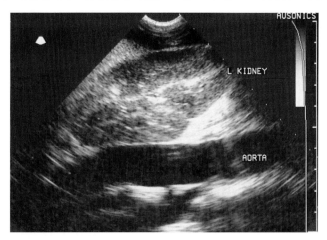

Figure 5.4. Sonogram of the normal left kidney of a neonatal foal visualized from the left flank region.

imaged from the appropriate flank area using a 7.5-Mhz (right kidney) or 5.0-Mhz (either kidney) transducer (1). The right kidney is imaged between the fourteenth and sixteenth intercostal spaces, whereas the left kidney is imaged between the seventeenth intercostal space and the paralumbar fossa medial to the spleen (1, 7). Either kidney may occasionally be seen from the caudoventral abdomen in small neonates, using the bladder as an acoustic window (Fig 5.3). The sonogram should be performed while angling and rotating the transducer so as many planes as possible are viewed. Kidney size varies with the age of the foal. As in the adult horse, the capsule is smooth and echogenic, the medulla is hypoechoic to anechoic, the cortex is slightly less echogenic than the liver, and the renal pelvis is echogenic with anechoic pelvic recesses (8). The difference in echogenicity between the cortex and medulla in the equine kidney is often not as pronounced as it is in small animal species (Fig 5.4). The ureters are generally not visible with ultrasound.

Umbilical Remnants

Sonographic evaluation of the internal umbilical remnants should be performed in foals with suspected umbilical infection. The umbilical vein, the umbilical arteries, and the sheath containing the umbilical arteries and urachus are easily visualized with diagnostic ultrasound in young foals. A 7.5-Mhz transducer generally provides optimal image quality, and a stand-off pad or built-in fluid bath may be necessary for adequate visualization of these structures. A wide strip of hair should be clipped along the midline, from the umbilical stump cranially to the liver and caudally to the bladder. The structures are imaged in a cross-sectional manner. Longitudinal views should also be performed in cases of urachal abscessation or gross enlargement of any of the structures. The transducer is placed immediately in front of the umbilical stump and is passed cranially toward the liver while the transducer is kept parallel to the body wall. The transducer is then passed from immediately caudal to the stump back toward the bladder in a similar fash-

ion, to evaluate the urachal sheath and the umbilical arteries. The umbilical vein is normally thin walled and measures 6±2 mm in diameter along its length from the stump to the liver (1). The contents of the lumen are often anechoic, although they may also be echogenic (Fig. 5.5). The

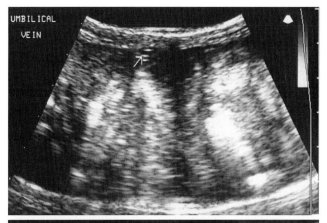

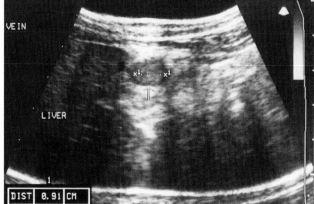

Figure 5.5. A, Cross-sectional view of a normal umbilical vein of a 4-day-old Thoroughbred foal (*arrow*). The thin echogenic parallel lines represent the walls of the vein. The anechoic lumen is seen. **B,** Cross-sectional view of the normal umbilical vein (between cursors) of a 4-day-old Thoroughbred foal at the level of the liver. The homogenous echogenicity of the contents of the lumen of the vein represent a clot.

urachal sheath, containing the two arteries, normally measures 17.5±4 mm in diameter at the apex of the bladder (1). A fluid-filled urachal lumen most often represents purulent material. The umbilical arteries may be visualized within the urachal sheath, depending on how far they retracted after birth, and they can be followed alongside the bladder (Fig 5.6). The umbilical arteries measure approximately 8.5±2 mm and have a thick wall (1). The lumen of the arteries may contain a clot ranging in echogenicity from anechoic to echogenic. The left and right umbilical arteries are often similar in sonographic appearance; however, noticeable differences in wall thickness, lumen diameter, and echogenicity of lumen contents can be seen in some normal foals. Both trauma and infection can result in minimal changes in the structures, such as thickening of the wall of the structure or overall enlargement, or in more obvious changes, such as large seromas or gross abscessation (see Chapter 35).

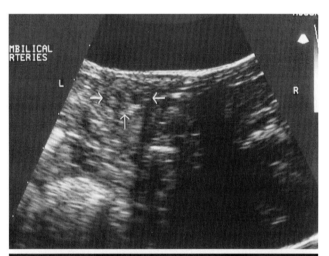

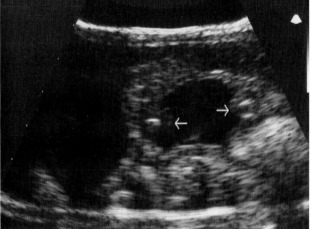

Figure 5.6. A, Cross-sectional view of a normal urachal sheath containing two normal umbilical arteries. The *arrows* delineate the walls of the urachal sheath. The left artery has a thicker wall with a small echogenic clot, whereas the right artery has a thinner wall and anechoic clot in its lumen. **B,** Cross-sectional view of normal umbilical arteries (*arrows*) at the level of the bladder. Again, notice the slight differences in the sonographic appearance of each artery.

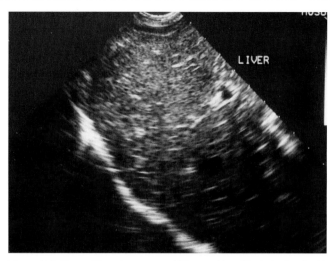

Figure 5.7. Normal liver in a neonatal Thoroughbred foal obtained with a 7.5-Mhz transducer.

Liver

Sonographic evaluation of the liver is performed in foals with hepatic disease (including ascending cholangitis secondary to gastrointestinal disorders), suspected liver laceration, and umbilical vein abscesses that extend into the liver. Portosystemic shunts may be diagnosed with ultrasound; however, the equine fetus does not have a ductus venosus, and any portosystemic shunt is likely to be extrahepatic and extremely difficult to visualize sonographically.

Combined use of both 7.5- and 5.0-Mhz transducers provides optimal image quality and adequate depth penetration. The procedure for imaging the neonatal liver is similar to that for the adult horse. The liver is identified just ventral to the lung margin, along the right side from the sixth to the fifteenth intercostal spaces (where it can be imaged alongside the right kidney) and on the left side from the seventh to the ninth intercostal spaces (at which point it is imaged alongside the spleen) (1, 6). The liver can be visualized from the cranioventral abdomen, just caudal to the xiphoid, in young foals less than 1 month of age. The neonatal liver often appears less echogenic with more parenchymal detail than the adult, because of enhanced image quality provided by the thinner and less fatty body wall of the neonate (Fig 5.7). As in the adult horse, the liver edges should appear sharp.

Spleen

Splenic disorders are uncommon in the foal, as in the adult. Sonographic evaluation of the spleen, however, is useful in a foal, or any animal, with abdominal trauma and suspected splenic fracture. A 7.5- or 5.0-Mhz transducer provides optimal image quality of the spleen, depending on the size of the foal and the size of the spleen. The spleen is identified on the left side of the abdomen and is echogenic. It can be imaged from the left paralumbar fossa (where it may be identified adjacent to the kidney) cranially and ventrally to the lung margin and liver border (6).

MUSCULOSKELETAL SYSTEM

Sonographic evaluation of distended joints, bursae, or tendon sheaths enables characterization of synovial fluid and permits an assessment of any synovial thickening. The presence of fibrin or of gas echoes (indicative of anaerobic infection) can be determined on the sonographic evaluation (Fig. 5.8). Sonography is also useful in determining whether joint swelling is solely periarticular or whether joint distention is also present.

Sonographic evaluation of the physes of foals with septic physitis enables delineation of any areas of gross fluid accumulation or abscessation. Fractures may be identified as a disruption in the bright linear echo of the bone surface. In particular, rib fractures lend themselves well to sonographic evaluation (Fig. 5.9). Edema, hemorrhage, or seroma may be identified at the fracture site. Fluid surrounding bone may also indicate osteomyelitis. The clinician should always compare the affected limb with the normal limb in foals with suspected sonographic abnormalities. Many bone surfaces and protuberances normally have a roughened contour.

Tendon and ligament injuries are as amenable to evaluation with diagnostic ultrasound in the foal as they are in the adult. If available, a 10-Mhz transducer can provide optimal image quality of the tendon and ligaments of the foal. The principles of sonography of these structures are no different from those in the adult.

Swellings, including umbilical swellings, can be evaluated with ultrasonography to determine whether the swelling

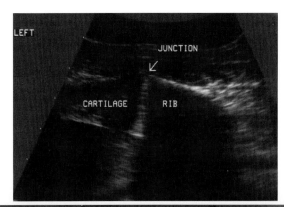

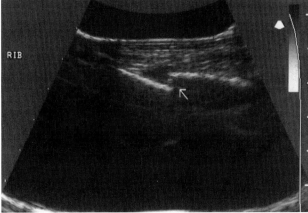

Figure 5.9. A, Sonogram of a normal rib at the level of the costochondral junction, longitudinal view. The cartilage is sonolucent, whereas the rib is echogenic, with acoustic shadowing below. The costrochondral junction is indicated. The vast majority of rib fractures occur just above the junction. Dorsal is to the right, ventral is to the left. **B**, Sonogram of the sixth rib of a 3-day-old Thoroughbred foal with numerous rib fractures. Notice the disruption of the suface of the rib at the fracture site (*arrow*). Dorsal is to the right and ventral is to the left. The costochondral junction is not shown (the transducer is not in contact with the skin suface at that level, as can be seen at the left of the image).

is due to an increase in soft tissue (fibrosis, neoplasia), fluid (serum, hemorrhage, or pus), edema, or herniation.

In general, a 7.5-Mhz transducer with a fluid offset is otherwise adequate for tendon and ligament evaluation, and it provides optimal image quality of joints, physes, ribs, and superficial bony surfaces. A 7.5-Mhz transducer without an offset can be used for deeper bony structures, for the hip joint, and for superficial structures in older foals.

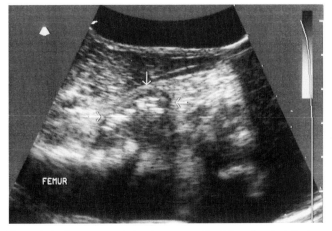

Figure 5.8. Sonogram of the femoropatellar joint of a foal (before arthrocentesis) with subsequently confirmed anaerobic (*Bacteroides fragilis*) septic arthritis. The joint capsule is delineated by *arrows*. The synovial membrane is thickened, and numerous echogenic bubbles (gas echoes) are within the joint. Proximal is to the left, distal is to the right. This sonogram was obtained with a 7.5-Mhz transducer with a built-in fluid off-set.

REFERENCES

1. Reef VB. Equine pediatric ultrasonography. Compend Contin Educ Pract Vet 1991;13:1277–1285.

2. Reimer JM. Noncardiac thoracic ultrasonography. In: Proceedings of the Second International Symposium of Veterinary Echography, Nice, France, 1993:136–137

3. Reef V B. Echocardiographic findings in horses with congenital cardiac disease. Compend Contin Educ Pract Vet 1991;13:109–117.

4. Reimer JM. Ultrasonography of the gastrointestinal tract of the foal. In: Proceedings of the Second International Symposium of Veterinary Echography, Nice, France, 1993:91–92.

5. Reef VB. Diagnostic ultrasonography of the foal's abdomen. In: McKinnon AO, Voss IL, eds. Equine reproduction. Philadelphia, Lea & Febiger,1993:1088–1094.

6. Rantanen NW. Diseases of the abdomen. Vet Clin North Am Equine Pract 1986;2:67–88.

7. Rantanen NW. Diseases of the kidneys. Vet Clin North Am Equine Pract 1986;2:89–103.

8. Pennick DG, Eisenberg HM, Teucsher EE, et al. Equine renal ultrasonography: normal and abnormal. Vet Radiol 1986;27:81–84.

6　Reproductive Ultrasonography

ANGUS O. McKINNON

THE MARE

Introduction

Few people predicted the impact that ultrasonography would have on equine reproductive management and understanding of reproductive physiology. The ability to examine a mare's reproductive tract noninvasively with ultrasonography provided the opportunity to diagnose pregnancy earlier than by rectal palpation, effectively manage twins, and detect impending early embryonic death (EED). However, ultrasonography has not been limited to these areas. As people became more familiar with the technique and clients accepted more widespread applications, the uses rapidly expanded. We now routinely use ultrasonography to diagnose uterine pathology such as intrauterine fluid, air, debris, cysts, and occasionally abscesses and neoplasia. In addition, ultrasonographic examination of the ovaries aids in determining stage of estrus cycle, status of preovulatory follicles, development and morphologic assessment of the corpus luteum (CL), and in interpreting ovarian irregularities such as anovulatory or hemorrhagic follicles, neoplasia, and peri-ovarian cysts. Recent applications to reproductive work are fetal sexing (Chapter 12) and transabdominal fetal monitoring or treatment (Chapter 13).

The costs of equipment can still result in rather limited applications to reproductive ultrasonography due to fees charged. Clients enthusiastically support ultrasonography to detect pregnancy. However, the same fee schedules for routine examination before and/or after breeding are not as easily accepted. An approach that allows multiple scanning while still keeping clients and farm managers happy is something all of us strive to achieve each year. A more logical and thus practical approach to diagnosis and treatment of physiologic and anatomic abnormalities of the mare's reproductive tract would be forthcoming if we could use the equipment more routinely. In addition, valuable information would be available from correlation of fertility data with normal and abnormal ultrasonographic observations. Regardless, informed clientele prefer routine ultrasonography and its use results in a more interactive approach to farm management with an increased awareness of the events associated with breeding, ovulation, and early fetal development. If there is a drawback with its use, then most commonly it is manifest as some clients wishing to purchase their own equipment and pursue their own diagnoses.

Equipment

The two major types of real-time ultrasonographic transducers used for reproductive examination of the mare are linear and sectorial. The physical arrangement of the crystals within the transducer determines the pattern by which sound waves are propagated from the transducer. With linear-array scanners, the width of the rectangular ultrasonic beam corresponds to the length of the active, crystallized portion of the transducer (Figs. 6.1 and 6.2). A linear-array transducer is oriented in the longitudinal plane with respect to the mare's body. Therefore, images of the cervix and uterine body are longitudinally oriented and those of the uterine horn are cross-sectional. Images of tissues closest to the transducer are at the top of the screen. Sector scanners produce a beam that is triangular in shape because sound waves radiate from a single point or source (Fig. 6.3). The sound beam generally travels transversely to the mare's body; consequently, images of the cervix and uterine body are cross-sectional, whereas images of the horns are longitudinal or oblique.

Resolution, which is the ability to detect small differences in tissue density, depends on the frequency of sound waves. High frequency provides greater detail, and lower frequency provides greater tissue penetration. Ultrasonographic frequencies are measured in megahertz (MHz; I hertz [Hz] = 1 sound wave/sec). The lower-frequency transducers (3 and 3.5 MHz) are suited for viewing larger structures at a greater distance from the transducer (Fig. 6.4) than the 5- or 7.5-MHz transducers. Higher-frequency transducers (5 to 7.5 MHz) are most useful for detailed study of structures close to the transducer. Most photographs of ultrasonographic images in this chapter and Chapters 10, 14, and 18, were recorded using a 5-MHz transducer from either the Aloka 210 DX or the Aloka 500. Image size will vary with equipment. A 5-MHz transducer can be used to detect a conceptus on day 10, follicles as small as 3 mm, and the presence of a CL throughout most of diestrus. In comparison, a 3- or 3.5-MHz transducer can be used to detect a conceptus at about day 13 to 15, follicles approximately 6 to 8 mm in diameter, and the presence of a CL for 5 to 6 days postovulation. The principal uses of lower-frequency transducers are to study an older fetus by either intrarectal or abdominal scanning, and pathologic conditions elsewhere in the body.

Most modern ultrasonographic equipment enables the operator to freeze and/or record images and automatically measure structures with a calliper-adjustment control. Some machines have split-frame capability with memory and various scanning frequencies. The equipment used in our practice is predominantly Aloka. We record images on Super VHS tapes and can review examinations later if necessary. Slides (35 mm) can be reproduced by playing the tape through a monitor using a good, still-frame holder (jog shuttle) and slowly advancing until the correct image is lo-

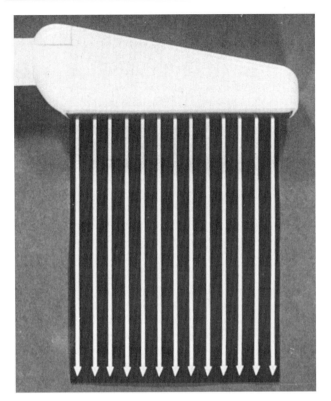

Figure 6.1. A linear-array transducer. Width of the rectangular sound beam corresponds to length of the active or crystallized portion of the transducer. (From McKinnon AO, Voss JL, eds. Equine reproduction. Philadelphia: Lea & Febiger, 1993, p. 212.)

cated. Images can be printed directly onto thermal printers or can be transferred by a frame grabber to a PC. Postrecording image processing can be performed by a variety of PC programs such as Corel Capture with Corel Photopaint or Image Pals Screen Capture with either Image Pals or Adobe Photoshop.

Procedures

The procedure and precautions for intrarectal ultrasonographic examinations are similar to those for rectal palpation, and no additional restraint is required. The transducer should be well lubricated and protected by the examiner's hand to prevent trauma to the rectal wall. Care should be taken to prevent fecal material from attaching to the transducer. After evacuating fecal material from the rectum, the probe is introduced and moved across the reproductive tract in the following pattern: uterine body, right uterine horn, right ovary, right uterine horn, uterine body, left uterine horn, left ovary, left uterine horn, uterine body, and cervix. Good contact must exist between the transducer and rectal wall. Air in the rectum or a gas or fluid-filled loop of bowel will result in a distorted image. To minimize scanning errors, principally those of omission, conduct the same scanning procedure during each examination. A brief, manual examination should precede all ultrasonographic procedures to facilitate proper orientation of the reproductive tract, to

enable repositioning of intestinal contents that are occasionally interposed between the rectum and uterus, and to assess tone and size of various components of the reproductive tract. With practice, ultrasonographic examination is expedient; however, caution is advised when examining mares in suboptimal conditions such as mares straining or in conditions of too much external light interference or inadequate restraint, for example, so that all parts of the reproductive tract are adequately visualized.

Environment

The surrounding environment influences the operators ability to utilize equipment properly and make correct interpretations. It is not acceptable to misdiagnose conditions such as twins due to inadequate examination conditions. There are good arguments for centralized examination areas that offer safety for the operator and good lighting conditions for interpretation of the ultrasonograms. It is also possible that in many situations the establishment of centralized facilities, particularly those that can handle multiple mares (Fig. 6.5) at one time, may attract decreased costs due to increased efficiency. The ideal scanning environment would be darkened to abolish reflections and glare and would keep mares restrained in a quiet and nontraumatic, nonthreatening en-

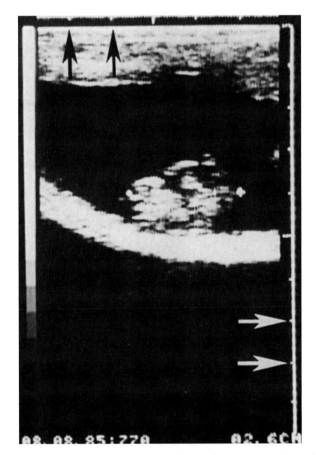

Figure 6.2. Ultrasonographic image from a linear-array scanner. Arrows delineate 10-mm markers. (From McKinnon AO, Voss JL, eds. Equine reproduction. Philadelphia: Lea & Febiger, 1993, p. 212.)

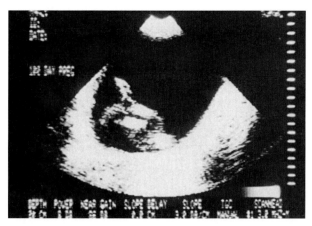

Figure 6.3. Ultrasonographic image from a sector scanner. Sector scanners produce a sound beam that is triangular in shape because the sound waves radiate from a single point or source in the transducer. (From McKinnon AO, Voss JL, eds. Equine reproduction. Philadelphia: Lea & Febiger, 1993, p. 213.)

vironment. To this end we have noticed that mares placed next to others (Fig. 6.5) tend to be calm for extended periods, particularly so if they are friends. If, however, they are left alone, these same mares frequently try to jump out of the crushes.

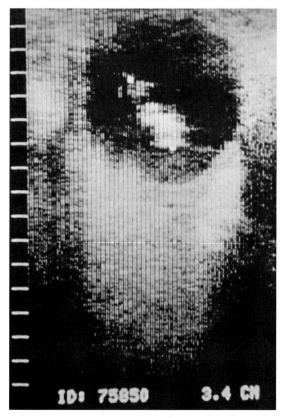

Figure 6.4. Ultrasonographic image from a 3-MHZ transducer. Lower-frequency transducers (3 MHZ) have less tissue resolution but greater tissue penetration. (From McKinnon AO, Voss JL, eds. Equine reproduction. Philadelphia: Lea & Febiger, 1993, p. 213.)

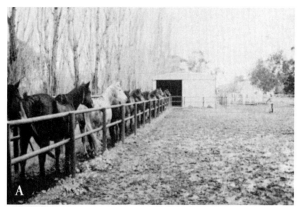

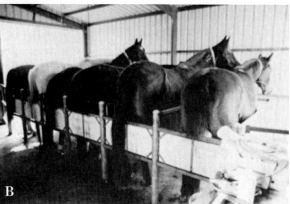

Figure 6.5. A. Mares can be individually teased while in the chute system. **B.** Side-loading stocks or crushes are designed to hold six mares, open either way, and are able to be loaded by one person without catching the mare. (From McKinnon AO, Voss JL, eds. Equine Reproduction, Philadelphia: Lea & Febiger, 1993, pp. 371–372.)

Uterus

A thorough knowledge of ultrasonographic anatomy and understanding of dynamic changes in the uterus are essential for ultrasonographic evaluation of the mare's reproductive tract. The dynamic changes visualized with ultrasonography mirror the ovarian hormonal influences and aid in estimating reproductive potential.

The relationship between orientation of a linear-array transducer and orientation of the mare's reproductive tract is shown in Figures 6.6 through 6.9. Because the probe is generally held in a sagittal plane, images of the cervix and uterine body are longitudinally orientated with the cervix to the left (or right) of the ultrasonographic picture. The orientation of craniad on the right and caudad on the left of the image remains constant throughout this chapter and Chapters 10, 14, and 18. Uterine horns are seen in cross-section as the transducer is moved left or right. Depending on orientation of the horn at a given examination, manipulation of the uterus may be necessary to obtain a true cross-section.

Ultrasonographic characteristics of the uterus during the anovulatory season, estrous cycle, and pregnancy may often be differentiated. During anestrus, the cross-section of the uterine horns (Fig. 6.10) and the longitudinal section of the

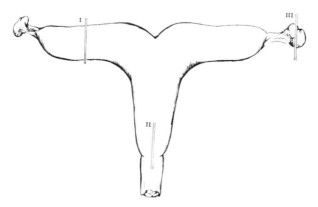

Figure 6.6. Diagrammatic view of the mare's reproductive tract. I, cross section of uterine horn; II, longitudinal section of uterine body and cervix; III, cross section of ovary. (From McKinnon AO, Voss JL, eds. Equine reproduction. Philadelphia: Lea & Febiger, 1993, p. 213.)

uterine body (Fig. 6.11) are often flat and irregular and may contour closely to surrounding abdominal organs. In estrus, uterine horns are well rounded and both horns and body commonly have an interdigitated pattern of alternating echogenic and nonechogenic areas (Figs. 6.12 and 6.13). The areas of decreased echogenicity are the edematous por-

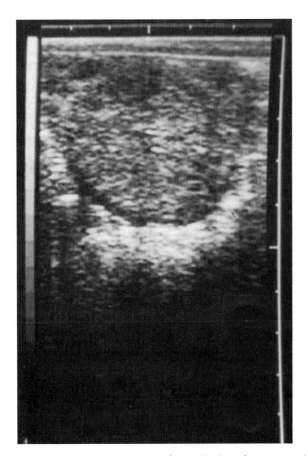

Figure 6.7. Ultrasonographic image of a uterine horn from a mare in diestrous (cross-sectional image from Figure 6.5 located at I). (From McKinnon AO, Voss JL, eds. Equine reproduction. Philadelphia: Lea & Febiger, 1993, p. 216.)

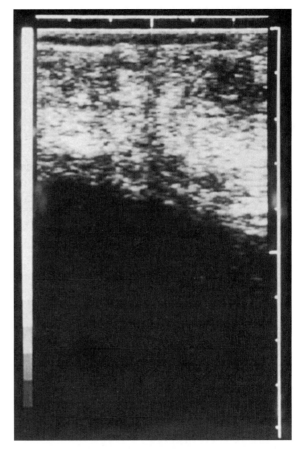

Figure 6.8. Ultrasonographic image of mare's uterine body and cervix (longitudinal section located in Figure 6.5 at II). (From McKinnon AO, Voss JL, eds. Equine reproduction. Philadelphia: Lea & Febiger, 1993, p. 216.)

tion of endometrial folds. The edema is caused by the effects of estrogen. This ultrasonographic pattern resembles the appearance of a sliced orange. Endometrial folds generally parallel estrogen production and are visible at the end of diestrus, become more prominent as estrus progresses, and decrease or disappear within 24 hours before the time of ovulation.

In one report (1) ultrasonographic properties of the uteri of 16 mares were determined each day of the cycle. Endometrial folds were not distinguishable during diestrus and were most prominent during estrus. The number of mares with intermediate folds or images characteristic of estrus increased gradually from day −7 (2 of 14) (day of ovulation equals day 0), to day −3 (11 of 16), to day −2 (10 of 16), and then declined between days −1 and +1 (0 of 12). From a preliminary study, involving 100 mare cycles, endometrial folds were graded from 0 (no folds) to 3 (prominent endometrial folds) and were most prominent 1 or 2 days before ovulation (Table 6.1) . A change to a lower grade could be used to predict ovulation. For example, a change from grade 3 to 0 was concomitant with ovulation. These changes are particularly important when breeding mares with frozen semen. Mares need to be examined regularly to determine

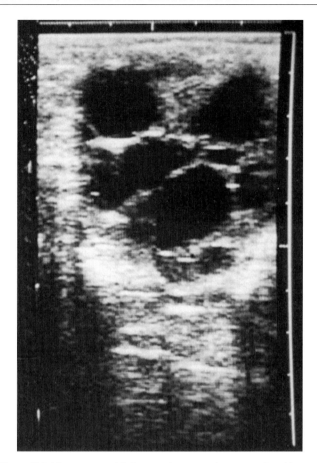

Figure 6.9. Ultrasonographic image of an ovary (cross-sectional image from Figure 6.5 at III). (From McKinnon AO, Voss JL, eds. Equine reproduction. Philadelphia: Lea & Febiger, 1993, p. 216.)

when they will ovulate. Failure to breed mares within a period of 12 hours prior to 6 hours after ovulation will result in decreased pregnancy rates (2).

Practitioners should be aware of the extent of change in height of endometrial folds between diestrus and early estrus. Prominence of endometrial folds during estrus (Figs. 6.12 and 6.13) should not necessarily be considered pathologic. Before the observation became common knowledge, some veterinary practitioners mistook prominent endometrial folds for endometritis and unnecessarily treated mares. Exceptionally prominent endometrial folds are associated with inflammation of the reproductive tract and may hide fluid within the lumen that subsequently becomes more obvious when the folding subsides. Ability to clearly observe endometrial folds depends on transducer frequency and resolution of ultrasonographic equipment. On occasion, impending early embryonic death is suspected when, during routine scanning for pregnancy, the embryonic vesicle is located in a uterus with prominent endometrial folds.

When a mare is in diestrus, individual endometrial folds are less distinct, or not discernible, and the echo texture is more homogeneous (see Fig. 6.7). When scanning the uterine body, the uterine lumen is often identified by a hyperechogenic white line. This is the result of apposition of en-

dometrial surfaces, and probably is caused by specular reflection. In general, during diestrus the entire uterine portion of the reproductive tract is well circumscribed and defined.

Ultrasonographic images of the pregnant uterus are often identical to those of diestrus with the exception that after day 16 slight endometrial folds may again be visualized. However, endometrial folds (Fig. 6.14) are not as prominent as during estrus and may be associated with increasing uterine tone. Another postulation is that they are associated with fetal estrogen production (4).

Ovaries

Ultrasonography is useful for monitoring dynamic follicular and luteal changes in equine ovaries, since it permits rapid, visual, noninvasive access to the reproductive tract. A 5-MHz transducer has greater resolution and is more suitable for evaluation of ovaries than a 3- or 3.5-MHz transducer. Follicles as small as 2 to 3 mm can be seen, and the CL can usually be identified throughout its functional life (5). Potential applications of ultrasonographic examination of the ovaries include (a) estimating stage of the estrous cycle, (b) assessing preovulatory follicles, (c) determining ovulation, (d) examining the CL, and (e) diagnosing ovarian abnor-

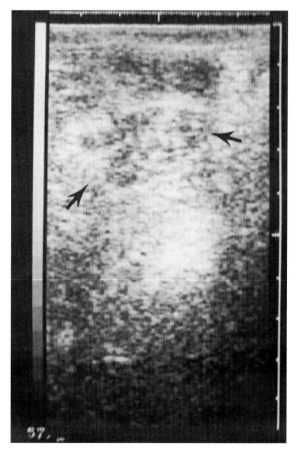

Figure 6.10. Ultrasonographic image of a uterine horn (*arrows*) from a mare in anestrus. Notice flat and irregular outline and close contour to surrounding organs. (From McKinnon AO, Voss JL, eds. Equine reproduction. Philadelphia: Lea & Febiger, 1993, p. 216.)

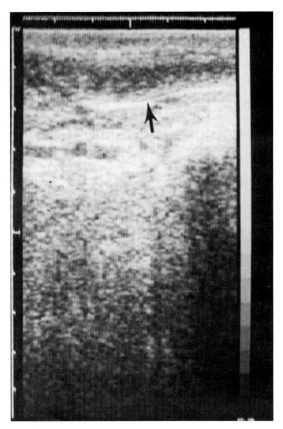

Figure 6.11. Ultrasonographic image of a uterine body (*arrow*) from a mare in anestrus. Structure is flat. (From McKinnon AO, Voss JL, eds. Equine reproduction. Philadelphia: Lea & Febiger, 1993, p. 217.)

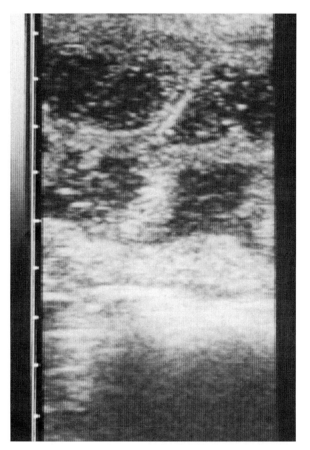

Figure 6.13. Ultrasonographic image of the uterine body from a mare in estrus. Body of uterus is rounded and has an interdigitated pattern of alternating echogenic and nonechogenic areas. (From McKinnon AO, Voss JL, eds. Equine reproduction. Philadelphia: Lea & Febiger, 1993, p. 217.)

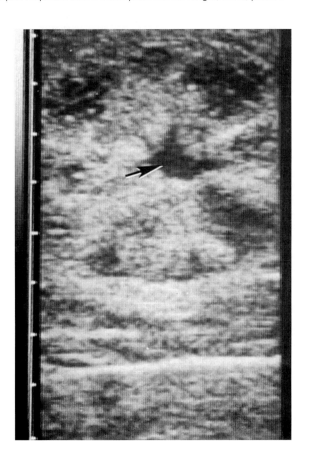

Table 6.1.
Number of Mares Displaying Endometrial Folds in Relation to Days of Ovulation

Grade of Endometrial Folds	Time From Ovulation (Days)				
	−3	2	−1	0	+2
0	73	27	33	64	95
1	3	17	24	24	4
2	18	35	27	12	1
3	6	21	16	0	0

Adapted from McKinnon AO, Squires EL, Carnevale EM, Harrison LA, Frantz DD, McChesney AE, Shideler RK. Diagnostic ultrasonography of uterine pathology in the mare. Proc AAEP 1987;605–622.

Figure 6.12. Ultrasonographic image of a uterine horn from a mare in estrus. Presence of endometrial folds in this image is not an indication of endometritis. However, fluid (*arrow*) within the lumen may be a sign of uterine infection. (From McKinnon AO, Voss JL, eds. Equine reproduction. Philadelphia: Lea & Febiger, 1993, p. 217.)

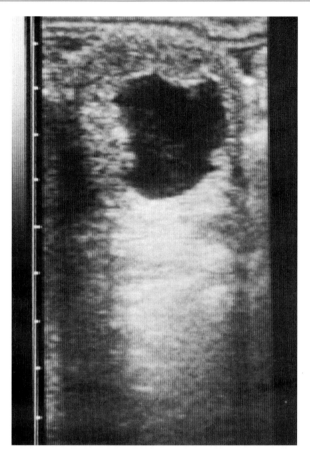

Figure 6.14. Ultrasonographic image of a 20-day pregnancy with slight endometrial folding. (From McKinnon AO, Voss JL, eds. Equine reproduction. Philadelphia: Lea & Febiger, 1993, p. 217.)

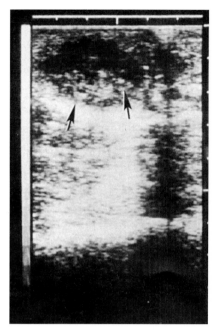

Figure 6.15. Ultrasonographic characteristics of an anestrous ovary (ovary delineated by arrows). (From McKinnon AO, Voss JL, eds. Equine reproduction. Philadelphia: Lea & Febiger, 1993, p. 285.)

malities and pathology. In our practice, clients have begun to request more and more frequent evaluation of mares for "stage of the reproductive cycle." Most useful are our abilities to accurately determine the following: the stage of the cycle, when to next examine the mare, if the mare is cycling, when the mare should receive $PGF_{2\alpha}$, and what the response to $PGF_{2\alpha}$ would be. These abilities have been fundamental to the expansion of our practice. The information available from ovarian examination should enable us to accurately determine the hormonal status of the mare.

Stage of the Estrous Cycle

Follicles, like other fluid-filled structures, are nonechogenic and appear as black, roughly circumscribed ultrasonographic images (Figs. 6.15 through 6.19). Compression by adjacent follicles, luteal structures, or ovarian stroma occasionally can result in irregular-shaped follicles. The apposed walls of adjacent follicles are often straight. Diameter can be estimated by adjusting an irregular-shaped follicle to an approximately equivalent circular form. Sequential monitoring of dynamic changes in a follicular population during the estrous cycle has been made possible by ultrasonography. During anestrus, inactive ovaries are readily differentiated from functional ovaries with ultrasonography. Occasional

small follicles (2 to 5 mm) may be present, but absence of an ultrasonographically visible CL is characteristic of anestrus (Fig. 6.15). Multiple, large follicles characteristic of transitional mares (Fig. 6.16), prior to their first ovulation of the year, are particularly frustrating to practitioners and researchers. Generally, follicular atresia and subsequent growth occur until one follicle becomes dominant and ovu-

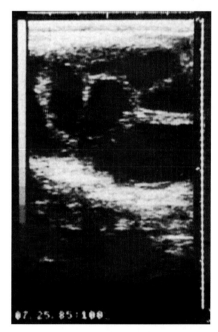

Figure 6.16. Ultrasonographic characteristics of multiple follicles in an ovary of a mare in transitional estrus. (From McKinnon AO, Voss JL, eds. Equine reproduction. Philadelphia: Lea & Febiger, 1993, p. 285.)

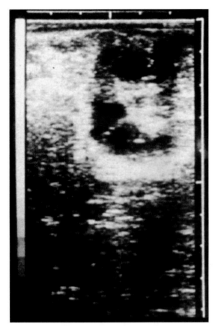

Figure 6.17. Ultrasonographic characteristics of small follicles in an ovary of a mare in early diestrus. (From McKinnon AO, Voss JL, eds. Equine reproduction. Philadelphia: Lea & Febiger, 1993, p. 285.)

lates. During transition, some ovulations are difficult to detect by palpation and in these cases ultrasonographic observation of a CL may confirm whether the mare has entered the ovulatory season. With the use of a 5-MHz transducer, the CL should be ultrasonographically visible for approximately 14 days after ovulating (5). Examination with ultrasonography has resulted in confirmation of the presence of many 5- to 10-mm follicles during early diestrus (Fig. 6.17); growth of large follicles at mid-cycle; observation of selective, accelerated growth of an ovulatory follicle beginning 6 days before ovulation; and regression of large, nonovulatory follicles a few days before ovulation (5, 6). Ultrasonographic examination of the ovaries should not replace sound management techniques such as regular teasing and rectal palpation to determine stage of estrous cycle; rather, it should be used as a powerful ancillary aid.

Preovulatory Follicles

The ability to accurately detect time of ovulation has significant practical applications. Selective growth of a single preovulatory follicle is initiated about 6 days before ovulation (6) (Figs. 6.19 and 6.20). Various characteristics can be used, within certain limitations, to predict time of ovulation. Softening of the follicle commonly occurs within 24 hours of ovulation in approximately 70% of mares. Ultrasonographically, this is frequently associated with a change in follicular shape from spherical to pear or irregular shapes (6), which may be due to disruption of ovarian stroma as the follicle progresses toward the fossa in preparation for ovulation. The mare's ovary is structurally inverted in comparison to most species with the exception of the ovulation fossa,

which is a 0.5- to 1-cm depression on the lesser curvature. The tunica albuginea and mesovarium forms a thick serosal coating covering the ovarian surface. Connective tissue tracts extend from the ovulation fossa to the periphery, which forces the follicle to grow centrally toward the fossa. These structural arrangements restrict ovulation to the ovulation fossa. Cinematographic and histologic studies have been used to determine the exact location of follicular rupture. However, time sequence and follicular changes during ovulation are not well characterized. Although stallion semen has been reported to survive for up to 5 days or longer in the mare's reproductive tract (7), it is more commonly accepted that a lapse before ovulation of greater than 48 hours between breeding and ovulation will result in decreased numbers of viable spermatozoa and reduced fertility (7). Use of frozen, cooled, or poor-quality semen may markedly hinder the life span of spermatozoa after insemination. Although no critical studies have been performed, the mare's oocyte probably begins to lose viability within 12 to 24 hours after ovulation (7, 8). In addition, semen deposited in the uterus after ovulation requires time to reach the oviduct (site of fertilization) and for capacitation. Breeding or insemination, particularly with semen of reduced longevity, just prior to ovulation would maximize pregnancy rates and prevent overuse of an individual stallion. Accurate predic-

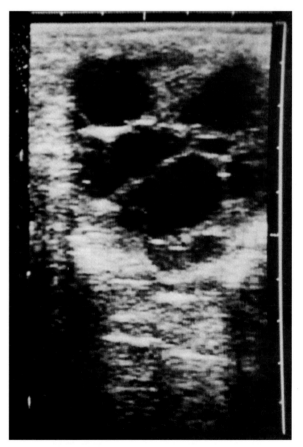

Figure 6.18. Ultrasonographic characteristics of follicles in an ovary of a mare during late diestrus. (From McKinnon AO, Voss JL, eds. Equine reproduction. Philadelphia: Lea & Febiger, 1993, p. 286.)

tion of impending ovulation would allow for collection of mature equine oocytes for in vitro fertilization or for gamete transfer from infertile mares (9, 10). In addition, recently ovulated oocytes or early cleavage embryos could be recovered from the oviduct at specific times postovulation. In one study (6), various criteria such as percentage change in shape, size of follicle, echogenicity of follicular fluid and wall, and thickness of follicular wall were evaluated in their ability to predict time of ovulation. Size of the preovulatory follicle was as accurate as any method in determining ovulation time. Generally, double, preovulatory follicles ovulated after attaining a smaller maximum diameter than single, preovulatory follicles. Thickening of the follicle wall occurs in most preovulatory follicles prior to ovulation (Fig. 6.21). However, it generally occurs too early to be an adjunct to predicting ovulation. Increased echogenicity of follicular fluid is sometimes seen prior to ovulation, perhaps due to degeneration and subsequent shedding of granulosa cells from the follicular wall (Fig. 6.22). This can be an indicator of impending ovulation, although it is neither common nor consistent enough to be particularly diagnostic. In general, the combination of softening of a large follicle, particularly when associated with pain as determined by rectal palpation, and a substantial change in shape of the follicle, as de-

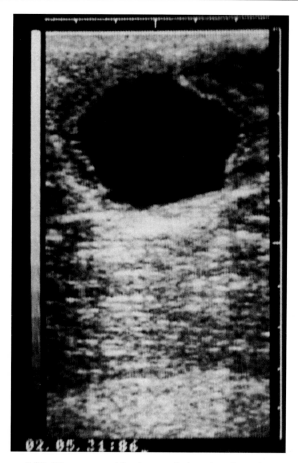

Figure 6.20. Ultrasonographic characteristics of an irregular-shaped preovulatory follicle. (From McKinnon AO, Voss JL, eds. Equine reproduction. Philadelphia: Lea & Febiger, 1993, p. 287.)

tected with ultrasonography, can be used to predict ovulation within a 24-hour period for most mares.

Characteristics of Ovulation

A study was performed to determine ultrasonographic characteristics of ovulation (11). Fifteen light-horse mares were assigned to the experiment upon acquiring the following preovulatory, follicular parameters: (a) diameter of >40 mm, (b) marked softening on palpation per rectum, (c) pain on palpation, and (d) a change in shape from round to irregular. Preovulatory follicles were observed at <1-hour intervals for 12 hours or continually when there were signs of impending ovulation. Ovulation was defined as a rapid decrease in follicular size characterized by disappearance of the large, fluid-filled, nonechogenic structure. A real-time, B-mode, linear-array scanner with a 5-MHz transducer was used for ultrasonographic examinations. Within the 12-hour examination period (mean = 85 minutes; range 15 minutes to 3 hours 37 minutes after beginning of observation) 13 of 15 mares ovulated. As ovulation approached, flattened or irregular images of the follicles were noted (Figs. 6.20 through 6.22), concomitant with reduced follicular tone. This was likely due to diminished tensile strength of

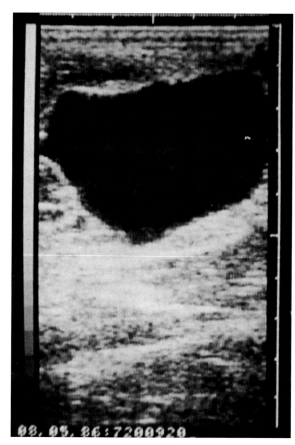

Figure 6.19. Ultrasonographic characteristics of a large preovulatory follicle. (From McKinnon AO, Voss JL, eds. Equine reproduction. Philadelphia: Lea & Febiger, 1993, p. 286.)

the follicular wall or perhaps a slow release of fluid from the follicle, although no fluid was visualized outside the follicle as ovulation approached. Prior to ovulation, 10 of 13 follicles developed a tear in the follicular wall, which was characterized by a jagged protrusion of the follicular border toward the ovulation fossa (Fig. 6.23). In seven mares, the tear or point was first observed an average of 41 minutes (range 15 to 77) prior to ovulation and was a consistent indicator of impending ovulation. A tear or pointed appearance, observed with ultrasonography just prior to ovulation, is likely due to breakdown of ovarian stroma and protrusion of the follicle toward the ovulation fossa. These observations probably parallel deterioration of the follicular wall, stigma formation, and protrusion of the basement membrane just prior to ovulation, as observed in other species. Ovulation (Fig. 6.24), defined as a rapid decrease in follicular size, occurred in an average of 42 seconds (range 5 to 90). Little or no follicular fluid remained in the follicle after ovulation. Two mares failed to ovulate within 12 hours after initiation of scanning and subsequently formed anovulatory hemorrhagic follicles (AHFs). This occurrence was possibly due to season (12). Abnormal ovulations such as AHFs and luteinized, unruptured follicles (13) may initially display a

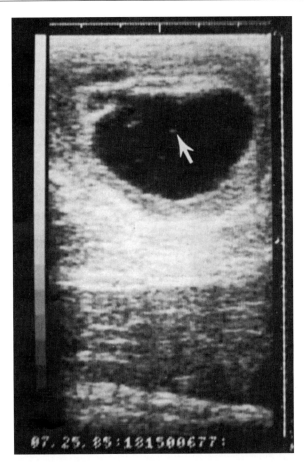

Figure 6.22. Echogenic (*arrow*) debris in follicular fluid. (From McKinnon AO, Voss JL, eds. Equine reproduction. Philadelphia: Lea & Febiger, 1993, p. 288.)

similar sequence of events as normal, preovulatory follicles without ovulation. Increased echogenicity of the follicular wall was visualized in all follicles prior to ovulation. Appearance of echogenic "spots" within the follicular fluid, probably due to dispersal of granulosa cells, was noted in 7 of 13 follicles (54%). However, echogenic "spots" within the follicular fluid, or a bright, echogenic follicular border, were not consistently useful in predicting time of ovulation. A bright echogenic border, an irregular shape, and a tear in the follicular wall were predictive of imminent ovulation.

Formation and Development of the Corpus Luteum

The CL is present during two-thirds of the mare's estrous cycle and for the first 4 to 6 months of pregnancy. Progesterone, a primary hormonal product from the CL, has a multitude of functions, including initiation and maintenance of pregnancy. Therefore, methods to evaluate the CL are extremely important. Because of the position of the CL within the ovary, palpation per rectum is of little value for identification and evaluation. However, ultrasonography has been shown to be an effective and accurate means of identifying this structure. Some of the reasons for ultrasonographic evaluation of corpora lutea are as follows:

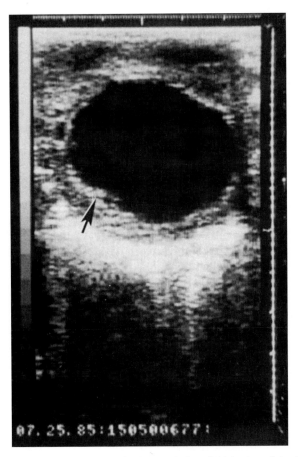

Figure 6.21. Ultrasonographic characteristics of thickening of the follicular wall (*arrow*) as sometimes seen before ovulation. (From McKinnon AO, Voss JL, eds. Equine reproduction. Philadelphia: Lea & Febiger, 1993, p. 288.)

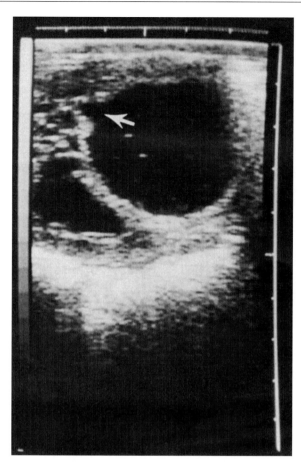

Figure 6.23. A follicle just before ovulation. Note the presence of a pronounced necklike process of the follicular wall (*arrow*), and increased echogenicity of follicular fluid. (From McKinnon AO, Voss JL, eds. Equine reproduction. Philadelphia: Lea & Febiger, 1993, p. 288.)

1. To detect ovulation
2. To evaluate CL formation
3. To determine size and characteristics of the CL
4. To determine if failure of a mare to display estrus is due to prolonged maintenance of a CL or absence of a CL and follicular activity
5. To distinguish between anovulatory hemorrhagic follicles, luteinized, unruptured follicles or CL
6. To determine if a mare has ovulated more than one follicle

After rupture of the follicle, a corpus hemorrhagicum is formed as a transient phenomenon in the development of the CL in the mare. However, it was demonstrated in an ultrasonographic study (5) that the equine luteal gland may involve two, ultrasonically distinct, luteal morphologies. Both types of luteal structures are uniformly echogenic on day 1. One type, classified as uniformly echogenic (Figs. 6.25 through 6.28), is seen in approximately 50% of the CLs, and the percent of echogenicity remains constant for the duration of diestrus. The other, classified as centrally nonechogenic or a corpus hemorrhagicum (Figs. 6.29 through 6.31), develops a nonechogenic center on day 0 or day 1. The percentage of CLs considered echogenic was lowest on day 3 and increased linearly throughout diestrus. In a

subsequent study (14), the time required for accumulation of fluid and formation of central clots (nonechogenic areas) was studied by ultrasonography. Examinations were conducted at 15-minute intervals for the first 2 hours after ovulation, again at 8 hours and thereafter at 12-hour intervals for 5 days. In two of ten mares, a nonechogenic area did not develop within the luteal gland, and in one mare only a small central area (0.5 cm^2) was detected at 20 and 32 hours, and not thereafter. In five mares, a nonechogenic central area developed within the luteal gland after expulsion of follicular fluid. The size of the nonechogenic area varied from 0.5 to 11.6 cm^2. For those mares with central nonechogenic areas, echogenic lines within the central area were detected. These were attributed to clotting and fibrinization of the contents. From the results of data collected at Colorado State University (12), it appeared that, when CL evaluations were made on days 5 to 7 postovulation, the number of centrally nonechogenic CLs was lower (9.2%, n = 192 cycles) than that reported previously (5). In addition, the incidence of at least one centrally nonechogenic CL increased with double ovulations (36%; n = 23 double ovulations). However, from the results of more recent data, a higher percentage of centrally nonechogenic CLs was observed (13). This is dependent, to some extent, on days postovulation. Comparative studies on duration of diestrus, concentrations of progesterone, and fertility data have been conducted to determine that both morphologic types of CLs are normal (15). Ginther reported on the accuracy of detecting a CL with ultrasonography. Location of the CL was established by daily palpation per rectum. Ultrasonographic examinations were done by another technician unaware of the site of ovulation. The ultrasonographer recorded the location of the CL, or indicated that one was not found or that there was uncertainty about identification. The ultrasonographer was correct in 88% of his examinations conducted on days 0 to 14 postovulation. In the remaining 12%, the ultrasonographer recorded the locations as uncertain. In addition, in all 12 mares that were in estrus, the location of the CL was recorded as uncertain. From these results it appeared that ultrasonography can be used to visualize a CL, even if the site of ovulation is unknown. Therefore, ultrasonography is an extremely valuable diagnostic tool for determining the presence or absence of the corpus luteum. The ultrasonographic image is affected by the amount of blood within the corpus luteum. Blood is nonechogenic, whereas luteal cells are echogenic. Generally, luteinization begins on the periphery of the structure and migrates medially. Normally, as the CL ages, blood is resorbed and a uniformly echogenic, luteal structure develops. Fibrinlike material can separate the blood clot into areas of dark, nonechogenic sections containing red blood cells, plasma, and/or perhaps follicular fluid. Lighter areas may be indicative of fibrin strands or developing luteal tissue. Although the ultrasonographic properties of the mature CL are similar to ovarian stroma, a CL can be distinguished by its defined borders. Ginther found that the ultrasonographic texture of the luteal gland

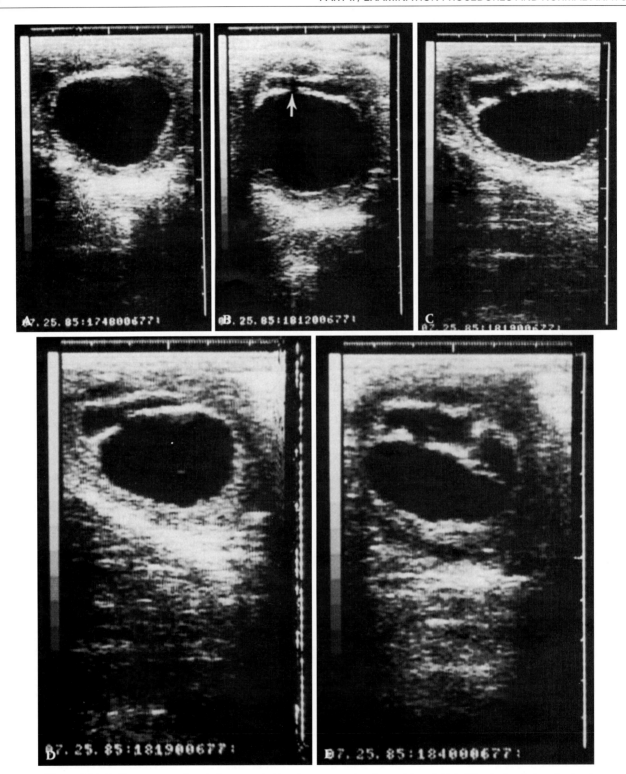

Figure 6.24. A. The process of ovulation recorded by ultrasonography. Preovulatory follicle 50 minutes before the beginning of ovulation. **B.** Preovulatory follicle 30 minutes before the beginning of ovulation. Note rent in dorsal follicular wall (*arrow*). **C.** Preovulatory follicle 20 minutes before the beginning of ovulation. Note decrease in follicular size. **D.** Preovulatory follicle 15 minutes before the beginning of ovulation. **E.** The beginning of ovulation. Ovulation has been defined as a rapid decrease in follicular size.

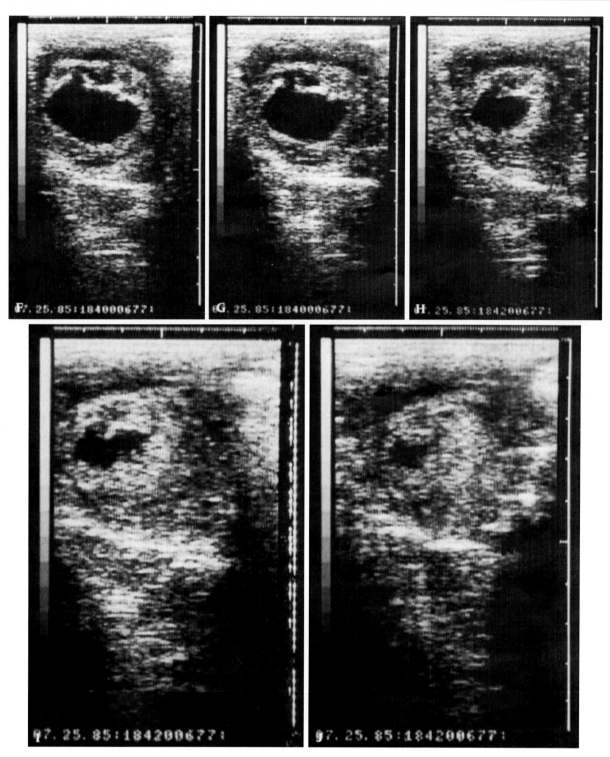

Figure 6.24. *(Continued)* **F–J.** The process of ovulation occurred over approximately 60 seconds. (From McKinnon AO, Voss JL, eds. Equine reproduction. Philadelphia: Lea & Febiger, 1993, pp. 289–290.)

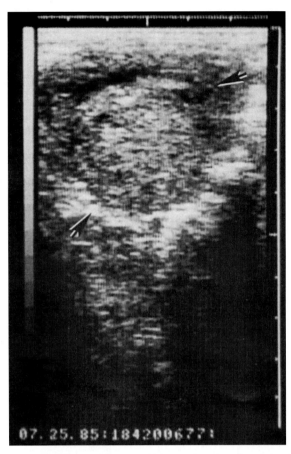

Figure 6.25. Uniformly echogenic CL (*arrows*) on day of ovulation (day 0). (From McKinnon AO, Voss JL, eds. Equine reproduction. Philadelphia: Lea & Febiger, 1993, p. 292.)

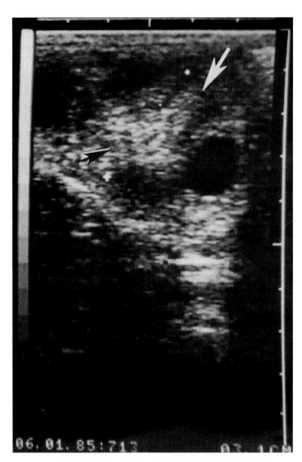

Figure 6.27. Uniformly echogenic CL on day 14 (*arrows*). (From McKinnon AO, Voss JL, eds. Equine reproduction. Philadelphia: Lea & Febiger, 1993, p. 292.)

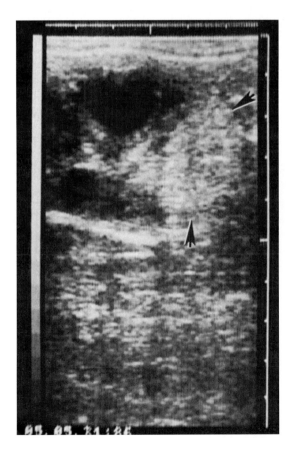

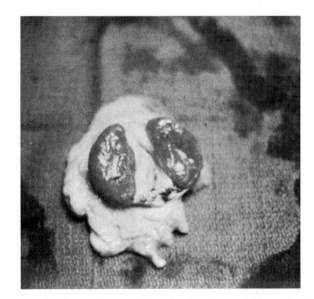

Figure 6.28. Gross characteristics of a CL that would be uniformly echogenic when visualized with ultrasonography. (From McKinnon AO, Voss JL, eds. Equine reproduction. Philadelphia: Lea & Febiger, 1993, p. 292.)

Figure 6.26. Uniformly echogenic CL on day 7 (*arrows*). (From McKinnon AO, Voss JL, eds. Equine reproduction. Philadelphia: Lea & Febiger, 1993, p. 292.)

was characterized by an echo pattern indicative of loosely organized, well-vascularized tissue, whereas ovarian stroma generally yielded brighter echoes in a pattern representative of dense tissue. Also, the majority of CLs had a distinct mushroom or gourd shape. In glands classified as centrally nonechogenic, the nonechogenic area was first visible on day 0 or 1 postovulation. These types of luteal structures were at their greatest echogenicity on the day of ovulation (75 to 100% of the gland). This probably was due to the ultrasonographic properties of collapsed follicular walls. The nonechogenic area, which was the central cavity, enlarged over days 1 to 3 due to enlargement of the blood clot. As the blood clot resorbed, that portion of the structure that was echogenic increased throughout the remaining portion of the cycle. In contrast, luteal glands that were characterized as uniformly echogenic did not change throughout the cycle, except the brightness (grey scale) changed throughout the life of the corpus luteum. Ginther also demonstrated that both types of glands change in echogenicity throughout the diestrous period. Initially, the CL is highly echogenic on the day of ovulation. At this time it is easiest to identify. The echogenicity decreases over the first 6 days of diestrus, remains at a minimum level for several days during the middle of diestrus, and then increases over days 12 to 16. The

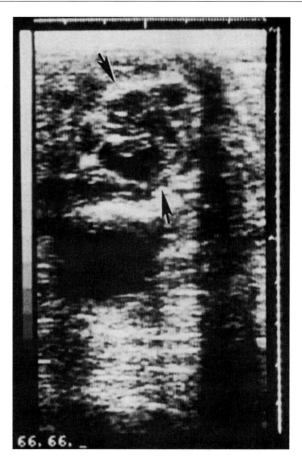

Figure 6.30. Corpus hemorrhagicum on day 9 postovulation. The borders of the luteal structure are designated by arrows. (From McKinnon AO, Voss JL, eds. Equine reproduction. Philadelphia: Lea & Febiger, 1993, p. 293.)

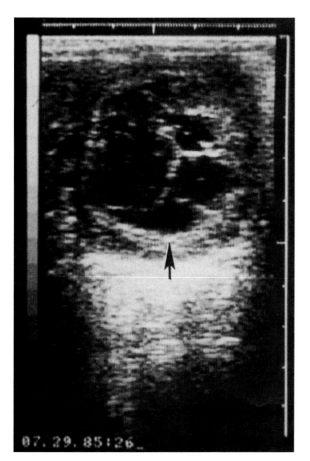

Figure 6.29. Corpus hemorrhagicum or central nonechogenic (*arrow*) CL on day 1 postovulation. (From McKinnon AO, Voss JL, eds. Equine reproduction. Philadelphia: Lea & Febiger, 1993, p. 293.)

very bright hyperechogenic echoes on day 0 may be due to apposition of collapsed follicular walls. There was also an increase in brightness of the CL during the time of CL regression. These ultrasonographic changes are apparently indicative of changes in luteal hemodynamics and changes in tissue density. With experience, the practitioner can become very accurate at using ultrasonography to confirm ovulation and to detect the presence of a corpus luteum. Ultrasonography can also be used to diagnose pseudopregnant mares. A persistent CL and absence of an embryonic vesicle are evidence of a pseudopregnant mare. Once these mares are identified, then prostaglandins can be safely given to induce estrus. Echogenicity of this structure can be used to determine to some extent the age of corpus luteum. Hyperechogenicity is typical of the first few days after ovulation or during CL regression. The first few days usually can be distinguished from the last few days on the basis of gland size. In the middle of diestrus, the CL will be lower on the grey scale than either at the beginning or the end. However, the structure will be at maximal size during the middle of diestrus. If the CL contains a central nonechogenic cavity, the ratio of luteal tissue to blood clot and degree of organization of the clot can be of assistance in estimating age of the gland. The blood clot develops during the first few days, then progressively becomes more organized and proportionally smaller.

Artifacts

Certain types or formations of tissue may cause waves to bend (refract), to bounce back and forth or re-echo (reverberate), or to become weakened or entirely blocked. These distortions may be mistaken for normal or pathologic structures or changes. Fluid-filled structures such as follicles, embryonic vesicles, and uterine cysts are common in the mare's reproductive tract and are responsible for causing the most notable artifacts. An intense echogenic formation beneath a fluid-filled structure is noted as an enhanced through-transmission artifact (Fig. 6.32). This artifact is common beneath images of follicles and embryonic vesicles. Sound waves passing through fluid are not as attenuated as waves passing through adjacent tissue. Therefore, a brighter echo exists beneath the fluid-filled structure when compared with echoes of corresponding depth beneath adjacent tissues. The intensity of echoes resulting from through-transmission can be reduced by proper adjustment of gain controls.

When an ultrasonic beam strikes the side of a curved structural boundary at less than 90°, it may bend or refract, causing a shadowing or lack of echo formation beyond the site of refraction. Refraction artifacts are especially common with images associated with follicles (Fig. 6.33).

When an ultrasonic beam strikes the upper and lower surface of a fluid-filled, spherical structure, a highly echogenic reflection is produced on the screen. This is termed specular reflection (Fig. 6.34). Specular reflection was originally confused and incorrectly identified as being embryonic structure.

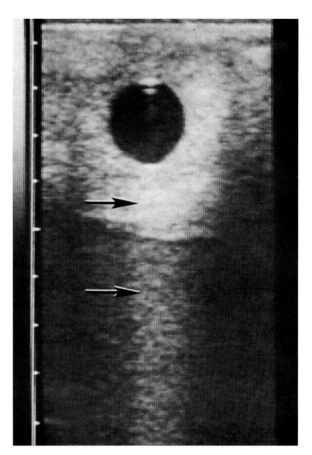

Figure 6.32. Ultrasonographic image of enhanced through transmission artefact (*arrows*) beneath the image of an embryonic vesicle. (From McKinnon AO, Voss JL, eds. Equine reproduction. Philadelphia: Lea & Febiger, 1993, p. 218.)

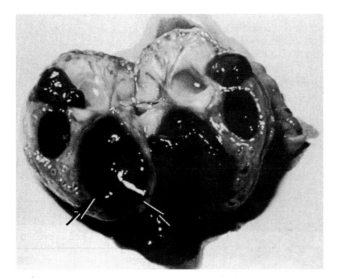

Figure 6.31. Gross characteristics of a developing corpus hemorrhagicum, which would appear as a centrally, nonechogenic CL when visualized with ultrasonography. (From McKinnon AO, Voss JL, eds. Equine reproduction. Philadelphia: Lea & Febiger, 1993, p. 293.)

Reverberation artifacts (Fig. 6.35) are commonly seen during intrarectal examination of the mare's reproductive tract because of gas-filled intestines around the area of interest. Reverberation occurs when waves encounter a highly reflective, gas-filled structure and bounce back and forth between intestine and transducer. Because of the lag time of each returning echo perceived by the transducer, bright echoes are recognized on the screen at deeper and deeper, evenly spaced intervals.

Shadowing is an artifact characterized by lack of an echo beneath a dense structure and is caused by complete reflection or absorption of ultrasonographic waves. This artifact is uncommon in images of the mare's reproductive system because of the relative lack of tissues with density comparable to bone. A notable exception is the occurrence of shadowing beneath fetal bone after death of the fetus, and occasionally from foreign bodies such as a tip of a uterine culturette (Fig. 6.36). The presence of fecal material on the transducer will also result in portions of the ultrasonographic image being obscured because of a shadowing artifact (Fig. 6.37).

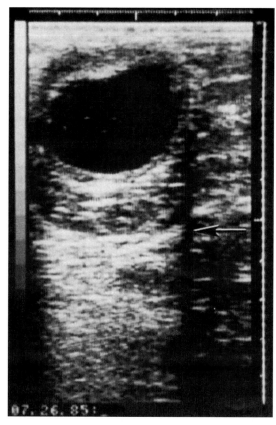

Figure 6.33. Ultrasonographic refraction creating an artefact beneath the edges of an ovary (*arrow*). (From McKinnon AO, Voss JL, eds. Equine reproduction. Philadelphia: Lea & Febiger, 1993, p. 219.)

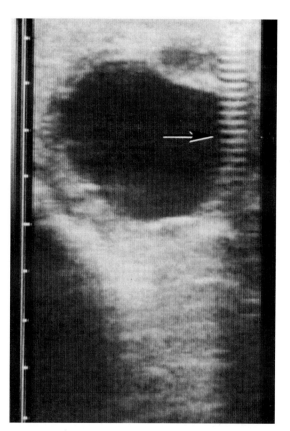

Figure 6.35. Ultrasonographic image of reverberation artefact (*arrow*). (From McKinnon AO, Voss JL, eds. Equine reproduction. Philadelphia: Lea & Febiger, 1993, p. 219.)

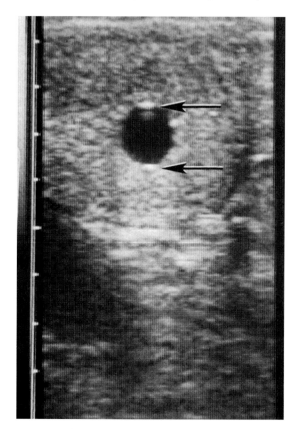

Figure 6.34. Ultrasonographic image of specular reflection (*arrows*). (From McKinnon AO, Voss JL, eds. Equine reproduction. Philadelphia: Lea & Febiger, 1993, p. 219.)

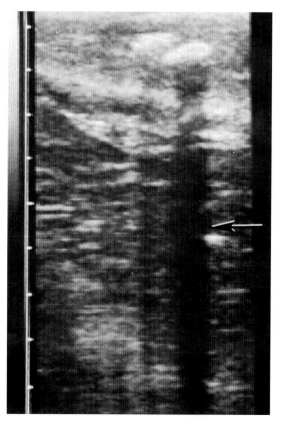

Figure 6.36. Ultrasonographic image of shadowing (*arrow*) from a foreign body (tip of a uterine culturette). (From McKinnon AO, Voss JL, eds. Equine reproduction. Philadelphia: Lea & Febiger, 1993, p. 219.)

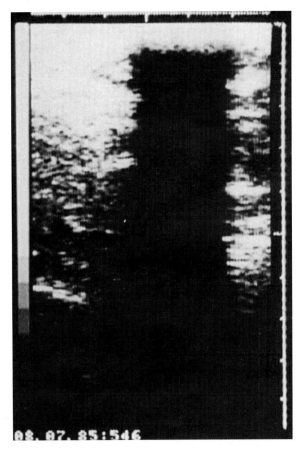

Figure 6.37. Ultrasonographic image of shadowing caused by fecal material on the transducer. (From McKinnon AO, Voss JL, eds. Equine reproduction. Philadelphia: Lea & Febiger, 1993, p. 220.)

THE STALLION

Ultrasonography of the stallion is only just beginning to become recognized as a source of good diagnostic information. Listed below are some conditions we routinely diagnose using ultrasonography.

Internal Reproductive Tract

Accessory sex gland and internal ring palpation are occasionally part of a stallion fertility examination. While the incidences of recognized accessory sex gland abnormalities are low (16), they are not always able to be diagnosed or even suspected from the history, a physical exam, or even semen evaluation. Stallions with high numbers of leukocytes or other abnormal cells in their ejaculates are good candidates for transrectal ultrasonography. This should be performed in conjunction with culture and cytology of semen, endoscopy, and palpation. A correlation between sexual development, hormonal environment, and accessory sex gland development has been demonstrated (17). Structures able to be identified by transrectal ultrasonography are the prostate gland, ampullae of the deferent ducts, vesicular glands, excretory ducts (all meet at the seminal colliculus), pelvic urethra, bulbourethral glands, and abdominally located testicles (Chapter 20).

Ampullae

The ampullae are enlarged, glandular portions of the terminal vas deferens (deferent ducts). They are readily located as they converge over the neck of the bladder and are well recognized as tubular structures that may have a nonechogenic center, particularly in aroused stallions. Transrectal ultrasonography should be performed in cases of suspected unilateral or bilateral duct obstruction. Blockage most commonly occurs in the ampulla and may occasionally be felt rectally. Ultrasonographically, the blockage can be seen as a hyperechoic mass in the ampullae. A 7.5-MHz probe is better for fine detail of smaller structures such as the ampullae and seminal vesicles (16, 18). At the GVEH we have been referred numerous cases of ampullary plugging or blockage. The common history is that the stallion has had normal fertility and at the begining of the subsequent breeding season does not get any mares (or very few mares) in foal. Seminal evaluation reveals markedly reduced sperm numbers compared with the stallions' testicular size. Quite often, none are identified at all and yet the testicles are of good consistency. Repeated administration of oxytocin followed by ejaculation 30 minutes to 1 hour later will clear the obstruction in most cases. Some refractory cases have needed xylazine tranquilization with rectal massage as well. When these stallions have been sexually stimulated prior to xylazine administration, many stallions will spontaneously ejaculate, most within 2 minutes (19). In our experience cases of ampullary blockage frequently reoccur.

Ejaculation can be visualized transrectally (20), and this technique has been able to demonstrate that the ampullae dilate rhythmically prior, during, and even after the ejaculation (21).

Vesicular Gland

The vesicular glands (seminal vesicles) are triangular sacs that produce and store the gel fraction of an ejaculate. The size and echotexture of the vesicular glands depend on the degree of sexual stimulation. Teasing dramatically increases the amount of gel produced (22). The incidence of seminal vesiculitis problems is much lower than bulls; however, we have identified some stallions with adenitis wherein the gel portion of the ejaculate has had large amounts of necrotic debris and even blood clots. We have seen this associated with hemospermia (23). Occasionally, rectal palpation does not demonstrate pain (24), and laboratory backup (white blood cells), fractionation of semen, expressed secretions, and even endoscopy of the vesicular gland openings are indicated to support the diagnosis. Recently, ultrasonography has been useful in diagnosis (25–27). In these cases ultrasonographic findings were an increase in overall size, thickened wall, and increased echogenicity when compared with the contralateral unaffected gland. In one case colic was the presenting clinical sign, and the stallion had discomfort on direct palpation of the seminal vesicle and when sexually aroused (27). Treatment is sometimes difficult and refractory cases are not uncommon. Presumably this is due to poor penetration of antimicrobials to the gland tissue (28). Long-term antibiotic administration (trimethoprim-sulfamethoxazole) has been successful; however, on occasion more aggressive therapy must be considered such as direct lavage through an endoscope or even surgical removal (29, 30). In some refractory cases, treatment of the semen with antibiotic laden extenders (28) and breeding after 30 minutes to 1 hour after mixing will prevent bacterial contamination (7).

Pelvic Urethra

The pelvic urethra runs from the neck of the bladder to the ischial arch. The urethra is difficult to see and may only be evident by specular reflection. There is a wider dilation to the urethra next to the colliculus that becomes visible ultrasonographically as the stallion becomes sexually aroused and releases pre-ejaculatory fluid. Few problems are visualized at the pelvic urethra apart from rare cases of rents in the urethra that communicate with the stratum cavernosum.

Inguinal Rings

At the GVEH, internal reproductive ultrasonography is always (mostly) performed in cases of suspected cryptorchidism (Fig. 6.38). It is quite easy to identify an abdominally retained testes (31) once the operator understands the normal echotexture of the testicle. The echotexture is slightly reduced in density compared with the external testis. In our experience no case of abdominally located testis has been misdiagnosed; occasionally, however, an extra-abdominal testes will not be identified in horses with excessive peri-inguinal fat. The advantages of presurgical identification of the testes are that it enables accurate scheduling of the following surgery (more quickly if the testes is extra-abdominal), that a definitive presurgical placement of the testicle provides confidence to enter the abdomen if difficulty is encountered during surgery, and that on occasion we have identified large neoplastic testicles in the abdominally retained testes. In one case of bilateral cryptorchidism, intraoperative transrectal ultrasonography was

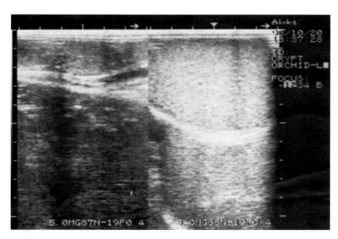

Figure 6.38. Split-screen ultrasonographic image of a cryptorchid testes (*left*) and a normal scrotal testes (*right*).

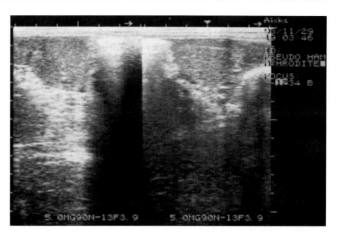

Figure 6.39. Split-screen ultrasonographic image of intra-abdominal testes from a male pseudohermaphrodite (left testicle on the left-hand side).

used to actually guide the surgeon's hand to the testicles through a dilated-inguinal-ring approach. Multiple cases of male pseudohermaphrodites have been identified at the GVEH, and in one instance a familial distribution was suspected with three siblings affected (JE Axon, personal communication). In all cases of male pseudohermaphrodites we have seen, the classical echotexture of testicular tissue was useful in confirming the diagnosis (Fig. 6.39). Male pseudohermaphrodites externally are females (64 XX), but have testicles that are almost exclusively abdominal cryptorchids. Behavior varies, but mostly is stallion like. The vulva is often displaced ventrally with varying degrees of enlargement of the clitoris to one resembling a short penis. Occasionally, chronic anabolic steroid administration may cause failure to cycle, male behavior, and an enlarged clitoris. It should be possible to differentiate these cases using ultrasonography.

External Reproductive Tract

External reproductive tract examination includes the scrotal contents (spermatic cords, testes, epididymides, vaginal cavities, and scrotum) and the external penis (Chapter 19). Commonly, a 5-MHz scan head is used; however, a 7.5 or even a 10 MHz would be preferable for many of the structures visualized. Due to the irritant nature of some lubricants special care of the sensitive scrotal skin is advised. We commonly use mineral oil and then later wash with a mild soap or detergent. The optimal time to evaluate most stallions is within a few minutes of ejaculation, which is when most stallions are relaxed.

SCROTAL CONTENTS

Vaginal Cavity

Ultrasonography is particularly useful in differentiating enlargements of the testes, the vaginal cavity, or the surrounding layer of the skin, tunic, and fascial layer. Fluid that accumulates between the testes and the parietal vaginal tunic (vaginal cavity) is termed a *hydrocele* if it is clear, a *hemato-*

cele if it contains blood, and a *pyocele* if it contains many white blood cells (Chapter 19). Hydroceles are the most common fluid accumulation (32). The epididymis, due to its ventral location and enlargement of the tail, is the area that is most commonly surrounded by fluid. This fluid often outlines the tail. Hydroceles are often transient and often reflect nonreproductive pathology such as low protein, abdominal neoplasia, and even on occasion chronic peritonitis with increased abdominal fluid. Hematoceles are generally associated with trauma and are recognized by fibrin strands and even swirling, nonclotted blood (Fig. 6.40). The visceral tunic should be evaluated for integrity if a hematocele is present and testicular removal contemplated if a rent is demonstrated. Pyoceles are less common and are seen with orchitis, peritonitis, secondarily infected hydroceles or hematoceles, and on occasion after a penetrating wound. Scrotal hernias (inguinal hernias, ruptured inguinal hernias, or inguinal ruptures) can also be diagnosed with ultrasonography (Fig. 6.41).

Scrotal Skin and Investments

Edema secondarily to trauma, allergic reactions, dependent edema, and after application of irritants are causes of scrotal skin thickening. Ultrasonography may be necessary to differentiate between firm scrotal edema and a hematocele, although many of these conditions may occur concurrently.

Spermatic Cord

The spermatic cord can twist within the scrotum if there is enough movement allowed by the caudal ligament of the epididymis or proper ligament of the testes. We assume most spermatic cord torsion is intravaginal (excluding the parietal layer of the vaginal tunic), although the relative frequencies of intravaginal versus extravaginal cord torsions

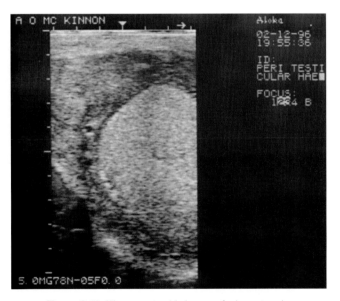

Figure 6.40. Ultrasonographic image of a hematocele.

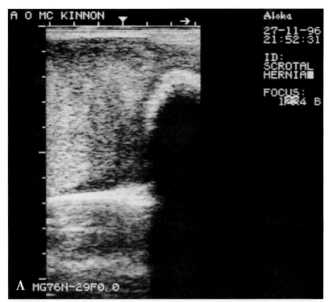

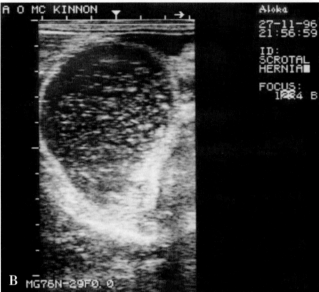

Figure 6.41. Ultrasonographic image of scrotal hernia depicting **(A)** loop of small intestine in the scrotum (external abdominal scan) and **(B)** dilated small intestine (internal scan).

have not been reported for horses (33). In addition, the term testicular torsion, although more commonly used, does not accurately describe the condition as it is the spermatic cord that has twisted. It is simple to diagnose a 180° torsion by location of the tail of the epididymis cranially. Our belief is that any stallion can develop a minor 180° torsion that can spontaneously correct, but that the older stallion is more likely to develop permanent 180° torsion due to stabilization of the testes by adhesions between the vaginal tunics that are presumably associated with strongylus edentatus migration (22, 34). Spermatic cord torsion of 180° has been associated with slightly reduced spermatozoal production (35). No attempt is made to correct a 180° torsion. Torsion of the spermatic cord of greater than 180° results in much more serious complications (33). Torsions of 360° or greater are treated as emergencies. Commonly, these are associated with thickening of the cord, edema, and painful enlargement of the scrotal contents. The primary differential diagnosis for spermatic cord torsion is inguinal/scrotal herniation. An edematous internal vaginal ring may occur with both conditions, and ultrasonography is useful in the differentiation. Other conditions that may mimic torsion are scrotal trauma, periorchitis, neoplasia, hematocele, varicocele, and thrombosis of the spermatic cord vasculature (36).

Another condition affecting the spermatic cords is the *varicocele*. A varicocele forms from abnormally distended and tortuous veins of the pampiniform plexus. The condition is well recognized in humans and rams. Their relationship to fertility has not been adequately studied in stallions. The source of infertility associated with varicoceles in men is disturbance of the thermoregulatory mechanisms. In sheep, breeding from affected rams is discouraged because of a possible inherited basis. In men, the condition may respond to surgery or, more commonly, thermoregulation with long-term commitment to water jacketed, cooled underpants.

Testicle

There are many conditions of the testicles that can be diagnosed or detected with ultrasonography. Cryptorchidism has been discussed above. Testicular neoplasia, although uncommon, may occur in any area of the testicle and can be visualized quite well due to different echogenicity. Germinal testicular tumors (originating from germ cells of the seminiferous epithelium) are in decreasing order of frequency: seminoma, teratoma, teratocarcinoma, and embryonic carcinoma (37). Somatic tumors (nongerminal derivation) are classified as parenchymatous such as Leydig and Sertoli-cell tumors and nonparenchymatous such as lipomas, fibromas, and leiomyomas (33). Most equine testicular tumors are unilateral and of germinal derivation. Seminomas accounted for 87% in one large survey (38). All are treated as potentially malignant. Tumors are more common in retained abdominal testes (39–44). In horses with testicular tumors growth is usually reported to be slow. The first sign is often a harder and slightly enlarged testicle that is discovered on routine examination such as for insurance. Intrascrotal masses may be identified as intratesticular or extratesticular and may be solid or cystic. Testicle tumors frequently have a decreased echogenicity; however, this depends on the amount of fluid within the tissue, the tissue type and the growth rate. Prompt orchidectomy is the only treatment. Prior to removal of the affected testicle, ultrasonography of the contralateral testicle and an internal reproductive tract examination must be performed to detect malignancy or other abnormalities. Semen evaluation will often remain almost unaffected early in the course of the disease. Following castration some testicular compensatory hypertrophy may occur, especially in young stallions (45, 46). Unilateral castration of stallions was associated with a sig-

nificant increase in serum LH and FSH concentrations and, perhaps, higher intratesticular testosterone, which may explain, in part, the compensatory hypertrophy noted in the remaining testis (45).

Testicular trauma may result in a testicular hematoma or chronic testicular degeneration. Testicular hematomas are discrete and rarely cause a rent in the visceral tunic. They are quite frequently painful on palpation and the scrotal contents enlarged. Because they are mostly traumatic in origin, other signs are also present such as scrotal edema. Testicular degeneration may be recognizable on palpation by a smaller and softer-feeling testicle than the contralateral one. Ultrasonographically, there is often an overall increase in echogenicity to the affected testicle, a reduction in size and a reduction in circulation to the testicular parenchyma as exemplified by loss of visibility of the central vein (47). Arteries that penetrate the tunica albuginea may also appear more prominent at the periphery of the testis due to a reduction in blood flow to the testicular parenchyma. Orchitis can be bacterial, viral, parasitic, or autoimmune in origin. Bacterial orchitis may be associated with hematogenous spread of *Streptococcus zooepidemicus, Streptococcus equi, Actinobacillus equuli, Pseudomonas mallei, Salmonella abortus equi,* or *Brucella abortus*. Local invasion of the testes can be secondary to peritonitis or a penetrating wound and frequently involve *Streptococcus* spp, *Staphylococcus* spp, and *E. coli* (37). Retrograde infection through the epididymis is also possible. Either unilateral or bilateral orchitis can develop. The affected testicle(s) is hot and painful. The horse frequently has an elevated temperature. Intratesticular and extratesticular edema is present, and frequently the horse will refuse to breed. If semen can be obtained, then frequently spermatozoal motility is decreased, morphological abnormalities are increased, and large numbers of leukocytes are present. On occasion, orchitis may develop into a testicular abscess. At the GVEH we had a 7-year-old stallion present with an enlarged scrotum and ultrasonography demonstrated an intratesticular abscess with periorchitis as well. Unilateral open castration resulted in the horse returning to breeding and successfully impregnating mares 120 days after the surgery. Medical management of bacterial orchitis should include appropriate antibiotics, anti-inflammatory medication, and even cold hydrotherapy. Viral orchitis is not as well understood and may be more important as a cause of testicular degeneration than we currently recognize. Equine influenza, viral arteritis, and EIA have been implicated (37). Parasitic orchitis has been associated with the migration of *Strongylus edentatus* causing testicular irritation and adhesions between the tunics (34). Autoimmune orchitis may result from testicular trauma and damage to the blood-testis barrier. Spermatozoa are highly antigenic, and it is postulated that developing spermatozoa are protected from the immune system by the blood-testis barrier. Localized granulomatous reactions and degeneration of the testicle are the sequelae to extravasation of spermatozoa from lacerations, biopsies, neoplasia, or trauma to the testicle. Antisperm an-

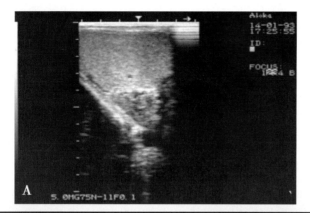

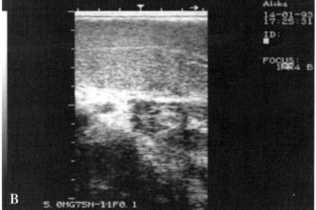

Figure 6.42. Ultrasonographic image of a testes demonstrating **(A)** cross-sectional scan with the central vein visible in the middle and **(B)** longitudinal scan.

tibodies have been documented for the stallion (48–50) and have a well recognized association with infertility in humans (51).

In addition to examination for disease processes, ultrasonography can be used to measure the length, width, and height (Fig. 6.42), as well as the cross-sectional area and the circumference at the widest part, of each testes (52). Using the formula for the volume of an ellipsoid (4/3 π abc, a = height/2, b = width/2, c = length/2), the volume of a testes can be measured (52) (Chapter 19).

Epididymis

Conditions detected in the epididymis are cysts, inflammatory reactions, and dilation of the tail lumen (Chapter 19). Epididymal cysts are round and generally smooth. They are not very common, and unless they become quite large, do not interfere with fertility. The cysts most commonly are located in the head and body. Occasionally, cysts form from extravasation of sperm in blind-ending, efferent ductules in the head of the epididymis. Infectious epididymitis is rarely seen as a primary entity and is most commonly associated with concurrent orchitis. The tail (cauda epididymis) is most commonly involved, although the head (caput epididymis) and body may also be affected (53). Acute epi-

didymitis can cause severe pain with swelling and edema that may later progress to abscessation, fibrosis, and periorchitis. Ultrasonographically, the diameter of the head and tail of the epididymis is often larger than normal, it is hyperechoic in relation to the testis, and an irregular border is detected (54). Several, bright, 1- to 5-mm-diameter, echogenic areas that alternated with less echogenic areas were seen in the head of the epididymis in one report (55). Ultrasonographic findings were interpreted as fibrosis attributable to chronic inflammation (55). Care in interpretation is needed as similar findings were also reported in a stallion with generalized lymphosarcoma (56). Examination of the ejaculate reveals increased abnormalities and abundant white blood cells. Culture of the ejaculate may help identify the bacteria. Treatment of infectious epididymitis is difficult and even unilateral castration is often unrewarding due to the likelihood that the other epididymis is involved (54, 55). Epididymal sperm granulomas are seen with loss of spermatozoa from the excurrent duct lumen (57). These are sequelae from a variety of causes such as parasite migration, lacerations, trauma, and epididymitis. Sperm granulomas may initially be painful, but become painless masses with time (53). Ultrasonographically, these are quite hyperechoic. Spermiostasis is seen with an abnormal accumulation of sperm in the tail of the epididymis. This is associated with sexual rest and some form of dysfunction of the epididymis. Ejaculates from these stallions frequently have very high numbers of spermatozoa (30 $\times$ 10^9) and have a high percentage of detached heads and concurrent poor progressive motility. We call these stallions accumulators. Quite often the ampullae are affected as well. Seven to eight ejaculates (sometimes more) are necessary to return spermatozoal transit time through the epididymis back to normal. Ultrasonography may be useful in determining abnormal gland storage.

Penis

Ultrasonographic diagnosis of penile trauma has been reported (58). Changes may be seen in several compartments after these insults. Edema may be seen between the tunica albuginea and in the preputial membrane. Blood clots may be visualized in the corpus cavernosum (59). Tears in the corpus can be detected as well as vascular shunts. Clots associated with phenothiazine-induced priapism can be imaged and then later the fibrosis that accompanies long-standing organization of thrombosis (58).

Prepuce

Ultrasonographic diagnosis of preputial lesions is limited to space-occupying problems such as posthitis (traumatic, etc.), edema, preputial abscesses, and neoplasia such as squamous cell carcinomas, papillomas, sarcoids, and melanomas (60). On occasion, it is useful to alert the clinician as to where the best place for drainage of an abscess or hematoma would be.

CONCLUSION

Ultrasonography has become indispensable to our practice. Fortunately, much of the equipment used for reproductive ultrasonography can be used to examine many other parts of the horse. Ultrasonography is now more fundamental than any other diagnostic technique. It has become so fundamental to our daily examination procedures that it would be difficult to practice veterinary medicine again without it.

REFERENCES

1. Ginther OJ, Pierson RA. Ultrasonic evaluation of the reproductive tract of the mare: principles, equipment and techniques. J Equine Vet Sci 1983;3:195–201.
2. McKinnon AO. Artificial insemination of cooled, transported and frozen semen. In: Equine Stud Medicine. Sydney: Post Graduate Foundation in Veterinary Science, 1996:319–337.
3. McKinnon AO, Squires EL, Carnevale EM, Harrison LA, Frantz DD, McChesney AE, Shideler RK. Diagnostic ultrasonography of uterine pathology in the mare. Proc AAEP 1987;605–622.
4. Ginther OJ, ed. Ultrasonic imaging and animal reproduction: horses. Cross Plains: Equiservices Publishing, 1995.
5. Pierson RA, Ginther OJ. Ultrasonic evaluation of the corpus luteum of the mare. Theriogenology 1985;23:795–806.
6. Pierson RA, Ginther OJ. Ultrasonic evaluation of the preovulatory follicle in the mare. Theriogenology 1985;24:359–368.
7. Pickett BW, Squires EL, McKinnon AO. Procedures for collection, evaluation and utilization of stallion semen for artifical insemination. Colorado State University: Animal Reproduction Laboratory, 1987.
8. Woods J, Bergfelt DR, Ginther OJ. Effects of time of insemination relative to ovulation on pregnancy rate and embryonic loss rate in mares. Equine Vet J 1990;22:410–415.
9. McKinnon AO, Wheeler M, Carnevale EM, Squires EL. Oocyte transfer in the mare: preliminary observations. J EquineVet Sci 1986;6:306–309.
10. McKinnon AO, Carnevale EM, Squires EL, Voss JL, Seidel GE Jr. Heterogenous and xenogenous fertilization of in vivo matured equine oocytes. J EquineVet Sci 1988;8:143–147.
11. Carnevale EM, McKinnon AO, Squires EL, Voss JL. Ultrasonographic characteristics of the preovulatory follicle preceeding and during ovulation in mares. J Equine Vet Sci 1988;8:428–431.
12. McKinnon AO, Squires EL, Voss JL. Ultrasonic evaluation of the mare's reproductive tract. I. Compend Con Educ PractVet 1987; 9:336–345.
13. McKinnon AO, Squires EL, Pickett BW. Equine diagnostic ultrasonography. Colorado State University: Animal Reproduction Laboratory; 1988.
14. Townson DH, Ginther OJ. Size and shape changes in the preovulatory follicle in mares based on digital analysis of ultrasonic images. Anim Reprod Sci 1989;21:63–72.
15. Townson DH, Pierson RA, Ginther OJ. Characterization of plasma progesterone concentrations for two distinct luteal morphologies in mares. Theriogenology 1989;32:197–204.
16. Little TV, Holyoak GR. Reproductive anatomy and physiology of the stallion. Vet Clin North Am Equine Pract 1992;8:1–29.
17. Holyoak GR, Little TV, Vernon M, McCollum WH, Timoney PJ. Correlation between ultrasonographic findings and serum testosterone concentration in prepubertal and peripubertal colts. Am J Vet Res 1994;55:450–457.
18. Little TV, Woods GL. Ultrasonography of accessory sex glands in the stallion. J Reprod Fertil Suppl 1987;35:87–947.
19. McDonnell SM, Love CC. Xylazine-induced ex copula ejaculation in stallions. Theriogenology 1991;36:73–76.
20. Weber JA, Woods GL. A technique for transrectal ultrasonography of stallions during ejaculation. Theriogenology 1991;36:831–838.
21. Weber JA, Woods GL. Ultrasonographic measurement of stallion accessory sex glands and excurrent ducts during seminal emission and ejaculation. Biol Reprod 1993;49:267–273.
22. Pickett BW, Amann RP, McKinnon AO, Squires EL, Voss JL. Management of the stallion for maximum reproductive efficiency. II. Colorado State University: Animal Reproduction Laboratory, 1989.
23. McKinnon AO, Voss JL, Trotter GW, Pickett BW, Shideler RK, Squires EL. Hemospermia of the stallion. Equine Pract 1988;10: 17–23.
24. Blanchard TL, Varner DD, Hurtgen P, Love CC, Cummings MR, Strezmienski PJ, Benson C, Kenney RM. Bilateral seminal vesiculitis and ampullitis in a stallion. J Am Vet Med Assoc 1988;192: 525–526.
25. Malmgren L, Sussemilch BI. Ultrasonography as a diagnostic tool in a stallion with seminal vesiculitis: a case report. Theriogenology 1992;37:935–938.
26. Malmgren L. Ultrasonography: a new diagnostic tool in stallions with genital tract infection? Acta Vet Scand Suppl 1992;88:91–94.
27. Freestone JF, Paccamonti DL, Eilts BE, McClure JJ, Swiderski CE, Causey RC. Seminal vesiculitis as a cause of signs of colic in a stallion. J Am Vet Med Assoc 1993;203:556–557.
28. Blanchard JL, Varner DD, Love CC, Hurtgen JP, Cummings MR, Kenney RM. Use of a semen extender containing antibiotic to improve the fertility of a stallion with seminal vesiculitis due to *Pseudomonas aeruginosa*. Theriogenology 1987;28:541–546.
29. Klug E, Deegen E, Martin J, Bader H, Lieske R, Freytag K. [Experimental uni- and bilateral extirpation of the seminal vesicle in the stallion (author's transl)] Experimentelle ein- und beidseitige Samenblasen-Exstirpation beim Pferd. Dtsch Tierarztl Wochenschr 1979;86:182–185.
30. Varner DD, Schumacher J, Blanchard TL, Johnson L. Diseases of the accessory genital glands. In: Diseases and management of breeding stallions. Goleta, CA: American Veterinary Publications, 1991;257–263.
31. Jann HW, Rains JR. Diagnostic ultrasonography for evaluation of cryptorchidism in horses. J Am Vet Med Assoc 1990;196: 297–300.
32. Varner DD, Schumacher J, Blanchard TL, Johnson L. Diseases of the scrotum. In: Diseases and management of breeding stallions. Goleta, CA: American Veterinary Publications, 1991;175–191.
33. Varner DD, Schumacher J, Blanchard TL, Johnson L. Diseases of the spermatic cord. In: Diseases and management of breeding stallions. Goleta, CA: American Veterinary Publications, 1991; 251–256.
34. Smith JA. The occurrence of larvae of *Strongylus edentatus* in the testicles of stallions. Vet Rec 1973;93:604–606.
35. Pickett BW, Voss JL, Bowen RA, Squires EL, McKinnon AO. Seminal characteristics and total scrotal width (TSW) of normal and abnormal stallions. Proc AAEP 1987;487–518.
36. Horney FD, Barker CAV. Torsion of the testicle in a standardbred. Can Vet J 1975;16:272–273.
37. Varner DD, Schumacher J, Blanchard TL, Johnson L. Diseases of the testes. In: Diseases and management of breeding stallions. Goleta, CA: American Veterinary Publications, 1991;193–232.

38. Reifinger M. Statistical investigations of testicular neoplasms in domestic mammals. J Vet Med Series A 1988;35:63–72.

39. Hunt RJ, Hay W, Collatos C, Welles E. Testicular seminoma associated with torsion of the spermatic cord in two cryptorchid stallions. J Am Vet Med Assoc 1990;197:1484–1486.

40. Smith BL, Morton LD, Watkins JP, Taylor TS, Storts RW. Malignant seminoma in a cryptorchid stallion. J Am Vet Med Assoc 1989;195:775–776.

41. Gelberg HB, McEntee K. Equine testicular interstitial cell tumors. Vet Pathol 1987;24:231–234.

42. Parks A., Wyn-Jones G, Cox JE, Newsholme BJ. Partial obstruction of the small colon associated with an abdominal testicular teratoma in a foal. Equine Vet J 1986;18:342–343.

43. Stick JA. Teratoma and cyst formation of the equine cryptorchid testicle. J Am Vet Med Assoc 1980;176:211–214.

44. Smyth GB. Testicular teratoma in an equine cryptorchid. Equine Vet J 1979;11:21–23.

45. Hoagland TA, Mannen KA, Dinger JE, Ott KM, Woody CO, Riesen JW, Daniels W. Effects of unilateral castration on serum luteinizing hormone, FSH, and testosterone concentrations in one-, two-, and three-year-old stallions. Theriogenology 1986;26:407–418.

46. Hoagland TA, Ott KM, Dinger JE, Mannen K, Woody CO, Riesen JW, Daniels W. Effects of unilateral castration on morphologic characteristics of the testis in one-, two-, and three-year-old stallions. Theriogenology 1986;26:397–406.

47. Love CC. Ultrasonographic evaluation of the testis, epididymis, and spermatic cord of the stallion. Vet Clin North Am Equine Pract 1992;8:167–182.

48. Lee C, Hunter AG, Joo HS. Effect of antisperm antibodies on ability of in-vitro capacitated stallion sperm to penetrate zona-free hamster eggs. Biol Reprod 1995;52:132 .

49. Teuscher C, Kenney RM, Cummings MR, Catten M. Identification of 2 stallion sperm-specific proteins and their autoantibody response. Equine Vet J 1994;26:148–151.

50. Nie GJ, Lee C, Momont HW, Joo HS. Equine antisperm antibodies (Easa)—preliminary study of the clinical response following breeding in immunized mares. Theriogenology 1993;40:1107–1116.

51. Gupta KG, Garg AK. Presence of antisperm antibodies in fertile and infertile persons. Acta Obstet Gynecol Scand 1975;54:407–410.

52. Love CC, Garcia MC, Riera FR, Kenney RM. Evaluation of measures taken by ultrasonography and caliper to estimate testicular volume and predict daily sperm output in the stallion. J Reprod Fertil Suppl 1991;44:99–105.

53. Varner DD, Schumacher J, Blanchard TL, Johnson L. Diseases of the epididymis. In: Diseases and management of breeding stallions. Goleta, CA: American Veterinary Publications, 1991;233–240.

54. Held JP, Adair S, McGavin MD, Adams WH, Toal R, Henton J. Bacterial epididymitis in two stallions. J Am Vet Med Assoc 1990;197:602–604.

55. Traub-Dargatz JL, Trotter GW, Kaser-Hotz B, Bennett DG, Kiper ML, Veeramachaneni DN, Squires E. Ultrasonographic detection of chronic epididymitis in a stallion. J Am Vet Med Assoc 1991;198:1417–1420.

56. Held JP, Mccracken MD, Toal R, Latimer F. Epididymal swelling attributable to generalized lymphosarcoma in a stallion. J Am Vet Med Assoc 1992;201:1913–1915.

57. Blue MG, McEntee K. Epididymal sperm granuloma in a stallion. Equine Vet J 1985;17:248–251.

58. Varner DD, Schumacher J, Blanchard TL, Johnson L. Diseases of the penis. In: Diseases and management of breeding stallions. Goleta, CA: American Veterinary Publications, 1991;273–320.

59. Hyland J, Church S. The use of ultrasonography in the diagnosis and treatment of a haematoma in the corpus cavernosum penis of a stallion. Aust Vet J 1995;72:468–469.

60. Varner DD, Schumacher J, Blanchard TL, Johnson L. Diseases of the prepuce. In: Diseases and management of breeding stallions. Goleta, CA: American Veterinary Publications, 1991;321–334.

7. Diagnostic Ultrasound: Applications in the Equine Limb

RONALD D. SANDE, RUSSELL L. TUCKER and GARY R. JOHNSON

Early development of diagnostic ultrasound in veterinary medicine focused on cardiology, theriogenology, and examination of the abdomen and thorax. Ultrasound examination of the soft-tissue structures of the limbs of horses developed more slowly. Diagnostic equipment that was designed for examination of the female genital tract and conceptus was not ideal for imaging the distal limbs of horses. The most suitable technology was expensive and difficult for most practitioners to justify, especially when applications had not fully been developed. Among the impediments to developing the applications were the difficulties in acquiring patients for suitable controlled studies and the relative inability to correlate pathologic changes with ultrasound images. Most of the significant initial publications regarding this subject originated with specialists and practitioners in the field who had the opportunity to examine large numbers of bowed tendons and suspensory desmitis (1–4).

Currently, the majority of ultrasound equipment used in equine practice utilizes linear-array transducer technology. The name is derived from the linear arrangement of piezoelectric crystals used to propagate and receive the sound beam. Two-dimensional image display with this technology is rectangular in shape and easily differentiated from the "pie-wedge" shaped display of the sector scanner.

The major advantage of linear-array technology is the lower purchase price and cost of maintenance when compared with sector technology. Disadvantages include difficulty focusing the sound beam and a cumbersome scan head that is difficult to fit to various body contours. At a tissue depth of less than 2 cm, standard linear-array transducers give a superior image. There is less distortion of the image in the "near" field and less artifact than occurs with sector transducers. Linear transducers give a larger tissue contact image or "footprint." Also, longitudinal images provide better visualization of the tissues where transducer contact is complete. However, near the carpus/tarsus or fetlocks the curvatures of the limb obstruct transducer-tissue contact. Transverse images (cross-section) are more difficult to acquire and may not provide a record of the total tissue anatomy on a single image because only a small section of the linear transducer can be kept in contact with the caudal surfaces of the equine limb in the transverse image planes.

Sector scanners use several forms of transducer technology. Mechanical sector scanners rotate a piezoelectric crystal about an axis to acquire a two-dimensional real-time image. The original advantage of this technology was that it included transducers with multiple crystals of different frequencies, allowing greater versatility in examination procedures. Phased-array sectors are more complex and more expensive. Multiple crystal-array transducers have several advantages, including the ability to "steer" the beam direction and electronic focusing of the beam giving better resolution, which ultimately translates to better image quality. Resolution and detail in deeper tissues are often superior when using sector technology and the beam shape enables the operator to make transverse scans of tendons and ligaments in the chosen focal zone. Edge artifacts are fewer on transverse images when using a sector transducer. The small footprint of a sector transducer facilitates imaging in contoured areas of limbs that are difficult to examine with a linear transducer. However, this characteristic requires continual repositioning of the transducer to make a complete longitudinal examination of the tendon. The major disadvantages of a sector transducer are the near-field artifact and decreased far-field lateral resolution resulting from the expanding beam transmitted by sector transducers. Regardless of the transducer technology, the operator must develop the skill and technique to make a systematic and repeatable examination.

Transducer frequency, type, and capabilities are often a function of availability. A multifrequency (7-10 MHz), small-footprint transducer (28 mm or 38 mm) has proven ideal for most equine limb applications; however, a 7.5-MHz transducer may be a suitable compromise. Economic considerations may force one to use a single transducer for multiple purposes (e.g., reproduction, tendons, ligaments, and deeper tissues) in which case 5.0-MHz linear-array transducer is probably the best compromise. The 5.0-MHz will lack the high resolution needed for superficial imaging and some subtle changes may be missed in the near field.

The near-field image is subject to loss of information resulting from a nonuniform wave front. The multiple sound waves, arising from the transducer, reinforce each other to form a continuous wave front at a distance from the transducer face that is determined by the ultrasound frequency and transducer design. Higher frequency results in the synchronous wave front being closer to the transducer. Even with a 7.5-MHz transducer, it may be necessary to use a standoff pad for suitable resolution of near-field structures. It is important that the standoff pad be acoustically similar to soft tissue. Various materials and commercially produced attachments have been used as a "standoff" spacer from the transducer (5–8). Early standoff pads were made from water-filled rubber gloves or plastic bags, breast prostheses, or other materials and were cumbersome or unreliable. Commercially available products marketed for the expressed use as standoff materials have proven effective (9). Various configurations and materials have been constructed to accommodate transducer design and act as a suitable acoustic coupler and conform to the unusual anatomy of the areas to be examined (10).

A 1-cm thickness of standoff material is suitable for use with most transducers. However, if one must use a transducer with a single, focused depth, there is an advantage to having two thicknesses available. One centimeter and two centimeter standoffs can be used to bring the optimum focus nearer the skin surface. Although some artifact may be encountered, the two thicknesses can be combined to give still a third focal depth. Using this procedure one can only reduce the focal depth in the tissues; the only ways to extend the focal depth are to apply pressure to the transducer and displace the more superficial tissues or to select a transducer with a longer focus. This is usually not a problem when scanning tendons and ligaments.

One may encounter a reverberation artifact when using standoff pads. The initial hyperechoic artifact will occur at a depth in the image equal to the thickness of the standoff pad, and it will continue at equal intervals deeper into the image. Usually, this does not present a problem since the standoff is used to acquire an image from the superficial tissues found at less depth than the thickness of the pad.

The patient must be restrained and properly prepared to allow thorough, systematic, and detailed exploration of the soft tissues of the distal limb. Patient preparation requires that hair and surface contamination be removed if one is to maximize image quality. Hair will scatter and attenuate the sound beam. In addition, the hair entraps air and solids, which cause serious image degradation. It is often with the most valuable patient and the most critical evaluation that one is challenged by an owner or trainer who is resistant to the removal of hair. Obviously, any blemish or evidence to suggest the horse may have a physical defect may affect public acceptance of a performance horse. Screening ultrasound examination of the horse may be made using cursory preparation of the area to be examined. However, for critical examination one must insist on proper application of this modality or risk erroneous interpretation of artifacts as meaningful detail. Adequate aqueous conducting gel should be applied to the skin surface. It is often helpful to wash the area with soap and water to remove oil and moisturize the skin as dry skin will absorb water from the conducting gel and compromise acoustical coupling.

Scab formation following shaving, subcutaneous emphysema at incisions, and healing incisions compromise image quality and may be a problem when short-interval progress exams are required (11).

Although controversial, screening examination may be performed on areas with thin hair and a well-groomed coat by wetting the hair with isopropyl alcohol (70% or less) followed by application of copious conducting gel. Image quality, although compromised, may be adequate to differentiate connective tissue disease from tendon and ligament disease. Removal of hair may be unnecessary to obtain the diagnosis,

and diseases of this nature may allow the horse to return to performance before hair could be regrown. Localization of areas of interest over body cavities may be obtained using the alcohol "wetting" technique; once located, only the significant area needs to be clipped or shaved. The more dilute the alcohol the less irritating it may be to both the horse and the transducer. Manufacturers' recommendations should be reviewed before applying any chemical to the transducer.

Aqueous coupling gels are commercially available. A suitable coupling gel must have acoustical transmission similar to tissue. Gels that are more viscous are better when scanning vertical surfaces and less frequent application of gel is required. During the early application of diagnostic ultrasound there was difficulty in obtaining commercial sources of aqueous coupling gel, and mineral oil or methyl cellulose (rectal lubricant) were used with some success. It was discovered that these materials had detrimental effects on the transducers and would permeate seams and contaminate electronics.

CREATING AN IMAGE

The brightest and most distinct leading edges are acquired when the ultrasound beam axis is perpendicular to an acoustical interface. Images acquired at less than or greater than the critical angle of reflection may have hypoechoic or anechoic areas since the "echo" does not return to the transducer. This is very important when scanning tendons and ligaments that have a highly organized texture. Transverse scans should be perpendicular to the longitudinal axis of the tendon fiber, and longitudinal scans require that the ultrasound scan plane be parallel to tendon fibers. Changing the angle of the incident ultrasound beam will result in decreased echogenicity of the tendon relative to that of muscle, a characteristic known as anisotropy (12). This characteristic may help the sonographer locate tendon tissue contained in larger volumes of connective tissue or tissue swelling. It is important, while scanning tendons, to continually explore the critical angle of reflection to acquire an accurate image and avoid interpreting hypoechogenic artifacts as areas of inflammation, edema, or hemorrhage.

Recognition of the anatomic location while scanning requires the sonographer to continuously move the scan head along the axis of the tendon. This movement is best made from proximal to distal, with the direction of the hair. Although the hair has been shaved, the protruding hair stubble is extremely abrasive and will cause unnecessary wear to the protective material used to cover many transducer contact surfaces. In addition, distal-to-proximal scanning movement exacerbates cutaneous hyperesthesia caused by clipping and shaving the area and may cause the horse discomfort. Concern for standardization of diagnostic ultrasound imaging has been expressed (13–14). The standardization of examination procedures and terminology has numerous advantages, but communication among veterinarians is perhaps most important. Diagnoses, prognoses, therapeutic regimen, client education, recovery progress, meaningful

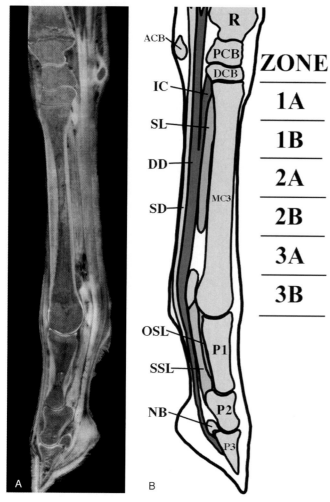

Figure 7.1. Sagittal view of the metacarpus. **A.** Frozen section. **B.** Schematic of frozen section. ACB = accessory carpal bone; DCB = distal row of carpal bones; DD = deep digital flexor tendon; IC = inferior check ligament; MC3 = third metacarpal bone; NB = navicular bone; OSL = oblique sesamoid ligament; P1 = first phalanx; P2 = second phalanx; P3 = third phalanx; PCB = proximal row of carpal bones; R = radius; SD = superficial digital flexor tendon; SL = suspensory ligament; SSL = straight sesamoid ligament.

have sufficient structural alteration to be recognized as abnormal must be carefully measured to establish a baseline record for charting the progress of healing. Improved resolution and advancements in diagnostic ultrasound technology have made it feasible for the practitioner to detect and monitor progress of most soft-tissue lesions. Diseases that result in swelling or enlargement may be documented by precise measurement. Normal values are available for transverse dimensions of tendons and ligaments (15), and total cross-sectional areas of the DD and SD flexor tendons have been compared between limbs and compared among different size horses (16). Documentation of the location of a scan image, standardized description of tissue echogenicity, and extent of changes have been reported (4, 13, 17–19). These parameters may be augmented in the future by quantitative analysis of ultrasonographic gray scale (20–22).

Several methods have been suggested for recording the location of interest on the limb. The length of the metacarpus of an average horse is about three widths of a person's hand; the metatarsus is about four widths. Originally these zones were numbered proximal to distal as Zone 1-3 on the front limb and Zone 1-4 on the hind limb. Soon the sophistication of the examination was improved and the zones were further divided into Zones 1A, 1B, 2A, 2B, etc. This method divides the metacarpus (tarsus) into six (eight) zones of nearly equal length (approximately 4 cm). Zone 1 of the metacarpus includes the origin of the suspensory ligament and the inferior check ligament and the deep and superficial flexor tendons emerging from the carpal sheath. Zone 2 is the middle one-third of the metacarpus and includes structures distal to the bifurcation of the suspensory ligament. Zone 3 is the distal one-third of the metacarpus from the bifurcation of the suspensory ligament to the fetlock joint (Fig. 7.1). The metatarsus is anatomically longer and is separated into four equal zones (Fig. 7.2).

Measuring from an anatomic reference provides a more exact location. A cloth or flexible tape can be affixed to the limb during the examination so areas of interest or lesions can be accurately documented during the scanning process. The "0" mark of the tape should be located at a palpable landmark (23). Using the accessory carpal bone in the front limb or the proximal lateral metatarsal bone in the hind limb provides a consistent reference location.

The length of the transducer can be used to document distance or the transducer and the cord can be indexed and marked, obviating the need for a separate measuring tape or one that is attached to the limb. While these latter methods are convenient for one's personal records, they do not fulfill the requirement for accurate communication among clinicians unless a systematic procedure is carefully followed.

A report of each examination with a clear description of the findings should appear in the patient's record. The format of a written report is not as critical as the information it contains. Standardized reports will facilitate communication and might make the practitioner's time profitability more efficient (13). Regardless of the format, the following

records, and sound scientific investigations depend on standardized terminology and procedures. A description of the scan plane should be included in the record for future reference. Conventional longitudinal and transverse scan planes should be used for examining tendons and ligaments. There are limited applications for oblique or complex scanning planes. Interpretation of nonstandard image planes is difficult and often causes confusion. Detailed descriptions of ultrasound lesions should always include the sonographic appearance of the abnormality in the longitudinal and transverse scan planes. If oblique scanning planes are required, an exact description of the scanning plane should be included in the record.

Diagnostic ultrasound mensuration of tissues is used to discriminate disease from normal tissues. Those lesions that

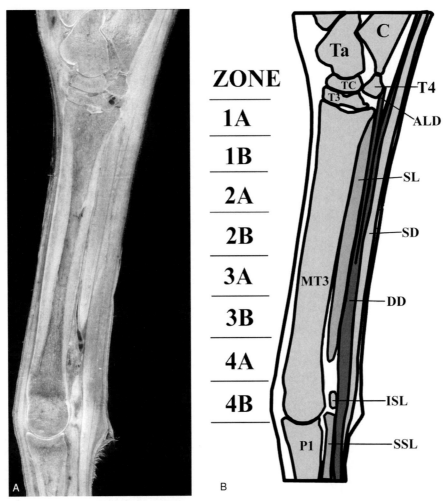

Figure 7.2. Sagittal view of the metatarsus. **A.** Frozen section. **B.** Schematic of frozen section. ALD = accessory ligament of deep digital flexor tendon; DD = deep digital flexor tendon; IC = inferior check ligament; ISL = suspensory ligament; MT3 = third metatarsal bone; P1 = first phalanx; SD = superficial digital flexor tendon; SL = suspensory ligament; SSL = straight sesamoid ligament; Ta = talus bone; TC = central talus bone; T3 = third tarsal bone; T4 = fourth tarsal bone.

information should be included: client name, name of the horse, date of examination, and a description of the findings, including the locations of lesions. The report should record the examining practitioner. Each image should have the examined structures identified (e.g., SD, DD, SL, ICL, etc.) and an accurate record of location, including the scan plane. Clear and concise records will provide better information than hard-copy records of the image. The sonographer's impression during the real-time examination is usually superior to any hard-copy records.

The moving, real-time image contains more information than can be displayed on the frozen image due to the technology of CRT display. This encourages the use of video recording of the examination to capture the real-time effect. Unfortunately, the storage of tapes and the acquisition of the desired images makes this practice less than profitable. Video recordings usually contain the entire examination, and often the viewer loses interest before the diagnostic images are found or the significant images are interspersed among those that are not recognizable or were not impor-

tant. Tape editors are expensive and the time required to edit tapes is not practical for clinical use. Repeat studies to document progress of healing will be facilitated if the record clearly shows the respective initial settings of power, gain, and dynamic range. The CRT adjustment should remain constant and any camera settings should be recorded. Artifacts due to technical errors are often interpreted as clinically significant lesions. The usual method of recording the ultrasound examination is by using a regular video camera recorder (VCR) connected to the video output. This has the added advantage of video recording the clinical appearance of the horse for future reference along with the ultrasound examination. Confusion and expense are added to this procedure when one tries to save cost by recording multiple exams of different animals on the same tape. One tape should be dedicated to a patient until the lameness is resolved and the case is archived. It is easier to copy each horse's complete record to an archive tape than it is to edit the daily exams, locate records, or review cases lost in the video tape. Another method of recording an examination is with Polaroid film, which is both expensive and outdated. Thermal-paper printers are quite effective and give excellent images. They do have the advantage of making multiple copies, and one can provide the clients with their own copy. Matrix cameras are used to record images on x-ray film and have been popular. This technology requires an automatic processor and will probably be phased out by digital images. Thermal printers and video camera recorders are currently the most practical and the most efficient for use in practice.

The potential for using diagnostic ultrasound to investigate changes in equine tendons and ligaments was recognized in the early development of the diagnostic ultrasound in veterinary medicine. However, the introduction of two-dimensional real-time gray-scale ultrasonography made

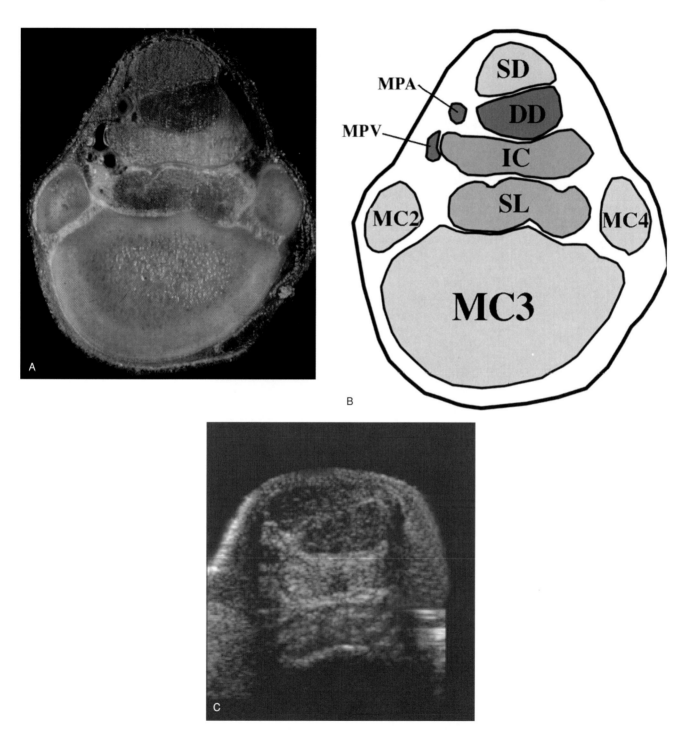

Figure 7.3. Transverse view of zone 1B. **A.** Frozen section. **B.** Schematic of frozen section. **C.** Sonogram. DD = deep digital flexor tendon; IC = inferior check ligament; MC2 = second metacarpal bone; MC3 = third metacarpal bone; MC4 = fourth metacarpal bone; MPA = medial palmar artery; MPV = medial palmar vein; SD = superficial digital flexor tendon; SL = suspensory ligament.

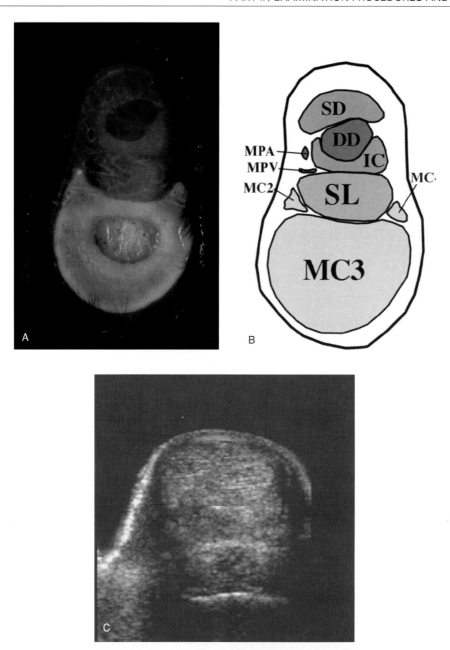

Figure 7.4. Transverse view of zone 2A. **A.** Frozen section. **B.** Schematic of frozen section. **C.** Sonogram. DD = deep digital flexor tendon; IC = inferior check ligament; MC2 = second metacarpal bone; MC3 = third metacarpal bone; MC4 = fourth metacarpal bone; MPA = medial palmar artery; MPV = medial palmar vein; SD = superficial digital flexor tendon; SL = suspensory ligament.

such examinations practical, and excellent ultrasound correlations with anatomy were published (9, 24, 25). Other publications emerged that were misleading and inaccurate (26). The following discussion includes material pertinent to the normal examination of the flexor tendons and ligaments of the distal limb of the horse.

FLEXOR TENDONS AND SUSPENSORY LIGAMENT

Superficial Digital Flexor Tendon (SD)

The superficial flexor tendon has its origin from the medial epicondyle of the distal humerus in the front limb. In the

hind limb, it has its origin from the supracondyloid fossa of the femur and consists of a strong tendon and little muscle located deep to the gastrocnemius muscle. The muscles differ significantly at their origin and insertions, but the area of interest through the metacarpus (tarsus) is essentially the same. An accessory ligament, commonly called the radial or superior check ligament, originates from a ridge on the posterior surface of the radius, at the distal diaphysis near the medial margin. The muscular part of the SD arises from the distal humerus and extends distally, becoming a multipennate tendinous structure at the distal one-third of the radius.

About 10 cm proximal to the carpus the accessory ligament joins the SD. The tendons of the SD and the deep digital flexor tendon (DD) continue distally through the carpal canal enveloped in the carpal synovial sheath (27). Proximal to the carpus the muscle and its tendon can be identified; however, the accessory ligament or radial check ligament can be difficult to image and must be identified by following the muscle tissue from the humeral head distally to its intersection with the accessory ligament. The accessory ligament is a "fan-shaped" band that is bordered on the medial margin by the tendon sheath of the flexor carpi radialis mus-

cle. Below the carpus the tendon remains immediately subcutaneous and may require the use of a standoff or a high-frequency transducer with built-in standoff for a satisfactory image. The SD is slightly hypoechoic to the DD; depending on gain, focal zone, and dynamic range adjustment, they may be isoechoic. The adjacent peritendon of the SD and the DD can usually be differentiated, especially if the limb is slightly extended by "rocking" the horse forward and back while the limb is supporting weight.

The SD emerges from the carpal canal toward the medial palmar quadrant. It is ellipsoid and approximately 7 to 10

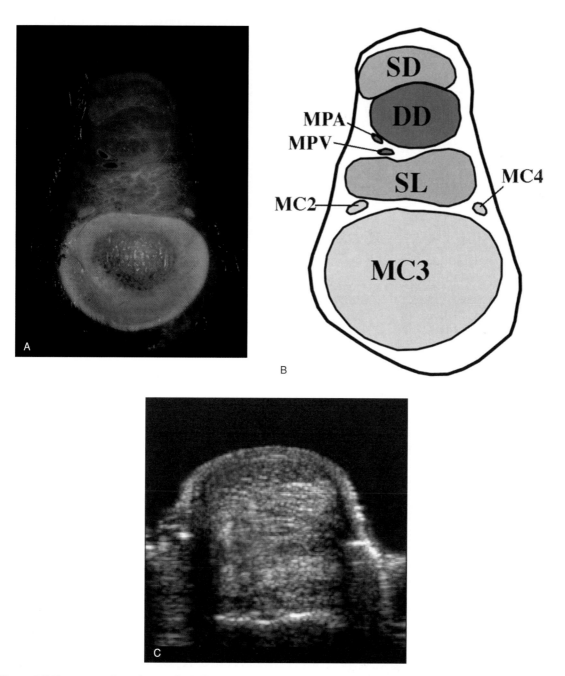

Figure 7.5. Transverse view of zone 2B. **A.** Frozen section. **B.** Schematic of frozen section. **C.** Sonogram. DD = deep digital flexor tendon; MC2 = second metacarpal bone; MC3 = third metacarpal bone; MC4 = fourth metacarpal bone; MPA = medial palmar artery; MPV = medial palmar vein; SD = superficial digital flexor tendon; SL = suspensory ligament.

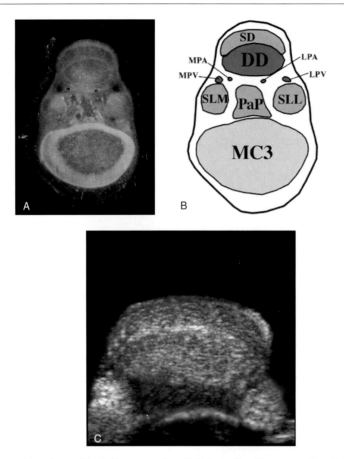

Figure 7.6. Transverse view of zone 3A. **A.** Frozen section. **B.** Schematic of frozen section. **C.** Sonogram. DD = deep digital flexor tendon; LPA = lateral palmar artery; LPV = lateral palmar vein; MC3 = third metacarpal bone; MPA = medial palmar artery; MPV = medial palmar vein; PaP = palmar pouch, metacarpophalangeal joint; SD = superficial digital flexor tendon; SLL = lateral branch of suspensory ligament; SLM = medial branch of suspensory ligament.

mm in dorsal palmar dimension. Through the first 8 cm (Zone 1) distal to the carpus the tendon begins to flatten, but its dorsal-palmar and medial-lateral axes remain approximately equal (Fig. 7.3). Through the middle of the metacarpus (Zone 2), the tendon continues flattening and wraps over the palmar margin of the DD in a "comma" shape with the lateral margin sharp and the medial margin rounded (Fig. 7.4). Complete imaging of the SD cannot be accomplished with any single position of the transducer, and the lateral and medial margins must be defined by repositioning the transducer over those margins. Longitudinal scans provide excellent information with regard to fiber continuity. However, significant core or margin lesions can be missed as a result of the narrow scanning slice of the beam. It is important to locate changes using the transverse scan and then carefully study these areas on longitudinal scans. The subcutaneous surface of the SD may be lost in the near-field artifact unless a standoff is used, and then the margins may be differentiated on both the transverse and longitudinal images. In Zone 2, the SD remains hypoechoic to the inferior check ligament (IC) and isoechoic to the DD (Fig. 7.5). Through the next 8 cm (Zone 3) the SD progressively

flattens, becomes symmetric, and forms a ring that surrounds the DD near the fetlock (Fig. 7.6).

Having encircled the DD, the two tendons pass through the intersesamoidean groove, bound down by the palmar annular ligament, which is essentially fused with the SD. The normal palmar annular ligament may be difficult to differentiate, even when using a standoff, and it should be only 2 to 3 mm thick (Fig. 7.7). Distal to the fetlock and near the distal end of the proximal phalanx the SD divides into two branches that insert on the distal aspect of the first phalanx palmar/plantar to the insertions of the collateral ligaments and at medial and lateral collateral eminence at the proximal margin of the second phalanx palmar/plantar to the insertion of the collateral ligaments of the proximal interphalangeal joint (Fig. 7.8).

Deep Digital Flexor Tendon (DD): Front Limb

The deep digital flexor muscle of the forelimb is the largest muscle of the flexor group and originates from the medial epicondyle of the humerus, the medial surface of the olecranon, and the caudal surface of the mid-diaphysis of the radius and ulna. The muscular tissue will be found deep to the other soft tissues and muscle, particularly the flexors of the

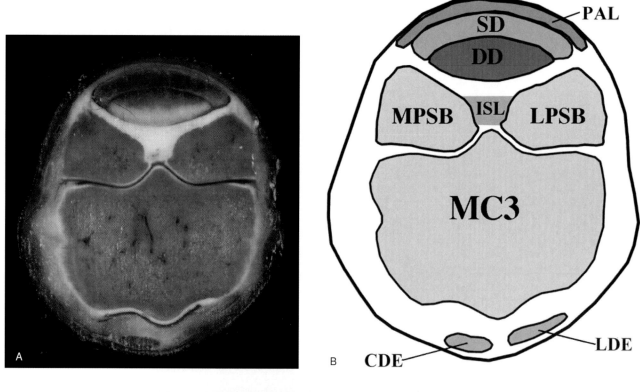

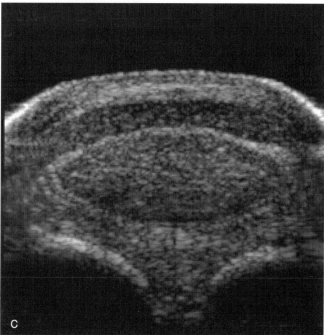

Figure 7.7. Transverse view of zone 3B. **A.** Frozen section. **B.** Schematic of frozen section. **C.** Sonogram. CDE = common digital extensor; DD = deep digital flexor tendon; ISL = intersesamoid ligament; LDE = lateral digital extensor; LPSB = lateral proximal sesamoid bone; MC3 = third metacarpal bone; MPSB = medial proximal sesamoid bone; PAL = palmar annular ligament; SD = superficial digital flexor tendon.

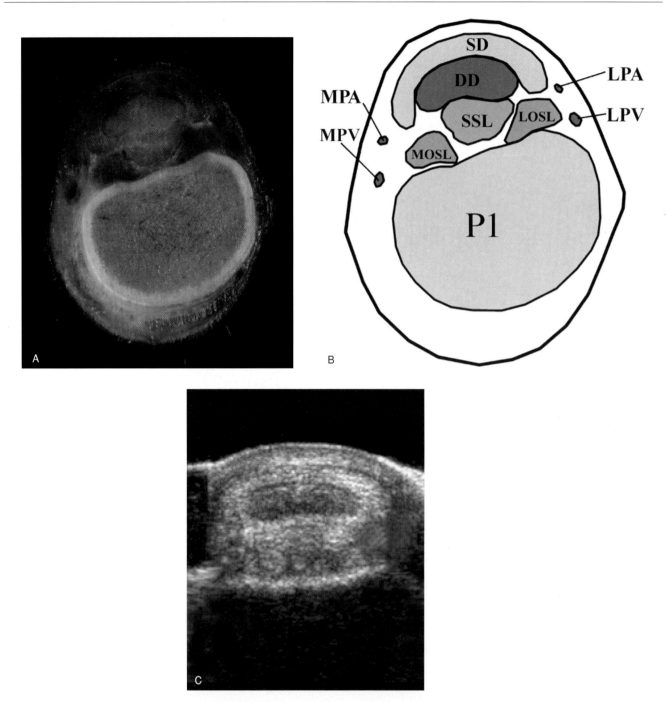

Figure 7.8. Transverse view of zone P1B. **A.** Frozen section. **B.** Schematic of frozen section. **C.** Sonogram. DD = deep digital flexor tendon; LOSL = lateral oblique sesamoid ligament; LPA = lateral palmar artery; LPV = lateral palmar vein; MOSL = medial oblique sesamoid ligament; MPA = medial palmar artery; MPV = medial palmar vein; P1 = first phalanx; SD = superficial digital flexor tendon; SSL = straight sesamoid ligament.

carpus and the superficial digital flexor muscle. The muscle comprises a large humeral head, intermediate ulnar head, and a small radial head (27). Each head has a tendon that emerges about 10 cm proximal to the carpus where they combine and are included with the tendon of the SD through the carpal canal. Emerging from the carpal canal in Zone 1, the DD has a triangular shape on a transverse image (Fig. 7.3). The DD becomes narrower and round as it

nears Zone 2B where it merges with the IC. The IC has its origin from the palmar ligaments of the carpus and may be regarded as the carpal or tendinous head of the DD (27). The IC is broad and rectangular near its origin (Zone 1A) and measures 4 to 7 mm thick and 14 to16 mm wide. It becomes narrower, cuboidal, and more consolidated in Zone 1B and 2A (Fig. 7.4). Through Zone 2 the DD and the IC converge and merge. The IC is hyperechoic to the DD, the

SD, and the suspensory ligament (SL). It becomes isoechoic with the DD as their fibers merge, and the DD becomes larger and rounder than the SD (Fig. 7.5).

Through Zone 3 the DD becomes elliptical as it is surrounded by the SD and compressed into the intersesamoidean groove where the SD and the palmar annular ligament make the bulk of the palmar tissues and the intersesamoidean ligament and the axial surfaces of the sesamoids

make the dorsal, medial, and lateral boundaries, respectively (Fig. 7.7). The DD is wider over the fetlock and narrows through the region of the proximal phalanx. Above the proximal interphalangeal joint the tendon emerges from between the branches of the SD and becomes the most superficial subcutaneous tissue as it separates into distinct medial and lateral bundles (Fig. 7.9). Distal to this area the tendon is difficult to image due to the contours of the superficial tis-

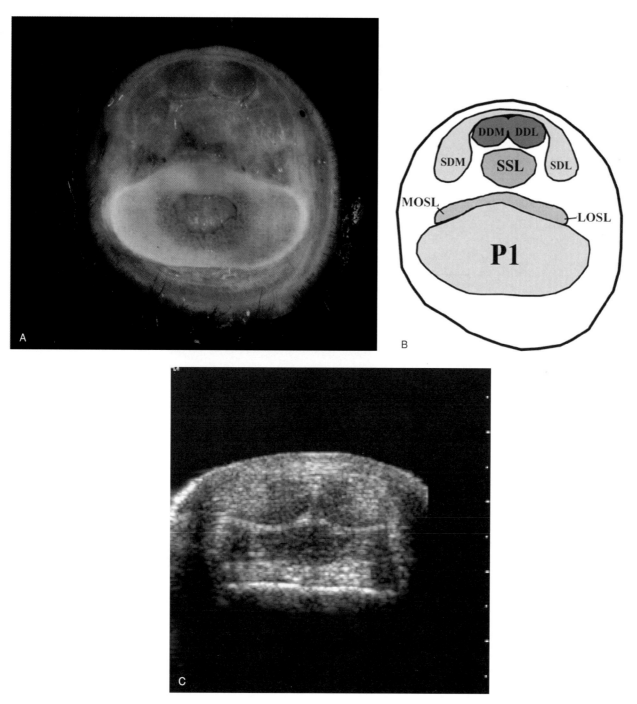

Figure 7.9. Transverse view of zone P1C. **A.** Frozen section. **B.** Schematic of frozen section. **C.** Sonogram. DDL = lateral branch of deep digital flexor tendon; DDM = medial branch of deep digital flexor tendon; LOSL = lateral oblique sesamoid ligament; MOSL = medial oblique sesamoid ligament; P1 = first phalanx; SDM = lateral branch of superficial digital flexor tendon; SDM = medial branch of superficial digital flexor tendon; SSL = straight sesamoid ligament.

sue and problems maintaining a critical angle of reflection. The DD continues over the distal sesamoid (navicular bone) to insert at the semilunar crest of the palmar margin of the third phalanx.

Deep Digital Flexor Tendon: Hind Limb

The DD in the hind limb has its origin from three muscle heads, a strong lateral flexor that has superficial and deep heads (*tibialis posterior and flexor hallucis longus*), respectively, and a smaller medial head (*long digital flexor*) (27). The tendons of the deep heads combine and form one tendon that passes over the sustentaculum tali within the tarsal sheath. The tendon of the medial head passes over the proximal tubercle of the talus and fuses with the lateral tendon in Zone 1 of the metatarsus. The accessory ligament (IC) is not as significant in the hind limb and merges with the DD in Zone 3A.

Suspensory Ligament (SL)

The suspensory ligament has similar origin and appearance in both the front and hind limbs, although it is more developed in the front limbs. The suspensory ligament is a modification of the muscles *Interossei*. They are three in number and originate from the proximal margin of the metacarpal bones. The medial and lateral muscles are small and have insignificant tendons that are lost in the palmar fascia. The *interosseus medius* muscle has its origin from the proximal palmar aspect of the third metacarpal and from the distal row of carpal bones. It has been modified into the ligamentous structure called the suspensory ligament or superior sesamoidean ligament (27). In most horses it contains very little muscular tissue, although the amount of muscle tissue remaining may vary between the forelimbs and the hind limbs of the same horse or among breeds; it was shown to be greater by 40% in Standardbreds than in Thoroughbreds (28). The remaining muscle may hypertrophy in well-trained and fit horses, giving some variability to the echoic texture of the structure. The SL has a more complex texture than the SD, DD, or IC due to the variable muscle it contains. Despite this, the SL is generally hyperechoic to the DD, the SD, and at least the proximal part of the IC. Distribution of muscle is more in the proximal portion of the ligament and diminishes distally. Anechoic or hypoechoic areas and complex patterns in the proximal SL may be a function of hypertrophy of the muscle fibers and may be bilateral. Similar areas in the distal ligament or branches should be considered abnormal.

The SL is broad and flat in Zone 1 and may not be distinctly separated from the third metacarpal (Fig. 7.3). The SL, in Zone 2, is distinctly separated from the third metacarpal bone and the IC/DD by hypoechoic connective tissue (Fig. 7.5). In the proximal part of Zone 3, the SL divides into diverging medial and lateral branches, each passing obliquely distally to the abaxial surface of the respective proximal sesamoid bone (Fig. 7.6). It can be quite difficult

to image the branches in transverse plane unless one palpates the branch and places the transducer while watching the horse's leg and not the ultrasound image. Near the branch, the ligament is oval and it becomes more triangular as it nears the proximal sesamoid. The branches contain essentially no muscle tissue and have a homogenous, hyperechoic texture. Both branches are approximately equal in diameter and should be less than 1 cm in the normal adult racehorse. The majority of insertion occurs at the abaxial surface of the proximal sesamoid bones, although some ligament tissue extends distally and dorsally to join the extensor tendon. The abaxial surface of the proximal sesamoid has a smooth, curved surface that forms a crisp interface at its junction with the suspensory ligament branch, especially on the longitudinal scan (Fig. 7.10). The intersesamoidean ligament (ISL) can be visualized as a hyperechoic tissue between the axial surfaces of the proximal sesamoid bones (Fig. 7.7). The suspensory ligament and its branches are essentially the same in the hind legs, except the shape is more rectangular and the ligament is usually slightly larger than in the front.

The palmar vasculature consists of the medial palmar artery and vein and the lateral palmar artery in Zones 1A to 3A, located in the connective tissue between the SL and the DD. Zone 3B and distal have paired vascular structures (medial and lateral palmar digital arteries and veins) located in the subcutaneous connective tissue superficial to the distal sesamoidean ligaments and the flexor tendons. Vascular structures are anechoic, circular in cross-section, and tubular in longitudinal planes. The arteries can be recognized by pulsation equivalent to the heart rate and the veins by compressibility under pressure from the transducer and distention when occluded. Blood flow may be detected as an intraluminal, composite, swirling motion when using high-resolution transducers.

Distal Sesamoidean Ligaments (DSL)

Diagnostic ultrasound examination of the equine limb distal to the metacarpo(tarso)phalangeal joint requires the same patient preparation, but may require additional restraint. Examination is made difficult by the position of the pastern relative to the ground. "End-fire" transducers may be difficult to position perpendicular to the palmar surface of the pastern due to interference with the floor. The examination may be made easier with the foot positioned more caudal as is done when proximal distal palmar radiographic projections of the navicular bone are made (e.g., flexor or tangential view). Also, the horse may be made to stand on a block, elevating the feet from the floor. It is best to make the initial examination with the horse bearing weight. The limb may then be flexed and extended and examined with no weight or tension on the stay apparatus, which will facilitate detection of adhesions.

Reference zones designated P1A, P1B, P1C, P2A, and P2B have been defined for the pastern (29). These zones are self explanatory in reference to the proximal, middle, and

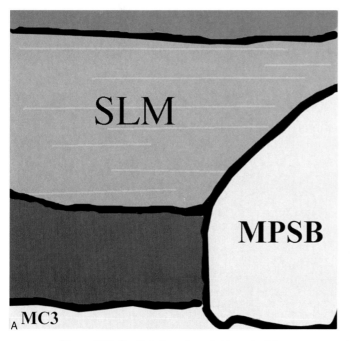
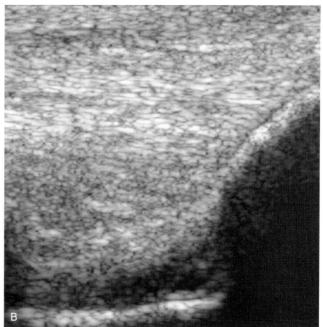

Figure 7.10. Sagittal view of medial branch of the suspensory ligament. **A.** Schematic of the insertion of the medial branch of suspensory ligament at the medial proximal sesamoid bone. **B.** Sonogram. MC3 = third metacarpal bone; MPSB = medial proximal sesamoid bone; SLM = medial branch of suspensory ligament.

distal one-third of the first phalanx (P1) and the proximal and distal one-half of the second phalanx (P2) (Fig. 7.11).

The DD and SD have previously been described as they pass through the fetlock canal to their respective insertions. There is essentially no major differences between the front limb and the hind limb distal to the fetlock joint. Below the fetlock joint, the SD forms a symmetric arc as it surrounds the DD. The SD progressively thins at the mid-pastern level in its central palmar/plantar-dorsal aspect as the medial and lateral abaxial branches become prominent (Fig. 7.8). In the distal aspect of the pastern, the SD is no longer visualized as the medial and lateral branches insert palmar/plantar to the collateral ligament insertions at the distal end of the proximal phalanx and on the palmar/plantar, proximal end of the middle phalanx. The DD tendon can be followed below the fetlock to the distal aspect of the pastern. Proximally, the DD is large, oval, and clearly visualized between the SD and the SSL (Fig. 7.8). The DD becomes bilobed in the mid-pastern and has distinct separation between the medial and lateral bundles (Fig.7.9). Distally the bilobed DD can be followed in transverse scanning planes to the level of the proximal second phalanx (P2). At this level the hyperechoic fibrocartilage of the middle scutum (MS) becomes a prominent feature deep to the DD. Sagittal planes can be used to image the pastern if a small transducer is available. The contour of the palmar/plantar pastern region usually limits sagittal imaging to the mid-zones (P1B-P2A) when using linear-array probes (Fig. 7.11). The most proximal and distal pastern regions can be examined in transverse image planes or with the use of a high-frequency sector probe.

Standoff pads can be used in the pastern, but the contours are complex and care must be taken to avoid misleading artifacts.

The distal sesamoidean ligaments (DSL) are continuations of the branches of the suspensory ligament, but are not true extensions of that tissue since the sesamoid bones are intercalated and serve an integral function in the continuity of the stay apparatus. The deep or cruciate sesamoidean ligaments (DDSL) are two, short bands of tissue that extend from the dorsal distal margin (base) of the respective sesamoid toward the opposite proximal palmar/plantar eminence of the proximal phalanx. These structures are small and closely associated with palmar tissues of the joint and the bone and are difficult to define during a routine ultrasound examination of the limb. The middle distal or oblique sesamoidean ligament (ODSL) originates as two, thick, triangular ligaments from the distal margins of the proximal sesamoids and a thin, central part from the distal margin of the intersesamoidean ligament. The medial oblique sesamoidean ligament (MOSL) and the lateral oblique sesamoidean ligament (LOSL) converge distally to insert on a triangular roughened surface on the palmar/plantar cortex of the proximal phalanx. This ligament is recognized by its triangular shape near the proximal sesamoids, which narrows rapidly distally as it approaches its insertion. It is the structure located adjacent to the underlying bone (Fig. 7.9).

The superficial or straight sesamoidean ligament (SDSL) is a flat, thin band that is wide at its origin from the distal margins of the sesamoids and becomes narrower near its in-

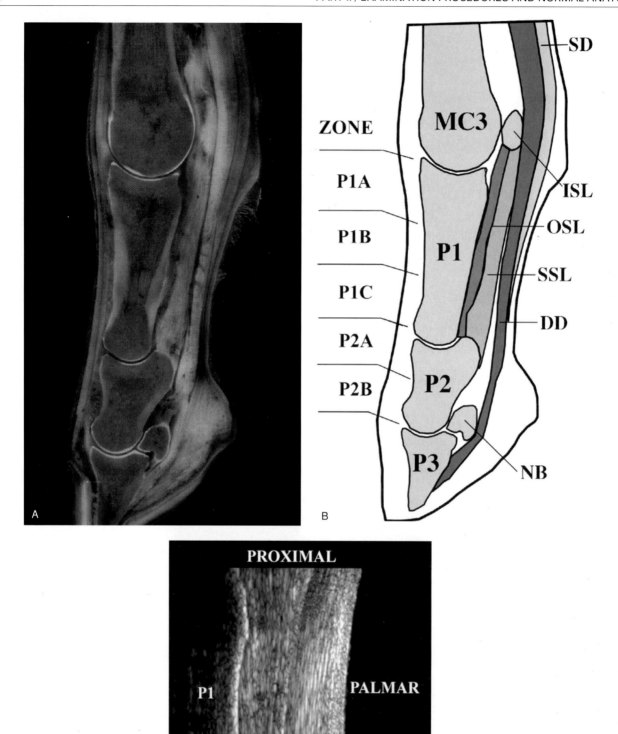

Figure 7.11. Sagittal view of the pastern. **A.** Frozen section. **B.** Schematic of frozen section. **C.** Sonogram of mid-pastern. DD = deep digital flexor tendon; ISL = intersesamoid ligament; MC3 = third metacarpal bone; NB = navicular bone; OSL = oblique sesamoid ligament; P1 = first phalanx; P2 = second phalanx; P3 = third phalanx; SD = superficial digital flexor tendon; SSL = straight sesamoid ligament.

sertion at the proximal palmar/plantar fibrocartilage eminence of the middle phalanx. This ligament is located between the DD and the ODSL. It is broad and flat near its origin and narrows slightly as it progresses distally to its insertion (Fig. 7.10). The distal sesamoidean ligaments are more easily recognized if the structures are tracked from origin to insertion. They are normally more coarse and slightly hyperechoic compared with the flexor tendons. The SDSL is surrounded by hypoechoic or anechoic tissue distally and is the most recognizable of the structures in the pastern.

Successful ultrasound examination of the flexor tendons and ligaments in the horse requires a combination of appropriate use of the ultrasound equipment and a good knowledge of normal anatomy. Tissue echogenicity and texture are important, but artifacts and improper equipment settings may lead to fictitious results and serious diagnostic errors.

REFERENCES

1. Rantanen NW, Genovese RL, Gaines R. The use of diagnostic ultrasound to detect structural damage to the soft tissues of the extremities of horses. J Equine Vet Sci 1983;3:134–135.

2. Hauser ML, Rantanen NW, Genovese RL. Suspensory desmitis: diagnosis using real-time ultrasound imaging. J Equine Vet Sci 1984;4:258–283.

3. Hauser ML, Rantanen NW, Genovese RL. Ultrasound anatomy and scanning technique of the distal extremities in the horse. Proc Am Assoc Equine Practitioners 1985;31:693–699.

4. Genovese RL, Rantanen NW, Hauser ML, et al. Clinical application of diagnostic ultrasound to the equine limb. Proc Am Assoc Equine Practitioners 1985;31:701–721.

5. Yeh HC, Wolf BS. A simple portable water bath for superficial ultrasonography. Am J Roentgenol 1978;130:257–258.

6. Claes HP, Reygaerts DO, Boven FA, et al. An echo-free silicon elastomer block for ultrasonography. Radiology 1984;150:596.

7. Chan B, Merton-Gaythorpe JV, Kadaba MP, et al. Acoustic properties of polyvinyl chloride gelatin for use in ultrasonography. Radiology 1984;152:215–216.

8. Pharr JW, Nyland TG. Sonography of the equine palmar metacarpal soft tissues. Vet Radiol 1984;25:265–273.

9. Biller DS, Myer W. Ultrasound scanning of superficial structures using an ultrasound standoff pad. Vet Radiol 1988;29:138–142.

10. Wood W, Newell WH, Borg RP. An ultrasonographic off-set system for examination of equine tendons and ligaments. Am J Vet Res 1991;52:1945–1947.

11. Henry GA, Patton CS, Goble DO. Ultrasonographic evaluation of iatrogenic injuries of the equine accessory (carpal check) ligament and superficial digital flexor tendon. Vet Radiol 1986;27:132–140.

12. Crass JR, van de Vegte GL, Harkavy LA. Tendon echogenicity: ex vivo study. Radiology 1988;167:499–501.

13. McClellan PD. A proposal for standardization in sonographic imaging. I. Metacarpus and metatarsus. J Equine Vet Sci 1986; 6:327–328.

14. Guidelines for performance of ultrasound examinations in large animals. Veterinary Ultrasound Society and American College of Veterinary Radiology, 1994, in preparation.

15. Craychee TJ. Ultrasonographic evaluation of equine musculoskeletal injury. In: Nyland TG, Matoon JS, eds. Veterinary diagnostic ultrasound. Philadelphia: WB Saunders, 1995.

16. Smith RKW, Jones R, Webbon PM. The cross-sectional areas of normal equine digital flexor tendons determined ultrasonographically. Equine Vet J 1994;26:460–465.

17. Cuesta I, Riber C, Pinedo M, et al. Ultrasonographic measurement of palmar metacarpal tendon and ligament structures in the horse. Vet Radiol Ultrasound 1995;36:131–136.

18. Reef VB, Martin BB, Elser A. Types of tendon and ligament injuries detected with diagnostic ultrasound: description and follow-up. Proc Am Assoc Equine Practitioners 1988;34:245–248.

19. Genovese RL, Rantanen NW, Hauser ML, et al. Diagnostic ultrasonography of equine limbs. Vet Clin North Am Equine Pract 1986;2:145–225.

20. Nicoll RG, Wood AKW, Martin ICA. Ultrasonographic observations of the flexor tendons and ligaments of the metacarpal region of horses. Am J Vet Res 1993;54:502–506.

21. Gillis CL, Meagher DM, Peal RR, et al. Ultrasonographically detected changes in the equine superficial digital flexor tendon during the first month of race training. Am J Vet Res 1993;54: 1797–1802.

22. Nicoll RG, Wood AKW, Rothwell TLW. Ultrasonographical and pathological studies of equine superficial digital flexor tendons: initial observations, including tissue characterisation by analysis of image grey scale, in a Thoroughbred gelding. Equine Vet J 1992;24: 318–320.

23. Pugh CR. A simple method to document the location of ultrasonographically detected equine tendon lesions. Vet Radiol Ultrasound 1993;34:211–212.

24. Hauser ML, Rantanen NW. Ultrasound appearance of the palmar metacarpal soft tissues of the horse. J Equine Vet Sci 1982; 2:19–22.

25. Hauser ML. Ultrasonographic appearance and correlative anatomy of the soft tissues of the distal extremities in the horse. Vet Clin North Am Equine Pract 1986;2:127–144.

26. MacKay-Smith M, Lieberman B. Aiding hands-on diagnosis: ultrasound's probing nature reveals the secrets of soft-tissue injuries. Equus 1985;94:26–29.

27. Sisson S, Grossman JD. The anatomy of the domestic animals. Philadelphia: WB Saunders, 1961.

28. Wilson DA, Baker GJ, Pijanowski GJ, et al. Composition and morphologic features of the interosseous muscle in Standardbreds and Thoroughbreds. Am J Vet Res 1991;52:133–139.

29. McClellan PD, Colby J. Ultrasonic structure of the pastern. Equine Vet Sci 1986;6:99–101.

8. Ultrasound Artifacts

ROBERT H. WRIGLEY

Image artifacts in ultrasound result from the display of erroneous returning echoes or the absence of echoes. Unfortunately, artifactual echoes arae displayed almost constantly during ultrasound imaging. Often, artifacts degrade the diagnostic information and make it more difficult to distinguish normal tissue from pathologic changes. A few artifacts exist, however, that provide important diagnostic information and should not be overlooked. The diagnostician needs to be able to distinguish between such false information and the true ultrasonographic display of the patient. To alleviate this continual problem, the ultrasonographer needs to recognize the artifactual display as it occurs and readjust the equipment or redirect the beam to achieve a more accurate display of the ultrasound characteristics of the underlying tissues.

Ultrasound machines have been designed to compute images using the following simple assumptions: sound travels only in a straight line; echoes result only from objects directly beneath the transducer; the intensity of the reflected echoes is directly proportional to the nature of the acoustic interface; and the speed of sound is constant in patient tissue.

Unfortunately, these assumptions do not hold up during ultrasonography of complex heterogeneous materials in living tissues. Erroneous echoes are detected; the relative intensity of these echoes may be incorrect and the location of the reflectors may be miscalculated, leading to an incorrect sonographic display of the patient (1).

ERRORS FROM SOUND REFLECTION

The echoes resulting from a single acoustic interface aligned perpendicular to the ultrasound beam are proportional to the difference in acoustic impedance between the two layers. However, in diagnostic ultrasonography acoustic boundaries are numerous, often one on top of another. The intensity of the returning echoes from the deeper boundaries is perturbed as the echo traverses back through the more superficial acoustic boundaries towards the transducer. As a result, the display of the echoes from deeper boundaries becomes less accurate. Also, the direction of reflected echoes depends on the angle of incidence to the acoustic interface. If the sound beam is perpendicular to an interface, then the generated echo returns directly towards the transducer. However, if the angle of insonation deviates from perpendicular, then the echoes move off in a path that makes them less likely to be received by the transducer. The echos generated by tissue boundaries scanned at oblique angles may never reach the transducer.

The echogenicity of uniform parenchymal tissue such as liver and spleen results from diffuse backscatter. The parenchyma is equally echogenic irrespective of the insonation angle because the backscatter is directionally independent. However, the echogenicity of parenchymal tissues made of orderly layering of parenchyma varies depending on the sound beam angle. Significant direction-dependent echogenicity was observed in the myocardium (2), skeletal musculature (3), tendons (4), and renal cortex (5). The echogenicity of equine tendons and ligaments depends on the ultrasound beam angle. Perpendicular alignment of the sound beam to the tendon and ligaments results in maximal backscatter and repeatable optimal images. Slight off perpendicular insonation leads to artifactual hypoechoic regions (Fig. 8.1A and B).

Echoes can also interact with several differently aligned reflectors and eventually return unexpectedly to the transducer. The relative intensity of such multipath echoes no longer represents the original acoustic interface; thus, the echoes are displayed by the computer with incorrect brightness. Also, the multiple reflections increase the distance of tissue through which the echo traveled and so delay the arrival of the echo. The computer then displays the echo with an incorrect intensity and incorrect location (6). Occasionally, mirrored duplicate images are observed in the far field. This can occur when an object is imaged close to a highly reflective curved surface such as the diaphragm or large bowel. A simultaneous display of the superficial object can be generated by additional reflections from deeper acoustic interfaces.

In heterogeneous living tissue, many acoustic interfaces are not perpendicular to the sound beam unless the ultrasonographer purposely realigns the sound beam to optimize the insonation angle of a selected boundary. Therefore, at any particular time during the examination some interfaces are optimally displayed and others suboptimally or not at all. Boundaries appear to come and go as the region is scanned. In addition, incorrect machine readjustment can introduce additional artifacts. In this way, the operator can compound the already difficult situation.

ERRORS FROM VARIATIONS IN SOUND VELOCITY

The speed of sound varies slightly in each tissue and fluid compartment. Slight bending (refraction) of the sound beam occurs as the sound traverses through regions of differing sound velocity. The refraction of the sound beam results in slight miscalculation of the source of returning echoes (6–8). Thus, variance in sound velocities result in reflectors being improperly positioned on the display.

Sound velocity is very different in air and bone than in the surrounding tissues. However, in the design of the ultrasound machine, it is assumed that the sound velocity is

119

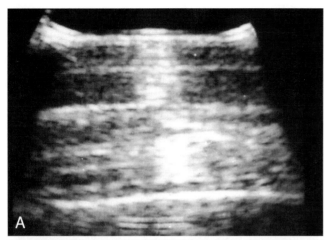

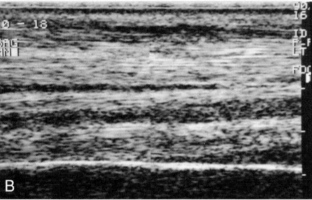

Figure 8.1. A, Longitudinal ultrasonogram made of equine tendons with a 7-MHz sector transducer and built in stand-off. The tendons directly under the center of the transducer were more echogenic than those in the proximal or distal regions. This artifactual varying echogenicity resulted from an optimal angle of incidence occurring in the center of the sweeping sector beam and suboptimal scan angles in the more proximal and distal tendons. **B**, Longitudinal ultrasonogram of equine metacarpal flexor tendons made by a 7-MHz linear transducer. The ultrasound beam was aligned at right angles throughout the length of the tendons and ligaments. Optimal angles of reflection occurred throughout the entire region and so echogenicity of proximal and distal structures remained constant.

constant throughout all patient tissues. When a constant sound velocity is assumed for soft tissues, the elapsed travel time of the returning echoes allows the computer to display the soft tissue echoes at the correct depth on the display screen. However, once the sound beam passes into gas pockets such as air in the lungs or bowel, the depth display of echoes is erroneous because the roundtrip travel time is lengthened by the slower speed of sound in gases. The converse occurs in bone, in which sound travels faster than it does in soft tissue. These errors introduced by gases and bone combined with the high reflectivity of the interface between soft tissue and gas and between soft tissue and bone result in erroneous information deep to layers of gas and bone. An important diagnostic principle is that once the sound beam interacts with gas and bone, then diagnostic information obtained from deeper layers is erroneous.

ERRORS RESULTING FROM BEAM SIZE

Beam size is a major limiting factor in the resolution of images obtained by scanning systems. Sound naturally diverges from its source spreading ever wider into the surrounding media. Unfortunately, the natural widening of the ultrasound beam reduces the resolution of the ultrasound images. To control beam size, additional sound is directed beside the main sound beam to help focus the main beam (9). These side, or grating, lobes beside the main sound beam can generate echoes if strong reflectors occur beside the main beam (9). These echoes appear above highly reflective curved surfaces and in the image of organs positioned beside intense reflectors such as gas or bone. The echoes are especially noticeable along curved edges or in anechoic fluid-filled structures (Fig. 8.2). Such echoes can create a diagnostic dilemma until the region is rescanned in another plane and true repeating structures become evident.

At depths at which the main sound beam is wider than the distance between individual reflectors, echoes from unrelated objects become summated and displayed erroneously as single objects on the image (1). Patient detail is lost. Resolution can be improved by improvement of beam focusing at the depth of diagnostic interest. Optimization of the beam focus is critical to obtaining high-resolution images. The ultrasonographer's options include changing to another transducer focused at the depth of maximal diagnostic interest or inserting acoustic stand-off materials between the transducer and the skin to raise the focal depth towards the surface. The most flexible approach is to use multicrystal transducers that allow adjustable focal depths because with these the ultrasonographer can optimize the resolution.

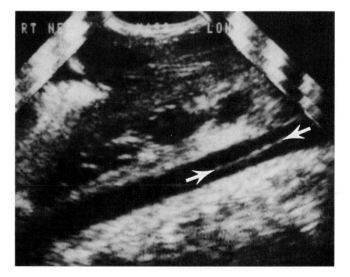

Figure 8.2. Sector scan ultrasonogram of an equine neck. Abscesses were present superficial to the carotid artery. An echogenic linear line (*arrows*) was evident within the carotid artery. This line would disappear when the transducer was moved slightly to the side or pressed downwards. The echogenic line was an artifact, most likely arising from beam sidelobes generating echoes from the adjacent air-filled trachea.

JUNCTIONAL ZONES BETWEEN ORGANS

When the ultrasound beam is centered over a vertical junction between two objects with greatly differing acoustic properties, erroneous echo intensities may be displayed. This results from averaging of the echo formation from each side of the boundary. This effect of section thickness causes a transient echogenic appearance that is uncharacteristic of either side of the boundary (10). Section thickness artifacts are especially noticeable on the edge of vertical fluid boundaries because increased echoes now appear within the fluid. The true echogenic nature of the region can be determined by redirecting the transducer so that the sound beam is perpendicular to the acoustic boundary.

RANDOM SPECKLE

The flickering display in an ultrasound image is, in part, the result of electronic noise in the ultrasound machine circuits, electrical power fluctuations, and the flicker of the televised display. In addition, random patterns of constructive and destructive interference occur in the returning wave fronts, resulting in transient echo patterns that do not accurately reflect the acoustic boundaries in the patient (11). The ultrasonographer may unintentionally exaggerate the random speckle by using too high a brightness setting on the television monitor or by excessive gain. Some ultrasound machines allow frame averaging memory to purposefully reduce the appearance of the random speckle.

REVERBERATION ARTIFACTS

Numerous overlying reflectors in the sound path may cause the sound to be reflected back and forth between them. This sound-trapping effect, known as *reverberation,* occurs between highly reflective acoustic interfaces (1). Reverberation occurs between the surface of the transducer and the skin, resulting in a constant set of echogenic lines being displayed at the top of the image irrespective of the placement of the transducer. This imaging dead zone prohibits visualization of very superficial structures. In addition, reverberation artifacts occur whenever the sound beam passes into gas cavities such as trapped air in the hair coat, lungs, or bowel. Such reverberation results in multiple echoes returning over and over again to the transducer. The ultrasound machine displays these erroneous echoes as banded lines or an echogenic haze over the boundaries of deeper reflectors (Fig. 8.3). When a great deal of sound becomes trapped in such gaseous resonate cavities, the sound beam may not be able to reach the underlying deeper structures. As a result, black areas (acoustic shadows) are observed deep to many reverberation artifacts. Less severe reverberation occurs at fluid–tissue and tissue–tissue interfaces. A haze of gray echoes may be observed in the superficial layers of water-filled cavities because of reverberation at the fluid–tissue interface. The appearance of such reverberation artifact can be suppressed by reducing the time gain setting at this depth level.

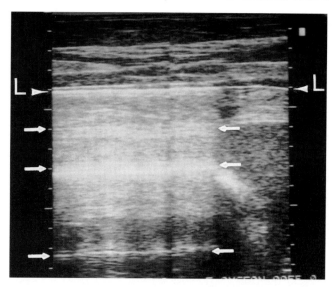

Figure 8.3. Transverse ultrasonogram made at the right fourteenth intercostal space of a horse. The echogenic surface of the lungs was identified (L). Repeating lines (*arrows*) occurred deep to the lung surface from reverberation artifacts resulting from repeated reflections between the lungs, subcutaneous fat, and the transducer. The reverberation echoes were superimposed over the echoes from the underlying tissue and prevented evaluation of the liver.

Recognition of reverberation in patient tissues is of diagnostic assistance because the lung or bowel gas can be located (Figs. 8.3 and 8.4). Unfortunately, reverberation prevents accurate imaging of the underlying tissues because reverberating echoes are superimposed over the real echoes and acoustic shadows occur (1). Successful imaging of underlying tissues can be achieved only by realignment of the

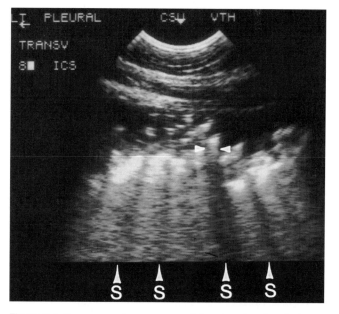

Figure 8.4. Transverse ultrasonogram of the pleural cavity of a horse with anaerobic bacterial pleuritis. The air bubbles resulted in hyperechoic foci with incomplete far field acoustic shadows (S). Unlike ribs, the shadows tend to begin as a transient echogenic region (*arrows*) and appear similar to a comet tail.

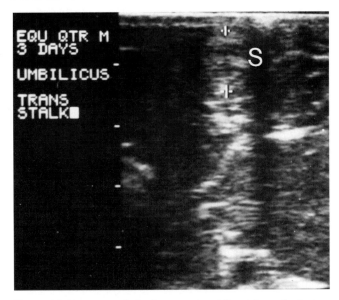

Figure 8.5. Sonogram of a foal's external umbilicus. Acoustic shadow (S) originated beside the umbilicus (marked with calipers). This artifact was from unequal transducer contact pressure and a small amount of air trapped beside the bulge of the umbilicus. Irregular transducer contact on the skin resulted in uneven transmission of sound into the patient and incomplete echo detection. Better acoustic coupling to the patient was achieved by clipping away the hair stubble and using additional ultrasound coupling gel.

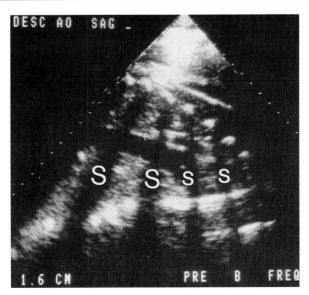

Figure 8.6. Transabdominal ultrasonogram of a third trimester foal. A series of multiple acoustic shadows arise from the ribs of the foal (S). Detection of the source of shadowing artifacts is a useful diagnostic tool because the shadows typically arise from calcified structures and larger foreign bodies. In this case the shadows identified the ribs and helped locate the foal's thorax.

sound beam or displacement of the gas (such as by transrectal manipulation) to achieve an alternative sound pathway. Reverberation artifacts from air can be eliminated and sound transmission improved by massaging acoustic coupling agents into the skin or by carefully shaving away hair stubble to remove air trapped on the skin (Fig. 8.5).

All water-based transducer standoffs create reverberation artifacts in the tissues at depths equal to the thickness of the stand-off. This limits applications of such transducers to organs that are no thicker than the stand-off. The problem is lessened, but not eliminated, by use of silicone or other stand-off pads that have acoustic properties more similar to those of soft tissues.

ATTENUATION ARTIFACTS

Acoustic shadowing results from the sound beam interacting with a highly reflective acoustic boundary such as bone, calculi, or gas. Such objects cause a high degree of reflection that markedly attenuates the ultrasound beam and blocks the pathway of echoes from the deeper layers. This shadowing phenomenon has diagnostic application because recognition of the blocked-out tissues (i.e., the shadow) helps localize bone (Fig. 8.6), calcification, calculi, and gas (see Fig. 8.4) (13). Differentiation between reverberation shadowing from gas and reflective shadowing is sometimes difficult. Careful evaluation of the transition between the reflector and the shadow is helpful. Reverberation shadows are preceded by a transitional zone of less intense echoes. Reflective shadows tend to arise abruptly. A calculus or bubble of gas smaller than the diameter of the sound beam may not cause

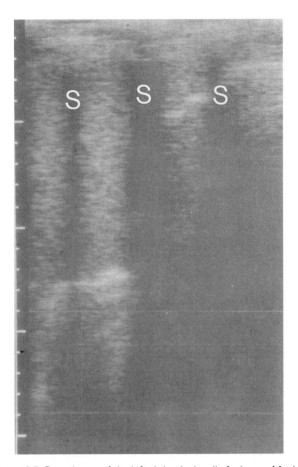

Figure 8.7. Dorsal scan of the left abdominal wall of a horse. Much of the underlying spleen tissue was not detected because large acoustic shadows (S) were present. These shadows resulted from the reflection and attenuation of the sound by the ribs. The shadows were eliminated when the transducer was turned to a transverse intercostal scan plane located between the ribs.

shadowing because all of the sound is not blocked. If the ultrasound beam can be narrowed by additional focusing, the characteristic shadows will occur and so help establish a diagnosis (14–16).

Far-field acoustic shadowing also occurs at the tangent to curved objects. This shadowing results from bending of the sound beam by reflection on the edge of the curved border and by refraction in the objects. The bending of the sound beam results in a sound void, leading to the shadow below the edge of the curved structure. Unfortunately, acoustic shadowing prevents evaluation of deeper structures. Often, underlying objects are momentarily hidden until the beam is realigned to direct the shadow into a different plane (Fig. 8.7).

ACOUSTIC ENHANCEMENT

Increased echogenicity is observed in the tissues deep to fluid-filled structures. This enhancement (far-field enhancement, or through transmission) results from relatively increased amplitude of the deeper echoes by an overlying structure of low attenuation (1). Most commonly this artifactual enhancement occurs deep to anechoic fluid (Fig. 8.8). The recognition of the far-field enhancement artifact helps characterize the fluid contents of the more superficial object.

LIMITS OF RESOLUTION

Deeper Tissue Visualization

In addition to shadowing from overlying bone or gas, excessive sound attenuation in overlying tissues may prevent visualization of deeper tissues because the region is mostly blocked out and anatomic structures are not displayed. Often this is a problem in evaluating the deeper thoracic and

abdominal organs in large horses. Low-frequency transducers (1.5 to 3.5 Mhz) are necessary to penetrate deeply; however, many veterinarians do not have low-frequency transducers. Additional visualization of the deeper regions may be obtained by shaving away hair stubble, setting the focus to the deepest setting, and maximizing the overall and far-field gain controls.

Tissue Fine Detail

The frequency of the transducer is an important determinant of the resolution of multiple overlying acoustic boundaries. When fine detailed images are required (i.e., tendons) higher frequency transducers (7 Mhz) should be selected. The focal depth of the beam should be in the level of maximal diagnostic interest to obtain best detail, and frame averaging should be activated to reduce the random speckle artifacts. Then it is important to stop patient motion and scan very slowly over the region of interest. For fast-moving objects such as heart valves, detail also depends on the scan frame rate. The machine should be reset to the highest frame rate and frame averaging turned off.

SUMMARY

Some artifacts (reverberation, shadowing, and far-field enhancement) are helpful because they aid in interpretation and diagnosis. Other artifacts degrade resolution and cause erroneous images that may lead to errors of interpretation. An understanding of the causes and appearance of ultrasonographic artifacts aids diagnosis.

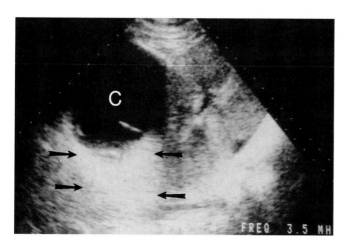

Figure 8.8. Dorsal ultrasonogram of an equine right kidney. A large fluid-filled cortical cyst (C) was present. The tissues directly deep to the cyst appeared artifactually echogenic (*arrows*). Such far-field acoustic enhancement occurs below water-filled structures and helps differentiate simple cysts from poorly echogenic tissues.

REFERENCES

1. Kremkau FW, Taylor JW. Artifacts in ultrasound imaging. J Ultrasound Med 1986;5:227–237.
2. Miller JO, Perez JE, Mottley JC, et al. Myocardial tissue characterization: an approach based on quantitative backscatter and attenuation. Proceedings of the Institute of Electrical and Electronic Engineers Ultrasound Symposium CH 1947-1, 1983, 782–793.
3. Mol CR, Breddels PA. Ultrasound velocity in muscle. J Acoust Soc Am 1982;71:455–461.
4. Fornage B. The hypoechoic normal tendon—a pitfall. J Ultrasound Med 1987;6:19–22.
5. Rubin JM, Carson PL, Meyer CR. Anisotropic ultrasonic backscatter from the renal cortex. Ultrasound Med Biol 1988;14:507–511.
6. Kremkau FW. Diagnostic ultrasound: principles, instrumentation and exercises. 2nd ed. Orlando: Grune & Stratton, 1984.
7. Muller N, Cooperberg PL, Rowley VA, et al. Ultrasonic refraction by the rectus abdominis muscles: the double image artifact. J Ultrasound Med 1984;3:515.
8. Buttery B, Davison G. The ghost artifact. J Ultrasound Med 1984; 3:49.
9. Laing FC, Kurtz AB. The importance of ultrasonic sidelobe artifacts. Radiology 1982;145:763–768.
10. Goldstein A, Madrazo BL. Slice-thickness artifacts in gray-scale ultrasound. J Clin Ultrasound 1981;9:365.

11. Wells PNT, Halliwell M. Speckle in ultrasonic imaging. Ultrasonics 1981;19:225.
12. Fried AM, Cosgrove DO, Nassiri DK, et al. The diaphragmatic echo complex: an in vitro study. Invest Radiol 1985;20:62.
13. Sommer FG, Taylor KJW. Differentiation of acoustic shadowing due to calculi and gas collections. Radiology 1980;135:399.
14. Jaffe CC, Taylor KJW. The clinical impact of ultrasonic beam focusing patterns. Radiology 1979;131:469.
15. Taylor KJW, Jacobson P, Jaffee CC. Lack of an acoustic shadow on scans of gallstones: a possible artifact. Radiology 1979;131:463.
16. Kirberger RM. Imaging artifacts in diagnostic ultrasound—a review. Vet Radiol Ultrasound 1995;36:297–306.

9. Pregnancy

DON R. BERGFELT, GREGG P. ADAMS, and ROGER A. PIERSON

Diagnostic ultrasonography has provided a window through which veterinarians and researchers can visualize, examine, and understand the interrelationships of the equine embryo and fetus during gestation in real time— that is, as it happens. This chapter is intended to review principal aspects of ultrasonography, embryology, and physiology with respect to diagnosis of pregnancy and monitoring of the conceptus and conceptus–uterine interactions. The intention is to provide a synopsis of key elements from previous reviews, particularly those of Ginther (1–3), which have eloquently detailed ultrasonographic techniques and reproductive biology in the mare. We hope that readers who are intrigued by this section study the specific references for further comprehension. In addition, a brief discussion of the frontiers of imaging technology, including color flow Doppler ultrasonography and three-dimensional image analysis of gestational events, is included to provide a glimpse of the future.

APPROACH

Detailed reviews of the basic principles and technique of transrectal ultrasonography in the mare are available (2, 4, 5) and are discussed elsewhere in this text. Only those aspects specific to pregnancy detection and subsequent monitoring of gestational events are presented here: transducers, preparation of the mare for transrectal examination, and technique of transrectal imaging of the uterus.

Transducer

Transducers are available in various types, such as linear-array and convex-array transducers, and several frequencies (i.e., 3.5, 5.0, 7.5 Mhz) and can be used intrarectally, intravaginally, and transabdominally. The approach and the type of transducer used are primarily dictated by the objective of the examination. Image resolution is a function of the frequency of acoustic pressure waves (sound waves) generated by the transducer. The higher the frequency of the transmitted sound waves, the higher the image resolution and the shallower the depth of penetration. Transrectal scanning has been the most common approach to ultrasonographic diagnosis of pregnancy in mares because accessibility through the rectum allows close proximity of the reproductive tract to the transducer. In addition, the broad, flat surface of the rectal mucosa is ideally suited for linear-array transducers. In this regard, a 7.5- or 5.0-Mhz linear-array transducer is generally used for approximately the first 80 days of gestation; thereafter, a 3.5-Mhz transducer may be used because of the depth of penetration required to visualize the large equine fetus. The transabdominal approach to fetal imaging has also been used to study developmental events during mid- to late gestation (6, 7). The transabdominal approach may also be useful for smaller horses, such as miniature horses, in which the operator's hand may be too large for intrarectal placement of the transducer. More recently, ultrasound examination of the conceptus has been approached transvaginally using a convex-array transducer for the purpose of allantocentesis (8).

Preparation

Selection of an examination area should include considerations for restraint of the mare, positioning of the ultrasound scanner, and ability to alter the ambient lighting. Proper restraint of the mare is necessary to protect the operator and the scanner. The scanner should be positioned close enough to the operator so controls can be reached for image adjustment and raised to eye level to allow scrutiny of image detail; subdued lighting is imperative for interpretation of image detail. Liquid contact between the transducer face and the rectal mucosa is required for the sound waves to be transmitted into the tissues. Air or bowel gas between the transducer face and the rectal wall completely blocks sound waves from penetration of tissues and is seen on the ultrasound screen as a bright echo with a shadow beneath it. Intervening fecal material can also cast a shadow or distort the image and should be removed. A coupling medium is essential; in most instances, standard lubricants used for transrectal palpation are satisfactory (e.g., methyl cellulose). Preparing the mare for a transrectal ultrasound examination is similar to preparation for rectal palpation; inserting the lubricated hand and transducer into the rectum requires the same degree of precaution to prevent rectal tears and ruptures. Transrectal ultrasonography is not necessarily any easier or more difficult than transrectal palpation. However, because of the ability to study sequential, sectional views of the conceptus and uterus in real time, a more in-depth knowledge of anatomy and physiology is required. One must be able to direct the transducer to the area of interest, such as the uterine body or uterine horns, and be able to interpret developmental changes associated with the conceptus, the uterus, and their interactions.

Technique

The uterus is the site of embryonic and fetal development, but it also serves as a guide for the location and orientation of the transducer during an ultrasound examination. The orientation of a linear-array transducer to the uterus is diagrammed in Figure 9.1. The diagram represents a dorsal view of the uterus, the shaded rectangular box represents

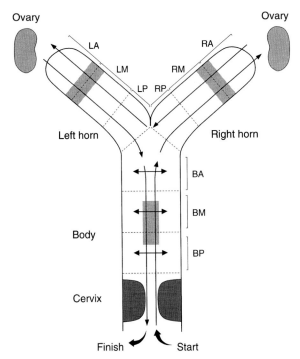

Figure 9.1. Diagrammatic representation of a dorsal view of the uterus. The shaded areas represent the face of the transducer over the uterine body and the left and right uterine horns, *arrows* represent the direction of movement of the transducer. Letters represent major portions of the uterus (B = body; L = left horn; R = right horn) and segments of respective portions (A = anterior; M= middle; P = posterior). Reprinted with permission from Ginther OJ. Ultrasonic imaging and reproductive events in the mare. Cross Plains, WI: Equiservices, 1986.

the face of the transducer, and the arrows represent the direction of movement of the transducer. On insertion of the transducer into the rectum, the uterine body can be seen in sagittal section on the ultrasound screen, and the uterine horns can be seen in cross-section as the transducer is moved or rotated laterally. When examining the uterus to diagnose early pregnancy, slow, methodical movements covering the entire uterine body and both uterine horns ensure proper diagnosis. Rapid movements may result in misdiagnosis because the ultrasound beam is thin (1 to 2 mm) and can quickly pass over small embryonic vesicles (3 to 4 mm on days 9 to 10) (9). Investigators have suggested (2), therefore, that a systematic routine be developed for examining the expanse of the uterus. An example of such a routine is indicated by the arrows in Figure 9.1. Beginning cranially to the cervix, the uterine body is viewed longitudinally; the transducer is rotated slightly side to side as it is advanced forward to view the entire width of the uterine body. At the corpus–cornual junction, the transducer is further rotated laterally to the right to view the uterine horn in cross-section. Scanning in this plane continues until the image of the tip of the horn disappears. Further lateral imaging allows visualization of the right ovary. Routine imaging of the ovaries during early pregnancy evaluation is recommended not only to allow assessment of the primary corpus luteum, but also to determine the presence of mul-

tiple corpora lutea. Detection of two functional corpora lutea before approximately 35 days of pregnancy necessitates careful scrutiny of the uterus for potential twin pregnancies. After inspection of the ovary, the transducer is rotated so the uterine horn is followed back toward the mid-line. Back at the corpus–corneal junction, the transducer is rotated laterally to the left to view a cross-section of the opposite uterine horn and ovary. On completion of the examination, the entire uterus has been examined twice. In addition to establishing a systematic approach to ultrasound examination of the uterus, the sonographer must establish a consistent record-keeping system. One approach (2) has been to divide the uterus into segments so location of the embryonic vesicle can be readily coded (see Fig. 9.1). Each major portion of the uterus (left horn, right horn, and body) can be subdivided into three segments (anterior, middle, and posterior). A segment is identified by moving the transducer from the structure of interest to each end of respective segments of the uterine body or horn. An example record entry may read LAEV12, indicating that a 12-mm embryonic vesicle was located in the left horn, anterior segment. Such recordings are useful for monitoring pregnancy status at subsequent examinations; that is, embryo growth or loss can be firmly documented if earlier recordings indicated that the structure identified as a vesicle changed in size or location. Occasionally, uterine cysts mimic the expected size and appearance of an embryonic vesicle (2). An embryonic vesicle can be differentiated from a cyst by documenting changes in size, location, or morphology of aberrant structures within the uterine lumen. The location and size of pathologic structures or conditions of the uterine lumen may be recorded as described for the embryonic vesicle.

YOLK SAC STAGE

When the conceptus enters the uterus approximately 6 days after ovulation (day 0), it is considered an early blastocyst (2). During the blastocyst stage (approximately days 6 to 10; Fig. 9.2), the embryonic vesicle is enveloped by a single layer of ectodermal cells (trophoblast). After day 10, an inner lining of endodermal cells encircles the blastocele, transforming the blastocyst into a bilaminar (two-walled) yolk sac (Fig. 9.2, day 12); the yolk sac stage extends from approximately day 11 to day 20. Ultrasonographic characteristics of the embryonic vesicle, vesicle mobility, fixation, and orientation within the uterine lumen are presented.

First Detection

Using the transrectal approach, the equine embryonic vesicle may be first detected at a diameter of 3 to 4 mm with a 5.0-Mhz linear-array transducer and at 6 to 7 mm with a 3.5-Mhz transducer (9). In one study, a vesicle was detected on day 9 in 10% of mares, on day 10 in 70%, and on day 11 in 98% using a 5.0-Mhz transducer. The use of a 7.5-Mhz transducer may allow a greater percentage of vesi-

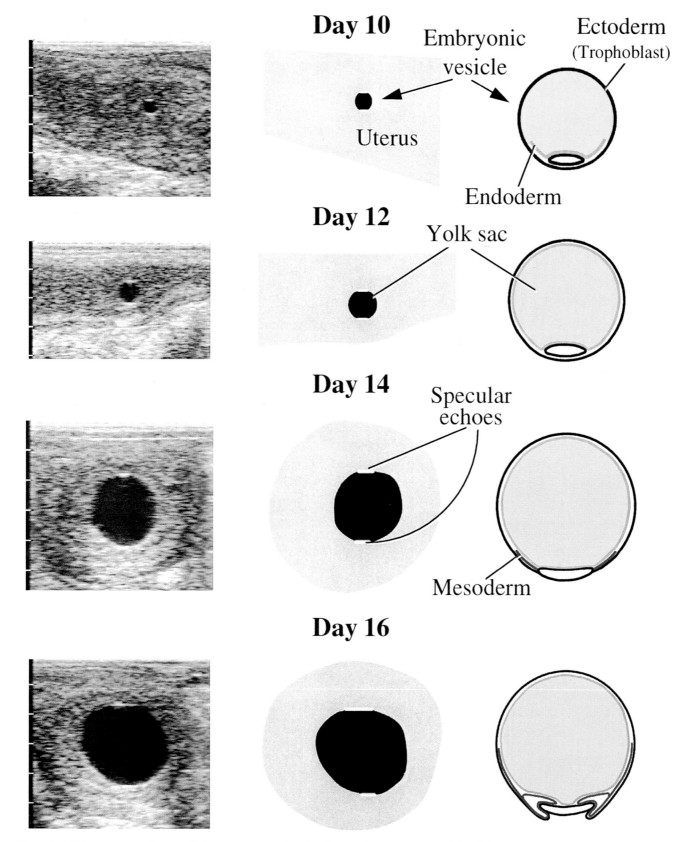

Figure 9.2. Ultrasonogram, diagram of ultrasonogram, and embryology of the conceptus on defined days of pregnancy. The day of pregnancy relative to ovulation is shown above each respective trio along with text indicating specific embryologic events that may be observed during an ultrasonographic examination. Embryology reprinted with permission from Ginther OJ. Reproductive biology of the mare: basic and applied aspects. Cross Plains, WI: Equiservices, 1979.

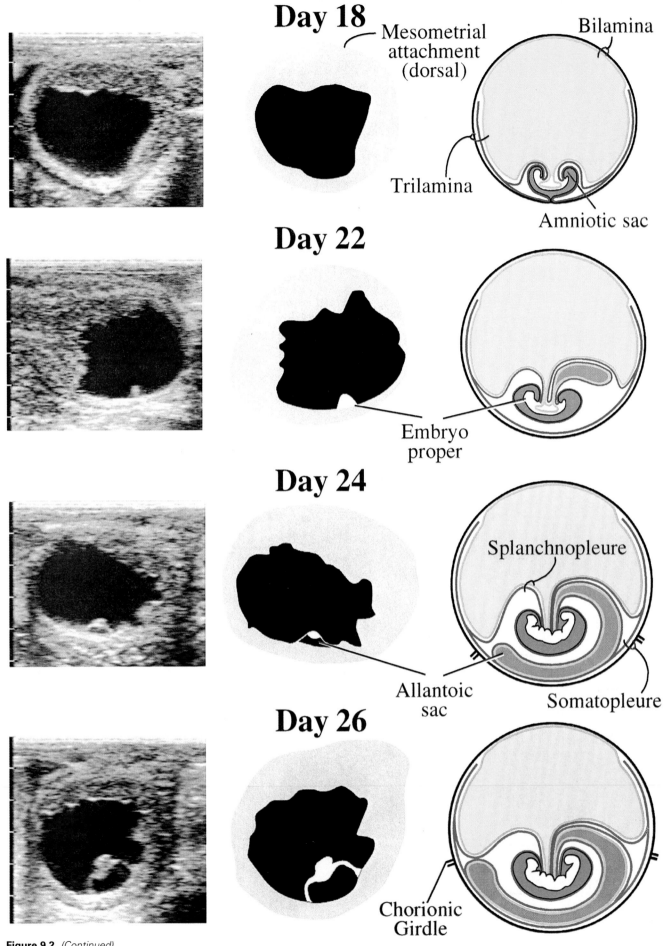

Figure 9.2. *(Continued)*

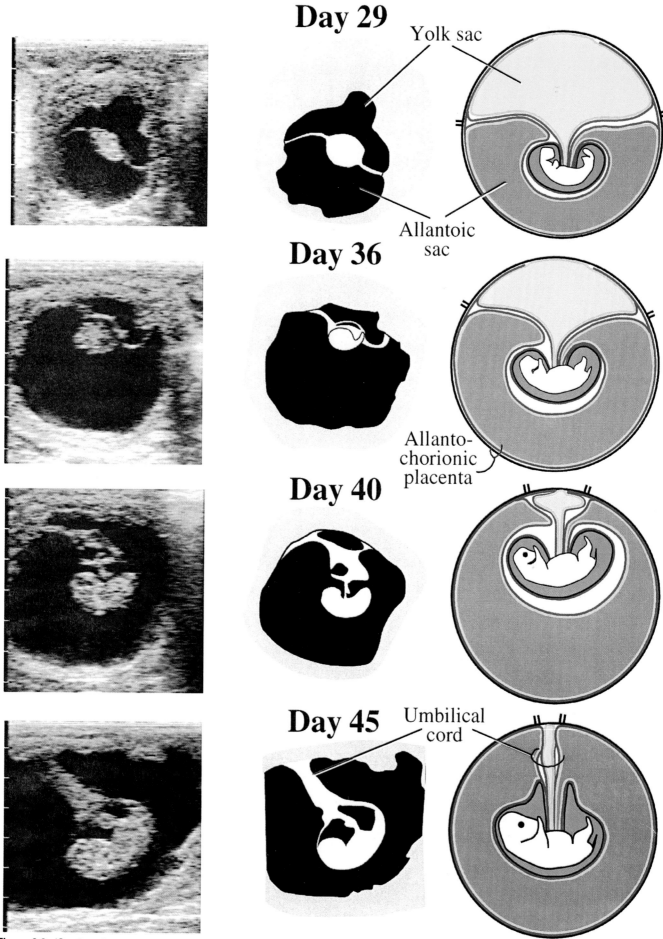

Day 29

Yolk sac

Allantoic sac

Day 36

Allanto-chorionic placenta

Day 40

Day 45   Umbilical cord

Figure 9.2. *(Continued)*

cles to be detected on or before day 9; however, the use of a 7.5-Mhz transducer for early pregnancy detection has not been critically evaluated. The early equine conceptus is spherical and fluid-filled, and it produces a black (anechoic) image on the ultrasound screen (Fig. 9.2, days 10 to 16). A bright white (hyperechoic) spot is frequently observed on the dorsal and ventral aspect of the yolk sac image. These spots are called specular reflections and are artifacts resulting from the interaction of the ultrasound beams with a smooth surface. Specular echoes can be a useful aid during the search for an early embryonic vesicle, but they should not be misinterpreted as the embryonic disc. Specular echoes are also characteristic of uterine cysts. In this regard, an early embryonic vesicle may be differentiated from a uterine cyst by growth and mobility of the embryo.

Mobility Phase

The phenomenon of transuterine migration of the early equine conceptus has been reviewed (2, 3, 10) and must be considered when searching the uterus for an early embryonic vesicle. Mobility of the equine conceptus, after it enters the uterus on approximately day 6, is essential for eliciting the first luteal response to pregnancy (i.e., maternal recognition of pregnancy) (3). Because the early vesicle is highly mobile (11), the uterus must be examined thoroughly and methodically from the cranial aspect of the cervix to the tip of each uterine horn (see Fig. 9.1). Mobility of the embryonic vesicle increases from first detection at day 9 or 10 to a maximum by day 11 or 12, at which time it may traverse the entire expanse of the uterus as much as 20 times in 1 day (mean 3.4 mm/minute) (10, 11). Maximum mobility is maintained until day 15 or 16 (fixation). Younger, smaller vesicles (3 to 6 mm, days 9 to 11) are found more frequently (>60%) in the uterine body (11, 12), and thereafter they are noted with increasing frequency traversing the uterine horns. Inherent characteristics of the conceptus and uterus favor embryo mobility: 1) spherical shape of the vesicle; 2) structural rigidity of the vesicle maintained by an outer acellular capsule; and 3) longitudinal orientation of endometrial folds.

The propulsive force behind embryo mobility is uterine contractility (13). Uterine contractions result in to-and-fro movements and expansion and compression of embryonic vesicles within the uterine body or horns. Uterine contractility is present at all stages of the estrous cycle and early pregnancy, but it is greatest during the mobility phase (days 11 to 14) (14, 15). Although progesterone is essential for uterine contractility (16), progesterone alone is not responsible for the profound degree of uterine contractility during maximum embryo mobility. In one study, physical isolation of the embryo to one of the uterine horns by surgical ligation resulted in increased uterine echotexture scores (enhanced endometrial edema and folding) in portions of the uterus exposed to the conceptus or its secretory products; decreased contractility was observed in the remainder of the uterus not exposed to the conceptus (17). The results

of this study indicated that the presence of the conceptus alters uterine contractility. In vitro culture of equine vesicles has indicated that the early conceptus is capable of estrogen production (18). In this regard, increased echotexture of the uterine endometrium in the presence of the conceptus is the basis for the hypothesis that the conceptus contributes to its own mobility by stimulating uterine contractility through its production of estrogen. Administration of estradiol in combination with progesterone to seasonally anovulatory mares did not alter uterine contractility scores from those obtained with progesterone alone (19), and injection of estradiol did not increase the extent of uterine contractility or embryo mobility in pregnant mares on day 10 or 12 (20). Although the conceptus has a local influence on uterine contractility, the biochemical or physical mechanisms involved are not known. Results of these studies (19, 20) failed to support a systemic role of estrogen; however, production of estrogens or other myometrial stimulants emanating from the early conceptus (e.g., prostaglandins such as PGF, PGE, and PGI_2) (21) may have a local role in uterine contractility and thus embryo mobility.

Fixation

Fixation of the embryonic vesicle has been defined (22) as cessation of intrauterine mobility as determined by failure to detect any intrauterine location changes during frequent serial ultrasonographic examinations. Movement of the embryonic vesicle from one intrauterine location to another should not be expected after fixation, with the exception of impending embryo loss (2, 23) in association with luteolysis (loss of uterine tone). In several experiments involving 100 mares, movement of the embryonic vesicle was not detected in daily examinations from the day of fixation (day 15 or 16) to day 40 (2). The mean day of vesicle fixation occurred earlier in ponies (day 15) than in horses (day 16) (2). The reason for the discrepancy of day of fixation between horses and ponies is not clear, especially because the daily growth profiles of the embryonic vesicle were similar between these two types of mares. Perhaps the smaller uterus in ponies (3) impedes vesicle mobility earlier and hastens fixation. Regardless, the latest documented day of fixation of a singleton embryo was day 17 (2). In barren (nonlactating and without pregnancy the previous year) and maiden mares, fixation occurred with greater frequency (63%) in the right uterine horn (24, 25). In postpartum mares, the vesicle was more likely (84%) to become fixed in the formerly nongravid horn (26–28). Corresponding to the approximate day of fixation, a transient period of enhanced endometrial folding has been described (17, 28). Endometrial echotexture appeared heterogeneous, beginning by approximately day 16 (Fig. 9.3a). The estrus-like echotexture was most likely due to exposure of the uterus to estrogen emanating from the conceptus (17, 18) or ovaries (2, 23). The transient increase in echotexture should not be confused with impending embryo loss and subsequent return to estrus. Other ultrasonographic characteristics of

Uterine Horn Characteristics
(n=5 mares)

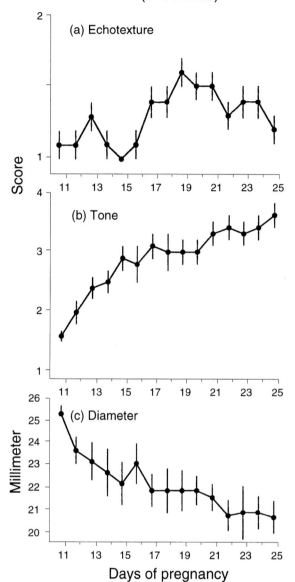

Figure 9.3. Mean (± SEM) uterine horn characteristics for endometrial echotexture (*a*), tone (*b*), and diameter (*c*). Endometrial echotexture was scored on a scale from 1 to 4, based on the degree of heterogeneity (minimal to maximal). Uterine tone was scored digitally on a scale from 1 to 4, based on the degree of turgidity (flaccid to tense). Adapted with permission from Griffin PG, Carnevale EM, Ginther OJ. Effects of the embryo on uterine morphology and function in mares. Anim Reprod Sci 1993;31:311–329.

the conceptus (2). Uterine horn diameter gradually decreases during early pregnancy, a phenomenon that corresponds temporally with increasing uterine tone (Fig. 9.3*b, c*) (2, 17). The close relationship between uterine turgidity and diameter supports the concept that the dramatic increase in uterine tone after day 12 is due to tonic contraction of the myometrium, thus decreasing uterine horn diameter. The factor most likely responsible for the extensive uterine tone of early pregnancy is estradiol emanating from the ovaries (3), conceptus, or both. Administration of a low dose of estrogen in combination with progesterone to cyclic mares beginning on day 10 mimicked uterine tone scores in a contemporary group of pregnant mares (29). The postulated mechanism of embryo fixation is a function of increasing size of the embryonic vesicle, combined with increasing intraluminal resistance to mobility caused by the development of tense uterine tone (22).

Orientation

Orientation refers to the rotation of the embryonic vesicle so the embryonic pole or disc assumes a specific position relative to the mesometrial attachment (2, 22). Beginning on approximately day 17, the vesicle begins to lose its spherical shape (see Fig. 9.2, day 18). The change in the shape of the vesicle is accounted for by reduced structural rigidity and accommodation of the expanding yolk sac to increasing uterine turgidity. The vesicle does not appear to increase in cross-sectional diameter over days 16 to 28 (Fig. 9.4*a*), but instead begins to elongate in response to continued uterine resistance to cross-sectional expansion. Changes in shape of the vesicle occur frequently during periods of continuous observation and are attributable to myometrial contractions exerting a kneading or massaging action on the fixed vesicle.

Initially, on the day of fixation, the conceptus appears to be centrally located in cross-sectional views of the uterine horn; a uniform thickness of the uterine wall encompasses the vesicle (see Fig. 9.2, day 16). After fixation of the embryonic vesicle and coupled with the shape change is a disproportional change in thickness of the uterine walls. The dorsolateral walls, adjacent to the mesometrial attachment, thicken. Conversely, the ventral uterine wall becomes thinner and smoother in cross-sectional image (see Fig. 9.2, day 18). At this stage of pregnancy, a third embryonic layer (mesoderm) has migrated from the embryonic disc, intervening between the ectoderm (trophoblast) and endoderm layers, to encompass approximately 50% of the yolk sac (see Fig. 9.2, day 18). Hence, the conceptus is a three-walled (trilaminar) structure where the mesoderm is present and a two-walled (bilaminar) structure where it is not. The morphologic arrangement of extraembryonic membranes is conducive to an orientation of the trilaminar portion (most rigid) forced into the ventral position by the massaging action of continued uterine contractions (10, 22). Consequently, the cross-sectional image of the vesicle often appears triangular, with the apex or bilaminar portion (least

the ovaries (e.g., regressing corpus luteum) and conceptus–uterus (e.g., failure of fixation) associated with embryo loss should be considered (2, 23).

The embryonic vesicle becomes fixed in a segment of the uterine horn near the corpus–cornual junction (2). Apparently, the sharp curvature or flexure of the uterine horns at this site represents the greatest impediment for vesicle mobility because continued uterine contractions force the vesicle against the ventral wall, thereby trapping

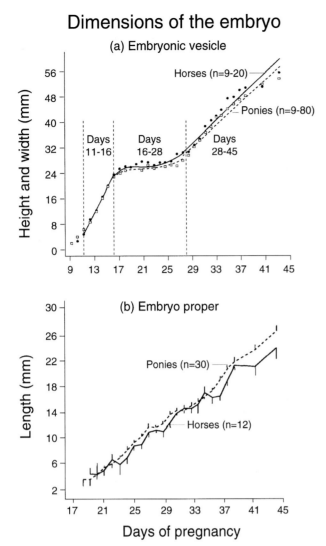

Figure 9.4. Growth profiles of the mean height and width of the embryonic vesicle (a) and mean (±SEM) crown-rump length of the embryo proper (b) in horse and pony mares as determined transrectally using a 5.0-Mhz linear-array transducer. Adapted with permission from Ginther OJ. Ultrasonic imaging and reproductive events in the mare. Cross Plains, WI: Equiservices, 1986.

rigid) oriented in the dorsal region of the uterine lumen adjacent to the mesometrial attachment. Thus, the embryonic disc is forced into a ventral position in which the embryo proper is initially detected.

ALLANTOIC SAC STAGE

Continued development of pregnancy can be viewed as the conceptus begins transition from the yolk sac stage to the allantoic sac stage after approximately day 20 (see Fig. 9.2, day 22) (3). Enlargement of the allantoic sac and regression of the yolk sac give rise to the ultrasonographic characteristics of ascent and descent of the embryo–amniotic unit and fetal–amniotic unit, respectively (see Fig. 9.2, days 22 to 45) (2). The term *embryo* is used to describe conceptus

development to day 40, and *fetus* describes development beyond day 40 (3).

Embryo–Amniotic Ascent

The embryo proper may first be detected by ultrasonography at approximately days 19 to 22 and is viewed as a small (approximately 4 mm) echoic spot along the ventral border of the vesicle (see Fig. 9.2, day 22) (2, 9). Development of the amniotic and allantoic sacs begins approximately the same time that the embryo proper is first visualized (see Fig. 9.2, days 18 and 22) (3). The amnion is formed by the union of the outer vesicle wall (trophoblast and mesoderm), which passes over the emerging embryo proper. The allantois emerges from the hindgut and moves into the exocoelom, which is a potential space or cavity located between the outer vesicle wall composed of trophoblast and mesoderm (somatopleure) and an inner vesicle wall composed of mesoderm and endoderm (splanchnopleure). By day 24, the allantoic sac has become prominent and is configured like a cup under the embryo–amniotic unit, lifting it from the ventral floor of the vesicle (see Fig. 9.2, days 24 and 26). The allantoic sac appears as a anechoic area beneath the embryo–amniotic unit; the echoic line represents the opposing walls of the yolk sac dorsally and the allantoic sac ventrally. The allantois eventually fuses with the amnion to form the allantoamniotic membrane. This membrane protects the embryo from the urine-like waste in the allantoic fluid. In addition, the allantois fuses with the somatopleure (chorion) to form the allantochorionic placenta, which is composed of ectoderm (trophoblast), mesoderm, and endoderm (allantoic membrane).

A circumferential band of specialized trophoblast cells at the region of allantoic sac–yolk sac apposition is termed the chorionic girdle (see Fig. 9.2, days 24 to 45). Girdle cells invade the uterine epithelium at approximately day 37 to form the prominent, gonadotropin-producing, decidua-like cells of endometrial cups (30). Over days 24 to 33, the allantoic sac enlarges and the yolk sac recedes; the embryo–amniotic unit and the echoic line separating the two placental sacs move toward the dorsal aspect of the embryonic vesicle (see Fig. 9.2, days 24 to 45). The horizontal orientation of the echoic line separating the two sacs can be a useful aid in differentiating a single pregnancy from unilaterally fixed twin pregnancies; the opposed walls of twin embryonic vesicles tend toward a vertical orientation (2, 3).

The allantoic sac continues to enlarge, eventually engulfing the vestige of the yolk sac dorsally by day 40 (see Fig. 9.2, days 40 and 45). The convergence of the opposing walls of the allantois and their subsequent fusion around the urachus, blood vessels, and yolk sac form the umbilical cord. Hence, the root of attachment of the umbilical cord is located dorsally near the mesometrial attachment, and the early fetus appears to dangle at the end of the umbilical cord in dorsal recumbency during ultrasonographic examinations (see Fig. 9.2, day 45).

Fetal–Amniotic Descent

Day 40 has been designated the approximate time of transition from the embryo stage to the fetal stage of development (3). The fetus is attached to the dorsal aspect of the vesicle by the umbilical cord, where the root of the cord is encircled by endometrial cups that have colonized the dorsal endometrial wall. As the umbilical cord begins to elongate, the fetal–amniotic unit descends toward the ventral pole (see Fig. 9.2, day 45). At approximately day 45, descent is about 50% complete, and by day 50, the fetal–amniotic unit has descended to the ventral aspect of the allantoic sac. The fetal–amniotic unit is mobile within the allantoic sac, and movement may be observed by gentle ballottement of the uterus with the transducer. Unlike in equids, the amnion in other farm species is fused to the allantochorion in certain areas, limiting intra-allantoic movement (31).

GROWTH CHARACTERISTICS

Serial imaging of the conceptus and its membranes has allowed construction of growth profiles for the vesicle, for the embryo proper, and for various anatomic structures of the embryo–fetus. Growth characteristics may be used as a means of estimating the stage of gestation and assessing the health and prenatal development of the conceptus.

Embryo Stage

Developmental events for estimating stage of pregnancy are indicated in Table 9.1. For accurate assessment of heart rate (beats/minute), an ultrasound scanner requires a frame rate of at least 20 frames/second (2). Maximum cross-sectional diameter of the embryonic vesicle in horse and pony mares has been determined for days 9 to 45 and is shown in Figure 9.4a. No differences in vesicle height on any day are noted between horse and pony mares. Cross-sectional growth or expansion of the vesicle was linear during days 11 to 16, at approximately 3.4 mm/day. During days 16 to 28, the S-shaped part of the curve represents a plateau in cross-sectional growth that is partly attributable to increasing uterine tone. Although cross-sectional expansion is not visible, the vesicle elongates up the uterine horn that can be detected by orientating the transducer longitudinally with respect to the uterine horn. After day 28, cross-sectional expansion of the vesicle is again linear but slower, occurring at 1.8 mm/day. Age of the conceptus can be estimated with 95% accuracy for 6- to 23-mm vesicles ($\pm$1.5 days) and for 27- to 56-mm vesicles ($\pm$4 days). During the S-shaped portion of the curve (days 16 to 28), the cross-sectional height does not change enough to be an adequate indicator of age; however, profound developmental events facilitate age determination (see Table 9.1). Length (from crown to rump) of the

Table 9.1.

Developmental Events of the Equine Conceptus Relative to the Number of Days Post-ovulation for Predicting the Stage of Pregnancy by Ultrasonography

Days of Pregnancy	Event
9–11	Embryonic vesicle first detected
11–14	Extensive transuterine migration
15–16	Cessation of mobility at caudal portion of uterine horn
17–19	Loss of spherical shape
19–22	Embryo proper first detected at ventrical pole and embryo heartbeat
22–24	Embryo-amniotic unit begins ascent to dorsal pole
25–27	Allantoic sac 25%; yolk sac 75%
28–30	Allantoic sac 50%; yolk sac 50%
31–33	Allantoic sac 75%; yolk sac 25%
34–36	Ascent complete and umbilical cord formation at dorsal pole
40–50	Umbilical cord elongation and descent of fetal-amniotic unit to ventral pole

embryo proper can also be a useful characteristic for estimating age of the embryo. Mean crown–rump length of the embryo in horse and pony mares was determined for days 19 to 45 and is shown in Figure 9.4b. No differences in embryo length on any day are noted between horse and pony mares. The appearance of the embryo proper at the ventral pole, the proportion of the vesicle that consists of yolk sac fluid versus allantoic sac fluid, the length of the umbilical cord, and the length of the embryo proper are perhaps the most useful characteristics for estimating age of the embryo during the first 2 months of pregnancy.

Fetal Stage

Ultrasonography of the fetus beyond day 40 has received only limited attention (32, 33). In one study (32), equine fetal development from 60 to 335 days of gestation was examined using transrectal imaging in which the fetus was visualized 75% of the time. Growth profiles of the fetal eye, cranium, ribs plus intercostal space, stomach, and trunk were developed, along with fetal heart rate (Fig. 9.5). Imaging of the head was possible 63% of the time, imaging of the thorax was possible 29% of the time, and the abdomen was visualized 18% of the time. The maximum diameter of the fetal eye and cross-section of the trunk showed the highest correlation to fetal age (Fig. 9.5a, e), and these characteristics may be valuable for estimating fetal age at later stages of pregnancy (>2 months). Transabdominal imaging also has been used to study characteristics of the late-gestation equine fetus (6, 7). The approach has particular potential for assessing fetal distress by monitoring fetal heart rate when the mare is under anesthesia during surgery or when the fetus is entrapped within the pelvis during the periparturient period.

Another anatomic feature readily accessible to ultrasonographic imaging is the genital tubercle (34; see also Chapter

Dimensions of the fetus

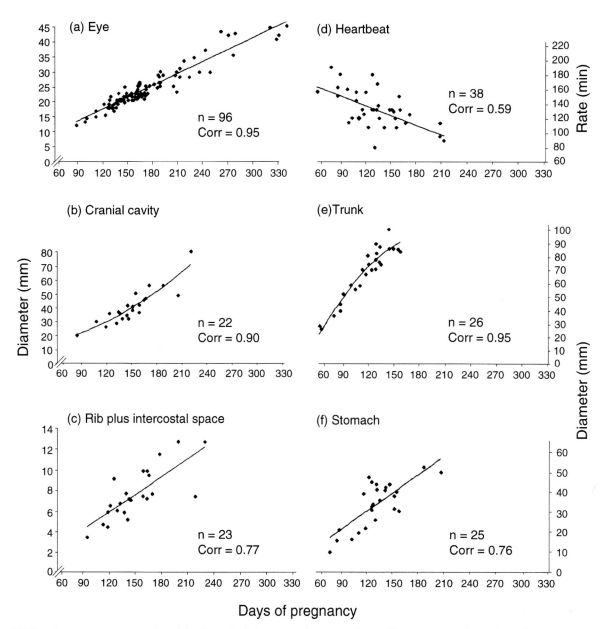

Figure 9.5. Developmental characteristics of the fetus depicting respective regression profiles correlating dimensions of the eye (*a*), cranial cavity (*b*), rib plus intercostal space (*c*), heart (*d*), trunk (*e*), and stomach (*f*) with days of pregnancy. Adapted with permission from Kahn W, Leidl W. [Ultrasonic biometry of horse fetuses in utero and sonographic representation of their organs] Die Ultraschall-Biometrie von Pferdefeten in utero und die sonographische Darstellung ihrer Organe. DTW. Dtsch Tierarztl Wochenschr 1987;94:509–515.

12), an embryonic process that differentiates into the penis (male) and clitoris (female). Ultrasonographic assessment of the tubercle can be used to determine fetal sex, optimally between days 60 and 70, by its relative location near the umbilical cord (male) or the tail (female).

FETAL KINETICS

Ultrasonographic imaging is the only available technology that permits in situ monitoring of fetal movement without

apparent interference. This approach has been used in studies to assess physical interactions between the fetus and the uterus involving fetal activity, mobility, recumbency, and presentation within the allantoic sac (35). Furthermore, this approach has been used to examine the interaction between uterine constrictions and subsequent intrauterine shifts in allantoic fluid. Ultrasonographic assessments of fetal–uterine interactions throughout gestation have required transducer frequencies ranging from 7.5 to 3.5 Mhz. The degree of penetration needed to image the deepest point of the uterus has dictated the frequency of transducer that must be used to obtain optimal fields of view and resolution.

Activity and Mobility

Fetal activity and fetal mobility are not mutually exclusive events, but they comprise a dynamic relationship resulting in movement of the fetus within the amniotic and allantoic sacs. Fetal activity refers to in-place movements of the head, limbs, and torso, whereas fetal mobility refers to location changes of the fetal–amniotic unit within the uterus. Studies (36,37) have shown that fetal activity occurs throughout the fetal stage and during parturition, with intermittent periods of quiescence. In these studies, activity of the fetal head, limbs, and torso was first detected on days 40 to 48 and increased over the next 2 months (36,37). At some times, activity involved simultaneous movement of the torso and appendages, whereas at other times, movement of the appendages was independent of the torso. Explosive whole-body movements appeared to suspend the fetus momentarily in the allantoic fluid and often resulted in intrauterine location changes (fetal mobility).

Studies showed that fetal mobility was indicated by the frequency of location changes among the uterine body and horns through weekly ultrasonographic examinations during months 2 to 11 (38). During months 2 to 3, cord horn (umbilical cord attachment) locations decreased while noncord horn and uterine body locations increased. By month 4, the fetus was equally likely to be found in the cord horn, noncord horn, or uterine body, but by months 5 to 7, the fetus was most frequently observed in the uterine body. After month 7, the fetus remained in the uterine body while the fetal hind limbs began to invade the cord horn. Mobility of the fetal–amniotic unit primarily depended on vigorous movements of the fetus rather than on uterine contractions, because injections of succinylcholine into the fetus to induce muscle paralysis resulted in a fivefold reduction in the number of fetal location changes without altering changes in diameter of the allantoic fluid compartment (i.e., uterine contractions) (39). Fetal mobility can also result indirectly from a floating response to allantoic fluid currents originating from extraneous movements by the mare, by the intestines, and by constrictions of the uterine horns. In summary, mobility of the fetal–amniotic unit among the uterine body and horns was maximal (five changes per hour) during early gestation (months 2 to 4), decreased during mid-gestation (months 5 and 7), and absent by late gestation (>month 7).

Uterine Constrictions and Allantoic Fluid Shifts

The expanding conceptus fills the umbilical cord horn and uterine body by days 60 to 80, as determined by transrectal palpation (40) or mid-ventral laparotomy (1); in one study, no apparent swellings were palpated to indicate when the conceptus invaded the noncord uterine horn. However,

with the use of ultrasonography (41), the chorioallantoic sac and attendant fluid were first detected in the uterine body at approximately day 41 and filled the uterine body at day 48. Arrival of the chorioallantoic sac and fluid at the tip of the cord horn occurred on approximately day 60, and entry into the noncord horn and arrival at the tip of the noncord horn occurred on days 53 and 65, respectively. Ultrasonographic imaging has revealed dynamic shifts in volume of allantoic fluid among the three major parts of the uterus (body and horns), with corresponding changes in diameter of the uterus during days 65 to 85 (37). At times, the uterine wall has been constricted around the fetal–amniotic unit with no detectable intervening fluid, whereas at other times, the uterus has been widely dilated in the same location (left or right horn; cord or noncord horn; fetus present or not present). In a study designed to inhibit myometrial contractions (39), uterine constrictions were not detected, and the height of allantoic fluid in the uterine horns increased as the uterus relaxed. Thus, shifts in allantoic fluid have been primarily attributed to active myometrial contractions.

After invasion of the cord horn and noncord horn by the chorioallantoic sac and fluid, frequent closures of both horns occur; in one study, the first complete closure of either horn occurred at approximately month 3 (41). During months 5 to 7, the frequency of both cord horn and noncord horn closures increased such that the fetus was confined predominantly to the uterine body. The frequency of closures of the noncord horn continued to increase until it was closed for the entire period of months 8 to 11. Complete closure of the noncord horn prevented entry of the fetus and its appendages. Conversely, complete closure of the cord horn did not occur until month 9, thereby allowing extension of the hind limbs of the growing fetus into the cord horn after month 7. During months 9 to 11, the cord horn was closed or constricted on the hind limbs such that retraction of the limbs did not occur even though the fetal limbs remained vigorously active. Investigators have suggested (41) that the role of uterine constriction about the fetal hind limbs is to maintain proper presentation as parturition approaches.

Recumbency and Presentation

Ultrasonographic assessment of fetal recumbency (lateral, dorsal, or ventral) has been described during frequent serial examination periods for days 70 to 80 (37). In this study, lateral recumbency was observed more frequently (74%) than ventral recumbency (3%), and the frequency of dorsal recumbency was intermediate (24%); recumbency changes occurred an average of 10 times per hour. Critical ultrasonographic assessment of fetal recumbency after day 80 has apparently not been done, although a preliminary study (see Chapter 12) indicated that the cranial half of the fetal torso was either in dorsal recumbency (61% of fetuses) or lateral recumbency (39%) after day 330. Similarly, the caudal portion of the fetus was either in dorsal recumbency (majority) or lateral recumbency (minority). Studies using radiography (42) or flank laparotomy (35) have revealed that the cranial portion of the fetus rotates into ventral recumbency during the first stage of labor, and the caudal portion follows the cranial portion in a screw-like fashion during the second stage delivery.

Fetal presentation (cranial, caudal, or transverse) has been described for months 2 to 11 during serial examination periods (37,38). Presentation has been defined as the predominant direction faced by the fetus as follows: cranial, fetal head toward cervix; caudal, fetal head away from cervix; transverse, fetal body perpendicular to sides of uterine horns or uterine body. In these studies, no presentation changes were detected during approximately the first half of month 2; however, a change of presentation was detected in 25% of the examinations during the second half. During months 3 to 5, presentation changes occurred approximately five times per hour; cranial and caudal presentations occurred with equal frequency, and transverse presentation occurred with less frequency. The proportion of examinations in which cranial presentation was detected did not begin to exceed that of caudal presentation until month 6, and, by month 7, nearly all presentations were cranial; only 6% of the observations during months 8 to 9 were noncranial. Investigators determined (38) that the length of the interval between presentation changes gradually increased from month 4 onward, such that only a few changes were detected during months 8 to 9, and none were noted during months 10 to 11. It appears, therefore, that after 7 months of gestation, the equine fetus has settled into a uterine location (body plus cord horn) and presentation (fetal head toward maternal cervix) conducive to successful delivery.

The mechanism for the gradual decrease in fetal mobility and positional changes as pregnancy progresses appears to be related to increasing physical restrictions of the growing fetus within the uterus. A limited study in pregnant pony mares found that the volume of amniotic fluid and weight of the fetus gradually increased over days 90 to 220 (approximately months 3 to 7), whereas the volume of allantoic fluid reached maximum at day 80 and gradually decreased thereafter (1). Thus, the gradual decrease in fetal mobility as parturition nears is a function of increasing physical restrictions. Physical restrictions consist of uterine horn constrictions and the increasing ratio in size of the fetus versus the allantoic fluid that challenge the inherent limitations of the uterus. The role of extensive fetal movement, especially during the first 4 months of gestation, is not known precisely; however, investigators have suggested (43) that movement is important for development of the musculoskeletal system so the fetus can adapt to the demands of parturition (i.e., recumbency and presentation) and early postnatal life.

THE FRONTIER

Gray-scale ultrasonography has provided an unheralded opportunity to visualize reproductive events in domestic animals in real time. Color flow Doppler ultrasonography has forever changed the practice of clinical obstetrics and gynecology in humans (44), and now the future is upon us regarding the application of this technology in theriogenology. Doppler interrogation of the vasculature and color flow imaging of the vessels of the reproductive tract and embryo–fetus offer new and exciting windows through which structural and functional events may be evaluated. In viewing the two-dimensional ultrasonographic image in real time, the experienced operator mentally constructs a three-dimensional image for comprehension. With advancing technologies in ultrasonography and in computer hardware and software, it may soon be possible to view reproductive organs in three dimensions and in real time (45). The purpose of this section is to provide a glimpse of what the application of advanced ultrasonographic imaging technologies may hold for the future in laboratories and hospitals.

Color Flow Doppler Ultrasonography

The flow of blood into various reproductive tissues can be quantitated while it is being visualized in real time using Doppler ultrasonographic imaging. A detailed appreciation of the physical principles of the Doppler effect and of ultrasound image formation are critical to the interpretation of the types of data generated by these modalities. The Doppler effect, as viewed during ultrasonographic evaluation of tissue vasculature, is a function of red blood cells moving within a vessel and the angle of intersection of the ultrasound beams with the vessel (46,47). The *spectral* Doppler signal is a waveform representing the Doppler shift created by circulating red blood cells during a cardiac cycle (i.e., systolic to diastolic). The ratio of systolic-to-diastolic flow, as measured by the amplitude of the waveforms, may be used to estimate resistance to blood flow. Doppler ultrasound data may be acquired and displayed in continuous-wave, pulsed-wave, or color flow imaging modalities. Although each modality has advantages and disadvantages, the ability to acquire quantitative data regarding vascular flow dynamics is common to each. Color flow Doppler imaging adds hues to standard gray-scale ultrasonography to indicate the direction of blood flow. The typical configuration for color display is blue for blood flowing away from the transducer and red for blood flowing toward the transducer. In addition, the intensity of color may be used to depict the velocity of blood flow (48). Differences in color intensity may also be used to indicate laminar or turbulent blood flow within a vessel. The direction (color) and velocity (intensity of color) of blood flow are calculated and displayed as a color overlay on the gray-scale image. Thus, the operator has simultaneous access to both structural and functional information. Color flow imaging is an exciting technique for the study of maternal and fetal hemodynamics during normal and abnormal pregnancies (44, 49, 50).

Two-dimensional ultrasonography, color flow Doppler ultrasonography, and spectral Doppler tracings are routinely used in human medicine, especially in assessment of reproductive status and fetal well-being (44, 51). The events related to maternal recognition of pregnancy and implantation dramatically alter the flow of blood to the uterus. In women, increased vascular flow into the uterine arteries and increased edema of the endometrium are among the first, although not definitive, signs of pregnancy (44,49). Little information is available on the application of color flow Doppler ultrasonography in domestic animals, especially with respect to reproductive events. In this regard, a preliminary study was done during early pregnancy to illustrate the power of color flow Doppler imaging in equine reproduction (GP Adams, DR Bergfelt, RA Pierson, unpublished data, 1994). Color flow Doppler images (Fig. 9.6) of a day 22 (**a**, **b**, and **c**) and a day 55 equine concep-

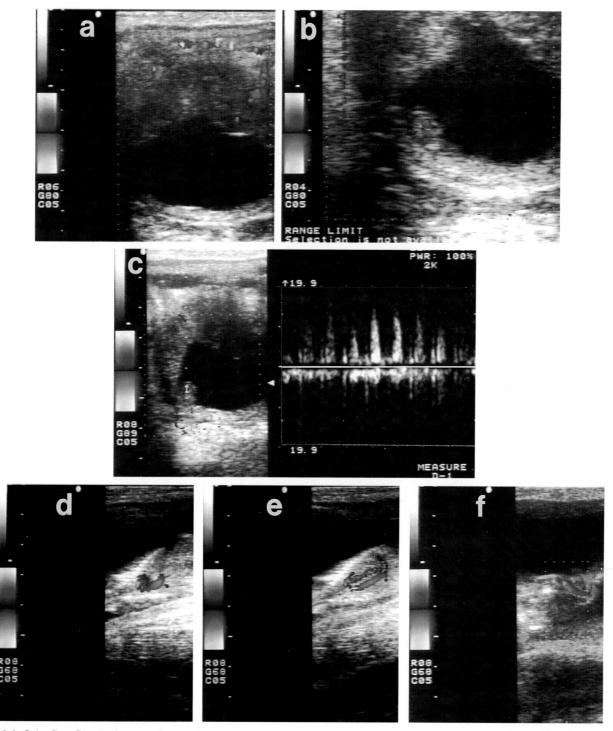

Figure 9.6. Color flow Doppler images of an equine conceptus on days 22 (*a-c*) and 55 (*d-f*). **a**, A branch of the uterine artery traversing the myometrium and penetrating into the endometrium. **b**, Cardiac activity of the embryo proper. **c**, A spectral Doppler signal showing systolic (*right*) and diastolic (*left*) wave-forms of the embryonic heart. **d**, Cardiac activity of the fetus. **e**, Vascular flow in the aorta and vena cava. **f**, Vascular flow in the umbilical cord.

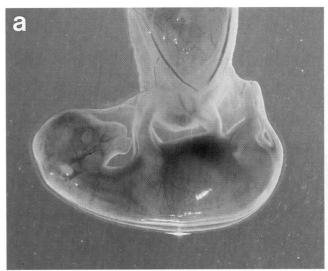 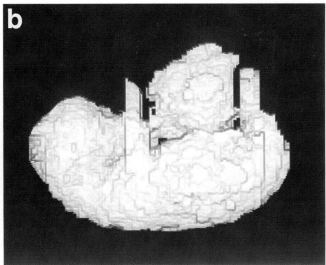

Figure 9.7. Three-dimensional reconstruction of a day 48 equine fetus done in vitro. **a**, Gross specimen. **b**, Three-dimensional image of reconstructed serial ultrasonographic images.

tus (**d**, **e**, and **f**) depict maternal and fetal vasculature and cardiac activity.

Three-Dimensional Image Reconstruction

Two-dimensional ultrasonography is a valuable research and clinical tool; however, the potential for three-dimensional visualization of structures in vivo is tantalizing. The current status of three-dimensional ultrasonography is of research application only; no practical or functional systems are capable of real-time three-dimensional imaging. Several independent research groups have developed off-line systems consisting of specialized ultrasound transducers in which information is directed to a high-speed graphics computer interfaced with a digital data acquisition board. These systems are capable of acquiring serial ultrasonographic images and converting them to a stack of parallel, equidistant images. The images may then be reconstructed in three dimensions and displayed to show surface structure. In addition, infrastructure may be displayed by selectively removing pixels of certain intensities or by peeling away portions of the stack of two-dimensional images that make up the three-dimensional image. Reconstructed three-dimensional images can also be oriented in any desired plane. Preliminary evaluation of the use of a three-dimensional imaging system was done in vitro using a day 48 equine fetus (RA Pierson, DR Bergfelt, GP Adams, unpublished data, 1994). The reconstructed image in Figure 9.7 illustrates the close association among structures (e.g., limb buds, cranium, umbilicus) of the gross specimen and the three-dimensional reconstruction. Many aspects of reproductive biology may be addressed with the application of three-dimensional imaging. Currently, volume documentation, "re-slicing" the reconstructed images in orthogonal or oblique planes, and development of advanced diag-

nostic techniques are being studied (52). Advanced computer image analysis algorithms may also be used in conjunction with three-dimensional imaging to reduce noise inherent in the initial ultrasonographic image and to enhance or accentuate biologically important structures after reconstruction (53–55). The potential for three-dimensional imaging is profound—development of integrated systems technologies will assist in the evaluation of internal and external organ structures in an automated and interactive fashion. Concurrent with development of three-dimensional imaging and color flow Doppler imaging, four-dimensional imaging is conceivable in which time becomes an aspect of the analysis.

REFERENCES

1. Ginther OJ. Reproductive biology of the mare: basic and applied aspects. Cross Plains, WI: Equiservices, 1979.
2. Ginther OJ. Ultrasonic imaging and reproductive events in the mare. Cross Plains, WI: Equiservices, 1986.
3. Ginther OJ. Reproductive biology of the mare: basic and applied aspects. 2nd ed. Cross Plains, WI: Equiservices, 1992:1–642.
4. Ginther OJ, Pierson RA. Ultrasonic evaluation of the mare reproductive tract: principles, equipment, and techniques. J Equine Vet Sci 1983;3:195–201.
5. Ligtvoet CM, Bom N, Gussenhoven WJ. Technical principles of ultrasound. In: Taverne MAM, Willemse AH, eds. Diagnostic ultrasound and animal reproduction. Amsterdam: Kluwer Academic, 1989:1.
6. Pipers FS, Adams-Brendemuehl CS. Techniques and applications of transabdominal ultrasonography in the pregnant mare. J Am Vet Med Assoc 1984;185:766–771.
7. Adams-Brendemuehl CS, Pipers FS. Antepartum evaluation of the equine conceptus. J Reprod Fertil 1987;35(Suppl):565–573.
8. Macpherson ML, et al. Transvaginal ultrasound-guided allantocentesis for pregnancy reduction in the mare. In: Proceedings of

the Annual Meeting of the Society of Theriogenology, Jacksonville, FL, 1993:168–177.

9. Ginther OJ. Ultrasonic evaluation of the reproductive tract of the mare: the single embryo. J Equine Vet Sci 1984;4:75–81.

10. Ginther OJ. Dynamic physical interactions between the equine embryo and uterus. Equine Vet J 1985;3(Suppl):41–47.

11. Ginther OJ. Intrauterine movement of the early conceptus in barren and postpartum mares. Theriogenology 1984;21:633–644.

12. Leith GS, Ginther OJ. Characterization of intrauterine mobility of the early equine conceptus. Theriogenology 1984;22:401–408.

13. Leith GS, Ginther OJ. Mobility of the conceptus and uterine contractions the mare. Theriogenology 1985;24:701–711.

14. Cross DT, Ginther OJ. Uterine contractions in nonpregnant and early pregnant mares and jennies as determined by ultrasonography. J Anim Sci 1988;66:250–254.

15. Griffin PG, Ginther OJ. Uterine contractile activity in mares during the estrous cycle and early pregnancy. Theriogenology 1990; 34:47–56.

16. Kastelic JP, Adams GP, Ginther OJ. Role of progesterone in mobility, fixation, orientation and survival of equine embryonic vesicles. Theriogenology 1987;27:655–663.

17. Griffin PG, Carnevale EM, Ginther OJ. Effects of the embryo on uterine morphology and function in mares. Anim Reprod Sci 1993;31:311–329.

18. Zavy MT, et al. An investigation of the uterine luminal environment of nonpregnant and pregnant pony mares. J Reprod Fertil 1979;27(Suppl):403–411.

19. Cross DT, Ginther OJ. The effect of estrogen, progesterone and prostaglandin$F_2\alpha$ on uterine contractions in seasonally anovulatory mares. Domest Anim Endocrinol 1987;4:271–278.

20. Bessent C, Cross DT, Ginther OJ. Effect of exogenous estradiol on mobility and fixation of the early equine conceptus. Anim Reprod Sci 1988;16:159–167.

21. Watson ED, Sertich PL. Prostaglandin production by horse embryos and the effect of co-culture of embryos with endometrium from pregnant mares. J Reprod Fertil 1989;87:331–336.

22. Ginther OJ. Fixation and orientation of the early equine conceptus. Theriogenology 1983;19:613–623.

23. Bergfelt DR, Woods JA, Ginther OJ. Role of the embryonic vesicle and progesterone in embryonic loss in mares. J Reprod Fertil 1992;95:339–347.

24. Ginther OJ. Effect of reproductive status on twinning and on side of ovulation and embryo attachment in mares. Theriogenology 1983;20:383–395.

25. Feo JCSA. Contralateral implantation in mares mated during postpartum estrus. Vet Rec 1980;106:368.

26. Allen WE, Newcombe JR. Relationship between early pregnancy site in consecutive gestations in mares. Equine Vet J 1981;13: 51–52.

27. Griffin G, Ginther OJ. Uterine morphology and function during the puerperium in mares. J Equine Vet Sci 1991;11:330–339.

28. Griffin PG, Ginther OJ. Dynamics of uterine diameter and endometrial morphology during the estrous cycle and early pregnancy in mares. Anim Reprod Sci 1991;25:133–142.

29. Hayes KEN, Ginther OJ. Role of progesterone and estrogen in development of uterine tone in mares. Theriogenology 1986;25: 581–590.

30. Steven DH. Placentation in the mare. J Reprod Fertil 1982; 31(Suppl):41–55.

31. Arthur GH. In: Veterinary reproduction and obstetrics. 4th ed. Baltimore: Williams & Wilkins, 1975.

32. Kahn W, Leidl W. [Ultrasonic biometry of horse fetuses in utero and sonographic representation of their organs] Die Ultraschall-Biometrie von Pferdefeten in utero und die sonographische Darstellung ihrer Organe. DTW Dtsch Tierarztl Wochenschr 1987;94:509–515.

33. McKinnon AO, Voss JL, Squires EL, et al. Diagnostic ultrasonography. In: McKinnon AO, Voss JL, eds. Equine reproduction. Philadelphia: Lea & Febiger, 1993:266–302.

34. Curran S, Ginther OJ. Ultrasonic diagnosis of equine fetal sex by location of the genital tubercle. J Equine Vet Sci 1989;9:77–83.

35. Ginther OJ. Equine physical utero-fetal interactions: a challenge and wonder for the practitioner. J Equine Vet Sci 1994;14: 313–318.

36. Ginther OJ, Adams PG. Equine fetal mobility observed by video-imaging endoscopy. Compend Contin Educ Pract Vet 1989;11: 1275–1280.

37. Griffin PG, Ginther OJ. Uterine and fetal dynamics during early pregnancy in mares. Am J Vet Res 1991;52:298–306.

38. Ginther OJ, Griffin PG. Equine fetal kinetics: presentation and location. Theriogenology 1993;40:1–11.

39. Griffin PG, Ginther OJ. Role of uterus in allantoic fluid shifts and fetal mobility in mares. Anim Reprod Sci 1993;31:301–310.

40. Allen WE. Palpable development of the conceptus and foetus in Welsh pony mares. Equine Vet J 1974;6:69–73.

41. Ginther OJ. Equine fetal kinetics: allantoic-fluid shifts and uterine-horn closures. Theriogenology 1993;40:241–256.

42. Jeffcott LB, Rossdale PD. A radiographic study of the fetus in late pregnancy and during foaling. Reprod Fertil 1979; 27(Suppl):563–569.

43. Fraser AF, et al. An exploratory ultrasonic study on quantitative foetal kinesis in the horse. Appl Anim Ethol 1975;1:395–404.

44. Jaffe R. Color Doppler imaging and assessment of early placental circulations. In: Jaffe R, Pierson RA, Abramowicz JS, eds.: Imaging in infertility and reproductive endocrinology. Philadelphia: JB Lippincott, 1994:345–354.

45. Steiner H, Staudach A, Spitzer D, et al. Three-dimensional ultrasound in obstetrics and gynecology: technique, possibilities and limitations. Hum Reprod 1994;9:1773.

46. Burns PN. Doppler flow estimations in the fetal and maternal circulation: principles, techniques and some limitations. In: Maulik D, McNellis D, eds. Doppler ultrasound measurements of maternal-fetal hemodynamics. New York: Perinatology Press, 1987.

47. Omoto R, Chihiro K. Physics and instrumentation of Doppler color flow mapping. Echocardiography 1987;4:467–483.

48. Meyer WJ, Jaffe R. Basic principles of Doppler ultrasonography. In: Jaffe R, Warsof S, eds. Color Doppler imaging in obstetrics and gynecology. New York: McGraw-Hill, 1992:1–16.

49. Kurjak A, Alfirevic Z, Miljan M. Conventional and color Doppler in the assessment of fetal and maternal circulation. Ultrasound Med Biol 1990;5:337–354.

50. Thaler I, et al. Changes in the uterine blood flow during human pregnancy. Am J Obstet Gynecol 1990;162:121–125.

51. Jaffe R, Warsof S, eds. Color Doppler imaging in obstetrics and gynecology. New York: McGraw-Hill, 1992.

52. Pierson RA, et al. Three dimensional ovarian ultrasonography in an in vitro model system. Int J Gynecol Obstet 1994;46(Suppl 2):37.

53. Muzzolini RE, Yang YH, Pierson RA. A framework for the evalu-

ation of feature detectors with application to diagnostic ultrasound images. Conference record of the Institute of Electrical and Electronic Engineers (IEEE), Nuclear Science and Medical Imaging Conference, Santa Fe, NM, 1991;3:2201–2204.

54. Muzzolini RE, Yang YH, Pierson RA. Three-dimensional segmentation of volume data. Institute of Electrical and Electronic Engineers (IEEE) Transactions on Medical Imaging Conference, Austin, TX, 1994;3:488–492.

55. Pierson RA, et al. New directions in imaging in infertility and reproductive endocrinology. In: Jaffe R, Pierson RA, Abramowicz, eds. Imaging in reproductive endocrinology and infertility. Philadelphia: JB Lippincott, 1994:389–398.

10 Twins

ANGUS O. McKINNON AND NORMAN W. RANTANEN

INTRODUCTION

Twins are important for a variety of reasons. Firstly, historically twins have been the single most important cause of abortion in Thoroughbreds (1, 2), and, secondly, regardless of the breed, twinning is a huge cause of reproductive wastage as most pregnancies terminate in early fetal resorption or loss, late-term abortions, or the birth of small, growth-retarded foals. Mares aborting twins in late gestation frequently have foaling difficulties, damage their reproductive tracts, and are difficult to rebreed, presumably due to delayed involution of an oversized uterus. Foals born alive are frequently small and demonstrate intrauterine growth retardation. Their survival rate is low, and for many of these foals long-term survival necessitates expensive, sophisticated critical care. For all of the above reasons twins are a disaster and should be avoided at all costs. An important philosophy that owners, stud managers, and veterinarians are all coming to grasp with is that *twins are preventable.*

Twins are linked with breed, season, nutrition, and a familial predisposition. More twins occur in Thoroughbreds, Draughthorses, and Warm-bloods compared with Standardbreds and Ponies. In early pregnancies diagnosed with ultrasonography, Thoroughbreds had an incidence of 97 of 629 pregnancies (15.4%) and Standardbreds an incidence of 39 of 634 (6.1%) (3). The number of abortions due to twins in one study was lowest in cold-blooded horses and in Arabian horses (4). In another study multiple ovulation rates were reduced in foaling mares (lactating) compared with barren mares and maidens and were more frequent in Thoroughbreds (19%) compared with Quarter horses (9%) and Appaloosa's (8%). Multiple ovulation rate is directly related to twinning and together with twinning was demonstrated as highly repeatable within mares. This study also showed that withholding breeding did not prevent twins (5). Twinning was the cause of 6.1% of equine abortions and stillbirths in central Kentucky during 1988 to 1989 (74 of 1211 fetuses) (6). Between 1986 and 1991 twins were associated with 221 of 3514 (6.3%) aborted fetuses, stillborn foals, or foals that died within 24 hours of birth (7). In cattle significant breed differences exist in ability to twin. Twinning increases from the first to the fourth calf and then plateaus. After the first twin calf is born, twinning is four to five times more likely compared with the normal population and, in addition, within season variability affects twin numbers (8). Twinning in mares was responsible for 4% of dystocias (9). Between 1968 and 1981 in West Germany twin pregnancies averaged 3.6% of a total population of 13,710 pregnancies. Eighty-five percent ended in last-trimester abortion, 5% as stillborn twins, and 10% produced either one or two live foals. Pascoe (1983) recorded that of 130 twin-pregnant mares (rectal palpation) only 17 gave birth to life foals (13%), and, furthermore, only 38 of 102 (37%) produced live foals the next year (10). A further study examining 1015 Standardbred mares from 2 to 24 years of age identified twin conception rate per cycle to be 15.3%, 8.8%, and 14% from maiden, lactating, and barren mares, respectively ($P < .01$) (11). In a study on abortion in Thoroughbred mares, twins accounted for 29% of an overall pregnancy loss of 12.8% (12). In a similar study twins accounted for a stillbirth percentage of 40.9% compared with 1.2% for the single group. Of twins born live, 30% died in the first week compared with 1% of singles. Thus only 25% of twins that had made it to the last month of pregnancy survived the first 8 weeks of life (13). High rates of eCG have been detected in mares with twin pregnancy (14), and these authors found twin pregnancy rates increased as the season progressed. The tendency for multiple ovulation and twinning to be familial was suggested by Urwin and Allen (15). Although improved nutrition did not increase the rates of multiple ovulation (16), it did appear to be related to a better display of estrus receptivity. Vandeplasshe (17) explained the high frequency of embryonic death and low vitality of twins as being caused by reduced blood supply associated with restricted uterine capacity in the later stages of pregnancy. He also noted interplacental vascular anastomoses were macroscopically visible in 25% of the cases, which resulted in blood chimerism. The chimerism did not interfere with subsequent fertility, and no freemartins were observed (17). More twins survive in Draught mares, and they have an incidence similar to Thoroughbreds (18). Twins were more common as the season progresses and in younger mares (19).

Because the expected outcome for mares with twins is so poor for either the mare or the resultant foal(s), it is our responsibility to successfully manage early pregnancies such that no mare delivers or aborts twin foals. In consultation with farm managers, owners, and clients we must utilize available equipment and technology commensurate with economic constraints and other owner/manager preferences to diagnose twin pregnancies as early as practically possible. It is the responsibility of a veterinary professional to adequately inform owners/managers/clients of the reasons why twins may not be diagnosed. *In the future it is possible that veterinarians will be held accountable for failure to diagnose twins, especially in circumstances where owners expect sophisticated reproductive services and mares are examined repeatedly.*

Reasons why twins may be missed despite repeated examination are as follows:

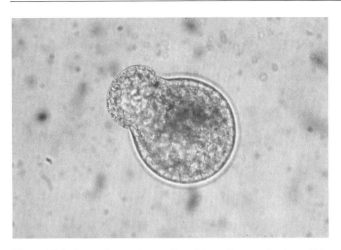

Figure 10.1. An equine embryo cultured from the morula stage. This embryo is hatching similar to other species because there is no capsule. The postulated mechanism for identical twin formation in *other species* is embryo bisection associated with hatching and pinching of an early embryo as the zona pellucida closes.

1. Difficulty distinguishing structures. This may be related to a poor scanning environment, that is, too much light, poor display characteristics of the ultrasound, or mare movement and/or lack of restraint.
2. Variable growth patterns.
3. Inability to detect heart beats of adjacent embryos.
4. Operator experience.
5. Resolution of the equipment.

In our experience the most common reason for misdiagnosing early twin pregnancy is scanning too early to be able to recognize a second pregnancy from an asynchronous ovulation. Another reason that frequently occurs is scanning too quickly.

Twin pregnancy has been a common cause of abortion (19). The incidence of abortion is decreasing (6) and in the German Thoroughbred industry has declined from 2.7% to 1.7% since the advent of ultrasonography (20). In our practice, when mares are examined according to our recommendations at day 15, 25, 35, and 45 postovulation, there have been no twin pregnancies or abortions from twin pregnancies (that we are aware of) after mares were initially diagnosed and subsequently recorded as having a single pregnancy.

ORIGIN OF TWINS

Many nonequine veterinarians would be surprised to learn that twins in the horse are almost, if not exclusively, associated with a double ovulation. Until recently, only one reference alluded to the identification of an identical twin (21). In this text Rooney states *"I have only seen one definite example of identical twinning (of some 600 such abortions examined); there were two amniotic sacs and a single allantochorion."* Recently, an article appeared that demonstrated that identical triplets had occurred (confirmed with DNA analysis), which were first suspected after video endoscopy

showed they were all in one chorionic sac (monochorionic) (22). This would appear to be an extremely unusual occurrence. Reasons for lack of identical twins in the horse may be related to the equine capsule. The capsule forms in embryos aged around 6 days, shortly after their entry into the uterus (23). When embryos were cultured prior to the formation of the capsule, hatching (Fig. 10.1) occurred similar to that which occurs in the bovine (23); however, when embryos were cultured after formation of the capsule, the zona pellucida continued to become progressively thinner and finally fell away from the developing conceptus (Fig. 10.2). The postulated mechanism for identical twin formation in other species is embryo bisection associated with hatching and pinching of an early embryo (A Trounson, personal communication—quoted by McKinnon et al. [24]). As an interesting aside, in one report 70 of 111 aborted twins (63%) were the same sex, which indicated to those authors (25) that perhaps splitting of the embryo occurs. However, this observation may be by chance alone. Another interpretation would be an improved efficiency of eliminating opposite-sex fetuses (earlier in gestation). A more recent study (26) recorded that of 35 twin pairs 65.7% were of opposite sexes. This study is in contrast to the previous one and serves to highlight dangers inherent in extrapolation from anything but large sets of data. The recent publication of identical horse triplets (22) stated that they did not arise from separation of blastomeres during early cleavage stages, as division at this time would have given rise to individual sets of extraembryonic membranes. *"Separation of the inner cell mass must have occurred prior to gastrulation in order to result in each embryo sharing the outermost chorion while at the same time having an individual amnion"* (22).

Originally, twins were hypothesized to have occurred more frequently from asynchronous ovulations (27). This author found that double ovulation and twins were seen more frequently in barren mares (11% and 6%, respectively) com-

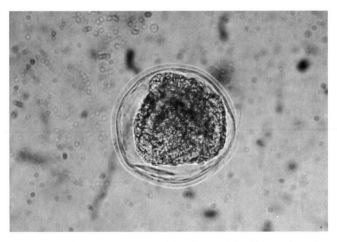

Figure 10.2. An equine embryo with collapse of the blastocele cavity (after freezing and thawing) showing clearly the capsule on the inside and the zona pellucida on the outside. In the horse we postulate that the capsule prevents identical twin formation by not allowing the embryo to hatch.

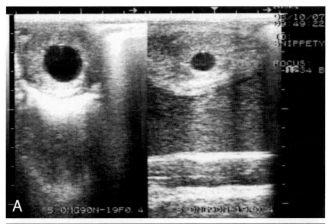

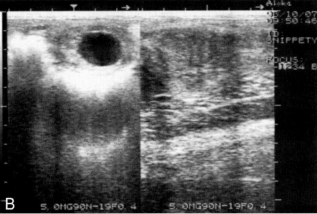

Figure 10.3. Split-screen image of **(A)** a 14-day (*left side*) and 12-day twin pregnancy, and **(B)** after crushing of the smaller vesicle, minimal fluid remains (*right*).

OUTCOME OF TWIN PREGNANCIES

Nonintervention

Prefixation

Days 11 Through 16. Embryo reduction before or on the day of fixation is not considered an important aspect of the natural correction of twins (31). Diameter and growth rates on days 11 through 16 were similar between singleton and twins, and the presence of two vesicles did not have a direct effect on diameter other than that attributable to their age. The probability of a mare loosing one or both vesicles of a set of twins from identification prior to fixation is minimal and approximates that of early embryonic death for the same time period (per vesicle). The recognition of twin pregnancies prior to fixation day (day 16) is dependent on the day of examination relative to the day of ovulation. Asynchronous ovulations occasionally result in a disparity in vesicle size (Fig. 10.3) sometimes as much as 5 days, that is, identification of a day-11 and a day-16 vesicle concurrently. In instances such as this, examination 1 day earlier most likely would have failed to detect the younger of the two pregnancies. Recognition that all twin pregnancies occur from multiple ovulations dictates mandatory reexamination of all mares that have two CLs and only a single vesicle detected prior to fixation (day 16). Recognition prior to fixation is also dependent on operator experience, resolution of the equipment (5 MHZ preferred), monitor capabilities, restraint and other facilities (ability to darken the environment), the presence of uterine cysts (Fig. 10.4), and the skill of the examiner.

Postfixation

Recognition. The recognition of unilaterally fixed twins from days 17 through 21 (prior to clear recognition of the developing fetus within the vesicle) may be the most difficult

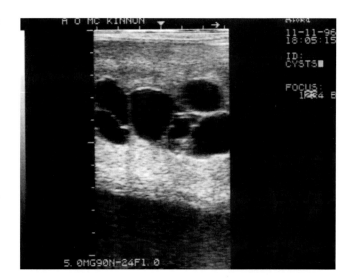

Figure 10.4. Multiple uterine cysts that are pedunculated and thus well circumscribed may confuse or create difficulty in diagnosis of either single or twin pregnancies.

pared with lactating mares (5% and 1%, respectively) and that nine twin pregnancies from 32 mares were associated with ovulations 2 days apart (asynchronous) compared with 0 of 19 for synchronous ovulations. Many of these original observations were made prior to ultrasonography and as a good example of these inherent diagnostic difficulties, the same author quoted 70% of twins arriving from one detected ovulation (based on analysis of multiple veterinarians' breeding-farm records) (27, 28). Subsequently, it was shown that twins were as likely to result from synchronous as asynchronous ovulation (29) and that the pregnancy rate per follicle from double ovulations on opposite ovaries was identical to that obtained per cycle from single ovulations, but was higher than the pregnancy rate per follicle when double ovulations occurred on the same ovary. These results indicated there was no embryo reduction prior to the first diagnosis of pregnancy with ultrasonography in bilateral ovulators, as each ovum had the same chance of developing into a day-11 conceptus as an ovum from single ovulators. In unilateral double ovulators the lower day-11 pregnancy rate per ovulation compared with bilateral ovulators and single ovulators was attributable to a greater frequency of mares with no embryonic vesicles rather than to a greater frequency of mares with one vesicle (30).

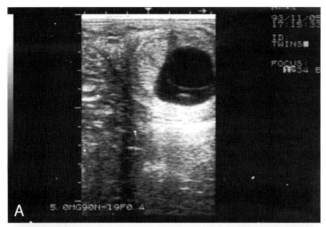

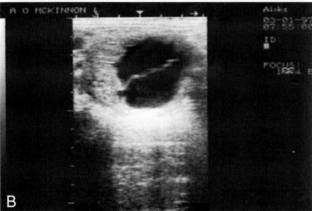

Figure 10.5. Unilaterally fixed twin pregnancies with an ultrasonographically visible line in between. **A.** Approximately 16-day twin vesicles with one larger. **B.** Approximately 19-day twin pregnancies.

time to determine if twins are present. Ultrasonographically, all that is present is a thin line (the apposition of the two yolk sacs) running approximately in the middle of a slightly oversized vesicle (Fig. 10.5). Recognition of the fetus(es) within the vesicle a few days later makes differentiation easier (Fig. 10.6). Occasionally, an inexperienced operator may confuse an abnormally orientated 28- to 30-day single pregnancy with 17- to 20-day unilaterally fixed twins. From days 22 to 60 the presence of multiple fetuses, umbilical cords, and a general excess in the number of visible membranes should alert the practitioner to the likelihood of more than one pregnancy. The junction between two developing fetuses (after 30 days) between the two allantochorions results in a common membrane from the area of apposition. This common membrane has been referred to recently as the *twin membrane* (32) and has diagnostic potential, particularly late in pregnancy when it might not be possible to view both fetuses transrectally (>100 days). After 100 days, careful transabdominal ultrasonography may be necessary to determine the presence of twins.

Days 17 through 39. The outcome of fetuses postfixation is dependent on the nature of their fixation. Unilateral (both fixed together at the same corpus cornual junction) fixation

reduction is much higher than bilateral (one on each side) fixation reduction. Fortunately, unilateral fixation is much higher (approximately 70%) compared with bilateral (30%). In one study of 31 mares with twin embryonic vesicles, unilateral fixation (71%) was more frequent ($P < .05$) than bilateral fixation (29%) (33). In 28 mares with known ovulatory patterns, synchronous ovulations did not affect the type of fixation (9 of 17 unilateral, 8 of 17 bilateral). However, for asynchronous ovulators the frequency of unilateral fixation (10 of 11) was greater ($P < .01$) than the frequency of bilateral fixation (1 of 11). The incidence of embryo reduction was greater ($P < .01$) for unilateral fixation (14 of 19) than for bilateral fixation (0 of 9) and was greater ($P < .05$) for asynchronous ovulators (9 of 11) than for synchronous ovulators (5 of 17) (33). When reduction occurs with unilateral fixation, it is most commonly detected early (prior to recognition of the fetus). In one study, 10 of 14 reductions occurred prior to detection of either embryo . The degree of synchrony of ovulation also affected reduction. Early reduction occurred in 8 of 11 mares with asynchronous ovulation, and for 17 synchronous ovulators none reduced early, 5 reduced late, and 12 did not reduce at all (33). In another study the incidence of reduction was higher for unilateral fixation (41 of 48) (85%). In cases of unilateral fixation 22 of 22 mares with vesicles of dissimilar size ($\geq$ 4 mm difference in diameter) had reduction compared with 19 of 26 (73%) with vesicles of similar size (34). As a result of work studying reduction of unilateral versus bilateral twin pregnancies in mares from days 17 to 40, Ginther proposed a deprivation hypothesis (33) that suggested that the nutrient intake from the larger vesicle (prefetal detection) prevented adequate nutrition of the smaller vesicle. Later the position of the embryo/fetus proper and its emerging allantoic sac seemed to determine whether a given conceptus survived or underwent late reduction. The embryo

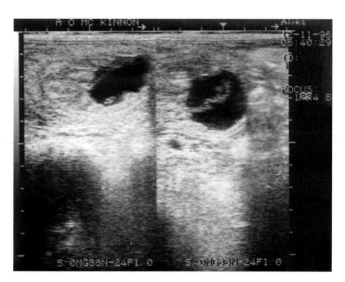

Figure 10.6. Split-screen image of a 22-day-old, unilaterally fixed, twin pregnancy with a detectable fetus and heart beat in each. The bottom pregnancy (*left side*) appears larger than the other (*right side*).

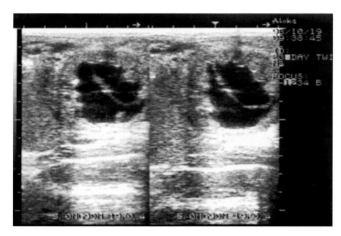

Figure 10.7. Split-screen image of a 22- and 20-day-old twin pregnancy that has been unilaterally fixed. A small fetus was seen in the upper pregnancy, and it had disappeared within 3 days of recording this picture. This supports the embryo reduction hypothesis.

proper, the vascularized wall of the yolk sac adjacent to the embryo proper, and the emerging allantoic sac were exposed to the endometrium (uterine lumen) in the surviving vesicles (Figs. 10.7 and 10.8). In the vesicles that underwent reduction, much of the corresponding area of the vesicle wall was covered by the wall of the adjacent survivor. Thus embryo reduction occurs when a major portion of the three-walled area of the yolk sac or the vascularized wall of the yolk sac or allantoic sac is in apposition with the wall of the adjacent vesicle rather than with the endometrium, and the vesicle is thus deprived of adequate embryonal-maternal exchange and therefore regresses.

In summary, dissimilarity in diameter increased the likelihood of unilateral fixation, increased the incidence of reduction for unilaterally fixed vesicles, hastened the day of occurrence of reduction, and shortened the interval from initiation to completion of reduction. The incidence of reduction for bilaterally fixed embryos was negligible and approximated that of standard early embryonic death in this period. Of the 85% of reductions by day 40 in cases of unilaterally fixed twin pregnancies, 59% of reductions had occurred between days 17 and 20, 27% between days 21 and 30, and 14% between days 31 and 38. The majority of early reductions occurred spontaneously (≤20 days) as compared with reductions after day 20 that were preceded by a gradual decrease in size of the eliminated vesicle. In addition, when twins were dissimilar in diameter (4 mm or more), they were more likely to undergo reduction by day 20 (34). Other studies have demonstrated similar results. Examination of 69 sets of twins revealed that the greater the disparity in size, the greater the chance of unilateral fixation (29). Differences of greater than 3 mm were associated with 83% unilateral fixation compared with 56% for those less than 3 mm (35). The hypothesis of an early embryo-reduction mechanism for elimination of excess embryos in mares was not new and had been suggested as early as 1982. However,

ultrasonography was necessary to adequately document the occurrence and nature of the reduction (36).

Day 40 Onward. Although many studies report the visible signs of later, twin pregnancies, that is, abortion, stillbirth, or production of live foals, apparently only one study has documented (using ultrasonography) the outcome of twin pregnancy after day 40 (32). Ginther and Griffin (1994) examined the natural outcome of bilateral twins (one in each horn) that were viable on day 40 in 15 pony mares. Readers should be aware that pony mares are not necessarily a good model for the Thoroughbred or other breeds, as the incidence of twins is low and evidence is suggestive that the larger the breed (Draught, Thoroughbred, and Warmblood), the higher the probability of maintaining twins. Fifteen pony mares were monitored by ultrasonography until the outcome of the pregnancy was determined. Sixty-six percent of the pregnancies resulted in either death of both fetuses (80%) or death of one fetus (20%) during months 2 or 3. Nothing occurred from then until month 8. Between months 8 and 11, two mares lost one fetus (one fetus became mummified and the other survived until term) and two mares lost both. The two mares that lost one pregnancy both delivered undersized weak foals at birth. One mare (7%) delivered live twins at term, and two normal foals were born from mares losing the one pregnancy in month 2. In this study six live foals were born (two of normal size) from a total of 15 mares and 30 fetuses. This incidence is similar to previous reports wherein of 130 twin-pregnant mares only 17 live foals (13%) were produced (10). An interesting observation from the later report was that from the 102 mares that delivered live or dead twins in the previous year, only 37 produced live foals the next seasons and thus over two seasons there was an average of 23% producing live foals (10). An earlier study (19) was extremely useful in categorizing the outcome of twins that managed to survive to later pregnancy. Twinning accounted for 22% of the cases of abortion and stillbirth between 1967 and 1970. Sixty-two sets of twins and their pla-

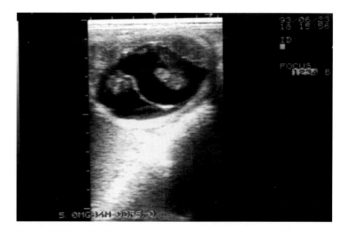

Figure 10.8. A 33-day twin pregnancy that persisted past 60 days of age. When first detected the embryos were at opposite poles of the vesicle.

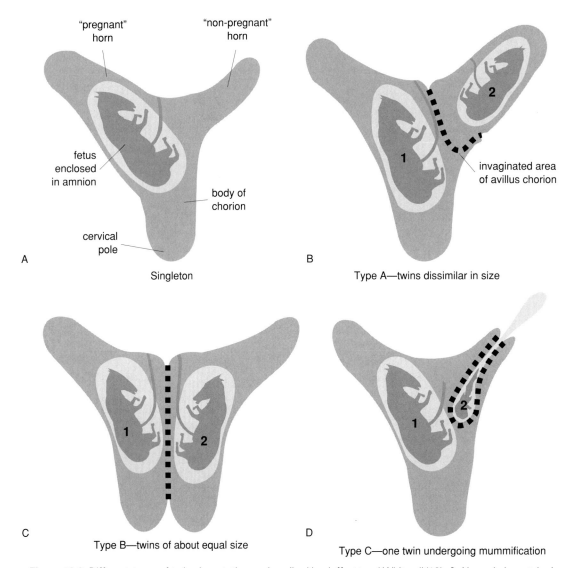

Figure 10.9. Different types of twin placentation as described by Jeffcott and Whitwell (19). **A.** Normal placental orientation of a singleton. The pregnant horn is slightly larger than the nonpregnant horn. **B.** Type A placentation. One fetus occupies one horn and most of the body, while the other twin occupies only one horn and usually only a small part of the adjacent body (see Fig. 10.10). **C.** Type B placentation. The placentas are orientated such that the villous surface areas are more or less equally divided and each fetus occupies one horn and half of the body (see Fig. 10.11). **D.** Type C placentation. There is a greater disparity between the surface area of the two chorions (see Fig. 10.12) (As observed at Goulburn Valley Equine Hospital.)

centas were examined from Thoroughbred mares. All were considered to be dizygous. Abortion or stillbirth of both twins from 3 months of gestation to term occurred in 64.5% of mares, although most (72.6%) slipped from 8 months to term. In the remaining cases one twin (21%) or both twins (14.5%) were born alive. Most foals at term were stunted and emaciated, and of the 31 alive at birth only 18 had survived to 2 weeks of age (19). In this study twin placentation was divided into three morphologic groups according to the disposition of the chorionic sacs within the uterus (Fig. 10.9). Type A placentation was seen in 79% of cases (48 sets of twins). One fetus occupied one horn and most of the body (mean 68% of the total functional surface area), while the other twin occupied only one horn and usually only a small part of the adjacent body.

Where the chorions abutted, there was a variable degree of invagination of the smaller chorion into the allantoic cavity of the larger twin. These pregnancies frequently ended in abortion or stillbirth of one or both twins (Fig. 10.10). The larger twin had a much greater chance of survival than the smaller one. In this group 31 of 48 lost their pregnancies between 3 and 9 months (64.5%). The gestation length in this group was frequently shorter, and at birth the larger twin had a much greater chance of survival than the smaller one. In this group only six foals of 48 sets were born alive. Of the six fetuses born alive, five were the larger twin. Type B placentation occurred in 11% of cases (seven sets), and the placentas were orientated such that the villous surface areas were more or less equally divided and each fetus occupied one horn and half of the body (Fig. 10.11). Both

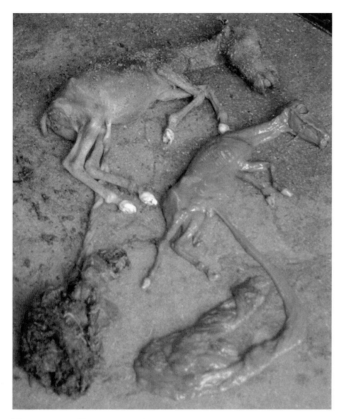

Figure 10.10. Two aborted fetuses demonstrating the type A placentation. The bottom fetus has begun to be mummified.

foals were usually similar in size (Fig. 10.11) and were usually born alive. Nine foals survived to 2 weeks from six sets of twins that made it to term. In this group (seven total) one aborted at 7 months. Type C placentation was seen in 10% of cases (six sets of twins). In this group there was a greater disparity between the surface area of the two chorions. The smaller twin that occupied only part of one horn died earlier on and became mummified (Fig. 10.12). The larger twin was usually born alive and had a fair chance of survival. In this group three foals were born alive from six pregnancies at term (19). The authors attributed the loss of twin fetuses and poor survival rates to placental insufficiency.

From the above discussion it would appear that nonintervention is probably only acceptable when twins are diagnosed as a unilateral occurrence between days 17 and day 40 and depends on factors such as the value of the foal, the potential for rebreeding, and the ability of the veterinarian to manually intervene. Intervention in twin pregnancies is strongly recommended in all other circumstances (see below).

Intervention

Prefixation

Days 11 Through 16. The first technique for manual crush of the conceptus during the mobility phase utilized manual reduction with good results (37) and was a variation from

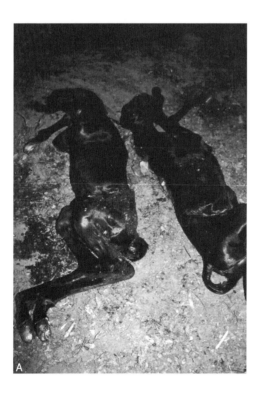
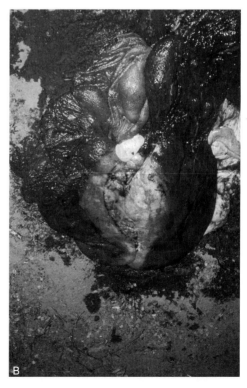

Figure 10.11. A. Twins that were carried to term and died due to dystocia. **B.** Membranes from a type B placentation twin pregnancy **(A)**. Note the avillous contact area and approximately even size of the villous placenta.

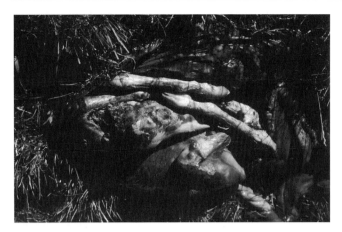

Figure 10.12. A mummified fetus delivered at term together with a slightly smaller than normal live foal.

previously reported techniques for twin pregnancies (38, 39). The technique involved gentle manipulation of the embryonic vesicle to the tip of one uterine horn and manual rupture. When applied to single pregnancies, it resulted in pseudopregnancy, and when applied to twin pregnancies, it resulted in a single pregnancy in seven of eight attempts (37). Later, utilizing the same techniques, mares were treated with single or multiple progesterone administration, an antiprostaglandin (flunixin meglumine) plus progesterone, or given no treatment prior to manual embryonic rupture in the mobility phase (40, 41). Results were 10 of 10 (100%) mares maintaining pregnancy in the control group (no treatment, just manual rupture) and 37 of 40 (92.5%) for treated mares. The amount of $PGF_{2\alpha}$ released was directly correlated with the pressure required to cause embryonic rupture. Flunixin meglumine inhibited $PGF_{2\alpha}$ release after embryonic rupture. Treatment with progesterone plus flunixin meglumine or progesterone singly or multiply was not better than no treatment at all (40, 41), although it was subsequently shown that the progesterone chosen (hydroxyprogesterone caproate) had no ability to maintain pregnancy in ovariectomized mares and did not bind to progesterone receptors in the horse (42). Another report (3) demonstrated that 60 of 66 mares (90.9%) maintained a single vesicle after manual reduction was attempted prior to fixation. Five of the six mares in which the procedure was not successful subsequently conceived when rebred.

Since 1984 we have used a modification (24) of the technique described originally by Ginther in 1983 (37). With this technique the ultrasound probe is used to manipulate the vesicles while keeping one or both vesicles in view during the manipulation and, more importantly, during the crushing or rupture of the vesicle (Fig. 10.13). Utilizing this technique, it is possible to more accurately and quickly separate vesicles (Fig. 10.14). It was originally proposed (37) that when vesicles were in apposition, mares be reexamined approximately 1 hour later. By utilizing the probe to ma-

nipulate vesicles, separation is achieved (prefixation) very quickly in most instances. Commonly, the smaller fetus is destroyed despite the lack of evidence to support prefixation reduction. Sometimes fluid from the destroyed vesicle surrounds the other (Fig. 10.15). This does not appear to be a problem with prefixation embryos. On occasion, it is necessary to revisit the mare 24 to 48 hours after the original examination if the smaller of the two vesicles is less than 1 cm in diameter since sometimes these can be more difficult to

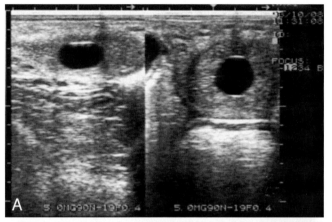

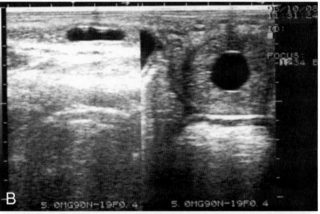

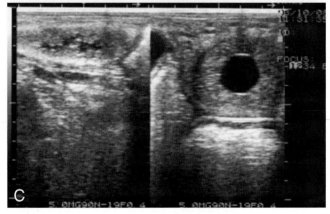

Figure 10.13. Split-screen image of prefixation twins. **A.** Approximately equal-sized 14-day twins that were separate (left and right horns). **B.** Gentle pressure with the probe has distorted the vesicle chosen to be ruptured (*left side*). **C.** Immediately after vesicle collapse (depending on its size), the fluid and membranes (*left side*) are commonly seen for around 5 to 30 seconds.

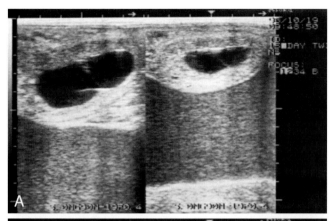

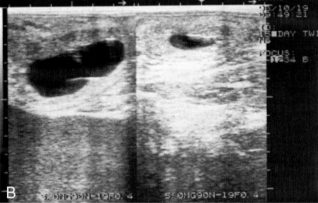

Figure 10.14. Split-screen image of twins fixed together at 16 and 15 days. **A.** On the left is the original configuration. On the right is the beginning of gentle pressure being applied between the two vesicles. **B.** By moving the probe back and forth slightly and gently, the vesicles can be separated (*right screen*).

destroy. At the GVEH (Goulburn Valley Equine Hospital) records are available for 3032 mares (1489 Thoroughbreds and 1543 Standardbreds) throughout the last three breeding seasons; 245 had twins diagnosed prefixation. After twin reduction (day 14 to 16) mares are not routinely examined until the next scheduled examination, that is 21 to 25 days postovulation (detection of the fetus). When mares were reexamined at day 25, 95.1% (233 of 245) were found to still be pregnant. The number of mares losing the pregnancy (4.9%) is similar to the normal rate of early embryonic death recorded on these farms during the same period (4.6%—117 of 2802), and of the 12 mares failing to maintain the single pregnancy after the elimination of the co-twin, 75% had demonstrable uterine inflammation (uterine infection) observed with ultrasonography at the next heat cycle. It is our contention that the procedure has developed to the stage that it is *always expected* that a single pregnancy will exist after manual prefixation embryo reduction is attempted. Unless a mistake occurs and the other vesicle is ruptured at the time of initial manipulation (this should not happen), we feel that any failure to survive the procedure is more likely a result of uterine inflammatory changes of infection rather than a result of the procedure. We believe that this is the

most reliable technique available, but feel it is important to highlight the experience of the personnel involved. From discussions with farm managers and other veterinarians it is clear that only veterinarians involved with sophisticated reproductive management such as the routine use of ultrasonography can expect to achieve these types of results. Our strong recommendation to veterinarians and clients is that all mares are examined within 14 and 16 days of breeding. Expected time to ovulation after breeding will depend on ovulation induction agents such as hCG or GnRH. Factors that may modify this decision are breed, mare value, ability of the stud master or owner to facilitate examination of the mare, and on occasion education of the owner. Another interesting observation to come out the study of our broodmare records was the significantly more frequent diagnosis ($P > .0001$) of twins (15.6 % of all pregnancies and 10 % of mare cycles) in Thoroughbred mares versus Standardbred mares (4.2 % of all pregnancies and 2.5 % of mare cycles). The percentage of mares loosing a pregnancy after twin ablation (negative at the next examination, $\sim$ day 25) was higher in the Standardbred population (8.8%, 5/57) versus the Thoroughbred mares (3.7%, 7/188) and most likely reflects the later timing of the first pregnancy diagnosis in the Standardbred population due to economic restraints. Another possible point of interest was the documentation of eight sets of triplets and one set of quadruplets. All but one were in Thoroughbreds, and all had a single pregnancy at the next examination period after vesicle ablation.

Postfixation

Days 17 Through 20. In all cases of bilaterally fixed twins one is destroyed immediately (Fig. 10.16); however, the mare has an extremely efficient biologic embryo-reduction mechanism that operates when twins are in apposition (unilaterally fixed) (33, 36, 43). In one study the incidence of embryo reduction after unilateral fixation was 14 of 19 (73.7%), which was significantly greater than 0 of 9 ($P < .01$) for bilateral fixation. In addition, asynchronous ovula-

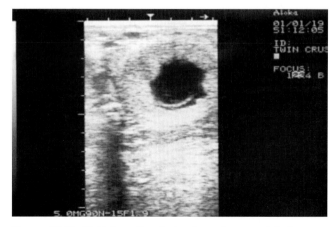

Figure 10.15. Fluid from the destruction of one vesicle has surrounded the other one. This does not appear to be a problem prefixation.

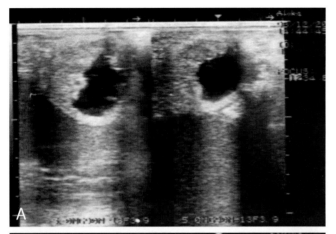

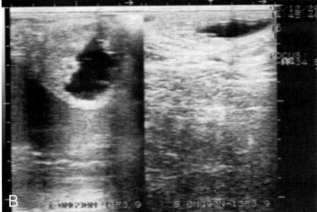

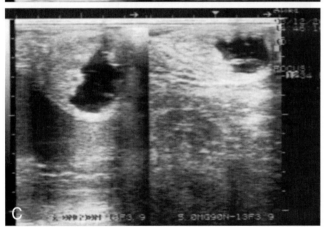

Figure 10.16. Splitscreen image showing bilaterally fixed 21-day-old twins. **A.** First examination. The fetus on the right side appears smaller and perhaps a little behind the one on the left. **B.** Pressure is being applied to the vesicle on the right side. **C.** Rupture of the vesicle has occurred and membranes and fetal fluid can be seen momentarily. In this case the remaining fetus survived. After fixation and probably more importantly after early invasion of the endometrium with the chorionic girdle cells, it appears that if the fluid from a crushed vesicle escapes and surrounds the other, the probability of a successful outcome is reduced.

tion resulted in 90% (9 of 10) embryo reduction after unilateral fixation. From the 14 mares that had embryo reduction, 10 (71.4%) had early embryonic reduction (17 to 20 days) (33). Other studies have confirmed these results. The

incidence of reduction was 41 of 48 (85%) following unilateral fixation (34). Reduction occurred in 100% of 22 mares with asynchronous ovulation (vesicles size greater than 4 mm in diameter) and 19 of 26 (73%) of mares with similar vesicle size (0 to 3 mm difference). Of all the reductions occurring, 59% of the reductions occurred between days 17 and 20, 27% between days 21 and 30, and 14% between days 31 and 38. In the early reductions the vesicles just simply disappeared. Reductions that occurred after day 20 were preceded by a gradual decrease in size of the vesicle that was lost. As the number of days after day 17 increased, the frequency of reduction decreased and the time required for completion of reduction increased. Because the rate of embryo reduction between days 17 and 20 is so high for unilateral fixation, equine practitioners frequently elect to leave these developing pregnancies and determine their outcome later. Our philosophies are that if the two vesicles have coalesced into one larger vesicle with an ultrasonographically visible line in division (Fig. 10.17), they are left totally alone; however, if the vesicles have still retained a spherical orientation or a spherical shape (Fig. 10.18), then they can be separated gently with the probe and crushed either in situ

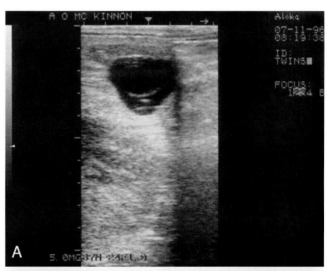

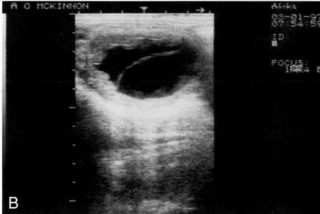

Figure 10.17. Unilateral fixation of twins postfixation. **A.** An 18- and 16-day set of twins. It would be difficult to separate these two. **B.** A 19- and an 18-day vesicle fixed.

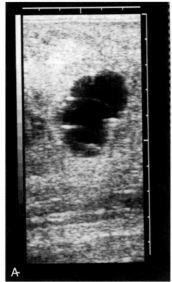

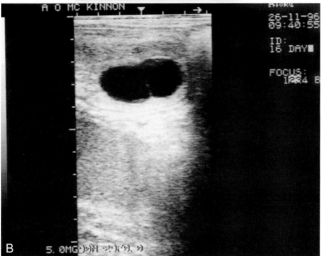

Figure 10.18. When vesicles retain a spherical shape they can commonly be manipulated apart at either **(A)** 17 days or **(B)** 15 days.

and days 25 to 30 (1/4—25%). Because of the high incidence of embryo reduction with unilateral fixation and the low incidence with bilateral fixation, we have clear recommendations with twins in the 17- to 20-day period. Those that have rounded-figure-8-shaped twins, still retaining their vesicle turgidity and that can be separated, are crushed either in situ or after being manipulated apart. In all cases where the vesicles have apparently coalesced into a larger vesicle with an ultrasonographically single line dividing the two, we leave them alone, more particularly so if there is any unevenness in vesicle size. In all cases of bilaterally fixed twins, one is destroyed immediately.

Days 21 Through 29. All cases of bilaterally fixed twins of this age group are manipulated and one destroyed immediately. In most cases we do not attempt to manually destroy one vesicle with unilaterally fixed twins of this age group until after day 30 and before day 35. At this age it is too easy to rupture both vesicles and the maximum success we believe we can expect is 50% (see previous section), which is less than or similar to the mares own biologic reduction mechanism.

Days 30 Through 35. During the period prior to the formation of endometrial cups, gentle pressure may be placed on one vesicle. We do not attempt total ablation at this time, as resulting fluid sometimes surrounds the other fetus and effectively separates early placental (chorionic girdle/trophoblast cells) attachments to the uterus. In these cases (total rupture of the vesicle), death of the remaining vesicle is very common. Between days 30 and 35 we attempt to pinch one vesicle and create a "snowflake" effect (Fig. 10.19), which is the shedding of cells from the membranes. Demonstration of this effect almost always results in gradual loss of the affected conceptus.

Days 36 Through 59. From day 36 onward it is a reasonable assumption that endometrial cup formation and subsequent eCG secretion will prevent many mares from returning to

or after being manipulated apart. Due to the nature of our practice, few mares present with this configuration in the Thoroughbred population; however, it is not uncommon in the Standardbred population wherein economics dictate that pregnancy diagnosis is often delayed past the time the mobility phase has ended (until after the time they normally would be expected to return to heat). Results from our practice with twins in this configuration are reduced compared with prefixation intervention procedures. Others have reported good results postfixation. One group reported success in 49 of 50 cases postfixation (40). The report from Bowman (3) more closely parallels our experiences. With bilateral embryo fixation and intervention, he reported almost no losses with 40 of 44 mares from days 16 to 30 (90.9%) having a single pregnancy detected on day 45. With unilateral fixation the results were as follows: days 16 to 17 (from breeding) (16/18—89%), days 18 to 19 (23/24—95.8%), days 20 to 21 (8/13—61.5%), days 22 to 24 (4/9—47.4%),

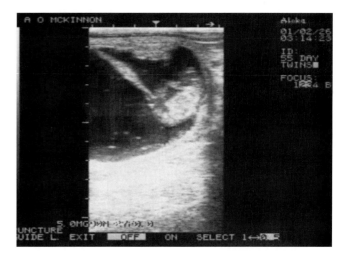

Figure 10.19. An image of a 44-day-old pregnancy that has the "snowflake" effect created by membrane damage associated with pinching.

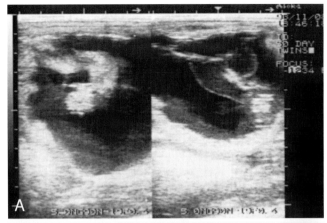

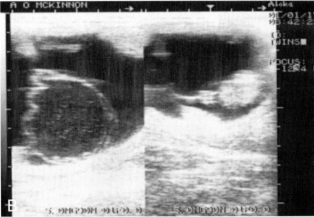

Figure 10.20. A. Split-screen image. On the left is a normally developing 50-day pregnancy and on the right is a pregnancy with no detectable heart beat and increased echogenicity of the fluid surrounding the fetus (amnionic cavity). This was created by multiple trauma to the selected fetus. **B.** Split-screen image. On the left side can be seen a circular membrane (twin membrane) within the fetal fluids of the dead twin have become quite echogenic. The fluids surrounding the live twin (*right side*) are quite clear.

heat after early embryonic death. Abortion after 35 days is commonly associated with difficulties recycling the mare (44, 45). In one study (46) when mares were aborted either between days 26 and 31 or between days 30 and 50, 8 of 11 became pregnant versus 2 of 7, respectively. This is similar to the work of Pascoe (10) who concluded that the administration of a prostaglandin analog less than 35 days of gestation was outstandingly successful as a method of treatment for twin pregnancy. Manual intervention at this time in our experience is approximately 50% successful. Success improves with use of more subtle pressure and damage to the chorioallantoic membrane rather than complete rupture in one attempt. Demonstration of the snowflake effect without vesicle rupture consistently results in a gradual (48 hour) stress of the fetus and ultimate loss of heartbeat for the conceptus. These pregnancies have fetal fluids that become progressively more hyperechoic (Fig. 10.20) and reduce in size without interfering with the survival of the other fetus. It is important with these fetuses to always attempt to damage the same one.

Multiple attempts, that is, every day or every other day for 5 to 10 sessions, may be necessary to elicit the correct response; however, quite frequently we are unable to create sufficient damage for fetal destruction. In these cases rather than creating major trauma (rupture of the vesicle) (Fig. 10.21), an alternative approach is sought after day 60. A variety of methods have been used to treat twins at this stage. Originally reported results of manual crushing (39) suggested that ear-

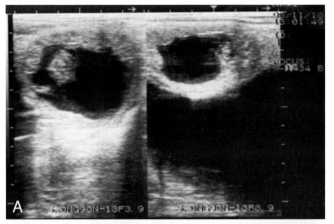

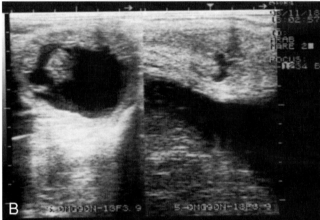

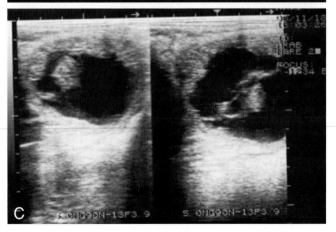

Figure 10.21. Split-screen image of a 36- and 34-day pregnancy fixed bilaterally. The pregnancy on the right-hand image in **A** is accidentally ruptured resulting in loss of fetal fluids **(B),** and subsequently they surround the other fetus **(C)** (*right side*). This pregnancy only survived for 2 days.

lier crushing was better and if possible crushing should occur prior to day 31 because after day 35 manual rupture was sometimes not possible. The author quoted the following results for manual intervention between day 35 and 45: 60% resorption of both, 20% single foaling, and 20% survival of both. One author (10) concluded recycling with prostaglandin prior to day 35 was an outstandingly successful method of treatment. This same author demonstrated that needle puncture of one twin combined with nonsteroidal, anti-inflammatory treatment (meclofenemic acid) resulted in no foals being born. More elaborate and invasive approaches, such as intrafetal injection with saline via a laparotomy (47) or removal of one fetus via a video endoscope (48), have been abandoned as being nonpractical. An interesting report was the surgical technique for removal of one conceptus from mares with twin concepti more than 35 days of gestational age (49, 50). Eight mares had bicornuate pregnancies and seven mares had unicornuate twin concepti. Five of six surviving mares with bicornuate twin concepti delivered a single viable foal, and none of the seven mares originally with unicornuate twin concepti produced a foal. The poor survival rate of unicornuate twin concepti was attributed to disruption of the remaining chorioallantois during surgery. Thirteen of fourteen mares are reported to have been successfully rebred. Transvaginal, ultrasound-guided, fetal puncture for destruction of one of a set of twin pregnancies has been reported (51). Fetal fluids from one fetus were aspirated while observing the relationship of the needle, fetus and yoke sac and/or allantochorion between days 20 and 45. Three of four bicornuate twin pregnancies resulted in a single pregnancy 10 days or more following interference (similar to our ability to manually destroy one conceptus in this configuration). Three of nine (33%) still had a viable single pregnancy after 10 days when twins were fixed together (between days 20 and 45). These results were disappointing; however, they may be improved with experience and/or antibiotic therapy at the time of intervention. Ultrasound-guided fluid withdrawal between days 50 and 65 was studied in single pregnancies (52); however, the study did not involve any twins. Our experiences with transvaginal, ultrasound-guided, fetal reduction are not good, as we found that between days 45 and 60 the fetus within the vesicle was difficult to position. We only have attempted to directly puncture the fetus (Fig. 10.22), not aspirate fluid, and are unlikely to persevere with this technique (fetal puncture at this age) due to difficulties involved. All cases ended in loss of both fetuses, usually within 3 days of interference.

Days 60 Through 99. Between days 60 and 100 it becomes more difficult to damage the chorioallantois. In these cases we identify the most conveniently located (always the smallest) of the twins and repeatedly traumatize it by oscillation or with multiple percussion attempts with the probe. Similar to the previous scenario, approximately 50% succumb to this procedure; however, it can be tedious and time consuming.

Day 100 Onward. Probably the most common reason for being presented mares at this late stage of gestation with twins is failure of the aforementioned techniques. Less frequently, twins have been missed in earlier diagnostic attempts. Frequently, mares have been identified with twins late in the breeding season and the owner has adopted a nonintervention approach. Because the possibility of fetal reduction after 100 days is low and the probability of abortion or stillbirth is high, an approach was developed to eliminate one pregnancy at a later stage of gestation (53). The technique involved transabdominal, ultrasonographic identification of the twins and intracardiac injection of a lethal substance. The smaller twin was always identified. Initial results with saline and air were unsuccessful, but when the solution was replaced with potassium chloride, 7 of 18 mares (39.9%) had single live foals. This rate has subsequently improved with current expectations of 50% being quoted to clients. This stemmed from the analysis of records of 84 mares in one practice (NWR). The procedure was performed on 59 mares after day 115, and 19 of 59 had single live foals (49.2%). The success difference prior to the day after 115 indicated that the younger pregnancies may not be able to withstand the trauma of adjacent twin loss. We (GVEH—Goulburn Valley Equine Hospital) have been utilizing this technique since 1988 and can report similar experiences. Initial success was not very promising (2 of 10 live foals) until the potassium chloride solution was replaced with 10 to 20 ml of procaine penicillin, which has resulted in eight live foals from the last 13 mares attempted. The current procedure at the GVEH is to tranquilize the mare with Detomidine (54) and to identify the smaller fetus or the one most accessible when they are evenly sized. A 6- to 10-inch, 16- or 18-gauge needle with a stylet and a tip designed for ultrasonographic enhancement (Cook, Australia) is passed

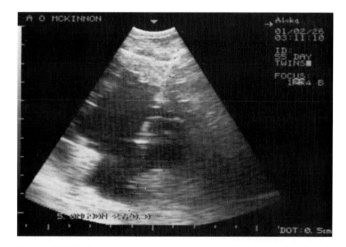

Figure 10.22. Ultrasonographic image from a specially designed vaginal probe, demonstrating the presence of a needle (*white line*), parallel to the left-hand side of the beam. The needle is about to puncture the fetus on the ventral floor. A special echoic needle tip can be seen within the hypoechoic fetal fluids. (Cook Veterinary Products, Brisbane, Australia.)

through the needle-guided biopsy channel into either the heart, lungs, or abdomen of the identified fetus (Fig. 10.23). Penicillin is injected and the fetus monitored for the next 5 to 10 minutes. If the needle is in the chest or abdomen, the demise of the fetus still occurs; however, it takes a little longer than after direct cardiac puncture. The apparent advantages of penicillin as we see them are (a) it reduces iatrogenic bacterial contamination, (b) it can be visualized ultrasonographically as it is injected, and (c) fetal death can still

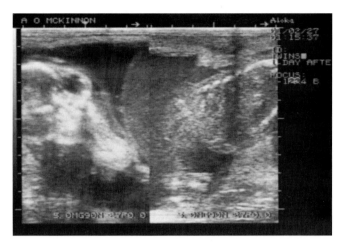

Figure 10.24. Split-screen image of a twin pregnancy 24 hours after induction of death using the transabdominal needle puncture technique. On the left-hand side the head (facing down and to the right) can be seen surrounded by clear fetal fluids. To the right of the head a membrane (the twin membrane) can be seen with hyperechoic fluid within it (surrounding the other pregnancy). On the right is the chest and associated structures of the dead fetus.

be obtained without intracardiac needle placement. We have attempted to place mares on Regu-Mate and long-term oral antibiotics; however, we have found no difference in fetal survival rates with either treatment compared with those that have received no treatment. At the time of needle puncture, mares are treated with systemic antibiotics for 3 days and intravenous phenylbutazone. After transabdominal needle puncture the pregnancy and mummification of the other twin can be monitored with serial ultrasonography (Fig. 10.24); however, it is interesting to note that an unsuccessful outcome is rarely apparent immediately. Most commonly, the mummification process begins and the other fetus appears to grow for the first few weeks. Final outcome is

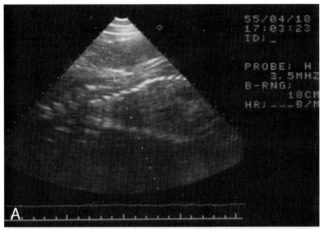

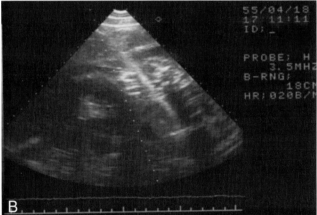

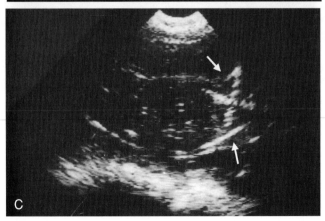

Figure 10.23. A. Transabdominal ultrasonography of a 100-day twin pregnancy. The dotted guideline of the expected path for needle entry is visible. **B.** The needle has entered the fetal chest and can be seen on the right-hand side of the dotted guide line. **C.** 18 gauge needle (upper arrow) inserted into the heart, thoracic wall (lower arrow).

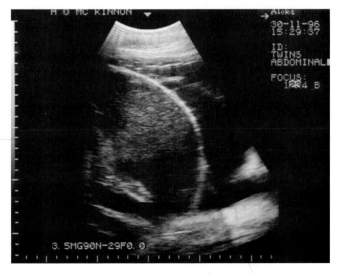

Figure 10.25. The apposition of the chorioallantois between twins results in an ultrasonographically identifiable line named the "twin membrane." It can be useful in identifying the presence of twins.

best predicted by waiting at least 3 and preferably 4 weeks after the needle puncture.

Late in gestation twins may be difficult to recognize with rectal ultrasonography except in those cases with observation of the twin membrane (32) (Fig. 10.25). Abdominal ultrasonography is useful to diagnose older twins (53, 55, 56) (see also Chapter 13). In the event of failure to diagnose twin pregnancies, occasionally abortion is heralded by lactation late in gestation (>7 months). There are reports of successful maintenance of pregnancy despite premature lactation (>1 month prior to foaling) in cases with twin gestation. Apparently, the premature lactation is induced by fetal death and the beginning of mummification of one fetus and thus is threatening to the remaining live fetus. In an initial report, four mares with apparent impending twin abortions were able to deliver live, single foals concurrent with a mummified twin after supplementation with progesterone was initiated on recognition of inappropriate lactation late in gestation (57, 58). In these cases, although foals were born small, they survived and thrived normally. Further work will be necessary to determine which mares with twins respond best or even at all to supplementation with progesterone after initiation of premature lactation.

Twinning is one of the most diagnostic and therapeutically challenging aspects of equine reproductive practice. Improved technology and understanding has resulted in earlier recognition and better success in elimination of one. From all of the preceding discussion it should be obvious to readers that in our opinion the best method of handling twins is early identification (days 11 to 16) and destruction of one before fixation, preferably by using the ultrasound probe to guide the separation and crushing. We feel confident that in time other techniques will be developed or refined to enable their successful use with twins when they have been diagnosed or presented after fixation.

REFERENCES

1. Acland HM. Abortion in mares: diagnosis and prevention. Compend Cont Educ Pract Vet 1987;9:318–326.
2. Acland HM. Abortion in mares. In: McKinnon AO, Voss JL, eds. Equine reproduction. Philadelphia: Lea & Febiger, 1993, pp. 554–562.
3. Bowman T. Ultrasonic diagnosis and management of early twins in the mare. Proc AAEP 1986;35–43.
4. Byszewski W, Gromnicka E. Results of reproduction of mares in the State Horse Stud Farms in 1983–1992. Med Weter 1994;50:493–495.
5. Ginther OJ, Douglas RH, Lawrence JR. Twinning in mares: a survey of veterinarians and analyses of theriogenology records. Theriogenology 1982;18:237–244.
6. Hong CB, Donahue JM, Giles RC, Petritesmurphy MB, Poonacha KB, Roberts AW, Smith BJ, Tramontin RR, Tuttle PA, Swerczek TW. Equine abortion and stillbirth in central Kentucky during 1988 and 1989 foaling seasons. J Vet Diagn Invest 1993;5:560–566.
7. Giles RC, Donahue JM, Hong CB, Tuttle, PA, Petrites-Murphy MB, Poonacha KB, Roberts AW, Tramontin RR, Smith B, Swerczek TW. Causes of abortion, stillbirth, and perinatal death in

horses: 3, 527 cases (1986–1991). J Am Vet Med Assoc 1993;203:1170–1175.
8. Johansson I, Lindhe B, Pirchner F. Causes of variation in the frequency of monozygous and dizygous twinning in various breeds of cattle. Hereditas 1974;78:201–234.
9. Leidl W, Stolla R, Schmid G. Equine dystocia. I. Etiology, conservative obstetrical methods and fetotomy. Tierarztl Umsch 1993;48:408–412.
10. Pascoe RR. Methods for the treatment of twin pregnancy in the mare. Equine Vet J 1983;15:40–42.
11. Pascoe RR, Pascoe DR, Wilson MC. Influence of follicular status on twinning rate in mares. J Reprod Fertil Suppl 1987;35:183–189.
12. Platt H. Aetiological aspects of abortion in the Thoroughbred mare. J Comp Pathol 1973;83:199–205.
13. Platt H. Etiological aspects of perinatal mortality in the Thoroughbred. Equine Vet J 1973;5:116–120.
14. Prohl VU, Busch W, Schuetzler H. Studies on how to step up PMSG formation in mare by induction of superovulation and twin pregnancy. Monatshefte Fuer Veterinaermedizin 1990;45:764–768.
15. Urwin VE, Allen WR. Follicle stimulating hormone, luteinising hormone and progesterone concentrations in the blood of thoroughbred mares exhibiting single and twin ovulations. Equine Vet J 1983;15:325–329.
16. Woods GL, Scraba ST, Ginther OJ. Prospect for induction of multiple ovulations and collection of multiple embryos in the mare. Theriogenology 1982;17:61–72.
17. Vandeplassche MM. Special features of twin gestation in the mare. Vlaams Diergeneesk Tijdschr 1993;62:151–154.
18. Vandeplassche M, Podliachouk L, Beaud R. Some aspects of twin-gestation in the mare. Can J Comp Med 1970;34:218–226.
19. Jeffcott LB, Whitwell K. Twinning as a cause of foetal and neonatal loss in the Thoroughbred mare. J Comp Pathol 1973;83:91–106.
20. Merkt H, Jochle W. Abortions and twin pregnancies in Thoroughbreds: rate of occurence, treatment and prevention. J Equine Vet Sci 1993;13:690–694.
21. Rooney JR, ed. The fetus and foal. In: Autopsy of the horse. 1st ed. Philadelphia: Williams & Wilkins, 1970, pp. 121–133.
22. Meadows SJ, Binns MM, Newcombe JR, Thompson CJ, Rossdale PD. Identical triplets in a Thoroughbred mare. Equine Vet J 1995;27:394–397.
23. McKinnon AO, Carnevale EM, Squires EL, Carney NJ, Seidel GE Jr. Bisection of equine embryos. Equine Vet J 8(Suppl):129–133.
24. McKinnon AO, Voss JL, Squires EL, Carnevale EM. Diagnostic ultrasonography. In: McKinnon AO, Voss JL. Equine reproduction. 1st ed. Philadelphia, London: Lea & Febiger, 1993, pp. 266–302.
25. Merkt H, Jungnickel S, Klug E. Reduction of early twin pregnancy to single pregnancy in the mare by dietetic means. J Reprod Fertil Suppl 1982;32:451–452.
26. Prohl HU, Busch W, Schutzler H. Studies on occurrence of spontaneous twin pregnancies in mares, with reference to PMSG formation. Monatsh Veterinarmed 1994;49:289–294.
27. Ginther OJ. Effect of reproductive status on twinning and on side of ovulation and embryo attachment in mares. Theriogenology 1983;20:383–395.
28. Ginther OJ. Twinning in mares: a review of recent studies. J Equine Vet Sci 1982;2:127–135.
29. Ginther OJ. Relationships among number of days between multiple ovulations, number of embryos, and type of embryo fixation in mares. J Equine Vet Sci 1987;7:82–88.

30. Ginther OJ, Bergfelt DR. Embryo reduction before day 11 in mares with twin conceptuses. J Anim Sci 1988;66:1727–1731.

31. Ginther OJ. Twin embryos in mares. I. From ovulation to fixation. Equine Vet J 1989;21:166–170.

32. Ginther OJ, Griffin PG. Natural outcome and ultrasonic identification of equine fetal twins. Theriogenology 1994;41:1193–1199.

33. Ginther OJ. The nature of embryo reduction in mares with twin conceptuses: deprivation hypothesis. Am J Vet Res 1989;50:45–53.

34. Ginther OJ. Twin embryos in mares. II. Postfixation embryo reduction. Equine Vet J 1989;21:171–174.

35. Ginther OJ. Transitory nature of twin pregnancy in mares. Proc Int Cong Anim Reprd AI 1984;10:116.

36. Ginther OJ, Douglas RH, Woods GL. A biological embryo-reduction mechanism for elimination of excess embryos in mares. Theriogenology 1982;18:475–485.

37. Ginther OJ. The twinning problem: from breeding to day 16. Proc AAEP 1983;11–26.

38. Pascoe RR. A possible new treatment for twin pregnancy in the mare. Equine Vet J 1979;15:40–42.

39. Roberts CJ. Termination of twin gestation by blastocyst crush in the broodmare. J Reprod Fertil Suppl 1982;32:447–449.

40. Pascoe DR, Pascoe RR, Hughes JP, Stabenfeldt GH, Kindahl H. Management of twin conceptuses by manual embryonic reduction: comparison of two techniques and three hormone treatments. Am J Vet Res 1987;48:1594–1599.

41. Pascoe DR, Pascoe RR, Hughes JP, Stabenfeldt GH, Kindahl H. Comparison of two techniques and three hormone therapies for management of twin conceptuses by manual embryonic reduction. J Reprod Fertil Suppl 1987;35:701–702.

42. McKinnon AO, Figueroa STD, Nobelius AM, Hyland JH, Vasey JR. Failure of hydroxyprogesterone caproate to maintain pregnancy in ovariectomized mares. Equine Vet J 1993;25:158–160.

43. Ginther OJ. Postfixation embryo reduction in unilateral and bilateral twins in mares. Theriogenology 1984;22:213–223.

44. Baucus KL, Squires EL, Morris R, McKinnon AO. The effect of stage of gestation and frequency of prostaglandin injection on induction of abortion in mares. Proc Equine Nutr Phys Soc 1987;255–258.

45. Squires EL, Bosu WTK. Induction of abortion during early to mid gestation. In: McKinnon AO, Voss JL, eds. Equine reproduction. Philadelphia, London: Lea & Febiger, 1993, pp. 563–566.

46. Penzhorn BL, Bertschinger HJ, Coubrough RI. Reconception of mares following termination of pregnancy with prostaglandin F2 alpha before and after day 35 of pregnancy. Equine Vet J 1986;18:215–217.

47. Hyland JH, Maclean AA, Robertson-Smith GR, Jeffcott LB, Stewart GA. Attempted conversion of twin to singleton pregnancy in two mares with associated changes in plasma oestrone sulphate concentrations. Aust Vet J 1985;62:406–409.

48. Allen WR, Bracher V. Videoendoscopic evaluation of the mare's uterus. III. Findings in the pregnant mare. Equine Vet J 1992;24:285–291.

49. Stover SM, Pascoe DR. Surgical removal of one conceptus from the mare with a twin pregnancy. Vet Surg 1987;16:87.

50. Pascoe DR, Stover SM. Surgical removal of one conceptus from fifteen mares with twin concepti. Vet Surg 1989;18:141–145.

51. Bracher V, Parlevliet JM, Pieterse MC, Vos PLAM, Wiemer P, Taverne MAM, Colenbrander B. Transvaginal ultrasound-guided twin reduction in the mare. Vet Rec 1993;133:478–479.

52. Squires EL, Tarr SF, Shideler RK, Cook NL. Use of transvaginal ultrasound-guided puncture for elimination of equine pregnancies during days 50 to 65. J Equine Vet Sci 1994;14:203–205.

53. Rantanen NW, Kincaid B. Ultrasound-guided fetal cardiac puncture: a method of twin reduction in the mare. Proc AAEP 1988;173–179.

54. McKinnon AO, Carnevale EM, Squires EL, Jochle W. Clinical evaluation of detomidine hydrocholoride for equine reproductive surgery. Proc AAEP 1988;563–568.

55. Pipers FS, Adams-Brendemuehl CS. Techniques and applications of transabdominal ultrasonography in the pregnant mare. J Am Vet Med Assoc 185:766–771.

56. McKinnon AO. Reproductive ultrasonography. In: Equine stud medicine. Sydney: Anonymous Post Graduate Foundation in Veterinary Science, 1996, pp. 395–430.

57. Roberts SJ, Myhre G. A review of twinning in horses and the possible therapeutic value of supplemental progesterone to prevent abortion of equine twin fetuses the latter half of the gestation period. Cornell Vet 1983;73:257–264.

58. Shideler RK. Prenatal lactation associated with twin pregnancy in the mare: a case report. J Equine Vet Sci 1987;7:383–384.

11. Early Embryonic Loss

EDWARD L. SQUIRES

Early embryonic loss in mares is costly to the breeder and limits the reproductive success of the breeding farm. Investigators often state that over half the conceptions are lost between fertilization and foaling. Baker and associates (1) reported the overall live-foaling rate was 58% for the entire Thoroughbred population during the 1987 and 1988 breeding seasons. The overall live-foaling rate per cycle was 42% for four well-managed Thoroughbred farms in Kentucky. These rates are in contrast to the high fertilization rates (96%) reported by Ball and colleagues (2). Most pregnancy losses occur early in gestation, with few losses occurring after day 40 (3). Therefore, the most recent studies of early embryonic loss focus on events occurring before the time of pregnancy detection with ultrasonography (days 10 to 14). Techniques such as ultrasonography, transvaginal ultrasound-guided follicular aspiration of oocytes, embryo recovery, and gamete intrafallopian tube transfer have provided critical information on the timing and causes of early embryonic death. Before the advent of ultrasonography, pregnancy detection was conducted by rectal palpation of the genital tract beginning at about day 20. Thus, many early embryonic losses had already occurred before the initial pregnancy diagnosis. Fortunately, with high-resolution ultrasound equipment, equine pregnancies can be detected with great accuracy early in gestation.

INCIDENCE

Ball and associates (2) reported that fertilization rates in young and old mares were similar, but the incidence of embryonic death between fertilization and day 14 was 9% for young mares and 62 to 73% for aged, subfertile mares. Numerous investigators have demonstrated low embryo recovery in subfertile mares, indicating that many embryonic deaths in subfertile mares occur before the embryo enters the uterus (4–6).

The reported incidence of embryonic death varies depending on the method of pregnancy detection, the time of initial pregnancy detection, and the reproductive history of the mares examined. Based on rectal palpation, the embryonic loss between approximately days 20 and 50 has varied from 8 to 16% (7). With the use of ultrasonography, the initial detection of pregnancy in most studies was on days 11 to 14, and the percentage of embryonic loss in these studies varied from 11 to 24% (7). Clients should be advised that earlier pregnancy detection results in higher pregnancy rates, but it also allows for greater detection of embryonic loss. Ginther (8) reported on embryonic loss between days 11 and 40 based on ultrasonic imaging. Embryonic losses were grouped into 5-day intervals from days 11 to 40. In

groups of apparently normal mares, the loss rate for each of the 5-day increments extending from day 11 to day 40 ranged from 1.1 to 2.1%, and no significant differences were noted among increments. In contrast, in a herd with a large proportion of subfertile mares, the loss rate on days 11 to 15 was 18.2%, significantly higher than that for reproductively normal mares (1.3%). The loss rates were also greater on days 15 to 20 in the subfertile mares than in the normal mares (3.1 versus 2.0%). On days 20 to 40, the loss rates were similar for the two groups.

In a study conducted at Colorado State University (3) over two breeding seasons, ultrasonography was performed every 5 days from days 15 to 50. The overall incidence of early embryonic death through postovulation day 50 was 17.3%. Most (77.1%) of early embryonic death occurred before day 35. Between postovulation days 15 and 35 days, a greater incidence of early embryonic death occurred than between postovulation days 15 and 20 and days 30 and 35, compared with other time periods.

ETIOLOGIC FACTORS

As stated previously, a high percentage of early embryonic deaths occurs before the time of ultrasonographic detection of the equine conceptus (day 10). Recently, Brinsko and colleagues (9) conducted a study to determine whether embryonic losses before exposure to the uterine environment are a result of prior embryonic defects or suboptimal oviductal environment. Their approach was to compare the development of equine embryos obtained 2 days after ovulation from young, fertile mares with that of embryos from aged, subfertile mares after co-culture with oviductal epithelium obtained from either young, fertile or aged, subfertile mares. No difference was noted in the ability of embryos from young mares or aged mares to reach blastocyst stage; however, embryos from aged mares were inferior to embryos from young mares based on embryo quality scores, embryo diameter, and total number of cells. In addition, the oviductal epithelial cells from aged mares appeared to have a detrimental effect on the development of embryos from young mares. The results of these studies suggested that failure to maintain pregnancy in aged, subfertile mares may be due to inherent developmental defects of the embryo or to an adverse oviductal environment. Ball and associates (10) transferred oviductal embryos on day 4 from normal, fertile mares, and from subfertile mares into the uteri of normal recipients. Significantly fewer embryos from subfertile mares than fertile mares resulted in pregnancy on day 14. In a series of experiments by Carnevale and colleagues (11), the percentage of ova that had cleaved on day 1.5 was significantly lower in old mares (>20 years) than in young mares (2 to 10 years). On day 3, oviductal embryos from old mares had significantly fewer cells and more morphologic abnormalities than embryos from young mares. Oviductal embryos from young and old donors were collected on day 1.5 and were transferred into the oviducts of young or old recipients. Embryos were recovered on day 3.5 and evaluated. Exposure of embryos to the oviductal environment of young versus old mares between days 1.5 and 3.5 did not seem to affect embryo development. However, none of these studies conclusively determined whether subfertility in old mares was due to reduced oocyte viability or to detrimental oviductal factors. Therefore, Carnevale and Ginther (12) conducted a study in which oocytes from young and old mares were collected from the follicle and were transferred into the oviduct of a normal mare that had been inseminated, that is, gamete intrafallopian tube transfer. Fertilization and embryo development occurred within the recipient; therefore, effects of a deleterious environment on fertilization or embryo development were avoided. Oocytes were collected by transvaginal ultrasonically guided follicular aspiration from young and old mares at 21 to 26 hours after administration of human chorionic gonadotropin. Oocytes were cultured for 16 to 20 hours and were then transferred into the oviducts of young recipients. Recipients were inseminated with semen from the same stallions. More oocytes from young than old donors resulted in embryonic vesicles, as imaged by ultrasound on day 12 (11 of 12, 92%; and 8 of 26, 31%, respectively). To obtain additional information, young and old mares were inseminated during the subsequent ovulatory cycle. After artificial insemination, the pregnancy rate for young mares was higher than that for old mares (83 versus 19%). Results demonstrated that oocytes from old mares were defective and that transfer of oocytes from old mares to young recipients did not eliminate age-associated subfertility. This high embryonic loss in the oviduct explains the reduced embryo recovery recorded for subfertile mares. Embryos recovered from subfertile mares by embryo recovery 6 to 9 days after ovulation are smaller in diameter and are associated with more morphologic defects (13).

The earliest time for ultrasonic detection of the equine conceptus is approximately day 9 or 10 (14, 15). However, in most cases practitioners perform the first ultrasound examination between days 14 and 20. The high embryonic loss between days 14 and 20, particularly for the aged mare, may be related to the uterine environment. The embryo at this time depends on protein secretions from the uterine glands (uterine milk) for its nourishment. During this time, the embryo must suppress prostaglandin $F_{2\alpha}$ secretion from the uterine endometrium, thus allowing continued secretion of progesterone from the primary corpus luteum (16). The embryo probably produces a factor responsible for suppression of prostaglandin $F_{2\alpha}$ secretion; however, at this time, the factor has not been identified. Recently, Sissener and associates (17) reported that this suppression of prostaglandin $F_{2\alpha}$ secretion occurs in equine embryos by day 12 to 13 but not by day 16.

Reduced progesterone secretion during early gestation has been implicated as a cause of early embryonic death. This reduced progesterone secretion could be a result of failure of maternal recognition of pregnancy, primary luteal insufficiency, or uterine-induced luteolysis. More than likely, primary luteal insufficiency does not occur, but luteal regression results from endometrial irritation that releases prostaglandin $F_{2\alpha}$. Luteolysis induced by inflammation of the uterus is a major cause of embryonic loss in the subfertile mare (18). In addition, periglandular fibrosis of the endometrium is associated with increased embryonic loss in the subfertile mare. Ricketts and Alanso (19) found a significant correlation between the severity of chronic degenerative endometrial disease and age of the mare. Therefore, the reduced fertility of older mares is related not only to oocyte and embryo defects, but also to an abnormal uterine environment.

Other causes of embryonic death are breeding mares on foal heat (20), stress (21), nutrition (22), environmental temperature (23), increased incidence of embryonic death associated with some stallions (24), chromosomal abnormalities (25), immunogenetic factors (26), and iatrogenic

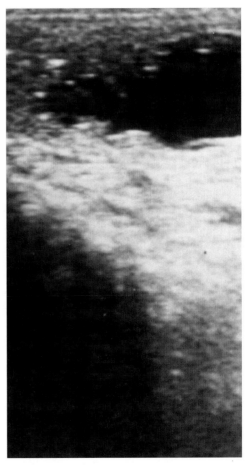

Figure 11.1. Grade 4 fluid in a mare's uterus.

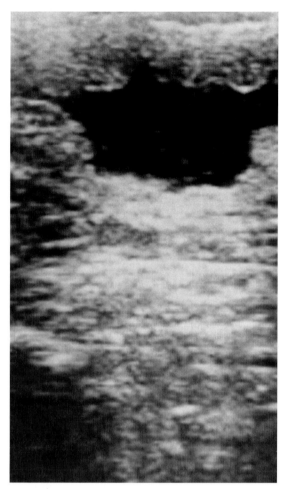

Figure 11.2. Grade 3 fluid in a mare's uterus. Evidence of echogenic spots.

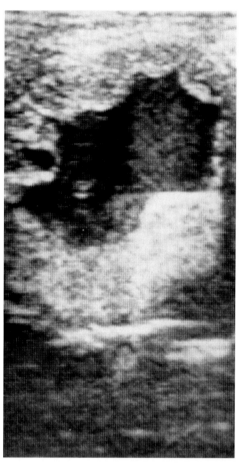

Figure 11.3. Grade 2 fluid in a mare's uterus. Increased gray scale and echogenicity.

factors such as palpation (27) and administration of anabolic steroids (28).

DIAGNOSIS

Ultrasonography has allowed the diagnosis of uterine problems associated with embryonic death. Numerous investigators have reported the reduced pregnancy rates and high embryonic death in mares diagnosed with intraluminal fluid (29, 30). Intraluminal fluid present during diestrus is generally associated with endometritis and premature luteal regression. McKinnon and colleagues (15) developed a grading system for uterine fluid (Figs. 11.1 through 11.4).

Grades 1 and 2 fluids were shown to be more detrimental to sperm survival and, more than likely, to embryo survival (15). The presence of numerous uterine cysts was also associated with a greater embryonic loss during early gestation (15, 29, 31). Although the presence of a uterine cyst smaller than 10 mm in diameter is of no consequence to pregnancy maintenance (Fig. 11.5), large cysts scattered throughout the uterus deprive the embryo of endometrial surface and often result in embryonic loss (Fig. 11.6). Additionally, large cysts may restrict embryo motility, thereby allowing prostaglandins to be secreted. Air in the uterus, as detected by ultrasonography, is generally an indication of poor reproductive anatomy (Fig. 11.7). Unfortunately, continual aspiration of air becomes an irritant to the endometrium and may result in luteolysis.

At Colorado State University, early embryonic death is diagnosed when an embryonic vesicle seen previously is not observed on two consecutive ultrasonographic scans or when only remnants of a vesicle are observed. In our laboratory at Colorado State University, mares are examined at days 14, 25, 35, and 50. Signs of impending early embryonic death at the initial examination (day 14) may include the presence of endometrial folds (Fig. 11.8), which indicate that the mare is undergoing luteolysis and that progesterone levels are low and estrogen levels are high, and the presence of embryonic vesicles of smaller diameter than normal for their age. Generally, these small embryonic vesicles experience embryonic death and are more commonly associated with older mares. However, accurate determination of ovulation is needed to determine whether vesicles are of normal size. Other indications of early embryonic death include reduced embryo mobility (32) and a greater incidence of embryonic vesicles detected in the uterine body versus uterine horn during days 10 to 16 (33). The ul-

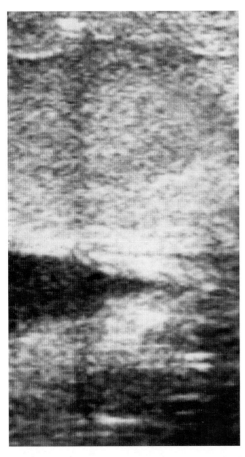

Figure 11.4. Grade 1 fluid in a mare's uterus. Increased echogenicity caused by white blood cells.

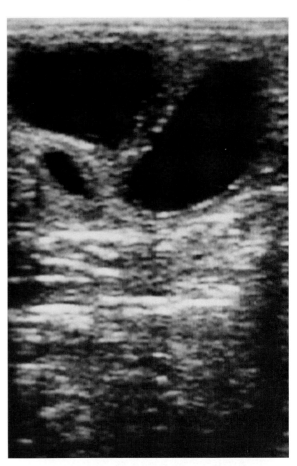

Figure 11.6. Large uterine cyst in mare's uterus.

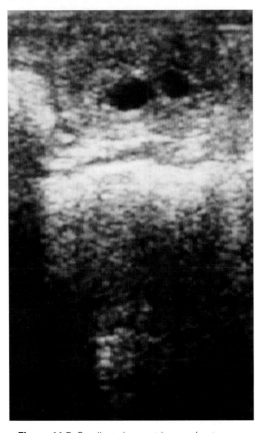

Figure 11.5. Small uterine cyst in mare's uterus.

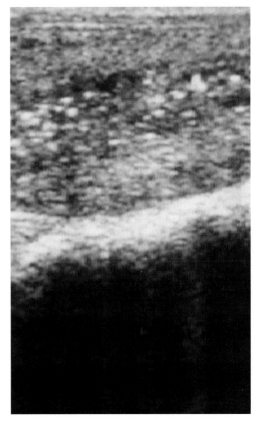

Figure 11.7. Air in mare's uterus.

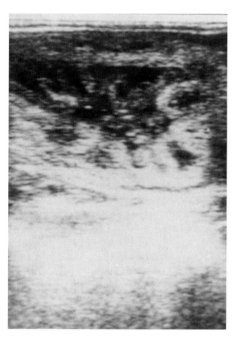

Figure 11.8. Prominent endometrial folds in mare's uterus.

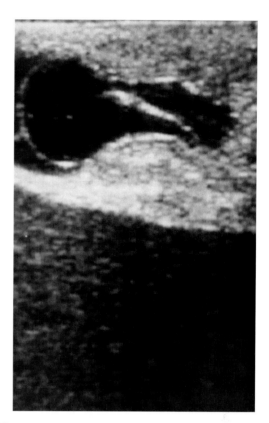

Figure 11.10. Dislodgement of vesicle into the uterine body.

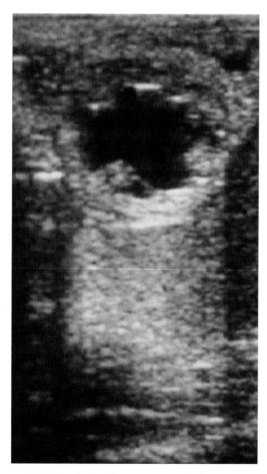

Figure 11.9. Twenty-five day pregnancy with fetus present.

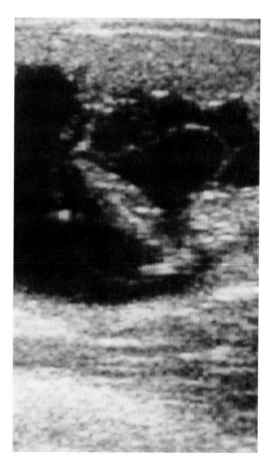

Figure 11.11. Echogenic mass of dead fetus and membranes floating in allantoic fluid.

trasound examination performed at day 25 is for the detection of a fetal heartbeat (Fig. 11.9). An embryonic vesicle may grow at a normal rate without development of a fetus. This phenomenon has been reported for embryos cooled to 5°C before transfer into recipients (34). In this report, more than likely, the inner cell mass was damaged such that a fetus did not develop. Before day 15, if an embryonic vesicle dies, the vesicle disappears rapidly, either because of resorption or as a result of expulsion through the cervix. In contrast, if the conceptus develops a heartbeat and later dies, approximately 12 days are required for disruption of the embryonic vesicle and release of its contents. Indications of embryonic death include failure of fixation, dislodgement of the vesicle after fixation (Fig. 11.10), an echogenic ring or mass floating in fluid (Fig. 11.11), an echogenic area in the dead embryo (Fig. 11.12), and disorganization of the conceptual membranes (Fig. 11.13) (35, 36)

MANAGEMENT

Because of the multifactorial nature of early embryonic death, no single therapy is effective. As shown by Carnevale and Ginther (12), if the oocyte is defective, then transfer of the oocyte to another environment, such as to a young mare, does not improve pregnancy rates. However, if the cause of

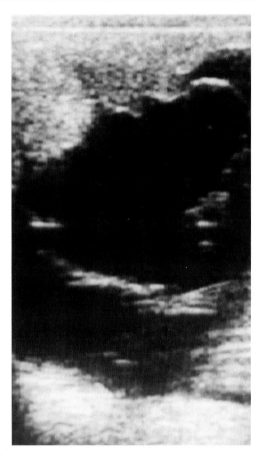

Figure 11.13. Disorganization of conceptus membranes.

possible early embryonic death is an unfavorable uterine environment and not a defective oocyte or embryo, then perhaps transfer of the embryo from that unfavorable environment into a more favorable uterine environment may allow the pregnancy to continue.

Other management tools that may decrease the incidence of embryonic death include correction of physical abnormalities, treatment of uterine infection, and artificial insemination, which limits the bacterial challenge to a mare's uterus, thus reducing the potential loss from endometritis. Prevention of recontamination is possible by using extended semen with antibiotics and minimizing the number of breedings. The efficacy of exogenous progesterone for decreasing early embryonic death is questionable. Although progesterone has been used clinically as a therapy for habitually aborting mares, conclusive studies demonstrating its effectiveness have not been conducted. Perhaps the changes most likely to decrease the incidence of embryonic death are improvements related to nutrition, environmental temperature, elimination of infectious diseases and other stresses, and postbreeding management.

REFERENCES

1. Baker CB, Little TV, McDowell KJ. The live foaling rate per cycle in mares. Equine Vet J 1993;15:28–30.

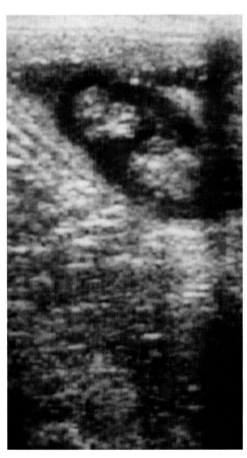

Figure 11.12. Echogenic area in dead fetus.

2. Ball BA, Little TV, Hillman RB, et al. Embryonic loss in normal and barren mares. In: Proceedings of the Thirty-First Annual Convention of the American Association of Equine Practitioners, 1985: 535–543.

3. Villahoz MD, Squires EL, Voss JL, et al. Some observations on early embryonic death in mares. Theriogenology 1985;23:915–924.

4. Douglas RH. Some aspects of equine embryo transfer. J Reprod Fertil Suppl 1982;32:405–408.

5. Squires EL, Imel KL, Iuliano MF, et al. Factors affecting reproductive efficiency in an equine embryo transfer programme. J Reprod Fertil Suppl 1982;32:409–414.

6. Vogelsang SG, Vogelsang MM. Influence of donor parity and age on the success of commercial embryo transfer. Equine Vet J 1989; 8:71–73.

7. Ball BA. Embryonic loss in mares: incidence, possible causes and diagnostic considerations. Vet Clin North Am Equine Pract 1988; 4:263–290.

8. Ginther OJ. Reproductive biology of the mare: basic and applied aspects. 2nd ed. Equiservices, Cross Plains, WI, 1991.

9. Brinsko SP, Ignotz GG, Ball BA, et al. Inherent factors contributing to early embryonic loss in aged subfertile mares. Sixth International Symposium on Equine Reproduction 1994:49-51.

10. Ball BA, Little TV, Weber JA, et al. Viability of day-4 embryos from young, normal mares and aged, subfertile mares after transfer to normal recipients. J Reprod Fertil 1989;85:187–194.

11. Carnevale EM, Griffin PG, Ginther OJ. Age-associated subfertility before entry of embryo into the uterus in mares. Equine Vet J 1993; 15:31–35.

12. Carnevale EM, Ginther OJ. Defective oocytes as a cause of subfertility in old mares. Biol Reprod Monogr Ser 1995;1:209–214.

13. Woods GL, Hillman RB, Schlafer DH. Recovery and evaluation of embryos from normal and infertile mares. Cornell Vet 1986;76: 386–394.

14. Ginther OJ. Ultrasonic imaging and reproductive events in the mare. Cross Plains, WI: Equiservices, 1986.

15. McKinnon AO, Squires EL, Carnevale EM, et al. Diagnostic ultrasonography of uterine pathology in the mare. In: Proceedings of the Thirty-Third Annual Convention of the American Association of Equine Practitioners 1987:605–622.

16. Berglund LA, Sharp DC, Vernon MW, et al. Effect of pregnancy and collection techniques on prostaglandin-F in the uterine lumen of pony mares. J Reprod Fertil Suppl 1982;32:335–341.

17. Sissener TR, Squires EL, Clay CM. Differential suppression of endometrial prostaglandin $F_{2\alpha}$ by the equine conceptus. Theriogenology 1996;541–546.

18. Ginther OJ. Embryonic loss in mares: incidence, time of occurrence and hormonal involvement. Theriogenology 1985;23:77–89.

19. Ricketts SW, Alonso S. The effect of age and parity on the development of equine chronic endometrial disease. Equine Vet J 1991; 23:189–192.

20. Merkt H, Gunzel A. A survey of early pregnancy losses in West German Thoroughbred mares. Equine Vet J 1979;11:256–258.

21. VanNiekerk CH, Morgenthal JC. Fetal loss and the effect of stress on plasma progestogen levels in pregnant Thoroughbred mares. J Reprod Fertil Suppl 1982;32:453–457.

22. VanNiekerk CH, VanHeerdon JS. Nutrition and ovarian activity of mares early in the breeding season. J S Afr Vet Assoc 1972;43: 351–360.

23. Ball BA. Embryonic death in mares. In: McKinnon AO, Voss, JL, eds. Equine reproduction. Philadelphia: Lea & Febiger, 1993: 523–524.

24. Platt H. Aetiological aspects of abortion in the Thoroughbred mare. J Comp Pathol 1973;83:199–205.

25. Romagnano A, King WA, Richer CL, et al. A direct technique for the preparation of chromosomes from early equine embryos. Can J.Genet Cytol 1985;27:365–369.

26. Shivers CA, Liu IKM. Inhibition of sperm biding to porcine ova by antibodies to equine zonae pellucidae. J Reprod Fertil Suppl 1982; 32:315–318.

27. Voss JL, Pickett BW, Back DG, et al. Effect of rectal palpation on pregnancy rate of nonlactating, normally cycling mares. J Anim Sci 1975;41:829–834.

28. Squires EL, Voss JL, Maher JM, et al. Fertility of young mares after long-term anabolic steroid treatment. J Am Vet Med Assoc 1985;186:583–586.

29. Adam, GP, Kastelic JP, Bergfelt DR, et al. Effect of uterine inflammation and ultrasonically detected uterine pathology on fertility in the mare. J Reprod Fertil Suppl 1987;35:445–454.

30. McKinnon AO, Squires EL, Harrison LA, et al. Ultrasonographic studies on the reproductive tract of mares after parturition: effect of involution and uterine fluid on pregnancy rates in mares with normal and delayed first postpartum ovulatory cycles. J Am Vet Med Assoc 1988;192:350–353.

31. Chevalier-Clements F. Pregnancy loss in the mare. Anim Reprod Sci 1989;20:231–244.

32. McDowell JK, Sharp DC, Grubaugh W, et al. Restricted conceptus mobility results in failure of pregnancy maintenance in mares. Biol Reprod 1988;39:340–348.

33. Ginther OJ. Embryonic loss in mares: Nature of loss after experimental induction by ovariectomy or prostaglandin $F_{2\alpha}$. Theriogenology 1985;24:87–98.

34. Carnevale EM, Squires EL, McKinnon AO. Comparison of Ham's FIO with CO_2 or Hepes buffer for storage of equine embryos at 5°C for 24 h. J Anim Sci 1987;65:1775–1781.

35. McKinnon AO, Squires EL, Pickett B. Equine reproductive ultrasonography. Animal Reproduction and Biotechnology Laboratory bulletin No.4. Fort Collins, CO: Colorado State University, 1988.

36. McKinnon AO, Voss OJ, Squires EL, et al. Diagnostic ultrasonography. In: McKinnon AO, Voss JL, eds. Equine reproduction. Philadelphia: Lea & Febiger, 1993:266–302.

12. Fetal Gender Determination

SANDRA CURRAN

Knowledge of the gender of an unborn foal may be beneficial for both research and commercial purposes. For example, results of a research project that characterizes differences between male and female fetuses can be determined 9 months before birth of the foals. Commercially, the value of a mare may be substantially increased if she carries a foal of the desired gender. Numerous techniques are being developed to determine embryonic or fetal gender in humans and domestic species and have been summarized (1). Some of these techniques have been applied to horses. Separation of X-chromosome and Y-chromosome sperm has been attempted with limited success (2). Detection of the male-specific H-Y antigen on the equine blastocyst has been demonstrated and the embryonic gender confirmed with karyotypes (3). Ultrasonography offers a noninvasive technique to determine the viability and gender of a fetus and has been used for this purpose in humans, cattle, and horses. In humans, gender is diagnosed by identification of fetal external genitalia after day 140 of gestation with accuracy nearing 100% (4). In cattle, fetal gender determination has been demonstrated by ultrasonic imaging of either the scrotum or the mammary glands (5) or by identifying and locating the genital tubercle (6). In horses, fetal gender can be accurately determined under research (7) or farm (8) conditions by identifying and locating the genital tubercle.

ANATOMY

The genital tubercle is the embryonic forerunner of the penis and clitoris (Fig. 12.1) (9). It can be identified by gross inspection of removed equine fetuses as small as 10 to 12 mm (approximately postovulation day 28). When first identified, the genital tubercle is located on the mid-line between the rear legs, and gender cannot be determined by gross inspection of the embryo. Fetal gender of removed specimens can be determined after days 40 to 45 (10). At this time, the clitoris is located along the posterior border of the perineal region in the female fetus; the penis is located in the anterior inguinal area in the male fetus. By day 55 after ovulation, the vulvar lips extend dorsally from the clitoris in the female fetus. By days 100 to 120, the clitoris recedes inside the ventral commissure of the labia, and the vulvar lips below the ventral commissure form the typical bulb appearance of the postnatal filly. In the male, a perineal raphe can be seen on mid-line from the base of the penis to the area of the future scrotum. The prepuce is first noted by day 77 and becomes pendulous by days 115 to 120. The scrotum is small (7.5 by 1 by 1 mm) and empty in the day-80 fetus. By day 150, the gubernacula are large and palpable in the scrotum. They may be mistaken for testes at this time but complete descent of the testes does not occur until the perinatal period. The mammary papillae are visible in both sexes by day 55 as small, pale dots (0.25 mm). In the female, the mammary gland becomes prominent by day 300. In the male, it is incorporated into the prepuce by day 120.

ULTRASONIC APPEARANCE

The ultrasonic appearance of the external genitalia from the time of first appearance throughout gestation has been described. The identification of these structures can be used to determine fetal gender.

Days 35 to 97

In one study (7), 26 pregnant mares were examined with a high-quality real-time ultrasound scanner equipped with a linear-array 5-Mhz transrectal transducer every other day from day 35 or 36 after ovulation (day of ovulation is day 0) until termination of the project (range; days 41 to 97). Each fetus was examined in its entirety in sequential cross-sectional, frontal, and sagittal planes, and the genital tubercle was identified. Location of the genital tubercle relative to surrounding structures was scored on a scale of 1 to 5 (1, in close proximity to the umbilical cord; 2, between the umbilical cord and hind limbs; 3, on the midline between the rear legs; 4, between the hind limbs and the tail; and 5, in close proximity to the tail), fetal gender was determined, and the degree of certainty of diagnosis was scored from 1 to 4 (1, sex not diagnosable; 2, 3, and 4, sex diagnosed with minimal, intermediate, and maximal certainty, respectively).

In this study, the genital tubercle could not be identified ultrasonically on day 35 or 36. After this time, the genital tubercle was identified with increasing frequency through day 54, at which time it was identified in all mares. The ultrasonic appearance of the genital tubercle in the younger fetuses was described as hyperechogenic and usually bilobed, with each lobe elongated and oval (Fig. 12.2). Fetal gender was determined by the ultrasonic location of the genital tubercle relative to surrounding structures. Before day 48, the genital tubercle was located on the mid-line between the rear legs (location score, 3). After day 48, the location of the genital tubercle relative to surrounding structures began to change; it moved toward the umbilicus in male fetuses and toward the tail in female fetuses. In males, the genital tubercle arrived at the area immediately caudal to the umbilical attachment (location score, 1) on day 62. In females, the genital tubercle was located under the tail (location score, 5) beginning on day 64 (Fig. 12.3).

Gender was not diagnosable (certainty score, 1) before

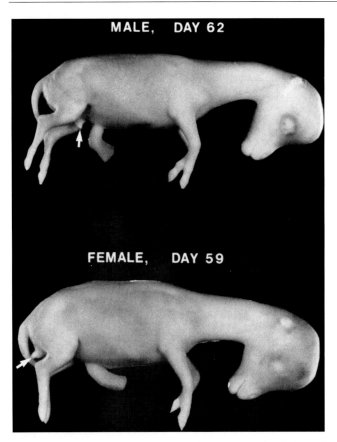

Figure 12.1. Location and appearance of the genital tubercle (*arrow*) in male and female equine fetuses. Reproduced with permission from Curran S, Ginther OJ. Ultrasonic diagnosis of equine fetal sex by location of the genital tubercle. J Equine Vet Sci 1989;9:77–83.

day 48 in all fetuses. As fetal age increased, certainty scores gradually increased, reaching an average of 3 on day 57. The average day on which the certainty first reached a maximum (certainty score, 4) was day 60. After day 70, the average certainty score began to fluctuate; gender could not always be determined. This was attributed to difficulty in obtaining an adequate view in the older fetuses. Accuracy of ultrasonic fetal gender determination was 100% on the first day of maximal certainty (certainty score, 4). Overall, 92 gender diagnoses were made in female fetuses, and all were correct. In male fetuses, 138 of 143 (97%) diagnoses were correct, with the errors all at minimal or intermediate certainty (certainty score 2 or 3, respectively). The optimal time for gender diagnosis was from days 59 to 68, at which time the genital tubercle was readily accessible and assignable to a location characteristic of its gender with a high level of certainty (see Fig.12.3).

Days 50 to 99 (Farm Conditions)

To assess the feasibility of the foregoing technique under farm conditions, fetal gender was determined with a single examination (8). Fetal age ranged from postovulation days 50 to 99 in 85 mares. End points included fetal gender diagnosis, certainty score, and time required to make a diag-

nosis after fecal removal. Certainty was rated from 50% (gender not diagnosable) to 99% (maximal certainty). Fetal gender was diagnosable in 75 of the 85 fetuses (88%) and was accurate in 73 of the 75 diagnoses (97%). Accuracy was 100% (44 of 44) when the certainty score was high (95 or 99%; Table 12.1). The average time required after fecal removal for fetal gender diagnosis was 1 minute 17 seconds. The optimal time for gender determination in this study was between days 55 and 64. Fetal gender diagnosis is limited in early pregnancy because of undifferentiated fetuses and in later pregnancy because of an inability to view the fetus adequately. However, in the older fetuses, when a diagnosis was made, it was accurate.

Months 5 to 11

A third study (11) was conducted to determine whether gender could be diagnosed in older fetuses (months 5 to 11 of gestation). The ultrasonic appearance of fetal external genitalia was described, and the reliability of gender determination was evaluated using a 3.5-Mhz transducer. Eighty five mares pregnant 5 to 11 months were examined once to ascertain fetal gender and to estimate expected accuracy. Fetal presentation (cranial, caudal, or transverse) was recorded, and the external genitalia were described.

Fetal gender was completed in 19 of 21 (90%) mares examined during months 5 to 6 of gestation. Ability to diagnose gender was independent of fetal presentation; that is, the appropriate areas to determine fetal gender were readily accessible at this age. During months 7 to 11, fetal gender could be diagnosed in only 4 of 64 (6%) attempts because of the size, depth, and presentation of the fetus. Ginther and Griffin (12) reported that fetuses are predominantly in a cranial presentation at this age of gestation;

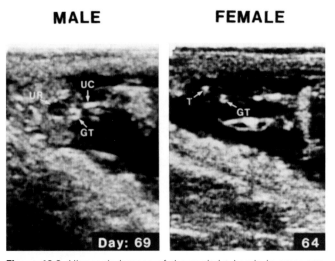

Figure 12.2. Ultrasonic images of the genital tubercle in cross-sectional views of male and female fetuses. Day of pregnancy is shown in the lower right corner of each image. GT = genital tubercle; T = tail; UC = umbilical cord; UR = urachus. Adapted with permission from Curran S, Ginther OJ. Ultrasonic diagnosis of equine fetal sex by location of the genital tubercle. J Equine Vet Sci 1989;9:77–83.

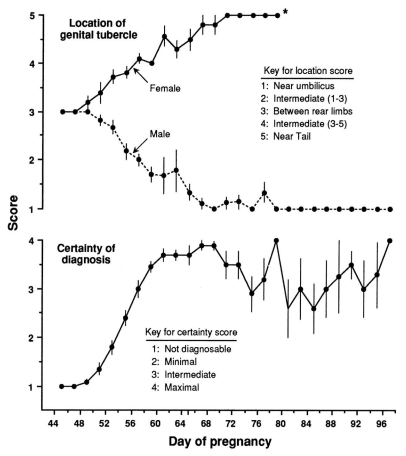

Figure 12.3. Mean (±SEM) changes in location of the genital tubercle in male and female fetuses and certainty scores of the ultrasonic diagnosis of fetal gender on various days of pregnancy. Adapted with permission from Curran S, Ginther OJ. Ultrasonic diagnosis of equine fetal sex by location of the genital tubercle. J Equine Vet Sci 1989;9:77–83.

therefore, only the head, neck, and chest could be viewed ultrasonically. Fetal gender could only be diagnosed in the older fetuses when they were in caudal presentation. Fetal gender diagnoses were correct for 16 of the 18 (89%) examinations in which the diagnosis was made and the gender of the foal was recorded.

During month 5, the penis/prepuce appeared as a trilobed, echogenic structure, as described for a day 97 fetus

viewed with a 5-Mhz transducer (7). No attempt was made to differentiate the penis from the prepuce in this study (11). During month 5, the penis/prepuce was located close to the body wall, but after this time, it often appeared pendulous. The penis/prepuce in cross-section was a hyperechogenic, circular structure with a central core that appeared more echogenic than the surrounding penile tissue. A cross-section of the umbilical cord was often imaged

Table 12.1.
Number of Correct Diagnosis and Expected Accuracy Rate for Diagnosis of Fetal Gender in Horses.

Expected Accuracy*		Number of Correct Diagnoses‡			
Score	No. of Animals	Male Fetus	Female Fetus	Undifferentiated Fetus	Total
50%†	10 (12%)	0/3	0/4	0/3	0/10 —
65–80%	9 (11%)	3/3	5/6	—	8/9 (89%)
85–90%	22 (26%)	9/10	12/12	—	21/22 (95%)
95%	9 (11%)	4/4	5/5	—	9/9 (100%)
99%	35 (41%)	19/19	16/16	—	35/35 (100%)
	85 (100%)				

* Degree of certainty in the diagnosis as recorded at the time of the ultrasonic examination.
† Certainty equivalent to a guess, and therefore diagnosis not made.
‡ Definitive diagnosis based on gross examination of removed fetuses.
With permission from Curran S, Ginther OJ. Ultrasonic determination of fetal gender in horses and cattle under farm conditions. Theriogenology 1991;36:809–814.

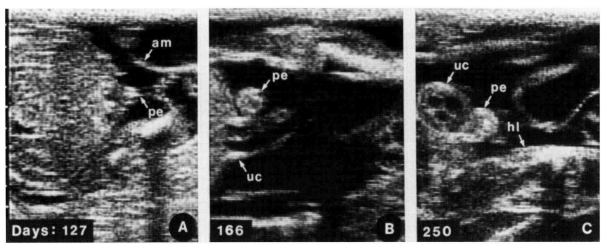

Figure 12.4. Ultrasonograms of the fetal penis/prepuce. Day of pregnancy is shown in the lower left comer of each image. Views are cross-sectional (**A** and **B**) or sagittal/oblique (**C**). **A**, The penis of the younger fetus is trilobed. **B**, The cross-section of the older penis/prepuce is circular and hyperechogenic. **C**, The cross-sectional diameter of the penis is smaller than that of the umbilical cord. am = amnion; hl = hind limb; pe = penis/prepuce; uc = umbilical cord.

in the same plane as the penis. The umbilical cord appeared as three nonechogenic, round areas (vessels) encircled by a wide, echogenic band. The umbilical cord was often larger in diameter than the penis, and it pulsated. Often, the penis could be seen moving at the same rate as the umbilical cord, presumably because of their close proximity (Fig. 12.4). The scrotum was not identified at any age, but the anogenital raphe appeared prominently as a hyperechogenic structure extending from the base of the penis to the area of the perineum. Anogenital raphe resembled, and could be mistaken for, the female fetal clitoris.

In the younger female fetuses, the ultrasonic appearance of the clitoris was similar to that of a penis/prepuce of the same age. When the entire perineal region was imaged, the labia were sometimes differentiated from the clitoris (Fig. 12.5). The mammary gland of the female fetus was

described as a triangular, hyperechogenic structure located between the hind limbs. As fetal age increased, echogenicity of the mammary gland also increased. The degree of echogenicity was similar to that of the anogenital raphe in the male; however, the mammary gland covered a larger area and was more triangular than the anogenital raphe. Individual teats could often be seen. The mammary gland was often more readily viewed than the clitoris or labia (Fig. 12.6). Although the mammary gland was the most obvious female gender characteristic, the reliability of fetal gender determination based on this feature alone was not studied.

In both genders, the anus was identified as a hyperechogenic structure protruding from the surface of the dorsal aspect of the perineal region. It resembled a fetal clitoris, except it was located in closer proximity to the attachment of the tail.

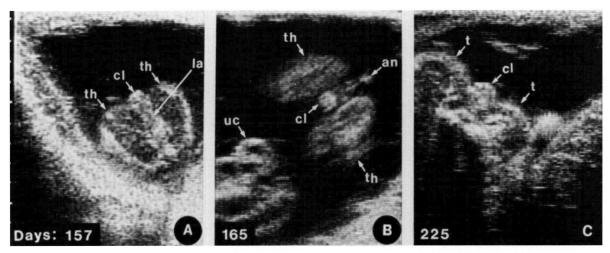

Figure 12.5. Ultrasonograms of the clitoris (cl). Views of the fetus are cross-sectional (**A** and **B**) or frontal (**C**). **A**, The clitoris is more echogenic than the labia (la). The clitoris appears trilobed and hyperechogenic. **B**, The anus (an) can be seen above and to the right of the clitoris. **C**, A cross-section through the clitoris is protruding from the caudal surface of the fetus. t = thigh; uc = umbilical cord. Adapted with permission from Curran S, Ginther OJ. Ultrasonic fetal gender diagnoses during months 5 to 11 in mares. Theriogenology 1993;40:1127–1135.

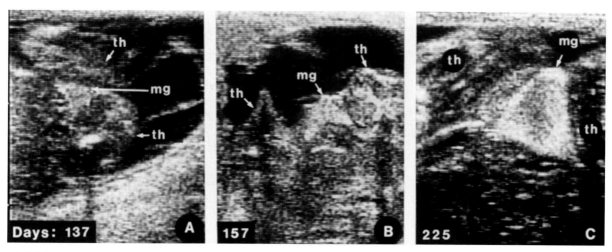

Figure 12.6. Ultrasonograms of the mammary gland (mg) of female fetuses. Views are frontal/oblique and the caudal aspect of the fetus is at the top of the image. **A**, The mammary gland of the younger fetus is a hyperechogenic triangle located between the rear limbs. **B**, Two distinct glands can be seen. **C**, The mammary gland of the older fetus is more echogenic than that of the younger fetus (F). th = thigh. Adapted with permission from Curran S, Ginther OJ. Ultrasonic fetal gender diagnoses during months 5 to 11 in mares. Theriogenology 1993;40:1127–1135.

CONCLUSION

In conclusion, equine fetal gender can accurately be determined by identifying and locating the genital tubercle. The optimal time for gender determination using a 5-Mhz transrectal transducer is between postovulation days 59 and 68. The upper age limit can be extended through the sixth month of gestation using a 3.5-Mhz transducer. After this time, the fetus lies predominantly in a cranial presentation, and the caudal aspect of the fetus is not accessible with ultrasound. Diagnosis of fetal gender requires differentiating the gender-specific external genitalia (genital tubercle, penis/prepuce, clitoris, mammary glands) from the surrounding structures (umbilical cord, anus, anogenital raphe, and tail).

REFERENCES

1. Betteridge KJ, Rieger D. Embryo transfer and related techniques in domestic animals, and their implications for human medicine. Hum Reprod 1993;8:147–167.
2. Amann RP. Treatment of sperm to predetermine sex. Theriogenology 1989;31:49–60.
3. Wood TC, White KL, Garza F Jr, et al. Detection of H-Y antigen on equine blastocysts. Theriogenology 1988;29:331.
4. Elejalde BR, De Elejalde MM, Heitman T. Visualization of the fetal genitalia by ultrasonography: a review of the literature and analysis of its accuracy and ethical implication. J Ultrasound Med 1985;4:633–639.
5. Müller E, Wittkowski G. Visualization of male and female characteristics of bovine fetuses by real-time ultrasonics. Theriogenology 1986;22:571–574.
6. Curran S, Kastelic JP, Ginther OJ. Determining sex of the bovine fetus by ultrasonic assessment of the relative location of the genital tubercle. Anim Reprod Sci 1989;19:217–227.
7. Curran S, Ginther OJ. Ultrasonic diagnosis of equine fetal sex by location of the genital tubercle. J Equine Vet Sci 1989;9:77–83.
8. Curran S, Ginther OJ. Ultrasonic determination of fetal gender in horses and cattle under farm conditions. Theriogenology 1991;36: 809–814.
9. Noden DM, De Lahunta A. The embryology of domestic animals: developmental mechanisms and malformations. Baltimore: Williams & Wilkins, 1985.
10. Bergin WC, Gier HT, Frey RA, et al. Developmental horizons and measurements useful for age determination of equine embryos and fetuses. In: Proceedings of the annual convention of the American Association of Equine Practitioners, New Orleans, 1967. 179–196.
11. Curran S, Ginther OJ. Ultrasonic fetal gender diagnoses during months 5 to 11 in mares. Theriogenology 1993;40:1127–1135.
12. Ginther OJ, Griffin PG. Equine fetal kinetics: presentation and location. Theriogenology 1993;40:1–12.

13 Fetal Ultrasonography

ANDREW MCGLADDERY

INTRODUCTION

The advent of diagnostic ultrasonography in the early 1980s has revolutionized the routine gynecological management of the mare. Transrectal ultrasonography is used routinely, often repeatedly, during the first weeks of pregnancy to identify and monitor the development of the early equine conceptus and subsequent fetus. This is in contrast to the current obstetric care regimen for pregnant women who normally have two midgestational scans, the first scan at approximately 16 weeks of pregnancy (essentially to confirm gestational age) and the second scan at about 22 weeks to detect any developmental abnormalities and confirm continued satisfactory growth. Further scans are not made unless there is a complication with the pregnancy, although an early dating and fetal anomaly scan at 11 to 12 weeks is being introduced in some centers. This difference, to a certain extent, reflects the differing priorities between the management of the pregnant mare and the pregnant mother and also the relative ease of diagnosis. In the latter, determining "dates" and identifying developmental abnormalities are the major priorities. In addition, in human obstetrics prepartum detection of fetal distress and disease has become an essential aspect of the management of the problem pregnancy. In these cases ultrasonography has proved invaluable, particularly where placental bleeding is present or where invasive procedures such as amniocentesis, chorionic villus sampling, and fetal blood or tissue sampling is necessary. With the improvement in the clinical management of the sick, newborn foal during the last 10 years, the need to develop techniques for assessing the status of the equine fetus in late term has become apparent. Hopefully, by detecting the distressed fetus and by diagnosing disease and prematurity, the management of the sick neonate will be further improved. To achieve this end a number of research workers have applied diagnostic ultrasonography to the assessment of the late gestational equine fetus (1, 2).

Indications for fetal ultrasonography in early to mid gestation include assessment of fetal viability and fetal sexing (3),which is best performed at about 60 days of gestation, and selective fetal reduction of twin pregnancies by lethal intracardiac injection using an ultrasound-guided technique commonly performed at about 120 days of gestation (4). Indications for fetal ultrasonography in mid to late pregnancy in the mare include vaginal discharge, premature mammary development and lactation, systemic maternal disease (colic, trauma, surgery), and a history of previous problems in late gestation such as abortion, stillbirth, prematurity, and neonatal septicemia or death.

FETAL IMAGING TECHNIQUES

Fetal imaging can be performed either from a transrectal or transabdominal approach. Both means of imaging the fetus have their own inherent limitations and advantages. Transrectal imaging only allows effective imaging of the fetus during the first 60 to 80 days of gestation; however, it is the preferred route for examining the fetus to determine fetal gender (60 to 70 days) and to measure the dimensions of the fetal orbit at more than 120 days. Most fetal ultrasonography is performed transabdominally because it allows the maximum visualization of the fetus and placenta. The fetus, often from as early as 60 days of gestation, can be visualized through the mare's ventral abdominal wall due to the close proximity the uterus adopts to the ventral abdomen. Both linear array and sector transducers can be used; however, the linear array transducer has the advantage of a rectilinear image that is easier to interpret, particularly as the fetus increases in size during the later stages of pregnancy. Sector transducers, which only need a small area of skin contact, are more useful in early pregnancy when accessibility within the inguinal area is important. In late gestation maximum penetration is important and therefore low-frequency transducers (e.g., 2.5 or 3 MHZ) are most suitable. However, higher-frequency transducers (e.g., 5 and 7.5 MHZ) have increased resolution and therefore are more appropriate for imaging fetal structures in the near field when fine detail is required. Good preparation of the mare is important to ensure high-quality images and to reduce artifacts. Ideally, the mare should be restrained in stocks and the skin closely clipped with a No. 40 surgical blade from the xiphoid sternum to the udder and on the lower flanks either side of midline. However, in many mares alcohol or scan gel alone may be sufficient without the need for extensive clipping. The mare should not be sedated as this will affect fetal activity and heart rate (5, 6). The skin surface is then coated with a high viscosity ultrasound coupling gel and the transducer placed in a longitudinal direction between the sternum and the mare's udder. The transducer is then moved systematically from side to side and up and down until the fetus is located. Usually, the relatively anechoic fetal fluids are most obvious along with the fetal thorax and contracting heart (Fig. 13.1). The ultrasound transducer can then be orientated to make sequential longitudinal or transverse images of the fetus as appropriate. In the later stages of pregnancy the fetus is most commonly in anterior presentation, in dorsal or dorsolateral recumbency, often slightly oblique in position. It may be possible to image the fetal head where the anechoic eyeball and orbit are the most prominent features. The fetal neck with tracheal rings and pulsatile carotid arteries can be recognized before joining the fetal thorax, where acoustic shadows are cast by the ribs and the contracting cardiac sil-

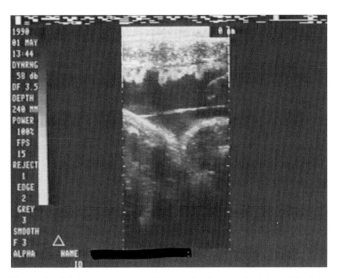

Figure 13.1. Ultrasonogram of the anterior thorax of a fetus. Allantoic and amniotic fluid can be seen separated by the amnion.

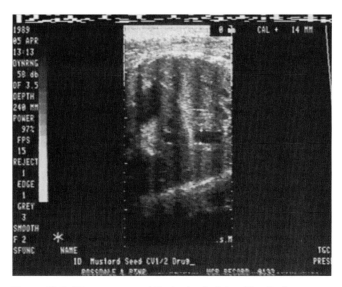

Figure 13.3. Ultrasonogram of the body of a fetus. The diaphragm can be seen separating the thorax from the abdomen.

houette is visible situated proximally in the thorax. If the fetus is appropriately positioned, it is occasionally possible to get good views of the cardiac chambers and valve movements. The aorta can be easily identified as it leaves the heart because of its echogenic walls and pulsatile nature; it is greatest in diameter proximal to the heart, becoming narrower more distally (Fig. 13.2). By scanning in a sagittal plane the regular-shaped, echogenic vertebrae are imaged. The diaphragm separates the thoracic and abdominal cavities (Fig. 13.3). The liver is homogenous in appearance and usually relatively more hypoechoic than the lung. The vena cava can be imaged passing through the liver (Fig. 13.4). The anechoic stomach bubble is a major feature of the abdomen (Fig. 13.5), and the fetal kidneys (Fig. 13.6) and gonads may be visualized from early in gestation. The umbil-

ical cord is normally imaged floating within the fetal fluids, highly coiled, and the vessel walls have a hyperechoic appearance. The two umbilical arteries, vein, and urachus are distinct (Fig. 13.7). Fetal breathing movements, that is, movements of the fetal ribs and diaphragm, can also be appreciated.

FETAL MEASUREMENTS

In pregnant women a number of different fetal measurements are commonly made. Crown-rump length is used in early gestation and is accurate prior to 13 weeks of gestation. Later in gestation the biparietal diameter, femur length, and abdominal circumference are measured and used to determine both fetal size and weight. The determined values are then compared, using growth charts, with the expected val-

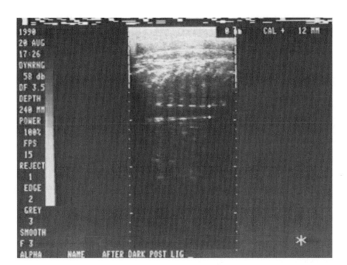

Figure 13.2. Ultrasonogram of the thorax of a fetus in a longitudinal plane through the descending aorta whose diameter decreases distally.

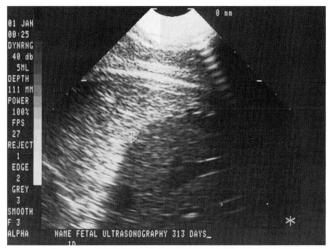

Figure 13.4. Ultrasonogram of a transverse section through the fetus. The lungs (*left*) are more hyperechoic than the liver (*right*), divided by the diaphragm (*arrow*).

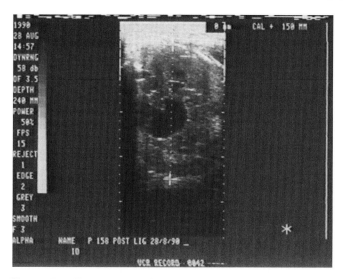

Figure 13.5. Ultrasonogram of a transverse section through the fetal abdomen. The anechoic stomach is centrally placed.

Figure 13.7. Ultrasonogram of a transverse section through the umbilical cord, which is surrounded by amniotic fluid.

ues for that age of fetus. A number of different growth charts are available to obstetricians to help them identify the growth-retarded fetus. Unfortunately, in the equine fetus its large size in the latter stages of pregnancy restricts the use of similar measurements. However, two structures that have been used, which are relatively small in size and can be measured sequentially, are the dimensions of the fetal orbit (7) and the diameter of the fetal aorta (1). The fetal eye is accessible either transabdominally (Fig. 13.8) or transrectally for most of the pregnancy. The orbital dimension in McKinnon's study was calculated from the sum of the width and length of the orbit; the 95% confidence limits are plus or minus 0.5 cm (+/−40 days). Unfortunately, this does still make the fetal eye a rather poor indicator of fetal age. Kahn and Leidl also studied growth of the fetus between 60 and 330 days of gestation and measured eye diameter amongst

other features (8). The diameter of the fetal aorta during systole at the level of the caudal border of the heart has been measured (Fig. 13.9) and has a range of 2.1 cm at 300 days to 2.7 cm at full term in light-breed mares (2). The results in Clydesdale foals and Arabian foals were greater and smaller, respectively, indicating a degree of breed variation. Aortic measurements were made in the Adams-Brendemuehl study during the last 7 days of pregnancy before parturition and had a good correlation with the weight of the foal and its girth and hip measurements. An estimate of the foal's newborn weight using this technique was accurate to within 2.5 kg. The use of aortic measurements in high-risk pregnancies has not been successful in identifying the compromised fetus and has been a poor predictor of birth weight. Fetuses found to be emaciated at delivery were thought to be normal in size from fetal ultrasonography (9).

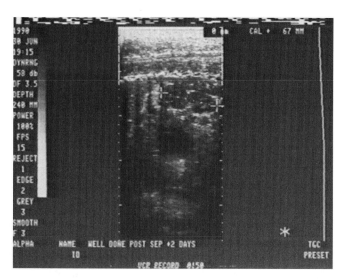

Figure 13.6. Ultrasonogram of a longitudinal section of a fetus. The fetal kidney is situated between the crosses.

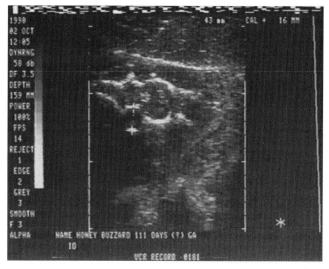

Figure 13.8. Ultrasonogram of a longitudinal section through the head of a 111-day fetus. The anechoic orbit is between the crosses.

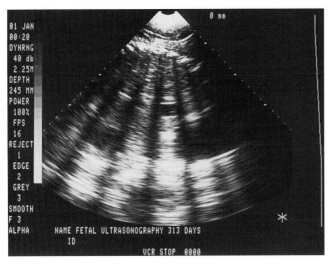

Figure 13.9. Ultrasonogram of a longitudinal section through the thorax of a 313-day fetus. The aorta at the level of the caudal border of the heart is between the crosses.

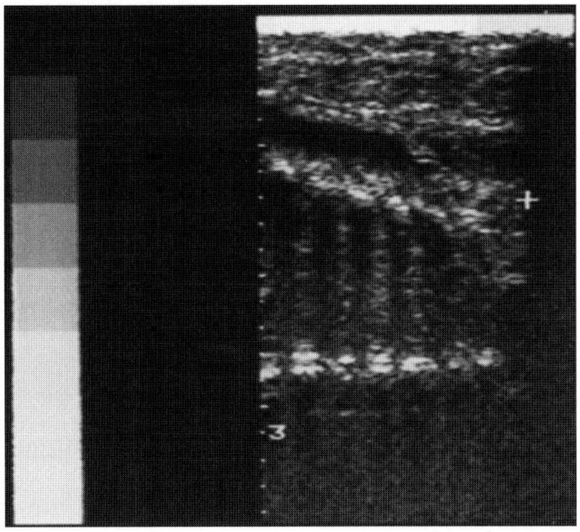

Figure 13.11. Ultrasonogram indicating localized area of placental separation (*cross*).

Imaging of the placenta and fetal fluids is best performed with a high-frequency transducer to ensure maximum resolution. It is not usually possible to differentiate between the uterus and the placenta as they both have a similar echogenic appearance. In late pregnancy the combined uteroplacenta is thin (Fig. 13.10), 1.26 cm thick $+/-0.33$ cm, especially where the fetal body overlies it. If greater than 2.0 cm, it should be considered abnormal (N.B. it will appear thicker and folded in areas more distant from the fetus toward the nonpregnant horn). Some workers have described hyperechoic foci within the placenta that have correlated with areas of mineralization found, following delivery, on the surface of the placenta. Placental blood vessels may be recognized distinct from the surface. Some workers have recognized apparent areas of placental separation (10) (Fig. 13.11). However, even in mares that are subsequently shown to have gross and extensive placentitis and separa-

tion, it is often difficult ultrasonographically to recognize its full extent. Placental thickening has been reported due to placental oedema associated with fescue toxicity (11).

The fetal fluids are readily identified because they are almost anechoic; however, the allantoic fluid in particular contains numerous hyperechoic foci. The amnion separating the two compartments appears as a thin, brightly echogenic membrane (Fig. 13.12). Amniotic fluid is usually most obvious around the fetal head, limbs, and neck. The depths of the pools of fluid can be measured, and the depth at the level of the scapulohumeral joint is 1.9 cm $+/-0.9$ cm (12). Although important in human obstetrics where oligohydramnios and polyhydramnios are problems, these conditions are rare in mares and associated with gross derangements in fluid volumes. Hydrops allantois can be confirmed clinically in mares that have developed a pear-shaped abdomen. The most striking feature identified by ultra-

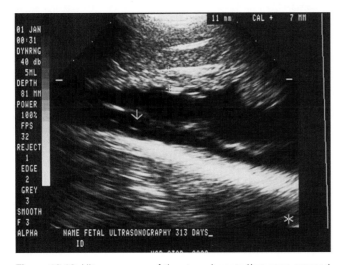

Figure 13.10. Ultrasonogram of the uteroplacenta (*between crosses*) of a 313-day fetus. The amnion (*arrow*) is also visible.

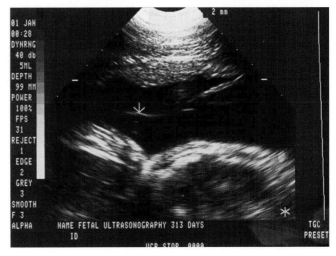

Figure 13.12. Ultrasonogram of amniotic and allantoic fluid separated by amnion (*arrow*).

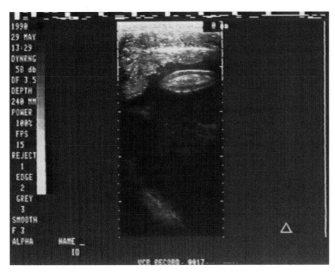

Figure 13.13. Ultrasonogram visualizing concentric, oval-ring appearance of hippomane within allantoic cavity.

sound examination is the very large quantities of fluid surrounding the fetus. Transrectal ultrasonography allows a similar view and the fetus normally cannot be palpated. Echogenic foci, particularly within the allantoic compartment, are due to desquamated cells and sebaceous secretions and appear in normal mares 10 to 40 days prior to delivery. Meconium and hemorrhage may also be responsible for similar-appearing particles in abnormal fetuses. Free-floating particles are positively correlated with pulmonary maturity in human fetuses; this has not been demonstrated in equines (12). The hippomane is usually readily identifiable as an oval, echogenic structure, sometimes with a concentric-ring appearance floating free in the allantoic cavity (Fig. 13.13).

The fetal heart is easily recognized due to the motion of the chamber walls and valves, and with high-resolution imaging it can, in some cases, be examined in great detail. Fetal heart rate (FHR) can be measured with 2-D imaging by counting the number of cardiac contractions over a known period or, more accurately, with M-mode by measuring the time between identical points on the cardiac cycle (Fig. 13.14). Both of these methods are relatively unhelpful as they do not, even with frequent repeated measurements, take accurate account of fetal heart rate variations over time. Consequently, in obstetric management continuous FHR monitoring utilizing Doppler heart rate monitors is undertaken. This equipment can be used in equines. It is easiest to locate the fetal heart first with 2-D imaging and then using the Doppler transducer. Regular relocation is necessary to maintain a reasonable trace, and the main limitation is an inability to measure rate if the heart is greater than about 20 cm from the skin surface. Numerous workers using different techniques have documented the decrease in fetal heart rate that occurs with increasing gestational age. This has been attributed to increasing parasympathetic tone in the developing fetus. Transient fetal heart

rate accelerations are associated invariably with fetal movement and activity. Abnormalities include persistent tachycardia, particularly prior to abortion; bradycardia; or heart rate patterns that show no variation. Assessment of fetal viability is the most common indication for FHR measurement, although studies on the effects of cardiotonic drugs have been performed (5, 6, 13). Human perinatologists study the fetus via nonstress and stress tests. A nonstress test involves simply observing FHR patterns over a period of 20 to 30 minutes during a single examination. A reactive (normal) pattern would require at least two accelerations of 15+ bpm for 15+ seconds with associated fetal body and limb movements.

Fetal movement is one of the most important means of assessing fetal health; an active fetus is essentially a healthy fetus. Studies between 64 and 84 days of gestation showed vigorous fetal mobility with movement between the horns and body occurring five times every hour (14). Another study by Ginther revealed that during 5-minute examinations the fetus was active at least 60% of the time, although there was a significant decrease during the seventh month of pregnancy when the fetus was only active for about 45% of the time (15). Equine fetal movements are complicated and have been studied in detail (16). Movements observed include simple extensions and flexions of the limbs and neck, which may be multiple and complex in their nature. More coordinated activities, including 360° rotations or less about the long axis, may also be noted. Increased fetal activity prior to parturition has also been noted (2). Most periods of inactivity or fetal sleep are for less than 10 minutes and rare for more than 40 to 60 minutes. One can attempt to arouse the fetus by vigorous palpation or sound stimulation per rectum (5). If there is little fetal response, reexamination is indicated within 24 hours.

Ginther and Griffin have shown in a study between 80 days of gestation and full term that there is an equal likeli-

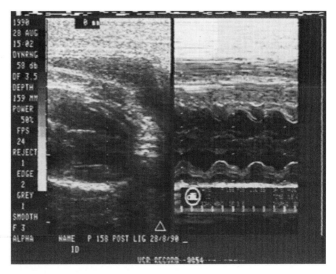

Figure 13.14. Ultrasonogram of longitudinal view through fetal heart. Two-dimensional image (*left*). The M-mode cursor can be seen passing through the ventricles giving an M-mode image (*right*).

hood of cranial or caudal presentation during the first 5 months and an increased likelihood of cranial presentation after 5 months of gestation. By 7 months more than 90% of fetuses were in cranial presentation. Maximum fetal mobility occurs between months 3 and 4, which is related to the relatively large amount of allantoic fluid present at this stage in proportion to the size of the fetus. Measurement of the ratio of the height of the fetus to the height of placental fluid is low. As the fetus increases in size, the relative proportion of fluid decreases, thus reducing mobility (17).

FETAL SEXING

In one study of 85 pony mares, up to 5 to 6 months, it was possible to detect gender in 90%; however, between 7 and 11 months it was only possible in 6% of mares. It was nearly always possible to detect fetal gender when the fetus was in caudal or transverse presentation. The diagnostic accuracy verified after birth was 100% when the expected accuracy estimated at the time of examination was greater than 80% (18).

FETAL BIOPHYSICAL PROFILE

This is a method of assessing fetal health by checking a number of biophysical features that will reflect both acute and chronic asphyxia of the fetus. These features arise from signals generated within the fetal central nervous system, generally with some inherent periodic rhythm. A variable such as fetal breathing movements arises from signals generated within the respiratory center of the medulla; if the biophysical variable is intact, then one can assume that the mechanisms that generate it are intact and functional. Neuronal tissues are very sensitive to oxygen supply; therefore if fetal breathing movements are present, it is not unreasonable to assume that the fetus is not hypoxic. Because of the periodic nature of these variables the use of multiple variables avoids the likelihood of false positives due to intrinsic rhythms. Some variables such as amniotic fluid volume determination reflect a more long-term constant which in this case depends on fetal regulation of production and elimination of amniotic fluid. Chronic asphyxia is known to reduce amniotic fluid volume. It is the combination of acute and chronic indices that produces a highly specific and sensitive profile of fetal health. In high-risk pregnancies in women the biophysical profile is used to determine when intervention (usually delivery) is necessary (19). Ultrasonographic examination is used in combination with FHR monitoring to construct the profile. The five parameters assessed are fetal breathing movements, gross body movement, fetal tone, reactive FHR, and qualitative amniotic fluid volume. A normal score = 2, and an abnormal score = 0 for each parameter. A total score of 8 or 10 of 10 is considered normal unless the amniotic fluid volume is abnormal, when a score of 8 of 10 indicates probable chronic fetal compromise. Abnormal scores usually require delivery. Human fetuses at risk are normally tested weekly from about 25 weeks (the lower limit of neonatal viability) until delivery, or if they go beyond full term, twice weekly testing is undertaken (19).

Adams-Brendemeuhl and Pipers developed a similar biophysical profile for use in late gestational mares that uses six parameters: aortic diameter, FHR, fetal movement, placental thickness, allantoic fluid volume, and particulate appearance of the fluid (2). The scoring in this system is slightly different and a negative (normal) profile would have no abnormal parameters. A positive (abnormal) profile would have at least one abnormal parameter. In their study of 17 mares in late gestation. Nine mares had normal profiles of which seven delivered normal foals, and eight mares had abnormal profiles of which seven delivered abnormal foals. The most common abnormal parameter was fetal bradycardia with heart rates between 48 and 58 per minute, followed by placental abnormalities. These results indicate that equine biophysical profiling has a reasonable degree of sensitivity in detecting fetuses at risk.

Biophysical profiling is a passive means of examining the fetus; a more active approach is stress testing where provocative tests on the fetus are employed. The oxytocin contraction test (OCT) is an intrapartum test used in human obstetrics. It is based on the principle that when blood flow is interrupted because of uterine contractions, the stressed fetus responds with late decelerations in heart rate that can be detected by FHR monitoring. In the OCT, contractions are induced by oxytocin infusion and the FHR effects monitored (20). Preliminary studies on the effects of oxytocin in normal pregnant mares showed that within 30 minutes of injection with 1 IU of oxytocin two to three major accelerations in FHR occurred with an increase of 18 to 50 bpm in baseline heart rate (5). It has been speculated that these accelerations are due to fetal activity associated with induced uterine contractions. Another test, which is considered by many assessing fetal health to be beneficial, is vibroacoustic stimulation, where FHR responses following sound stimulation of the fetus are determined. Several different heart rate patterns have been described, including sustained tachycardia, accelerations, combined accelerations and decelerations, and no change. All but the latter are predictive of a nonacidotic fetus (21). A preliminary study in pregnant mares, where the normal equine fetus was exposed to sound from a device placed per rectum, resulted in fetal heart rate patterns similar to those observed in healthy human fetuses. However, a deceleration pattern suggesting possible distress was also observed, in some fetuses, without any adverse outcome. Further work is needed before the possible usefulness of this test in determining equine fetal health will be known (5).

DOPPLER ULTRASOUND

Doppler ultrasound is now commonly available as an added application on many modern real-time ultrasound scanners. Rather than producing a two-dimensional image, the Doppler ultrasound transducer is used by the operator in an identical fashion but instead analyzes the information it collects to detect and measure the velocity of blood flow in the

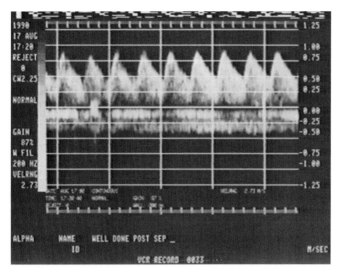

Figure 13.15. Spectral Doppler of a typical flow velocity. Waveforms of the umbilical artery above baseline and vein below baseline.

body's vessels. The technique makes use of the Doppler shift and measures the change in frequency that occurs when ultrasound strikes moving red blood cells within a vessel. The technique was first used to examine the human fetal circulation in 1977 (22), and they suggested it might be useful for in utero investigations of the fetal cardiovascular changes that occur with intrauterine growth retardation and preeclampsia. Doppler is used primarily to measure the velocity of blood flowing within a blood vessel. When ultrasound of known frequency *(f)* insonates a vessel, it is scattered by the blood cells it strikes. This results in a backscattered echo that is higher in frequency than the incident beam; if the angle of the beam *(cos 0)* is constant, *the variation in velocity of blood within the vessel is directly proportional to the change in frequency (fd)* as determined by the Doppler equation (below) where *(c)* is a constant representing the velocity of sound through body tissues.

$$\text{velocity} = v = \frac{fd/cos0}{2fc} \qquad (13.1)$$

The frequency shift that occurs is within the audible range so that the operator can use this feature to achieve the clearest signal. It is possible to discriminate very subtly using this feature and, when sufficiently skilled, to identify the type of blood vessel being interrogated. The technique has become widespread in obstetric management because of its noninvasive nature. The simplest form of Doppler ultrasound is continuous wave (CW), which analyzes echoes from all structures in the path of the ultrasound beam. The second type of Doppler ultrasound is pulsed wave (PW), which uses a range gate so that only echoes originating from within the gate are analyzed. When PW is combined with two-dimensional imaging, a duplex system is created that allows the source of the Doppler signal (the gate) to be placed under visual control. The flow velocity waveform (FVW) is

the term applied to the Doppler-shifted signal obtained when the vessel is insonated over one cardiac cycle. This FVW varies depending on the vessel under interrogation. Initially, the work centered on the desire to measure blood flow in an attempt to measure fetal cardiac output; however, the FVW changes its appearance in various disease states, and therefore in recognition of this and because of the development of indices that compare the velocities in systole and diastole, the more difficult volume measurements have largely been abandoned. The simplest of these indices is the systolic : diastolic ratio or A : B ratio. Others that are somewhat more complex include the resistance index and the pulsatility index. However, all enable objective analysis of blood flow without the need to measure the exact angle between the blood vessel under study and the incident ultrasound beam. In human pregnancy the fundamental change occurring with increasing gestational age is the decrease in peripheral resistance of the placental circulation. Most abnormalities of the FVW are associated with a pathologic increase in the peripheral resistance with most notably a decrease occurring in the flow of blood during diastole, leading to, in some cases, a loss of end diastolic flow or even reverse diastolic flow.

A number of studies in pregnant women have demonstrated the poor fetal outcomes associated with fetuses demonstrating abnormal indices, such as an increased number of perinatal deaths, small for gestational age fetuses, or operative deliveries for fetal distress (23, 24). The most widely studied vessel is the umbilical artery; however, examination of the fetal aorta and carotid arteries gives similar results.

The technique has been applied to equine umbilical vessels; however, the size of the mare is a limitation and does create difficulties because signals can only be obtained if the vessel is within 20 cm of the transducer. Thus poor fetal positioning in large-type mares, in late pregnancy, can result in great difficulty in obtaining signals. Studies in pregnant pony mares (25) have shown a similar decrease in peripheral resistance (Fig. 13.15) with increasing gestational age as seen in both the human and sheep fetus. The A : B ratio fell from a mean of 3.1 between 151 and 182 days of gestation to a mean of 2.0 at 298 to 326 days of gestation. Considering the high incidence of abortions that are attributed to umbilical cord abnormality, this technique may have some potential in the investigation of this condition. To date, in a number of abnormal pregnancies that have resulted in the delivery of compromised foals, no abnormalities in the FVW or indices have been detected. This is an area that may warrant further investigation.

ULTRASOUND-GUIDED TECHNIQUES

Amniocentesis is a well-developed technique in obstetric practice where it is most commonly used for prenatal diagnosis of fetal karyotype, for measurement of *a*-feto-protein (associated with neural tube defects), and in the assessment of hemolytic disease and pulmonary maturity. It can also be used for the detection of mecomium, bacteria, and inflammatory cells in amniotic fluid. In pregnant women it carries a risk of abortion of approximately 1% (26). In polyhydramnios, where excess fluid is present, fluid can be removed, or in oligohydramnios, where insufficient fluid is present, saline can be added. Amniocentesis/allantocentesis has been adapted for the pregnant mare (27). It is relatively straightforward with the mare, ideally, sedated and prepared as if for a routine transabdominal ultrasound scan; a suitable pool of amniotic fluid and allantoic fluid separated by amnion is identified. The skin surface at the appropriate point is surgically prepared, and local anaesthetic is infiltrated into the skin and abdominal muscle layer. With a sterile sleeve covering the ultrasound transducer and a 15-cm 18-gauge spinal needle held within the channel of the needle guide attachment, the needle is advanced under continuous ultrasound guidance into the pool of amniotic fluid. The stylet is then removed and a 10- to 20-ml sample collected by gravity flow. The needle is then withdrawn into the allantoic fluid compartment, and a similar quantity of fluid is collected. The needle is then completely withdrawn. If the procedure is performed carefully, only a single puncture of the uterus and placenta should be necessary. Various groups of research workers have analyzed fetal fluids for biochemical, hormonal, and phospholipid concentrations. Biochemical analysis of amniotic and allantoic fluids reveals variations in the concentration of the different biochemical constituents between the two fluid compartments (28–31), which allows them to be distinguished and also indicates their probable origin. The Na and Cl values are higher in amniotic than allantoic fluid and the concentrations tend to increase in allantoic fluid during gestation. The concentrations of Na, K, and creatinine remain relatively constant in amniotic fluid. Allantoic K concentrations peak at 200 days in Thoroughbred mares and then decline as gestation progresses. Creatinine concentrations increase through gestation also and are significantly higher in allantoic than amniotic fluid. Urea concentrations are similar in both fluid compartments. Amniotic fluid resembles adult or foal plasma, whereas allantoic fluid resembles urine reflecting their probable origins.

Hormonal analysis indicates that relatively high levels of cortisol can be measured in amniotic fluid just prior to parturition, which corresponds to the levels present in fetal plasma and supports the concept of maturation of the fetal adrenocortical axis (32). The assessment of phospholipids to determine pulmonary maturity has been to date relatively unrewarding. The L : S ratio (lecithin : sphingomyelin ratio) and percentage of phosphatidylglycerol (% PG) is commonly measured in amniotic liquor in pregnant women and is a useful determinant of fetal pulmonary maturity. In the equine fetus the L : S ratio does not appear to correlate well with fetal outcome and has produced inconsistent results. In a study by Williams (33) the ratio was >4 : 1 in all foals from 292 days of gestation until full term, although the % PG did alter significantly with gestational age. In a study by Paradis (34) the L : S ratio in 12 normal foals had a mean of 2.2 : 1 and in six premature foals measured between 1.5:1 and 3.9 : 1, again suggesting that it does not help identify premature foals at risk. However, in this study a positive % PG was indicative in 85% of foals of pulmonary maturity. Although there is a relatively low incidence of neonatal respiratory distress syndrome in the equine neonate and because, compared to human obstetrics, preterm delivery is rarely considered an option, the need to determine pulmonary maturity as an indicator of overall maturity still remains an important goal. The safety of the technique in the equine has been questioned by some workers. In Williams' study (33) 25% aborted; however, a further two foals were also treated for dysmaturity and sepsis and survived. This study did involve serial sampling, and therefore the risk may be significantly reduced if only single samples are taken. Other workers have experienced fewer problems even with numerous serial amnio/allantocenteses (McGladdery AJ, Rossdale PD, unpublished data). This is in contrast to the human situation where the abortion rate was less than 1% in the only large randomized trial performed so far (26). The author has experienced complications in a number of cases where damage to the amnion has been initiated, which has led to mixing of fluids and the creation of effectively a single compartment. One foal had conjunctivitis associated with the apparent irritant nature of the fluids. The potential for disrupting the environment of the fetal foal is likely to be heightened if serial sampling is undertaken, and the validity of subsequent fluid analyses becomes questionable.

In addition to sampling of fetal fluids, the technique can be very simply adapted to allow access to and manipulation of the fetal environment by injecting drugs into the compartments surrounding the fetus or directly into the fetus itself. In one study precocious maturation of the fetal adrenal cortex as evidenced by a premature rise in maternal plasma progestagens was produced by injecting CRH (corticotropin-releasing hormone), ACTH (adrenocorticotropic hormone), or betamethasone either subcutaneously or intramuscularly into the fetus in late pregnancy (35). These results may have clinical benefit in that it may be a means of deliberately shortening gestation, for example, when serious maternal disease exists. This has yet to be demonstrated. Allantocentesis has been used in studies by Sertich and Vaala (36) to measure the concentrations of penicillin/gentamicin or trimethoprim in treated mares to determine the efficacy against diseases such as bacterial placentitis. Similarly, drugs injected into the allantois, such as antibiotics, may enter the fetal circulation and can be measured in foal plasma after delivery (37).

Fetal twin reduction has also been discussed in Chapter 10 and can be performed transvaginally (38) by aspiration of allantoic fluid or transabdominally by a lethal intracardiac injection (4). The success rate of the transabdominally method is in the author's experience relatively low with only a 40% (live foal) success rate, although the success rate in one large series was over 50% (Rantanen N, personal communication).

FUTURE TECHNIQUES

Modern techniques such as chorionic villus sampling are used in women to detect genetic disorders, but are not applicable to the mare due to their lower incidence and have therefore not been investigated. Fetal blood sampling is used in human obstetrics mainly for detecting genetic blood disorders, for rapid chromosome analysis from fetal lymphocytes, for acid-base evaluation, for determining the extent of fetal anemia in alloimmunization, and for diagnosing viral infections. Blood samples are taken using ultrasound guidance from the umbilical vein close to its insertion into the placenta (39, 40). This technique has not been reported to date in the equine; however, in performing twin reductions fetal blood sampling is possible, and because it has proved difficult to kill the fetus by exsanguination, cardiocentesis may be a potential source of fetal blood. Ultrasound-guided cardiocentesis is considered the most efficient technique for obtaining blood samples in the nonhuman primate fetus, and although it carries some risk, serial studies have been performed (41). Therefore this technique may merit investigation in the pregnant mare.

REFERENCES

1. Pipers FS, Adams-Brendemuehl C. Techniques and applications of transabdominal ultrasonography in the pregnant mare. J Am Vet Med Assoc 1984;185:766–771.
2. Adams-Brendemuehl C, Pipers PS. Antepartum evaluations of the equine fetus. J Reprod Fertil Suppl 1987;35:565–573.
3. Curran S, Ginther OJ. Diagnosis of equine fetal sex by location of the genital tubercle. J Equine Vet Sci 1989;9:77.
4. Rantanen NW, Kincaid B. Ultrasound guided fetal cardiac puncture: a method of twin reduction in the mare. Proceedings of the 34th Annual Convention of the American Association of Equine Practitioners, 1988, pp. 173–179.
5. Smith LJ, Schott H. Xylazine-induced fetal bradycardia. In: Rossdale PD, ed. Proceedings of the 2nd International Conference on Veterinary Perinatology, 1990; p. 36.
6. McGladdery AJ, Rossdale PD. Responses of the equine fetus to maternal drug administration and acoustic stimulation. Proceedings of the 37th Annual Convention of the American Association of Equine Practitioners, 1991; pp. 223–228.
7. McKinnon AO, Squires EL, Pickett BW. Equine reproductive ultrasonography. Fort Collins: Colorado State University Animal Reproduction Laboratory, 1988.
8. Kahn W, Leidl W. Ultrasonic measurement of the fetus in utero and ultrasonographic imaging of fetal organs. Disch Tierarztl Wscher 1987;94:509–515.
9. Adams-Brendemuehl C. In: Koterba AM, Drummond WH, Kosch PC, eds. Fetal assessment. Malvern, PA: Lea & Febiger, 1990; pp. 16–33.
10. Reef VB, Vaala W, Worth LT. Transabdominal fetal ultrasonography: a biophysical profile for the equine fetus. Proceedings of the 2nd European Association of Veterinary Diagnostic Imaging—Annual Congress, 1993; p. 32.
11. Green EM, Loch WE, Messer NT. Maternal and fetal effects of endophyte fungus infected fescue. Proceedings of the 37th Annual Convention of the American Association of Equine Practitioners, 1991; pp. 29–44.
12. Gross TL, Wolfson RM, Kuhnert PM, Sokol RJ. Sonographically detected free-floating particles in amniotic fluid predict a mature lecithin-sphingomyelin ratio. J Clin Ultra 1985;13:405.
13. Card CE, Wood MR. The effects of acute administration of clenbuterol on uterine tone and equine fetal and maternal heart rates.

14. Griffin PG, Ginther OJ. Uterine and fetal dynamics during early pregnancy in mares. Am J Vet Res 1991; 52:298–306.
15. Ginther OJ. Ultrasonic imaging and animal reproduction in horses. Book 2. Cross Plains, WI: Equiservices Publishing, 1995; p. 223.
16. Frazer AF, Hastie H, Callicott RB, Brownlee S. An exploratory ultrasonic study on quantitative foetal kinesis in the horse. Appl Anim Ethol 1975;1:395.
17. Ginther OJ, Griffin PG. Equine fetal kinetics: presentation and location. Theriogenology 1993;40:1–11.
18. Curran S, Ginther OJ. Ultrasonic fetal gender diagnoses during months 5–11 in mares. Theriogenology 1993; 40:1127–1135.
19. Manning FA. The biophysical profile. In: Spencer J, ed. Fetal monitoring. Castle House Publications, 1989; p. 73–77.
20. Freeman RK. The use of the oxytocin challenge test for antepartum clinical evaluation of uteroplacental respiratory function. Am J Obstet Gynecol 1975;121:481–489.
21. Polzin GB, Balkemore KJ, Petrie RH, et al. Fetal vibroacoustic stimulation: magnitude and duration of fetal heart rate accelerations as a marker of fetal health. Obstet Gynecol 1988;72: 621–626.
22. Fitzgerald DE, Drumm JE. Non-invasive measurement of human fetal circulation using ultrasound: a new method. Br Med J 1977; 2:1450.
23. Trudinger BJ, Cook CM. Umbilical and uterine flow velocity waveforms in pregnancy associated with major fetal abnormalities. Br J Obstet Gynaecol 1985;92:666–670.
24. Fleischer A, Schulman H, Farmakides G, Bracero L, Blattner P, Randolph G. Umbilical artery velocity waveform and intrauterine growth retardation. Am J Obstet Gynecol 1985;151:502–505.
25. McGladdery AJ, Ousey JC, Rossdale PD. Serial Doppler ultrasound studies of the umbilical artery during equine pregnancy. Proceedings of the 3rd International Conference on Veterinary Perinatology, Davis, CA, 1992; p. 37.
26. Tabor A, et al. Randomised control trial of genetic amniocentesis in 4606 low risk women. Lancet 1986;1:1287–1293.
27. Schmidt AR, Williams MA, Carlton CL, Darien BJ, Derksen FJ. Evaluation of transabdominal ultrasound guided amniocentesis in the late gestational mare. Eq Vet J 1991;23:261–265.
28. Holdstock NB, McGladdery AJ, Ousey JC, Rossdale PD. Assessing methods of collection and changes in selected biochemical constituents of amniotic and allantoic fluid throughout equine pregnancy. Biol Reprod Mono 1995;1:21–38.
29. Paccamonti D, Swiderski C, Marx B, Gaunt S, Blauin D. Electrolytes and Biochemical enzymes in amniotic and allantoic fluid of the equine fetus during late gestation. Biol Reprod Mono 1995;1:39–48.
30. Williams MA. Amniotic fluid analysis for evaluation of equine foetal development. In: Rossdale PD, ed. Proceedings of the 2nd International Conference on Veterinary Perinatology, 1990; p. 38.
31. Schott HC, Mansmann RA. Biochemical profiles of normal equine amniotic fluid at parturition (abstract). Eq Vet J 1988;5(Suppl):52.
32. Bennett SD, et al. Equine amniocentesis (abstract). Eq Vet J 1989; 8(Suppl):86.
33. Williams MA, Goyert NA, Goyert GL, Sokol RJ. Preliminary report of transabdominal amniocentesis for the determination of pulmonary maturity in an equine population. Eq Vet J 1988;20:457–458.
34. Paradis MR, Altmaier KR, Schelling SH, Lamb C. Assessment of lung maturity in normal and premature foals. Proceedings of Havermeyer Foundation International Workshop on Disturbances in Equine Foetal Maturation: Comparative Aspects, 1992; p. 48.

Proceedings of the 6th International Symposium on Equine Reproduction, 1994; pp. 1–2.

35. Rossdale PD, McGladdery AJ, Ousey JC, Holdstock N, Grainger L, Houghton E. Increase in plasma progestagens concentrations in the mare after foetal injection with CRH, ACTH or betamethasone in late gestation. Eq Vet J 1992;24(5):347–350.

36. Sertich PL, Vaala W. Preliminary study of post treatment antibiotic concentrations in pregnant mares, foals and fetal fluids. Proceedings of the 12th Animal Reproduction Congress, Netherlands, 1992; pp. 1921–1923.

37. McGladdery AJ, Rossdale PD, Callingham B, Houghton E, Ousey JC. Placental transfer of drugs adminstered to the pregnant mare either intravenously or via the allantois and their effects on the fetus. Proceedings of the 4th International Conference on Veterinary Perinatology, 1995; p. 33.

38. Bracher V, Parlevliet JM, Pieterse MC, Vos PLAM, Taverne MAM, Colenbrander B. Transvaginal guided twin reduction in the mare. Vet Rec 1993;133:478–479.

39. Daffos F, Capella-Pavlovsky M, Forestier F. Fetal blood sampling during pregnancy with the use of a needle guided by ultrasound: a study of 606 consecutive cases. Am J Obstet Gynecol 1985;153: 655–660.

40. Nicolaides K, Soothill P, Rodeck C, Campbell S. Ultrasound guided sampling of umbilical cord and placental blood to assess fetal well being. Lancet 1986;1:1065–1067.

41. Tarantal A. Interventional ultrasound in pregnant macaques: embryonic/fetal applications. J Med Primat 1990;19:47–58.

14. Uterine Pathology

ANGUS O. McKINNON

With ultrasonography, the uterus can be examined noninvasively for detection of pathologic changes and for monitoring therapeutic regimen(s). The three most common forms of uterine pathology detected by ultrasonography are accumulations of intrauterine fluid, air, and cysts. Less commonly, fetal remnants, debris, abscess, and neoplastic conditions are observed. Recent applications of ultrasonography to medical conditions have demonstrated its usefulness in examining mares with problems prepartum and postpartum.

INTRAUTERINE FLUID

Ultrasonography is extremely valuable for estimating quantity and quality of fluid in the uterine lumen. Rectal palpation is only accurate when the quantity of intrauterine fluid is large ($>$100 ml) and/or when uterine tonicity changes. Confirmation of intrauterine fluid, without invasive techniques such as lavage and cytologic analysis, was difficult until direct, noninvasive visualization was made possible with ultrasonography. Volumes of fluid within the uterine lumen are estimated (graded as very small, small, medium, large, or excessive) with ultrasonography, and quality is graded from 1 to 4 according to degree of echogenicity (1) (Figs. 14.1 through 14.4). Degree of echogenicity is related to amount of debris or white blood cell infiltration into the fluid. Grade 1 fluid has large numbers of neutrophils and grade 4 has very few neutrophils. Observations on quality and quantity of uterine fluid have been used to assess efficacy of various therapeutic procedures on individual animals treated for naturally occurring endometritis (2). Experiments (1, 3, 4) have been conducted to determine the relationship of intrauterine fluid to fertility and are discussed below.

Some areas where recognition of intrauterine fluid may be of particular value are (a) evaluation of the postpartum mare, (b) diagnosis and treatment of endometritis, and (c) effects on pregnancy rate and early embryonic death (EED).

ULTRASONOGRAPHIC STUDIES OF THE UTERUS AFTER PARTURITION

In the equine industry, economic incentives influence breeders to attempt a foaling interval of 12 months or less. This commonly necessitates breeding of mares during the first postpartum ovulation. However, fertility has been reported lower in mares bred during the first postpartum ovulatory period compared with mares bred during subsequent cycles (5), and early embryonic death has been reported higher for mares bred at this time (5–7). This decreased fertility may be due to failure of elimination of microbes during uterine involution (5, 7) or their introduction at breeding. In addition, presence of uterine fluid during estrus and diestrus (3, 4) has been shown to reduce fertility of mares. A study (1) was conducted to evaluate two hypotheses: (a) uterine involution and fluid accumulation could be effectively monitored with ultrasonography and used to predict fertility of mares bred during the first postpartum ovulatory cycle, and (b) delaying ovulation with a progestin would result in improved pregnancy rates in mares bred during the first postpartum ovulatory period. The previously gravid horn was larger than the nongravid horn for a mean of 21 days (range 15 to 25) after parturition. Uterine involution was most obvious at the corpus cornual junction. When the results of three ultrasonographic scans were similar, over a 5-day period, the uterus was considered to be involuted. On the average, uterine involution was completed by day 23 (range 13 to 29). Quantity and quality of uterine fluid were not affected by progestin treatment. Number of mares with detectable uterine fluid decreased after day 5 postpartum. Uterine fluid generally decreased in quantity and improved in quality between days 3 and day 15. Fewer ($P < .005$) mares became pregnant when uterine fluid was present during the first postpartum ovulatory period (3 of 9, 33%), compared with mares that had no fluid detected (26 of 31, 84%). Mares with uterine fluid during breeding did not have appreciably larger uterine dimensions, compared with those mares not having fluid. There was no relationship between uterine size on day of ovulation and pregnancy rate. Ovulation was delayed, and pregnancy rates improved in progestin-treated mares. More ($P < .05$) mares became pregnant (23 of 28, 82%) when they ovulated after day 15, in the first postpartum ovulatory period, than mares that ovulated before day 15 (6 of 12, 50%). This study demonstrated that ultrasonography was useful in detecting mares with postpartum uterine fluid. Further, it now can be used to aid in determining whether a mare should be bred, treated, or not bred during the first postpartum ovulatory period. During estrous, uterine fluid may be spermicidal and/or an excellent medium to support bacterial proliferation. In addition, fluid may indicate poor uterine involution. When fluid is present during diestrus, it may cause premature luteolysis or early embryonic death (4). Quantity of uterine fluid during the first postpartum ovulatory period appeared to be related to stage of uterine involution and was reduced or eliminated by delaying the ovulatory period with progestins. Progestin treatment not only allowed time for elimination of uterine fluid before the first postpartum ovulation, but it also significantly delayed the first postpartum ovulation. Results of this study concurred with those of others in which it was concluded that progestin treatment de-

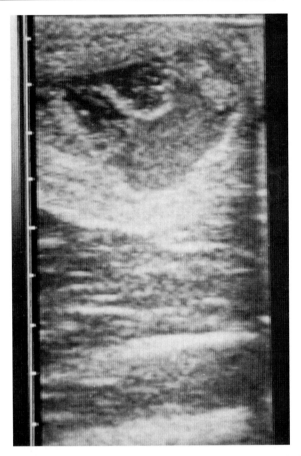

Figure 14.1. Grade 1 intrauterine fluid. The fluid is very echogenic (almost white) and represents large amounts of suspended debris. On occasion it may be difficult to see the junction of the fluid and the uterine wall clearly. (From A.O. McKinnon and J. L. Voss, eds. Equine reproduction. Philadelphia: Lea & Febiger, 1993; p. 281, with permission of Williams & Wilkins, Baltimore.)

treatment in the immediate postpartum period, and our aims should be to identify those that do need treatment. Mares managed by personnel at the GVEH are routinely examined between day 2 and day 4 after foaling. The purpose of the examination is to detect those mares that may develop postfoaling problems such as delayed involution and metritis. Prompt action may prevent the mare from becoming a problem breeder (2). Examination at day 9 or 10 is performed on all mares when stud masters wish to breed on foal heat. Those mares with uterine fluid are treated and then recycled. Mares that have already ovulated are recycled with $PGF_{2\alpha}$ 6 days later. Mares that are developing a follicle and are not showing signs of delayed involution are bred if they meet criteria such as being less than 12 years old and an expected ovulation day of day 11 or later.

DIAGNOSIS OF ENDOMETRITIS

There are numerous techniques to diagnose endometritis. However, no technique is completely reliable. The common, currently accepted techniques are as follows:

1. Rectal palpation
2. Vaginal-speculum examination

layed onset of the first postpartum ovulatory period, but did not affect rate of uterine involution (8–10). Long-term progestin administration to normal, cycling mares has not been shown to adversely affect fertility (11). However, treatment with progestins will affect uterine defense mechanisms (12, 13), and thus care is recommended before prolonged progestin treatment is administered to postpartum mares or mares susceptible to infection. Since there were decreased pregnancy rates associated with uterine fluid, and increased pregnancy rates as ovulation was delayed, it was suggested both techniques could be used to manipulate breeding strategies and improve pregnancy rates from normal mares bred during the first postpartum ovulatory period.

Other authors have indicated that the results of clinical, microbiologic, and hormonal examinations performed during the puerperal period provide useful information when deciding whether to use the foal heat for breeding or to initiate a therapy during this period of time (14). Interpretation of results of lavage or other postpartum treatments (15, 16) should be viewed with caution when all mares are treated in different groups, because most mares do not need

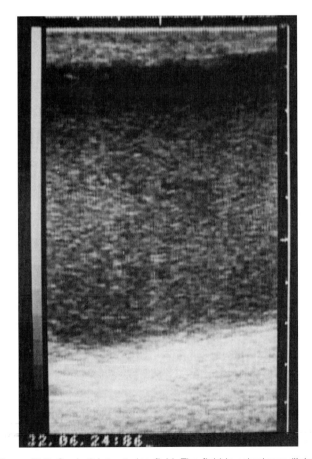

Figure 14.2. Grade 2 intrauterine fluid. The fluid is echodense (light gray) but less so than grade 1. (From A.O. McKinnon and J. L. Voss, eds. Equine reproduction. Philadelphia: Lea & Febiger, 1993; p. 281, with permission of Williams & Wilkins, Baltimore.)

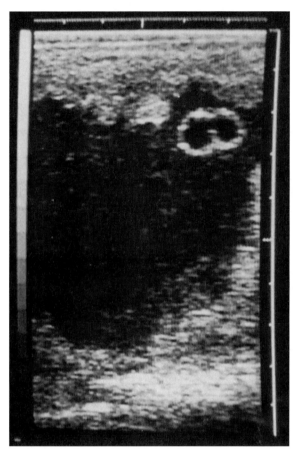

Figure 14.3. Grade 3 intrauterine fluid. The fluid is dark gray in color due to a few hyoechoic foci suspended in an anechoic medium. (From A.O. McKinnon and J. L. Voss, eds. Equine reproduction. Philadelphia: Lea & Febiger, 1993; p. 281, with permission of Williams & Wilkins, Baltimore.)

3. Bacterial culture of uterine contents
4. Cytologic examination of uterine contents
5. Endometrial biopsy
6. Ultrasonography

A study was conducted (3) to examine the efficacy of individual diagnostic techniques to predict endometritis. The experimental model involved sixty intact mares that were treated with progesterone for 31 days, and 50 were inoculated with a broth of *Streptococcus zooepidemicus*. Reproductive evaluations were performed the day progesterone treatment began, 13 days after progesterone treatment began, and 2 and 7 days after various therapeutic regimens. Thus, for the 60 experimental mares, there were 240 individual examinations for endometritis. The following criteria were used to assess the degree of endometritis:

1. Ultrasonographic detection of intraluminal fluid accumulation
2. Vaginal speculum examination
3. Cytologic examination of uterine contents
4. Culture of uterine contents
5. Acute and chronic inflammatory changes detected by endometrial biopsy

Each individual parameter was assigned a score from 0 to 3. The total index score of 0 to 18 calculated from summation of each component of reproductive evaluation was used as a standard to determine if the mare had endometritis. To determine the efficacy of each individual diagnostic test, a predictive value for each test (for each score >0) was calculated against a positive diagnosis of endometritis obtained from the total index score (at two different levels of diagnosis).

Results from this experimental model indicated support for two conclusions: (a) bacterial culture was not as accurate in predicting endometritis as other diagnostic tests, *and* (b) ultrasonographic detection of any uterine fluid accumulation was an accurate indicator of endometritis (3).

This study had several limitations: (a) The model of endometritis was progesterone-dependent and may not accurately reflect the naturally occurring condition of endometritis. A progesterone-dependent model may result in increased bacterial proliferation, decreased neutrophil numbers and function, and decreased drainage of uterine contents. (b) Without an independent standard to determine endometritis (i.e., used to compare the individual tests against a positive or negative diagnosis of endometritis), the

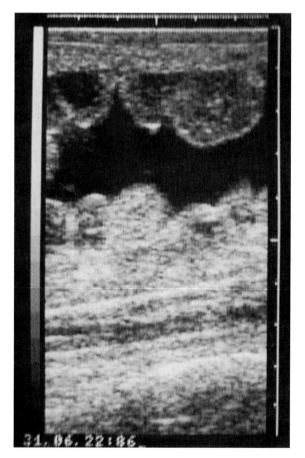

Figure 14.4. Grade 4 intrauterine fluid. The fluid is black or anechoic. (From A.O. McKinnon and J. L. Voss, eds. Equine reproduction. Philadelphia: Lea & Febiger, 1993; p. 281, with permission of Williams & Wilkins, Baltimore.)

predictive value in this study may have more accurately reflected each individual component's influence on the total index score.

Despite these drawbacks, the study demonstrated the usefulness of ultrasound to diagnose endometritis. The application of ultrasonography becomes even more apparent when considering that it is noninvasive. All 10 uninoculated control mares developed endometritis most likely induced in progesterone-treated mares from repeated invasion into the uterus to collect data during the study. It can also be concluded that despite accepted hygienic techniques, invasion of the uterus in progesterone-dominated mares resulted in endometritis. More recently, other authors have made similar associations (17).

BREEDING PROBLEM MARES

Prebreeding Assessment

At the GVEH ultrasonography is fundamental to our problem-mare breeding program (2). The primary goal of the prebreeding assessment period is to have a uterine environment capable of supporting spermatozoa long enough so they can reach the oviduct in a condition capable of initiating fertilization. It only takes a few hours for spermatozoa to pass through the utero-tubule junction and remain relatively free from toxic products in the uterus. However, fluid inflammatory products, when mixed with spermatozoa, cause an immediate decline in spermatozoal motility that is proportional to the amount of inflammatory products (18). Also, the addition of uterine fluid of grades 1–3 (3) to spermatozoa prior to breeding mares by AI resulted in a decreased embryo recovery ($P < .05$) (19). Decline in spermatozoal motility "in vitro" can be arrested by the addition of an extender to the uterine fluid prior to addition of spermatozoa (19). However, it appears that for best fertility, the removal of inflammatory products from the uterus prior to the introduction of spermatozoa is the most logical approach. To meet these objectives, mares are examined in early estrus. Ultrasonographic identification of uterine fluid and culture and sensitivity results are used to determine whether uterine lavage, ecbolic agents (2, 20–22), local antibiotics, or a combination of all of the above are necessary to obtain a uterus free from inflammatory products at the time of breeding. It is an inappropriate use of time and finances to breed mares destined to return to estrus; thus mares with abnormal uterine fluid accumulations detected at the time of breeding may have to be recycled as soon as PGF$_2\alpha$ is capable of causing luteolysis.

Breeding Management

If the uterine environment is prepared properly at the time of breeding, then our goal is to prevent contamination at, or immediately after, breeding. Clearly, breeding contamination is more easily controlled with AI than with natural service. However, both techniques result in introduction of bacteria. Research in this area was originally reported by Kenney et al. in 1975 (23). They demonstrated that hygienically collected semen from "noninfected" stallions contained numerous types of aerobic bacteria and fungi. The total number of aerobic microorganisms in each of eight ejaculations from five stallions collected ranged from 0.09 to 36 million. However, the addition of raw semen to nonfat-dry-milk seminal extenders containing either penicillin-streptomycin (1500 IU/ml and 1500 μg/ml, respectively) or gentamicin sulfate (1 mg/ml) resulted in no growth on any of the subcultures from treated samples, including zero time, which was after about 5 minutes of exposure. There was heavy growth in all subcultures from raw semen (23). Aerobic bacteria commonly isolated from the urethra, semen, and prepuce of stallions are *E. coli* and other coliforms, *Pseudomonas aeruginosa,* beta-hemolytic and nonhemolytic streptococci *(S. zooepidemicus), Klebsiella sp.,* hemolytic and nonhemolytic staphylococci, *Proteus sp.,* and *Corynebacterium.* Further experimentation has demonstrated effective elimination of bacteria without affecting motility using seminal extenders containing either penicillin-gentamicin or polymyxin B sulfate (1000 IU/ml). Thus it appears that the addition of raw semen to appropriate antibiotic-containing seminal extenders is one method of ensuring minimal contamination at the time of breeding (24–29). It is important to remember that some antibiotics affect spermatozoal motility at high concentrations and may adversely affect fertility (30, 31).

Artificial Insemination

If possible, mares are inseminated without disturbing reproductive surgeries such as the Caslick procedure. The perineum is diligently cleaned and dried as previously described (30) and 500 × 10^6 progressively motile spermatozoa (PMS) mixed with the appropriate antibiotic-containing extender are inseminated. Proper technique to ensure cleanliness of the stallion and collection equipment is important (30). To ensure that the antibiotics have had adequate time to eliminate bacterial growth, it is best to allow at least 15 minutes at 37°C prior to insemination. If a longer interval is required, extended semen may be cooled to 20°C and stored for at least 12 hours (32) and often considerably longer at 4°C (30, 33). To reduce contaminating organisms to an absolute minimum, a method was devised (23) to "wash" spermatozoa by dilution with an antibiotic-containing extender, followed by centrifugation (300 G) to produce a "soft" pellet, decantation of the supernatant, and resuspension of the resulting pellet in fresh, warm extender. This technique has the added advantage of removing much of the seminal plasma, which reduces motility after prolonged incubation (30), with minimal damage to spermatozoa (34); however, it is time consuming and may not be necessary.

Natural Service

Regardless of whether AI or natural service is used to breed mares, if a Caslick has to be opened, it should be immediately apposed after breeding. Temporary apposition may be achieved with Michelle clips; however, mares often become irritated by their continual reinsertion. Another technique is placement of breeding stitches that allow the penis or forearm to penetrate the vagina without damaging the labial commissures. Unfortunately, in many instances they are not effective because the vaginal lips are often not joined far enough ventrally to provide a good barrier to pneumovagina. Effective management often involves immediate replacement of stitches into the vulvar lips post service. Mares and stallions to be bred by natural service should be well cleaned. It is wise to avoid strong disinfectants that may cause overgrowth of potentially pathogenic bacteria after prolonged use. A technique of minimizing contamination by prebreeding infusion of 100 to 300 ml of antibiotic-enriched seminal extender has been described (19). This technique has advantages; however, caution should be advised. For maximum reproductive efficiency, 500×10^6 PMS should be deposited into the reproductive tract (30). However, lower spermatozoal numbers are quite effective in highly fertile stallions (30). This information was derived from AI with small volumes of semen or semen plus extender. Recent information has indicated that spermatozoal concentration or volume of inseminate may be important factors in fertility. When mares were bred with 250×10^6 PMS in 100 ml of extender, embryo recovery rate was significantly depressed (13.6%, $P < .001$) compared with mares bred with these same spermatozoal numbers from the same ejaculates in 10 ml of extender (70.6%) (19). This finding becomes important when mares are bred naturally to stallions that, due to frequent breedings, may have low spermatozoal numbers in normal ejaculate volumes (30 to 150 ml). Our approach for mares bred by natural service is to use ultrasonographic detection of quality and quantity of fluid combined with culture and sensitivity results to determine optimum treatments. For instance, if mares have a large volume of fluid detected, then voluminous lavage of the uterus with a physiologic solution such as Dulbecco's phosphate buffered saline that is not expected to be detrimental to spermatozoal survival is instituted immediately prior to breeding. Increased temperature (41 to 45°C) of infused fluids seems to aid in evacuation of uterine contents by increasing uterine tone. This procedure is slightly irritating; however, the aim is to clear the uterus of inflammatory products and enable spermatozoa to have a relatively safe passage into the oviduct before further inflammatory products are released. If small quantities of uterine fluid are detected, then intrauterine antibiotics are infused prebreeding (>12 hours). If uterine fluid is detected at the time of scheduled breeding, depending on the type and volume of fluid, the mare is either recycled, a small volume of antibiotic-containing extender (<50 ml) is infused immediately prebreeding, or oxytocin is administered intravenously and the mare reexamined in 1 to 2 hours (35, 36). When organizing timing of breeding the problem mare, much effort is directed toward trying to breed only once, just prior to ovulation

(<12 hours). Induction of ovulation with human chorionic gonadotropin (hCG) is routine (37), although difficulties may be encountered with precise time of ovulation after the initial injection for the season. This is presumably mediated by antibody formation (38) and becomes important because many mares are bred on subsequent cycles. Mares are treated with hCG on the second and third day of estrus when a follicle >30 and <40 mm is detected and when endometrial folds are prominent (3). Following this strict guideline for induction results in most mares ovulating between 36 to 48 hours after treatment (37). Recent developments have shown that other drugs such as GnRH analogs (39–41) are capable of precise, timed ovulation and are now commercially available for routine induction of ovulation in cycling mares (39, 42). Use of GnRH is expected to be associated with less immunogenicity because of its smaller molecular weight, and could be used as a primary induction agent or between cycles when hCG was administered. Mares are bred regardless of the number of preovulatory follicles and multiple ovulations are actively encouraged. There are few effective, commercially available drugs to increase the number of ovulations per cycle. Follicle stimulating hormone, although effective, is very expensive for equine use, and crude pituitary extracts are not commercially available. Recently, immunization against recombinant bovine inhibin subunit has been demonstrated effective in increasing ovulation rates in mares (43, 44). Conception rates are proportional to ovulation rates (45), thus treatment by immunization against inhibin should improve pregnancy rates in normal and subfertile mares and in mares bred to subfertile stallions. With intensive reproductive management, multiple pregnancies when diagnosed early present little difficulty in reduction (see chapter 10) to a singleton (46, 47).

Postbreeding Management

The aim of therapies in the immediate period after breeding is to (a) reduce infection and inflammation to create a uterine environment capable of supporting pregnancy, and (b) prevent further contamination. Spermatozoa are safely in the oviduct within 4 hours of breeding (46) and are protected from inflammatory products in the uterus and/or uterine treatments by the utero-tubule junction after this time (48). The embryo will not be released into the uterus until around 6 days after ovulation; however, because most intrauterine therapies have an attendant degree of inflammatory response, and to allow time for foreign material to be expelled or absorbed, no treatments are administered after day 4. The cervix begins to exhibit increasing tone and improves as a barrier to infection within 2 days of ovulation, although it remains more relaxed when inflammation of the reproductive tract is present. In addition, the corpus luteum remains resistant to $PGF_2\alpha$ released from local inflammatory responses until at least day 5 after ovulation. Approximately 12 to 24 hours after breeding, the uterine response to breeding and contamination is assessed by ultrasonography.

If fluid is absent, then plasma, intravenous oxytocin, and antibiotics are administered as indicated daily for 2 additional days. If small amounts of fluid are detected, the same treatment is applied after first lavaging the uterus with buffered saline (pH ~ 7.0). Saline is quite an irritant, especially with low pH (49). Usually, only 1 or 2 litres are necessary to remove inflammatory products. When large amounts of fluid are detected, the fluid is recultured and removed by voluminous lavage until returning fluid is free from debris. Oxytocin is added (20 to 40 IU/L) to flushing solutions and given intravenously. Oxytocin increases myometrial contractions in estrogen dominated reproductive tracts (50, 51) and aids in expulsion of material.

EFFECT OF INTRAUTERINE FLUID ON PREGNANCY RATE AND EARLY EMBRYONIC DEATH

A study was designed to determine the influence of intrauterine fluid on pregnancy rate and early embryonic death (3). It was concluded from this study that (a) the presence of small quantities of intrauterine fluid during estrus in cycling mares did not affect pregnancy rates at either day 11 or 50; (b) intrauterine fluid, detected 1 or 2 days after ovulation, did not affect day 11 pregnancy rates, but was associated with a significant increase in EED and reduced day-50 pregnancy rates; and (c) the presence of intrauterine fluid during diestrus was associated with a significant decrease in day-50 pregnancy rates. Another study revealed that the incidence of intrauterine fluid collections during dioestrus (12/43,28%) represented the presence of an inflammatory process as indicated by a high biopsy score, reduced progesterone concentrations, and a shorter interovulatory interval (4). Mares with fluid collections at dioestrus had a lower pregnancy rate at day 11 and a higher embryonic loss rate by day 20 than did mares without collections. The progesterone profile and length of interovulatory interval for mares with uterine inflammation suggested that embryonic loss in this herd was due to uterine-induced luteolysis rather than primary luteal inadequacy (4).

The effects on pregnancy rate of three different treatments to remove intrauterine fluid were assessed in 1267 mares (20). The mares were mated and allocated, in strict rotation, to four treatment groups: (1) untreated controls, (2) intrauterine infusion of broad spectrum antibiotics, (3) intravenous injection of oxytocin, and (4) intravenous injection of oxytocin followed by intrauterine antibiotics. The pregnancy status of the mares was determined 13 to 15 days and 27 to 30 days after ovulation by ultrasonography. The pregnancy rate of group 4 (72%) was higher than that of group 2 (64%, P < .01) or group 3 (63%, P < .01). The pregnancy rates of groups 2 and 3 were higher than that of group 1 (56%, P < .01). The treatment with antibiotics and oxytocin appeared to have an additive beneficial effect that suggested two different modes of action of the combination treatment, namely, antibacterial activity and fluid drainage. In the untreated mares more fluid accumulated in the uter-

ine lumen after mating, and this was the most likely reason for their lower pregnancy rate (20).

At the GVEH the amount and quality of fluid detected is the determinant of how to treat the mare. Large volumes of poor-quality (grade 1 or 2) fluid are treated with voluminous saline lavage, while small volumes of grade 4 fluid quite often are treated with local antibiotics and oxytocin. When fluid is detected after ovulation, then treatments such as intravenous, nonsteroidal, anti-inflammatory agents; intrauterine antibiotics; and systemic oxytocin are directed at reducing the fluid and inflammation.

UTERINE CYSTS

Prior to ultrasonography, uterine cysts were most commonly diagnosed from postmortem examination and occasionally by rectal palpation (52). More recently, they have been diagnosed by hysteroscopy and ultrasonography (3, 53). Cysts in the uterus are fluid-filled and apparently have two origins. The histologic structures of uterine cysts have been described. Endometrial cysts arise from endometrial glands and are usually <10 mm in diameter. Their incidence and significance are largely unknown. The second form of uterine cysts is lymphatic in origin (Fig. 14.5), and these generally are larger than endometrial cysts. They are common in older mares (4) and have been associated with both normal and abnormal uterine biopsies (52). Size of uterine cysts may be indicative of origin. No data have been reported on the growth rate of uterine cysts. Despite the occasional large cysts, it is unlikely that they grow at a rate similar to the early embryonic vesicle (days 10 to 20). When visualized with ultrasonography, cysts are commonly rounded (Figs. 14.6 and 14.7), sometimes with irregular borders, and occasionally are multiple or compartmentalized (lymphatic

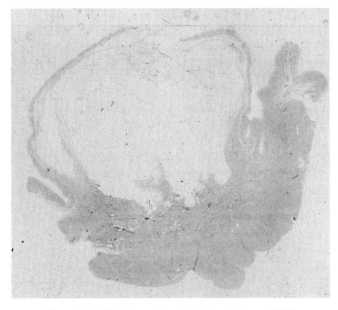

Figure 14.5. Histology of a uterine lymphatic cyst (X5).

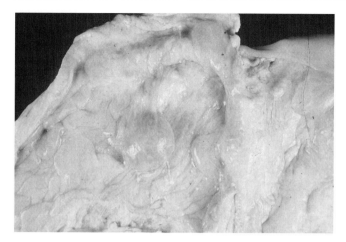

Figure 14.6. A large, single, rounded and pedunculated uterine cyst on the surface of the endometrium. (Courtesy of Dr. V. E. Osbourne.)

lacunae) (Figs. 14.8 and 14.9). Most cysts are luminal; however, occasionally transmural (Fig. 14.10) and subserosal cysts (Fig. 14.11) are detected. Movement of the early equine conceptus (days 10 to 16), the presence of specular reflection, a spherical appearance, and the growth rate of the embryo should aid in its differentiation from uterine cysts. The relationship between infertility and uterine cysts is axiomatic. Cysts may impede movement of the early conceptus, restricting the reported ability of the vesicle to prevent luteolysis after day 10 (54). Later in pregnancy, contact between the cyst wall and yolk sac or allantois may prevent absorption of nutrients (Fig. 14.12). This may be more important when considering the recognition that large uterine cysts are more commonly located at the junction of the uter-

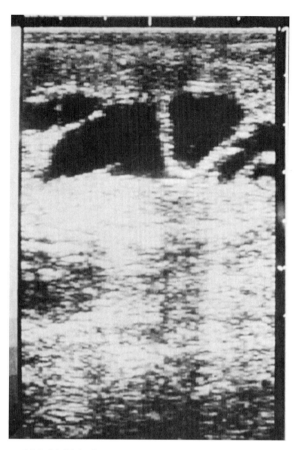

Figure 14.8. Multiple, large, compartmentalized uterine cysts sometimes are termed lymphatic lacunae. (From A.O. McKinnon and J. L. Voss, eds. Equine reproduction. Philadelphia: Lea & Febiger, 1993; p. 282, with permission of Williams & Wilkins, Baltimore.)

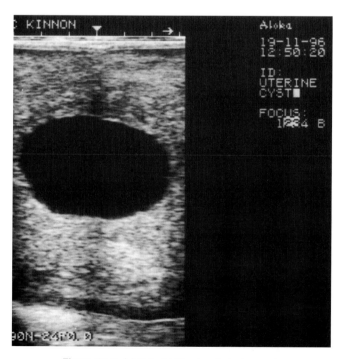

Figure 14.7. A large, single, round uterine cyst.

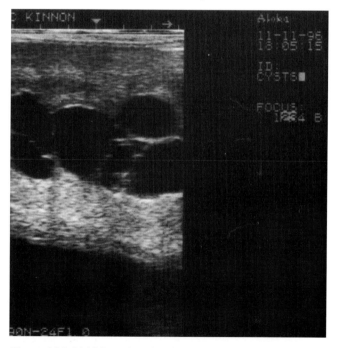

Figure 14.9. Multiple pedunculated cysts together at the corpus cornual junction.

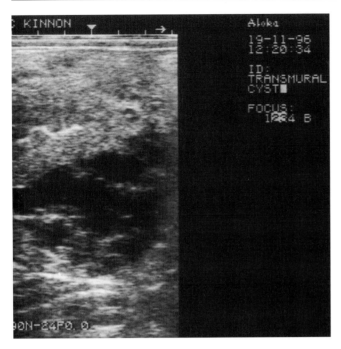

Figure 14.10. A large transmural cyst. Uterine tissue can be seen around the cyst and a white line denoting the uterine lumen above.

ine horn and body (55), which is the most common site of vesicle fixation (56). Finally, cysts are commonly indicative of uterine disease. They may reflect senility or be associated with endometritis. It has been reported (4) that there is an association between number of uterine cysts, age of the mare, and endometrial biopsy. The number of treatments proposed for uterine cysts probably reflects the inability of any individual treatment to consistently be useful. Rupture

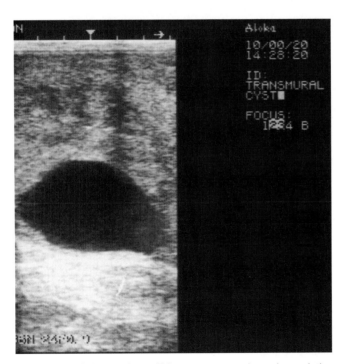

Figure 14.11. Subserosal cyst. This cyst appears to be underneath the serosa.

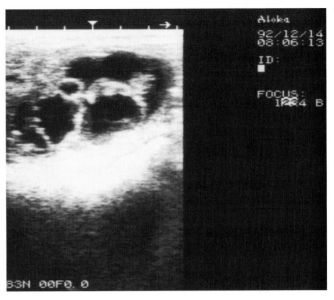

Figure 14.12. An approximate 30-day fetus with multiple surrounding cysts. It is possible that nourishment of the fetus may be affected when the number of cysts present is high.

of the fluid-filled structures has been attempted via uterine-biopsy forceps (52), surgery, fine needle aspiration, and puncture via hysteroscopy. Electrocoagulative removal of cysts has also been described. Endometrial curettage and repeated lavage with warm saline (40 to 45°C) have also been advocated (52). Although there are no reports on respective efficiency of these treatments, endometrial curettage and saline lavage are frequently applied to treat the primary problem, which would appear to be lymphatic blockage. The following were concluded from one study (3):

1. Uterine cysts, when detected by ultrasonography, were lymphatic in origin.
2. Uterine cysts did not change rapidly in size or shape, although they were more difficult to detect during estrus.
3. Treatment with infrared radiation was not effective.
4. There was no consistent location for uterine cysts.
5. Uterine cysts were commonly associated with chronic, infiltrative, lymphocytic endometritis.

Another study on 259 normal fertile Thoroughbred mares (55) revealed the incidence of uterine cysts was 22.4%. Of the 95 cysts observed during the trial, 87.4% were located in the middle and posterior segments of both uterine horns. The size of all cysts ranged between 3 and 48 mm. When all mares were assigned to three age groups, <7 years (n = 116), 7–14 years (n = 117), and >14 years (n = 26), a significant ($P < .01$) increase in the number of cysts was observed with advancing age (4.3%, 29.1%, and 73.1%, respectively). The pregnancy rates at days 14 and 40 were significantly ($P < .01$) lower in mares with cysts (77.6% and 71.4%) compared with mares without cysts (91.5% and 88.0%). This suggested to the authors that the presence of uterine cysts plays an important role in the reduction of fertility of Thoroughbred mares (55).

slightly cranial to the cervix, although it can be present in the cranial body or uterine horns. When air is present <24 hours after artificial insemination (Fig. 14.16), we consider it normal. However, we do not expect it to be detected in normal mares >24 hours after breeding. The observation of air in the uterus of mares that have not been bred recently is an indication of pneumo-uterus (Fig. 14.17) and reflects failure of the competency of the vaginal labia, vestibulovaginal sphincter, and/or cervix (3). In our experience it has been of use in determining when some mares may need to be caslicked, particularly so when a clinical examination did not suggest the procedure. Occasionally, air may be detected in a pregnant mare (Fig. 14.18). In these cases the prognosis for pregnancy maintenance is poor.

FOREIGN BODIES

On occasion, strongly echogenic areas in the uterine lumen are observed with a concomitant echo shadow, such as is seen with dense tissue like fetal bone. This might be expected after mummification. We have also identified a similar ultrasonographic image that was confirmed subsequently as the tip of a uterine culturette (Fig. 14.19). Another substance that creates a strong echo shadow is the

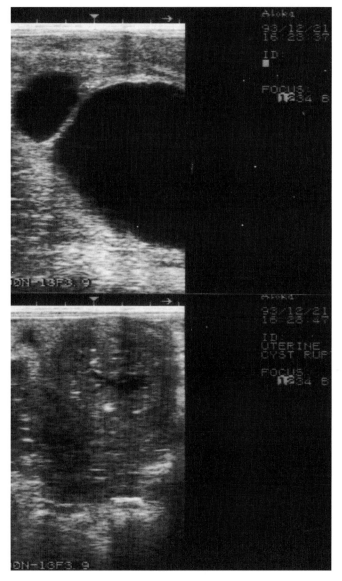

Figure 14.13. A large uterine cyst **A**, that was manually ablated **B**.

At the GVEH we recognize cysts more commonly in older mares. Cysts are also more commonly recognized in the immediate postpartum period and at the corpus-cornual junction. Uterine cysts are more commonly pedunculated and luminal; however, transmural and nonpedunculated cysts are seen. Our treatment for uterine cysts has varied over the years; however, for the last 8 years whenever we have believed treatment to be necessary, we have dilated the mare's cervix while in heat and ablated the cyst(s) manually (Fig. 14.13). Nonpedunculated cysts may be more difficult to destroy this way; however, they seldom appear to cause many problems.

INTRAUTERINE AIR

Air is recognized as multiple, hyperechogenic reflections (Fig. 14.14) (occasionally, a ventral reverberation artifact is present [Fig. 14.15]), and it appears to be more prevalent

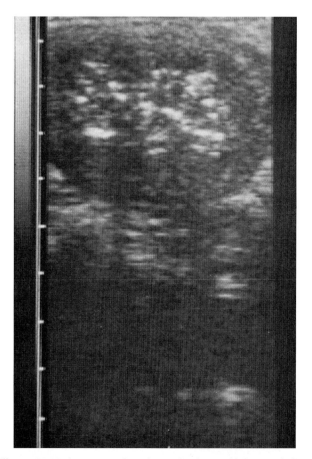

Figure 14.14. A cross-section of a uterine horn with hyperechoic reflections representing intraluminal air. (From A.O. McKinnon and J. L. Voss, eds. Equine reproduction. Philadelphia: Lea & Febiger, 1993; p. 284, with permission of Williams & Wilkins, Baltimore.)

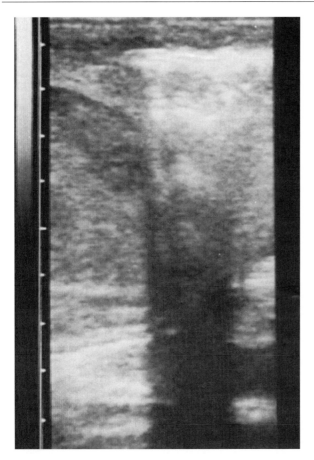

Figure 14.15. Caudal uterine body with a large reverberation artifact characteristic of air. (From A.O. McKinnon and J. L. Voss, eds. Equine reproduction. Philadelphia: Lea & Febiger, 1993; p. 283, with permission of Williams & Wilkins, Baltimore.)

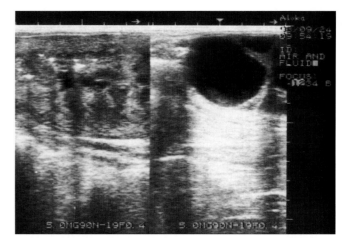

Figure 14.16. Split-frame view. On the left is air and fluid, and on the right is a preovulatory follicle. Small amount of air and fluid such as this immediately after artificial insemination would be normal.

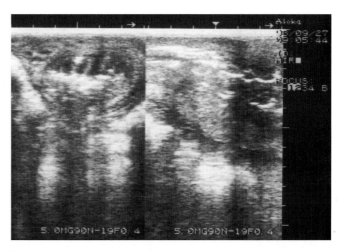

Figure 14.17. Split-frame view. On the left is an excessive amount of air in the uterine horn, and on the right is a longitudinal view demonstrating air in the uterine body.

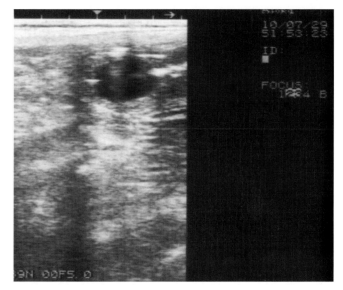

Figure 14.18. A 14-day pregnancy with air surrounding it. The prognosis for these pregnancies is poor.

presence of chronically retained fetal membrane (Fig. 14.20). These cases are usually first recognized at the first postpartum examination (see later); however, they may not be apparent until the echogenicity increases. In addition, we have seen a few interesting cases such as calcification on the uterine epithelial surface (Fig. 14.21), suture material after a cesarean section (Fig. 14.22), and post-treatment debris after multiple antibiotic suspension treatments into the uterus of a mare that had poor uterine clearance abilities (Fig. 14.23). In a normal pregnancy the endometrial cups are not detected; however, on occasion after EED and expulsion of fetal fluids they become visible (Fig. 14.24).

UTERINE ADHESIONS

Occasionally, after severe trauma to the reproductive tract or even after irritation from endometritis, uterine adhesions will form (Fig. 14.25). Because of continuing secretions from the oviduct or endometritis in the horn proximal to the adhesions, fluid will accumulate in the tip of the affected horn (Fig. 14.26). This fluid is well localized and should make the examiner suspicious of a complete adhesion. Diagnosis can be confirmed manually after first gently dilating the cervix, or, if that is not possible, infusions of fluid (i.e.,

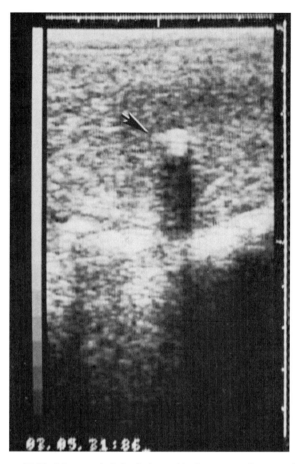

Figure 14.19. A hyperechoic body *(arrow)* in the uterus of a mare that later was demonstrated to be a tip from a uterine culturette.

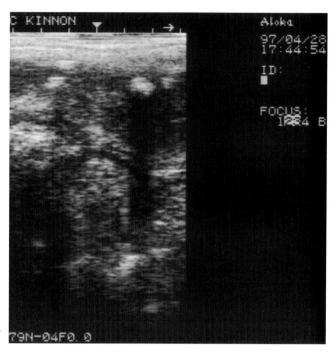

Figure 14.21. Hyperechoic spots in the caudal uterine body from fibrosis and calcification possibly secondary to trauma.

respond better to either an oil-based corticosteroid cream or rest from treatment for at least 3 weeks.

Undoubtedly, there are many other forms of less commonly recognized uterine pathology such as uterine neoplasia, abscesses, and hematomas that will be recognized as ultrasonography of the uterus becomes more routine.

1 L of saline) into the uterus should be visible immediately. When adhesions exist, it is not possible to dilate the tip of the affected horn because the fluid has restricted or denied entry. Adhesions may respond to manual breakdown and multiple infusions of an antibiotic extender; however, some appear to get worse with the irritation of treatment and may

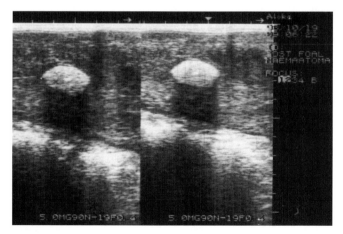

Figure 14.20. Hyperechoic mass resulting from a small piece of chronically retained fetal membrane that had become imbedded in the uterine wall.

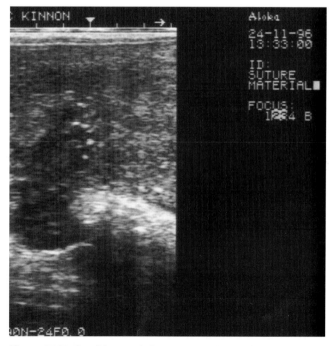

Figure 14.22. Small hyperechoic spots associated with suture material in a mare after cesarean section.

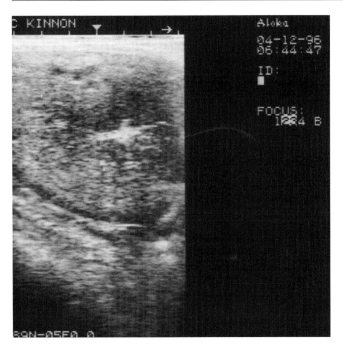

Figure 14.23. Intraluminal debris from repeated intrauterine infusions of an antibiotic suspension into a mare with poor uterine clearance.

PERIPARTURIENT MATERNAL DISORDERS

A variety of injuries and disorders develop around the time of foaling and in the immediate postpartum period that can have serious consequences for the mare. The age and breed of the dam have some influence on the incidence of these complications, but many are purely accidents associated with the rapid and often violent birth process. Frequently, diagnosis is difficult because the clinical signs of many post-partum problems are nonspecific. Early recognition of peripartum disorders may improve the success rate of treatment.

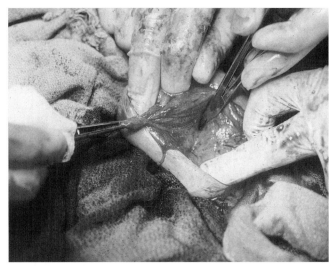

Figure 14.25. The tip of this uterine horn has an adhesion that will not let fluid escape. Manual breakdown was attempted through an incision.

If not quickly recognized and treated, some of these conditions will be life threatening, some will seriously compromise the future reproductive career of the mare, and some will cause considerable delay in the establishment of a healthy pregnancy. Ultrasonography has become an indispensable tool for the diagnosis and in some cases the monitoring of these conditions.

PREPARTURIENT PROBLEMS

Mummification and Maceration

Mummification is not uncommon when one twin dies and the other continues to develop. Mummification of a single

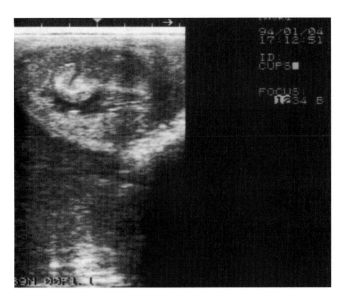

Figure 14.24. After EED occasionally endometrial cups may become obvious.

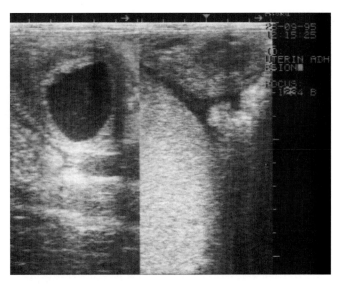

Figure 14.26. Ultrasonographically, a uterine adhesion may be suspected when fluid accumulates at the tip of one horn and is repeatable on different occasions. In this image the affected horn is on the left of the slip screen, and the other horn is on the right.

pregnancy is rare and has been reported (57). Occasionally, lactation in a late-pregnant mare may suggest mummification; commonly, however, no clinical signs are recognized. Mummified fetuses are most commonly seen at birth or abortion. Maceration most commonly occurs when a single pregnancy dies and is not aborted. External signs of discharge may lead to the diagnosis. Treatment for both is gentle relaxation of the cervix and then delivery. We have seen three mummified fetuses with transabdominal ultrasonography. In all cases the mares were late in gestation and had started to lactate. The diagnosis of mummification was not easy as all had an additional viable pregnancy present. In our limited experience it appears that identification of the fetal head or ribs as a separate entity from the live fetus are the easiest and most consistent fetal parts to find. As the mummification process proceeds, it is harder to see fetal parts because they all assume a similar echogenicity. Only one case had a demonstrable "twin membrane," which probably was related to the more recent demise of that fetus.

Hydrops

Ultrasonography is useful for diagnosis of excessive accumulation of fluid in the uterus of a pregnant mare. Hydroallantois is a rare condition that occurs during the last trimester of pregnancy in primarily pluriparous mares after an otherwise uneventful gestation. Clinical signs include an enormous increase in abdominal size over 10 to 14 days due to a rapid accumulation of allantoic fluid. Other clinical signs result from the pressure exerted by the excess amount of fluid. Mares may have anorexia, tachycardia, tachypnea, dyspnea, ventral edema, colic, and difficulty in defecating and walking. Horses with advanced cases may show evidence of ventral abdominal hernia or prepubic tendon rupture.

Evaluation of the genital tract per rectum reveals a huge, fluid filled uterus, and it may be difficult to palpate the fetus. Prognosis for obtaining a live foal is poor, and management of the case should be directed at saving the mare's life (58). Parturition should be induced to relieve the pressure on the mare's internal organs. Removal of the allantoic fluid slowly by rupture of the allantochorion should be attempted, as should siphoning of the fluid while supporting the mare with intravenous fluids and corticosteroids to prevent shock. Rather than fluid loss causing shock, we believe that the fluid loss removes the pressure on the abdominal vessels, and pooling and hypovolemic shock may follow when it occurs to quickly. Oxytocin may be administered to aid in evacuation of the uterine contents, although in mares with uterine inertia the uterus may not respond to treatment.

Hydrops amnii is an excessive accumulation of amniotic fluid in the amniotic cavity and it has a low incidence in all species. Hydrops amnii in the mare is reported less frequently than hydroallantois (59). The normal volume of amniotic fluid in the mare near term is between 3 to 7 L. Hydrops amnii tends to develop gradually over several weeks or months during the latter half of gestation. The normal amniotic cavity has a direct communication with the digestive system by way of the mouth and anus. The fetus swallows fluid and may keep levels constant as fetal monsters with gut abnormalities often have excessive fluid (8 to 10 times normal) in the amniotic cavity (hydrops amnii). Amniotic fluid is composed of saliva and secretions of the nasopharynx of the fetus. Although the swallowing fetus may play a role in the maintenance of fetal fluid balance, other mechanisms may be important. In cases of hydrops amnii, prognosis for the pregnancy is poor, because abortion and premature delivery are quite common. Fortunately, the prognosis for future fertility is fair to good, because the dam's genital tract usually is normal after termination of the pregnancy.

Prepubic and Abdominal Wall Rupture

A breakdown in the body wall of pregnant mares is common in older draft mares (58), but it also has been reported in other breeds. Conditions causing severe distention of the body wall, such as hydrops, twins, severe ventral edema, or trauma, may result in rupture of the prepubic tendon or an abdominal hernia; however, many cases occur with no apparent reason. Mares usually present very close to foaling with severe, ventral edema running cranially from the udder and in many cases involving the udder itself. Unilateral edema may suggest partial rupture of the prepubic tendon or damage to the ventrolateral body wall. Affected mares have difficulty rising and are reluctant to move. Acute progression of either condition may result in severe distress, colic, tachypnea, tachycardia, sweating, internal hemorrhage, shock, and death.

Although the causes of these conditions are similar, the clinical appearance may help differentiate them. A mare with prepubic tendon rupture will have an elevated tail head and tuber ischii, due to the lack of ventral support of the pelvis, that results in lordosis and a sawhorse stance. The mammary gland will be shifted cranially from its normal position. Although a mare with an abdominal hernia or rupture may have an enlarged abdomen, her tail head and tuber ischii will be in a normal position.

A diagnosis of prepubic tendon rupture or ventral body wall hernia may be difficult to confirm. In heavily pregnant mares, the presence of the fetus often makes palpation of the defect per rectum very difficult and palpation transabdominally is usually impossible because of the amount of edema in the area. In our experience ultrasonography can be useful in identifying body-wall defects and herniation of intestine, but the extent of the damage may not be clearly defined until after parturition when most of the edema is resolved. On occasion, a diagnostic differential is severe edema in the prepartum mare. In cases of rupture the secretions in the mammary gland will commonly be blood stained (Fig. 14.27), while prepartum edema will not have any. This has important diagnostic significance as exercise is useful in the former condition.

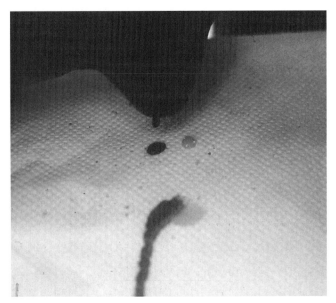

Figure 14.27. Udder secretions from a mare with a prepubic tendon rupture. The cranial quarter is blood stained, and the caudal quarter has normal colostrum.

Uterine Torsion

Uterine torsion in the mare occurs late in gestation (>8 months), more frequently in draft breeds than light horses, and is not usually associated with parturition, unlike in the cow. A low incidence of uterine torsion in mares is attributed to the sublumbar attachment of the ovaries and the dorsal insertion of the broad ligaments in the uterus. The causes of uterine torsion in the mare are not well defined, but include factors such as vigorous fetal movements, sud-

den falls, relative fetal oversize, diminished volume of fetal fluids, lack of tone in the pregnant uterus, long mesometrium, and the presence of a large, deep abdomen. Clinical signs are related to the severity of the torsion and include signs of abdominal pain such as restlessness, sweating, anorexia, frequent urination, sawhorse stance, looking at the flank, and kicking the abdomen. Signs may present for a variable duration (from few hours to 3 days or more), and they can mimic those of the early stages of parturition.

The uterus may twist 90 to 540° on its long axis (60) (Fig. 14.28). In the mare the twist typically involves the uterine body, not the cervix or the vagina, as occurs in the cow. If the torsion is less than 180° and blood flow to the uterus is not compromised, correction may not be required. Clinical signs may be more severe if the intestines are involved in the torsion. The mare may show signs of shock if uterine rupture has occurred. Diagnosis is made by clinical signs and palpation by rectum of the gravid uterus; vaginal examination is only occasionally diagnostically useful. Palpation per rectum reveals tense broad ligaments, spiraling in the direction of the torsion. If the torsion is counterclockwise, the left broad ligament will be taut and be felt to traverse under the uterus, while the right broad ligament will stretch dorsally over the distended uterus. The small colon undergoes a variable amount of constriction, due to the compressive forces of the displaced broad ligaments, and may impede the ability of the palpator to perform a complete rectal examination. In such cases it is difficult to evaluate fetal viability or uterine integrity, and it may even be impossible to determine which direction the uterus is rotated. Ultrasonography has not been useful for diagnosis of uterine torsion in our clinic; however, it has been useful for determining if the fetus is still alive. In cases where the fetus

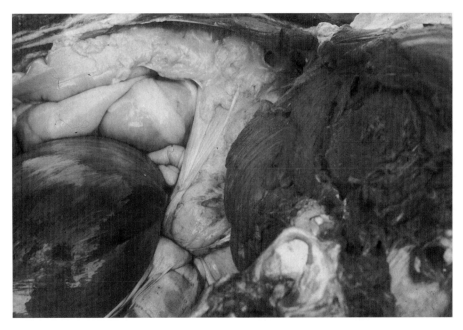

Figure 14.28. A 360° torsion of the uterus confirmed at postmortem. The mare was euthanized because ultrasonography demonstrated that the fetus had died prior to admission.

has already died, management is different and frequently more aggressive.

The prognosis for cases of equine uterine torsion depends on the degree of the circulatory disturbance resulting from involvement of the broad ligaments and uterine vessels. When the fetus is alive, the uterine wall not severely congested and edematous, and the treatment prompt, the prognosis for maternal survival and the birth of a normal, live foal at term is good.

Uterine Rupture (Preparturient)

Uterine rupture usually occurs in the peripartum period as a result of manual intervention or fetotomy or possibly because of violent intrapartum movement. However, in cases of uterine torsion or hydrops, the uterus can rupture before term. When the uterus ruptures before term, the mare may not show much pain, and, if the fetus escapes into the abdomen and hemorrhage is not severe, uterine involution may occur without external signs.

Diagnosis of uterine rupture may be facilitated by palpation of the uterus per rectum, by fetal examination, abdominal centesis, and a history of moderate to severe abdominal pain during the last trimester of pregnancy. Once the uterus has ruptured and its contents have escaped, the uterine wall may feel thickened and corrugated, because the uterus contracts and begins to involute quite quickly. The site of rupture may be equally difficult to demonstrate by transrectal ultrasonography. However, transabdominal ultrasonography may reveal the presence of the dead fetus on the abdominal floor with excessive free abdominal fluid.

Placental Preview/Placentitis

Detachment of a significant portion of the allantochorion from the endometrium constitutes an emergency for the foal owing to failure of adequate exchange of oxygen, carbon dioxide, and nutrients. Premature placental separation may

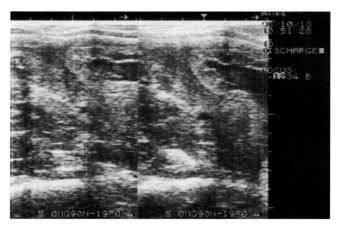

Figure 14.29. Split-screen ultrasonographic image of a mare with ascending placentitis. Note on both images the presence of a thickened caudal placenta and hyperechoic fluid outside the placenta but inside the uterus. The mare had an external discharge.

occur in two forms in pregnant mares: acutely at parturition and more chronically during gestation, usually associated with placentitis. Chronic placentitis may be recognized by transabdominal ultrasonography; however, rectal ultrasonography is necessary to examine the cervix region in cases of ascending placentitis (Fig. 14.29). Chronic ascending placentitis or edema may result in separation and thickening of the placenta over the cervical region.

Prolonged Gestation

Gestation usually lasts for 310 to 374 days, but normal pregnancies can be as long as 399 days (61). Foals born from such pregnancies are not usually oversized and do not predispose the mare to dystocia (61). Little is known of this syndrome, but prolonged gestation has been attributed to delayed embryonic development, especially during the first 2 months of gestation (61). The duration of gestation is partly controlled by nutrition and the genotype of the foal, but mares themselves may also control the duration of gestation (58). Based on the finding that average gestational durations were longer for mares bred earlier in the season, Ginther suggested that mares may be able to make limited adjustments, so that their foals are born with an optimal chance for survival (62). The physiologic control of this phenomenon is unknown, but it may be related to photoperiod.

Owners and farm managers are often concerned about pregnancies extending beyond the expected parturition date and begin to exert pressure on the veterinarian to induce foaling. If no mammary development has occurred and fetal well-being has been assessed by ultrasonography, this practice should be discouraged even if the duration of gestation is longer than 1 year. Patience and waiting for parturition to be initiated without intervention are indicated in most cases of prolonged gestation; however, fescue toxicosis also causes prolonged gestation and very large foals and requires specific intervention (63). Tall fescue grass, parasitized by the endophytic fungus *Acremonium coenophialum,* when ingested by pregnant mares can have serious deleterious effects on the latter stages of equine pregnancy. Fescue toxicosis causes not only prolonged gestation, but also dystocia and hypogalactia. In affected foals, toxicosis causes dysmaturity and poor chances of survival (63).

Placentas from affected mares are thick and edematous, and placental edema and premature separation of the chorioallantois have both been observed on ultrasound.

POSTPARTURIENT PROBLEMS

Perivaginal Hematomas

Intrapelvic perivaginal bleeding that results in perivaginal hematoma formation should not be difficult to diagnose with ultrasonography. Large hematomas can be drained 2 to 3 days postpartum, after clot formation has occurred. If hematomas do not regress or do not become progressively firm, abcessation should be suspected.

Abcessation

Abcessation can be confirmed by ultrasound and by needle biopsy. The abscess should be incised and drained. Occasionally, large intrapelvic hematomas may leave permanent lumps of scar tissue that are palpable ventrally in the pelvic canal and, unless marked vaginal stenosis occurs, the ability to deliver a fetus per vagina is not compromised.

Periparturient Hemorrhage

Hemorrhage from the middle uterine, utero-ovarian, or, less frequently, external iliac arteries is a significant cause of peripartum colic syndrome and death, usually in older, multiparous brood mares. Hemorrhage from these vessels is often fatal, especially if the hemorrhage is into the abdominal cavity. The incidence of periparturient hemorrhage increases with age. Although it may occur before, during, or after parturition, it is most common during or within the first 24 hours postpartum. Dystocia does not seem to influence the incidence of the disease, and it is often seen in mares after an apparently problem-free delivery. Fatal hemorrhage has also been reported after periparturient accidents such as uterine torsion or uterine prolapse. The clinical signs associated with periparturient hemorrhage depend on the site and severity of the hemorrhage and whether the bleeding is contained within the broad ligaments or freed into the abdomen. Mares that bleed into the broad ligaments will exhibit variable signs of abdominal discomfort as a result of tension on the ligament and uterine serosa. Sometimes the signs may be overlooked because observers expect mares to show some abdominal discomfort immediately postpartum, which is usually associated with uterine contractions. As blood loss and broad-ligament distention increase, signs of abdominal pain, sweating, weakness, tachycardia, tachypnea, ataxia, and pale mucous membranes become more apparent. Continued blood loss may lead to rapid onset of hemorrhagic shock with prostration, cold extremities, extreme paleness of membranes, and death. The course of clin-

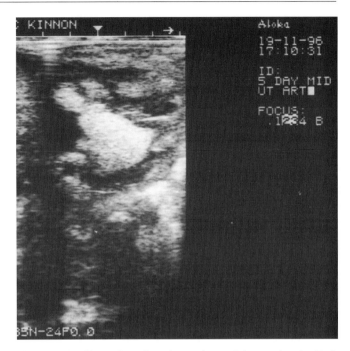

Figure 14.31. Hemorrhage into the uterine wall detected at day 5 after parturition. There was a baseball-sized hematoma in the dorsal uterine wall.

ical signs may be extremely rapid in cases in which complete rupture occurs and hemorrhage is directly into the abdomen. Death often ensues within minutes to hours after the appearance of the first signs of discomfort. In other cases mares may have exhibited mild signs initially (associated with containment of hemorrhage within the broad ligament), only to collapse later. Mares suffering from uterine hemorrhage are sometimes just found dead. In addition to the above, sometimes hemorrhages contained within the

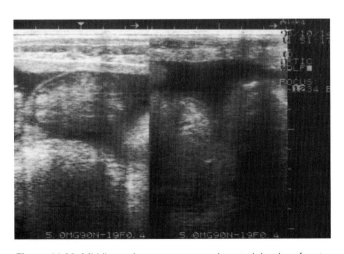

Figure 14.30. Middle uterine artery rupture detected the day of parturition. Large clots are present together with free hemorrhage.

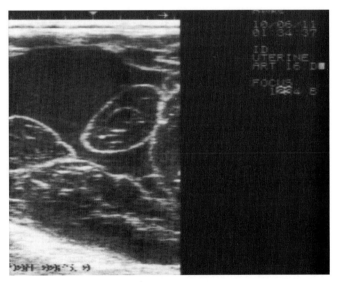

Figure 14.32. Middle uterine artery rupture in a mare visualized 16 days after parturition. The mare had been distressed in the immediate postpartum period, and ultrasonography was used to diagnose and monitor the condition.

broad ligament may go undetected unless a prebreeding examination of the reproductive tract is performed. Right uterine or utero-ovarian artery rupture apparently occurs more commonly than left. Mares that show persistent signs of abdominal pain or blood loss soon after parturition, should be evaluated by rectal palpation of the uterus and broad ligaments. Both linear and sector scanning ultrasonography are useful in the diagnosis and management of cases of abdominal, mesometrial, and mural hemorrhage in the mare (Figs. 14.30 through 14.32).

Retained Placental Membranes/ Metritis-Endotoxemia-Laminitis Syndrome

The fetal membranes are usually expelled 30 minutes to 3 hours after parturition. Horses in a natural environment may retain fetal membranes in the uterus for up to 24 to 48 hours without complications. These mares may produce a foal the same time the following year without treatment, which suggests that treatment is not always necessary. In an intensive management environment, mares may experience complications (endometritis, metritis, laminitis, and even death) that are related to retention of the fetal membranes for 8 hours or less. The percentage of postparturient mares with retained fetal membranes is believed to range from 2 to 10% (64, 65). The probability of retained placenta increases after dystocia, probably as result of trauma to the uterus or myometrial exhaustion. Disturbance of the normal uterine contractions at parturition also might make retained placenta more likely. Retention is particularly likely if severe placentitis was present. Placental retention is more common in the nongravid uterine horn, perhaps because of a progressive increase in the degree of placental folding and attachment from the gravid to the nongravid horn. Partial placental retention is also more likely to occur in the nongravid uterine horn (66) because the chorioallantoic membrane is thinner, resulting in easier tearing.

A variable portion of the placenta may be exposed through the vulvar opening. Occasionally, the veterinarian is alerted to the possibility of retained fetal membranes, when no placenta is found after foaling. Aseptic intrauterine examination may reveal the presence of the placenta in the uterine cavity. Alternatively, part of the placenta may remain in the uterus and continue to initiate mild straining or colic after most of the placenta has been removed. Not uncommonly, fetal membranes may be found days later when the mare has signs of discharge. Sequel of retained placenta vary from none to the development of toxic metritis, septicemia or endotoxemia, laminitis, and death (67). On occasion, fetal membranes may be detected with ultrasonography, days or even weeks after foaling (Fig. 14.33). In addition, ultrasound examination will provide information regarding uterine involution and the presence of fluid within the uterine lumen.

Retained placenta and serious sequel are reportedly more common in draft horses than in Thoroughbreds or Standardbreds, and mares with retained placenta after dystocia

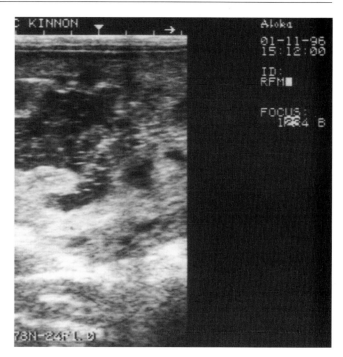

Figure 14.33. Fluid and fetal membranes in a mare presented for breeding at 25 days after foaling.

are at greater risk of developing toxic metritis and laminitis (67). Severe toxic metritis and laminitis after dystocia are believed to result from damage to the uterine lining that subsequently promotes absorption of endotoxins associated with the common bacterial proliferation in the postpartum mare. In patients with toxic metritis after dystocia and retained placenta, the uterine wall becomes thin and friable or

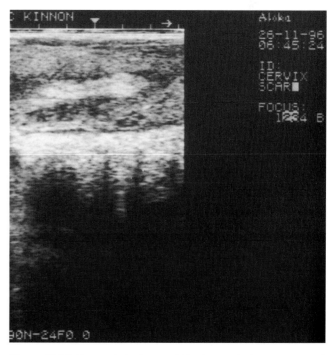

Figure 14.34. Hyperechoic tissue within the cervix that represented damage and scarring after foaling.

even necrotic. Absorption of bacteria and bacterial toxins probably follows disruption of the endometrium and precipitates the peripheral vascular changes that lead to laminitis (67).

EVALUATION OF THE CAUDAL REPRODUCTIVE TRACT

Ultrasonography has not been particularly useful for diagnosis of cervical conditions; however, on a few occasions we have identified pathology such as cysts or scarring of the cervix (Fig. 14.34). In general, manual or speculum examination are more useful. Once the reproductive tract is fully involuted and the mare is in diestrus (when the cervix should be completely closed), the cervix can be evaluated to determine whether it is capable of closing (68). Many cervical tears early in the postpartum period do not prevent the cervix from closing sufficiently once involution is complete, particularly when the tear is located in the caudal portion of the cervix. It the cervix remains open during diestrus after uterine involution is complete, surgical repair can be performed to ensure that the cervix will be capable of closing

and maintaining a pregnancy following repair. Involution is also necessary to allow identification of the muscular and mucosal layers that must be debrided and sutured. We commonly find unidentified cervical tears when referred cases of problem mares. In addition, it is surprising how many mares with cervical defects will become pregnant.

Occasionally, ultrasonography can be useful in diagnosing cases of vaginal hematomas and abscesses. Careful evaluation may even reveal urine or other fluid in the vagina/vestibule in mares with reproductive problems (Fig. 14.35). Recently there has been some interest in stage of cycle examinations being augmented by transrectal ultrasonography of the cervix. Size and echotexture were useful in evaluating hormonal changes to the organ (69).

ACKNOWLEDGMENT

Portions of this chapter were compiled from notes originally prepared by Dr. Stephania Bucca.

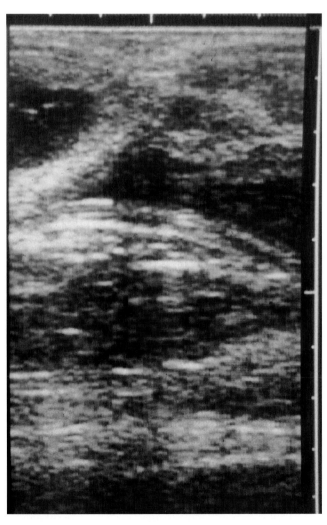

Figure 14.35. Ultrasonography was useful to visualize urine in the cranial vagina of this mare with vesicovaginal reflux.

REFERENCES

1. McKinnon AO, Squires EL, Harrison LA, Blach EL, Shideler RK. Ultrasonographic studies on the reproductive tract of mares after parturition: effect of involution and uterine fluid on pregnancy rates in mares with normal and delayed first postpartum ovulatory cycles. J Am Vet Med Assoc 1988;192:350–353.
2. McKinnon AO, Voss JL. Breeding the problem mare. In: McKinnon AO, Voss JL, eds. Equine reproduction. 1st ed. Philadelphia and London: Lea & Febiger, 1993:368–378.
3. McKinnon AO, Squires EL, Carnevale EM, Harrison LA, Frantz DD, McChesney AE, Shideler RK. Diagnostic ultrasonography of uterine pathology in the mare. Proc AAEP 1987:605–622.
4. Adams GP, Kastelic JP, Bergfelt DR, Ginther OJ. Effect of uterine inflammation and ultrasonically detected uterine pathology on fertility in the mare. J Reprod Fertil Suppl 1987;35:445–454.
5. Merkt H, Gunzel AR. A survey of early pregnancy losses in West German thoroughbred mares. Equine Vet J 1979;11:256–258.
6. Lieux P. Comparative results of breeding on first and second post-foaling heat periods. Proc AAEP 1980;129–132.
7. Platt H. Aetiological aspects of abortion in the Thoroughbred mare. J Comp Pathol 1973;83:199–205.
8. Loy RG, Evans MJ, Pemstein R, Taylor TB. Effects of injected ovarian steroids on reproductive patterns and performance in postpartum mares. J Reprod Fertil Suppl 1982;32:199–204.
9. Pope AM, Campbell DL, Davidson JP. Endometrial histology and postpartum mares treated with progesterone and synthetic GnRH (AY-24,031). J Reprod Fertil Suppl 1979;27:587–591.
10. Sexton PE, Bristol FM. Uterine involution in mares treated with progesterone and estradiol-17beta. J Am Vet Med Assoc 1985;186:252–256.
11. Squires EL, Heesemann CP, Webel SK, Shideler RK, Voss JL. Relationship of altrenogest to ovarian activity, hormone concentrations and fertility of mares. J Anim Sci 1983;56:901–910.
12. Evans MJ, Hamer JM, Gason LM, Graham CS, Asbury AC, Irvine CHG. Clearance of bacteria and non-antigenic markers following intra-uterine inoculation into maiden mares: effect of steroid hormone environment. Theriogenology 1986;26:37–50.
13. Winter AJ. Microbial immunity in the reproductive tract. J Am Vet Med Assoc 1982;181:1069–1073.
14. Glatzel PS, Belz JP. Fertility in mares after disturbed or undis-

turbed puerperal periods—significance of clinical, microbiological and hormonal examinations. Berl Munch Tierarztl Wochenschr 1995;108:367–372.

15. McCue PM, Hughes JP. The effect of postpartum uterine lavage on foal heat pregnancy rate. Theriogenology 1990;33:1121–1130.

16. Blanchard TL, Varner DD, Brinsko SP, Meyers SA, Johnson L. Effects of postparturient uterine lavage on uterine involution in the mare. Theriogenology 1989;32:527–536.

17. Hinrichs K, Spensley MS, McDonough PL. Evaluation of progesterone treatment to create a model for equine endometritis. Equine Vet J 1992;24:457–461.

18. Nishikawa Y, ed. Studies on reproduction in horses: singularity and artificial control in reproductive phenomena. Tokyo: Japan Racing Association, 1959; 1.

19. Squires EL, Barnes C, Rowley HS, McKinnon AO, Pickett BW, Shideler RK. Effect of uterine fluid and volume of extender on fertility. Proc AAEP 1989;35:25–30.

20. Pycock JF, Newcombe JR. Assessment of the effect of 3 treatments to remove intrauterine fluid on pregnancy rate in the mare. Vet Rec 1996;138:320–323.

21. Leblanc M, Neuwirth L, Mauragis D, Klapstein E, Tran T. Oxytocin enhances clearance of radiocolloid from the uterine lumen of reproductively normal mares and mares susceptible to endometritis. Equine Vet J 1994;26:279–282.

22. Pycock JF. Assessment of oxytocin and intrauterine antibiotics on intrauterine fluid and pregnancy rates in the mare. Proc AAEP 1994;40:19–20.

23. Kenney RM, Bergman RV, Cooper WL, Morse GW. Minimal contamination techniques for breeding mares: technique and preliminary findings. Proc AAEP 1975;21:327–335.

24. Danek J, Wisniewski E, Krumrych W, Dabrowska J. Prevalence and sensitivity to antibiotics of facultative pathogenic bacteria isolated from the semen of stallions. Med Weter 1994;50:385–387.

25. Vaillancourt D, Guay P, Higgins R. The effectiveness of gentamicin or polymyxin-b for the control of bacterial-growth in equine semen stored at 20°C or 5°C for up to 48 hours. Can J Vet Res 1993;57:277–280.

26. Padilla AW, Foote RH. Extender and centrifugation effects on the motility patterns of slow-cooled stallion spermatozoa. J Anim Sci 1991;69:3308–3313.

27. Blanchard TL, Varner DD, Love CC, Hurtgen JP, Cummings MR, Kenney RM. Use of a semen extender containing antibiotic to improve the fertility of a stallion with seminal vesiculitis due to Pseudomonas aeruginosa. Theriogenology 1987;28:541–546.

28. Arriola J, Foote RH. Effects of amikacin sulfate on the motility of stallion and bull spermatozoa at different temperatures and intervals of storage. J Anim Sci 1982;54:1105–1110.

29. Timoney PJ, O'Reilly PJ, Harrington AM, McCormack R, McArdle JF. Survival of Haemophilus equigenitalis in different antibiotic-containing semen extenders. J Reprod Fertil Suppl 1979; 27:377–381.

30. Pickett BW, Squires EL, McKinnon AO, eds. In: Procedures for collection, evaluation and utilization of stallion semen for artifical insemination. 2nd ed. Fort Collins, CO: Colorado State University Animal Reproduction Laboratory, 1987; p. 1.

31. Jasko DJ, Bedford SJ, Cook NL, Mumford EL, Squires EL, Pickett BW. Effect of antibiotics on motion characteristics of cooled stallion spermatozoa. Theriogenology 1993;40:885–893.

32. Francl AT, Amann RP, Squires EL, Pickett BW. Motility and fertility of equine spermatozoa in a milk extender after 12 or 24 hours at 20°C. Theriogenology 1987;27:517–526.

33. Douglas-Hamilton DH, Osol R, Osol G, Driscoll D, Noble H. A field study of the fertility of transported equine semen. Theriogenology 1984;22:291–304.

34. Pickett BW, Sullivan JJ, Byers WW, Pace MM, Remmenga EE. Effect of centrifugation and seminal plasma on motility and fertility of stallion and bull spermatozoa. Fertil Steril 1975;26:167–174.

35. Neuwirth L, LeBlanc MM, Mauragis D, Klapstein E, Tran T. Scintigraphic measurement of uterine clearance in mares. Vet Radiol Ultrasound 1995;36:64–68.

36. LeBlanc MM, Neuwirth L, Asbury AC, Tran T, Mauragis D, Klapstein E. Scintigraphic measurement of uterine clearance in normal mares and mares with recurrent endometritis. Equine Vet J 1994; 26:293–298.

37. Voss JL. Human chorionic gonadotropin. In: McKinnon AO, Voss JL, eds. Equine reproduction. Phildelphia and London: Lea & Febiger, 1993:325–328.

38. Roser JF, Kiefer BL, Evans JW, Neely DP, Pacheco DA. The development of antibodies to human chorionic gonadotrophin following its repeated injection in the cyclic mare. J Reprod Fertil Suppl 1979;27:173–179.

39. McKinnon AO, Nobelius AM, Figueroa STD, Skidmore J, Vasey JR, Trigg TE. Predictable ovulation in mares treated with an implant of the gnrh analog deslorelin. Equine Vet J 1993;25: 321–3233.

40. Harrison LA, Squires EL, McKinnon AO. Comparison of hCG, Burserelin and Luprostiol for induction of ovulation in cycling mares. J Equine Vet Sci 1991;11:163–166.

41. Meinert C, Silva JF, Kroetz I, Klug E, Trigg TE, Hoppen HO, Jochle W. Advancing the time of ovulation in the mare with a short-term implant releasing the GnRH analogue deslorelin. Equine Vet J 1993;25:65–68.

42. Jochle W, Trigg TE. Control of ovulation in the mare with ovuplant (tm)—a short-term release implant (sti) containing the GnRH analog deslorelin acetate—studies from 1990 to 1994. J Equine Vet Sci 1994;14:632–644.

43. McKinnon AO, Brown RW, Pashen RL, Greenwood PE, Vasey JR. Increased ovulation rates in mares after immunisation against recombinant bovine inhibin alpha-subunit. Equine Vet J 1992;24: 144–146.

44. McCue PM, Carney NJ, Hughes JP, Rivier J, Vale W, Lasley BL. Ovulation and embryo recovery rates following immunization of mares against an inhibin alpha-subunit fragment. Theriogenology 1992;38:823–831.

45. Squires EL, McKinnon AO, Carnevale EM, Morris R, Nett TM. Reproductive characteristics of spontaneous single and double ovulating mares and superovulated mares. J Reprod Fertil Suppl 1987; 35:399–403.

46. McKinnon AO, Voss JL, Squires EL, Carnevale EM. Diagnostic ultrasonography. In: McKinnon AO, Voss JL, eds. Equine reproduction. 1st ed. Philadelphia and London: Lea & Febiger, 1993: 266–302.

47. Pascoe DR, Pascoe RR, Hughes JP, Stabenfeldt GH, Kindahl H. Comparison of two techniques and three hormone therapies for management of twin conceptuses by manual embryonic reduction. J Reprod Fertil Suppl 1987;35:701–702.

48. Brinsko SP, Varner DD, Blanchard TL. The effect of uterine lavage performed four hours post insemination on pregnancy rate in mares. Theriogenology 1991;35:1111–1120.

49. Pascoe DR, Stabenfeldt GH, Hughes JP, Kindahl H. Endogenous prostaglandin F$_2$ alpha release induced by physiologic saline solution infusion in utero in the mare: effect of temperature, osmolarity, and pH. Am J Vet Res 1989;50:1080–1083.

50. Jones DM, Fielden ED, Carr DH. Some physiological and pharmacological factors affecting uterine motility as measured by electromyography in the mare. J Reprod Fertil Suppl 1991;39:357–368.

51. Liu IKM, Troedsson MHT, Williams DC, Pascoe JR. Electromyography of uterine activity in the mare: comparison of single vs multiple recording sites. J Reprod Fertil Suppl 1991;44:744 (abstr).

52. Kenney RM, Ganjam VK. Selected pathological changes of the mare uterus and ovary. J Reprod Fertil Suppl 1975;23:335–339.

53. McKinnon AO, Squires EL, Voss JL. Ultrasonic evaluation of the mare's reproductive tract. II. Compend Cont Educ Pract Vet 1987;9:472–482.

54. McDowell KJ, Sharp DC, Grubaugh W, Thatcher WW, Wilcox CJ. Restricted conceptus mobility results in failure of pregnancy maintenance in mares. Biol Reprod 1988;39:340–348.

55. Tannus RJ, Thun R. Influence of endometrial cysts on conception rate of mares. J Vet Med [A] (Zbl Vet [A] Physiol) 1995;42:275–283.

56. Ginther OJ. Fixation and orientation of the early equine conceptus. Theriogenology 1983;19:613–623.

57. Barber JA, Troedsson MHT. Mummified fetus in a mare. J Am Vet Med Assn 1996;208:1438.

58. Lofstedt RM. Miscellaneous diseases of pregnancy and parturition. In: McKinnon AO, Voss JL, eds. Equine reproduction. Philadelphia and London: Lea & Febiger, 1993:596–603.

59. Sertich PL, Reef VB, Oristaglioturner RM, Habecker PL, Maxson AD. Hydrops amnii in a mare. J Am Vet Med Assn 1994;204:1481–1482.

60. Vasey JR. Uterine torsion. In: McKinnon AO, Voss JL, eds. Equine reproduction. Philadelphia and London: Lea & Febiger, 1993:456–460.

61. Vandeplassche M. Obstetrician's view of the physiology of equine parturition and dystocia. Equine Vet J 1980;12:45–49.

62. Ginther OJ, ed. Reproductive biology of the mare: basic and applied aspects. 2nd ed. Cross Plains, WI: Equiservices, 1992.

63. Green EM, Loch WE, Messer NT. Maternal and fetal effects of endophyte fungus-infected fescue. Proc AAEP 1991;29–44.

64. Vandeplassche M, Spincemaille J, Bouters R. Aetiology, pathogenesis and treatment of retained placenta in the mare. Equine Vet J 1971;3:144–147.

65. Threlfall WR. Retained placenta. In: McKinnon AO, Voss JL, eds. Equine reproduction. Philadelphia and London: Lea & Febiger, 1993:614–621.

66. Perkins NR, Frazer GS. Reproductive emergencies in the mare. Vet Clin North Am Equine Pract 1994;10:643–670.

67. Blanchard TL , Elmore RG, Varner DD, Garcia MC, Orsini JA, Youngquist RS. Dystocia, toxic metritis and laminitis in mares. Proc AAEP 1987;641–648.

68. McKinnon AO, Arnold KS, Vasey JR. Selected reproductive surgery of the broodmare. Proceedings of the Post Graduate Committee in Veterinary Science, Sydney. Equine reproduction: a seminar for veterinarians.1991;174:109–125.

69. Day WE, Evans JW, Volgelsang MM, et al. Characterization of the cervix in cycling mares using ultrasound. Biol Reprod Mono 1995;1:519–526.

15. Folliculogenesis and Ovulation

ELAINE M. CARNEVALE

Monitoring ovarian activity is an important component of reproductive management in mares, because the ovaries serve both gametogenic and endocrine functions. Ultrasonography is an accurate and rapid method to evaluate ovarian follicular and luteal activity. Applications of ovarian ultrasonography include 1) stage of cycle determination, 2) detection of luteal tissue, 3) detection of multiple ovulations, 4) prediction of ovulation, 5) detection of ovulatory abnormalities, and 6) evaluation of ovarian pathology.

INTEROVULATORY INTERVAL

Mares are seasonally polyestrus with estrous cycles between 19 and 24 days (mean 22 days) of length during the ovulatory season (1). The estrous cycle is defined by behavioral changes in sexual receptivity; a more accurate description of the estrous cycle, based on ultrasonic imaging, is the period between ovulations or the interovulatory interval (IOI). The IOI is composed of luteal and follicular phases, corresponding to behavioral diestrus and estrus, respectively. The luteal phase extends from ovulation until lysis of the corpus luteum (CL) and is associated with progesterone secretion. During the luteal phase, circulating concentrations of follicle-stimulating hormone (FSH) increase and initiate growth of the ovulatory wave of follicles; mean daily concentrations of FSH significantly increase 6 days before emergence of the primary, or ovulatory, wave of follicles (2). Concomitant with behavioral estrus, the follicular phase extends from luteolysis until the subsequent ovulation. Estrus in the mare is long (approximately 7 days) (1) when compared with most other species and is associated with growth of the ovulatory follicle and regression of subordinate follicles. For 7 days before ovulation, the mean diameter of the ovulatory follicle (average of length and width) increases by 3 mm/day (1); however, growth of the ovulatory follicle is slower in older mares (15 to 19 years or 20 years and older, 2 mm/day) than in young mares (5 to 7 years, 3 mm/day) (3) and is slower before the first ovulation than before the second ovulation of the year (4). Concentrations of luteinizing hormone (LH) increase during the follicular phase until peak concentrations are obtained on the day of ovulation or the day after ovulation. Mares typically display estrous behavior for 1.5 to 2 days after the day of ovulation (5). An example of circulating concentrations of FSH, LH, and progesterone during an IOI is displayed in Figure 15.1.

A series of experiments was done to characterize follicular activity in the mare. Follicles as small as 2 or 3 mm were accurately detected with ultrasonic imaging (6), and indi-vidual follicles were sequentially monitored (6, 7). The number of follicles in different size categories varied with the stage of the cycle. Many small follicles (2 to 5 mm) were present during early diestrus. The number of small follicles increased before ovulation, reached a maximum approximately 5 days after ovulation, and decreased until approximately day 14 (day 0 = day of ovulation). The mean number of medium-sized follicles (16 to 20 mm and 20 mm or larger) began to increase between days 6 and 10. Selective growth of the dominant (ovulatory) follicle began 5 days before ovulation, whereas subordinate (nonovulatory) follicles regressed in size before ovulation. To summarize, small follicles were observed early in the luteal phase; follicles increased in size until luteolysis. During the follicular phase, one follicle became dominant and continued to grow while the other follicles underwent atresia and regressed in size. An example of follicular activity during an IOI is depicted in Figure 15.1; ovarian scans during different stages of the cycle are shown in Figure 15.2.

The ovary serves endocrine functions: estrogen is secreted by follicles, and progesterone is secreted by the CL. The steroid hormones influence tone of the uterus and cervix, and ultrasonic characteristics of the uterus will reflect ovarian activity. The pattern of echogenicity, or echotexture, of the uterus changes relative to ovarian production of estrogen or progesterone. When circulating progesterone concentrations are elevated (luteal phase), uterine echotexture is a homogeneous gray. Because uterine tone is firm, uterine horns appear circular when imaged with ultrasonography. In contrast, uterine echotexture during early estrus demonstrates an alternating echogenic (white) and nonechogenic (black) pattern; the edematous uterine folds can be palpated. The echotexture associated with estrus is caused by edema of the uterine folds from estrogen stimulation. As ovulation approaches, uterine echotexture becomes less prominent and is imaged as variations in gray tones (Fig. 15.3). The uterus before ovulation has poor tone; therefore, a cross-sectional image of the horn is more oblong than circular. Because changes in the tubular genitalia mirror ovarian function, appearance of the uterus and palpable tone of the uterus and cervix should also be determined when monitoring ovarian activity. This provides additional information and confirms findings from ovarian scans.

PREOVULATORY FOLLICLE

Characteristics of the preovulatory follicle (e.g., size, echogenicity and thickness of the wall, pain and softness on palpation, and shape) can aid in predicting the time to ovu-

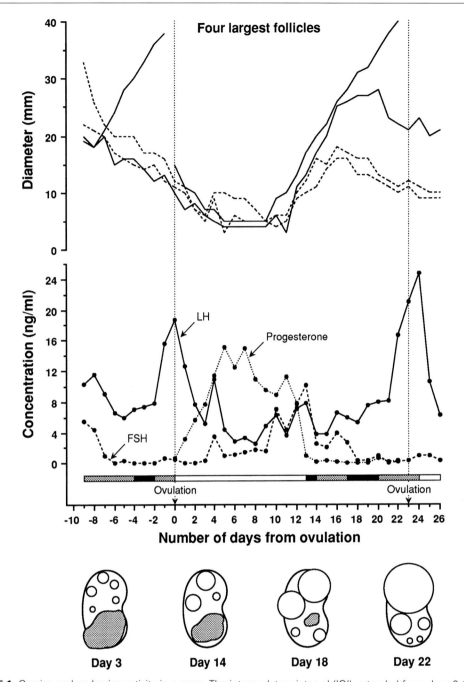

Figure 15.1. Ovarian and endocrine activity in a mare. The interovulatory interval (IOI) extended from days 0 to 23. **Top**, The two largest follicles of each ovary (solid line = left ovary; dotted line = right ovary). **Center**, Circulating concentrations of follicle-stimulating hormone (FSH), luteinizing hormone (LH), and progesterone. The bar designates uterine echotexture (white = homogeneous, diestrus; gray = heterogeneous gray pattern, estrus; black = heterogeneous black and white pattern, early estrus). **Bottom**, Diagram of follicular activity of the left ovary on days 3 (early diestrus), 14 (early estrus), 18 (mid-estrus), and 22 (late estrus). Gray areas are luteal structures imaged by ultrasound: on day 3, the corpus luteum (CL) was not yet functionally mature and progesterone concentrations were increasing; on day 14, the CL was regressing and progesterone concentrations were minimal; on day 18, a corpus albicans was present.

lation; for the most accurate prediction, information obtained from ultrasonography and from palpation should be integrated.

The preovulatory follicle of the mare can be accurately measured (average of height and width) with ultrasonography. In a review of studies performed at the University of Wisconsin (8), the mean diameters of preovulatory follicles were 43 ± 6 mm and 45 ± 5 mm. None of the follicles ovulated at less than 35 mm in diameter, and the largest follicle was 70 mm before ovulation. When size of the preovulatory follicle was measured at intervals (12 hours or less), no significant differences in diameter were recorded during the 48 hours before ovulation (9) (Table 15.1) (10). The size of the preovulatory follicle can be influenced by

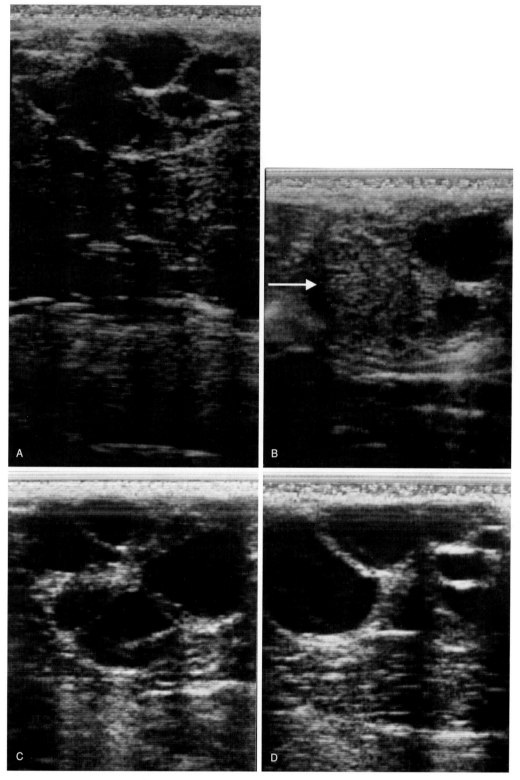

Figure 15.2. Ultrasonograms of ovaries during different stages of the estrous cycle. **A**, Small follicles during estrus; a large follicle was present on the opposite ovary. **B**, Follicles and corpus luteum (*arrow*) during mid-diestrus. **C**, Medium-sized follicles during late diestrus. **D**, Medium-sized follicles with one larger follicle (dominant) during early estrus.

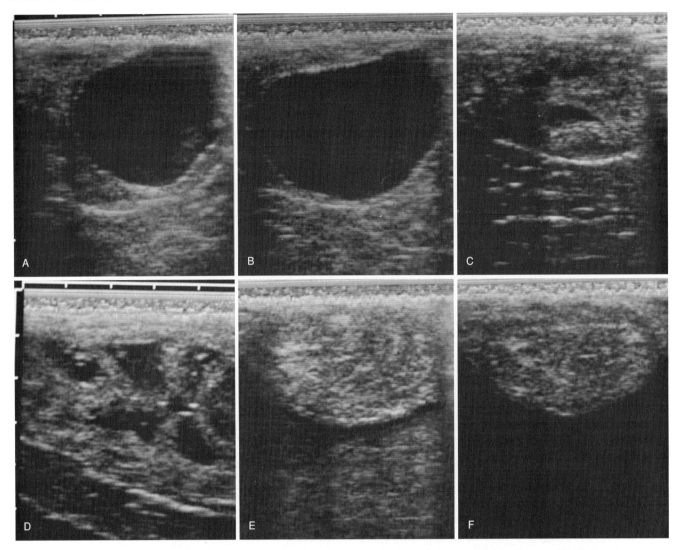

Figure 15.3. Sequential follicular scans during estrus in the same mare. Ultrasound images of the ovary (**A**, **B**, **C**) and uterus (**D**, **E**, **F**) on days −3, −1, and 0 (day 0 is the day of ovulation), respectively. On day −3, the dominant follicle is round and uterine echotexture is prominent; an image of the opposite ovary is depicted in Figure 15.2**A**. On day −1, the preovulatory follicle has become slightly oblong and an echogenic border is present; uterine echotexture is less pronounced. The ovulation site is imaged on day 0, and the uterus is a homogeneous gray.

various factors. None of 181 single preovulatory follicles, but 11 of 24 double preovulatory follicles, ovulated before obtaining a diameter of 35 mm (8). The mean diameter of the largest follicle during the IOI was greater in May through July than in August through October (7), and the mean diameter of the preovulatory follicle was larger in April (46 mm) and May (48 mm) than in July (40 mm) (11). The preovulatory follicle for the first ovulation of the year was larger than that of the second ovulation of the year (4). In one study (3), pony mares 15 to 19 years of age ovulated significantly smaller follicles than mares 5 to 7 years or those at least 20 years old (mean diameters of 35, 40, and 40 mm, respectively). Therefore, although most follicles were at least 35 mm in diameter before ovulation, the size of the preovulatory follicle varied. Within 48 hours before ovulation, the size of the follicle did not predict ovulation.

A study (10) was conducted to examine changes in follicular characteristics before ovulation (see Table 15.1). Light-horse mares ($n = 84$ cycles) were scanned and palpated at 12-hour intervals during estrus, and the following characteristics of the preovulatory follicle were scored: 1) echogenicity of the wall; 2) thickness of the wall; 3) pain on palpation; 4) softness on palpation; and 5) shape. Mean scores for echogenicity and thickness of the follicular wall significantly increased within 24 hours before ovulation; changes were noted in 60 and 70%, respectively, of individual cycles. Less than 12 hours before ovulation, mean scores for softness and pain of the follicle were significantly increased; increases were recorded in 77 and 75% of cycles, respectively. The mean score for shape was significantly greater less than 12 hours before ovulation; a change in shape of the preovulatory follicle occurred in 21% of cycles.

Table 15.1.
Changes in Ultrasonic Characteristics of the Preovulatory Follicle for 48 Hours Before Ovulation

Hours Before Ovulation	Size (mm)[1]	Follicular Border		Palpation		Shape[6]
		Echogenicity[2]	Thickness[3]	Softness[4]	Pain[5]	
72	37.3 ± 5.5^b	1.4 ± 0.8^d	1.3 ± 0.7^b	1.2 ± 0.8^d	1.1 ± 0.8^d	1.0 ± 0.1^b
60	38.4 ± 4.4^b	1.6 ± 0.7^{cd}	1.3 ± 0.6^b	1.4 ± 0.7^{dc}	1.4 ± 0.6^{cd}	1.0 ± 0.0^b
48	40.3 ± 5.1^a	1.7 ± 0.6^{bd}	1.5 ± 0.6^b	1.5 ± 0.6^{dc}	1.5 ± 0.6^c	1.0 ± 0.0^b
36	41.1 ± 5.3^a	1.8 ± 0.6^{bc}	1.5 ± 0.6^b	1.6 ± 0.7^{bc}	1.6 ± 0.6^c	1.0 ± 0.0^b
24	41.6 ± 5.5^a	2.1 ± 0.7^{ab}	1.9 ± 0.7^a	1.8 ± 0.7^{bc}	1.9 ± 0.7^b	1.0 ± 0.2^b
12	41.5 ± 5.4^a	2.2 ± 0.7^a	2.1 ± 0.7^a	2.3 ± 0.7^a	2.3 ± 0.8^a	1.2 ± 0.4^a

[abcd] Values within columns with different superscripts are different ($P < 0.05$).
[1] Average of height and width.
[2] Scored from 0 (minimum, gray) to 3 (maximum, hyperechogenic).
[3] Scored from 0 (minimum, no border) to 3 (≥3 mm border).
[4] Scored from 0 (firm) to 3 (flaccid).
[5] Scored from 0 (no reaction) to 3 (very painful).
[6] Scored 1 (round) or 2 (irregular).
(Reproduced with permission from McKinnon AO, Carnevale EM. Characteristics of the preovulatory follicle during the 48 hours prior to ovulation [unpublished].)

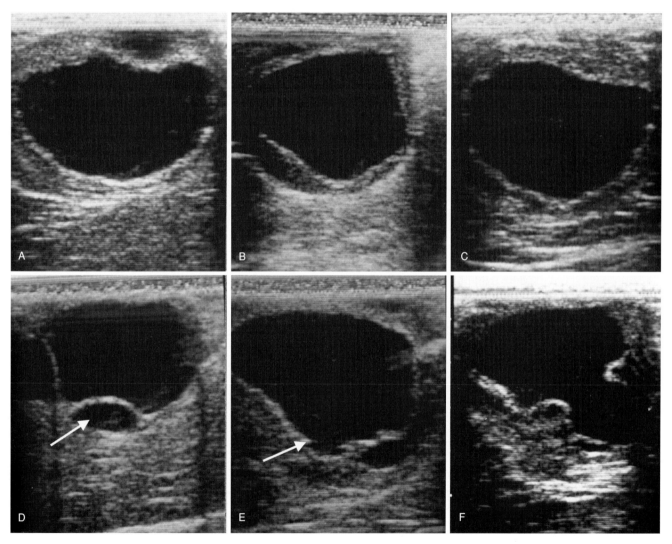

Figure 15.4. Ultrasound images of preovulatory follicles. **A**, **B**, **C**, The follicles are oblong, and follicular borders are echogenic and thick. **D**, A small follicle (*arrow*) is impinging into the preovulatory follicle; this has been attributed to a decline in follicular fluid pressure within the larger follicle as ovulation approaches. **E**, A small rent (*arrow*) is present on the ventral border of the follicle, indicating imminent ovulation. **F**, The follicle is protruding into the ovulation fossa as ovulation approaches.

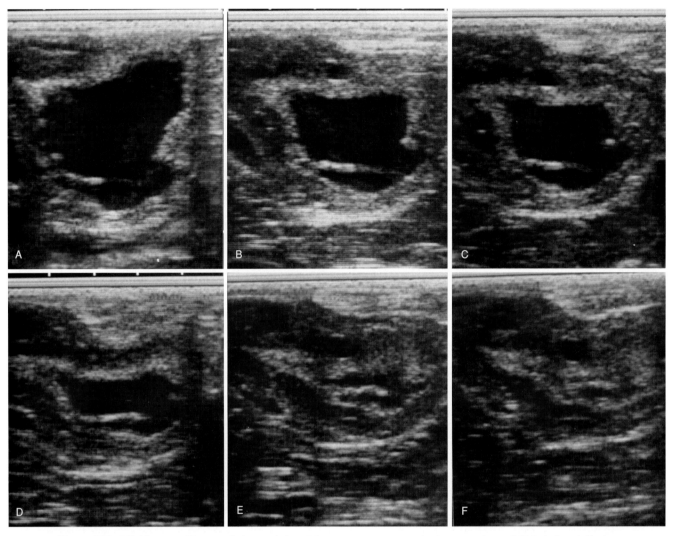

Figure 15.5. A-F, Ultrasound images during ovulation. A large rent was present in the preovulatory follicle before follicular evacuation. The follicle was evacuated in less than 5 minutes.

In a study by Townson and Ginther (9), changes in shape of the preovulatory follicle during the 48 hours before ovulation were detected using computerized digital analysis of ultrasonic images. The first significant change in shape occurred between 12 and 3 hours before ovulation; an additional change in shape occurred half an hour before ovulation. Differences in shape were due to a gradual change in the cross-sectional image of follicles from circular to oblong as ovulation approached (Fig. 15.4A–C). The change in shape of the preovulatory follicle before ovulation seemed to be associated with reduced pressure in the follicular antrum (Fig. 15.4D). When evaluating the shape of a follicle, it is important to realize that compression by adjacent follicles, luteal tissue, or stroma can result in an irregular shape that is not associated with impending ovulation; however, in these instances, the apposing follicular borders are often linear, and the follicle is firm on palpation.

In conclusion, ultrasonic characteristics of the preovulatory follicle can be used to predict ovulation; however, the most accurate assessment is made by integrating results

from ultrasonography, palpation, and teasing. Although the size of the preovulatory follicle is an important parameter for breeding management in the mare, the time of ovulation cannot be predicted within 48 hours by the size of the follicle. In approximately 70% of cycles, the appearance of the follicular wall (e.g., increased thickness and echogenicity) changes within 24 hours before ovulation; and less than 12 hours before ovulation, the follicle increases in softness and painfulness on palpation. Finally, a change in shape from round to oblong or irregular may precede ovulation by less than 12 hours; because changes in shape usually occur close to the time of ovulation, they may not be observed if scanning is done at intervals of 24 hours or longer.

OVULATION

When compared with most species, the mare's ovary is structurally inverted with a superficial medulla and internal cortex. A thick serosal lining composed of the tunica albuginea and mesovarium covers the ovarian surface except at

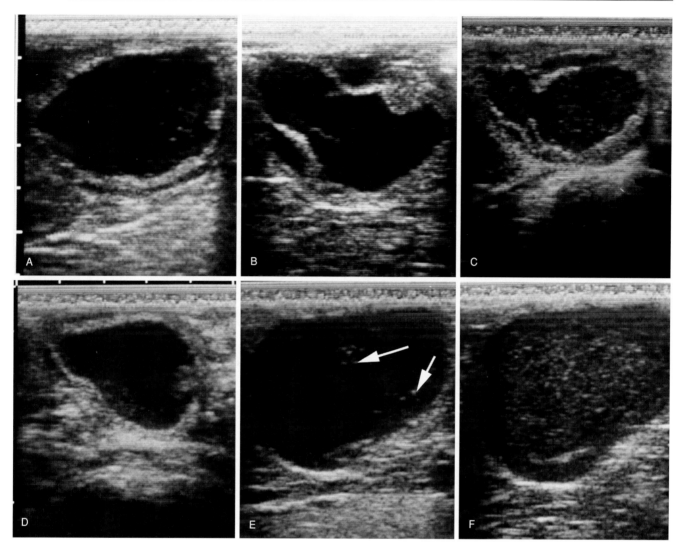

Figure 15.6. Ultrasonograms from mares that did not ovulate normally. **A**, An oblong follicle with an extremely thickened border and echogenic areas within the antrum. The follicle filled with echogenic debris, then collapsed a few days later. **B** and **C**, Irregularly shaped follicles in two old mares. Follicular aspiration was attempted in a few follicles with a similar appearance and the oocytes were recovered. **D**, An apparent preovulatory follicle; the follicle is pointed and soft with an echogenic border. The mare did not ovulate within the next 2 hours. **E**, Two days later, the follicle had enlarged and was firm; a few echogenic spots were detected within the antrum (*arrows*). **F**, After ballottement, echogenic debris filled the antrum. The echogenic debris probably represented blood. Failure of the blood to clot indicated that follicular fluid was present within the follicle because follicular fluid has anticoagulatory properties. The mares shown in **A** through **D** were bred; however, no pregnancies resulted.

the ovulation fossa, a 0.5- to 1-cm depression on the lesser curvature of the ovary lined with germinal epithelium. Connective tissue tracts extend from the ovulation fossa to the periphery of the ovary, thereby restricting follicular growth toward the ovulation fossa.

Ultrasonic characteristics of ovulation have been studied using continual monitoring of the ovulatory follicle. In one study (12), 15 mares were assigned to the experiment when the preovulatory follicle became painful and soft on palpation and changed from round to irregular. Thirteen of the mares ovulated between 15 minutes and 3 hours, 37 minutes after the beginning of observation (mean, 85 minutes). Two mares did not ovulate within 12 hours after the initiation of scanning and formed anovulatory hemorrhagic fol-

licles. Before ovulation, 76% (10 of 13) of the follicles developed a rent or tear in the follicular wall with a jagged protrusion of the follicular border toward the ovulation fossa (Fig. 15.4E). A pointed appearance of the follicle was noted in the remaining 3 follicles, with the border remaining smooth (Fig. 15.4F). The rent or point was observed between 77 and 15 minutes (mean, 41 minutes) before ovulation in 7 mares and served as an indicator of imminent ovulation. The remaining mares had a rent or point at the initial time of observation; these mares ovulated between 3 and 27 minutes later. The rent or pointed appearance of the preovulatory follicle is likely due to protrusion of the follicle toward the ovulation fossa as ovarian stroma is broken down.

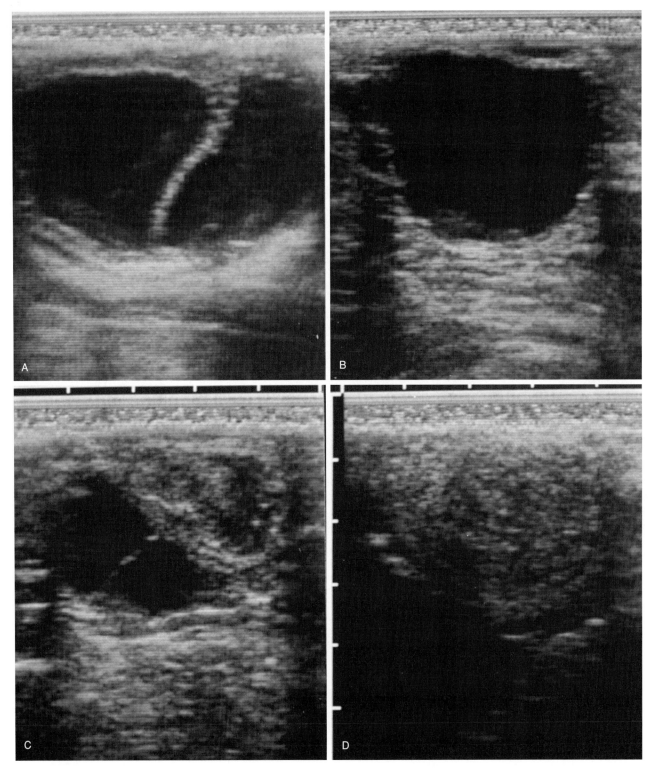

Figure 15.7. Ultrasonograms from a mare with a large diestrous follicle. **A**, Ultrasonic image of double preovulatory follicles. **B**, The right ovary with a large follicle. **C**, Smaller follicles and a corpus luteum on the left ovary. **D**, Homogeneous grey echotexure of the uterine horn is consistant with diestrus. Ultrasonic images associated with the diestrous follicle should be compared with those of a mare in estrus with a similar-sized follicle (see Figs. 15-2**A**, 15-3**A**, and 15-3**D**).

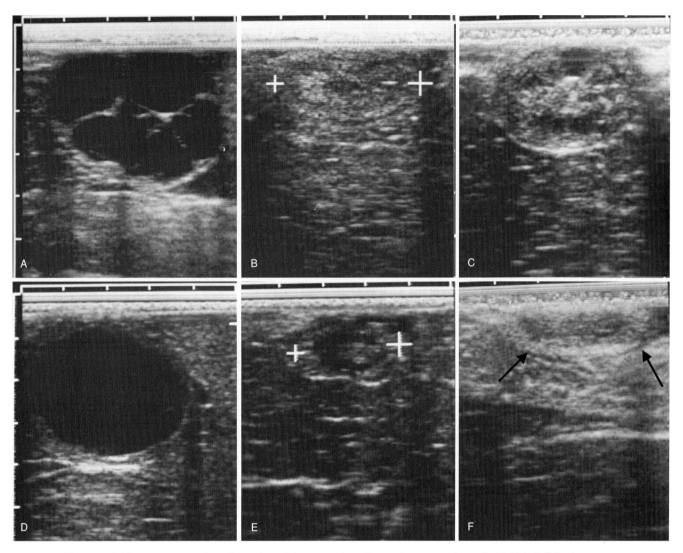

Figure 15.8. Ultrasonograms of ovaries and uteri demonstrating effects of season and age. **A,** Multiple follicles in an ovary during vernal transition. **B,** Cross-sectional image of the uterine horn of a transitional mare. Uterine tone is flaccid (cursors delineate the lateral borders of the uterus). **C,** An ovary during winter anestrus. **D** and **E,** A single large follicle in the left ovary of a mare less than 20 years of age, and the inactive right ovary of the same mare (cursors designate ovarian borders). The mare ovulated only twice between February and October; no follicles other than the ovulatory follicles were present. **F,** The uterus of a mare in reproductive senescence; (*arrows*) the ovaries appeared similar to the ovary pictured in **E.** Uteri in noncycling, aged mares are flaccid and often appear flat when imaged with ultrasonography; a similar image would be obtained during anestrus.

In the study by Carnevale and colleagues (12), ovulation was defined as a rapid decrease in follicular size. Ovulation occurred in an average of 42 seconds (range, 5 to 90 seconds). Little or no follicular fluid remained in the follicle after ovulation; follicular fluid was not visualized in the oviduct or uterine horn immediately after ovulation. In another study (13), follicular evacuation during ovulation was studied in 11 mares. Eighty percent of the antral area disappeared in 90 seconds. However, in this study, two forms of follicular evacuation were observed: a rapid decrease to less than 10% of the original antral area within 60 seconds; and a slower decrease to half of the antral area by 60 seconds. No fluid was detected in the oviduct during

or immediately after follicular collapse. The process of ovulation as imaged by ultrasound is shown in Figure 15.5.

In the foregoing study, an intensely echogenic border, irregular shape, and a rent in the follicular wall were predictive of imminent ovulation (12). Ova probably retain maximum viability until approximately 12 hours after ovulation (14). Significantly fewer pregnancies resulted when mares were inseminated 18 to 24 hours than 0 to 6 hours after ovulation (15). Therefore, mares with follicular changes suggestive of imminent ovulation should be bred or inseminated as soon as possible to allow sperm transport, capacitation, and fertilization before loss of oocyte viability.

Because follicular fluid is evacuated rapidly, imaging the

follicle during ovulation is unusual. Follicles that probably do not ovulate, but form abnormal structures such as anovulatory hemorrhagic follicles (14) or luteinized unruptured follicles (16), may initially display an appearance similar to that of an ovulating follicle (Fig. 15.6) (12, 17). The incidence of hemorrhagic follicles increases during the transition from cyclicity into winter anestrus. More ($P <$ 0.001) hemorrhagic follicles occurred in pony mares during the autumnal months of September and October than during April through August (1 of 139, 1%, and 19 of 92, 21%, respectively). During September and October, hemorrhagic follicles occurred in more ($P < 0.025$) mares 20 years old or older than in mares 2 to 20 years of age (10 of 28, 36%, and 9 of 64, 14%, respectively; Carnevale and Ginther, unpublished data). The occurrence of atypical ovulations, in which follicular evacuation appeared to be delayed or incomplete, was significantly greater for mares 20 years old or older than for mares 5 to 7 or 15 to 19 years old (17). Follicles that appear to be ovulating should be scanned within a few hours or the following day to determine whether ovulation occurred.

ALTERATIONS IN FOLLICULAR DYNAMICS

Multiple Ovulations

Most mares ovulate one follicle during an estrus cycle. The frequency of multiple ovulations is influenced by breed; Thoroughbred, warm blood, and draft mares have the highest incidence of multiple ovulations (18). Double ovulations may be synchronous (occurring on the same day) or asynchronous. Multiple preovulatory follicles may be difficult to detect by palpation, especially when follicles are located on the same ovary. When imaged by ultrasonography, follicles may be separated only by the apposing follicular walls, and adjacent borders may be flattened (Fig. 15.7A).

Diestrous Ovulations

Large follicles are occasionally imaged during the luteal phase and may result in diestrous ovulations. Diestrous follicles can be differentiated from ovulatory follicles by the presence of a CL, by uterine echotexture, by the tone of the uterus and cervix, and by the mare's behavior (Fig. 15.7B–D).

Season

Reproductive activity in the mare is influenced by season. The mare does not ovulate during periods of short daylight; transitional periods exist between winter anestrus and cyclicity. Before the first ovulation of the year, the ovaries characteristically contain numerous follicles that undergo growth and regression without ovulating (Fig. 15.8A and B). Mares may display estrous behavior for an extended period during the vernal transition, making breeding management difficult. The echotexture of the uterus fluctuates in intensity during this period in association with the growth and regression of follicles. The use of ultrasonography can help to determine whether an ovulatory-sized follicle is present or whether ovulation has occurred. The autumnal transition from cyclicity into anestrus has been studied (19). Mares entered anestrus after one of three ovarian states: luteolysis of a normal CL, spontaneously prolonged CL, or follicular atresia.

During anestrus, inactive ovaries may contain small follicles (Fig. 15.8C). Because circulating concentrations of estrogen and progesterone are negligible, the uterus is typically flaccid and may appear flattened when imaged with ultrasound.

Age

In one study, follicular activity was affected by increasing age in mares; cycling pony mares 5 to 7, 15 to 19, and 20 years old or older were compared (3). Length of the luteal phase was not different among groups. However, mares 20 years old or older had a longer follicular phase and a longer interval from a luteolytic dose of prostaglandin until ovulation than younger mares; this was associated with smaller follicles in mares 20 years old or younger than in the younger groups at the time of natural or induced luteolysis. Because mares 20 years old or older usually require more time to obtain a preovulatory follicle than do younger mares, age differences should be considered when synchronizing young and old mares for procedures such as embryo transfer.

Reproductive failure has been reported in old mares (17, 20, 21). The progression into reproductive senescence in pony mares seems to occur in the following sequence: 1) sequential ovulations with elongation of the follicular phase in association with reduced ovarian activity; 2) sporadic ovulations with elevated concentrations of FSH and LH when progesterone is low; and 3) persistent ovarian inactivity with no ovulations and maintenance of elevated concentrations of FSH and LH (17). In these studies, mares in a persistent state of ovarian inactivity had plasma concentrations of FSH and LH similar to ovariectomized mares, indicating a failure of ovarian feedback on the pituitary gland. Potentially, lack of ovarian activity was due to an age-associated insufficiency in the number of primordial follicles.

The ovaries of noncycling animals are small, with little or no follicular development (Fig. 15.8E and F), and the uterus and cervix are flaccid. Before the complete failure of follicular growth and ovulation, old mares may ovulate at extended intervals. A single follicle may result in ovulation (Fig. 15.8D and E) and in the formation of an apparently normal CL (17).

REFERENCES

1. Ginther OJ. Reproductive biology of the mare. Cross Plains, WI: Equiservices, 1986.

2. Bergfelt DR, Ginther OJ. Relationships between FSH surges and follicular waves during the estrous cycle in mares. Theriogenology 1993;39:781–796.

3. Carnevale EM, Bergfelt DR, Ginther OJ. Aging effects on follicular activity and concentrations of FSH, LH, and progesterone in mares. Anim Reprod Sci 1993;31:287–299.

4. Ginther OJ. Folliculogenesis during the transitional period and early ovulatory season in mares. J Reprod Fertil 1990;90:311–320.

5. Pickett BW, Squires EL, McKinnon AO, et al. Management of the mare for maximum reproductive efficiency. Animal reproduction laboratory bulletin 6. Fort Collins, CO: Colorado State University, 1989:42.

6. Ginther OJ., Pierson RA. Ultrasonic anatomy of equine ovaries. Theriogenology 1984;21:471–483.

7. Pierson RA, Ginther OJ. Follicular population dynamics during the estrous cycle of the mare. Anim Reprod Sci 1987;14: 219–231.

8. Ginther OJ. Ultrasonic imaging of equine ovarian follicles and corpora lutea. Vet Clin North Am 1988;4:197–213.

9. Townson DH, Ginther OJ. Size and shape changes in the preovulatory follicle in mares based on digital analysis of ultrasonic images. Anim Reprod Sci 1989;21:63–71.

10. McKinnon AO, Carnevale EM. Characteristics of the preovulatory follicle during the 48 hours prior to ovulation, unpublished.

11. Ginther OJ., Pierson RA. Regular and irregular characteristics of ovulation and the interovulatory interval in mares. Equine Vet Sci 1989;9:4–12.

12. Carnevale EM, McKinnon AO, Squires EL, et al. Ultrasonographic characteristics of the preovulatory follicle preceding and during ovulation in mares. Equine Vet Sci 1988;8:428–431.

13. Townson DH, Ginther OJ. Ultrasonic characterization of follicular evacuation during ovulation and fate of the discharged follicular fluid in mares. Anim Reprod Sci 1989;20:131–141.

14. Ginther OJ. Reproductive biology of the mare. 2nd ed. Cross Plains, WI: Equiservices, 1992.

15. Woods J, Bergfelt DR, Ginther OJ. Effects of time of insemination relative to ovulation on pregnancy rate and embryonic-loss rate in mares. Equine Vet J 1990;22:410–415.

16. McKinnon AO, Squires EL, Pickett BW. Equine reproductive ultrasonography. Animal reproduction laboratory bulletin 4. Fort Collins, CO: Colorado State University, 1988:56.

17. Carnevale EM, Bergfelt DR, Ginther OJ. Follicular activity and concentrations of FSH and LH associated with senescence in mares. Anim Reprod Sci 1994;35:231–246.

18. Ginther OJ. Twinning in mares: a review of recent studies. J Equine Vet Sci 1992;2:127–135.

19. King SS, Neumann MS, Nequin LG, et al. Time of onset and ovarian state prior to entry into winter anestrus. J Equine Vet Sci 1993;13:512–515.

20. Wesson JA, Ginther OJ. Influence of season and age on reproductive activity in pony mares on the basis of a slaughterhouse survey. J Anim Sci 1981;52:119–129.

21. Vanderwall DK, Woods GL. Age-related subfertility in the mare. Proceedings of the 36th annual convention of American Association of Equine Practitioners, Lexington, KY, 2–5 December 1990:85–89.

16. Ultrasound-Guided Follicular Aspiration

EDWARD L. SQUIRES and NANCY L. COOK

Progress in technology such as in vitro fertilization, oocyte maturation, and cryopreservation of oocytes depends on a supply of viable oocytes. In most studies, oocytes were obtained from slaughterhouse animals. However, this approach does not allow for genetic improvement. In the mare, progress in oocyte maturation and in vitro fertilization has been slow because of an inadequate number of equine oocytes. The collection, maturation, and fertilization of equine oocytes in vitro may be the only procedure that will allow foals to be obtained from old, infertile mares. Unfortunately, in the old mare, the rate of embryo recovery from the uterus is extremely low, making conventional embryo transfer techniques inefficient; to date, only two foals have been produced from in vitro fertilization (1).

Tremendous advances have been made in both human and bovine medicine regarding oocyte collection, maturation, and in vitro fertilization. Many laboratories routinely mature and fertilize bovine oocytes in vitro. In fact, Pieterse and colleagues (2) suggested that nonsurgical follicular aspiration of immature oocytes can be used successfully for in vitro production of embryos and that this procedure offers a competitive alternative to conventional superovulation–embryo collection procedures. In humans, follicular aspiration was initially performed by laparoscopic visualization of the follicle. Steptoe and Edwards (3) first reported on laparoscopic aspiration of follicles in humans. For many years, this technique was widely accepted as a means of obtaining oocytes for human in vitro fertilization programs (4). However, in the early 1980s, ultrasound was introduced as an alternative method for oocyte collection in humans (4, 5). Subsequently, various techniques using ultrasound were developed as alternatives to laparoscopically guided oocyte retrieval. These techniques included transabdominal–transvesical, transvaginal, and perurethral–transvesical methods, as well as a transvaginal approach using an abdominally placed ultrasound transducer. Several investigators have compared the efficacy of transvaginal ultrasonically guided follicular aspiration (TVA) with that of laparoscopically guided follicular aspiration (4, 5). Seifer and associates (4) reported a similar number of oocytes obtained with laparoscopy, abdominal ultrasound, and transvaginal ultrasound. In addition, Gonen and colleagues (5) reported that fewer follicles were aspirated using laparoscopy than using transvaginal ultrasonography. The mean number of oocytes recovered and the number of embryos transferred did not differ between the two groups. Investigators in both studies concluded that laparoscopy had no proved advantage for oocyte recovery over ultrasonically directed techniques. However, the disadvantage of laparoscopy was significant postoperative patient discomfort, some morbidity, the need for general anesthesia, and increased costs. Therefore, most human in vitro clinics now use TVA as the means of obtaining oocytes.

OOCYTE COLLECTION IN HORSES

Follicular oocytes were collected from mares primarily by inserting a needle through the mare's flank and into the follicle or by using ovaries obtained from a slaughterhouse. Vogelsang and associates (6) conducted a series of experiments to develop a procedure for consistent, repeatable collection of oocytes from the preovulatory follicle of mares. From 37 aspirations performed by insertion of a needle through the mare's flank, only 4 oocytes were recovered. In a second experiment, ovaries were visualized by standing flank laparotomy, and a needle and syringe used to aspirate 7 follicles. Only 1 of 7 attempts provided an oocyte. In contrast, when a continuous irrigation system was used and vacuum was applied, 6 of 10 attempts were successful. McKinnon and colleagues (7) also reported on collection of oocytes by syringe and needle when the ovary was exposed (5 of 13 oocytes), or percutaneous needle aspiration (1 of 5). Palmer and associates (8) described a nonsurgical method for oocyte recovery in mares. Follicles were punctured 36 hours after administration of human chorionic gonadotropin (hCG). Sixteen aspirations resulted in the recovery of 9 oocytes. Six oocytes were transferred into oviducts of recipient mares, but no pregnancies resulted. McKinnon and colleagues (9) recovered 45 equine oocytes matured in vivo from 63 follicular aspiration attempts. Fifteen oocytes were transferred into the oviduct of inseminated recipient mares, and 15 oocytes plus equine spermatozoa were transferred into rabbit oviducts. Ten oocytes (3 fertilized) were recovered from the oviducts of recipient mares following removal and flushing 2 days after transfer. Eight oocytes (nonfertilized) were recovered from rabbit oviducts. Oviductal transfer of the 3 embryos into separate recipients resulted in 2 pregnancies and 1 live foal. Hinrichs and Kenney (10) reported on a slight variation in technique for oocyte collection. In their study, the ovary was held against the mare's internal abdominal wall by the operator's hand inserted into the abdomen by a vaginal incision, and the follicle was flushed after aspiration. Recovery rates were 9 of 13 for mares treated with hCG and 15 of 21 for unstimulated mares. The major disadvantages of needle puncture by the flank are possible trauma and adhesions created by repeated puncture.

ULTRASOUND-GUIDED METHODS FOR COLLECTION OF EQUINE OOCYTES

Because of the limitations of laparoscopy and follicular aspiration by needle puncture through the flank, techniques of transvaginal follicular aspiration in both cattle and horses have been developed. Bruck and associates (11) were the first to report on the procedures for follicular aspiration in the mare using a TVA technique. However, only 4 follicles were punctured by this method, and only 1 oocyte was obtained. Cook and colleagues (12, 13), in our laboratory, described a procedure for routine collection of equine oocytes using TVA. This study evaluated the efficacy of collection of equine oocytes matured in vivo from preovulatory follicles, collection of immature oocytes from diestrous follicles, and recovery of oocytes from superovulated mares. Thirty normally cycling light-horse mares of mixed breed were used as oocyte donors during at least 4 consecutive cycles of the 1992 breeding season. Before the first follicular aspiration, each mare experienced a normal estrus accompanied by ovulation. At 7 days after ovulation, mares received 10 mg of prostaglandin $F_{2\alpha}$ ($PGF_{2\alpha}$) to induce luteal regression. Follicular aspirations were performed on each estrus and every diestrus in which sufficient follicular activity was present (at least 4 follicles 10 to 20 mm). Throughout the study, mares were teased daily for signs of behavioral estrus, and follicular activity was monitored at least every 3 days by routine rectal palpation and ultrasonography. When in estrus, mares were examined daily, and changes in size and shape of the preovulatory follicle determined. For follicular aspiration performed during estrus, the following criteria were met: 1) 1 or more follicles greater than 35 mm; and 2) estrus displayed or the presence of endometrial folds or a soft cervix. Mares were then given an intravenous injection of 3300 IU of hCG or a subcutaneous injection of 2.2 mg of a gonadotropin-releasing hormone (GnRH) analog, deslorelin (Peptide Technology, Sydney, Australia), and the preovulatory follicles were aspirated 36 ± 6 hours later. Preovulatory follicles were aspirated by 1 of 3 techniques. In technique 1, a 12-g single-lumen needle, with an internal diameter of 0.091 inch, lancet bevel 20 to 30° (Cook OBG, Spencer, IN), was used with repetitive filling and evacuation of the follicle (minimum of 3 repetitive flushes). Technique 2 was the same as technique 1, except a wire-loop device (Hobb Medical, Stanford Springs, CT) was threaded through the needle and rotated to dislodge cumulus cells. In technique 3, a 12-g double-lumen needle (Veterinary Concepts, Spring Valley, WI) was used with continuous rinsing of the follicle over 2 to 4 minutes. The rinse solution, a modified Dulbecco phosphate-buffered saline solution with 1% heparin and 10% fetal calf serum, was delivered using a pressurized (300 mm Hg) intravenous fluid system.

During diestrus, follicular aspirations were performed between days 7 and 10 after ovulation. Two techniques were evaluated: A) a 16-g, single-lumen needle, internal diameter 0.059 inch, lancet beveled 20 to 30° (Cook OBG, Spencer, IN) with simple aspiration of follicular fluid; and B) a 16-g, double-lumen needle (Veterinary Concepts, Spring Valley, WI) with continuous rinsing of the follicle. Because of the frequent presence of blood when aspirating diestrous follicles, frequent removal and rinsing of the needle with heparinized, Dulbecco's phosphate-buffered saline was necessary to minimize clotting.

During the last estrous cycle, 15 mares were given crude equine pituitary extract (40 mg daily) beginning more than 7 days after ovulation, when mares had acquired more than 4 follicles 10 to 15 mm in diameter. Daily injections were continued until 2 follicles larger than 35 mm in diameter were obtained, and then mares received 3300 IU of hCG intravenously, 2.2 mg deslorelin subcutaneously, or 80 mg of equine pituitary extract intramuscularly, and all aspirations of the preovulatory follicles were performed 36 ± 6 hours later. Technique 3 (double-lumen needle) provided the highest oocyte recovery in mares during estrus, and therefore, it was used for recovery of oocytes from superovulated mares.

All aspirations were performed with mares in a breeding stanchion. The mares were sedated with xylazine (0.45 mg/kg), acepromazine (0.05 mg/kg), and butorphanol tartrate (0.22 mg/kg) intravenously about 20 minutes before the aspiration attempt. The perineal region was scrubbed with povidone–iodine (Betadine) surgical scrub. For all aspirations, the transvaginal probe containing a 5-Mhz curvilinear transducer was used, attached to an Aloka 500 console (Fig. 16.1) (Corometrics, North Wallingford, CT). A sterile lubricant was placed on the transducer, and the transducer was placed into the vagina alongside the cervix, ipsilateral to the ovary containing the follicles to be aspirated (Fig. 16.2). With the other hand, the technician then entered the mare's rectum and positioned the ovary against the serosal surface of the vagina such that the follicle could be visualized on the screen. A puncture-line guide on the ultrasound screen was used to align the follicle optimally for aspiration. The needle was then inserted through the probe guide, the cranial vaginal wall, and directly into the follicle being aspirated (Fig. 16.3). A vacuum aspiration pump (Model 1180, Gomco, St. Louis, MO) with pressures between 100 and 300 mm Hg was used to evacuate the follicular contents. After all aspiration procedures, mares were monitored for signs of pain, colic, fever, and shock related to potential blood loss.

For aspirations performed during estrus, two methods were used to identify oocytes. With techniques 1 and 2, large volumes of aspiration fluid were commonly obtained. If not contaminated with blood, the fluid was centrifuged in 250-mL collection bottles for no more than 10 seconds. Fluid was withdrawn from the bottom of the conical bottle, placed on a search dish, and examined under a stereoscope at 7× magnification. When an oocyte was present, it was always found in the initial fluid pipetted from the centrifuge tube. With technique 3, small amounts of aspiration fluid were obtained (approximately 80 mL) because

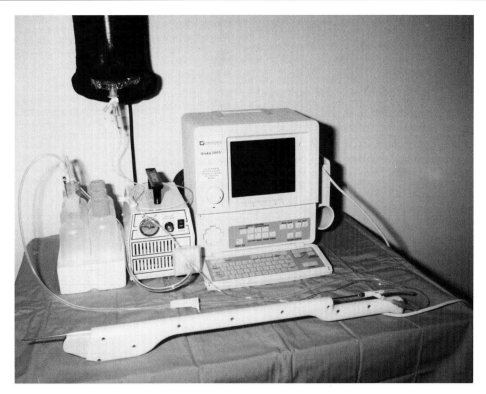

Figure 16.1. Transvaginal probe containing a 5-Mhz curvilinear transducer attached to an Aloka 500 console (Corometrics Medical Systems, North Wallingford, CT).

of the limited fluid-influx rate. If not contaminated with blood, these samples were searched in a square 10 × 15 mm plastic dish (Fig. 16.4). The large, cumulus masses could be easily identified, drawn into a pipette, and searched for an oocyte. Fluid from aspirations during diestrus was placed in a plastic dish and searched for oocytes. If the contents of any aspirates contained blood,

rinsing and filtration of the aspirate through an Emcon 75-μg filter was necessary before searching the fluid for oocytes. Oocytes were graded at the time of collection as either excellent, good, or poor (13).

The recovery rate of oocytes from preovulatory follicles aspirated during estrus is presented in Table 16.1. Technique 2, which incorporated the wire loop within the nee-

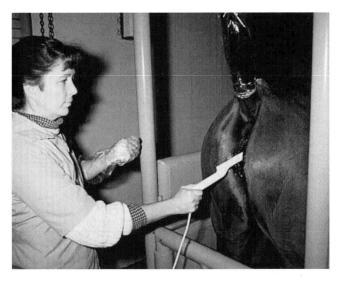

Figure 16.2. The probe was introduced into the mare's vagina and the transducer positioned alongside the cervix.

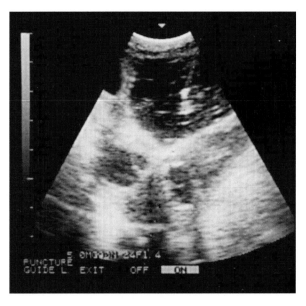

Figure 16.3. The needle was inserted into the follicle and fluid is being aspirated. Echogenic area in follicle is tip of needle.

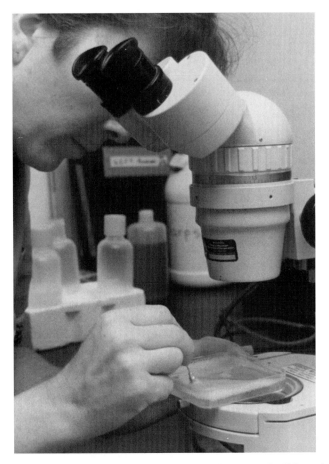

Figure 16.4. Aspirated fluid was poured into search dish and examined for oocytes.

Table 16.2.
Recovery of Oocytes from Follicles of Mares in Diestrus

	Technique A	Technique B Follicle Size (mm)		
		≤15	≥20	Total
Number of aspirations	167	118	38	156
Number of oocytes	32	36	3	39
Recovery rate (%)	19	31	8	25

(Adapted from Cook NL, Squires EL, Ray BS, et al. Transvaginal ultrasound-guided follicular aspiration of equine oocytes. Equine Vet Sci 1993;15(Suppl):71–74.)

blood was observed, the procedure was terminated. Recovery of oocytes from follicles of mares in diestrus was lower than that for preovulatory follicles (Table 16.2). For aspirations during diestrus, techniques A and B provided similar oocyte recovery rates, but more oocytes were recovered with technique B for follicles less than 15 mm than those from follicles 20 mm in diameter or larger. The overall recovery rate for diestrous follicles was 22%. Aspiration of follicles during diestrus required a longer period of time, and after several follicles were aspirated on an ovary, the procedure appeared to become painful. The smaller follicles were often positioned deep within the ovary and therefore required penetration of the stroma before follicular puncture. Presented in Table 16.3 are oocyte recovery rates from mares given pituitary extract during estrus. Overall recovery was 61% per follicle punctured. Approximately three preovulatory follicles developed per mare, but in some mares, follicles ovulated before follicular aspiration, and therefore, only two to three follicles were aspirated per mare.

Twenty-nine oocytes recovered from preovulatory follicles were examined to assess the extent of in vitro maturation. Eight of 10 (80%) and 13 of 19 (68%) oocytes recovered from estrous and superovulated mares, respectively, were in later stages of meiosis (late anaphase I through metaphase II). The mean interval between treatment with the ovulatory agent (either hCG or GnRH) and subsequent aspiration of preovulatory follicles was 31 hours. Perhaps closer timing of aspiration before ovulation may increase the percentage of oocytes in metaphase II.

Each mare in this study experienced about five follicular aspiration procedures. No signs of fever, infection, or abscess formation were observed. These authors concluded that a 12-g, double-lumen needle with continuous rinse al-

dle, resulted in the lowest oocyte recovery and was discontinued. Technique 3 was the most efficient method. The double-lumen needle allowed fluid to drip into the follicle continuously while suction was applied. Movement of the needle within the follicle assisted in fluid recovery and, perhaps, in dislodgment of the oocyte. A steady flow of fluid accompanied by the presence of thick, cellular masses in the collection tubing was a common indicator of a successful aspiration with this technique. About half the aspirates were tinged with blood, but oocyte recovery did not appear lower in these samples. However, when a steady flow of frank

Table 16.1.
Recovery of Oocytes from Preovulatory Follicles of Mares in Estrus

	Technique		
	1	2	3
Number of aspirations	47	9	43
Number of oocytes	24	2	36
Recovery rate (%)	51	22	84

(Adapted from Cook NL, Squires EL, Ray BS, et al. Transvaginal ultrasound-guided follicular aspiration of equine oocytes. Equine Vet Sci 1993;15(Suppl):71–74.)

Table 16.3.
Oocyte Recovery from Mares Induced to Superovulate During Estrus

Number of Follicles Aspirated	Number of Oocytes	Recovery Rate (%)
36	22	61

(Adapted from Cook NL, Squires EL, Ray BS, et al. Transvaginal ultrasound-guided follicular aspiration of equine oocytes. Equine Vet Sci 1993;15(Suppl):71–74.)

lowed recovery of oocytes from a high percentage of pre-ovulatory follicles (84%). However, additional studies are needed to evaluate various intervals between administering an ovulatory agent and aspiration of the preovulatory follicle to determine the most appropriate timing for in vivo maturation.

More recently, in our laboratory, Ray and associates (14) modified slightly the technique that Cook and colleagues (12) reported for TVA of equine oocytes. The objective of the study by Ray and associates was to develop the technique of gamete intrafallopian tube transfer in mares using oocytes obtained by TVA. The modification of Cook's procedure included the use of an infusion and suction pump (Cook Veterinary Products) and of a 16-g double-lumen needle (Cook Veterinary Products). In this study, 26 oocytes were obtained from preovulatory follicles and were transferred into the oviducts of 8 bred recipients. Two mares were confirmed pregnant based on ultrasound examination, 12 and 17 days after transfer. Pregnancy resulting from possible fertilization of recipient oocytes was ruled out in each case by DNA fingerprint analysis. In a subsequent study in our laboratory, Dippert and colleagues (15) attempted to maximize ultrasound-guided retrieval of equine oocytes by eliminating the dominant follicle present during diestrus. The hypothesis was that the dominant follicle inhibited development of smaller follicles, and, if eliminated, a greater number of follicles would be available for follicular aspiration. Unfortunately, the hypothesis was not substantiated. However, these investigators did report a greater oocyte recovery for mares during diestrus in which the dominant follicle was eliminated (30 of 85, 35%, versus 17 of 77, 22%). Oocyte recovery was greater from follicles 13 to 17 mm (35%) versus those larger than 27 mm (13%). In addition, higher maturation rates were obtained for oocytes collected from mares 3 days after elimination of the dominant follicle.

Bracher and associates (16) also reported on a study to investigate the suitability of TVA as a technique for puncturing multiple ovarian follicles in the mare. Five normally cycling Dutch warm-blood mares were used for repeated follicular aspiration from July to September 1992. In the first 6 weeks of the study, mares were injected with $PGF_{2\alpha}$ analog when at least one follicle reached a diameter of 30 mm. Twenty-four hours later, follicle aspirations were performed. In the second 6 weeks, the same mares were injected intravenously with 3300 IU of hCG 36 hours before aspiration. For their aspiration procedure, the mares were sedated and restrained in stocks, and intestinal relaxation was achieved with an intravenous injection of 20 mg hyoscine-N-butylbromide and an interrectal instillation of 50 mL of lidocaine (2%). An ultrasound sector scanner with a vaginal transducer (7.5 Mhz) was fitted into a specially designed handle (50 cm). Puncture needles with an internal diameter of 1.0 and 1.2 mm were used. Follicles at least 15 mm in diameter were flushed 1 to 3 times during the aspiration procedure. In the PGF-treated group, a total of 38 follicles were punctured during 7 attempts. Follicle sizes ranged from 7 to 44 mm. Only 1 oocyte was recovered from a follicle with a diameter of 16 mm. In the hCG-treated group, 3 oocytes were recovered from 13 attempts.

Not only has oocyte retrieval been attempted in estrous, diestrous, and superovulated mares, but also this technique has been used for oocyte retrieval in pregnant horse and pony mares (17). Follicles of pregnant mares were aspirated when the largest follicle of each mare reached a diameter of at least 25 mm. This procedure was performed 2 or 3 times between days 22 and 66 of gestation. The equipment and procedures used for follicular aspiration in their study were similar to those reported by Cook and associates (12). A 12-g, single-lumen, 50-cm needle was used to aspirate each follicle. Once the follicle was evacuated with negative pressure, flushing medium was introduced into the follicle with a plastic hand pump. Depending on the size of the follicle, 50 to 500 mL of medium was washed through the follicle. The follicle was flushed 5 or more times. During the lavage procedure, the needle was slowly rotated, and the follicle was rectally massaged to create intrafollicular turbulence. The flushing medium consisted of Dulbecco's phosphate-buffered saline with 1% calf serum, 100 IU of penicillin G, 100 mg streptomycin, and 2 IU heparin/ mL of medium. Thirty-three follicles were aspirated from pregnant mares, yielding 25 oocytes (75.8%). No pregnant mares aborted after the follicular aspiration procedures. These authors concluded that the pregnant mare's follicle may be a source of oocytes for subsequent in vitro maturation and fertilization.

REPEATED FOLLICULAR ASPIRATION

Although limited data are available on ultrasonically guided retrieval of equine oocytes, numerous studies have been published on aspiration of bovine oocytes using transvaginal ultrasound scanning. Pieterse and colleagues (2, 18, 19) at Utrecht have been leaders in developing the techniques for aspiration of bovine oocytes. In preparation of cattle for TVA, 0.1 mL/100 kg of domosedan was given intravenously to sedate the cows. In addition, an epidural injection of lidocaine plus epinephrine was given to prevent abdominal straining. A Foley catheter was placed in the bladder, and the standing cow was restrained in such a way that little movement of the animal was possible during oocyte recovery. An ultrasound sector scanner (SDR 1550, Phillips) was used with a vaginal transducer with a frequency of 5 Mhz; the transducer was extended to a length of 50 cm. Needles used were either 1.2 or 1.5 mm in external diameter (0.8 and 1.0 mm in internal diameter). These needles had a bevel of approximately 25° and a roughened area near the tip to enhance reflection. Of 197 follicles, 54 oocytes were recovered (27.4%). More oocytes were recovered from cows that had received superovulatory hormonal treatment. These cows had larger ovaries, and there were more follicles 5 to 10 mm in size.

In a subsequent study by Pieterse and colleagues (2), follicular aspirations using TVA were performed in 21 cows over a 3-month period. All visible follicles larger than 3 mm in diameter were punctured and aspirated 3 times during the estrous cycle on days 3 or 4, 9 or 10, and 15 or 16. The mean estrous cycle length after repeated follicular puncture was within normal range (22.2 days). The total number of punctured follicles per estrous cycle was 12.6. The largest number of follicles punctured for ovum pickup was on day 3 or 4 of the estrous cycle. The overall recovery of 541 punctured follicles was 55%. Most oocytes were aspirated from follicles smaller than 10 mm. After in vitro maturation and fertilization, 104 oocytes were transferred to sheep oviducts. Six days later, 75 ova or embryos were recovered after flushing the oviducts of the sheep; 24% of these ova or embryos developed into transferable morula and blastocysts. These investigators concluded that a nonsurgical, follicular aspiration procedure had been developed for repeated collection of immature oocytes. These immature oocytes could be used for in vitro production of embryos as a competitive alternative to conventional superovulation and embryo collection procedures. Several other investigators (20, 21) have also reported on repeated bovine oocyte collection by ultrasound-guided follicular aspiration. Kruip and associates (20) evaluated the use of this procedure in several different breeds of beef cattle. In some breeds, several thousand follicles were punctured, whereas, in other breeds, several hundred follicles were punctured. In general, the oocyte recovery rate varied from 47 to 57%. No significant difference due to breed was noted. No detrimental effects were observed by clinical and postmortem examination. The overall efficiency of producing blastocysts from oocytes matured in vitro was 18.3% (6.6 to 30.%). This resulted in an average yield of 2.2 embryos per animal per week. Based on the embryo production of 8.8 blastocysts per month, these investigators concluded that ovum pickup is a technique competitive with embryo production in vivo by superovulation.

Limited studies are available in which the effects of repeated oocyte collections in the horse were examined. Cook and colleagues (13) reported no adverse effects when oocytes were collected transvaginally during four to five consecutive cycles. However, fewer mares had sufficient follicular activity (at least four follicles, 10 to 20 mm during diestrus) to warrant aspiration during cycles 4 and 5 versus earlier cycles. This finding appeared to be related to suppressed concentrations of follicle-stimulating hormone (22). Unfortunately, these investigators were unable to determine whether suppressed follicular development was due to repeated oocyte retrieval or to repeated injection of a GnRH analog used to induce ovulation during each estrus. However, the interovulatory interval was not altered by repeated aspiration of follicles during estrus or during estrus and diestrus.

FACTORS AFFECTING OOCYTE COLLECTION

TVA of oocytes in cattle appears to be an effective means of obtaining both oocytes matured in vivo and immature oocytes. This procedure will likely continue to be used as a source of oocytes for in vitro production of embryos. The procedure is particularly valuable for cows that do not respond to superovulatory treatment. Unfortunately, this procedure in horses needs to be refined. Some factors that affect the success of obtaining equine oocytes with the TVA procedure include restraint of the animal, the sharpness and strength of the needle, vacuum pressure and the ability to flush the follicle. Equipment used for follicular aspiration in the mare is generally a 5-Mhz, curvilinear transducer with a 50- to 60-cm handle containing a needle guide. However, several ultrasound equipment companies do provide a handle that can be used with a 5- or 7.5-Mhz linear transducer. We use a 60-cm, double-lumen needle obtained from Cook Veterinary Products. These needles are used 20 to 30 times and are then discarded. Attempts to sharpen the needles have been less than satisfactory. In general, 16-g, double-lumen needles are used for follicles during diestrus, and 12-g needles are used for aspiration of preovulatory follicles. Other investigators have not used a double-lumen needle, but rather, they have used single-lumen needles in which the fluid is evacuated from the follicle and then either follicular fluid or flushing medium is injected into the follicle. This procedure is repeated 3 to 5 times in an attempt to loosen the oocyte from the follicle wall.

Recovery rates of oocytes from preovulatory follicles of mares in estrus are comparable to, or possibly higher, than those previously reported for needle puncture of the follicle by the flank. If mares are examined daily with ultrasonography and if follicular aspiration is performed 30 to 36 hours after either hCG or GnRH analog treatment, then recovery rates for oocytes are high. Unfortunately, in vitro fertilization of equine oocytes matured in vivo is extremely poor. Therefore, at the present time, equine oocytes matured in vivo should be transferred into the oviduct of bred recipients in an attempt to produce gamete intrafallopian transfer pregnancies. Workers in Wisconsin reported over a 90% pregnancy rate when oocytes matured in vivo collected transvaginally were transferred into oviducts of bred recipients (Carnevale, personal communications). Aspiration of several follicles on the mare's ovary at one time would increase the number of oocytes available for maturation and subsequent fertilization. Certainly, in cattle, aspiration of follicles three times each cycle provided numerous oocytes for subsequent in vitro fertilization and maturation. Overall, the recovery rate for oocytes collected transvaginally from cattle during the luteal phase (30 to 35%) is slightly higher than that obtained for the same procedure used in mares (20 to 30%). Rinsing the follicle of the mare during the aspiration procedure would appear to increase the oocyte recovery rate. The oocyte is embedded more firmly in the follicular cells of the mare's follicle than that in cattle (23). The use of TVA will provide a source of equine oocytes that can be used to develop the techniques of in vitro maturation.

OTHER USES OF TRANSVAGINAL ULTRASOUND-GUIDED ASPIRATION

Transvaginal ultrasound has been used to obtain amniotic and allantoic fluid from both cattle (24) and horses (25, 26). Mcpherson and colleagues (26) reported on the use of this TVA approach for reduction of single pregnancies in mares. Twenty-eight light-horse mares were used in their study. Pregnant mares were randomly assigned to 1 of 4 treatment groups at days 40 to 50 of gestation: 1) needle puncture of allantois without aspiration of fluid (sham controls); 2) aspiration of allantoic fluid; 3) sham control and exogenous progestin treatment once a day for 30 days; and 4) aspiration of allantoic fluid and exogenous progestins. A Corometrics UST 974-V-5 equine–bovine intravaginal 5-Mhz curvilinear transducer was used. The transducer was coupled to the Corometrics Aloka 500V ultrasound unit. Before each procedure, the transducer and transducer casing were sterilized in 2% glutaraldehyde solution. A 4 × 30 cm sterile transducer cover was filled with 2 oz of sterile lubricating jelly and slipped over the end of the transducer. Wearing a sterile obstetric sleeve, the operator introduced the transducer into the most cranial aspect of the mare's vagina. The operator's arm was removed from the vagina and placed in the mare's rectum for manipulation of the reproductive tract. A puncture guide on the ultrasound screen was utilized to select the path for needle placement in the allantoic sac, in an attempt to avoid damage to the fetus. An assistant placed a sterile, 18-g, 60-cm spinal needle with an echogenic tip, through the needle channel in the transducer casing. After positive identification of the echogenic needle tip in the allantoic sac, the allantoic fluid was aspirated using a 60-mL Luer tip syringe. Aspiration was discontinued when the fetus approached the needle tip, when fetal membranes approached the needle tip, when resistance developed to fluid aspiration, when the image was lost because of fluid removal, or when it was no longer possible to obtain fluid. Seven of 14 sham-treated mares (needle puncture without aspiration of allantoic fluid) maintained viable pregnancies throughout the treatment period. Twelve of 14 aspirate-treated mares lost viable pregnancies within 30 days after treatment. Two mares in the aspirate-treated group maintained viable pregnancies for 30 days after treatment. The incidence of fetal loss was not different between aspiration versus needle puncture alone. However, day of treatment was an important factor in considering the most successful treatment in managing a twin pregnancy. Among aspirate-treated mares, pregnancy outcome did not differ significantly in mares treated between days 40 and 44 and days 45 and 50 of gestation. In contrast, pregnancy loss for sham-treated mares between 40 and 44 days of gestation (6 of 6) was significantly greater than for mares treated between days 45 and 50 of gestation (1 of 8).

In a similar study conducted in our laboratory (25), 14 mares at 50 to 65 days of gestation were randomly assigned to 1 of 2 treatments: 1) aspiration of allantoic fluid; or 2) injection of procaine penicillin into the allantoic fluid. A 5-Mhz transvaginal probe attached to an Aloka 500 console was used for this study. A 16-g, double-lumen needle was introduced through the vaginal wall and into the allantoic cavity. For mares in treatment 1, an attempt was made to aspirate all allantoic fluid, whereas, for mares in treatment 2, 2.5 million U of potassium penicillin suspended in 10 mL of saline was injected into the allantoic cavity. Jugular blood samples were obtained on the day of treatment and every other day for 2 weeks after treatment to determine concentrations of progesterone. Mares were examined with ultrasonography every other day for 2 weeks after treatment. Based on rectal palpation, the tone of the cervix and uterus was scored from 1 to 3: 1, extremely tight; 3, flaccid. The quality of uterine fluid was graded 1 to 4, as described by McKinnon and associates (27): grade 1, echogenic, grade 4, nonechogenic. The quantity of uterine fluid was designated as small, moderate, or large. The number of days to loss of heartbeat and the number of days to progesterone concentrations lower than 1 ng/mL were also determined. Elimination of pregnancy occurred in 7 of 7 mares in which aspiration of allantoic fluid was accomplished. Six of 7 pregnancies were eliminated after injection of potassium penicillin into the allantoic sac. Concentrations of progesterone decreased after day 6 in 5 of 7 mares in groups 1 and 2. Decreases in concentrations of progesterone generally persisted for only 2 to 4 days, and concentrations seldom decreased below 1 ng/mL. Seven of 14 mares had a slight softening of cervical tone 6 to 12 days after treatment. Three additional mares had considerable softening of cervical tone during this same period. Tone of uterus also decreased in 9 of 14 mares during days 6 to 12 after treatment. Two days after treatment, fluid was noted in the uterus of 12 of 14 mares. Fluid was detected in the uterus of the majority of mares on days 2, 4, 6, 8, and 10. By day 12, fluid was still detected in 8 of 14 mares. The quality of fluid varied over time, with increased echogenicity of fluid on days 4, 6, and 8, compared with all other sampling days. In 11 of 14 cases, the fetal heart stopped beating 2 days after treatment. In the remaining mares, loss of fetal heartbeat occurred at days 4, 6, and 14. In the present study, both treatments produced adverse reactions that question the use of this procedure for reduction of twin pregnancies to singletons. The decrease in concentrations of progesterone for 2 to 4 days apparently was responsible for decreased cervical tone in 7 of 14 mares and decreased uterine tone in 9 of 14 mares. Decreased concentrations of progesterone was likely due to uterine secretion of $PGF_{2\alpha}$. However, in no cases did the corpus luteum appear to regress completely, because serum concentrations of progesterone increased within 2 to 4 days. Mcpherson and colleagues (26) administered a synthetic progestin, altrenogest, to mares in which puncture of the allantoic sac had been performed. Of 16 altrenogest-treated mares with terminated pregnancies, 14 mummified fetuses were found. Perhaps progestin therapy after twin elimination would be a means of maintaining high progesterone levels needed for cervical and uterine tone and perhaps mummification of one of the fetuses. However, improved methods are needed such that the uterine environment after elimination of a fetus is conducive to survival of the remaining fetus.

Transvaginal ultrasound-guided puncture can also be used for obtaining fetal fluids for sex determination or perhaps for determination of the viability of the fetus. Amniocentesis in the bovine was utilized in our laboratory to confirm whether the fetus was transgenic (Seidel, unpublished data). Vos and associates (24) used a TVA puncture technique for collection of bovine fetal fluid several times during 30 to 100 days of gestation. Unfortunately, repetitive puncture resulted in fetal death in most of the animals. Apparently, improved procedures are needed before TVA can be used to obtain fetal fluids safely. Other uses of TVA that have not been reported may include injection of material into the ovary, follicle, or embryo, or perhaps removal of fluid or tissue from the ovary, follicle, or embryo. Numerous applications for TVA certainly will be reported in the literature during the next decade.

REFERENCES

1. Palmer E, Bezard J, Magistrini M, et al. 1991. *In vitro* fertilization in the horse: a retrospective study. J Reprod Fertil Suppl 1991;44:375–384.
2. Pieterse MC, Vos PLAM, Kruip TAM. Transvaginal ultrasound guided follicular aspiration of bovine oocytes. Theriogenology 1991;35:857–861.
3. Steptoe P, Edwards RG. Laparoscopic recovery of preovulatory human oocytes after priming of ovaries with gonadotropins. Lancet 1970;1:683–692.
4. Seifer DB, Collins RL, Paushter DM. Follicular aspiration: a comparison of an ultrasonic endovaginal transducer with fixed needle guide and other retrieval methods. Fertil Steril 1988;49:462–467.
5. Gonen Y, Blanker J, Casper R. Transvaginal ultrasonically guided follicular aspiration: a comparative study with laparoscopically guided follicular aspiration. J. Clin Ultrasound 1990;18:257–261.
6. Vogelsang MM, Kreider JL, Bowen MJ. Methods for collecting follicular oocytes from mares. Theriogenology 1988;29:1007–1018.
7. McKinnon AO, Wheeler MB, Carnevale EM, et al. Oocyte transfer in the mare: preliminary observations. Equine Vet Sci 1987;6:306–309.
8. Palmer E, Hajmeli G, Duchamp G. Non-surgical recovery of follicular fluid and oocytes of mares. J. Reprod Fertil Suppl 1987;35:689–690.
9. McKinnon AO, Carnevale EM, Squires EL. Heterogenous and xenogenous fertilization of *in vivo* matured equine oocytes. Equine Vet Sci 1988;8:143–147.
10. Hinrichs K, Kenney RM. A colpotomy procedure to increase oocyte recovery rates on aspiration of equine preovulatory follicles. Theriogenology 1987;27:237–238.
11. Bruck I, Raun K, Synnestvedt B, et al. Follicle aspiration in the mare using a transvaginal ultrasound-guided technique. Equine Vet J 1992;24:58–59.
12. Cook NL, Squires EL, Ray BS. Transvaginal ultrasonically guided follicular aspiration of equine oocytes: preliminary results. J Equine Vet Sci 1992;12:204–207.
13. Cook NL, Squires EL, Ray BS, et al. Transvaginal ultrasound-guided follicular aspiration of equine oocytes. Equine Vet Sci 1993;15(Suppl):71–74.
14. Ray BS, Squires EL, Cook NL, et al. Pregnancy following gamete intrafallopian transfer in the mare. J Equine Vet Sci 1994;14:27–30.
15. Dippert KD, Ray BS, Squires EL. Aspiration of the dominant follicle and its effect on subsequent follicular development in mares 3 and 6 days later. Anim Reprod Sci 1995;40:77–88.
16. Bracher V, Parlevliet J, Fazeli AR. Transvaginal ultrasound-guided follicle aspiration in the mare. Equine Vet Sci 1993;15(Suppl):75.
17. Meintjes M, Bellows MS, Paul JB. Transvaginal ultrasound guided oocyte retrieval in cyclic and pregnant horse and pony mares for in vitro fertilization. Biol Reprod Monogr Ser 1995;1:281.
18. Pieterse MC, Kappen, KA. Aspiration of bovine oocytes during transvaginal ultrasound scanning of the ovaries. Theriogenology 1988;30:751–762.
19. Pieterse MC, Vos PLAM, Kruip TAM. Characteristics of bovine estrous cycles during repeated transvaginal, ultrasound-guided puncturing of follicles for ovum pick-up. Theriogenology 1991;35:401–413.
20. Kruip TAM, Boni R, Wurth YA, et al. Potential use of ovum pick-up for embryo production and breeding in cattle. Theriogenology 1994;42:675.
21. Van der Schans A, Van der Westerlaken LAJ, de Wit AAC, et al. Ultrasound-guided transvaginal collection of oocytes in the cow. Theriogenology 1991;35:288 (abstract).
22. Cook NL, Squires EL, Jasko DJ. Repeated transvaginal follicular aspiration in cyclic mares. Equine Vet J 1994 (accepted).
23. Hawley LR, Enders AC, Hinrichs K. Comparison of equine and bovine oocyte-cumulus morphology within the ovarian follicle. Biol Reprod Mono 1995;1:243–252.
24. Vos PLAM, Pieterse MC, Van der Weyden GC, et al. Bovine fetal fluid collection: transvaginal, ultrasound-guided puncture technique. Vet Rec 1990;17:502–504.
25. Squires EL, Tarr SF, Shideler RK, et al. Use of transvaginal ultrasound probe for elimination of equine pregnancies during days 50 to 65. J Equine Vet Sci 1994;14:203–206.
26. Mcpherson M, Homco LD, Varner DD, et al. Transvaginal ultrasound-guided allantocentesis for pregnancy elimination in the mare. Biol Reprod Mono 1995;1:215.
27. McKinnon AO, Squires EL, Voss JL. Ultrasonic evaluation of the mare's reproductive tract. Part 1. Compend Contin Educ Pract Vet 1987;9:336–345.

17. Form and Function of the Corpus Luteum

DON R. BERGFELT, ROGER A. PIERSON, AND GREGG P. ADAMS

The luteal gland (corpus luteum) is a temporary endocrine gland that forms at the site of ovulation and progresses through a growth, maturity, and regression stage in both pregnant and nonpregnant mares. The primary corpus luteum is the sole source of progesterone during the estrous cycle and for approximately the first 40 days of pregnancy. Thereafter, supplemental luteal glands (secondary and accessory corpora lutea) contribute to systemic levels of progesterone until approximately the sixth month of gestation; a placental source of progesterone gradually replaces the ovarian source beginning at approximately the second month of gestation.

The ovary of the adult mare is structured so ovulation occurs at a defined location or depression known as the ovulation fossa (1). Although an ovulation papilla may be seen in the fossa, it does not typically project from the surface of the ovary as in other domestic species (e.g., cattle, sheep). In mares, the entire luteal gland is contained within the ovarian stroma. Consequently, transrectal palpation of the corpus luteum is difficult. In this regard, ultrasonography is a particularly powerful tool in that it allows immediate, visual assessment of the luteal gland throughout its life span.

Ultrasonographic anatomy of the equine luteal gland (2–4) and its physiology (1, 4, 5) have been previously described. This chapter is intended to consolidate the principal elements from previous publications on equine luteal dynamics and to discuss the technical aspects of detection and monitoring luteal glands in situ. Functional aspects of luteogenesis are included to emphasize and elucidate the structural dynamics of corpora lutea during the estrous cycle and early pregnancy. In addition to gray-scale ultrasonography, this chapter discusses other technologies (i.e., computer-assisted image analysis and color flow Doppler ultrasonography) that may aid both the clinician and scientist in understanding luteal development (growth, maturity, and regression) in the mare.

TERMINOLOGY

The synthesis and secretion of progesterone by luteal glands occur during the luteal phase of the estrous cycle and early gestation. If the mare is not pregnant, the luteal gland regresses just before final growth and maturation of the preovulatory follicle during the follicular phase. Conversely, if pregnancy is established, the gland is maintained for approximately the first 180 days of gestation. The period of expected luteal dominance is subject to the relationship of the ovaries with the uterus through prostaglandin $F_{2\alpha}$ ($PGF_{2\alpha}$). Before delving into the technical aspects and the

methodology of using ultrasonography to assess luteal gland development, the veterinarian should become familiar with the current terminology used to describe luteal glands and the concept of prolonged luteal activity (6). Precise terminology has evolved from observations made using ultrasonography and is necessary to communicate the origin of luteal glands resulting from ovulations or luteinization of anovulatory follicles during the estrous cycle and pregnancy. In addition, precise terminology is needed to differentiate the origin of prolonged or abbreviated luteal function in association with uterine disease or embryo loss.

Luteal Glands

The *primary corpus luteum* results from ovulation of the dominant follicle of the primary follicular wave terminating the estrous cycle (1). Luteal glands that result from ovulation of dominant follicles of a secondary follicular wave during diestrus or from large follicles present at the time of equine chorionic gonadotropin (eCG) production in early pregnancy are termed *secondary corpora lutea*. Secondary corpora lutea result from ovulations occurring during periods of progesterone dominance (i.e., diestrus, pregnancy) and need to be differentiated from primary corpora lutea that develop from synchronous or asynchronous double ovulations in association with estrus (1).

Primary and secondary corpora lutea can develop with or without a fluid-filled central cavity (2). Luteal glands with a central blood-filled cavity may be referred to as *corpora hemorrhagica*. Luteinization of anovulatory follicles, especially during the period of eCG production associated with pregnancy, are termed *accessory corpora lutea*. The term *supplemental corpora lutea* has been coined to include both secondary and accessory corpora lutea (1). A regressed luteal gland that occurs during the estrous cycle or pregnancy may be referred to as a *corpus albicans*. Luteal gland terminology is summarized in Table 17.1.

Luteal Irregularities

The term *prolonged luteal activity* was used previously to indicate luteal persistence without regard to cause (6). Ultrasonographic studies have revealed specific conditions of ovarian (i.e., secondary ovulations and hemorrhagic follicles) and uterine (i.e., pyometra, mucometra) origin that have resulted in prolonged luteal function. Severe uterine inflammation may be associated with extensive loss of surface epithelium; therefore, pyometra is often associated with luteal maintenance because of the absence of release of $PGF_{2\alpha}$ from the endometrium (7). The phrase *uteropathic*

Table 17.1.
Luteal Gland Terminology Used During the Estrous Cycle and Early Pregnancy

Luteal Structure	Definition
Primary corpora lutea	Result from single or multiple ovulations during the follicular phase (*estrogen dominance*)
Secondary corpora lutea	Result from ovulations during the luteal phase (diestrus ovulation; >2 days from the primary ovulation) or early pregnancy (*progesterone dominance*)
Accessory corpora lutea	Result from luteinization of anovulatory follicles during early pregnancy
Supplemental corpora lutea	Include secondary and accessory corpora lutea that develop during early pregnancy
Corpora hemorrhagica	Primary or secondary corpora lutea that develop a central blood-filled cavity subsequent to ovulation
Corpora albicantia	Regressed corpora lutea

(Adapted and summarized from Ginther OJ. Reproductive biology of the mare: basic and applied aspects. 2nd ed. Cross Plains, WI: Equiservices, 1992:1–642.) (1)

persistence of the corpus luteum has been suggested for the purpose of differentiating and communicating luteal persistence associated with uterine disease (6). In the absence of any apparent ovarian or uterine irregularity, *idiopathic persistence of the corpus luteum* has been suggested (6).

The term *pseudopregnancy* was initially used in conjunction with transrectal palpation to describe a prolonged interestrous interval in nonpregnant mares, especially if early embryo loss was suspected (1). Misuse of the term pseudopregnancy arose when it was adopted to describe prolonged interestrous intervals in nonbred mares. With the advent of ultrasonography, pseudopregnancy has been more strictly defined as a prolonged interval to ovulation that occurs in association with luteal persistence and tense uterine tone after embryo loss (6). The critical period during which the embryo must be present to block luteolysis is approximately 11 to 16 days after ovulation (1); embryo loss after the critical period results in a prolonged interval to ovulation (luteal persistence). Uterine tone during pregnancy is much greater than during diestrus (1). In this regard, if embryo loss occurs after maximal uterine tone has been achieved, immense uterine turgidity is maintained. Because considerable confusion has emerged with the use of the term pseudopregnancy, *pseudopregnancy* should be reserved to describe a prolonged interval to ovulation in association with tense uterine tone that has occurred in association with confirmed loss of pregnancy. Idiopathic persistence of the corpus luteum may be used to describe prolonged interovulatory intervals (i.e., interestrous intervals) in nonpregnant and nonbred mares if the origin of persistence is unknown.

In addition to prolonged luteal function, ultrasonographic studies have revealed uterine and ovarian irregularities that have resulted in abbreviated luteal function. Premature release of $PGF_{2\alpha}$ associated with endometritis

has resulted in early regression of the corpus luteum and, consequently, shortened estrous cycles (8, 9). In a study done under field conditions (10), 81% of the mares without a detectable corpus luteum on day 13 or 14 after ovulation showed clinical signs of uterine infection and a shortened luteal phase; mean cycle lengths were 15.7 to 17.9 days. The term *uteropathic* can also be used to describe abbreviated luteal function as a result of uterine disease (6). Shortened luteal function has also been associated with gonadotropin-releasing hormone (GnRH)–induced ovulation during the anovulatory season, especially in mares that had quiescent ovaries (diameter of the largest follicle 15 mm or less) at the start of treatment (11). Circulating concentrations of progesterone were significantly lower on days 11, 15, and 18 after ovulation, and the embryo loss rate was significantly greater (64%) in GnRH–treated mares compared with mares during the ovulatory season.

APPROACH

Detailed discussions of the transrectal technique of ultrasonographic imaging of the ovary in the mare are given elsewhere in this text (12) and in other publications (4, 13, 14). The following section focuses on the technical aspects and methodology of gray-scale ultrasonography for assessing luteal gland development. In addition, we discuss the use of color flow Doppler ultrasonography for assessing vascular dynamics associated with luteal development.

Technical Aspects

Makes and models of ultrasound instruments vary widely in their imaging capabilities and incidental provisions. Transducers are available in various types (e.g., linear-array, convex-array) and frequencies (e.g., 3.5, 5.0, 7.5 Mhz), and can be used intrarectally, intravaginally, and transabdominally. Transrectal scanning with a linear-array transducer has been the most common approach to ultrasonographic imaging of the ovaries of the mare. A transducer with a 5.0-Mhz frequency is typically used for detection and assessment of the corpus luteum throughout its functional life span (approximately 17 days during the estrous cycle) (2). Use of a 3.5-Mhz transducer dramatically limits detectability of the corpus luteum to approximately 6 days (8).

The transvaginal approach to ultrasonographic imaging of the corpus luteum using either a linear-array or a convex-array transducer fastened to a hand-held extension is also possible, and it has been used most recently for the aspiration of ovarian follicles for oocyte collection (15). This approach, however, is not routinely employed as a method to monitor ovarian dynamics sequentially because of the necessity of sanitary preparation of the transducer and the perineal area. The transabdominal approach may be used for viewing the ovaries, especially in young and miniature horses, the size of which preclude intrarectal insertion of a gloved hand. However, this approach has not been critically evaluated in small equids. Moreover, detectability of ovarian structures would be limited by the use of a 3.5-Mhz transducer—a frequency needed to penetrate the abdomen to the depth of the ovaries. Alternatively, transrectal ultrasonographic imaging of the ovaries in young and miniature horses can be done by affixing semirigid tubing to the transducer cord similar to that used for scanning sheep (16) and prepubertal cattle (17). The leverage provided by the rigid tubing allows the operator to manipulate the intrarectally placed transducer externally. Extreme caution must be taken with this approach, because the transducer is unguarded in the rectum and may increase the potential for rectal injury.

Location of either ovary by the transrectal approach may initially be frustrating, but it is quickly grasped with a few examination attempts. Identification of the ovary may be facilitated by first viewing a cross-section of a uterine horn and, second, by rotating the transducer laterally toward the tip of the uterine horn. The ovary should come into view just beyond the tip of the uterine horn. At times, the ovary is difficult to view or the image is not clear because of intervening tissue (e.g., intestines) between the rectal wall and the ovary. In this regard, it may be necessary to locate and reposition the ovary digitally.

The ovary is mobile in its suspension from the mesovarium, and often the position of the ovary changes during examination. As the transducer is rotated laterally or medially, great care must be taken to ensure that the entire ovary is scanned, especially if the ovary has changed its orientation during the examination.

Methodology

The luteal gland undergoes morphologic as well as functional changes during its life span. Frequent or periodic ultrasonographic assessment of luteal changes has been accomplished by measuring the cross-sectional diameter or area of the luteal gland (18–22), by estimating the percentage of echoic versus nonechoic tissue (2), by assessing grayscale values (2, 18, 19, 22) and by using computer-assisted image analysis (19) during various reproductive states. Quantitative data generated by these approaches have been used to characterize structural and functional dynamics of the luteal gland.

Luteal glands can be distinguished from ovarian stroma by a well-defined border (2). The distinct demarcation between the highly vascularized luteal tissue of a mature corpus luteum and the dense connective tissue of the stroma results from a difference in acoustic impedance at the tissue interfaces (4). However, as luteal glands regress, they become more difficult to distinguish from the ovarian stroma (2). Corpora albicantia become increasingly echoic as a result of decreased vascularization and increased tissue density. Occasionally, they may be visualized in subsequent cycles surrounded by a group of small follicles (2).

Luteal glands resulting from ovulation follow one of two paths of development (Fig. 17.1). Approximately 50 to 70% of luteal glands form a central fluid-filled cavity (blood clot; corpora hemorrhagica) that is relatively hypoechoic (2, 18); an outer wall of echoic luteal tissue encompasses the central cavity. The formation of a central blood-filled cavity appears to be a random event (2); repeatability was not detected within mares from one ovulation to the next. Moreover, in mares that have had multiple ovulations, morphologic features of the luteal gland were as likely to be similar as dissimilar. The ratio of luteal to nonluteal tissue of newly formed corpora hemorrhagica is approximately 10%:90% (see Fig. 17.1; early diestrus). Through its life span, the central cavity of corpora hemorrhagica increases in echogenicity as a result of an increase in fibrin and it decreases in size as a result of organization of the fibrin into a clot. Still, the central cavity can be typically identified throughout diestrus (see Fig. 17.1; late diestrus). Concomitant with the decrease in size of the central cavity, the ratio of luteal to nonluteal tissue increases (see Fig. 17.1; mid-diestrus). Alternatively, luteal glands can develop without a central cavity (see Fig. 17.1). Approximately 30 to 50% of luteal glands remain relatively uniform throughout their life span and do not develop from a classic corpus hemorrhagicum.

In situ ultrasonographic measurements of luteal glands have been determined during the estrous cycle (18, 19, 22), in early pregnancy (20, 22), and subsequent to embryo loss (19, 20). The ultrasonographic image of the luteal gland was frozen at its maximum height and width, and dimensions were measured. Height and width measurements were used to give an overall cross-sectional diameter (mm) or area (mm^2) of the luteal gland. In corpora hemorrhagica, the central cavity was measured and subtracted from the overall luteal area to adjust for the nonluteinized area of the central blood clot. Ultrasonographic images of luteal glands with and without a central cavity often resemble mushrooms or gourds in shape (2). The gourdlike shape was attributed to the constraints of the surrounding connective tissue of the ovarian stroma as the luteal glands formed in the pathway to the ovulation fossa. The irregular shape of luteal glands and the mobility of the loosely suspended ovary make it difficult to obtain the same plane of scan on subsequent examinations. In this regard, measurement of the luteal gland often included only the body of the gland and not the necklike process leading to the ovulation fossa. This approach seemed to decrease the variation of point measurements between examinations.

Gray-scale values have been assigned to the corpus luteum throughout the luteal phase to characterize the extent of luteal tissue echointensity associated with growth, maturity, and regression (Fig. 17.2) (2, 19, 22). The degree of echointensity or brightness that luteal tissue exhibits appears to correspond inversely to luteal hemodynamics; that is, very high to high values seen during early diestrus (growth) correspond to minimal or increasing vascularity, low to very low values observed during mid-diestrus (maturity) correspond to maximal vascularity, and high to very high values recorded during late diestrus (regression) corre-

OVULATION

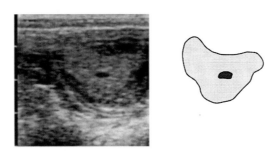

LUTEAL GLAND DEVELOPMENT

with central cavity   *without central cavity*

Early Diestrus

Mid-Diestrus

Late Diestrus

Figure 17.1. Ultrasonograms and corresponding diagrams depicting the site of ovulation and the primary corpus luteum during various stages of the luteal phase. The scale bars at the left portion of the ultrasonograms represent 10-mm increments.

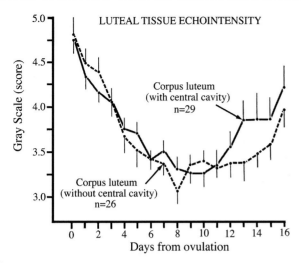

Figure 17.2. Mean (± SEM) gray-scale score subjectively assigned to luteal tissue of glands with and without a central cavity. Luteal tissue echointensity profiles of the two morphologies were not different statistically.

spond to decreasing vascularity. The degree of luteal gland echointensity may also be related to changes in luteal cell hypertrophy or atrophy during development. Nonetheless, changes in luteal tissue echointensity during the luteal phase may be used in combination with diameter or area of the corpus luteum as an aid for estimating the stage of the estrous cycle (4). Corresponding changes in luteal morphology and luteal tissue echointensity during the luteal phase are illustrated in Figures 17.1 and 17.2, respectively.

Subjective interpretation of ultrasonographic images has the potential for inconsistencies within and among operators. Hence, a more objective and quantitative approach is needed to assess changes in echogenicity of ultrasonographic images. Computer-assisted analysis of pixel intensities associated with ultrasonographic images of ovarian dynamics has been done in women (23), cattle (24), and horses (19, 25). Ultrasound images are composed of pixels (picture elements) of varying brightness or shades of gray. The number of shades of gray determines the gray-scale resolution of an ultrasound scanner. High-quality scanners have as many as 256 levels of gray shades, whereas lesser-quality scanners may have only 16. Although only 16 to 32 shades of gray can be reasonably distinguished by the human eye, a computer can quantitatively distinguish all shades displayed in an ultrasonographic image. Image analysis is a procedure in which selected ultrasonographic images are digitized and pixel intensities are evaluated. Digitization is the procedure in which each pixel of an image is assigned to a computer file for brightness. Once digitized, the pixel intensity information may be used as discrete pieces of information and analyzed. In one study (19), the results of computer-assisted pixel analysis of equine luteal tissue echointensity closely paralleled the more subjective, visual assessment of gray-scale scoring. Only a slight difference in the time interval was detected when luteal echointensity first significantly

declined after reaching maximal values at 24 hours after ovulation (72 versus 108 hours by computer analysis and visual scoring, respectively). When daily changes in echointensity of the luteal gland are evaluated subjectively or objectively, gain settings (near, far, and overall fields) on the ultrasound scanner console need to be standardized. The similarity in results between subjective and objective evaluations is encouraging for the practicing veterinarian who may choose to use visual gray-scale scoring as a diagnostic tool for assessing luteal gland development; however, a more objective and quantitative approach (computer-assisted pixel analysis) may be required for accurate clinical diagnoses and for testing scientific hypotheses.

Color Flow Doppler

Gray-scale ultrasonography is a simple, noninvasive method for evaluation of the dynamics of ovarian, uterine, and embryonic events in real time. Now, with color flow Doppler ultrasonography, we can begin to examine the dynamics of vascularity in the reproductive organs and conceptus without surgical intervention.

The flow of blood into various reproductive tissues can be quantitated during visualization in real time using color flow Doppler ultrasonography. Doppler ultrasound data may be acquired and displayed in color flow imaging or spectral modalities (Fig. 17.3). A detailed appreciation of the physical principles of the Doppler effect is critical for the interpretation of the types of data generated by these modalities. The Doppler effect, as discerned during ultrasonographic evaluation of tissue vasculature, is a function of red blood cells moving within a vessel and the angle of intersection of the ultrasound beams with the vessel (26, 27). Color flow imaging adds hues to standard gray-scale displays that indicate the direction of blood flow. The typical configuration for color display is blue for blood flowing away from the transducer and red for blood flowing toward the transducer. In addition, the intensity of the color displayed may be used to depict the velocity of blood flow (28). Differences in color intensity may indicate laminar or turbulent blood flow within a vessel. The direction (color) and velocity (intensity of color) of blood flow are calculated and are displayed as a color overlay on the gray-scale image. Spectral Doppler signals are waveforms created by the interaction of moving red blood cells during a cardiac cycle (systole to diastole). The ratio of systolic to diastolic flow, as measured by the amplitude of the waveforms from the spectral trace patterns, may be used to estimate resistance to blood flow. With the use of Doppler ultrasonography, the operator has simultaneous access to both structural and functional information, especially regarding the perfusion of organs of interest.

The newly formed luteal gland undergoes profound angiogenesis during its early growth and exhibits degradation of the vascular supply during its regression. At the onset of luteogenesis in women, the walls of the evacuated follicle become vascularized 48 to 72 hours after ovulation

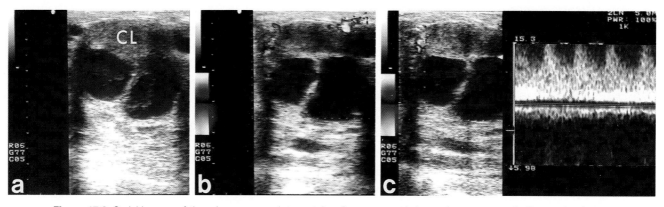

Figure 17.3. Serial images of the primary corpus luteum taken from a mare during early pregnancy. **A**, Conventional gray-scale image of the corpus luteum and surrounding follicles. **B**, Color flow Doppler image overlaid on a gray-scale image showing arterial and venous blood flow associated with the luteal gland in the upper left portion of the image (the ovarian artery is seen in the upper right portion of the image). **C**, Placement of the spectral Doppler gate on the arterial supply to the luteal gland (*left panel*) and the generated spectral trace (*right panel*).

(29). Blood and lymphatic vessels colonize the newly developing luteal gland. In women, one typically sees a pronounced ring of vascularity that encompasses the former preovulatory follicle, becoming more apparent as the corpus luteum matures (29, 30). Color flow Doppler ultrasonography was used to examine the primary corpus luteum in a mare during early pregnancy (see Fig. 17.3**B**). Although there was no obvious vascular ring encompassing the primary corpus luteum, distinct vascular areas about and within the corpus luteum were detected. In women, during the period of maximal progesterone production at maturity of the corpus luteum, resistance to vascular flow is relatively low (29–31). In contrast, during the period of decreasing progesterone production at regression, resistance to flow increases. Changes in luteal gland vascularization can be determined by examining spectral trace patterns. A spectral trace pattern of blood flow associated with the primary corpus luteum in a mare is shown in Figure 17.3**C**.

In the mare, critical studies using color flow Doppler ultrasonography to evaluate the vascular dynamics associated with development of the primary and secondary or accessory corpora lutea have not been done. Nonetheless, we expect that this technology will be utilized in both applied and basic situations to enhance our understanding of the role of the corpus luteum during the estrous cycle, early pregnancy, and embryo or fetal loss.

FORM AND FUNCTION

The intimate relationship between follicle granulosa and theca cells provides the foundation for steroidogenesis in the ovary. Concurrent with and subsequent to ovulation, granulosa cells undergo biochemical and morphologic changes (luteinization). In its simplest form, luteinization involves morphogenesis of estrogen-secreting granulosa cells to progesterone-secreting luteal cells. Microscopic characteristics of the corpus luteum in mares have been reported (32–34), and the ultrasonographic characteristics have been reviewed (1, 4). This section focuses on consoli-

dating the ultrasonographic morphology (form) of the primary corpus luteum with its physiology (function) from ovulation to ovulation (i.e., the estrous cycle). Luteal glands that form from ovulations during diestrus and pregnancy (secondary corpora lutea) and those that form from luteinization of anovulatory follicles during early pregnancy (accessory corpora lutea) are also discussed.

Estrous Cycle

Ovulation is discussed elsewhere in this text (35) and is mentioned here only as a prelude to the discussion of luteal gland formation. Ovulation is the process of follicular rupture that includes evacuation of follicular fluid along with the ovum. The day of ovulation (day 0) may be defined by the disappearance of a large follicle that was present at a recent previous examination (14). If daily examinations (once every 24 hours) are done to detect ovulation, day −1 is as close to the time of ovulation as day 0, on average, because ovulation occurs sometime between day −1 and day 0. Nevertheless, day 0 is reserved to indicate the day of ovulation as a point of reference for communicating other reproductive events. The interval between ovulations of successive ovulatory periods is termed an *interovulatory interval*; this interval is used to specifically indicate the length of the estrous cycle from ovulation to ovulation. Some of the studies that follow involved ultrasonographic imaging at intervals less than 24 hours to critically examine the ovulatory process and luteal gland formation immediately after follicular rupture.

An ovulation site can usually be detected ultrasonographically on the day of follicle rupture by the intense echocity at the site (see Fig. 17.1; ovulation). In one study, hyperechocity was seen in 88% of newly forming glands on day 0 and persisted until approximately day 3 or 4 (2). In a more recent study (22), luteal tissue hyperechocity was maximal at day 1 in horses and at day 2 in ponies; gray-scale scores gradually decreased thereafter. Equine luteal cells appear to be derived primarily, if not exclusively, from granulosa cells (32–34). Theca cells begin degenerating just before ovulation and are near complete degeneration by 24 hours after ovulation. Within 24 hours of ovulation, granulosa cells increase from approximately 10 to 15 μm in diameter. Microscopically, the nuclei are vesiculated, and the cytoplasm contains fine vacuoles, indicating luteinization and secretory activity. Concurrent with luteinization, neovascularization is observed, with proliferation of capillaries accompanied by the invasion of folds of stromal tissue into the luteinizing tissue (32, 33). Hence, the apposition of the collapsed follicular walls and the initial phases of luteinization and vascularization are likely contributors to the high degree of echocity at the ovulation site.

Development of corpora lutea with (corpora hemorrhagica) or without a central fluid-filled cavity was first evident by ultrasonography (2) on day 0 (28%), day 1 (62%), day 2 (6%), and day 3 (4%). Subsequent studies (18, 19) were designed to examine in detail the time and incidence of fluid accumulation within the central cavity of newly forming corpora hemorrhagica. Fluid or blood accumulation was first detected approximately 24 hours (day 1) after ovulation. Blood accumulation continued, and the central cavity increased in size to maximal size at 72 hours (day 3); the maximum size of the central cavity varied from 8 to 38 mm in diameter. Organization of the accumulated blood into a clot was first noticed on approximately day 2 (44 hours) by detection of echoic spots, bands, or a network of fibrinlike material (see Fig. 17.1; early diestrus). Throughout diestrus, the blood clot becomes progressively more organized and smaller in diameter (see Fig. 17.1; mid-diestrus), but it is usually distinguishable throughout the luteal phase (see Fig. 17.1; late diestrus) (2). Continued maintenance of the luteal gland during early pregnancy allows the central blood

clot eventually to become indistinguishable; luteal glands that initially formed a central cavity may become relatively uniform, resembling luteal glands that developed without a central cavity.

The overall size of corpora lutea that develop a central cavity is usually larger than that of corpora lutea without a central cavity. Averaged over days 0 to 5, corpora lutea with a central cavity had a mean diameter of 32.8 mm, whereas corpora lutea without a central cavity had a mean diameter of 26.0 mm. Despite the difference in the overall size of luteal glands with or without a central cavity, no difference in absolute luteal tissue area was noted after subtraction of the nonluteinized area of the central cavity. Correspondingly, profiles of daily plasma concentrations of progesterone (36), the degree of luteal tissue echocity (2, 19), and the length of the interovulatory interval were similar between the two luteal morphologies. In spite of distinct morphologic differences, the presence of a central cavity has been suggested to be functionally incidental (2). Irrespective of the type of luteal morphology, mean plasma progesterone concentrations increased on day 1, continued to increase on day 5, and reached an apparent plateau at day 6. The plateau extended from day 6 through day 11, with high diestrus concentrations of progesterone maintained at approximately 11 ng/mL. After day 11, concentrations declined to a nadir at day 17 (Fig. 17.4).

The association of form (morphology) and function (physiology) of the equine corpus luteum during the luteal phase approximates a growth stage during early diestrus (days 0 to 5), a maturity stage during mid-diestrus (days 6 to 11), and a regression stage during late diestrus (days 12 to 17), as shown in Figure 17.4. Daily concentrations of plasma progesterone are closely associated with daily

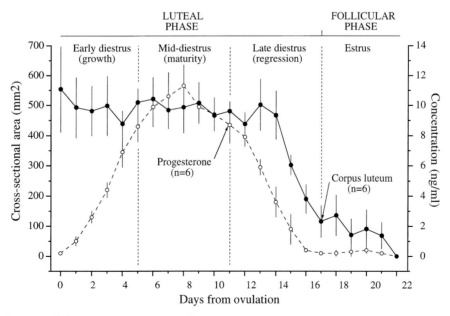

Figure 17.4. Mean (± SEM) cross-sectional area of the primary corpus luteum and circulating concentrations of progesterone during various stages of the estrous cycle. Values were normalized to a mean interovulatory interval of 22 days.

changes in luteal tissue area. Because of the high degree of parallelism between luteal morphology (luteal tissue area) and function (progesterone production), ultrasonographic determination of luteal tissue area may be used as an indirect measure of luteal productivity (i.e., progesterone-producing capability). Regardless of luteal gland morphology, maximal luteal area is attained by approximately day 5 or 6 concurrent with maximal progesterone output. However, functional regression of the corpus luteum precedes morphologic regression by 2 days; that is, progesterone begins to decline after approximately day 12, whereas luteal area begins to decline after approximately day 14. Hence, the lag time between a decrease in progesterone and a corresponding decrease in luteal tissue area bears consideration when one attempts to use luteal tissue area as an indirect measure of luteal productivity.

Ovarian irregularities are defined as a deviation from the conventional dynamics of ovarian function (1). Some irregularities include multiple primary ovulations, secondary ovulations, rupture of small or regressing follicles, and hemorrhagic follicles. Multiple primary ovulations (i.e., double synchronous or asynchronous ovulations) may occur simultaneously or 1 to 2 days apart in association with estrus (i.e., follicular phase), whereas secondary ovulations occur more than 2 days after the primary ovulation in association with elevated levels of progesterone during diestrus (i.e., luteal phase). In addition to ovulation of large secondary follicles during diestrus, apparent rupture of small or regressing follicles (17 to 28 mm in diameter) also has been reported; however, no detectable corpora lutea formed after the disappearance of such follicles (37).

Hemorrhagic follicles bear a distinct resemblance to the original description of "autumn" follicles (38, 39) and are likely one and the same. As the name implies, autumn follicles were reported to occur more commonly during the months of October and November (38); however, a seasonal incidence is equivocal (1). Hemorrhagic follicles are an ovarian irregularity well described (40, 41) in ultrasonographic studies. Because some of the developmental characteristics of a hemorrhagic follicle are similar to those exhibited by a corpus hemorrhagicum, awareness of differential characteristics using ultrasonography is essential. Hemorrhagic follicles appear to result from a failure to ovulate, as indicated by 1) a dramatic increase in size (60 to 90 mm in diameter) without a preceding decrease, 2) fluidity of antral contents for several days (scattered free-floating echoic specks that swirl during ballottement), and 3) maintenance of a relatively spherical shape during increasing organization and loss of fluidity of antral contents (not gourdlike in appearance as contents become increasingly echoic from an increase and organization of fibrinous tissue). Ultrasonographic morphology of hemorrhagic follicles has indicated the formation of an outer wall 4 to 7 mm thick (40) that may be luteinized tissue. Although investigators have indicated that some hemorrhagic follicles produce progesterone (5), critical studies to evaluate proges-

terone productivity by these structures have not been done. Nevertheless, hemorrhagic follicles eventually regress, albeit gradually, and typically are no longer detected approximately 1 month after formation.

Pregnancy

Prevention of regression of the primary corpus luteum in the presence of an embryo is often called maternal recognition of pregnancy, but it may be more appropriately termed *luteal response to pregnancy* (1). Unlike other domestic species, the mare exhibits a first, second, and third luteal response to pregnancy. The first luteal response to pregnancy is *continued maintenance of the primary corpus luteum* during the expected time of luteal regression in a nonpregnant mare. The second luteal response to pregnancy is *resurgence of the primary corpus luteum,* and the third response is *development of supplemental corpora lutea,* both occurring during the period of eCG production.

An ovarian source of progesterone is essential for maintenance of pregnancy until approximately days 50 to 70. Thereafter, the fetal–placental unit begins producing sufficient progestogens to support pregnancy (42). Progesterone from the primary corpus luteum is needed for physical embryo–uterine interactions (i.e., embryo mobility, fixation, and orientation) and uterine secretions, whereas the functional role of supplemental corpora lutea is not clearly understood. It is not unusual to find mares at 60 to 160 days of pregnancy without supplemental corpora lutea.

Contrary to the dogma that persisted for approximately 40 years (1930 to 1970), the primary corpus luteum of pregnancy does not regress at the end of the first month (2). Instead, the primary corpus luteum regresses along with supplemental corpora lutea by days 180 to 200 of gestation (approximately 6 months). In a landmark experiment (43), the primary corpus luteum was injected with India ink by laparotomy to allow differentiation of the primary corpus luteum from supplemental corpora lutea. Subsequently, mares were slaughtered on selected days of pregnancy (24 to 220 days), and their ovaries were collected at necropsy. Although there was a gradual, progressive decrease in weight of the primary corpus luteum after approximately day 60, the primary corpus luteum and supplemental corpora lutea were well vascularized, as indicated by their pink coloration. In a separate study (44), both primary and supplemental luteal tissues taken from mares at day 100 were capable of in vitro production of progesterone. By approximately 180 to 220 days of gestation, all luteal glands were in advanced stages of regression, as indicated by their orange-brown and pale coloration (43). In vitro production of progesterone also decreased markedly after day 160 (45).

The use of ultrasonography to study luteal development during pregnancy has received limited attention. In two separate studies (20, 22), ultrasonography was used to characterize the first and second luteal responses to pregnancy (Fig. 17.5). Daily changes in mean diameter of the primary corpus luteum and circulating concentrations of proges-

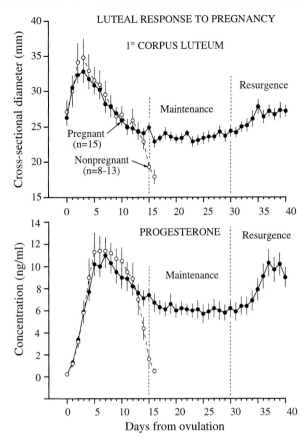

Figure 17.5. Mean (± SEM) cross-sectional diameter of the primary (1°) corpus luteum and circulating concentrations of progesterone in nonpregnant mares (open circles) during the luteal phase and in pregnant mares (closed circles) during luteal maintenance and resurgence.

terone were similar between nonpregnant and pregnant mares for days 0 to 14. Divergence in luteal diameter and plasma progesterone concentrations was evident at day 15. Luteal diameter and systemic progesterone levels continued to decrease in nonpregnant mares, but, in pregnant mares, the corpus luteum and progesterone concentrations were maintained (*first luteal response to pregnancy*). Although luteal diameter and progesterone concentrations were reduced in pregnant mares, they were maintained at an apparent plateau until approximately day 30. Thereafter, both luteal diameter and progesterone concentrations increased. The increase in systemic levels of progesterone was not confounded by the contribution of additional progesterone from the formation of supplemental luteal tissue; secondary and accessory luteal glands formed after day 40. The phenomenon of a decrease followed by an increase in luteal diameter, concurrent with similar changes in progesterone output during pregnancy, is referred to as resurgence of the primary corpus luteum (*second luteal response to pregnancy*). Investigators hypothesized (20) that resurgence of the primary corpus luteum occurred in pregnant mares between days 30 and 40 and that the resurgence was a response to the release of eCG into the circulation. When plasma concentrations of progesterone were normalized to

first detection of systemic eCG levels (mean, day 35), an increase in progesterone was not evident before eCG was detected. However, on the first day that eCG was detected, progesterone concentrations increased and were significantly elevated by 2 days after eCG detection. A corresponding increase in luteal area paralleled the increase in progesterone. Further support of the hypothesis was obtained by comparing pregnant mares and mares with embryo loss in which the primary corpus luteum was maintained (21). Both the size of the corpus luteum and systemic progesterone levels were greater on day 36 in mares that maintained pregnancy than in mares with embryo loss. Because embryo loss occurred before endometrial cup formation, the primary corpus luteum did not resurge but gradually regressed in the absence of eCG. In summary, form and function of the primary corpus luteum of pregnancy are similar to those observed during diestrus over approximately days 0 to 14; thereafter, luteal regression continues in nonpregnant mares, but is abated in pregnant mares. At approximately day 30, resurgence of the primary corpus luteum occurs in response to eCG.

Formation of supplemental luteal glands in pregnant mares occurs during eCG production (*third luteal response to pregnancy*) (1). Initially, formation of supplemental luteal glands results from luteinization of ovulatory follicles (*secondary corpora lutea*; Fig. 17.6, *upper panel*) and, later, from luteinization of unovulated follicles (*accessory corpora lutea*; Fig. 17.6, *lower panel*). Based on transrectal palpation, the mean number of days to the first secondary ovulation was 56.2 (range, 34 to 70 days) and to the last ovulation was 74.1 (43). Luteal gland formation after approximately day 70 resulted primarily from luteinization of anovulatory follicles. The mean number of supplemental corpora lutea was 2.8 at 70 days and 10.2 at 140 days of pregnancy. Not only is eCG involved in the formation of supplemental corpora lutea, but also it assists in maintaining their function. Addition of eCG to cultured slices of luteal tissue from primary, secondary, and accessory corpora lutea resulted in a significant increase in progesterone production that was similar among the three types of luteal tissue (44). Although the gross morphologic appearance of supplemental luteal glands has been described using excised ovaries (43), information regarding supplemental luteal gland development in situ using ultrasonography is scarce. Ultrasonographically, secondary corpora lutea appear to go through a developmental stage similar to that of the primary corpus luteum (see Fig. 17.6, *upper panel*). Some secondary corpora lutea are solid, whereas others form central blood-filled cavities (corpora hemorrhagica) of various sizes and shapes (43). Because accessory corpora lutea develop from unovulated follicles, they inherently have a central fluid-filled cavity (see Fig. 17.6, *lower panel*). In both secondary corpora lutea with a central cavity and accessory corpora lutea, the central cavity becomes increasingly organized concurrent with luteinization; that is, the central cavity decreases in size and becomes relatively solid.

Supplemental Corpora Lutea

with central cavity   *without central cavity*

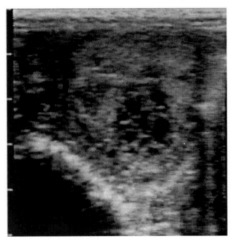 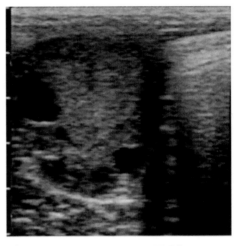

Secondary corpora lutea (< Day 70)

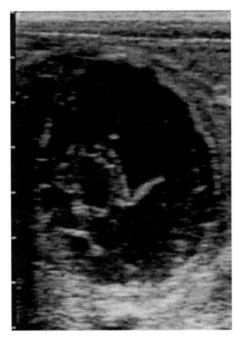 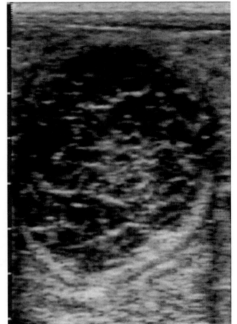

Accessory corpora lutea (> Day 70)

Figure 17.6. Ultrasonograms of secondary corpora lutea (*upper panel*) and accessory corpora lutea (*lower panel*) from pregnant mares on different days of gestation. The scale bars at the left portion of the ultrasonograms represent 10-mm increments. Note the morphologic diversity (with and without a central cavity) of supplemental luteal glands that result from ovulatory follicles (secondary corpora lutea) compared with the consistent morphology (that is, central cavity) of luteal glands that result from luteinization of unovulated follicles (accessory corpora lutea).

The extent of follicular activity during early pregnancy is closely associated with the extent of formation of supplemental corpora lutea, and it varies greatly within and among mares (1). Consequently, ultrasonographic monitoring of individual structures in the maternal ovaries during supplemental luteal gland formation can be complicated; ultrasonographically, the primary corpus luteum cannot be differentiated from secondary corpora lutea (without a central cavity) with a single examination. In this regard, examination before luteal gland formation and frequent or periodic examinations thereafter may assist in maintaining individual identity of ovarian structures. In addition, ultrasonographic images of the ovaries may be recorded and stored on videotape for later scrutiny. Diagrams depicting relative location, size, and morphology of individual luteal glands can be made for each ovary on successive days. Quantitative data can also be generated by determining luteal area, estimating the percentage of echocity, assigning gray-scale values, or digitizing for computerized pixel analysis.

SUMMARY

Ultrasonographic imaging allows immediate detection and assessment of luteal glands. Morphologic changes (size, echointensity) associated with luteal gland development closely parallel physiologic changes (progesterone production) during the estrous cycle and early pregnancy. As such, gray-scale ultrasonography is an invaluable diagnostic and research tool. Computerized image analysis and color flow Doppler ultrasonography are newer technologies that can complement conventional ultrasonographic imaging in domestic species. Through the use of these technologies, clinicians and scientists can objectively evaluate ovarian function in situ. Previous concepts of luteal dynamics in the mare are being challenged by critically derived information. Traditional terminology is being replaced with words and phases that will communicate and differentiate more accurately typical or atypical luteal growth, maturation, and regression. This new knowledge base will provide veterinarians with information to update reproductive management practices in the mare and will provide researchers with alternative modeling systems to investigate ovarian dynamics further in equids and other species, including humans.

REFERENCES

1. Ginther OJ. Reproductive biology of the mare: basic and applied aspects. 2nd ed. Cross Plains, WI: Equiservices, 1992:1–642.
2. Pierson RA, Ginther OJ. Ultrasonic evaluation of the corpus luteum of the mare. Theriogenology 1985;23:795–806.
3. Ginther OJ. Ultrasonic imaging of equine ovarian follicles and corpora lutea. Vet Clin North Am Equine Pract 1988;4:197–213.
4. Ginther OJ. Ultrasonic imaging and reproductive events in the mare. Cross Plains, WI: Equiservices, 1986:1–378.
5. Ginther OJ. Reproductive biology of the mare: basic and applied aspects. Cross Plains, WI: Equiservices, 1979:1–412.
6. Ginther OJ. Prolonged luteal activity in mares: a semantic quagmire. Equine Vet J 1990;22:152–156.
7. Hughes JP, et al. Pyometra in the mare. J Reprod Fertil Suppl 1979;27:321–329.
8. Ginther OJ, et al. Embryonic loss in mares: pregnancy rate, length of the interovulatory interval and progesterone concentrations associated with loss during days 11 to 15. Theriogenology 1985;24:409–417.
9. Adams GP, Kastelic JP, Bergfelt DR, et al. Effect of uterine inflammation and ultrasonically detected uterine pathology on fertility in the mare. J Reprod Fertil Suppl 1987;35:445–454.
10. Newcombe JR. Identification of the corpus luteum in nonpregnant mares at days 13 to 16 using ultrasound. J Equine Vet Sci 1994;14:655–657.
11. Bergfelt DR, Ginther OJ. Embryo loss following GnRH-induced ovulation in anovulatory mares. Theriogenology 1992;38:33–43.
12. McKinnon AO. Reproductive ultrasonography. In: Rantanen NW, McKinnon AO, eds. Equine diagnostic ultrasonography. Philadelphia: Williams & Wilkins, 1997.
13. Ginther OJ, Pierson RA. Ultrasonic anatomy of equine ovaries. Theriogenology 1984;21:471–483.
14. Ginther OJ, Pierson RA. Ultrasonic evaluation of the mare reproductive tract: ovaries. J Equine Vet Sci 1984;4:11–16.
15. Squires EL, Cook NL. Ultrasound-guided follicular aspiration. In: Rantanen NW, McKinnon AO, eds. Equine diagnostic ultrasonography. Philadelphia: Williams & Wilkins, 1997.
16. Ravindra JP, Rawlings NC, Evans ACO, et al. Ultrasonographic study of ovarian follicular dynamics in the ewe. J Reprod Fertil 1994;101:501–509.
17. Adams GP, Evans ACO, Rawlings NC. Follicular waves and circulating gonadotrophins in 8-month-old prepubertal heifers. J Reprod Fertil 1993;100:27–33.
18. Townson DH, Ginther OJ. The development of fluid-filled luteal glands in mares. Anim Reprod Sci 1988;17:155–163.
19. Townson DH, Ginther OJ. Ultrasonic echogenicity of developing corpora lutea in pony mares. Anim Reprod Sci 1989;20:143–153.
20. Bergfelt DR, Pierson RA, Ginther OJ. Resurgence of the primary corpus luteum during pregnancy in the mare. Anim Reprod Sci 1989;21:261–270.
21. Bergfelt DR, Woods JA, Ginther OJ. Role of the embryonic vesicle and progesterone in embryonic loss in mares. J Reprod Fertil 1992;95:339–347.
22. Bergfelt DR, Ginther OJ. Ovarian, uterine and embryo dynamics in horses versus ponies. J Equine Vet Sci 1996;16:27–33.
23. Pierson RA, Adams GP. Computer-assisted image analysis, diagnostic ultrasonography and ovulation induction: strange bedfellows. Theriogenology 1995;43:105–112.
24. Adams GP, Pierson RA. Bovine model for study of ovarian follicular dynamics in humans. Theriogenology 1995;43:113–120.
25. Townson DH, Ginther OJ. Size and shape changes in the preovulatory follicle in mares based on digital analysis of ultrasonic images. Anim Reprod Sci 1989;21:63–71.
26. Burns PN. Doppler flow estimations in the fetal and maternal circulation: principles, techniques and some limitations. In: Maulik D, McNellis D, eds. Doppler ultrasound measurements of maternal–fetal hemodynamics. New York: Perinatology Press, 1987.
27. Omoto R, Chihiro K. Physics and instrumentation of Doppler color flow mapping. Echocardiography 1987;4:467–483.
28. Meyer WJ, Jaffe R. Basic principles of Doppler ultrasonography. In: Jaffe R, Warsof S, eds. Color Doppler imaging in obstetrics and gynecology. New York: McGraw-Hill, 1992:1–16.

29. Backstrom T, Nakata M, Pierson RA. Ultrasonography of normal and aberrant luteogenesis. In: Jaffe R, Pierson RA, Abramowicz JS, eds. Imaging in infertility and reproductive endocrinology. Philadelphia: JB Lippincott, 1994:143–154.

30. Pierson RA. From ovulation to implantation. In: Jaffe R, Warsof S, eds. Color Doppler imaging in obstetrics and gynecology. New York: McGraw-Hill, 1992:35–60.

31. Pierson RA, Chizen DR. Transvaginal ultrasonographic assessment of normal and aberrant ovulation. In: Jaffe R, Pierson RA, Abramowicz JS, eds. Imaging in infertility and reproductive endocrinology. Philadelphia: JB Lippincott, 1994:129–142.

32. Harrison RJ. The early development of the corpus luteum in the mare. J Anat 1946;80:160–166.

33. Van Niekerk CH, Morgenthal JC, Gerneke WH. Relationship between the morphology of and progesterone production by the corpus luteum of the mare. J Reprod Fertil Suppl 1975;23: 171–175.

34. Watson ED, Sertich PL. Secretion of prostaglandins and progesterone by the cells from corpora lutea of mares. J Reprod Fertil 1990;88:223–229.

35. Carnevale EM. Folliculogenesis and ovulation. In: Rantanen NW, McKinnon AO, eds. Equine diagnostic ultrasonography. Philadelphia: Lea & Febiger, 1995.

36. Townson DH, Pierson RA, Ginther OJ. Characterization of plasma progesterone concentrations for two distinct luteal morphologies in mares. Theriogenology 1989;32:197–204.

37. Sirois J, Ball BA, Fortune JE. Patterns of growth and regression of ovarian follicles during the oestrous cycle and after hemiovariectomy in mares. Equine Vet J 1989;8(Suppl):43–48.

38. Burkhardt J. Some clinical problems of horse breeding. Vet Rec 1948;60:243–248.

39. Stangroom JE, Weevers RG. Anticoagulant activity of equine follicular fluid. J Reprod Fertil 1962;3:269–282.

40. Carnevale EM, Squires EL, McKinnon AO, et al. Effect of human chorionic gonadotropin on time to ovulation and luteal function in transitional mares. J Equine Vet Sci 1989;9:27–29.

41. Ginther OJ, Pierson RA. Regular and irregular characteristics of ovulation and the interovulatory interval in mares. J Equine Vet Sci 1989;9:4–12.

42. Holtan DW, Squires EL, Lapin DR, et al. Effect of ovariectomy on pregnancy in mares. J Reprod Fertil Suppl 1979;27:457–463.

43. Squires EL, Douglas RH, Steffenhagen WP, et al. Ovarian changes during the estrous cycle and pregnancy in mares. J Anim Sci 1974; 38:330–338.

44. Squires EL, Stevens WB, Pickett BW, et al. Role of pregnant mare serum gonadotropin in luteal function of pregnant mares. Am J Vet Res 1979;40:889–891.

45. Martin JL, Salteil A, Evans JW. Progesterone synthesis by different types of corpora lutea during the first 198 days of pregnancy. J Equine Vet Sci 1989;9:84–87.

18. Ovarian Abnormalities

ANGUS O. McKINNON

Recognition of when an ovary has an abnormality or is abnormal may not always be obvious. Examination must include relevant history and seasonal information. Some cases of apparent abnormalities are reflections of hormonal status, that is, transitional ovaries early in the breeding season or accessory corpora lutea in pregnant mares between days 40 and 120. The ability to noninvasively examine the mare's ovaries using ultrasonography permits diagnosis of various forms of ovarian abnormalities and pathology. However, the principles of good examination should remind us to consider the whole animal, that is, to interpret not just obvious abnormalities but the behavior of the animal, to examine both ovaries, and to use ancillary diagnostic tests such as hormonal analysis before reaching an accurate diagnosis. Some ovarian abnormalities that have been recognized with ultrasonography are (a) functional irregularities, (b) physical irregularities, (c) neoplasms, and (d) periovarian abnormalities.

FUNCTIONAL IRREGULARITIES

Multiple Preovulatory Follicles

Since the mare normally ovulates only one follicle during each estrous cycle, multiple ovulations may be considered an abnormality. Difficulty in interpretation of terminology may influence previous reports. We record double or multiple ovulation as being primary when they are 2 days or less apart. An exception to this is the occasional split cycle wherein mares will ovulate a second follicle 4 or more days after the first, while continuing to demonstrate estrus in the intervening period. In our experience with these cases, the first ovulation is unlikely to be fertile. Even with ultrasonography it may be difficult to determine that a second follicle is likely to continue and grow and increase the likelihood of twins (see Chapter 10). Breed influences the incidence of multiple ovulation. For example, Thoroughbreds, warm bloods, and draft mares have been shown to have the highest incidence of multiple ovulation; whereas quarter horses, Appaloosas, and ponies have the lowest incidence with Standardbreds being intermittent (1). Multiple, preovulatory follicles or ovulations may be particularly difficult to detect by rectal examination, especially when they are in close apposition on one ovary. In one study more embryos were obtained from multiple ovulating mares that bilaterally ovulated than from those in which multiple ovulations were unilateral (2). Multiple ovulation appears to be quite repeatable, as mares previously diagnosed as having twins have a greater chance of them occurring again (3) (Chapter 10),

and if the previous cycle was associated with a double ovulation, then the probability of subsequent cycle multiple ovulation was doubled (4). Multiple ovulation is less common in the first postpartum ovulatory period (4); however, they increase with age (5). Although improved nutrition did not increase the rates of multiple ovulation (6), it did appear to be related to a better display of estrus receptivity. Originally, twins were hypothesized to have occurred more frequently from asynchronous ovulations (7). This author found double ovulation and twins were seen more frequently in barren mares (11 and 6%, respectively) compared with lactating mares (5 and 1%, respectively) and that nine twin pregnancies from 32 mares were associated with ovulations 2 days apart (asynchronous) compared with 0 out of 19 for synchronous ovulations. Many of these original observations were made prior to ultrasonography, and as a good example of these inherent diagnostic difficulties, the same author quoted 70% of twins arriving from one detected ovulation (based on analysis of multiple veterinarians' breeding-farm records) (1, 7). Subsequently, it was shown that twins were as likely to result from synchronous versus asynchronous ovulation (8) and that pregnancy rate per follicle was identical for double ovulations on opposite ovaries to that obtained per cycle from single ovulations, but was higher than the pregnancy rate per follicle when double ovulations occurred on the same ovary. In unilateral, double ovulators the lower, day-11 pregnancy rate per ovulation compared with bilateral ovulators and single ovulators was attributable to a greater frequency of mares with no embryonic vesicles rather than to a greater frequency of mares with one vesicle (9).

Multiple ovulations (Figs. 18.1 and 18.2) should be encouraged when ultrasonography is available to eliminate one of two developing vesicles at 14 days, because multiple ovulations increase the probability of conception (10). The ability to collect and transfer multiple embryos from a donor mare has the potential of improving efficiency of an equine embryo-transfer program. The viability of embryos collected from naturally and induced, multiply ovulating mares versus naturally, singly ovulating mares is similar (2). Recovery of embryos from singly ovulating mares was 53% compared with 106% for naturally, doubly ovulating mares. Pregnancy rates, 50 days after surgical transfer, were 68 and 129%, respectively. Treatment of normally, singly ovulating mares with equine pituitary extract resulted in two embryos recovered per donor compared with 0.65 for control (2). Nonsurgical pregnancy rates for embryos collected from superovulated mares were identical to those obtained for untreated controls.

233

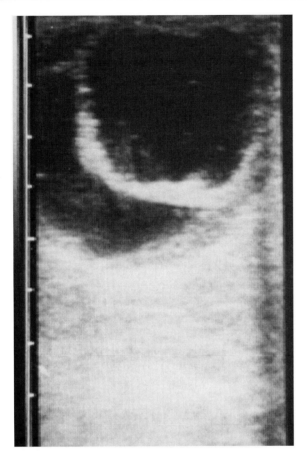

Figure 18.1. Ultrasonographic image of double preovulatory follicles. (From A.O. McKinnon and J. L. Voss, eds. Equine reproduction. Philadelphia: Lea & Febiger, 1993; p. 295, with permission of Williams & Wilkins, Baltimore.)

Follicles in the Transition

During the nonbreeding season many mares enter a period of anestrus defined by lack of ovarian activity, associated decreased production, and storage of gonadotropin-releasing hormone (GnRH) (11). As transition back into the cycling season progresses, multiple follicles grow and regress (Fig. 18.3). Later, when luteinizing hormone (LH) increases (12, 13), ovulation ensues. This period of follicular waxing and waning has occasionally been referred to as cystic ovarian disease. This term is unfortunate, and its use should be discouraged as it does not accurately reflect the mare's ovarian status and has nothing in common with cystic ovarian disease recognized in other species (14). Occasionally, the shape and echo texture of the uterus may be useful in determining if the mare has entered the cyclic season. When ovulation has occurred, even if the mare is currently in estrus, the mare's reproductive tract has a more pronounced tubularity to it when compared with the atonic anestrous or transitional mare's uterus.

Diestrus Ovulation

The normal cycle involves an ovulation during estrus with further follicular waves in diestrus. Occasionally, ovulation of a large follicle occurs in diestrus associated with progesterone concentrations >1 ng/ml (Fig. 18.4). This was first reported by Hughes et al. in California in 1972 (15). They demonstrated that the mares were not in estrus and had a tight, pale cervix. In addition, mares had normal progesterone secretion from the diestrous ovulation (15) and could be come pregnant if artificially inseminated (16). There is some disagreement about the rate of diestrous ovulation. Originally, they were reported as occurring in 21% of cycles (15); however, ultrasonography has suggested the rate may be quite lower, around 4% (17). It is also possible there may be breed differences to explain this discrepancy. Diestrous ovulations are important only for their effect on prolonging luteal activity and increasing the interovulatory interval.

Ovarian Inactivity

Anestrus-associated ovarian inactivity is normal during the nonbreeding season; however, it is quite uncommon 1 to 2 months on either side of the summer solstice. If the mare has a history of never producing a foal, then gonadal dysgenesis may be suspected (Fig. 18.5). The most common chromosomal abnormality detected is the 63 XO karyotype (18–20). The common expression reported is a small mare

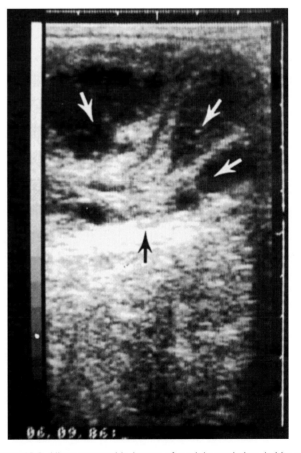

Figure 18.2. Ultrasonographic image of a triple ovulation *(white arrows)*. All ovulations have tracts to the ovulation fossa *(black arrow)*. (From A.O. McKinnon and J. L. Voss, eds. Equine reproduction. Philadelphia: Lea & Febiger, 1993; p. 295, with permission of Williams & Wilkins, Baltimore.)

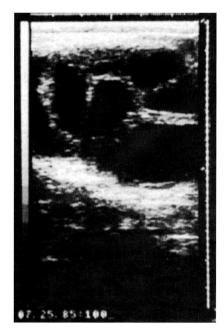

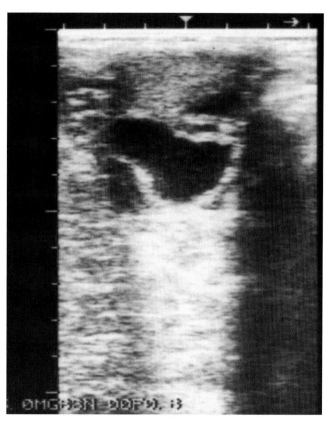

Figure 18.3. Ultrasonographic characteristics of multiple follicles in an ovary of a mare in transitional estrus. (From A.O. McKinnon and J. L. Voss, eds. Equine reproduction. Philadelphia: Lea & Febiger, 1993; p. 285, with permission of Williams & Wilkins, Baltimore.)

Figure 18.4. Active corpus luteum and ovulating follicle present together in a mare undergoing a diestrous ovulation.

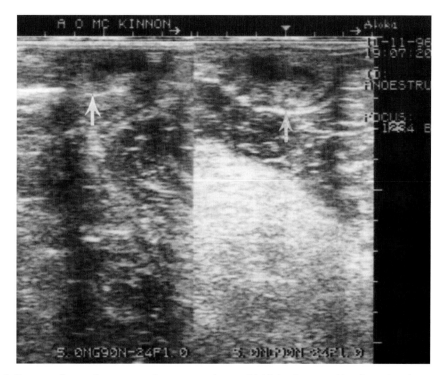

Figure 18.5. Split-screen image from a mare in anestrus. Arrows highlight the ventral borders of each ovary. This image came from a 6-year-old mare with a history of never becoming pregnant despite three seasons at stud. The mare had demonstrated variable and subtle signs of estrus. The mare was presented at the height of the breeding season and so was most likely a mare with gonadal dysgenesis. Reevaluation 2 months later revealed the same structures.

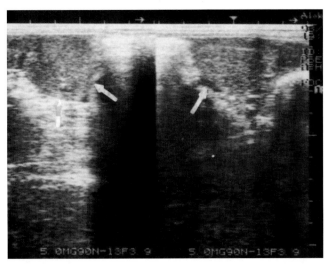

Figure 18.6. Intra-abdominal scan produced these images of a left and right testes in a case of male pseudohermaphrodite. The animal was retained as a teaser.

with inactive pea-sized ovaries with a dilated, flaccid cervix. In our experience the size of the mare has not been always useful in predicting the mare was a 63 XO. Other chromosomal abnormalities occur and have varying expressions of ovarian activity (21–26) and even fertility (24).

> An inherited genetic disorder causes XY embryos of the horse to develop as mares. On the basis of our study of 38 such mares, we have identified four grades or classes of XY sex reversal according to this scheme: class I, nearly normal female, of which some are fertile; class II, female with gonadal dysgenesis, normal mullerian development; class III, intersex mare with gonadal dysgenesis, abnormal mullerian development, enlarged clitoris; class IV, virilized intersex characterized by high levels of testosterone. In general, class I and class II mares were typed H-Y antigen-negative, whereas class III and class IV mares were typed H-Y antigen-positive (24).

The term of gonadal dysgenesis means defective embryonic development; it does not indicate the type of disorder or whether the defective gonad is an ovary or testes (14). The term includes gonadal aplasia, agenesis, and hypoplasia, as well as hermaphroditic and streak gonads (14). Male pseudohermaphrodites externally are females (64 XX), but have testicles that are almost exclusively abdominal cryptorchids. Behavior varies, but mostly is stallion like. The vulva is often displaced ventrally with varying degrees of enlargement of the clitoris to one resembling a short penis. There is one report on a stallion that sired 15 intersex foals from different mares (27) (quoted in Ref. 14). Multiple cases of male pseudohermaphrodites have been identified at the GVEH, and in one instance a familial distribution was suspected with three miniature pony siblings affected (JE Axon, personal communication). It is possible in this latter instance that the condition was really testicular feminization, which is an inherited form of male pseudoher-

maphroditism that is transmitted from females to half of their offspring (14). In all cases of male pseudohermaphrodites that we have seen, the classical echo texture of testicular tissue was useful in confirming the diagnosis (Fig. 18.6). Occasionally, chronic anabolic steroid administration may cause failure to cycle, male behavior, and an enlarged clitoris. Most of these cases can be differentiated using ultrasonography.

If the mare has produced a foal before, then some form of acquired abnormality should be suspected. In older mares with long hair coats (hirsutism) (Fig. 18.7), it is common to find ovarian inactivity due to an adenoma of the pars intermedia. Other conditions to consider would be ovarian neoplasia (see later). Adenomas of the pars intermedia of the hypophysis are manifested primarily in middle-aged to older horses as lethargy, muscle wasting, polyuria, polydipsia, hirsutism, recurrent infections, skin abnormalities, voracious appetite, and recurrent bouts of laminitis. In addition, numerous clinical pathology variations are reported in horses and ponies (28). Hyperglycemia, hyperlipemia, neutrophilia, lymphopenia, electrolyte alterations, and anemia or chronic disease are predominate findings in many cases (28). Occasionally, affected animals will show clinical signs with normal complete blood counts and equine chemistry panel results (29). Many pituitary function tests such as adrenocorticotropin hormone (ACTH) stimulation, thyroid-stimulating hormone (TSH) stimulation, dexamethasone suppression, and glucose tolerance, as well as measurements for proopiolipomelanocortin peptides (POLMC), melanocyte-stimulating hormone (MSH), or ACTH, are used to aid diagnosis (29). The treatment for laboratory-confirmed cases has included nutritional and management support, as well as drug therapy. Cyproheptadine, an antiserotonergic drug, has had limited success. The dopaminergic agonist agents—bromocriptine and pergolide—have been used, but with a concern for potential vasoconstriction

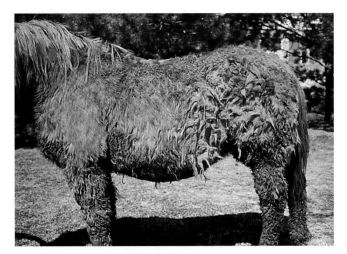

Figure 18.7. Abnormally long hair coat, termed hirsutism, may alert the clinician of a suspected pituitary adenoma. It is quite common for these mares to have ovarian inactivity.

and the possible exacerbation of laminitis at recommended doses. Additionally, long-term therapy at the present recommended dosage can be cost prohibitive. The adrenocorticolytic drug mitotane, or op'-DDD, although effective in small animals, has not been of benefit in horses (29). Recently, a study of the efficacy of low-dose pergolide therapy in horses and ponies with adenomas of the pituitary gland concluded that it was a safe and efficacious treatment (29).

Ovulation Failure

Once mares have entered the ovulatory season, they are unlikely to fail to ovulate and then regress. A few exceptions exist, and they are generally heralded by an enlarging ovary (see below). Prior to the advent of ultrasonography, mares frequently were reported to have undergone follicular atresia during the later part of estrus, and accompanying the regression of the follicle was a change to diestrous behavior. Ultrasonography demonstrated that in these cases it was the formation of a corpus hemorrhagicum that had similar physical characteristics to the previously identified follicle that had created the confusion. Prior to the first ovulation in the recognized ovulatory season, many mares will undergo a transition or recrudescence to cyclicity. This period is well documented for large follicles failing to ovulate and becoming atretic.

Prolonged Luteal Phase

Rectal palpation of the mature CL, although possible on occasion, is generally unrewarding. Prolonged maintenance of the CL, sometimes termed "pseudopregnancy," can be differentiated from an anovulatory or anestrous condition by ultrasonography. However, it is not possible, apart from serial examination, to differentiate a prolonged CL from a diestrous ovulation or even a silent heat with ovulation. In those cases, rather than a failure of response to PGF$_{2\alpha}$, or failure of, it may be that the CL of another ovulation is too immature to respond. The CL is first visible on the day of ovulation (day 0) as a strongly echogenic, circumscribed mass of tissue (30) (see chapter 17). The echogenicity gradually decreases throughout diestrus. However, just prior to regression of the CL, echogenicity increases. This may reflect changes in luteal hemodynamics. In one study (30), the CL could be observed for a mean of 17 days (n = 55). On occasion, the presence of a CL may be seen as a circumscribed, highly echogenic area of tissue in the ovary in mares that failed to return to estrus at the expected time. Prolonged maintenance of the CL is more commonly recognized in normally cycling mares that have been bred. Generally, the mare fails to return to estrus at the expected time, even though she is not pregnant (31). Perhaps pregnancy is initiated and the embryo prevents secretion of PGF$_{2\alpha}$ prior to undergoing early embryonic death. In one study (32) removal of the conceptus early in pregnancy (days 7 to 11) re-

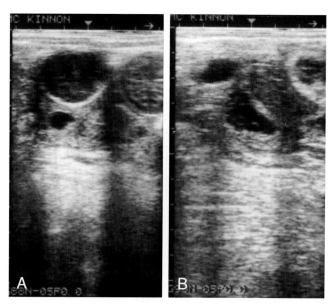

Figure 18.8. A and **B,** Ultrasonographic images from a mare with secondary and accessory CL that develop in pregnancy between days 40 and 120.

sulted in return to estrus at the expected time or slightly earlier, while removal later (days 14 to 16) resulted in prolonged maintenance of the CL or pseudopregnancy. In our practice ultrasonography became more commonly accepted due to our abilities to diagnose retained CLs and predict the mare's response to PGF$_{2\alpha}$. These stage-of-cycle exams are now routinely performed on all mares arriving at stud late in the breeding season and on any mares not showing heat within 3 weeks of arriving.

Secondary and Accessory Corpora Lutea

The initial response of luteal tissue to pregnancy is maintenance and resurgence of the primary CL (33). Later in pregnancy supplemental progesterone is provided by the secondary and accessory CL (34–36). Secondary CLs form by ovulation between days 40 and 70, and accessory CLs form from luteinization of follicles between days 40 and 150 (4). Ultrasonographically, the accessory CLs will appear unusual to people who have not had the opportunity to see or study them (Fig. 18.8). It has not been uncommon for mares to be referred with ovarian abnormalities when in fact it was accessory CLs that were making the ovaries look so different.

PHYSICAL IRREGULARITIES

Anovulatory Hemorrhagic Follicles

Anovulatory hemorrhagic follicles (AHFs) are the result of preovulatory follicles growing to an unusually large size (70 to 100 mm), failing to ovulate, then filling with blood, and gradually receding. This phenomenon may be recognized as

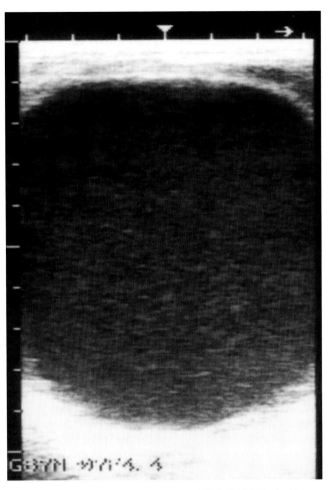

Figure 18.9. An anovulatory hemorrhagic follicle (AHF) filled with non-clotted blood.

an entity distinct from a corpus hemorrhagicum by its size and by ultrasonographic characteristics (Fig. 18.9). The blood in an AHF is distinctly echogenic, whereas normal development of the corpus hemorrhagicum results in a generally nonechogenic central blood clot (15 to 35 mm in diameter) (Fig. 18.10). However, both may have criss-crossing fibrinlike strands (Fig. 18.11). Strange things happen to follicles when blood enters, and presumably they are related to an anticoagulant identified in follicular fluid (37). If the mare has ovulated, then a corpus hemorrhagicum forms with a typical peripheral luteal gland. If the follicle has not ovulated by the time bleeding occurs, then the follicle becomes unusually large and echodense from the blood (Fig. 18.12). Careful bouncing of the follicle will elicit a swirling motion of the blood in the AHF. However, if an abnormal bleed has occurred after ovulation (within a few hours), there is not enough anticoagulant to stop clotting; thus the follicle will not have a swirling motion on bouncing (38). The formation of luteal tissue around the periphery of an AHF follicle is variable. We have noted in some mares the development and subsequent ovulation during the same es-

trous cycle of another follicle after formation of an anovulatory hemorrhagic follicle. In these mares behavioral signs of estrus persisted throughout an unusually long cycle of approximately 12 days, or 5 days after recognition of an anovulatory hemorrhagic follicle. Unfortunately, serum progesterone has not been measured in these animals. It is possible that AHFs are the previously reported "autumn" follicles, since most have occurred toward the end of the ovulatory season. Perhaps AHFs develop because of insufficient stimulus for ovulation from gonadotrophin-releasing hormones. After the last ovulation of the year, mares may develop a large follicle at the expected time, but the follicle does not ovulate and the mare enters the anovulatory season. Studies at the GVEH (39) have demonstrated that as the transition into the nonbreeding season begins, one of two scenarios occur. If a CL is present, it takes ~5 weeks for it to disappear. During this time the mare has a tight, closed cervix. The other scenario is that a primary follicle grows, but fails to ovulate and slowly (~3 weeks) regresses. After these changes have occurred, mares demonstrate no folding of the endometrium and have a flaccid cervix with little or no ovarian activity (39).

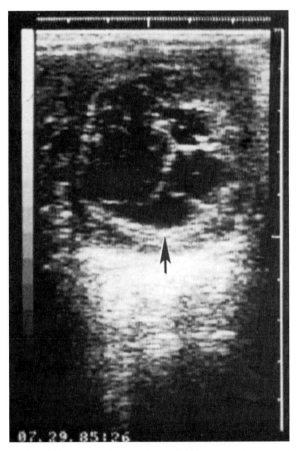

Figure 18.10. A 1-day-old corpus hemorrhagicum that has organizing criss-crossing fibrin strands. (From A.O. McKinnon and J. L. Voss, eds. Equine reproduction. Philadelphia: Lea & Febiger, 1993; p. 293, with permission of Williams & Wilkins, Baltimore.)

Luteinized Unruptured Follicles

Although anovulatory estrous periods are common during the anovulatory season, they are rare during the ovulatory season. An incidence of 3.1% was reported in Thoroughbreds and quarter horses (40), and even these may have been misdiagnosed because palpation was used. Luteinized, unruptured follicles have been reported in women and mice. This phenomenon is thought to be associated with reproductive senility. In one study that was initiated to recover embryos from oviducts of old, infertile mares, on some occasions, when the oviducts were flushed 2 days postovulation, no embryos or unfertilized ova were recovered, and from close examination of the ovulation fossa it appeared that recent ovulation had not occurred (41). Surgical removal of two ovaries from two mares confirmed that ovulation into the ovulation fossa had not occurred, and from prior ultrasonographic examination it appeared that an atypical corpus hemorrhagicum had formed (Fig. 18.13). Both mares ceased displaying signs of estrus within 1 day of the suspected ovulation. These structures may have been luteinized, unruptured follicles similar to those in

women and mice and may be associated with senility. Luteinization without ovulation occurs quite commonly in pregnant mares in association with formation of accessory CLs (42).

Follicular Cysts

Despite the lack of association with the bovine follicular cyst complex and our denial that the transitional mare has follicular cysts, we believe at the GVEH that occasionally mares form follicular cysts. They are not common; however, we have instances wherein a large (>70 mm) fluid-filled anechoic structure (Figs. 18.14 and 18.15) forms and persists. If nothing is done, occasionally they disappear, but the majority persist. Some mares continue to cycle on the other ovary and some do not. Our treatment has been to drain them via flank or vaginal ultrasonographic, needle-guided aspiration. After drainage is complete, they are injected with antibiotics. Unfortunately, we have not taken fluid for hormonal analysis. Some of these structures may be variations of a granulosa-theca cell tumor or other neoplasms (see below); however, some are simply follicular cysts, and removal of the fluid results in return to normal function. Failure to remove the fluid results in compression atrophy of the ovary. A syndrome of induced follicular cysts has been reported in the mare (43).

Epithelial Inclusion Cysts

Epithelial inclusion cysts arise from surface epithelium becoming pinched off from the ovarian surface and becoming embedded in the peripheral part of the ovarian cortex following ovulation (14). They form in proximity to the ovulation fossa in mares and have been termed "ovulation fossa cysts" (44, 45). They are seen in most ages of mares but were more common in mares greater than 15 years of age and not seen in young fillies (44). Grossly, they are variable in size, ranging from microscopic to a few millimeters; contain clear, serous fluid; and have a tough, white, fibrous capsule (Fig. 18.16). Ultrasonographically, the cysts can be recognized by their number and location (Figs. 18.17 and 18.18). Originally, we incorrectly identified them as multiple, small follicles and on occasions have even thought that they were early granulosa-theca cell tumors. Microscopically, the cysts are lined by ciliated, low, cuboidal cells, which suggested to Prickett that the cysts originated from the fimbrial epithelium (44). These cysts have also been referred to as "germinal inclusion cysts" (44); however, this is a misnomer (14).

Clinically, the cysts may interfere with fertility due to their location near the ovulation fossa. Occasionally, they provide obstruction or even obliteration of the ovulation fossa (44). In advanced cases the ovary may be obliterated (14).

Ovarian abscesses have been associated with needle aspi-

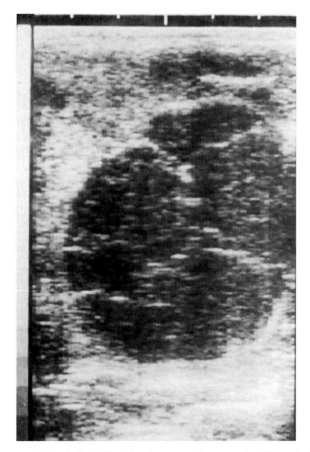

Figure 18.11. A day-5 AHF that has started to organize. (From A.O. McKinnon and J. L. Voss, eds. Equine reproduction. Philadelphia: Lea & Febiger, 1993; p. 296, with permission of Williams & Wilkins, Baltimore.)

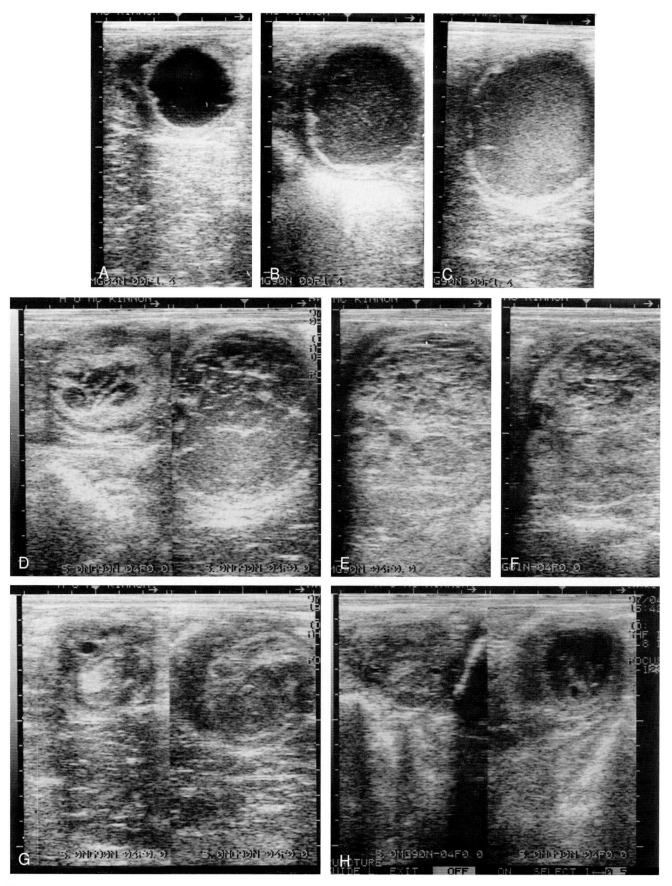

Figure 18.12. A sequential view of development and resolution of an AHF. **A,** Day 1. The potential for an AHF was first recognized. Another follicle had ovulated the day before, and this follicle was developing thickening of the follicular wall and slight echogenicity to the follicular fluid. **B,** Day 2. The follicle was monitored closely to determine that no fluid escaped. Later, it fills with blood and enlarges. **C,** Day 3. The follicle is still being distended with blood. There is no clotting as ballotment causes swirling. (*continued*)

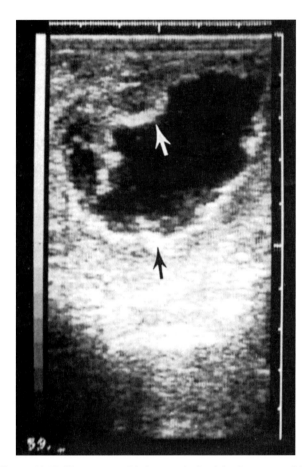

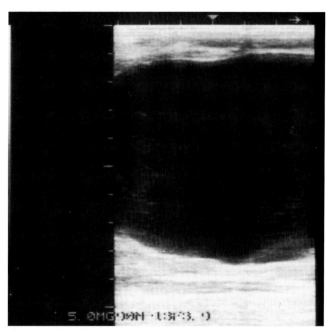

Figure 18.14. The large, persistent, fluid-filled structure was diagnosed as a follicular cyst. The ovary was removed.

Figure 18.13. Ultrasonographic image of a luteinized unruptured follicle (LUF). The fluid did not appear to escape, and ovariectomy failed to reveal any sign of ovulation. Luteal tissue appears to be forming around the outside of the LUF. (From A.O. McKinnon and J. L. Voss, eds. Equine reproduction. Philadelphia: Lea & Febiger, 1993; p. 297, with permission of Williams & Wilkins, Baltimore.)

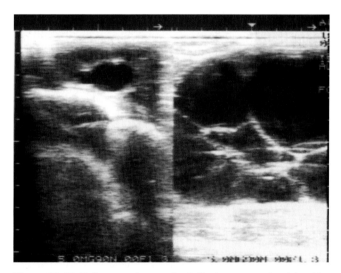

Figure 18.15. Split-screen image of a follicular cyst on the right side. The cyst had been present for at least three cycles before referral. Drainage resulted in return to function of that ovary.

Figure 18.12. *(Continued)* **D,** Day 4. Split-screen image demonstrating that the follicular fluid is starting to organize. On the left is the CL that formed from the ovulation on day 0. **E,** The follicle fluid can no longer be induced to swirl, and no further growth has been detected with the maximum diameter reaching approximately 80 mm. **F,** On day 7 the mare is treated with $PGf_{2\alpha}$. The day before a normal day-7 embryo was recovered by uterine flush for embryo transfer. **G,** Day 9. The CL *(left side)* is starting to regress, and the AHF is becoming smaller. **H,** On day 15 the CL was no longer visible, and the AHF *(right side)* was becoming rapidly smaller. At no time was luteal tissue detected in the AHF by ultrasonography.

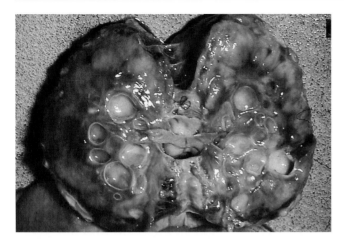

Figure 18.16. Gross characteristics of epithelial inclusion cysts. In this specimen the ovary has been cut down the longitudinal axis to leave the ovulation fossa and the cysts in the center.

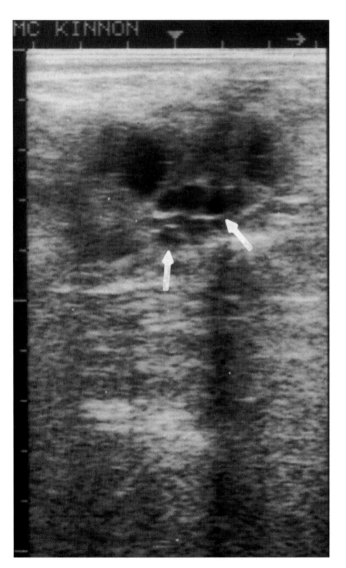

Figure 18.17. Ultrasonographic characteristics of epithelial inclusion cysts. Arrows highlight the cysts in the ovulation fossa.

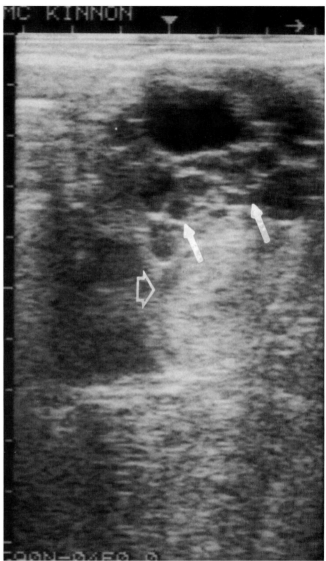

Figure 18.18. Ultrasonographic characteristics of epithelial inclusion cysts in the ovulation fossa *(closed arrows)* with a surrounding CL *(open arrows)*.

ration for diagnostic purposes (46) or as the cause of an ovarian enlargement (47). They have not been detected by us, despite performing over 300 follicular aspirations for oocyte retrieval in both research and clinical situations. Perhaps it is just a matter of time before they become more common with the current interest in IVF and assisted reproductive technologies. Ultrasonography should be useful in differentiating abcessation from hemorrhage or other abnormalities (48).

Ovarian hematomas are not seen frequently (Figs. 18.19 and 18.20). We distinguish them by the presence of blood clots rather than either frank, nonclotted hemorrhage as in the AHF, an absence of blood in the case of a LUF or a follicular cyst, and no evidence of a serum fibrinized clot in the follicle as with an corpus hemorrhagicum. They regress quite slowly.

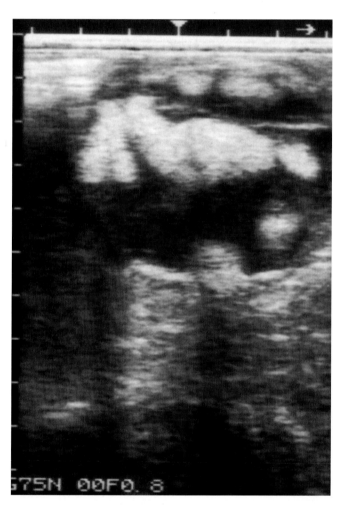

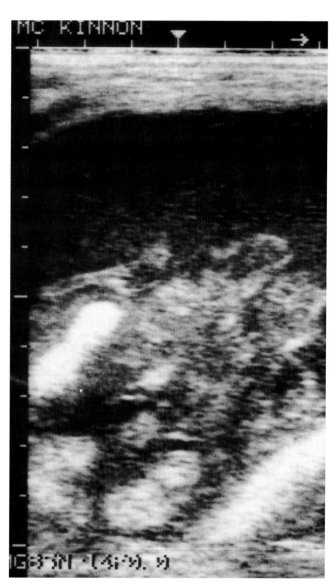

Figure 18.19. An ovarian hematoma. This mare would form these structures at least twice each season. She was 21 years old and became pregnant once in 3 years.

Figure 18.20. A large ovarian hematoma. This mare was pregnant at around 45 days when this was first detected (previous routine examinations for breeding were normal). The mass gradually disappeared.

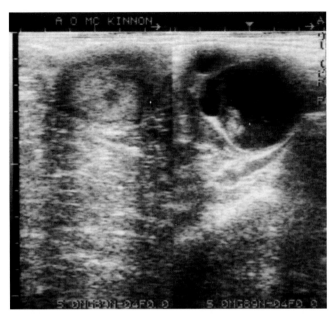

Figure 18.21. Fibrin strands had coalesced to lie on the ventral surface of the follicle on the right side. On the left is a recent CL. The structure gradually receded, but the mare had multiple similar occurrences.

Unusual Follicular Structures

From time to time we see strange and as yet unidentified ovarian structures. Unfortunately, their etiology will be slow forthcoming as they mostly are non–life threatening and are not always repeatable in the same mare at the next or subsequent cycles. Into this category we place *fibrin strands* (Fig. 18.21) or *clumps* (Fig. 18.22) appearing in preovulatory follicles. On occasion, mares will ovulate these follicles and quite frequently they will have similar occurrences again.

OVARIAN NEOPLASIA

The incidence of ovarian tumors is relatively common in mares when compared with other domestic species. The incidence of ovarian tumors in horses has been reported to be as high as 5.6% of all neoplasms. By far the two most common tumors are granulosa-theca cell tumors and teratomas. Rarely, ovarian enlargements associated with a cystadenoma may be detected (49). Ovarian tumors are often classified according to their tissue origin as either gonadal stroma, germ cells, or epithelial.

Gonadal stromal tumors are tumors of granulosa and theca cells and their luteinized counterparts (50). Granulosa and theca cells frequently coexist together in these tumors (50).

Granulosa-Theca Cell Tumors (GTCT)

GTCT are usually large, benign, steroid-producing tumors often associated with behavioral changes and poor reproductive performance. The most common history is a barren, anestrous mare. Other clinical signs are intermittent or continuous estrus, nymphomania, or stallion-like behavior. GTCT are most commonly detected in the middle-aged, anestrous, barren mare; however, they have been detected in

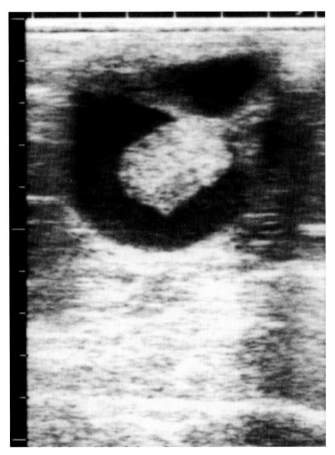

Figure 18.22. A large clump of pedunculated tissue in a follicle that was detected as an incidental finding. The mare was aged 15 and became pregnant and lost to further follow-up.

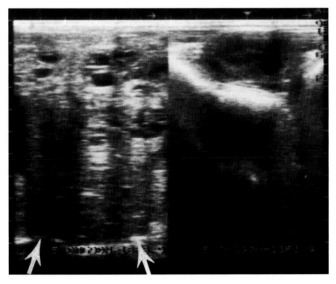

Figure 18.23. Split-screen image of a mare with a relatively solid GTCT on the left side (*arrows delineate the ventral border*) and an inactive ovary on the right side.

foals (51) and weanlings (52), as well as in maiden (53), pregnant (46), and foaling mares (53, 54). Unusual clinical signs such as lameness (55), colic (56, 57), or hemoperitoneum (56) have also been reported.

The ultrasonographic characteristics of granulosa-theca cell tumors will vary, as they may be solid or cystic (41, 58-62) (Figs. 18.23 and 18.24). Palpation may reveal a smooth surface or a knobby, hard surface. When the ovary is large (Fig. 18.25), the ovulation fossa may not be palpable, as it has been obliterated by the developing tumor. One of the most useful criteria to diagnose GTCTs is the recognition of a small and inactive contralateral ovary (Fig. 18.26). There are reports of contralateral and ipsilateral cyclicity despite the presence of a GTCT (63, 64); however, these findings are usually associated with early diagnosis and recognition prior to contralateral ovarian suppression. In the 1995 breeding season we had the opportunity to diagnose a GTCT after watching the mare ovulate on both ovaries for three cycles and then finally cease cycling altogether (Fig. 18.27). The affected ovary enlarged to three to four times its normal size over a 2-month period, and the unaffected ovary became totally quiescent. Bilateral GTCTs are rare (65, 66). We have seen one mare with a bilateral GTCT. The mare

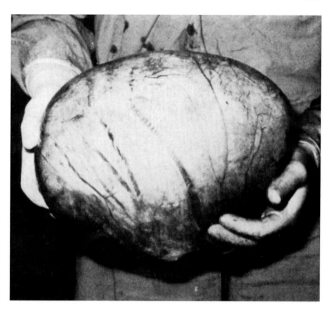

Figure 18.25. Gross characteristics of a large GTCT. (From A.O. McKinnon and J. L. Voss, eds. Equine reproduction. Philadelphia: Lea & Febiger, 1993; p. 297, with permission of Williams & Wilkins, Baltimore.)

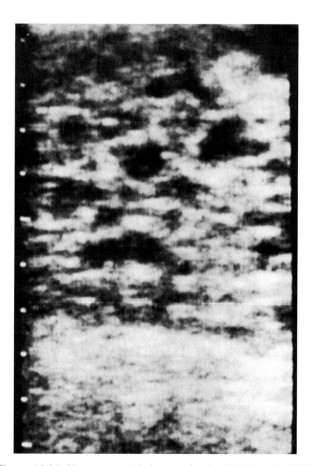

Figure 18.24. Ultrasonographic image of a (multiple) cystic GTCT. (From A.O. McKinnon and J. L. Voss, eds. Equine reproduction. Philadelphia: Lea & Febiger, 1993; p. 298, with permission of Williams & Wilkins, Baltimore.)

acted as an aggressive stallion intermittently, with periods of estrous behavior in between. The larger ovary was removed. The other ovary (which was identical ultrasonographically) was left in situ. Follow-up 3 years later revealed it had not grown at all in size, and the mare remained free from behavioral abnormalities. GTCTs are commonly steroidogenic, and this characteristic has led to hormonal diagnostic techniques. Testosterone is elevated in many cases of GTCT (67, 68). Male behavior is seen when testosterone concentrations exceed 100 pg/ml (50, 68). However, in one study (64) elevated testosterone was only diagnostic in 21 of 39

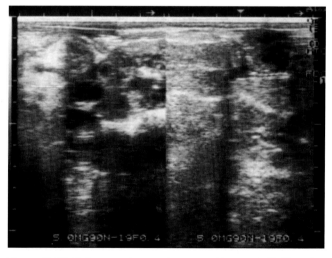

Figure 18.26. Split-screen image of a mare with a small GTCT on the left side and an inactive ovary on the right side. The GTCT was removed through a colpotomy.

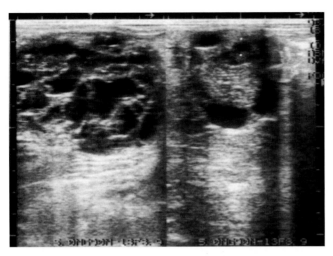

Figure 18.27. Split-screen image of a GTCT on the left side and a CL on the right side. After three cycles the ovary on the right became inactive and the ovary on the left became quite enlarged.

cases (53.8%). Originally, contralateral ovarian atrophy was thought to be associated with androgen production; however, other androgen-producing tumors are not associated with follicular suppression (50). In the normal cycling animal granulosa cells produce inhibin (69) to regulate FSH secretion through negative feedback. Equine GTCTs were recently reported to express mRNA for inhibin (70), and in one study elevated inhibin was useful in diagnosing GTCTs in 34 of 39 cases (64) (87.2%). At the GVEH inhibin is routinely evaluated and is considered suspicious when levels of >0.8 ng/ml are detected. As inhibin is elevated in mares with a dominant follicle in estrus, care is needed to avoid sampling mares with a large, growing follicle (Fig. 18.28) (71). Further evidence that GTCTs produce inhibin is presented in Figure 18.29, which demonstrates a half-life of ap-

proximately 40 minutes and rapid decline of serum inhibin when an ovary with a GTCT is removed (72).

Surgical excision is the treatment of choice, and most mares will return to normal reproductive performance within 2 to 16 months after surgery. At the GVEH we prefer to remove tumors less than 10 cm by colpotomy (73). Larger tumors of approximately 10 to 20 cm are removed via flank laparotomy, either standing in quiet mares or mostly under general anesthesia. The largest tumors are removed through a ventral midline approach. In one case a large tumor was removed through a standing, flank incision after first being ecrasuered by colpotomy. Tension on the ovarian pedicle caused by manipulation can cause serious blood pressure complications for the horse and anesthetist. All cases are very carefully desensitized with topical application of local anesthetic before any major manipulations. Of use in some cases, regardless of the approach, is the drainage of any cystic compartments as this will reduce the diameter of the mass to be removed.

The previously reported arrhenoblastoma (74) was probably just a slight variation and thus an incorrect classification of a GTCT (14).

Germ cell tumors arise from germ cells and usually divided into the two main categories of teratomas and dysgerminomas (50). Ovarian *teratomas* are benign and nonsecretory. The tumors arise from germ cells and are usually nondescript, epithelial tissue, but may contain cartilage, skin, bone, hair, nerves, sebaceous material, and even teeth (50) (Fig. 18.30). They may be solid or cystic (50). They generally do not interfere with fertility and are most commonly discovered during routine rectal palpation (46), unless they become extremely large and affect other organs. Ultrasonographically, they may be expected to have echo-shadowing from denser tissues such as teeth or cartilage. Occasionally, hard structures may be detected by palpation.

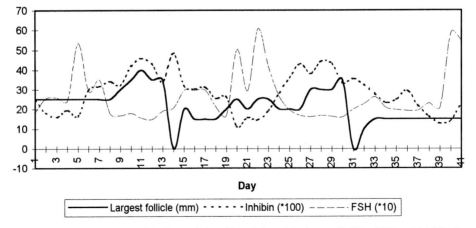

Figure 18.28. Graphical representation of the interrelationships of size of the largest follicle, FSH, and inhibin. Data collected was consistent for all mares examined, and it was collected at the GVEH in March and April, which in the southern hemisphere is toward the end of the cycling season. (From McKinnon AO, Irvine CHG, Dekretser DM, Baffy M, Perkins NR. Studies on the temporal relationship of FSH, inhibin, and day of ovulation. Unpublished data, 1993.)

GTCT removal

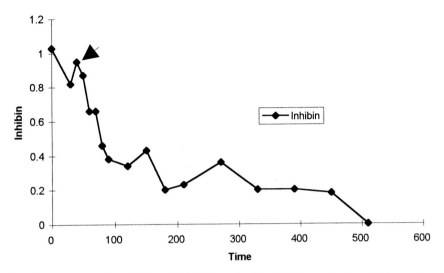

Figure 18.29. Graphical representation of change in inhibin levels after GTCT removal. Arrow indicates time of ovarian removal. The first data point is at the beginning of surgery. (From McKinnon AO, Dekretser DM. Studies on the half-life of equine inhibin. Unpublished data, 1993.)

Dysgerminomas are reported in mares (46, 75) and are the female counterparts to seminomas of stallions (14, 76–80). Dysgerminomas commonly metastasize (75) and have an association with hypertrophic osteopathy (14, 75). The association with hypertrophic osteopathy is most likely related to metastatic masses in the lung (75, 81–85) rather than an effect of the tumor. Weight loss, inappetance, or intermittent lameness were presenting signs. However, in two cases (14, 46) the mares were in continual estrus for 1 month, and this was apparently associated with an estradiol concentration of 67.3 pg/ml in one mare (quoted in Ref. 14), which is approximately double that expected for a mare in estrus.

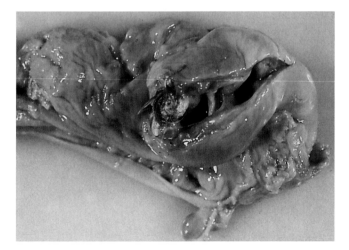

Figure 18.30. Gross specimen of an ovarian teratoma. Pieces of hair and teeth can be visualized in an otherwise nondescript ovary. This was an incidental postmortem finding.

Epithelial tumors arise from both surface and subsurface epithelial structures to give rise to the papillary and cystic adenomas and less frequently papillary adenocarcinomas (50).

Findings of large cystic ovaries have later been determined to be *serous cystadenomas*. These appear to arise from the surface epithelium of the ovulation fossa (67, 86). In most cases the contralateral ovary has continued to function normally despite high testosterone levels (49, 67, 87). They have also been detected in pregnant mares (67, 87).

Occasionally *ovarian adenocarcinomas* develop in mares (88, 89). These would appear to be highly metastatic and serve to highlight how an accurate diagnosis is essential in deciding the reproductive potential of the mare. Occasionally, they can have multiple cell origins (89, 90).

Miscellaneous Neoplasms

Hamartomas (91, 92) and *lymphosarcomas* (14, 93) have been reported in association with the equine ovary. They are rare.

PERIOVARIAN ABNORMALITIES

Periovarian Cysts

Embryonic vestiges and cystic accessory structures associated with the ovary and oviduct are quite common in mares. These cysts, although often small, may occasionally be confused with an ovarian follicle. Rectal palpation in these circumstances is generally more accurate than ultrasonography (Fig. 18.31) in determining whether the structure is part of the ovary. Small fimbrial cysts (<10 mm) probably do not

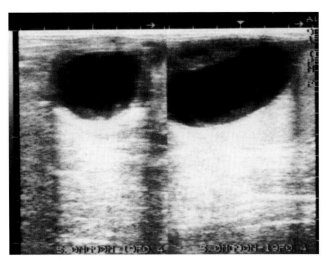

Figure 18.31. Split-screen image of ultrasonographic identification of a large epoophoron cyst or hydatid of Morgagni in cross-section *(left side)* and longitudinal section *(right side)*.

cause infertility; however, on occasion, cystic remnants of the mesonephric tubules and ducts may grow quite large (30 to 60 mm in length and 10 to 15 mm in diameter). One such recognized epoophoron cyst is the hydatid of Morgagni (Fig. 18.32).

Ectopic adrenal cortical tissue has been described as a postmortem finding (94) (quoted in Ref. 14). It is more common in pregnant mares (14), and they may produce detectable quantities of progesterone (95). These nodules were found in 59% of 271 mares (94). Their location is variable, but is usually the mesovarium, and the size was up to 2.5 cm (94) (Fig. 18.33). It is unlikely that they would be detected by either rectal palpation or ultrasonography.

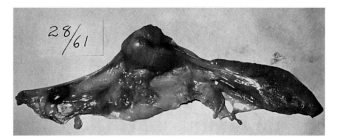

Figure 18.33. Gross characteristics of ectopic adrenal cortical tissue. (Courtesy of Dr. V.E. Osborne.) The tissue is on the ovarian fimbria.

Varicose veins develop on the surface of the ovary in aged mares (14). Mares may be more susceptible due to the peripheral location of the veins (14). Ultrasonographically, these would be expected to be thin-walled, anechoic structures at the periphery of the ovary and difficult to distinguish from small developing follicles.

Hydrosalpinx is not common in mares, but since it is a fluid-filled structure (Fig. 18.34), it may be detected with ultrasonography. Definitive diagnosis will probably require laparoscopy or exploratory surgery.

Oophoritis in mares, presented as adhesions between the ovulation fossa and fimbria, are quite commonly detected in older mares. These may be associated with migration of *Strongylus endentatus* larvae (14).

CONCLUSION

Ultrasonography is an exceptional tool for diagnosis of ovarian problems. It should be reiterated that a correct diagnosis of ovarian abnormalities will be more accurate when all factors are taken into consideration. Ultrasonographic examination may help differentiate between ovarian abnormalities; however, in general, definite diagnosis will rely on histologic or gross examination of the affected ovary.

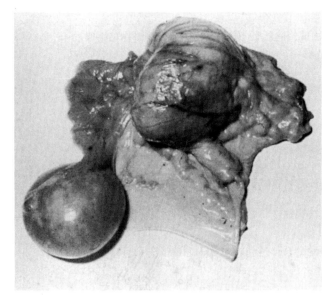

Figure 18.32. Gross characteristics of an epoophoron cyst or hydatid of Morgagni. (Courtesy of Dr. V.E. Osborne.) (From A.O. McKinnon and J. L. Voss, eds. Equine reproduction. Philadelphia: Lea & Febiger, 1993; p. 298, with permission of Williams & Wilkins, Baltimore.)

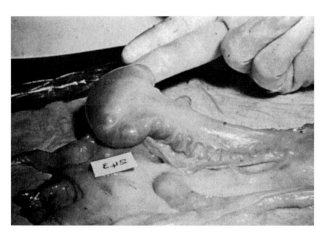

Figure 18.34. Gross characteristics of a mare with hydrosalpinx. (Courtesy of Dr. V.E. Osborne.) (From A.O. McKinnon and J. L. Voss, eds. Equine reproduction. Philadelphia: Lea & Febiger, 1993; p. 299, with permission of Williams & Wilkins, Baltimore.)

REFERENCES

1. Ginther OJ. Twinning in mares: a review of recent studies. J Equine Vet Sci 1982;2:127–135.

2. Squires EL, McKinnon AO, Carnevale EM, Morris R, Nett TM. Reproductive characteristics of spontaneous single and double ovulating mares and superovulated mares. J Reprod Fertil Suppl 1987; 35:399–403.

3. Ginther OJ, Douglas RH, Lawrence JR. Twinning in mares: a survey of veterinarians and analyses of theriogenology records. Theriogenology 1982;18:237–244.

4. Ginther OJ, ed. Reproductive biology of the mare: basic and applied aspects. 2nd ed. Cross Plains, WI: Equiservices, 1992.

5. Henry M, Coryn M, Vandeplassche M. Multiple ovulation in the mare. Zentralbl Veterinarmed [A] 1982;29:170–184.

6. Woods GL, Scraba ST, Ginther OJ. Prospect for induction of multiple ovulations and collection of multiple embryos in the mare. Theriogenology 1982;17:61–72.

7. Ginther OJ. Effect of reproductive status on twinning and on side of ovulation and embryo attachment in mares. Theriogenology 1983;20:383–395.

8. Ginther OJ. Relationships among number of days between multiple ovulations, number of embryos, and type of embryo fixation in mares. J Equine Vet Sci 1987;7:82–88.

9. Ginther OJ, Bergfelt DR. Embryo reduction before day 11 in mares with twin conceptuses. J Anim Sci 1988;66:1727–1731.

10. McKinnon AO, Brown RW, Pashen RL, Greenwood PE, Vasey JR. Increased ovulation rates in mares after immunisation against recombinant bovine inhibin alpha-subunit. Equine Vet J 1992;24: 144–146.

11. Silvia PJ, Johnson L, Fitzgerald BP. Changes in the hypothalamic-hypophyseal axis of mares in relation to the winter solstice. J Reprod Fertil 1992;96:195–202.

12. Silvia PJ, Squires EL, Nett TM. Pituitary responsiveness of mares challenged with GnRH at various stages of the transition into the breeding season. J Anim Sci 1987;64:790–796.

13. Silvia PJ, Squires EL, Nett TM. Changes in the hypothalamic-hypophyseal axis of mares associated with seasonal reproductive recrudescence. Biol Reprod 1986;35:897–905.

14. McEntee K. Reproductive pathology of domestic mammals. San Diego, CA: Academic Press, 1990:31–93.

15. Hughes J P, Stabenfeldt GH, Evans JW. Clinical and endocrine aspects of the estrous cycle of the mare. Proc AAEP 1972;18: 119–151.

16. Hughes JP, Stabenfeldt GH. Conception in a mare with an active corpus luteum. J Am Vet Med Assoc 1977;170:733–734.

17. Ginther OJ, Pierson RA. Regular and irregular characteristics of ovulation and the interovulatory interval in mares. J Equine Vet Sci 1989;9:4–12.

18. Makinen A, Katila T, Kuokkanen MT. XO syndrome in the mare. Nord Vet Med 1986;38:16–21.

19. Trommershausen-Smith A, Hughes JP, Neely DP. Cytogenetic and clinical findings in mares with gonadal dysgenesis. J Reprod Fertil Suppl 1979;27:271–276.

20. Hughes JP, Benirschke K, Kennedy PC, Trommershausen-Smith A. Gonadal dysgenesis in the mare. J Reprod Fertil Suppl 1975;23: 385–390.

21. Pailhoux E, Cribiu EP, Parma P, Cotinot C. Molecular analysis of an XY mare with gonadal-dysgenesis. Hereditas 1995;122: 109–112.

22. Kubien EM, Pozor MA, Tischner M. Clinical, cytogenetic and endocrine evaluation of a horse with a 65,XXY karyotype. Equine Vet J 1993;25:333–335.

23. Hinrichs K, Riera FL, Klunder LR. Establishment of pregnancy after embryo transfer in mares with gonadal dysgenesis. J In Vitro Fert Embryo Transf 1989;6:305–309.

24. Kent MG, Shoffner RN, Hunter A, Elliston KO, Schroder W, Tolley E, Wachtel SS. XY sex reversal syndrome in the mare: clinical and behavioral studies, H-Y phenotype. Hum Genet 1988;79: 321–328.

25. Bowling AT, Millon L, Hughes JP. An update of chromosomal abnormalities in mares. J Reprod Fertil Suppl 1987;35:149–155.

26. Power MM. XY sex reversal in a mare. Equine Vet J 1986;18: 233–236.

27. Levens H. Einige Falle von Pseudohermaphroditismus beim Pferd. Monatsh Prakt Tierheilkd 1911;22:267–273.

28. Beech J. Tumors of the pituitary gland (pars intermedia). In: Robinson NE, ed. Current therapy in equine medicine. 2nd ed. Philadelphia: WB Saunders, 1987:182–185.

29. Peters DF, Erfle JB, Slobojan GT. Low-dose pergolide mesylate treatment for equine hypophyseal adenomas (Cushing's syndrome). Proc AAEP 1995;41:154–155.

30. Pierson RA, Ginther OJ. Ultrasonic evaluation of the corpus luteum of the mare. Theriogenology 1985;23:795–806.

31. Stabenfeldt GH, Hughes JP, Evans JW, Neely DP. Spontaneous prolongation of luteal activity in the mare. Equine Vet J 1974; 6:158–163.

32. Hershman L, Douglas RH. The critical period for the maternal recognition of pregnancy in pony mares. J Reprod Fertil Suppl 1979;27:395–401.

33. Bergfelt DR, Pierson RA, Ginther OJ. Resurgence of the primary corpus luteum during pregnancy in the mare. Anim Reprod Sci 1989;21:261–270.

34. Holtan DW, Squires EL, Ginther OJ. Effect of ovariectomy on pregnancy in mares. J Anim Sci 1975;41:359.

35. Squires EL, Douglas RH, Steffenhagen WP, Ginther OJ. Ovarian changes during the estrous cycle and pregnancy in mares. J Anim Sci 1974;38:330–338.

36. Squires EL, Wentworth BC, Ginther OJ. Progesterone concentration in blood of mares during the estrous cycle, pregnancy and after hysterectomy. J Anim Sci 1974;39:759–767.

37. Stangroom JE, Weevers RdG. Anticoagulant activity of equine follicular fluid. J Reprod Fert 1962;3:269–282.

38. Ginther OJ, ed. Ultrasonic imaging and animal reproduction: horses. Cross Plains, WI: Equiservices, 1995:1

39. McKinnon AO, Perkins NR. Studies on follicular and luteal development as mares enter the transitional period into the nonbreeding season. Unpublished data, 1994.

40. Hughes JP, Stabenfeldt GH, Evans JW. Estrous cycle and ovulation in the mare. J Am Vet Med Assoc 1972;161:1367–1374.

41. McKinnon AO, Squires EL, Pickett BW. Equine diagnostic ultrasonography. Fort Collins: Colorado State University Animal Reproduction Laboratory, 1988.

42. Squires EL, Douglas RH, Steffenhagen WP, Ginther OJ. Changes during the oestrus cycle and pregnancy in mares. J Anim Sci 1974; 38:330–338.

43. Bowen JM. An induced cystic ovarian condition in the mare. Int Cong Anim Reprod Artif Insem (Paris) 1968;2:1559–1561.

44. Prickett ME. Pathology of the equine ovary. Proc AAEP (San Francisco) 1966:145.

45. O'Shea JD. A histological study of nonfollicular cysts in the ovulation fossa region of the equine ovary. J Morph 1968;124:313–320.

46. Bosu WTK, Van Camp SC, Miller RB, Owen RR. Ovarian disorders: clinical and morphological observations in 30 mares. Can Vet J 1982;23:6–14.

47. Nie GJ, Momont H. Ovarian mass in three mares with regular estrous cycles. J Am Vet Med Assoc 1992;201:1043–1044.

48. Frazer GS, Threlfall WR. Differential diagnosis of enlarged ovary in the mare. Proc AAEP 1986:21–28.

49. Hinrichs K, Frazer GS, deGannes RV, Richardson DW, Kenney RM. Serous cystadenoma in a normally cyclic mare with high plasma testosterone values. J Am Vet Med Assoc 1989;194:381–382.

50. Jubb KVF, Kennedy PC, Palmer NC. The female genital system. In: *Pathology of domestic animals.* 4th ed. Vol 3. New York: Academic Press, 1993:358–370.

51. Green SL, Specht TE, Dowling SC, Nixon AJ, Wilson JH, Carrick JB. Hemoperitoneum caused by rupture of a juvenile granulosa cell tumor in an equine neonate. J Am Vet Med Assoc 1988;193:1417–1419.

52. Hultgren BD, Zack PM, Pearson EG, Kaneps AJ. Juvenile granulosa cell tumour in an equine weanling. J Comp Pathol 1987;97:137–142.

53. Stickle RL, Erb RE, Fessler JF, Runnels LJ. Equine granulosa cell tumors. J Am Vet Med Assoc 1975;167:148–151.

54. Schmidt GR, Cowles RR, Flynn DV. Granulosa cell tumor in a broodmare. J Am Vet Med Assoc 1976;169:635.

55. Gift LJ, Gaughan EM, Schoning P. Metastatic granulosa cell tumor in a mare. J Am Vet Med Assoc 1992;200:1525–1526.

56. Gatewood DM, Douglass JP, Cox JH, DeBowes RM, Kennedy GA. Intra-abdominal hemorrhage associated with a granulosa-thecal cell neoplasm in a mare. J Am Vet Med Assoc 1990;196:1827–1828.

57. Wilson DA, Foreman JH, Boero MJ, Didier PJ, Lerner DJ. Small-colon rupture attributable to granulosa cell tumor in a mare. J Am Vet Med Assoc 1989;194:681–682.

58. Hinrichs K. Ultrasonographic assessment of ovarian abnormalities. Proc AAEP 1990:31–40.

59. Hinrichs K, Hunt PR. Ultrasound as an aid to diagnosis of granulosa cell tumour in the mare. Equine Vet J 1990;22:99–103.

60. White RAS, Allen WR. Use of ultrasound echography for the differential diagnosis of a granulosa cell tumor in a mare. Equine Vet J 1985;17:401–402.

61. McKinnon AO, Squires EL, Shideler RK. Diagnostic ultrasonography of the mare's reproductive tract. J Equine Vet Sci 1988;8:329–333.

62. McKinnon AO. Reproductive ultrasonography. In: Equine stud medicine. Sydney: Post Graduate Foundation in Veterinary Science, 1996:395–430.

63. Hinrichs K, Watson ED, Kenney RM. Granulosa cell tumor in a mare with a functional contralateral ovary. J Am Vet Med Assoc 1990;197:1037–1038.

64. McCue PM. Equine granulosa cell tumors. Proc AAEP 1992:587–593.

65. McCoy DJ. Diabetes mellitus associated with bilateral granulosa cell tumors in a mare. J Am Vet Med Assoc 1986;188:733–735.

66. Turner TA, Manno M. Bilateral granulosa cell tumor in a mare. J Am Vet Med Assoc 1983;182:713–714.

67. Hughes JP, Kennedy PC, Stabenfeldt GH. Pathology of the ovary and ovarian disorders in the mare. 9th Int Cong Anim Reprod AI 1980;9:203–222.

68. Stabenfeldt GH, Hughes JP, Kennedy PC, Meagher DM, Neely DP. Clinical findings, pathological changes and endocrinological secretory patterns in mares with ovarian tumours. J Reprod Fertil Suppl 1979;27:277–285.

69. Burger HG, Igarashi M. Inhibin: definition and nomenclature, including related substances. Biomed Tech (Berlin) 1988;122:1701–1702.

70. Piquette GN, Kenney RM, Sertich PL, Yamoto M, Hsueh AJW. Equine granulosa-theca cell tumors express inhibin alpha- and beta A–subunit messenger ribonucleic acids and proteins. Biol Reprod 1990;43:1050–1057.

71. McKinnon AO, Irvine CHG, Dekretser DM, Baffy M, Perkins NR. Studies on the temporal relationship of FSH, inhibin and day of ovulation. Unpublished data, 1993.

72. McKinnon AO, Dekretser DM. Studies on the half-life of equine inhibin. Unpublished data, 1993.

73. McKinnon AO, Arnold KS, Vasey JR. Selected reproductive surgery of the broodmare. Post Graduate Committee in Veterinary Science, Sydney. Equine reproduction: a seminar for veterinarians. 1991:109–125.

74. Mills JH, Fretz PB, Clark EG, Ganjam VK. Arrhenoblastoma in a mare. J Am Vet Med Assoc 1977;171:754–757.

75. McLennan MW, Kelly WR. Hypertrophic osteopathy and dysgerminoma in a mare. Aust Vet J 1977;53:144–146.

76. Smith BL, Morton LD, Watkins JP, Taylor TS, Storts RW. Malignant seminoma in a cryptorchid stallion. J Am Vet Med Assoc 1989;195:775–776.

77. Hunt RJ, Hay W, Collatos C, Welles E. Testicular seminoma associated with torsion of the spermatic cord in two cryptorchid stallions. J Am Vet Med Assoc 1990;197:1484–1486.

78. Becht JL, Thacker HL, Page EH. Malignant seminoma in a stallion. J Am Vet Med Assoc 1979;175:292–293.

79. Pandolfi F, Roperto F. Seminoma with multiple metastases in a zebra (Equus zebra) X mare (Equuscaballus). Equine Vet J 1983;15:70–72.

80. Trigo FJ, Miller RA, Torbeck RL. Metastatic equine seminoma: report of two cases. Vet Pathol 1984;21:259–260.

81. Leach MW, Pool RR. Hypertrophic osteopathy in a Shetland pony attributable to pulmonary squamous cell carcinoma metastases. Equine Vet J 1992;24:247–249.

82. Lavoie JP, Carlson GP, George L. Hypertrophic osteopathy in three horses and a pony. J Am Vet Med Assoc 1992;201:1900–1904.

83. Godber LM, Brown CM, Mullaney TP. Polycystic hepatic-disease, thoracic granular-cell tumor and secondary hypertrophic osteopathy in a horse. Cornell Vet 1993;83:227–235.

84. Long MT, Foreman JH, Wallig MA, Chambers MD, Losonsky JM, Muhlbauer MC. Hypertrophic osteopathy characterized by nuclear scintigraphy in a horse. Vet Radiol Ultrasound 1993;34:289–294.

85. Chaffin MK, Ruoff WW, Schmitz DG, Carter GK, Morris EL, Steyn P. Regression of hypertrophic osteopathy in a filly following successful management of an intrathoracic abscess. Equine Vet J 1990;22:62–65.

86. Held JP, Buergelt C, Colahan P. Serous cystadenoma in a mare. J Am Vet Med Assoc 1982;181:496–498.

87. Bridges ER. Serous cystadenoma in a pregnant mare. Equine Pract 1994;16:15–17.

88. Morris DD, Acland HM, Hodge TG. Pleural effusion secondary to metastasis of an ovarian adenocarcinoma in a horse. J Am Vet Med Assoc 1985;187:272–274.

89. Van Camp SD, Mahler J, Roberts MC, Tate LP, Whitacre MD.

Primary ovarian adenocarcinoma associated with teratomatous elements in a mare. J Am Vet Med Assoc 1989;194:1728–1730.

90. Frazer GS, Robertson JT, Boyce RW. Teratocarcinoma of the ovary in a mare. J Am Vet Med Assoc 1988;193:953–955.

91. Rhyan JC, D'Andrea GH, Smith LS. Congenital ovarian vascular hamartoma in a horse. Vet Pathol 1981;18:131.

92. Foley GL, Johnson R. A congenital interstitial cell hamartoma of the equine ovary. Vet Pathol 1990;27:364–366.

93. Lock TF, Macy DW. Equine ovarian lymphosarcoma. J Am Vet Med Assoc 1979;175:72–73.

94. Ono H, Satoh H, Miyake M, Fujimoto Y. On the development of "ovarian adrenocortical cell nodule" in the horse. Exp Reprod Equine Hlth Lab 1969;6:59–90.

95. Kenney RM, Ganjam VK. Selected pathological changes of the mare uterus and ovary. J Reprod Fertil Suppl 1975;23:335–339.

19. Ultrasonography of the Scrotal Contents and Penis of the Stallion

CHARLES C. LOVE AND DICKSON D. VARNER

The scrotal contents, including the paired spermatic cords, testes, epididymides, vaginal cavities, and scrotum, can be evaluated by ultrasonography. Using a 5- or 7.5-MHz transducer, pathologic changes in these structures may not be as easily detected as in other organ systems, due to the small size of the structures and the limited resolution of the instruments used. Nevertheless, when changes in these structures are pronounced, ultrasonographic examination can be a useful aid in the diagnosis of abnormalities involving the scrotum and its contents. The size of the testes, in terms of the length, width, height, and volume, can be estimated using measures derived during the ultrasound examination. This volume estimate can then be used to estimate expected daily sperm output (DSO) from any particular stallion. In addition, the ultrasound can be used to evaluate the extra-abdominal penis. In this chapter we will present the normal appearance of the scrotal contents and penis, as well as several pathologic conditions associated with these structures and how testis measures can be used to estimate DSO.

Ultrasonography has been previously used in the stallion to aid in the diagnosis of cryptorchidism (1), epididymitis (2–4), and sperm granuloma (5), as well as spermatic cord torsion, varicocele, testicular neoplasia, spermatocoele, hydrocoele, and inguinal hernia (4, 6). Ultrasonography has also been used to estimate the total testicular volume and, from that estimate, predict daily sperm output (7, 8). In dogs, ultrasonography has been used to aid in the diagnosis of testicular tumors (9, 10), epididymal cysts, and spermatic cord torsion, as well as to locate cryptorchid testes (11). In the bull, it has been used to detect the accumulation of rete testis fluid (12). Epididymitis, spermatocoele, testicular cysts, testicular abscesses, and scrotal hernias have been described, using ultrasonography in the ram (13). In humans, ultrasonography has been used to diagnose epididymitis, neoplasia, spermatic cord torsion, and varicocele (14, 15). Evaluation of the testes by ultrasonography has been used to describe the appearance of the testicular parenchyma and measure the size of the testes in bulls (16), rams (17), boars (18), stallions (6, 19), and dogs (20, 21).

Examination of the scrotal contents can be performed in the standing stallion. If performed as part of the routine breeding soundness evaluation, it is usually best performed following the last ejaculation when the stallion is more relaxed and tolerant of the procedure. Sedation of the animal is usually not necessary and in fact may increase the likelihood of spontaneous striking with the hind legs if xylazine is used! The stallion should be examined in an environment free of distractions, and its movement should be restricted, so that the scrotal contents can be completely evaluated. Placement of the stallion in a stocks is preferred to minimize the risk of injury to the examiner or equipment.

Prior to the use of the ultrasound, the scrotal contents should be examined manually, so as to allow the stallion to become familiar with the examination procedure, as well as to allow the clinician to know if the stallion will tolerate the procedure. More obvious defects may also be identified when performing this preliminary physical examination.

Either a linear array or a sector 5.0- or 7.5-MHz ultrasound transducer can be used for the evaluation. Because of improved resolution, the authors prefer a 7.5-MHz frequency to more accurately evaluate the scrotal contents; however, a 5.0-MHz transducer may be needed to perform measurements of the testes. A lubricant designed for use with the ultrasound transducer is preferred, and lubricants that have air bubbles (such as those prepared for per rectum evaluation) or those that easily form a lather when in contact with a sweaty surface (such as sterile, water-soluble lubricants) should be avoided because of the associated reduction in resolution. If a lather is formed on the scrotal skin during the evaluation, the skin should be cleaned to ensure optimal resolution at all times.

The evaluation should be performed in a systematic way to ensure that all the scrotal structures are evaluated. The ultrasonographically relevant structures and anatomy of the scrotal contents are presented in Figure 19.1 and can be compared with the fresh specimen presented in Figure 19.2.

The ultrasound probe is placed vertically on the craniolateral surface of the testis and passed caudally to the region of the tail of the epididymis. This should result in a cross-section of the testicular parenchyma. At the most cranial position the central vein will be largest and easiest to visualize (Fig. 19.3). In addition, the head and body of the epididymis, as well as the spermatic cord, can be evaluated (Fig. 19.4). As the probe is passed caudally, the spermatic cord will no longer be seen, but the body of the epididymis will still be present (Fig. 19.5). The head and body of the epididymis may be difficult to visualize because of their small cross-sectional size, in addition to the fact that it is ultra-

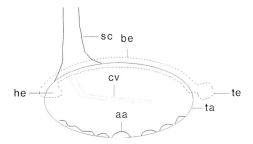

Figure 19.1. Schematic showing the scrotal content structures that can be imaged with the ultrasound. SC = spermatic cord; he = head epididymis; be = body epididymis; te = tail epididymis; cv = central vein; aa = arcuate artery; ta = tunica albuginea.

sonographically similar in texture to the testis. In the live animal, the body of the epididymis does not always lie in the horizontal position depicted in Figures 19.1 and 19.2, but may be elevated so that it assumes a half-circle shape rather than a straight line above the testicle. Elevation may render this structure difficult to locate, both manually and with the ultrasound.

Throughout the cross-sectional scan of the testis, the parenchyma should appear relatively homogenous (Fig. 19.6). The echodense reflections in the normal testis are due to the connective tissue trabeculae that support the seminiferous tubules. While these are present in all testis, they tend to be more prominent in the testes of younger animals and in older animals in which the testes are undergoing degenerative atrophy, wherein the amount of seminiferous tubule tissue is reduced in proportion to the amount of connective tissue. The relative increase of connective tissue may be difficult to appreciate unless the scan is directly compared with that of a normal testis.

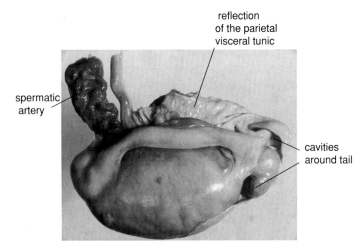

Figure 19.2. Picture showing the appearance of a freshly mounted testis and associated structures. Notice the tortuous spermatic artery, the reflection of the parietal visceral tunic, the attachment of the cauda epididymis to the testis and to the parietal visceral tunic, and the small cavity formed around the cauda epididymis allowing for the accumulation of small amounts of fluid.

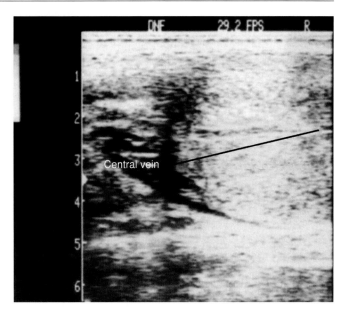

Figure 19.3. Image showing the central vein, which is most easily visualized at the cranial aspect of the testis.

When the caudal aspect of the testis is reached, the tail of the epididymis can be visualized. There are at least two approaches to examine the cauda epididymis. One is to place the probe on the most caudal aspect of the scrotum with the beam pointing cranially. The second approach is to maintain the probe in the lateral position used to examine the testis, but to angle the probe in an oblique manner to include the cauda epididymis, in effect, using the testis as a "standoff" to examine the cauda epididymis. The latter technique is the one preferred by the authors.

The cauda epididymis should be easily identified, but it should be kept in mind that the position can vary. If the scrotum is not completely relaxed, the proper ligament of the tail of the epididymis, which connects the tail to the dorsal parietal vaginal tunic (Fig. 19.2), may elevate the tail dorsally. In addition, the cauda epididymis can move from side to side, and therefore the clinician should not expect it to be located at the most extreme caudal aspect of the testis at all times. The ultrasound image of the cauda should have a "Swiss-cheese" appearance (Fig. 19.7) similar to the spermatic cord, only the lumina should be smaller. The lumen of the caudal-most aspect of the tail, prior to ascent into the ductus deferens, is larger than the cranial portion (Fig. 19.8). This difference may be difficult to appreciate in all images.

The primary arterial supply to the testis is from the testicular artery that winds through the pampiniform plexus as it leaves the external inguinal ring. Because of its prominent lumen, it is the vessel that is most easily identified when the spermatic cord is evaluated. The spermatic cord should have the appearance of "Swiss cheese" when it is evaluated in cross-section, and each hole in the section should be of equal size (Fig. 19.9). Both spermatic cords should be evaluated

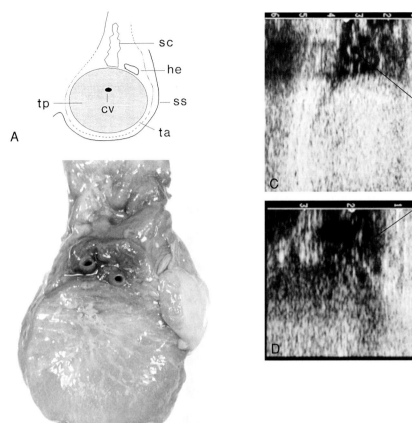

Figure 19.4. Schematic **A,** fresh mount **B,** and images **C, D,** showing a cross-section through the testis in the region of the spermatic cord.

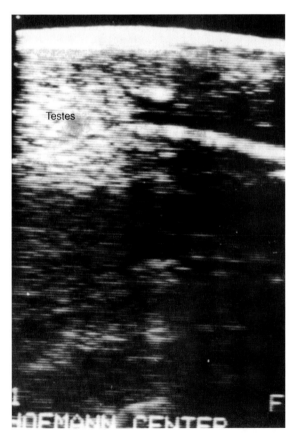

Figure 19.5. Normal appearance of the body of the epididymis associated with the testis.

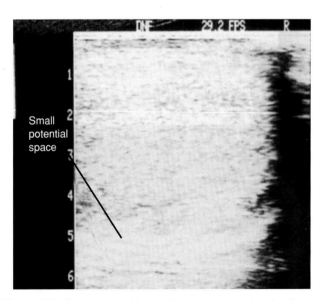

Figure 19.6. Cross-sectional image of a normal testis showing the homogenous parenchyma, and the small potential space between the visceral and parietal vaginal tunics.

255

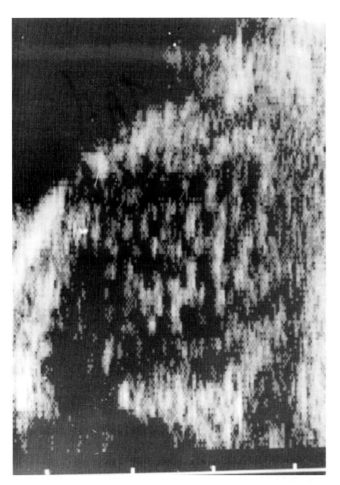

Figure 19.7. Normal image of the epididymal tail with the characteristic "Swiss-cheese" appearance.

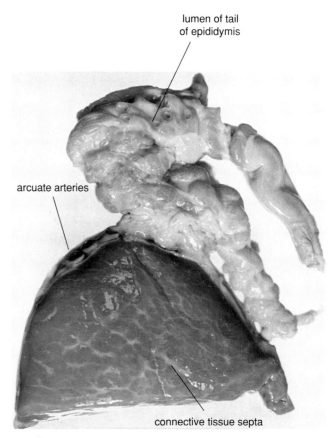

Figure 19.8. Longitudinal section of the testis, corpus, and cauda epididymis. Notice prominent arcuate arteries, lumen of cauda epididymis, and the connective tissue septa in the testis.

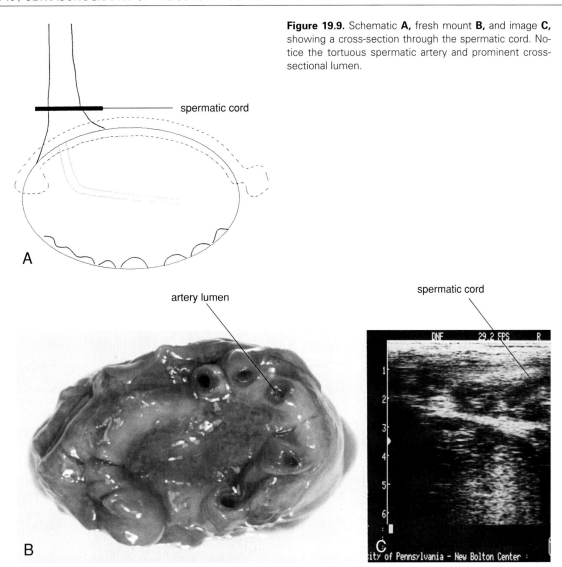

Figure 19.9. Schematic **A,** fresh mount **B,** and image **C,** showing a cross-section through the spermatic cord. Notice the tortuous spermatic artery and prominent cross-sectional lumen.

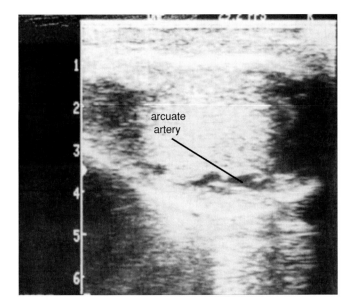

Figure 19.10. Image showing the appearance of the arcuate artery around the tunica albuginea.

side by side on the ultrasound screen and should be approximately of equal size. When the artery reaches the level of the testis, it travels dorsally to the caudal region of the testis before it divides and penetrates the tunica albuginea. These branches can be most easily visualized on the caudal surface of the testis (Figs. 19.8 and 19.10).

DIAGNOSIS OF THE ENLARGED SCROTUM

Evaluation of the enlarged scrotum is an important diagnostic challenge facing the clinician and can be aided by the use of the ultrasound. In general, there are three compartments involving scrotal contents in which the enlargement can occur: the testis, the vaginal cavity, or the scrotum itself, which includes the skin, tunica dartos, and fascial layer of the scrotum.

Often the scrotum is enlarged, and one is unable to palpate the scrotal contents due to the distention of the scrotal skin. To determine the site of the enlargement in this situation, the use of ultrasound greatly facilitates the examination. As a general rule, the most common sites involved in the enlargement involve the scrotum itself or the vaginal cavity, while the testis is seldom enlarged, probably due to the thick tunica albuginea that covers its surface and restricts expansion of the testis in all but extreme cases of vascular impairment. Therefore, when the scrotum is traumatized or the circulation to the testis is compromised, enlargement tends to occur in those spaces that are more easily distensible.

Free fluid can accumulate between the testis and the parietal vaginal tunic in the vaginal cavity and is termed a hydrocoele if the fluid is essentially clear, a hematocele if blood is present, and a pyocele if white blood cells are present. Hydrocoeles are the most common type of fluid accumulation that occurs. The amount of fluid that accumulates can vary greatly from only a few milliliters to enough fluid to fill and distend the entire vaginal cavity. The presence of a small amount of fluid probably does not affect the function of the testis, but is probably a sign of a minor disturbance in the circulation in the testis, probably involving drainage by the lymphatics. The most common location for the accumulation of a small amount of fluid is in the region of the tail of the epididymis because of its ventral location, as well the space that is created by the bulging of the tail (Fig. 19.2). When the fluid accumulates in this location, the outline of the tail is easily visualized (Fig. 19.11). When a large amount of fluid grossly distends the scrotum, it is usually related to a more serious primary problem affecting the venous circulation from the testis, such as an inguinal hernia (Fig. 19.12) or a space-occupying lesion, such as generalized lymphosarcoma in the peritoneum, that impinges on the internal inguinal ring (Fig. 19.13). Often the underlying cause of the hydrocoele cannot be definitively diagnosed. Some hydrocoeles are only transient and may be either unilateral or bilateral in occurrence.

In the case of the inguinal hernia (Fig. 19.12), the intestine that passes through the inguinal canal causes enough re-

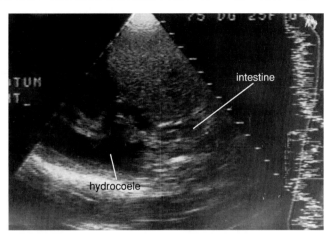

Figure 19.12. Inguinal hernia showing the intestine in a prominent hydrocoele next to the testis. The lumen of the intestine can be visualized.

striction of the venous supply to result in a hydrocoele. The intestine is characterized by an echolucent lumen, and the examiner, using real-time ultrasound, may be able to see intestinal peristaltic waves.

A more severe restriction of the venous supply, such as a diffuse lymphosarcoma that covers the internal inguinal ring, may result in enlargement of the spermatic cord (Fig. 19.13A); congestion of blood in the testis, especially in the center of the testis where the blood is draining into the central vein (Fig. 19.13B); an overall increase in the echogenicity of the affected testis when compared with the opposite testis (Fig. 19.13C); and enlargement of the cauda epididymis (Fig. 19.13D).

Generalized edema of the scrotum can result from topical skin irritants (such as insecticides), allergies, any condition that results in dependent edema (such as equine viral arteritis), any hypoproteinemic condition, or blunt trauma. Scrotal edema can be distinguished from hydrocoele due to the thickened scrotum and the presence of echolucent fluid in the vaginal cavity in the latter (Fig. 19.14). These two conditions may occur concurrently. Based on manual palpation, scrotal edema feels very firm, while the hydrocoele feels like fluid surrounding the testis; however, a hematocele may feel very firm if a blood clot has formed in the vaginal cavity.

Torsion of the spermatic cord (often incorrectly referred to as testicular torsion) may result in an edematous scrotum; however, there are other ultrasonographic signs associated with this condition that are not present with simple edema of the scrotum. A change in the location of the tail of the epididymis has been suggested as a clinical sign to use in the diagnosis of this condition; however, the tail may be very difficult to locate even with the aid of the ultrasound and therefore may not be a reliable indicator of the condition. Other more consistent signs associated with torsion of the spermatic cord include enlargement of the ipsilateral sper-

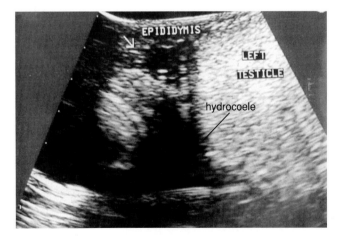

Figure 19.11. Hydrocoele due to a small amount of accumulated fluid in the vaginal cavity. The fluid is in the caudal region of the cavity outlining the cauda epididymis.

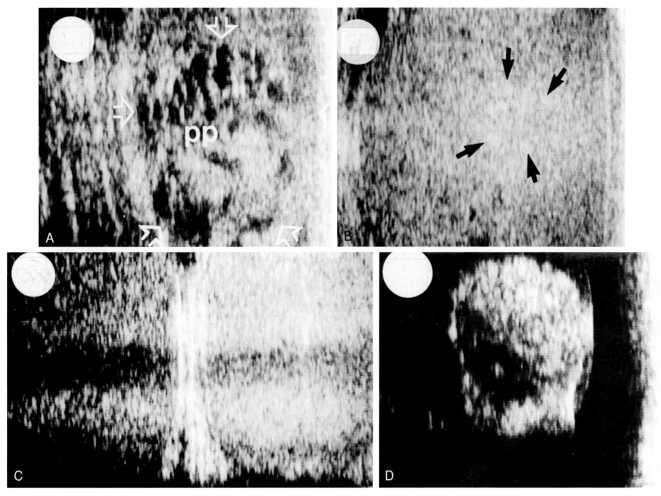

Figure 19.13. Images showing generalized changes that occur in the scrotal contents resulting from impaired circulation to the testis. **A,** Enlarged spermatic cord with circulation. **B,** Increase in echogenicity of the central region of the testis due to venous congestion in the region of the central vein. **C,** The affected testis has an overall increase in echogenicity when compared with the opposite. **D,** Enlarged cauda epididymis in a large hydrocoele.

matic cord when compared with the opposite cord (Fig. 19.15A). This enlargement of the cord may be localized ventral to the torsion itself, as a result of venous congestion in the pampiniform plexus. There will be an increase in echodensity and size of the affected testis when compared with the contralateral testis (Fig. 19.16).

Spermatic cord torsion can be manifest in several ways. The condition can present in the subclinical form in which there is usually a 180° torsion of the cord. This is usually detected on routine evaluation of the testes, and it may spontaneously return to the normal position. The other form occurs when the torsion is greater than 180° and results in restriction of the venous blood flow from the testis. Most of these cases of spermatic cord torsion presented to these authors have been permanent with the exception of one case in which the torsion had occurred prior to examination and had lasted up to the point where the above clinical signs occurred but then subsided, so at the time of the evaluation the cord was no longer twisted. Three days later this cord ex-

hibited the normal pattern and size of the opposite cord (Fig. 19.15B). The one difference between this case and those that are permanent is that blood could be seen passing through the enlarged affected cord (Fig. 19.16). The spermatic cord from a case of a permanent torsion would show

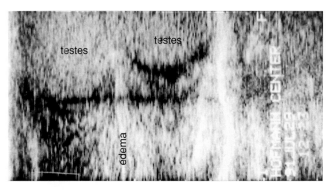

Figure 19.14. Image showing scrotal edema, the echodense image extending ventrally from the image of the testes.

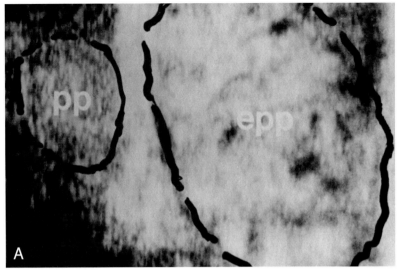

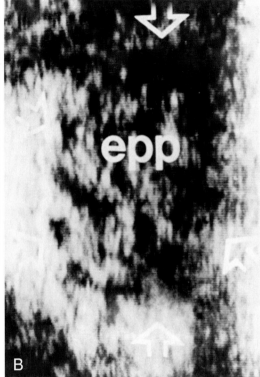

Figure 19.15. A, Comparison of an enlarged spermatic cord *(epp)* resulting from a transient spermatic cord torsion with the contralateral cord *(pp)*. In real-time viewing evidence of circulation was visualized in the enlarged cord (in the lucent areas in epp). **B,** The same cord *(epp)* 3 days later after most of the edema was gone and it had returned to normal size.

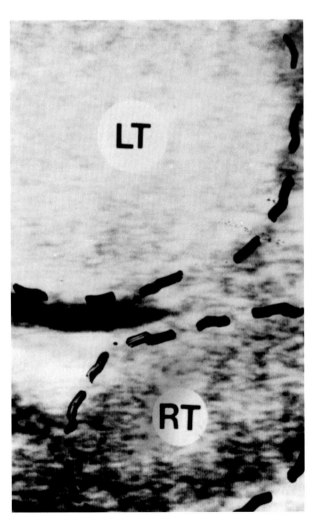

no signs of circulation (Fig. 19.17A) such as the normal "Swiss-cheese" appearance previously described. In addition, a clot may form ventral to the twist and, depending on the maturity of the clot, may appear somewhat echolucent when compared with the surrounding tissue (Fig. 19.17B), similar to a recent corpus hemorrhagicum on a mare ovary. Therefore, when examining a possible case of spermatic cord torsion, it is important to determine that the cord has not spontaneously untwisted. The initial sign of spermatic cord torsion is transient colic, and if the scrotum is not examined and the animal is treated as if the pain was of gastrointestinal origin, the condition may not be presented to the clinician until several hours to days following the loss of circulation to the testis. If this occurs, the chance of salvaging the testis is low. In humans there is an 80 to 100% salvage rate if the surgery is performed within 5 hours after the onset of pain, but is reduced to only 20% if surgery is performed 12 hours after the onset of pain. Therefore, to maximize the chance of saving an affected testis, diagnosis must be made at the time of the initial clinical signs.

As described above, changes in the size of the spermatic cord are usually secondary to another condition. The spermatic cord is usually an easy structure to evaluate regardless of the overall condition of the scrotum; therefore it can supply useful information about the primary cause of an enlarged scrotum.

Figure 19.16. Comparison of the testes from the transient spermatic cord torsion. The affected testis *(LT)* is larger and has a more hyperechoic image than the opposite testis.

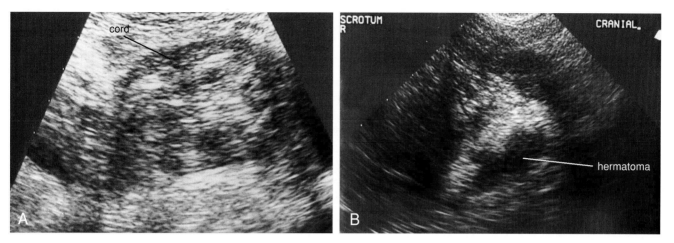

Figure 19.17. Spermatic cord from a permanent spermatic cord torsion (360°) in which no evidence of circulation can be imaged in the cord **A,** and in which a hematoma has formed in the region of the torsion **B.**

The only primary condition that affects the spermatic cord that is detectable by ultrasound is a varicocele. The condition results from the dilation of the pampiniform plexus and is due to a defect or absence of valves in the vein. In men varicoceles may affect 8 to 20% of the adult population, but their effect on fertility is unclear (22–25). The incidence of this condition in the stallion is probably less or it may just not be diagnosed. The image of the cord shows echolucent circles of different sizes (Fig. 19.18), which is considerably different than the normal image, which consists of echolucent circles of similar size. The varicocele in the spermatic cord may also be accompanied by distention and possibly a varicocele of the central vein in the ipsilateral testis (Fig. 19.18B).

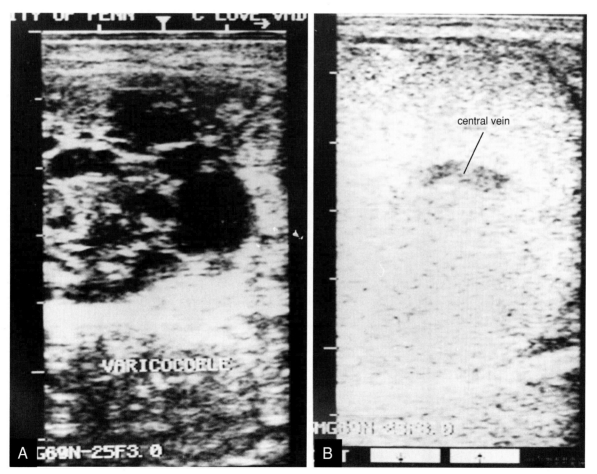

Figure 19.18. Varicocele of the pampiniform plexus **A,** associated with varicocele of the central vein **B.**

EXAMINATION OF THE TESTES

There are several primary conditions of the testis that can be detected with the ultrasound, including testicular tumors and lesions resulting from trauma to the testis. Testicular tumors may occur in any area of the testis and may appear as echolucent areas. These areas may be very obvious (Fig. 19.19A) or have a more discrete, mottled appearance (Fig. 19.19B).

Trauma to the testis, such as may occur as a result from a kick from a mare at the time of breeding, can result in a chronically firm testis, due to testicular degeneration. When compared with the normal testis (Fig. 19.20B), there is often an overall increase in the echogenicity of the testis and a reduction in circulation to the testicular parenchyma, as exemplified by the loss of the central vein. Arteries that penetrate the tunica albuginea may also appear more prominent at the periphery of the testis due to a reduction in blood flow to the testicular parenchyma (Fig. 19.20A).

The ultrasound can also be used to determine the location of a nonscrotal testis. The clinician can be presented with a colt/stallion without one or both scrotal testes and therefore must determine if and where the testis is located. For identification of a testis located within the inguinal canal, the ultrasound can be placed in the inguinal region with the beam directed toward the inguinal canal. For identification of an abdominal testis, the ultrasound can be used per rectum, as previously described. The manual identification tends to be different for the nonscrotal testis because it is smaller and softer and tends to be more hypoechoic than a normal, scrotal testis.

EXAMINATION OF THE EPIDIDYMIDES

Conditions affecting the epididymis include cysts, inflammation, and dilation of the lumen of the tail. Cysts are usually first recognized during palpation of the scrotum by their firm, round feel. They are usually located in the region of the caput and proximal body of the epididymis. Their image may appear either as an echolucent fluid-filled structure (Fig. 19.21) or may be echodense (Fig. 19.22). When these cysts reflect a dense image, they are difficult to distinguish from the surrounding structures and are best diagnosed by palpation. These cysts may result from a granulomatous reaction due to the extravasation of sperm in blind-ended, efferent ductules in the caput epididymis. If this occurs, there is the potential that sperm flow through the epididymis will

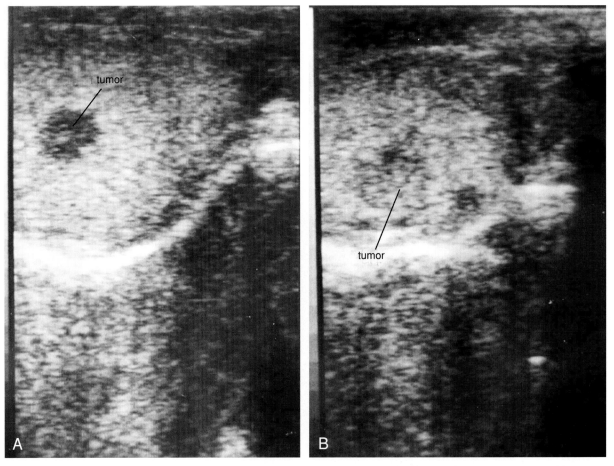

Figure 19.19. Testicular tumor may be manifest as a discrete hypoechoic area **A,** or more heterogeneous image **B.**

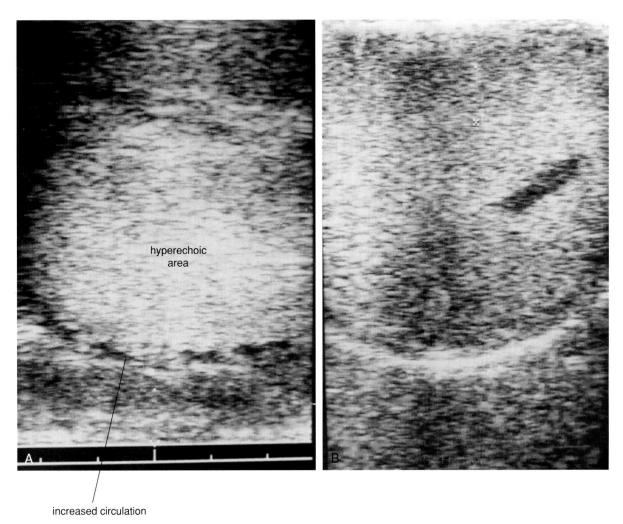

increased circulation

Figure 19.20. Image of a degenerated testis **A,** Notice the hyperechoic parenchyma associated with the absence of central vein, and a prominent increase in circulation at the periphery of the testis. The outline of the testis is irregular when compared with the opposite **B,** an earlier image of the same horse.

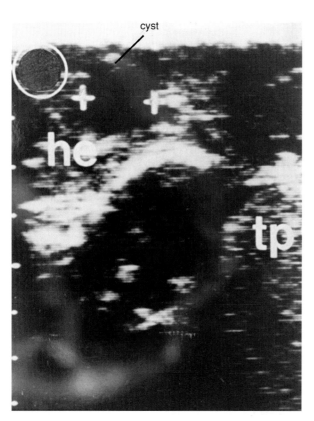

Figure 19.21. Hypoechoic cyst in the region of the body of the epididymis.

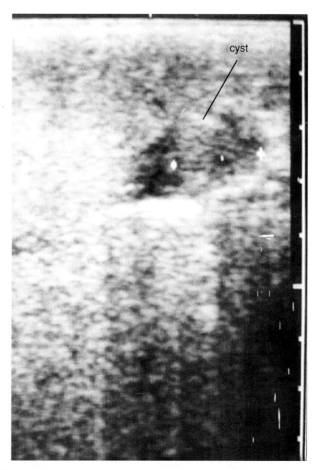

Figure 19.22. Hyperechoic cyst in the region of the body of the epididymis.

be impaired or stopped. However, this was not the case in either horse presented in Figures 19.21 and 19.22.

The lumen of the cauda epididymis can become dilated due to inflammation (epididymitis) or due to excessive accumulation of sperm. Epididymitis results in enlargement of the epididymis and a more heterogeneous image with hyperechoic areas when compared with the normal image of the epididymal body (Fig. 19.5) and tail (Fig. 19.7). This condition may be associated with scrotal pain and pyrexia in contrast to most other conditions of the scrotum, which are relatively free of pain and systemic signs. Cystic dilations of the epididymis may also be detected. The image of these dilatations may either be echodense or echolucent (Fig. 19.23), depending on the amount of white blood cells or debris in the contents.

Dilation of the cauda epididymis resulting in excessive sperm accumulation may occur secondary to occlusion of the ampullae, or in rare cases may accumulate sperm in the absence of occlusion of the ampullae. Primary distention of the lumen of the cauda is an unlikely event because of the thick, smooth muscle that surrounds the lumen, thereby restricting expansion; nevertheless, there is the potential for it to occur (Fig. 19.24). Whether the site of the primary problem is the ampullae or, less commonly, in the cauda epididymis, the condition may be characterized by a large percentage of detached heads, supraphysiologic levels of sperm in the ejaculate (30 to 70 billion sperm), and immotile sperm (19).

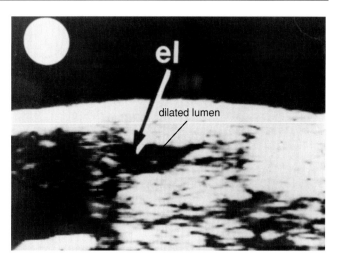

Figure 19.24. Dilated lumen in the tail of the epididymis.

EXAMINATION OF THE PENIS

The ultrasonographically relevant structures in the penis are illustrated in Figures 19.25 and 19.26. In the erect penis the veins that drain the penis are prominent dorsally. The paired corpus cavernosum penis is the largest blood-filled body in the shaft of the penis of the stallion and accounts for the elongation and overall increase in size of the penis. It is supported by fibrous trabeculae that account for the more hyperechoic areas in this space.

Directly beneath the corpus cavernosum lies the urethra, surrounded by the corpus spongiosum penis, which is a smaller trabeculated space that is responsible for the passage

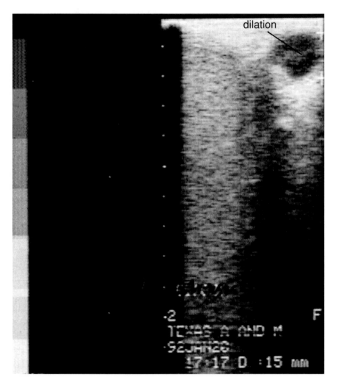

Figure 19.23. An example of epididymitis showing an image of the cauda epididymis showing an echolucent dilation with echodense areas in the lumen.

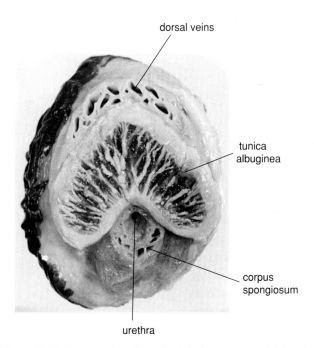

Figure 19.25. Cross-section of the distal shaft of the penis. Notice the prominent dorsal veins, the tunica albuginea of the corpus cavernosum, and the corpus spongiosum that surrounds the urethra.

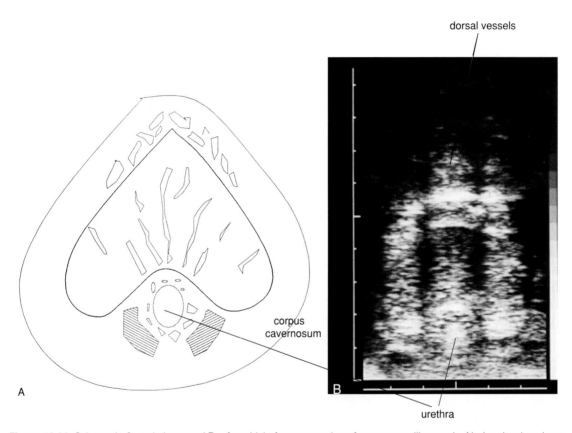

Figure 19.26. Schematic **A,** and ultrasound **B,** of a midshaft cross-section of an erect stallion penis. Notice the dorsal vessels, the corpus cavernosum, corpus spongiosum, and urethra.

of blood, immediately prior to ejaculation, to the glans penis.

Trauma to the penis, resulting from a kick, malalignment with the mare or artificial vagina at the time of breeding, or administration of phenothiazine tranquilizers, can result in paraphimosis or the inability to retract the penis. Changes may be seen in several of the compartments of the penis following these insults. Edema can be imaged between the tunica albuginea and the preputial mucous membrane (Fig. 19.27). Blood clots may form within the corpus cavernosum if the paraphimosis is not treated immediately. If the condition becomes chronic, the corpus cavernosum probably becomes fibrotic due to the deposition of fibrin from the clot. At this time the corpus cavernosum penis takes on a more hyperechoic appearance (Fig. 19.28). This fibrotic change usually occurs first in the distal part of the penis. The transition from normal cavernous tissue to abnormal tissue can be imaged. This transition is usually evident clinically because the stallion is unable to develop an erection beyond this point.

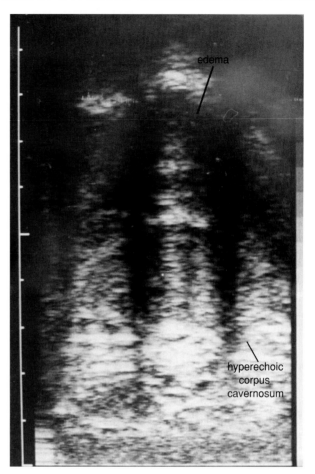

Figure 19.28. Image of the midshaft cross-section of a nonerect penis from a stallion with a chronic paraphimosis. This image is more distal than Figure 19.27. Notice the edema as well as the increase in echogenicity in the corpus cavernosum, probably reflecting increased fibrotic changes.

MEASUREMENT OF THE TESTES

The ultrasound can be used to measure the length, width, and height, as well as the cross-sectional area and the circumference at the widest point of each testis. The linear measures can be used to approximate the volume of each testis using the estimate for the volume of an ellipsoid, which is $4/3 \times$ length/2 $\times$ width/2 $\times$ height/2 or 0.523 $\times$ length $\times$ width $\times$ height. The combined volume of both testis can then be used to determine the expected daily sperm output (DSO) from that stallion (Fig. 19.29) when the excurrent ducts have been cleared of sperm following seven daily ejaculations. This evaluation is possible because each cubic centimeter (cc) of testicular parenchyma produces approximately 16×10^6 sperm/24 hours. The regression formula to estimate DSO from the testes volume is y (DSO in billions) = 0.024 (total testes volume) − 0.76. The regression coefficients for the relationship between DSO and total testicular cross-sectional area and total testicular circumference are presented in Figures 19.30 and 19.31.

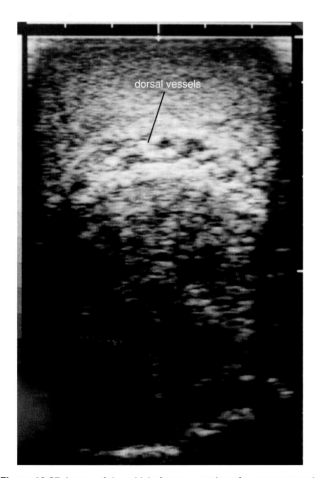

Figure 19.27. Image of the midshaft cross-section of a nonerect penis from a stallion with a chronic paraphimosis. Notice the prominent dorsal vessels and the edema. The corpus cavernosum appears relatively normal at this level.

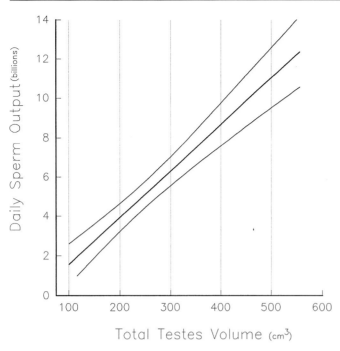

Figure 19.29. Relationship between DSO and total testes volume.

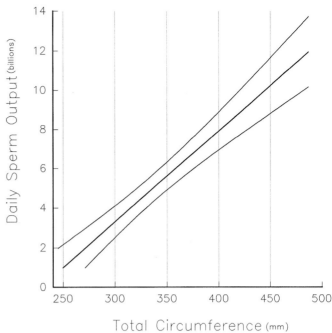

Figure 19.31. Relationship between DSO and total testes circumference.

The area and circumference can only be determined by ultrasonography, whereas the linear measures can be determined either by caliper or ultrasound. It is recommended that the linear measures, as well as the area and circumference, be performed. This allows the clinician to have several measures by which the estimated DSO can be determined. Therefore, when one performs all the measures, the ex-

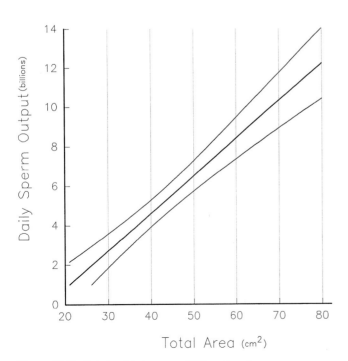

Figure 19.30. Relationship between DSO and total testes cross-sectional area.

pected DSO should be similar. If it is not, one should suspect that one or several of the measures is discrepant and should be performed again, if possible, until there is general agreement between the different measures.

The estimated DSO value can then be compared with the total number of sperm collected from the stallion. This comparison should be performed when the suspect stallion is at DSO. In the event the stallion is not at DSO, but rather at sexual rest, the total number of sperm in the second of two ejaculates can be used as the comparison value. If the total number of sperm is less than expected, further steps should be taken to determine the reason behind the discrepancy between testes size and sperm output. This discrepancy is one of the early signs of testicular stress that occurs well in advance of the more common clinical signs associated with end-stage testicular degeneration, such as a reduction in testes size and the change in consistency of the testicular parenchyma.

Ultrasonic evaluation is a very useful aid in the diagnosis of pathologic conditions of the testes, epididymides, spermatic cord, vaginal cavity and scrotum, and penis. The ultrasound can also be used effectively to estimate testicular volume to determine if the parenchyma is producing the proper number of sperm for that volume.

REFERENCES

1. Jann HW, Rains JR. Diagnostic ultrasonography for evaluation of cryptorchidism in horses. JAVMA 1990;196:297–300.
2. Traub-Dargatz JL, Trotter GW, Kaser-Hotz B, Bennett DG, Kiper ML, Veeramachanemi NR, Squires E. Ultrasonographic detection of chronic epididymis in a stallion. JAVMA 1991;198:1417–1420.

3. Held JP, Adair S, McGavin MD. Bacterial epididymitis in two stallions. J Am Vet Med Assoc 1990;197:602–604.

4. Varner DD, Schumacher J, Blanchard TL, Johnson L. Diseases and management of breeding stallions. Goleta, CA: American Veterinary Publications, 1991; p. 349.

5. Held JP, Prater P, Toal RL, et al. Sperm granuloma in a stallion. J Am Vet Med Assoc 1989;194:267–268.

6. Love CC. Ultrasonographic evaluation of the testis, epididymis, and spermatic cord of the stallion. Vet Clin North Am Equine Pract (Stallion Management) 1992a;8:167–182.

7. Love CC, Riera FL, Garcia ML, et al. Use of testicular volume to predict daily sperm output in the stallion. In: Proceedings of the 36th American Association Equine Practitioners, Lexington, KY, 1991a; pp. 15–21.

8. Love CC, Riera FL, Garcia ML, et al. Evaluation of measures taken by ultrasonography and calipers to estimate testicular volume and predict daily sperm output in the stallion. J Reprod Fertil Suppl 1991b;44:99–105.

9. Pugh CR, Konde LJ. Sonographic evaluation of canine testicular and scrotal abnormalities: a review of 26 case histories. Vet Radiol 1991;32:243–250.

10. Eilts BE, Pechman RD, Hedlund CS, Kreeger JM. Use of ultrasonography to diagnose Sertoli cell neoplasia and cryptorchidism in a dog. JAVMA 1988;192:533–534.

11. Johnston GR, Feeney DA, Rivers B, et al. Diagnostic imaging of the male canine reproductive organs. Vet Clin North Am Small Anim Pract 1991;21:553–589.

12. Andersson M, Alanko M. Ultrasonography revealing the accumulation of rete testis fluid in bull testicles. Andrologia 1991;23:75–78.

13. Ahmad N, Noakes DE, Subandrio AL. B-mode real time ultrasonographic imaging of the testis and epididymis of the sheep and goats. Vet Rec 1991;128:491–496.

14. Feld R, Middleton WD. Recent advances in sonography of the testis and scrotum. Radiol Clin North Am (Ultrasonography of Small Parts) 1992;30:1033–1051.

15. McAlister WH, Sisler CL. Scrotal sonography in infants and children. Curr Probl Diagn Radiol 1990;19:203–242.

16. Cartee RE, Gray BW, Powe TA, Hudson RS, Whitesides J. Preliminary implications of B-mode ultrasonography of the testicles of beef bulls with normal breeding soundness examinations. Theriogenology 1989;31:1149–1157.

17. Cartee RE, Rumph PP, Abuzaid S, Carson R. Ultrasonographic examination and measurement of ram testicles. Theriogenology 1990;33:867–875.

18. Cartee RE, Powe TA, Gray BW, Hudson RS, Kuhlers DL. Ultrasonographic evaluation of normal boar testicles. Am J Vet Res 1986;47:2543–2548.

19. Love CC, Kenney RM. Sperm occluded (plugged) ampullae in the stallion. Proceedings of the Society for Theriogenology, San Antonio, TX, August 14–15, 1992b; pp. 117–125.

20. Pugh CR, Konde LJ, Park RD. Testicular ultrasound in the normal dog. Vet Radiol 1990;31:195–199.

21. Eilts BE, Williams DB, Moser EB. Ultrasonic measurement of canine testes. Theriogenology 1993;40:819–828.

22. Vermeulen A, Vandeweghe M, Deslypere JP. Prognosis of subfertility in men with corrected or uncorrected varicocele. J Androl 1986;7:147–155.

23. Costabile RA, Skoog S, Radowich M. Testicular volume assessment in the adolescent with varicocele. J Urol 1992;147:1348–1350.

24. Kupeli S, Arikan N, Aydos K, at el. Multiparametric evaluation of testicular atrophy due to varicocele. Urol Int 1991;46:189–192.

25. Weiss AJ, Kellman GM, Middleton WD, et al. Intratesticular varicocele: sonographic findings in two patients. AJR 1992;158:1061–1063.

20. Accessory Sex Gland and Internal Reproductive Tract Evaluation

THOMAS V. LITTLE

Transrectal palpation of the internal reproductive tract is often performed as part of a clinical fertility evaluation of the stallion (1–3). This examination typically includes evaluation of the accessory sex glands and the internal inguinal rings. The accessory sex glands of the stallion comprise the ampullae of the deferent ducts, the prostate gland, the vesicular glands, and the bulbourethral glands (Fig. 20.1). Their small size, soft consistency, and muscular investments make palpation a rather subjective exercise. In the case of some structures, such as the excurrent ducts of the accessory sex glands, the seminal colliculus, and the pelvic urethra, direct palpation may be impossible. Transrectal ultrasonography has proved to be a useful adjunct to palpation in evaluating the anatomic relationships, physical dimensions, and acoustic characteristics of the stallion's accessory sex glands and related structures (4).

This chapter describes the indications for a transrectal ultrasound examination, the recommended imaging equipment and procedures, the relevant anatomy, and the ultrasonographic appearance of the internal reproductive tract of the stallion.

INDICATIONS

Some clinicians believe that internal reproductive examinations are justified only when the breeding history or the results of semen analysis suggest a specific problem. Although the incidence of recognized accessory sex gland abnormalities is admittedly low, such abnormalities are not always evident from the history or semen evaluation. Furthermore, some abnormalities defy detection by palpation. A complete internal reproductive examination should include transrectal ultrasonography.

Transrectal ultrasonography is specifically indicated when the history suggests reproductive tract infection or the semen evaluation reveals an abnormally high number of leukocytes. For this indication, ultrasonography should be used in conjunction with culture and cytology of semen fractions, rectal palpation, and endoscopy to identify the source of inflammation or infection. Transrectal ultrasonography is also indicated in suspected unilateral or bilateral excurrent duct obstruction (5), hemospermia, and emission or ejaculation failures. Ultrasonographic findings associated with these conditions are discussed later in this chapter.

Transrectal ultrasonography may be beneficial in conjunction with palpation for differentiating abdominally from inguinally retained testes (6). When a retained testis is suspected on behavioral grounds but cannot be located, ultrasonographically determined accessory sex gland dimensions may be useful in discriminating between an abdominal cryptorchid and a true gelding.

Transrectal ultrasonography can also be used to evaluate the effects of sexual stimulation and ejaculation on the size and appearance of the accessory sex glands (7) and to examine the sequence and timing of selected events associated with emission and ejaculation (8). As the use of transrectal ultrasonography for evaluating the reproductive tract of the stallion becomes more frequent, additional indications will undoubtedly arise.

IMAGING PROCEDURE

Equipment Requirements

A 7.5-Mhz transducer is highly recommended to provide optimal resolution of small structures, but a 5-Mhz transducer has been used successfully for some purposes (9). The highest quality images are obtained with short focal distances because structures are generally within 4 cm of the transducer face and a suitable stand-off for transrectal use is lacking. Ultrasound units in which focal distances can be selected are ideal.

For complete internal examinations, the orientation of the transducer, the dimensions of the transducer housing, and the flexibility of the transducer cable should allow the operator to obtain both transverse and longitudinal scanning planes within the confines of the pelvic cavity. The transverse plane is particularly useful in evaluations of the pelvic urethra, seminal colliculus, and excretory ducts of the ampullae prostate and vesicular glands.

Restraint

Although stallions and geldings are generally not accustomed to rectal palpation, many tolerate the procedure with minimal restraint. The temperament of the stallion may dictate the use of a safe, secure palpation chute and perhaps tranquilization to ensure the safety of both clinician and patient. In contrast to the risks reported for rectal palpation of male horses examined for colic (10), transrectal ultrasonography of the internal reproductive tract involves little risk because the glands are rapidly located and the depth of penetration required is minimal. The accessory sex glands are almost entirely within the pelvic cavity and are generally in close proximity to the rectal wall. Depth of penetration

271

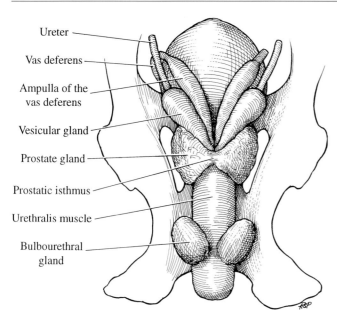

Ureter

Vas deferens

Ampulla of the
vas deferens

Vesicular gland

Prostate gland

Prostatic isthmus

Urethralis muscle

Bulbourethral
gland

Figure 20.1. Schematic dorsal view of the pelvic organs of the mature stallion.

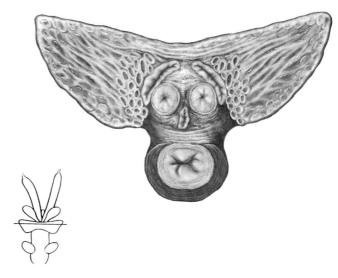

Figure 20.2. Transverse section of the urethralis muscle and enclosed structures immediately proximal to the seminal colliculus. Plane of section is depicted by bold line in schematic diagram. (Adapted from Little TV, Holyoak GR. Reproductive anatomy and physiology of the stallion. Vet Clin North Am Equine Pract 1992;8:1–30, with permission from WB Saunders Company, Philadelphia.)

rarely exceeds 12 inches and little downward pressure is required.

Technique

Imaging the stallion's reproductive tract is similar to scanning that of the mare. The rectum is evacuated and the tract

palpated manually. After application of coupling gel, the transducer is introduced into the rectum with the beam directed downward. The best anatomic landmark for palpating or imaging the accessory sex glands is the prominent, tubular urethralis muscle found on the floor of the pelvis be-

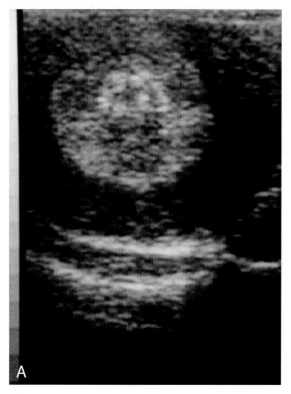

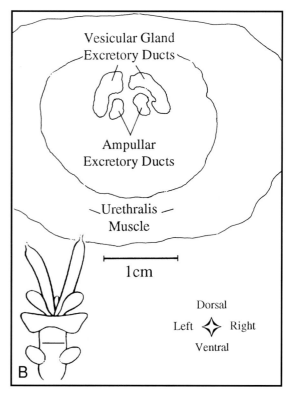

Vesicular Gland
Excretory Ducts

Ampullar
Excretory Ducts

Urethralis
Muscle

1cm

Dorsal

Left ◇ Right

Ventral

Figure 20.3. A, Transverse ultrasonogram of the urethralis muscle and enclosed structures. Transducer placement is depicted by a bold line in the schematic diagram. **B**, Image orientation is shown by compass key.

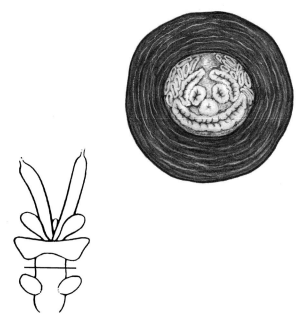

Figure 20.4. Transverse section of the prostate gland and excurrent ducts at the level of the prostatic isthmus. Plane of section is depicted by bold line in schematic diagram. (Adapted from Little TV, Holyoak GR. Reproductive anatomy and physiology of the stallion. Vet Clin North Am Equine Pract 1992;8:1–30, with permission from WB Saunders Company, Philadelphia.)

tween the bladder neck and the ischial arch (see Fig. 20.1). This thick muscle surrounds the excretory ducts of the accessory sex glands and the pelvic urethra (Fig. 20.2) (11). When imaged in a transverse plane, this muscle is readily demonstrated as an echolucent ring approximately 3 to 4 cm

in diameter (Fig. 20.3). If the urethralis muscle is identified first and then followed to its cranial extent, the prostate gland, the ampullae, and the vesicular glands can be readily located and imaged in their entirety.

ANATOMIC RELATIONSHIPS AND ULTRASONOGRAPHIC APPEARANCES

Prostate Gland

The pyramid-shaped lobes of the prostate gland are located on either side of the midline at the cranial border of the urethralis muscle (see Fig. 20.1). They are connected to one another by a thin band of prostatic parenchyma, the prostatic isthmus. The ampullae, the vesicular gland necks, and the bladder neck all converge and pass under the prostatic isthmus (Fig. 20.4), where they are joined by multiple excretory ductules that emerge from the ventromedial aspect of each prostate lobe. The excretory ducts of all three glands travel together to the seminal colliculus within the confines of the urethralis muscle (see Fig. 20.2). The distance from the prostatic isthmus to the colliculus is approximately 4 cm.

Ultrasonographically, the glandular parenchyma of the prostate is largely homogeneous in the nonstimulated state (Fig. 20.5). Small pockets of accumulated secretion may be evident. Sexual stimulation produces rapid fluid accumulation within the parenchyma of the prostate and a 20% increase in the dorsoventral dimension of each lobe (12). Accumulated fluid is visible as echolucencies that converge near the medial border of each lobe (Fig. 20.6), where the prostatic ductules are located. Recognized abnormalities of the stallion's prostate are rare. Some older horses exhibit

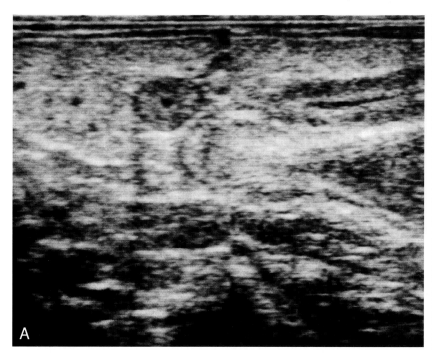

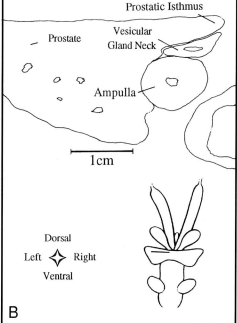

Figure 20.5. A, Transverse ultrasonogram of the wing of the prostate gland from nonstimulated stallion. The terminal ampulla and vesicular gland neck are also visible. **B,** Image orientation is shown by compass key.

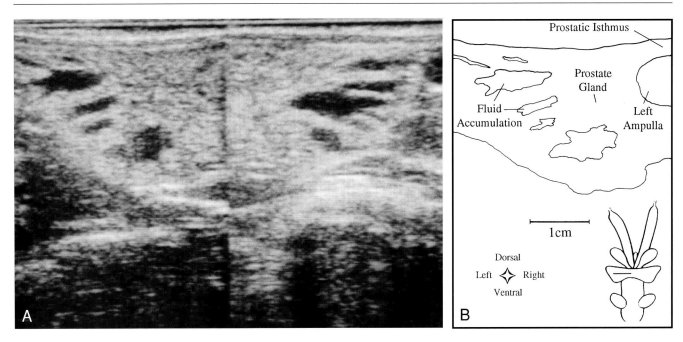

Figure 20.6. A, Transverse ultrasonogram of the wing of the prostate gland from a sexually stimulated stallion. Hypoechoic accumulations of fluid are visible within the prostatic parenchyma. **B**, Image orientation is shown by compass key.

pockets of accumulated fluid even in the nonsexually stimulated state.

Ampullae of the Deferent Ducts

The ampullae are enlarged, glandular portions of the terminal vasa deferentia (deferent ducts). They are readily located as they converge over the neck of the bladder and pass under the prostatic isthmus (see Fig. 20.1). From this point they can be traced either proximally to their junction with the nonglandular part of the vas or distally under the prostatic isthmus to their terminations as excretory ducts at the seminal colliculus. Ultrasonographically, the ampullae are readily identified in transverse images obtained immediately proximal to the prostatic isthmus. The ampullae are round in cross-section and range from 1.0 to 2.5 cm in diameter in the mature stallion. The ampullar lumen is generally evident as a result of specular reflection or fluid accumulation (Fig. 20.7). The lumen is particularly evident in sexually stimulated stallions, in whom fluid accumulation may double the lumen diameter (12).

The parenchymal portion remains unchanged after sexual stimulation (7) and normally exhibits a homogeneous texture. In some apparently normal stallions, the ampullar parenchyma may assume a highly mottled or cystic appearance as the result of dilated tubuloalveolar glands within the parenchyma (Fig. 20.8). Another variation is a pattern of hyperechoic spots throughout the parenchyma. When the latter is seen in conjunction with increases in ampullar tone

or diameter, it may be indicative of a sperm-occluded ampulla (5).

Other cases of sperm-occluded ampullae are associated with cystic structures in the area between the terminations of the ampullar excretory ducts within the colliculus seminalis (Fig. 20.9). In men, similar cysts have their origin in müllerian duct remnants or the vesicular glands and are referred to as *prostatic utricles*. They are reported to be responsible for cases of ejaculatory duct obstruction, hemospermia, dysuria, and ejaculatory dysfunction (13). In stallions, these cysts are typically unilocular and teardrop-shaped and may occupy more than 50% of the cross-sectional area encompassed by the urethralis muscle at the level of the seminal colliculus. Located between the ampullar excretory ducts and within the confines of the surrounding urethralis muscle, a noncompressible cyst may interfere with the loss of unejaculated spermatozoa during micturition or with the transport of sperm during emission. The resulting accumulation of sperm could eventually result in excretory duct occlusion. In one stallion exhibiting long-term ampullar excretory duct obstruction associated with a müllerian duct cyst, the ampullar lumen became grossly distended (Fig. 20.10). This stallion also exhibited apparent discomfort immediately preceding ejaculation and often required multiple jumps to obtain a collection. These cysts are seen more frequently in older horses, which suggests that they are an acquired problem. They are not detectable by palpation. Endoscopically, even large cysts are evident only as a prominence or asymmetry to the colliculus seminalis. Cystic müllerian duct remnants are also commonly seen in the urogen-

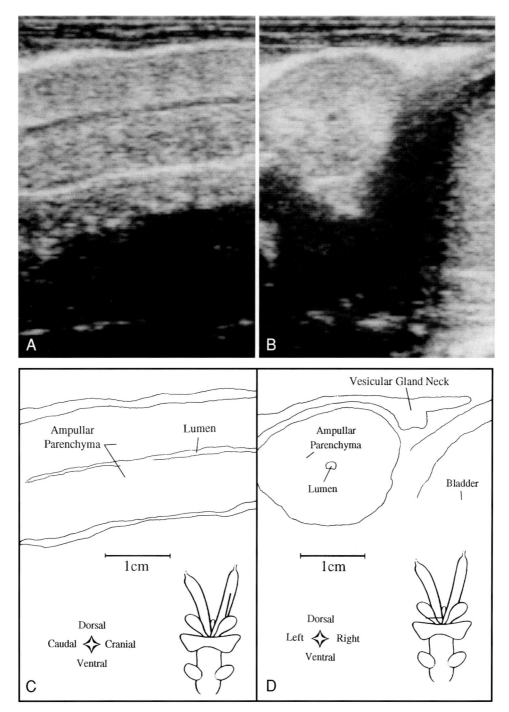

Figure 20.7. A and **B**, Longitudinal (*left side*) and transverse (*right side*) ultrasonograms of the ampulla of the vas deferens in a mature stallion. **C** and **D**, Image orientation is shown by compass key.

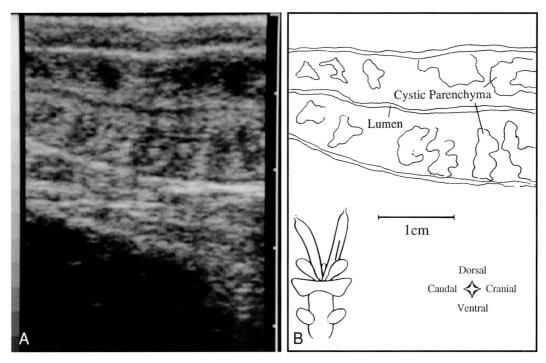

Figure 20.8. A, Longitudinal ultrasonogram of the ampulla from a mature stallion exhibits hypoechoic areas within the parenchyma that are typical of dilated tubuloalveolar glands. **B**, Image orientation is shown by compass key.

ital fold between converging ampullae, where they are apparently of no clinical significance.

Vesicular Glands

The vesicular glands are pyriform sacs that produce, store, and emit the gel fraction of the stallion ejaculate. They are found dorsolateral to the bladder and the ipsilateral ampullae (see Fig. 20.1). Each gland consists of a neck, body, and fundus. Their size depends primarily on the duration of sexual stimulation and the season of the year.

In nonstimulated stallions, the vesicular glands are typically almost empty, easily compressed, and closely opposed to the rectal wall; their mucosal surface is less echogenic. These characteristics make both palpation and ultrasonography more difficult. In nonstimulated stallions, the vesicular glands are best evaluated by identifying the gland neck in transverse section, dorsolateral to the ipsilateral ampulla, and following the neck cranially to the fundus.

After sexual stimulation, echolucent fluid accumulates in the fundus, the echogenicity of mucosal folds increases, and the glands are readily identified ultrasonographically (Fig. 20.11). Manual redistribution of gel from the fundus to the neck can be used to highlight the neck region from surrounding soft tissue. The vesicular glands are the most frequent site of bacterial infection among the accessory sex glands of the stallion. Diagnosis of vesicular adenitis relies on rectal palpation, culture, and cytology of fractionated ejaculates or expressed secretions and perhaps endoscopy of the vesicular gland lumen (14). In at least one report, palpa-

tion findings were unremarkable (15). Recently, transrectal ultrasonography has been used to support the diagnosis made by traditional means (16,17). Ultrasonographic findings reported in these cases were increased overall size, thickened wall, and increased echogenicity when compared with the contralateral, unaffected glands.

Excretory Ducts

The excretory ducts of the ampullae, vesicular glands, and prostate course to the seminal colliculus within the core area surrounded by the urethralis muscle. If the transducer is positioned for a transverse image at the cranial border of the urethralis muscle and slid caudally, the excretory ducts may be evident (see Fig. 20.3). When visible, the vertical crescents represent the seminal vesicle excretory ducts and the white dots medial to these crescents are the excretory ducts of the ampullae. Lateral or dorsolateral to the seminal vesicles, the area occupied by bundles of prostatic ductules from the ipsilateral prostate lobe is occasionally evident (Fig. 20.12). Experimentally, this core region has been useful in evaluating the sequence and timing of events associated with emission and ejaculation (8) because fluid passing through the ampullar and vesicular gland excretory ducts is clearly visible ultrasonographically (Figs. 20.13 and 20.14).

Pelvic Urethra

The pelvic urethra runs from the bladder neck to the ischial arch, also within the core area surrounded by the urethralis

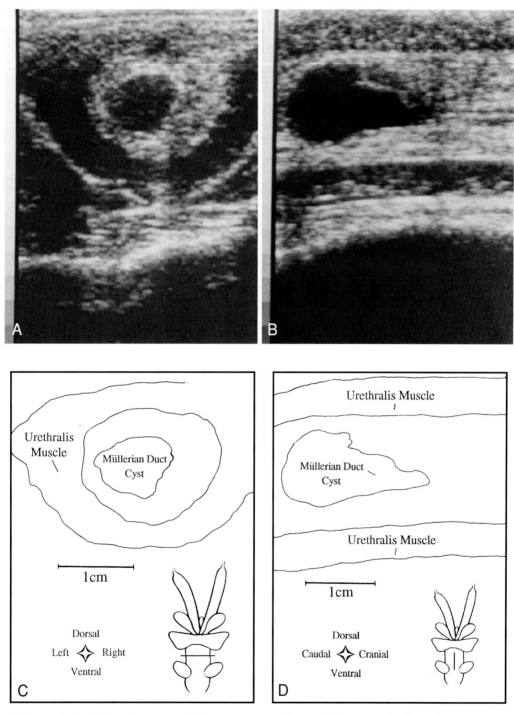

Figure 20.9. Longitudinal (**A**) and transverse (**B**) ultrasonograms at the level of the seminal colliculus from a mature stallion with obstructive azoospermia. A hypoechoic structure is evident at the colliculus. Dissection proved this structure to be a cystic Müllerian duct remnant. **C** and **D**, Image orientation is shown by compass key.

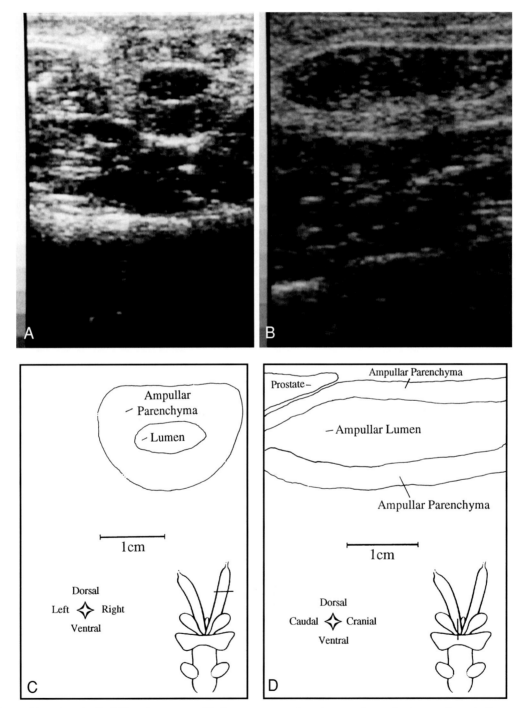

Figure 20.10. Longitudinal (**A**) and transverse (**B**) ultrasonograms of an obstructed ampulla show a distended lumen. **C** and **D**, Image orientation is shown by compass key.

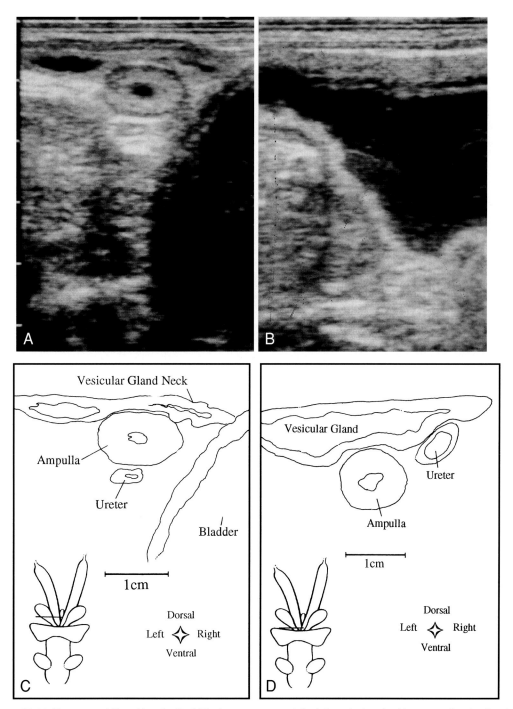

Figure 20.11. Transverse (**A**) and longitudinal (**B**) ultrasonograms of the left vesicular gland in a sexually stimulated mature stallion. The vesicular gland neck contains a small amount of fluid and lies dorsal to the ampulla. The ureter is imaged obliquely as it courses to the neck of the bladder, ventral to the ampulla. The distended body of the vesicular gland is evident in longitudinal section. **C** and **D**, Image orientation is shown by compass key.

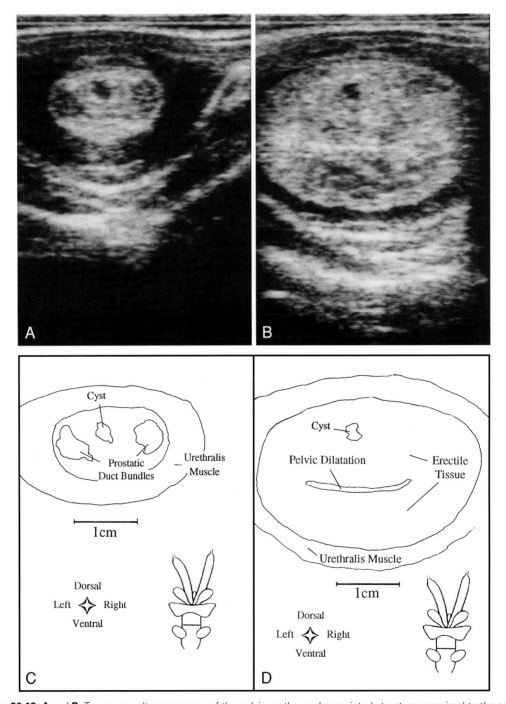

Figure 20.12. A and **B**, Transverse ultrasonograms of the pelvic urethra and associated structures proximal to the seminal colliculus. The prostatic ducts are visible as hypoechoic bundles on each side of a small cystic structure. The seminal vesicle necks and ampullar excretory ducts are not readily visible in this photograph. **C** and **D**, Image orientation is shown by compass key.

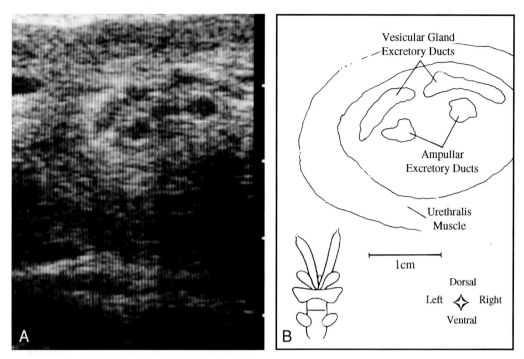

Figure 20.13. A, Transverse ultrasonogram of the excretory ducts of the ampullae and vesicular glands from a mature stallion during the late stages of emission and early ejaculation. The ampullar excretory ducts are fully open and emitting the last epididymal and vasal contributions to the ejaculate. The vesicular gland excretory ducts carrying the gel fraction are just beginning to open. In most ejaculates the ampullar contribution is complete before the vesicular gland contribution begins. **B**, Image orientation is shown by compass key.

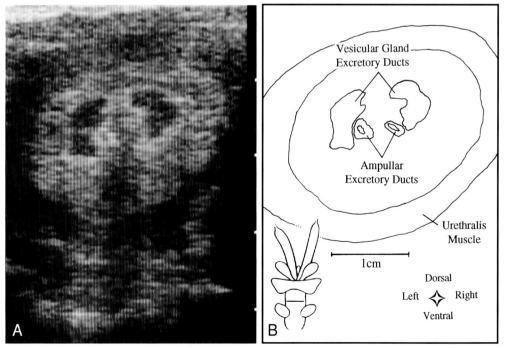

Figure 20.14. A, Transverse ultrasonogram of the excretory ducts of the ampullae and vesicular glands from a mature stallion during the final stages of emission. The ampullar excretory ducts are closed and the vesicular gland excretory ducts are distended with the gel fraction. **B**, Image orientation is shown by compass key.

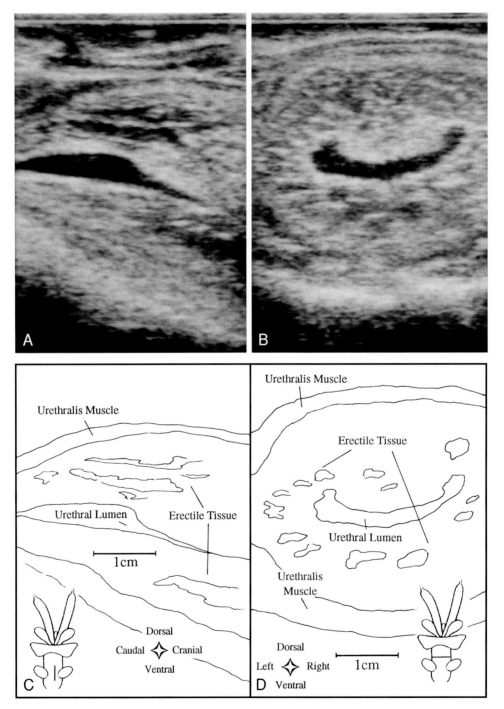

Figure 20.15. A and **B**, Longitudinal (*left side*) and transverse (*right side*) ultrasonograms of the pelvic urethra and surrounding erectile tissue in a sexually stimulated stallion. Preejaculatory fluid in the dilated portion of the pelvic urethra highlights the seminal colliculus protruding from the dorsal wall. The erectile tissue surrounding the urethra is filled. This stretches and thins the urethralis muscle. **C** and **D**, Image orientation is shown by compass key.

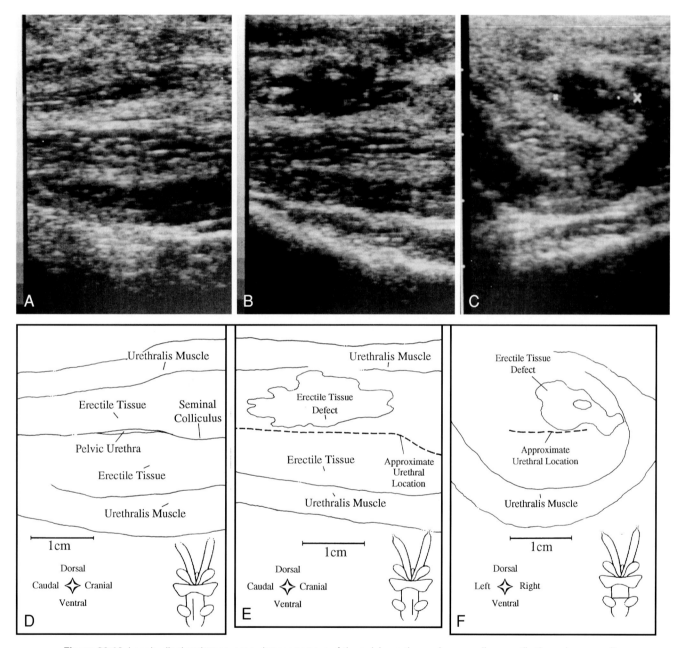

Figure 20.16 Longitudinal and transverse ultrasonograms of the pelvic urethra and surrounding erectile tissue in a sexually stimulated, hemospermic stallion. **A**, The longitudinal image (*left*) shows normal erectile tissue just left of the midline. The urethral lumen and the caudal portion of the seminal colliculus are evident. **B**, This image was taken from just right of midline and reveals an irregular, hypoechoic region within the erectile tissue immediately above the urethra. **C**, The same defect is visible in the transverse image (*right*). Endoscopy revealed that this defect was immediately adjacent to a small rent in the urethral mucosa. **D–F**, Image orientation is shown by compass key.

muscle. The urethra is ventral to the excretory ducts and is usually evident only by specular reflection. The initial segment is quite narrow but widens at the seminal colliculus to form the pelvic dilatation of the urethra. An erectile tissue layer, the stratum cavernosum, begins just proximal to the seminal colliculus and surrounds the pelvic dilatation of the urethra, where emitted semen fractions are deposited immediately before ejaculation. Distally, this erectile cavity is continuous with the corpus spongiosum surrounding the penile urethra. Fluid waves generated along these erectile cavities

by rhythmic contractions of the urethralis muscle rapidly propel semen through the urethra during ejaculation (18). After sexual stimulation, preejaculatory fluid accumulates within the dilated portion of the urethra and is evident as a crescent-shaped echolucency in transverse sections (Fig. 20.15). The crescent shape is the result of the seminal colliculus protruding downward from the roof of the urethra. The coarse trabecular pattern of the blood-filled stratum cavernosum also becomes evident.

In hemospermic stallions in whom rents or lacerations in

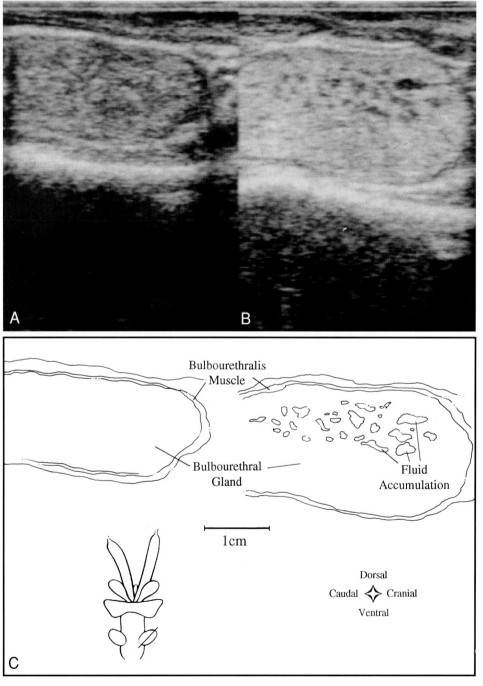

Figure 20.17. A and **B**, Longitudinal ultrasonograms of the same bulbourethral gland from a mature stallion before (*left*) and after (*right*) sexual stimulation. Note the increased size, enhanced echogenicity, and fluid accumulation in the stimulated gland. **C**, Image orientation is shown by compass key.

the urethra communicate with the stratum cavernosum, disruption of the normal trabecular pattern in this erectile layer may be evident (Fig. 20.16). These stallions show profound hemospermia that often begins after intromission, as pressure in the stratum cavernosum and corpus cavernosum urethra increases (18). These rents occur most frequently near the level of the bulbourethral gland openings, where the erectile cavities narrow as they pass around the ischial arch.

Bulbourethral Glands

The bulbourethral glands are paired structures located dorsolateral to the pelvic urethra at the ischial arch. They produce preejaculatory fluid, which enters the caudal pelvic urethra via multiple openings on either side of the midline. The bulbourethral glands may be difficult to palpate, particularly in the young stallion, but they are readily evaluated by ultrasonography.

For imaging of the bulbourethral glands, the transducer should be inserted into the rectum in a longitudinal orientation and directed by only two or three fingers. By leaving the rest of the hand outside the anus, the operator achieves better contact between the transducer and the rectal wall and minimizes straining by the stallion. For in-line transducers, the glands are located by rotating the probe around its longitudinal axis alternating between the 5 and 7 o'clock positions until the glands are visualized. The bulbourethral parenchyma is ovoid in longitudinal section and surrounded by a thin, echolucent layer of muscle. The parenchyma is homogeneous in appearance in the nonstimulated state (Fig. 20.17).

After sexual stimulation, fluid accumulates rapidly in echolucent pockets. These pockets contrast sharply with the parenchyma, which concurrently increases in echogenicity. In transverse scans after stimulation, the general course of the bulbourethral gland excretory ducts over the urethralis muscle to the dorsal midline may be appreciated. The trabecular pattern of the stratum cavernosum surrounding the narrow urethra is also apparent at this level after sexual stimulation (Fig. 20.18).

Accessory Sex Gland Dimensions

The stallion's accessory sex glands depend on the presence of androgens for their development and maintenance (19). After castration, ultrasonographically determined gland dimensions are reduced (20), resulting in measurable differences in gland dimensions between mature stallions and geldings (Table 20.1)(Fig. 20.19).

These differences may be useful in appraising the endocrine status of horses that exhibit stallion-like behavior but have no palpable testes. Many of these horses are abdominal cryptorchids, but in one study, just as many were previous castrates (21). Since many cryptorchid testes are capable of producing testosterone at levels similar to those of the normal stallion (22,23), a presumptive diagnosis of retained testicular tissue may be made ultrasonographically by comparing the accessory sex gland dimensions of the suspect cryptorchid to those of true geldings. Ampullar dimensions in particular may be useful in this regard because they exhibit the least variability between readings and the greatest percent decrease in diameter after castration. Ampullar dia-

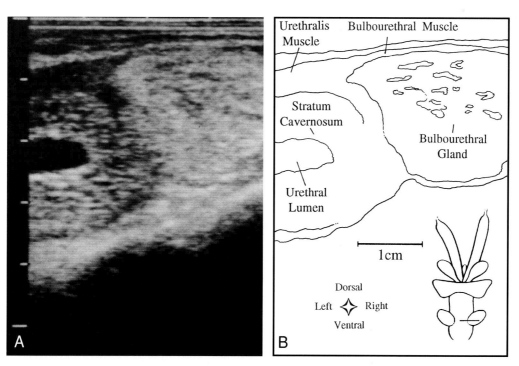

Figure 20.18. A, Transverse ultrasonogram of the caudal pelvic urethra and right bulbourethral gland of a mature, sexually stimulated stallion. The distended stratum cavernosum surrounding the urethra is evident. **B**, Image orientation is shown by compass key.

Table 20.1.
Maximum Dorsoventral Gland Diameter (mm)
in Nonstimulated Stallions and Geldings

Group	Ampulla		Prostate		Bulbourethral	
	Mean	SD	Mean	SD	Mean	SD
Stallions[a]	15.7	2.4	32.9	6.4	23.1	3.0
Geldings[b,c,d]	5.1	0.9	12.8	3.1	12.3	2.5

[a] Values are from 20 stallions more than 3 years of age, right and left sides.
[b] Values are from 12 geldings more than 3 years of age, right and left sides.
[c] Two castrated at maturity; age at time of castration for others unknown.
[d] Little, Timoney, and McCollum, unpublished data.

meters exceeding 6 mm at their widest point are suspect cryptorchids. An inherent advantage to the ultrasonographic diagnosis is that the pulsatile nature of testosterone secretion is not a source of error. Caveats to this approach are that before the spring of their 3-year-old year, cryptorchid colts may still have low testosterone levels and insufficient accessory sex gland development to reliably differentiate them from true geldings. Also, recent castrates may require up to 2 months for glands to fully regress.

SUMMARY

In summary, transrectal ultrasonography offers a useful adjunct to palpation in evaluating the internal reproductive tract of the stallion. It facilitates rapid identification and evaluation of the accessory sex glands, provides objective assessments of gland dimensions, and offers unique information on structures that are not readily palpated. Transrectal ultrasonography is specifically indicated in suspected cases of reproductive tract inflammation or infection, excurrent duct obstruction, hemospermia, and ejaculatory dysfunction. Ultrasonographically determined accessory sex gland dimensions may be useful in establishing the presence of testicular tissue in suspect cryptorchids. As the use of transrectal ultrasonography becomes more commonplace, additional indications are anticipated.

REFERENCES

1. Kenney RM. Clinical fertility evaluation of the stallion. Proceedings of the Annual Convention of the American Association of Equine Practitioners 1975:336–355.
2. Kenney RM, Hurtgen J, Pierson R, et al. Theriogenology and the equine. Part II, the stallion. J Soc Theriogenology 1983;9:7–100.
3. Varner DD. Introduction of the stallion breeding soundness examination form of the Society for Theriogenology. Proceedings of the Annual Meeting of the Society for Theriogenology 1992:113–116.
4. Little TV, Woods GL. Ultrasonography of the accessory sex glands in the stallion. J Reprod Fertil 1987;35(Suppl):87–94.
5. Love CC, Riera FL, Oristaglio RM, et al. Sperm occluded (plugged) ampullae in the stallion. Proceedings of the Annual Meeting of the Society for Theriogenology 1992:117–127.
6. Jann HW, Rains JR. Diagnostic ultrasonography for evaluation of cryptorchidism in horses. J Am Vet Med Assoc 1990;196:297–300.
7. Weber JA, Geary RT, Woods GL. Changes in accessory sex glands of stallions after sexual preparation and ejaculation. J Am Vet Med Assoc 1990;196:1084–1089.
8. Weber JA, Woods GL. Ultrasonographic measurement of stallion accessory sex glands and excurrent ducts during seminal emission and ejaculation. Biol Reprod 1993;49:267–273.

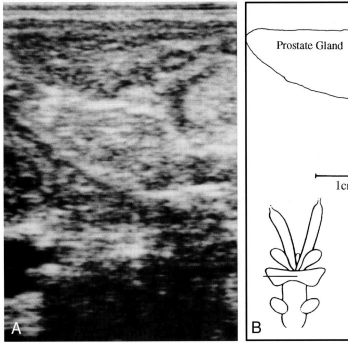
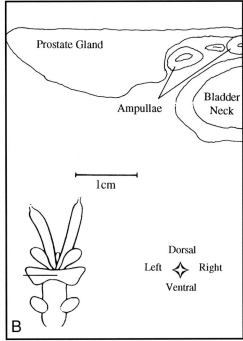

Figure 20.19. A, Transverse ultrasonogram of the wing of the prostate gland from a 4-year-old gelding castrated 6 months previously. **B**, Image orientation is shown by compass key.

9. Varner DD, Schumacher J, Blanchard TL, et al. Diseases and management of breeding stallions. Goleta: American Veterinary Publications, 1991:1–349.

10. Arnold JS, Meagher DM, Lohse CL. Rectal tears in the horse. J Equine Med Surg 1978;2:55.

11. Little TV, Holyoak GR. Reproductive anatomy and physiology of the stallion. Vet Clin North Am 1992;8:1–30.

12. Weber JA, Woods GL. Ultrasonographic studies of accessory sex glands in sexually rested stallions and bulls, sexually active stallions and a diseased bull. Proceedings of the Annual Meeting of the Society for Theriogenology 1989:157–165.

13. Pryor JP, Hendry WF. Ejaculatory duct obstruction in subfertile males: analysis of 87 patients. Fertil Steril 1991;56:725–730.

14. Varner DD, Taylor TS, Blanchard TL. Seminal vesiculitis. In: McKinnon AO, Voss JL, eds. Equine reproduction. Philadelphia: Lea & Febiger, 1993:861–863.

15. Blanchard TL, Varner DD, Hurtgen JP, et al. Bilateral seminal vesiculitis and ampullitis in a stallion. J Am Vet Med Assoc 1988; 192:525–526.

16. Malmgren L, Sussemilch BI. Ultrasonography as a diagnostic tool in a stallion with seminal vesiculitis: a case report. Theriogenology 1992;37:935–938.

17. Freestone JF, Paccamonti DL, Eilts BE, et al. Seminal vesiculitis as a cause of signs of colic in a stallion. J Am Vet Med Assoc 1993; 203:556–557.

18. Beckett SD, Walker DF, Hudson RS, et al. Corpus spongiosum penis pressure and penile muscle activity in the stallion during ejaculation. Am J Vet Res 1975;36:431–433.

19. Thompson DL, Pickett BW, Squires EL, et al. Sexual behavior, seminal pH, and accessory sex gland weights in geldings administered testosterone and (or) estradiol-17β. J Anim Sci 1980;51: 1358–1366.

20. Little TV, Holyoak GR, McCollum WH, et al. Output of equine arteritis virus from persistently infected stallions is testosterone-dependent. Proceedings of the Sixth International Conference on Equine Infectious Diseases 1992:225–229.

21. Cox JE. Behavior of the false rig: causes and treatments. Vet Rec 1986;118:353–356.

22. Cox JE, Redhead PH, Dawson FE. Comparison of the measurement of plasma testosterone and plasma oestrogens for the diagnosis of cryptorchidism in the horse. Equine Vet J 1986;18:179–182.

23. Stabenfeldt GH, Hughes JP. Clinical aspects of reproductive endocrinology in the horse. Compend Contin Educ Pract Vet 1987; 9:678–684.

21. The Superficial Digital Flexor Tendon

RONALD L. GENOVESE AND NORMAN W. RANTANEN

INTRODUCTION

Two-dimensional equine musculoskeletal diagnostic ultrasound was first reported in the veterinary literature in 1982 (1). A second report followed shortly, (2) and four reports were published in 1983 (3–6). There were 22 reports of its use in equine musculoskeletal disorders from 1983 to 1986 (7). From those humble beginnings, considerable expertise has been developed in lesion detection and management (8–11). The first report of quantitative analysis of superficial digital flexor tendon injuries in racehorses appeared in 1990 (12). Those investigations have developed treatment recommendations and rehabilitation programs for injured horses (13, 14). These programs monitor tendon healing and the surrounding tissues ultrasonographically. The objective measurements have been proven prognostically and diagnostically.

The experimental drug, Beta-aminoproprionitrile (BAPN or BAPTEN®, Alaco Inc., Tuscon, AZ), is being investigated as an aid to more organized tendon healing because of its inhibition of collagen cross-linking. This clinical research has spawned a new science of scar manipulation as it applies to connective tissue healing in the horse (15, 16). Tendon treatment regimens, rehabilitation protocols, and long-term tendon injury management are peripheral benefits of the BAPTEN® research (17–19). Ultrasonography is the primary imaging modality supporting this clinical research. See Chapter 27 for more on treatment.

Considering the short time that has passed since the first reports, tendon and ligament ultrasonography has come a long way. Tendon examination has gone beyond finding the "black hole." When most practitioners saw their first "black hole" on a Polaroid picture in the early 1980s, conventional tendon treatment suddenly lost its meaning. Since that time, tendons and ligaments have been viewed differently. No longer were the heat, pain, and swelling the only "bad guys;" tendon lesions had to be reckoned with because they were now visible. One author (RLG) presented a talk to a group of trainers 11 years ago demonstrating the "black holes." When he was introduced, the host commented that he "wanted to hear this talk because, in his long training career, when a horse bowed, he got rid of it." Luckily, this attitude is changing. Progress has been made and more horses with tendon injuries are returning to competition, many at or above their previous performance levels. Sonography has contributed significantly to this progress, providing earlier diagnosis, better case management, and improved treatment; thereby returning more horses to competition.

The purpose of this chapter is two-fold: 1) to introduce the basic application principles of tendon sonography for those who may be unfamiliar with the technology; and 2) to present the successes and failures of tendon injury management (and the reasons why) and to share our opinions with those more experienced clinicians who have also stared at sonograms and wondered what was going on. The chapter has been divided into several sections that allow readers to concentrate on specific interest areas. These sections begin with the basic principles of application and end with clinical case presentations. Two goals of this chapter are to help the reader improve technical skills and sonographic interpretation. New quantitative assessment methods are explored that will hopefully improve tendon injury management.

NORMAL EQUINE LIMB SONOGRAPHY

To better appreciate the abnormal, it is essential to properly master normal superficial digital flexor tendon sonography (SDFT). To become proficient at equine limb sonography, one should begin with proper limb preparation. State of the art imaging equipment should be used for all studies. The sonogram displays specific morphologic features that help the clinician confirm and support clinical impressions.

SDFT evaluation includes five basic sonographic parameters: size, shape, texture, position, and fiber alignment. These parameters are used to identify sub-gross abnormalities that can confirm SDFT disease or the repair status. Valid conclusions can be made only from good quality sonograms. Sonography, unlike some aspects of radiology, is user-specific. Only through examiner expertise can accurate sonographic information be obtained. Improper use can lead to recording artifacts that can cause misdiagnosis. For instance, improper limb preparation causes poor transducer contact, resulting in an SDFT image that is diffusely or focally hypoechoic. This may lead to the false impression of SDFT injury. A special effort should be made to produce excellent quality hard copy images that correlate with the real time image viewed during scanning. Printed copies that are too bright or too dark or that improperly represent the lesion lead to misdiagnoses. The beginner sonographer must become proficient at image making to interpret the information properly. Data obtained in real time must be recorded accurately for the patient record, for future review, and for comparison of serial images. It is advantageous to give real time diagnostic impressions and to review the hard copies later. There are many interpretive options available at

289

the hard copy review session that are not accomplished easily during real time examination. For instance, a zone-by-zone comparison to a contralateral normal limb can be accomplished more efficiently by comparing images after the examination. A comparison of tendon texture on previous scans is done more accurately from images. There are many innovative quantitative SDFT measurements made on the images that can contribute diagnostic and prognostic information. We have found that in clinical practice, it is preferable to give a preliminary stall side diagnosis, but to withhold a final evaluation until the images have been reviewed thoroughly. We strongly advise this approach as a means to reduce diagnostic errors.

PATIENT PREPARATION AND SCANNING TECHNIQUE

In most circumstances, horses should be sedated before sonographic examination. The sonographer usually does the examination in a sitting or kneeling position. The examiner must focus his or her center of attention on transducer placement and on viewing the monitor. Because of this positioning, a fractious horse can inadvertently injure the sonographer or damage the equipment. Proper sedation and restraint allow the sonographer to concentrate on the examination. Some of the most questionable sonographic data is obtained when horses are difficult to manage during scanning.

The skin surface can be prepared in two basic ways: First, the area can be clipped with #40 clipper blades and then shaved. This provides the best preparation and skin contact for the transducer. A second method is to wash the limb with soap and water and to apply rubbing alcohol before applying the contact gel. This method works well and avoids clipping the hair. Some clients prefer not to have their horse's legs clipped. However, the equipment manufacturer should be consulted to verify that alcohol will not damage the transducers.

The horse should stand squarely on the limb being studied to assure proper SDFT tension. Tendon laxity can produce artifacts and misdiagnoses. However, to assess the flexor tendon gliding movement and to determine relative flexor tendon motion, an assistant can hold the limb in flexion during scanning while flexing and extending the metacarpophalangeal joint. This study may be useful in locating restrictive adhesions between the flexor tendons and the surrounding soft tissues or tendon sheath. It is useful for determining whether palmar or plantar annular ligament constriction is present (historically referred to as volar annular ligament [VAL] constriction). Palmar or plantar annular ligament (AL) constriction would be the more correct terminology according to the Anatomica Medica.

The SDFT should be scanned through a standoff device which allows tendon surface visualization. It is possible to miss SDFT surface tears because of artifacts created by the transducer and skin interface and because of the difficulty in focusing the crystals within the first centimeter.

A systematic scanning procedure should be developed by each sonographer to ensure thorough tendon evaluation. Furthermore, a complete metacarpal/metatarsal examination should be included. During scanning, a survey of all structures should be made, including vasculature, subcutis, ligaments, and tendons. It is common to find lesions in multiple structures that may influence treatment options and prognosis. Our systematic scanning approach continues from proximal to distal while viewing all structures. A second series of scans targets the area(s) of interest, and appropriate zone hard copies are made. The beginner should do a general metacarpal/metatarsal survey before recording images. This step ensures a complete evaluation without the distraction of identifying precise limb levels and trying to make prints. Once the survey is done and general impressions are gained, the limb is rescanned to obtain images of the appropriate zones. The recorded levels contain the most meaningful data. When scanning the metacarpus/metatarsus, the sonographer should make a cross-sectional and sagittal print of each zone regardless of the SDFT appearance. These prints allow for quantitative measurements like cross sectional area (CSA) or the hypoechoic fiber path volume (T-HYP), which are discussed later in the chapter.

Both superficial flexor tendons should be scanned in horses with minimal tendon abnormalities. Images of comparable zones from each tendon should be recorded so that comparisons can be made. Presently, we include both limbs routinely and include at least six identical (preferably seven zones) in the forelimb, and at least seven levels (preferably nine matching levels) in the hindlimb, for CSA data.

SONOGRAPHIC EQUIPMENT AND HARD COPY PROCEDURE

The ultrasound machine should be in good working order and positioned at stall side on a firm base, cart, or table. A 7.5-MHz transducer is preferable for tendon and ligament scanning because of its superior lateral resolution. A 5.0-MHz transducer is not recommended because subtle lesions cannot be seen due to inadequate lateral resolution.

As with good radiographic technique, special attention should be given to proper image identification and labeling. Each print represents valuable diagnostic and prognostic information that is a part of the patient record. Many clinical decisions, primarily based on morphologic abnormalities, are influenced by the horse's age, use, exercise level, and other factors. Attempting to recall this information from memory several months after the scan is difficult, if not impossible. If this information is included on the image, it is readily available at any time during case review and greatly improves case management. Furthermore, if properly-labeled scans are submitted for a second opinion, the additional information improves communication. The following information should be included on each hard copy whenever possible:

1. Patient name
2. Owner or trainer
3. Name of the examining clinician or veterinary group

4. The scanned limb
5. Age, use, breed
6. Predominant exercise level preceding the scan
7. The image zone or level

In the developmental stages of equine limb sonography, a system of level identification was proposed by Genovese et al. (20). The metacarpus was originally divided into six zones and the metatarsus into eight zones. Since the original zones were defined, others have expanded the metacarpus to seven zones and the metatarsus to nine zones. The scan level "zone" designation was established to assist the practitioner scanning in the field without a ruler. Often, a ruler is not available, and it is difficult to manipulate the transducer, standoff, and contact gel while measuring each scan level at the same time. Therefore, the "zone" designation on the print level is a practical labeling method. For more precise level identification, one can use an ordinary ruler or a specially designed attachable one. In the forelimb, metacarpal measurements are recorded in centimeters (cm) distal to the accessory carpal bone base (DACB). In the hindlimb, metatarsal measurements are recorded in cm distal to the tuber calcaneous (DTC).

If one uses the "zone" method of metacarpal level identification, the most proximal zone is Zone 1A. This zone encompasses the most proximal 4 cm of the metacarpal starting at the DACB. Zone 1B is approximately 4–8 cm DACB. Zones 2A and 2B span 8 cm of the middle third of the metacarpal. The zones in the distal third of the metacarpal are 3A and 3B. Zone 3C includes the metacarpophalangeal joint palmar surface. Zone 3A includes the digital tendon sheath origin (seldom seen in the normal horse) and the distal most suspensory ligament body (third interosseous muscle). Zone 3B includes the medial and lateral suspensory ligament branches distally from the bifurcation. In Zone 3B, the digital tendon sheath is seen. Zone 3C includes the proximal sesamoid bone axial surfaces and the palmar annular ligament (AL).

In the hindlimb, the most proximal zones are along the plantar talus surface. Zone 1A is the proximal half of the plantar talus (7 cm), and Zone 1B is the distal half of the talus (7 cm). Zone 2A is the first metatarsal zone and, like the forelimb, the zones are 4 cm in length in the average 15.2-hand Thoroughbred (TB) horse. Zone 2B is in the proximal third of the metatarsus. Zones 3A and 3B are the middle 8 cm of the metatarsus, and zones 4A and 4B are the distal third of the metatarsus. Zone 4C includes the plantar metatarsophalangeal joint surface.

THE NORMAL SDFT SONOGRAM

Sonographic SDFT examination should include a survey of the entire metacarpus/metatarsus. Relationships of the various structures should be noted, and the vasculature and subcutaneous tissue should be evaluated. Periligamentous and peritendinous tissues should be assessed along with the bone surface contour. For specific structures, the transducer must

be directed at 90° to view the size, shape, texture, density, position, and fiber alignment. Seldom can more than one structure be in the perfect scanning position perpendicular to the soundbeam.

Figure 21.1 is a normal cross-sectional and sagittal left metacarpal Zone 1A sonogram made 4 cm DACB. At this level, the SDFT is oval shaped and is in intimate contact with the skin and subcutis on the medial, lateral, and palmar surfaces, and the DDFT dorsally. In the normal metacarpus, it may be difficult to differentiate the SDFT and DDFT interface. The tendon size, or CSA, is measured in the cross-sectional plane. In the normal horse, the flexor retinaculum is not sonographically distinguishable from the skin and subcutis. However, in some SDFT Zone 1A injuries, flexor retinaculum fibrosis can be seen and may compromise the SDFT gliding motion in the carpal canal.

Currently, there are several methods to measure tendon cross-sectional area (CSA). The first and least accurate, but most practical, method is to measure the palmar/plantar to dorsal dimension (thickness) and the medial to lateral dimension (width) and multiply. This product is a rectangular CSA or, in some instances, a square. Although the SDFT cross-section is neither of these shapes, this simple technique provides valid comparative measurements. This technique is done easily at minimal cost. As long as technique is consistent, tendon size can be compared in both limbs, or the size of one tendon can be determined serially and compared at different times. However, one would not be able to compare cross-sectional area measurements obtained in this manner to other, more accurate methods that trace the tendon perimeter. The same method should be used in each case. In our example (15.1-hand five-year-old thoroughbred gelding in Figure 21.1), the thickness is 9 mm and the width is 12 mm. The product (CSA) is 108 mm². This number is greater than the "actual" CSA, but if the same method is used in the same zone of the opposite normal leg, valid, relative comparisons can be made.

The second method requires tracing the SDFT perimeter

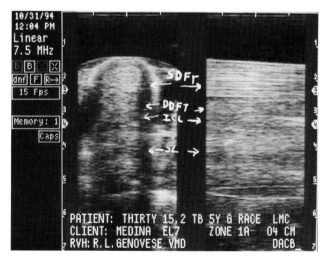

Figure 21.1.

on a digitizing pad. Software programs are used to record the data. This method is more accurate, but more time consuming and more costly. The example Zone 1A, analyzed by this method, was 69mm^2 compared to 108 mm^2 in the previous example.

The third CSA measurement method is done on the ultrasound machine's video screen with built in calipers and software programs. The CSA is displayed on the screen and is recorded on the hard copy. This method provides accurate CSA measurements during the examination; however, it requires more time. Any of the previously mentioned methods can be used if consistency is maintained and values from different methods are not compared.

A similar fourth method is to download the image into a personal computer and use software programs to measure the image. This method is possible directly with the Classic Medical 200 scanner or through an external floppy disk drive used for image capture.

Figure 21.2 is a normal cross-sectional left metacarpal Zone 1A SDFT trace made at 7.5 MHz with a Classic Medical 200 scanner (Classic Medical Supply, Inc., Tequesta, FL) at a 7 cm field depth from the example horse. The CSA determined with the electronic calipers is 72 mm^2.

Figure 21.3 is a normal cross-sectional and sagittal Zone 1A SDFT sonogram at a 4-cm field depth scan made with the same scanner. The digitizing pad method was used to measure this tendon, and the CSA was 82 mm^2.

Figure 21.4 is a normal cross-sectional and sagittal Zone 1A SDFT sonogram made at 7.5 MHz with an ATL 4600 sector scanner (Advanced Technology Laboratories, Inc., Bellevue, WA). The CSA was 81 mm^2 by the digitizing pad method. It is obvious from these examples that measurement error exists and may depend on several factors. Suboptimal image quality or a small tendon image on the dis-

play may be more difficult to trace than a larger one. A digitizing pad may be more accurate than an onscreen tendon tracing during the examination. Different ultrasound machines may have differences in software that might influence tendon tracing accuracy, and differences between operators must be taken into account. Cross-sectional area measurements are useful for SDFT evaluation; however, care should be taken to minimize the error.

To this point, we have illustrated CSA data for one zone. This quantitation can be expanded and summed for any number of tendon levels. By doing this, the clinician can get an idea of a working SDFT "volume." To be accurate, at least six zones, and preferably seven zones, should be included. This "total volume" is referred to as total cross-sectional area (T-CSA).

Figure 21.5 is the computer-generated reproduction of seven SDFT cross-sectional zones of the normal horse using the 7 cm field depth with the Classic Medical 200 Scanner. The seven-level CSA sum is 558 mm^2. Figure 21.6 is the same data obtained from Fig. 21.5 at the 4 cm field depth. The seven-level T-CSA is 602 mm^2. Figure 21.7 is a seven-level T-CSA calculated from images made with the ATL 4600 scanner. The SDFT "volume" is 590 mm^2.

Variation does exist just as it does for the single level determination. However, the T-CSA can be used to detect subtle, diffuse SDFT enlargement without detectable fiber tearing. It can also be used during rehabilitation to monitor tendon repair. Preliminary data from research done on intralesional therapy with experimental BAPTEN® indicates that decreasing T-CSA during rehabilitation suggests a more favorable athletic outcome, and increasing T-CSA during repair could indicate an unfavorable sonographic repair or low-grade inflammation.

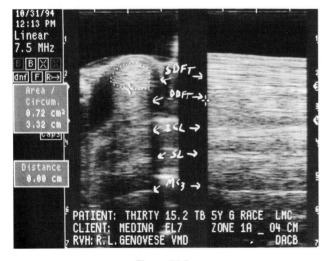

Figure 21.2.

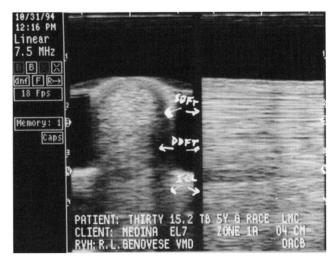

Figure 21.3.

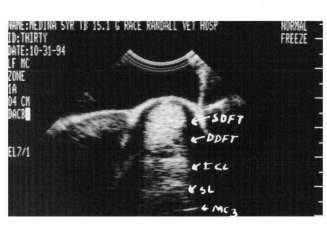

Figure 21.4.

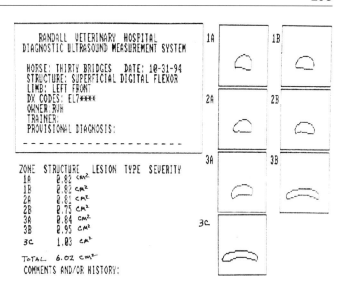

Figure 21.6.

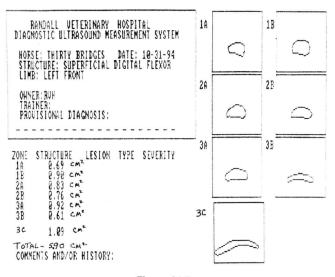

Figure 21.5.

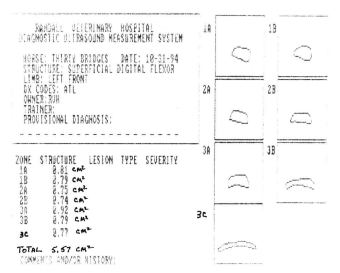

Figure 21.7.

Figure 21.8 is a normal cross-sectional and sagittal left metacarpal Zone 1B SDFT sonogram made 8 cm DACB. At this level, the tendon is slightly crescent shaped. The lateral border has a sharper curve than the more rounded medial border. According to Denoix, the lateral SDFT border is more cellular than the medial border (21). The texture is uniform and referred to as isoechogenic or isoechoic. The palmar, lateral, and medial borders are in contact with the skin and subcutis. The dorsal border is in contact with the DDFT. In the normal horse, the caliper thickness is 8 mm and the width is 14 mm. The digitizing pad CSA is 79 mm^2.

The sagittal view of each SDFT zone (normal or abnormal) should always be included in the examination to confirm lesions, and a quantitative fiber alignment assessment can be made by determining a fiber score (FS). Fiber align-

ment quantitation provides additional important sonographic data for SDFT assessment. Fiber alignment evaluation is useful during healing to assess the sonographic quality of repair (SQR). Fiber alignment scoring was developed during the BAPTEN® field trials to evaluate the remodeling repair phase. In that study, SDFT fiber alignment was scored as the percentage of parallel tendon fibrils in the "target" fiber tract. The "target" tracts are those that have been injured or are under repair. A zero score is given when the "target" area viewed in the sagittal plane has 76–100% parallel fiber alignment. A score of one is given for 51–75%, two for 26–50%, and 3 for 0–25% fiber alignment. In the example 1B sagittal sonogram, there is 100% parallel SDFT fibers scoring zero.

Figure 21.9 is a normal cross-sectional and sagittal Zone

2A SDFT sonogram (10 cm DACB) made with a Classic Medical 200 scanner with a 7.5-MHz linear array transducer displaying a 7.0 cm field depth. The density is isoechogenic, the shape is slightly crescent, and the positioning is the same as in Zone 1B. The short axis and long axis caliper measurements are the same as Zone 1B (8 × 14 mm). The computer-generated CSA is 75 mm². On the longitudinal view, the tendon fibers are nearly all parallel (FS = 0).

It is important to note other pertinent clinical information included on this properly labeled sonogram. The date and time of the study is displayed by an internal clock. The transducer type (linear, 7.5 MHz), field size (7 cm), and the number and focal zone location (3 cm and 4 cm) are displayed. A centimeter ruler borders two sides to allow caliper measurements. These measurements clearly define the sonographic technical settings and are recorded on each hard copy. The sonographer has added vital patient information for this study, including: the name (Thirty), size, age, breed, sex and use (15.2-hand five-year-old Thoroughbred gelding racehorse), owner (Medina), anatomic site [LMC Zone 2A (10 cm DACB)], sonographer (R L Genovese) and finally, the exercise level before the sonogram. When one interprets tendon sonograms, it must be based on the performance level. Therefore, each print contains the important technical and clinical information. This information is essential when serially monitoring tendon injuries. For example, if a tendon had a large hypoechoic lesion 5 months post-injury at stall rest and handwalking only, this would be an unfavorable, SQR. However, a horse with a similar lesion that was galloping daily might have a more favorable prognosis and may respond favorably to a reduction in exercise level. In the BAPTEN® clinical trials, exercise level management, based upon sonographic findings, proved to be extremely important, influencing return to training. All exercise level increases or decreases were strictly guided by prior sonographic findings. For the BAPTEN® research, a practical exercise level sequence was developed so that each sonogram would include this information. The most currently used exercise levels are designed to be practical for the athletic horse.

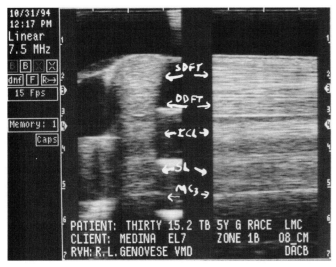

Figure 21.8.

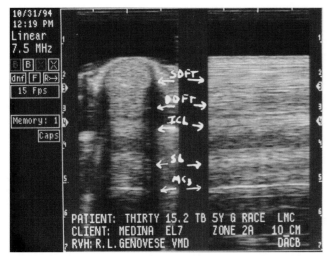

Figure 21.9.

EXERCISE LEVELS

Exercise Level		Activity
EL 1	ALL	walk 30 minutes per day (in hand/mechanical walker).
EL 2a	1.	TB/SH (sport horse)—swim/pony/trot lunge 5–10 min/trot under saddle 5–10 min.
	2.	STD—swim/pony/trot lunge 5–10 min.
EL 2b	1.	TB/SH—swim/pony/trot lunge 10–15 min.
	2.	STD—swim/pony/trot lunge 15 min/*walk* only in bike 30 min.
EL 3a		ALL—small paddock equivalent to round pen.
EL 3b		ALL—regular paddock exercise.
EL 4		TB—DO NOT GO ON TRACK!
		TB/SH—hack in arena w/t/c/ 15–20 min. 3 days/week.
		STD—jog 1 mile *over* 6 min., 5 days/week.
EL 5		TB—normal galloping 1–2 miles on track.
		STD—normal multiple mile jogging on track.
		SH—normal arena work, limited low fence jumping.
EL 6		TB—normal gallop plus *slow* breezes.
		STD—normal jog miles plus *slow* training miles (over 2:20).

SH—normal hacking and practice round jumps.

EL 7   TB—works/racing.

STD—training miles under 2:20/qualifiers/racing.

SH—regular show ring/events.

BAPTEN® RESEARCH PROTOCOL

In our example case, the exercise level before this sonogram was EL-7. It is important to know that this horse is in maximum work and its sonogram is normal at that exercise level.

Figure 21.10 is a normal cross-sectional and sagittal Zone 2B SDFT sonogram (12 cm DACB). The tendon is more crescent-shaped and the thickness is decreased to 7 mm. The width increased to 16 mm, and the computer generated CSA is 76 mm². The density is isoechogenic, positioning is normal, and the fiber alignment is parallel.

Figure 21.11 is a normal cross-sectional and sagittal Zone 3A SDFT sonogram (16 cm DACB). Normally, this level has the distal segment of the suspensory ligament (SL) main body. The proximal digital tendon sheath reflection is normally not seen in this zone. The density is isoechogenic. The tendon is 7.0 mm thick and 19 mm wide. The computer generated CSA is 92 mm². The fiber alignment continues to be parallel and is scored FS-0.

Figure 21.12 is a normal cross-sectional and sagittal Zone 3B SDFT sonogram (21 cm DACB). The medial and lateral suspensory ligament branches (SLB) and the proximal digital tendon sheath (TS) reflection are in this zone. Normally, the dorsal, medial and lateral digital tendon sheath borders can be seen as a 1- to 2-mm echogenic structure, but the sheath palmar to the SDFT is seldom seen. The SDFT tendon is 6.0 mm thick and 26 mm wide. The computer generated CSA is 95 mm² and the fiber alignment is parallel (FS-0).

Figure 21.13 is a normal cross-sectional Zone 3C SDFT sonogram (24 cm DACB). This zone includes the sesamoid bone apices, median sagittal metacarpal ridge, and intersesamoidean ligament, but it is called the most distal metacarpal segment. The palmar annular ligament (AL) can be seen in this zone in some normal horses. The annular ligament appearance has been reported by Dik. In his work, he classified tendon and tendon sheath diseases and added Zone 3C to include the annular ligament (22). Normally, the annular ligament and digital tendon sheath are approximately 2 mm thick when they can be seen. The SDFT is 5 mm thick and 30 mm wide. The computer generated CSA is 109 mm² and the fibers are parallel. Because the SDFT is wide in Zone 3C, the medial and lateral margins may be "cut-off." It may be necessary to scan the tendon margins from oblique directions.

The forelimb zones of a normal 15.2-hand Thoroughbred are as follows:

Zone 1A —0–4 cm DACB (palmar metacarpal)

Zone 1B —4–8 cm DACB (palmar metacarpal)
Zone 2A —8–12 cm DACB (palmar metacarpal)
Zone 2B —12–16 cm DACB (palmar metacarpal)
Zone 3A —16–20 cm DACB (palmar metacarpal)
Zone 3B —20–24 cm DACB (palmar metacarpal)
Zone 3C —24–28 cm DACB (palmar metacarpophalangeal joint)

THE NORMAL HIND SDFT

The hind SDFT can be imaged from its origin to its insertion. The following discussion includes the tendon at the plantar talus, metatarsus, and metatarsophalangeal joint. The plantar hind limb is divided into zones and centimeter measurements are made distal to the tuber calcis (DTC).

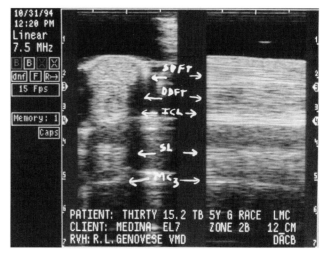

Figure 21.10.

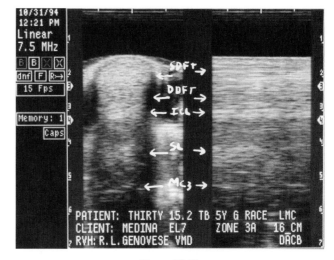

Figure 21.11.

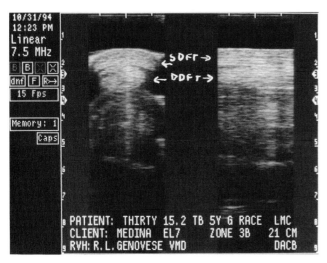

Figure 21.12.

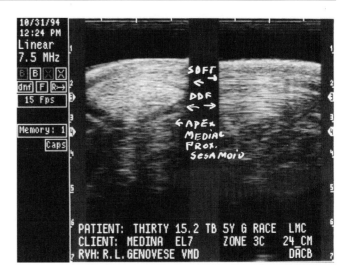

Figure 21.13.

Figure 21.14 is a normal cross-sectional and sagittal Zone 1A SDFT hind limb sonogram made with a Classic Medical 200 scanner with a 7.5-MHz transducer. This level is in the proximal plantar half of the talus (fibular tarsal bone). In this horse, the plantar talus is approximately 15 cm long, making Zones 1A and 1B about 8 cm each in length. This scan is in the most distal Zone 1A, and the tendon is midline. The plantar, medial, and lateral borders contact subcutaneous tissue and skin. The dorsal border opposes the plantar ligament (PL) with a visible interface between them. The tendon is isoechogenic and slightly crescent shaped. It is 10 mm thick and 22 mm wide (CSA = 10 × 22 = 220 mm²). The computer generated CSA measured on the 7.0 cm field depth is 164 mm². At this level, the deep digital flexor tendon (DDFT) is not visible on midline scans, and the transducer must be moved or directed medially to image it. The sagittal sonogram has a parallel SDFT fiber alignment (FS-0).

Figure 21.15 is a normal cross-sectional and sagittal Zone 1B SDFT (11 cm DTC) hind limb sonogram. The image is displayed at a 4 cm field depth. The dorsal SDFT border apposes the DDFT medially and the PL laterally. Normally, there is a 1- to 2-mm wide, vertical, anechoic shadow between the DDFT and the PL. In Zone 1B, the SDFT has an ovoid shape. The density is isoechogenic and fiber alignment is parallel (FS-0). The tendon is 10 mm thick and 19 mm wide (10 × 19 = 190 mm²). The computer generated CSA is 115 mm².

Figure 21.16 is a normal cross-sectional and sagittal Zone 2A (16 cm DTC) hind limb sonogram. This level is the most proximal metatarsal zone which starts approximately 16 cm DTC. This is a difficult zone to scan, especially when trying to evaluate the suspensory ligament origin caused by fiber angle variation and the large, artifact-producing blood vessels. The SDFT contacts the skin and subcutis except on its dorsal surface and images are relatively easy to obtain. The dorsal border contacts the DDFT that has progressively coursed from a medial position to the midline. The inferior check ligament (ICL) is located on the dorsal DDFT surface

and often is not identified easily. It is a more rudimentary structure than in the forelimb. The suspensory ligament (SL) origin and body are roughly rectangular in shape and are commonly, artifactually, partly hypoechoic. The SDFT is oval, isoechogenic, and sagittally has parallel fiber alignment. It is 11 mm × 15 mm (11 × 15 = 165mm²). The computer-calculated CSA for this horse is 113 mm².

Figure 21.17 is a normal cross-sectional and sagittal Zone 2B SDFT (20 cm DTC) hindlimb sonogram. The SDFT has an oval shape and is correctly positioned. It is isoechogenic, 10 mm thick, and 15 mm wide (10 × 15 = 150 mm²). The calculated CSA is 150 mm². The on-screen measured CSA is 107 mm². The fibers are parallel.

Figure 21.18 is a normal cross-sectional and sagittal Zone 3A SDFT (24 cm DTC) hind limb sonogram. This level is in the most proximal aspect of the middle third of the metatarsus. At this level, the SDFT is slightly crescent shaped. The SDFT contacts the skin and subcutis except on its dorsal border. The DDFT opposes the dorsal SDFT border, and the interface is visible. It is isoechogenic and the fibers are parallel. The tendon is 9.0-mm thick and 14-mm wide (9 × 14 = 126 mm²). The computer generated CSA is 104 mm².

Figure 21.19 is a normal cross-sectional and sagittal Zone 3B (28 cm DTC) hindlimb sonogram. The SDFT is isoechogenic and slightly crescent shaped. The fibers are parallel. The caliper dimensions are 8 × 18 mm (8 × 18 = 144 mm²). The calculated CSA is 144 mm². The computer generated CSA is 118 mm².

Figure 21.20 is a normal cross-sectional and sagittal Zone 4A SDFT (32 cm DTC) hindlimb sonogram. This zone, as in the forelimb Zone 3A, is near the suspensory ligament bifurcation. The digital tendon sheath is normally not seen at this level. In this zone, the SDFT is crescent shaped and the texture is isoechogenic. The positioning is normal. The caliper measurements are 8 × 32 mm (8 × 32 = 256mm²). The calculated CSA is 168 mm². The computer generated CSA is 123 mm².

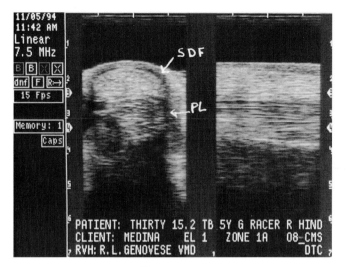

Figure 21.14.

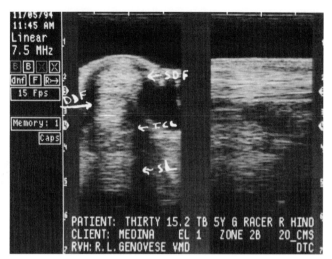

Figure 21.17.

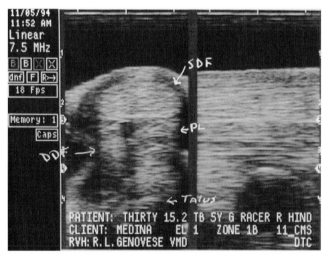

Figure 21.15.

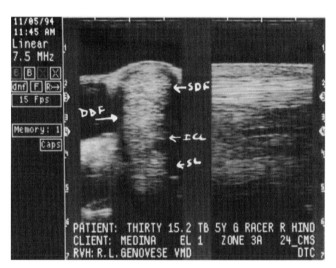

Figure 21.18.

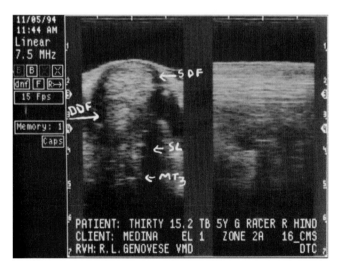

Figure 21.16.

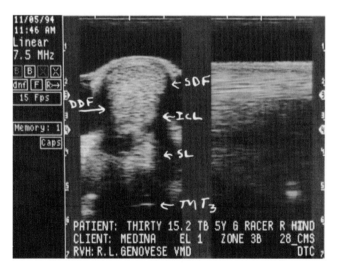

Figure 21.19.

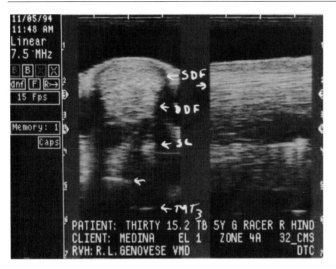

Figure 21.20.

Figure 21.22 is a normal cross-sectional and sagittal right hind sonogram made of the plantar metatarsophalangeal joint. The scan level is Zone 4C (42 cm DTC). This zone contains the proximal sesamoid bone apical outlines, the intersesamoidean ligament, and the AL. As in Zone 4B, it may be difficult to include the entire SDFT on one midline image because of the tendon's width and shape. Multiple images may be needed to document the medial and lateral border morphology. In this example case, the SDFT is isoechogenic, crescent shaped, and properly positioned, and the tendon fibers are parallel (FS-0). The caliper dimensions are 6 mm × 30 mm (6 × 180 = 180mm^2), and the computer generated CSA is 117 mm^2. Figure 21.23 is a computer printout of the nine level hind limb CSA. The total cross-sectional area (T-CSA) is 10.98 cm^2.

Figure 21.21 is a normal cross-sectional and sagittal Zone 4B (40 cm DTC) hindlimb sonogram. At this level, the suspensory ligament has branched. The SDFT is thinner than in the more proximal levels and is isoechogenic. It contacts the skin and subcutis on its plantar, medial, and lateral borders. The dorsal border contacts the DDFT. Normally, the digital tendon sheath can be seen as a 1- to 2-mm curved echogenic structure on the dorsal DDFT. The medial and lateral tendon sheath borders are normally seen. The SDFT is wide and the lateral border is hypoechoic because of scanning artifact. It is difficult to contact the skin in Zone 4C and image the entire SDFT. Therefore, multiple prints may be necessary to document the total texture and medial and lateral SDFT borders. The tendon is narrow and crescent shaped and the caliper measurements were 6 × 27 mm. The calculated CSA is 162 mm^2. The computer generated CSA is 137 mm^2.

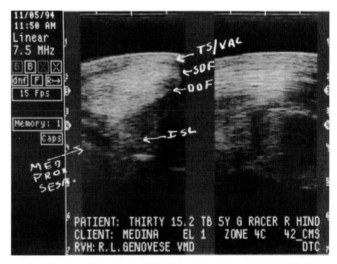

Figure 21.22.

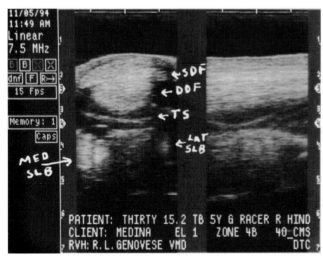

Figure 21.21.

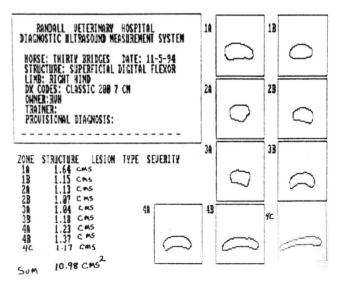

Figure 21.23.

BASIC FUNDAMENTALS OF SONOGRAPHIC EVALUATION OF SDFT INJURY

Introduction

Once the normal SDFT sonographic morphology is familiar, the next step is identifying sonographic abnormalities consistent with injury or disease. Tendon tissue responds to injury in a finite number of ways. Injuries cause abnormalities in size, shape, texture, density, positioning, fiber alignment, and appearance of surrounding soft tissue structures. Tendonitis can be caused by trauma, infection, and adverse chemical reaction; however, the most common cause is over-stretching from athletic use. For the most part, throughout this chapter, use-related injury is our primary concern. Many factors, including conformation defects, improper shoeing, hazardous athletic surfaces, improper or excessive training, and poor rider skills, have been suggested as tendon injury causes. Others in this field have suggested that these factors cause the final insult, but physiologic factors, such as central collagen fiber aging, increased tendon "core" temperature, cyclic loading, collagen/collagen matrix degeneration, or a basic physiologic small tolerance level to overstretching, are the basic tendonitis causes (23). In other words, some athletic activities that horses are forced to perform exceed the tendon's physiologic tolerance. Since racehorses have the highest tendon injury incidence, repetitive, fast works apparently are a significant insult to the SDFT. In our experience, most racehorse tendon injuries have a gradual onset.

An acutely ruptured racehorse SDFT should not pose a diagnostic challenge. However, tendonitis, in the early stages, may present the sonographer with interpretive diagnostic challenges that may cause difficulty in differentiating sonographic abnormalities from normal tendons. Once tendonitis has been diagnosed, a deluge of owner, trainer, and veterinary medical decisions must be made. Underinterpreting sonographic findings can result in more severe, career-ending, or career compromising injuries; conversely, overinterpretation can lead to premature retirement of an equine athlete, causing the owner economic loss. Sonographic SDFT injury assessment is in its infancy compared to radiographic diagnosis of bone disease. Uniform agreement is lacking regarding the clinical significance of some morphologic SDFT abnormalities.

Relating sonographic abnormalities and clinical tendonitis is challenging and at times equivocal. However, as tendon ultrasonography is evaluated over time, its value will be established as interpretive skills improve. This will improve the accuracy of ultrasonographic SDFT injury diagnoses and provide the basis for sensible clinical management of the injured horse. Our present knowledge of tendon injury diagnosis is derived from 14 years' experience. It has provided a template for daily clinical diagnosis, prognosis, and management of SDFT injuries. As diagnostic ultrasound progresses, it will adapt to or dictate changing principles of tendon injury diagnosis and management.

Before diagnostic ultrasound, the clinical approach to an athletic SDFT injury was a clinician's response to the horse attendant's report of palmar/plantar metacarpal/metatarsal swelling that may or may not have a lameness history. Most of the time, lameness is not a complaint associated with mild to moderate tendon injury. The trainer may report a gradual or sudden onset of swelling. The clinician would then examine the horse and attempt to establish a diagnosis of the injury by visual inspection, gait evaluation, and digital palpation. From this examination, a diagnosis, treatment plan, and prognosis would be offered. Regardless of the clinician's palpation skills, a lack of imaging allows room for error in SDFT injury diagnosis. Error could be made in confirming the injury or in assessing the injury's extent. The examination and the subsequent conclusions have significant economic impact for the owner and the horse's well-being.

Hypothetically, if a racehorse completely ruptures the SDFT in a race, the physical examination would not represent a diagnostic challenge. The horse would be lame, most likely there would be increased distal metacarpophalangeal joint deflection at the walk, and palpation would readily reveal a gross tendon tear. This scenario, however, is the least common clinical presentation of horses with SDFT injuries. More commonly, subtle, equivocal tendon injury signs are the presenting complaint. There may be slight vascular distention along the medial metacarpal, or there may be a focal mid-metacarpal "lump," commonly referred to as a "bandage pinch" or "corded" tendon. Without imaging, the clinician cannot make an accurate diagnosis of the injury and offer proper treatment. One author (RLG) has experienced this dilemma in the prediagnostic ultrasound era. He examined a horse with a small swelling and treated it symptomatically, only to discover after the next race or two that the SDFT had completely ruptured.

Ultrasonographic assessment of SDFT healing can be error prone, and an inaccurate judgment of SQR can allow premature training and subsequent reinjury. However, sonography has allowed more accurate tendon injury diagnosis and has helped the practitioner solve these dilemmas. Advances in equine limb sonography over the past decade have shown conclusively that veterinary intervention can redirect and improve the management of metacarpal/metatarsal soft tissue injury.

Any new medical technology initially creates more questions than it answers. Diagnostic ultrasound was no exception to that rule, but the questions and the search for answers helped improve patient care. The most pressing question clinicians ask is the clinical significance of tendon abnormalities. For example: "Does this small focal hypoechoic tendon fiber path mean this horse is 'bowed' or is it just an incidental, nonclinical finding?" or, "If I treat this horse symptomatically and continue use, is it likely that there will be a severe SDFT injury?" With clinical experience and continued research, definite answers will be found for these questions.

A series of physiologic and biochemical events occur at

the time of a tendon injury. Some of these occur at a chemical and not grossly apparent level (23). Many structural changes are sonographically identifiable and others are readily detected grossly. Obviously, a sonogram cannot image a chemical event or a small microscopic event. In the quest to detect chemical differences at this level, attempts are being made to identify blood markers as early evidence of SDFT injury (24). Tendon biopsy is not a practical diagnostic option; however, ultrasound is a practical, noninvasive method of detecting early and small subgross tendon lesions. Subtle inflammation between fiber bundles or small focal fiber tears can be identified and recorded. Minor changes in shape or slight malpositioning are early signs of SDFT injury.

Abnormal SDFT Sonography

Texture, Density and Lesion Types

By definition, tendon density is the degree of brightness (white) or darkness (gray or black). Terms used to describe density include: echogenic (white), echodense (white), echolucent (black), anechoic (black), and hypoechoic (various gray shades). Texture—the pattern configuration that makes up the tendon cross section image or the linear pattern seen on sagittal scans—can have a variable density. Terms used to describe texture include: coarse, fine, linear, cystic, and homogeneous. Texture and density are usually evaluated subjectively.

Texture evaluations are the sonographer's opinion of the tissue pattern, and they usually include a descriptive narrative. For example, one might describe chronic tendonitis texture as follows: "the tendon had a mottled appearance with homogeneous areas interspersed between linear echoes and smaller zones of amorphous dot pattern."

Density has been assigned five brightness (or darkness) levels in an attempt at standardization. The density reflects the degree of collagen fiber echodensity, inflammatory fluids, cellular infiltrates, or a combination of tissue components, depending on the chronicity. This has been called the lesion *type*. Our logic is that normal collagen fiber tracts have a geometric configuration made up of fibers, fluid, and cells that produce an echodensity resulting in a specific brightness that can be recognized as "normal" by the sonographer. This indicates that the fiber constituents are mature collagen (echogenic and dense) and closely packed fiber tracts (i.e., small dot size texture). Immature collagen that has a larger number of cells and more fluid with a scant, immature matrix is less echogenic, resulting in a decreased brightness or whiteness (less dense). Consequently, fewer mature collagen fibers produce a less dense, darker image. Furthermore, if fiber tracts are intact yet spread apart by interstitial fluid accumulation, echogenicity is reduced because of the fluid, and the texture is characterized by a mottled, variable-sized echo pattern surrounded by homogeneous fluid spaces.

The lesion densities or types are as follows:

Type 0: Isoechogenic density; the area in question is a normal, expected brightness.

Type 1: Hypoechoic density; the area in question is mostly echogenic and is viewed as having a slightly reduced but recognizable brightness or whiteness.

Type 2: Hypoechoic density; the area in question would have equal bright and dark areas. This type is less dense than Types 0 and 1.

Type 3: Hypoechoic density; the area in question would be mostly dark or black. Most new lesions with significant fiber tearing or inflammatory infiltrate fall into this category. The predominate shade is dark, but low amplitude echoes are seen within the lesion.

Type 4: Anechoic density; the area in question totally lacks identifiable echoes.

The rationale for grading tissue density is to provide the sonographer with a useable scale to objectively evaluate the severity of morphologic change. The more echoes that are present, the less fiber tearing, hemorrhage, inflammation, or all three. Grading new lesion density can be used as an injury severity parameter. Obviously, an anechoic Type 4 lesion would have a greater amount of collagen disruption than a slightly hypoechoic, Type 1 lesion. In evaluating lesion density as a repair quality measure, a Type 1 repairing lesion would be more favorable than a Type 3. Furthermore, in repair, an increasing visible density or a decrease in the score indicates collagen production. This correlates with improving tendon tensile strength.

Finally, when the repairing scar tissue is more dense than normal tendon, it is referred to as *hyperechoic*. We do not score this density per se, but it represents dense scar formation or mineral deposition and is usually an unfavorable finding. An excessive scar or mineral deposition indicates an inelastic repair that may not be compatible with athletic function.

A large number and wide variety of case examples follow, which we hope demonstrate the gamut of morphologic SDFT abnormalities. Scans were made with 7.5-MHz transducers, using linear array and sector scanheads. The basic objective in this chapter is to address the practical questions: Now that I have detected this sonographic abnormality, what does it imply clinically? What do I tell the client about the tendon's health?

Figure 21.24 is a cross-sectional and sagittal left metacarpal Zone 2B SDFT sonogram of a Thoroughbred race horse with slight swelling along the mid-lateral tendon border. There was no lameness reported at any exercise level, but the swelling persisted despite treatment. The cross-sectional view reveals a focal, round, 7-mm, Type 1 tendon fiber tract along the palmar-lateral tendon border. This lesion was confirmed on the longitudinal view. The pertinent information from these scans is that a rounded, lateral tendon swelling is present and the density is slightly less echogenic than that of the surrounding fiber tracts. The texture is characterized by echolucent spaces separating fiber bundles in both planes. Because the decrease in density and fiber separation is slight, it would follow that many collagen bundles exist and minimal inflammatory infiltrate is present. This would be interpreted as relative minor fiber pattern and tendon strength compromise. The interpretation takes into account the fact that this is a "new" lesion. If this scan was reviewed without any history or clinical findings, one would not be able to differentiate this from an old lesion in repair or an old lesion in an "inactive" state. The sonographer placed all pertinent clinical information on the scan. The exercise level and date of onset are essential information for lesion assessment. In this case, one can comfortably interpret this lesion as having low-grade fiber disruption and minor inflammatory infiltration. This would be diagnosed as a slight SDFT injury or tendonitis.

Figure 21.25 is a cross-sectional left metacarpal Zone 3A SDFT sonogram of a Thoroughbred racehorse with a diffuse Type 1 lesion. Compared with the focal lesion shown in Figure 21.24. The tendon is 7.0 mm by 20 mm and the lesion is 5 mm by 17 mm. The texture is mottled and collagen fascicles are separated. The texture is compatible with an inflammatory infiltrate rather than fiber tract disruption and hematoma formation. Peritendonous palmar anechoic fluid space. This fluid accumulation supports an inflammatory reaction and recent injury. The clinical significance of this appearance is that fiber tearing is probably not a major problem. Systemic anti-inflammatory treatment should be started, the exercise level should be reduced, and the tendon should be scanned again in 2 to 3 weeks, after the inflammation is under control. This allows a more accurate prognosis and confirms any significant fiber tearing. In this horse, it is realistic to advise a short-term interruption in athletic activity and serial sonographic monitoring as a management option. Once again, it is imperative that the clinical presentation be known because it is difficult to distinguish sonographically between a subacute tendonitis and a healing injury that is older and more serious.

Figure 21.26 is a cross-sectional and sagittal left metacarpal zone 1A SDFT sonogram with a small, rounded Type 1 core lesion. This lesion's unique feature is the echolucent inflammatory "halo" around the central injured fiber tract.

Figure 21.27 is a cross-sectional right metacarpal zone 2A SDFT sonogram of an event horse with an acute Type 2 central core lesion measuring 9 mm by 15 mm. Moderate inflammatory infiltrate and fiber disruption are present. In our opinion, there is more strength loss and greater fiber compromise than the Type 1 lesion. Therefore, it is a more serious injury and more careful management is necessary.

Figure 21.28 is a cross-sectional and sagittal right metacarpal zone 3B SDFT sonogram of a racing Thoroughbred with a 7.0 by 15 mm Type 2 injury similar in distribution to the injury shown in Figure 21.27. A linear array scanner was used that displays 64 gray levels compared with 32 gray levels in Figure 21.27. The increased number of gray levels reduces the injured tendon's contrast, causing the tendon and the lesion density to appear more gray instead of black.

Figure 21.29 is a cross-sectional and sagittal left metacarpal Zone 2B SDFT sonogram of a Thoroughbred racehorse with a 5 mm by 7 mm round, focal core lesion. The lesion density is echolucent (dark) with some low amplitude echoes present (Type 3). The surrounding tendon texture and density is relatively normal. The sagittal scan density is similar to the cross-section, confirming that this lesion has more fluid content. There is significantly more fiber bundle disruption and hemorrhage, making this a more serious injury than the Type 2 lesions discussed earlier.

Figure 21.30 is a cross-sectional right metacarpal zone 3A SDFT sonogram of a Thoroughbred racehorse with a recent, diffuse rectangular lesion measuring 10 mm by 16 mm. The density is primarily echolucent; however, echogenic fiber tracts were scattered throughout, making this a Type 3 lesion.

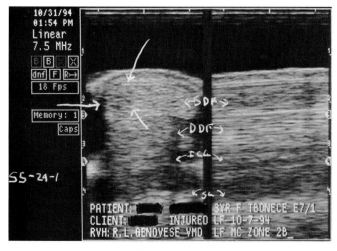

Figure 21.24.

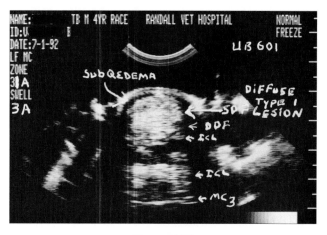

Figure 21.25.

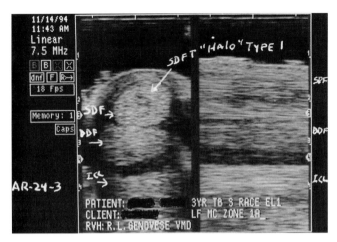

Figure 21.26.

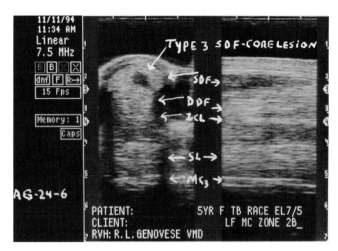

Figure 21.29.

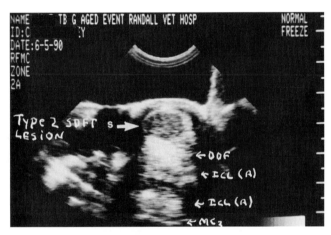

Figure 21.27.

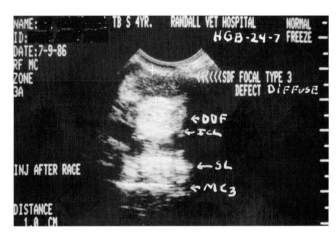

Figure 21.30.

Figure 21.31 is a cross-sectional left metacarpal zone 3A SDFT sonogram of a Standardbred racehorse with a recent focal, rectangular dorsal border lesion. It is graded a Type 4 because the density is totally anechoic and no texture is seen.

Figure 21.32 is a cross-sectional right metacarpal zone 3A SDFT sonogram of a Thoroughbred racehorse with a recent large Type 4 fiber disruption. The tendons in this figure and in Figure 21.32 have total fiber disruption, and the echolucency is primarily hemorrhage, inflammatory infiltrate, and damaged, necrotic collagen fibers. Type 4 tendon lesions are considered the most serious fiber pattern loss. If a significant percentage of the tendon is damaged, considerable tendon strength is lost.

On the infrequent occasions when dense scar and intratendinous mineral deposition are found, they indicate that the tendon damage is chronic. These findings would most likely be detected on a follow-up scan from the sixth to twelfth month after injury. It may be difficult to decide whether the abnormal tract is hyperechoic or isoechogenic

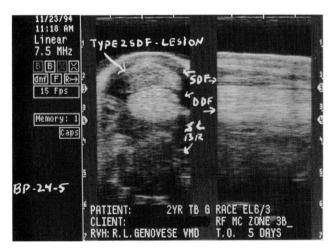

Figure 21.28.

relative to the surrounding echolucent inflammatory infiltrate. The texture of the DDFT can be compared to that of the SDFT, or normal contralateral limb scans can be compared. Other injured tendon zones may also help determine if hyperechoic scar tissue is present. Bright echoes amidst a disorganized tendon fiber pattern might indicate nothing more than tendon fibers or scar segments that are oriented at 90° to the sound beam, generating brighter echoes than the surrounding tissue. Conversely, hypoechoic areas may be created by improper beam angle. The principal reflection angle at the sound–tissue interface is an important factor dictating the reflected sound beam percentage returning to the crystal. Interfaces perpendicular to the sound beam produce high amplitude echoes. Interfaces not oriented at 90° appear more echolucent or, at times, anechoic, depending on the orientation. Diagnosing dense mineral deposition, however, is straightforward because acoustic shadows are present deep to the mineral.

Hyperechoic scar tissue is of concern because of future healing tendon elasticity. Presently, few therapeutic approaches result in excessive, restrictive intratendinous fibrosis. The most likely situation for this to occur is during SDFT injury repair secondary to a laceration or secondary infection. It has been our experience that excessively dense scar tissue creates a tendon repair that is too "stiff," and when loading increases, injury recurs. Excessive peritendinous scarring is discussed later in this chapter.

For example, Figure 21.33 is a cross-sectional right metatarsal zone 4B SDFT sonogram of a Thoroughbred racehorse with a laceration (arrows) that is several months old. The sonogram reveals two focal potential hyperechoic tendon fiber tracts along the mid-plantar and plantar medial borders. The majority of the repairing tendon is hypoechoic relative to these two areas. Because the scar tissue density is similar to the DDFT and normal zones more proximal to this area, we conclude that these two tracts are isoechogenic and the remaining cross-sectional area is hypoechoic.

Figure 21.34 is a dual cross-sectional left metatarsal zone 1B SDFT sonogram of a Standardbred racehorse with a central horizontal hyperechoic scar (arrows). This horse had a long-standing lameness seen at racing speeds and a chronic plantar talus swelling (curb). This intratendinous scar is hyperechoic relative to the isoechogenic SDFT in the right image and it produces an incomplete acoustic shadow.

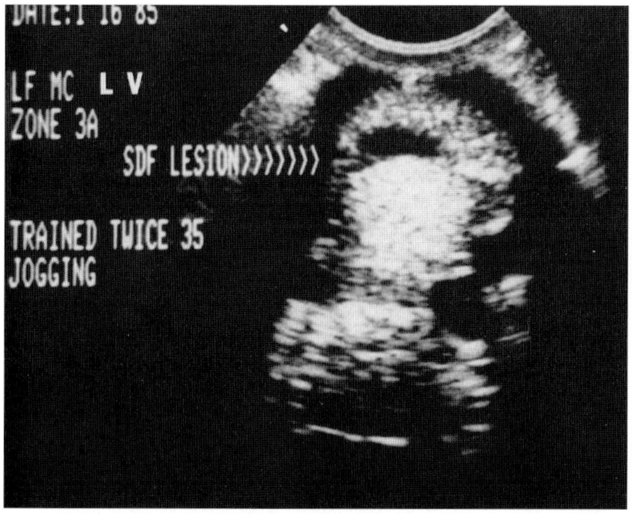

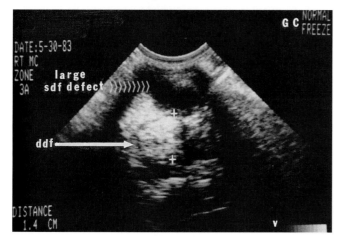

Figure 21.31.

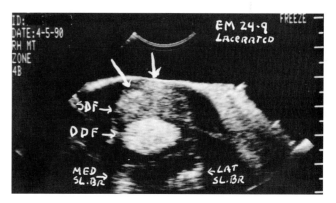

Figure 21.33.

Figure 21.32.

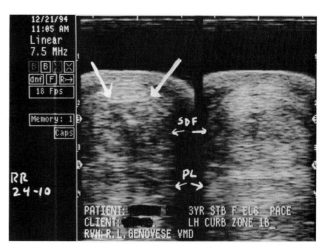

Figure 21.34.

Figure 21.35 is a cross-sectional and sagittal left metacarpal zone 2A SDFT sonogram of a Thoroughbred racehorse with a subtle focal hyperechoic fibrosis. A large core lesion was diagnosed 10 months earlier. The tendon was split and blistered externally, and the horse was allowed pasture rest. Examination of this sonogram reveals several rounded, focal hyperechoic fiber tracts. The surrounding tendon borders are isoechogenic. This hyperechoic fibrous tissue is readily apparent when compared with the normal DDFT density. Fortunately, this hyperechoic scar did not extend very far proximally or distally and will most likely not influence future training.

Figure 21.36 is a cross-sectional left metacarpal zone 3A SDFT sonogram of a Standardbred racehorse with a long history of recurring SDFT injuries. Peritendinous corticosteroid or corticosteroid/hyaluronic acid combination injections were given on various occasions. A horizontal, hyperechoic central SDFT density measuring 5 mm casts a large shadow that is consistent with mineral deposition. The shadow prevents imaging of the remaining tendon from the palmar surface and requires a different transducer location that avoids the highly reflective mineral.

Figure 21.37 is a dual cross-sectional left metatarsal zone 1B SDFT sonogram of a Standardbred racehorse with a large mineral density casting an acoustic shadow. Mineral deposition varies slightly compared with that in Figure 21.36. The mineral is deposited in several adjacent focal sites and the acoustic shadow is not as complete.

Position

Superficial digital flexor tendon displacement is not a common finding in horses. Gross displacement is usually found during physical examination. Subtle medial SDFT displacement secondary to stretching beyond the elastic limit may be overlooked grossly and is usually found during ultrasonographic examination. However, it is worthwhile to present the sonographic appearance of gross tendon displacement because it emphasizes the value of systematic evaluation of sonograms. Also one may be asked to review sonograms with no history and a significant tendon displacement may have been overlooked.

The most common SDFT malpositioning is luxation from the tuber calcaneous. This injury would be easily diagnosed grossly, but if one only had the plantar talus sonogram and had not physically examined the horse, an oversight might occur. Figure 21.38 is a cross-sectional and sagittal left metatarsal zone 1A SDFT sonogram of a Thoroughbred racehorse with displaced tendons (TC = tuber calcaneous). As one proceeds from the skin surface towards the talus bone echo only one soft tissue structure is visible, the plantar ligament (PL). This structure is crescent shaped and attaches to the plantar talus surface. The sagittal scan confirms the plantar ligament origin and a small enthesis can be seen. Normally, the SDFT is midline on the plantar PL surface. The tendon is luxated medially and is not visible on this midline sonogram.

Figure 21.39 is a dual cross-sectional right metacarpal zone 2B (left) and 3B (right) SDFT sonogram of a Standardbred with chronic injury. In right fore zone 3B, the SDFT is in its normal palmar midline position, opposing the DDFT. However, in zone 2B, the tendon is medially displaced. The significance and cause are speculative, but stretching of this tendon beyond its elastic limit, allowing medial displacement, is the most likely cause. Because no preinjury sonograms were available, this malpositioning could possibly have been a preexisting conformation abnormality. It is interesting to speculate whether congenital malpositioning would predispose to injury with increasing workloads. The contralateral limb was normal. Like many pacing Standardbreds, this horse had a varus conformation. If the horse did not have previous SDFT displacement, then it is injury induced. This would allow a more guarded prognosis to return to racing speeds. Because we are unaware of research addressing SDFT positioning and injury predisposition, it is not known if a varus conformation increases the risk of tendon injury in racehorses.

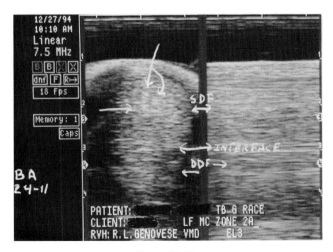

Figure 21.35.

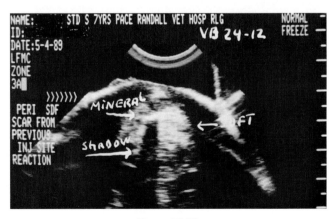

Figure 21.36.

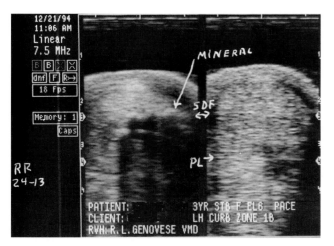

Figure 21.37.

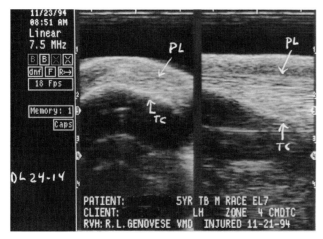

Figure 21.38.

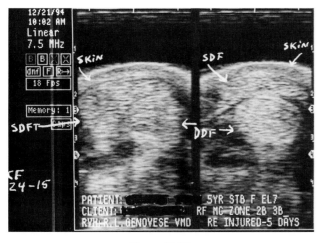

Figure 21.39.

Figure 21.40 is a cross-sectional right metacarpal zone 3A SDFT sonogram of a Thoroughbred racehorse. In addition to other obvious tendon abnormalities, medial displacement is present. The displacement occurred only in zone 3A and proximal zone 3B (arrows), which is unusual.

Shape

Although the cross-sectional SDFT shape is not as significant as its texture, density, size, and fiber alignment, it can be indicative of subtle SDFT injury and may be useful in evaluation of SQR evaluation. Changes in shape are directly related to changes in size. As the cross-sectional area at any given level increases or decreases, tendon shape usually changes concomitantly. Shape is readily perceptible during the real-time examination and any change should prompt measuring of the CSA of the tendon. Since shape is related to cross-sectional area, it is not numerically graded. Subtle changes in tendon shape without changes in density can be early signs of tendonitis. From a clinical perspective, detection of early changes provides a major service and may preclude a serious injury. If a chronically enlarged, healed tendon has an abnormal shape, serial monitoring may allow detection of an early reinjury based on an additional shape change. Injured tendons that return to a near normal shape have a more favorable prognosis.

Figure 21.41 is a cross-sectional right metacarpal zone 1A SDFT sonogram of a Thoroughbred racehorse with low-grade metacarpal swelling. Overall, subtle cross-sectional SDFT enlargement is present, but there are no areas of decreased density and no change in tendon shape. This is compatible with the least amount of fiber path disruption. The prognosis is favorable with time off from training and racing.

Figure 21.42 is a cross-sectional right metacarpal zone 1A SDFT sonogram of a Standardbred racehorse with metacarpal swelling. A focal Type 3 core lesion is present and CSA is increased, but SDFT shape is not changed. The shape did not change because the lesion is centrally located and the inflammatory reaction caused uniform swelling. The SDFT is normally oval or round in zone 1 and little shape change would occur with a core lesion.

Figure 21.43 is a cross-sectional right metacarpal zone 1A SDFT sonogram. The horse is a racing Thoroughbred with SDFT swelling. CSA is increased, Type 1 density is present, and the shape of the medial border is changed. This is a more serious tendonitis because fiber path alignment is altered. The shape change of the medial border indicates that this area has morphologic fiber tract abnormalities.

Figure 21.44 is a cross-sectional right metacarpal zone 2B SDFT sonogram of a Thoroughbred in race training with low-grade SDFT swelling. The scan reveals slight subcutaneous swelling, which the trainer believed was the result of overapplying leg liniment. Sonographic evidence of subcutaneous edema/hemorrhage might substantiate the trainer's suspicion; however, further review revealed an SDFT shape change. The normal SDFT is crescent shaped, but this tendon had a slight "hump" on the palmar-medial aspect . This subtle change in shape indicates fiber tract swelling caused by strain with focal tendon fiber injury. This Type of focal lesion is slightly more significant than subtle diffuse enlargement.

Figure 21.45 is a cross-sectional left metacarpal zone 3B SDFT sonogram of a Thoroughbred racehorse with moderate distal tendon sheath (TS) swelling. Distal tendon sheath swelling is addressed later in this chapter. This case is included to illustrate the SDFT shape change with increased intrathecal fluid pressure. There is tendon sheath effusion surrounding the DDFT and palmar SDFT surface. The normal crescent-shaped SDFT is more horizontal and the medial and lateral borders are displaced abaxially from their normal position. The palmar SDFT surface is still smooth and gently curved. Obviously, the increased intrathecal fluid pressure altered the normal SDFT shape. It is not known if the fluid pressure places the tendon at a higher risk of injury. Although no supporting data exist, caution should be used during training. Serial sonography and careful clinical observations are indicated during symptomatic treatment and return to competition. If other signs of SDFT injury are present, then cessation of training and a long-term therapy program should be considered.

Figure 21.46 is a cross-sectional left metacarpal zone 3B SDFT sonogram of a Thoroughbred racehorse with distal TS swelling. The scan reveals an increased intrathecal fluid; however, minimal fluid surrounded the DDFT. The SDFT shape is normal, indicating less sheath pressure than seen in Figure 21.45. A slight midline "bulge" is present in the normally smooth, curved palmar contour. This subtle shape alteration is abnormal and if it is a recent finding, the tendon should be carefully monitored.

As the severity of SDFT injury increases, shape abnormalities become more obvious and more serious sonographic abnormalities are usually present. Figure 21.47 is a cross-sectional right metacarpal zone 2B SDFT sonogram of a Standardbred pacer with a history of tendinitis for more than 1 month. The medial tendon border was more square than normal and enlarged. Focal hypoechoic fiber disruption was present within the medial half. This is in contrast to the more normal curved, tapering shape.

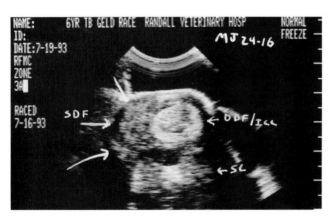

Figure 21.40.

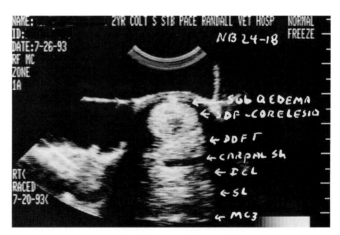

Figure 21.42.

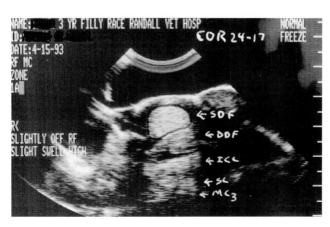

Figure 21.41.

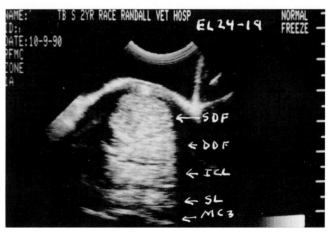

Figure 21.43.

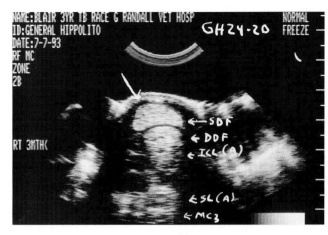

Figure 21.44.

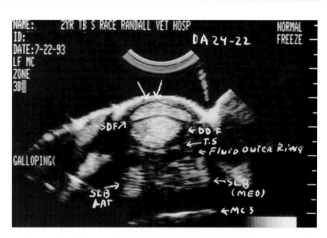

Figure 21.46.

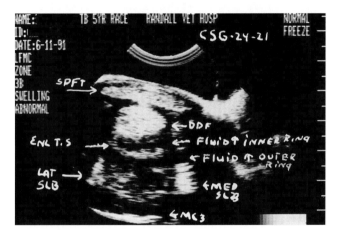

Figure 21.45.

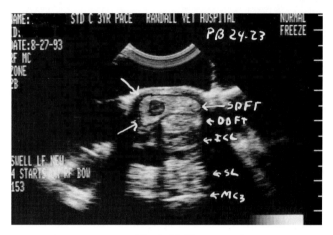

Figure 21.47.

Figure 21.48 is a cross-sectional left metacarpal zone 3B SDFT sonogram of a Standardbred pacer. The tendon had a chronic, actively inflamed core lesion. Irrespective of the obvious fiber disruption, shape is markedly changed from a narrowed crescent to a large oval-shaped tendon.

Return of the injured SDFT to a more normal shape may indicate a favorable SQR. It is not proven whether a normal tendon shape has a more functional repair compared with a tendon equally healed but abnormal in shape. We believe that healing tendons that regain their normal shape have a more favorable prognosis. Further research must be conducted to substantiate this belief.

Figure 21.49 is a cross-sectional left metacarpal zone 2B SDFT sonogram of a Thoroughbred racehorse with a recent large Type 3 core lesion. The SDFT changed from slightly crescent to oval. Training was stopped and treatment begun.

Figure 21.50 is a cross-sectional left metacarpal zone 2B SDFT sonogram of the same horse shown in Fig. 21.49 made 6 months after injury. Although the CSA is enlarged, the SDFT has returned to a crescent shape.

Figure 21.51 is a cross-sectional left metacarpal zone 2B SDFT sonogram of the same horse shown in Figures 21.49 and 21.50 made 10 months after injury at EL-3. The SDFT shape is oval compared with the 6-month scan. This shape

regression during a subtraining exercise level is an unfavorable sonographic finding.

Figure 21.52 is a cross-sectional left metacarpal zone 3A SDFT sonogram of a Thoroughbred racehorse with a large, Type 3 core lesion. Although the CSA is increased as expected, the SDFT shape is still slightly crescent.

Figure 21.53 is a cross-sectional left metacarpal zone 3A SDFT sonogram of the same horse shown in Figure 21.52 made 6 months after injury. Although a persistent increased CSA is present, the SDFT shape is still crescent.

Figure 21.54 is a cross-sectional left metacarpal zone 3A SDFT sonogram of the same horse shown in Figures 21.52 and 21.53 made 10 months after injury at EL-3. The SDFT has a more normal crescent shape than it did 6 months after injury. This return to normal shape is a favorable SQR.

Size

The size, or CSA, can be used for sonographic SDFT assessment. Cross-sectional area measurements can be used to confirm subtle tendinitis and tendon injury. Serial measurements reflect the SQR. During the past 5 years of BAPTEN clinical trials, it has become apparent that reduction in CSA of a healing SDFT injury is a more functional repair. Conversely, increases in CSA with increasing exercise levels during recovery suggest low-grade reinjury.

Our routine approach, when measuring the CSA of forelimb or hind limb SDFT injury, is to record cross-sectional images of at least six (and preferably seven) forelimb zones and at least seven (and preferably nine) hindlimb zones. This provides the sonographer with a "tendon volume."

Similar measurements are made of the contralateral normal limb. Occasionally, both limbs have an abnormal SDFT, making comparison inaccurate. For reasons mentioned earlier, it is not reliable to compare CSA data derived by different methods. However, most (more than 85%) SDFT injuries are unilateral. The contralateral limb serves as a normal baseline for comparison.

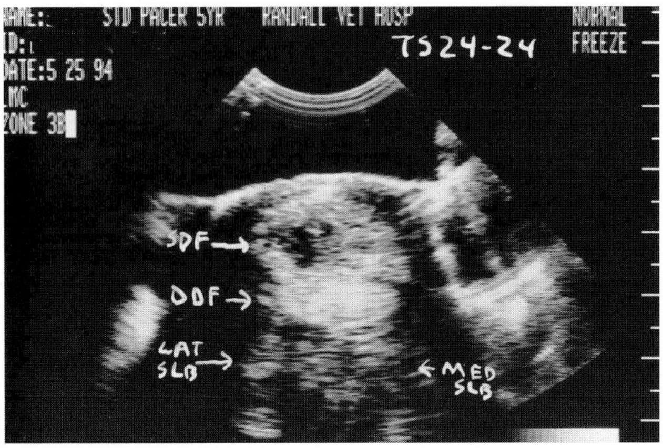

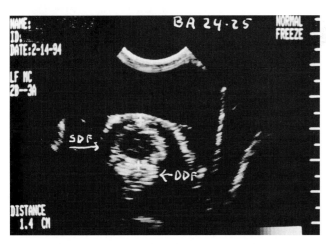

Figure 21.48.

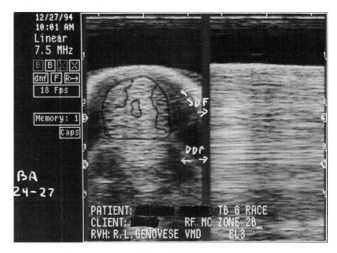

Figure 21.51.

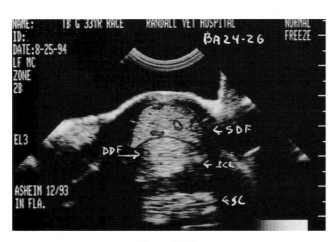

Figure 21.49.

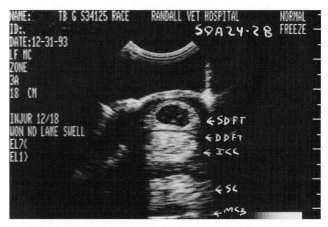

Figure 21.52.

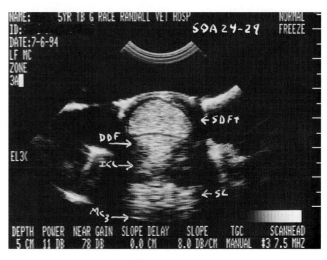

Figure 21.50.

Figure 21.53.

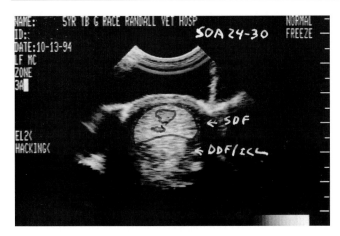

Figure 21.54.

The individual zone with the greatest increase and the tendon's total increase above normal both can be determined from the CSA data. SDFT injury usually is seen in two forms. The first is enlargement without evidence of fiber tearing (subtle tendon enlargement), and the second is fiber tearing with or without significant enlargement. The most common form has variable amounts of fiber tearing with tendon enlargement. In this form, the sonographer identifies some normal CSA levels without fiber tearing, a level or two of increased CSA without fiber tearing, and then some zones with fiber tearing and an increase in CSA. When an injured SDFT is evaluated, one zone is designated as the most compromised zone. This identifies the tendon's "weakest link," which is referred to as the maximum injury zone (MIZ). The MIZ in SDFT injuries *without* identifiable fiber tearing is the zone with the greatest percent CSA increase. For example, if when compared with the normal tendon, the injured tendon is 10% larger in zone 1B, 14% larger in zone 2A, 27% larger in zone 2B, and 16% larger in zone 3A, then zone 2B would be considered the MIZ. The CSA for this zone would be recorded as the maximum injury zone CSA (MIZ-CSA). In the tendon with fiber tearing at various levels, the MIZ is the zone that has the largest hypoechoic fiber percentage regardless of the density. For example, if zone 1B has 12% Type 3 fibers, zone 2A has 22% Type 2 fibers, zone 2B has 29% Type 1 fibers, and zone 3A has 16% Type 2 fibers, then zone 2B is the MIZ and the CSA for that zone would be designated the MIZ-CSA.

The next step in CSA evaluation would be to estimate the extent of injury by summing the zones for a total cross-sectional area "volume" (T-CSA). The T-CSA is used for both forms of SDFT injury (with or without identifiable fiber tearing). If no fiber tearing is present, the T-CSA is the most sensitive measurement indicating subtle tendinitis. For example, assume a 2-year-old Thoroughbred racehorse has slight metacarpal swelling. The trainer suspects an injured tendon. Limb palpation is not conclusive the limb is evaluated sonographically. During the examination, no fiber tearing is found (no black holes). However, the T-CSA of the possibly injured SDFT is 798 mm^2. The contralateral normal limb T-CSA is 638 mm^2. The T-CSA increase is 25%.

Because slight variations exist in zone selection and scanning techniques from zone to zone and because slight measurement error occurs, a small variation is seen between normal tendons when the MIZ-CSA and T-CSA are measured. One author refers to this as sonographic "vibration" caused by technical error (RL Genovese, personal communication). When the CSA of normal tendons is compared, this technical vibration ranges between 5 and 15% for the T-CSA and 10 and 20% for the MIZ-CSA. Therefore, tendon measurements in this range are equivocal. However, increases in MIZ that approach 25 to 30% are compatible with tendinitis. T-CSA increases approaches 20 to 25% also indicates tendinitis. Therefore, in the example case, the T-CSA increase of 25%, even without sonographically identifiable fiber tearing, is an indication of low-grade tendon injury. An accompanying MIZ increase of 25 to 30% or more is even more positive for tendinitis, and this magnitude of increase identifies the "weak link."

In tendons that have hypoechoic or anechoic lesions, the compromised tendon fiber path CSA is recorded for each zone in absolute volume and as a percent of the total CSA. For example, in zone 2A, the CSA is 100 mm^2 and the hypoechoic fiber "volume" is 10 mm^2. The percent abnormal is 10%. Furthermore, the density is scored as follows: 0 (isoechogenic), 1 for Type 1 (mostly echogenic but not isoechogenic), 2 for Type 2 (mixed echogenicity), and 3 for Type 3 (mostly anechoic) or 4 (mostly anechoic or anechoic). The zone with the largest percent of compromise is designated the MIZ and the percent of hypoechoic or anechoic tendon fiber paths for the MIZ is designated the MIZ-HYP, regardless of the density. This is carried one step further to determine the extent of the injury by summing all zones with compromised fiber paths and recording the total hypoechoic tendon "volume" (T-HYP). Once the T-CSA and the T-HYP "volumes" have been determined, the total percent compromised fiber paths is determined (percent T-HYP). This represents the third "volumetric" determination used to establish a baseline for quantitative assessments of injured SDFT. These volumetric determinations are used during rehabilitation to monitor the SQR.

The percent T-HYP can also be used to establish a practical means to categorize the severity of an injured SDFT. We have found that this not only provides practical communication with the client but also serves as a means to compare similar injuries for clinical research purposes. Based upon our clinical experiences in the BAPTEN field trials, the following categorization is used: *slight* SDFT injuries are those with more than 15 to 20% T-CSA increase without fiber tearing or SDFT injuries that are 1 to 15% T-HYP; *moderate* SDFT injuries are 16 to 25% T-HYP; *severe* SDFT injuries are more than 25% T-HYP.

These quantitative assessments are easily performed, greatly improve the objectivity of SDFT injury identification classification, and are extremely useful in case management during rehabilitation. From these data, one can easily determine the SQR with a given treatment program. Most importantly, these data guide changes in exercise level during recovery and indicate stability or instability of the tendon when training and high level competition resume.

For example, a Thoroughbred racehorse is presented for left forelimb SDFT swelling after a morning breeze 3 days earlier. Ultrasonographic findings included the following:

Normal Right Forelimb SDFT

Zone	CSA	Absolute Hypoechoic Fibers
1A	101 mm^2	0 hypoechoic fibers
1B	91 mm^2	0 hypoechoic fibers
2A	109 mm^2	0 hypoechoic fibers
2B	95 mm^2	0 hypoechoic fibers
3A	94 mm^2	0 hypoechoic fibers
3B	105 mm^2	0 hypoechoic fibers
3C	128 mm^2	0 hypoechoic fibers

T-CSA = 723 mm^2 T-HYP = 0 %

This is the normal SDFT baseline data for comparison.

Abnormal Left Forelimb SDFT

Zone	CSA	Absolute Hypoechoic Fibers (% HYP)	%CSA Increase/ Decrease (+/-)
1A	116 mm^2	5 mm^2 Type 1 hypoechoic (4%)	+15
1B	155 mm^2	88 mm^2 Type 2 hypoechoic (54%)	+70
2A	115 mm^2	51 mm^2 Type 2 hypoechoic (44%)	+00.06
2B	160 mm^2	86 mm^2 Type 2 hypoechoic (54%)	+68
3A	153 mm^2	103 mm^2 Type 3 hypoechoic (67%)	+62
3B	164 mm^2	84 mm^2 Type 3 hypoechoic (51%)	+56
3C	126 mm^2	0 hypoechoic	−2

T-CSA = 989 mm^2 417 mm^2 hypoechoic fibers T-HYP = 42% (severe injury)

T-CSA increase = 37% The maximum injury zone is 3A

From these quantitative data, the clinician can more fully appreciate the injury's extent, and this baseline information helps in the formulation of a management program.

Figure 21.55 is a cross-sectional left forelimb zone 1A SDFT sonogram of a Thoroughbred racehorse with slight swelling. Sonographic examination did not reveal any variation from normal texture, density, shape, or fiber alignment of six metacarpal zones. The most proximal zones had an increased CSA when compared with contralateral normal tendon. The CSA increase was greatest in zone 1A; the variation from normal gradually decreased distally and no appreciable difference was found at zone 3A. In this case, four abnormal CSA levels were found that decreased in severity proceeding distally. This confirmed the diagnosis of low-grade tendinitis without significant fiber disruption. In addition, the finding that the proximal two-thirds of the tendon had an 18% CSA increase suggested that more serious injury might occur if training continued.

Figure 21.56 is a cross-sectional left forelimb zone 2B SDFT sonogram of a 2-year-old Thoroughbred racehorse with low-grade swelling. Density, texture, shape, and fiber alignment were normal. In this instance, there is good evidence, based on CSA data alone, that SDFT fiber tract disruption might occur if training continued. The prognosis is favorable for recovery because no significant fiber tearing was found.

Most SDFT injuries have several abnormalities, and some sonographic variables are more applicable than others. In the next section, the emphasis is on appreciation of the impact on case management that CSA alone can have in different clinical scenarios, not on the integration and prioritization of the variables.

Figure 21.57 is a cross-sectional left metacarpal Zone 3A SDFT sonogram of a Thoroughbred racehorse with a recent large Type 2 central lesion. Fibers were damaged in all six levels; Zone 1A had the least damage. Training was stopped and time off was given to repair the tendon. Zone 3A was selected as the MIZ because 67% of the cross-sectional area had textural changes.

Figure 21.58 is a left metacarpal zone 3B sonogram of the same horse shown in Figure 21.57 made 2 months after injury at EL-3. The sonogram reveals significant improvement in lesion density and texture. Mature collagen was not produced in 2 months, and the increased echogenicity can be attributed to hematoma resolution and decreased inflammatory infiltrate. Originally, the large core lesion was a Type 2 density, which indicates the presence of viable fiber tracts. The SDFT shape is becoming more crescent, and the CSA increased to 350 mm^2.

A significant increase has occurred in total tendon "volume." There are two possible explanations for the CSA increase: either EL-3 was too much activity for the injury (persistent low-grade inflammation), or the fibrous tissue production was excessive and randomly oriented. The CSA data indicate an unfavorable SQR at this time.

Figure 21.59 is a cross-sectional left metacarpal zone 3B SDFT sonogram of the same horse shown in Figures 21.57 and 21.58 made 5 months after injury. The horse was ridden at a walk (EL-2) and was also being turned out into pasture (EL-3). Scattered focal hypoechoic areas were present, but no indication to suggest the low level exercise was excessive. The tendon had a trapezoid shape. The MIZ-CSA decreased to 323 mm^2. However, this is still 16% larger than the original CSA. Based on our experience, a 25% size increase is a less than satisfactory finding. Note that only CSA was measured in the above tendon evaluation; other significant sonographic parameters were not considered in this example.

Figure 21.60 is a cross-sectional right metacarpal zone 3A SDFT sonogram of a Thoroughbred racehorse that sustained an injury during a race. Five levels had varying degrees of textural change. A large, Type 3 lesion is at zone 3A along the palmar medial tendon. The CSA is 244 mm^2.

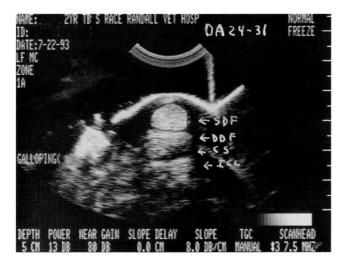

	CSA		
	Abnormal Left Forelimb	Normal Right Forelimb	% CSA increase
Zone 1A	104 mm^2	79 mm^2	32
Zone 1B	97 mm^2	86 mm^2	13
Zone 2A	93 mm^2	76 mm^2	22
Zone 2B	95 mm^2	88 mm^2	8
Zone 3A	93 mm^2	92 mm^2	0
Zone 3B	95 mm^2	94 mm^2	0
Total (1A–2B)	389 mm^2	329 mm^2	% Change 18% T-CSA increase
Total (1A–3B)	577 mm^2	515 mm^2	% Change 12% T-CSA increase

Figure 21.55.

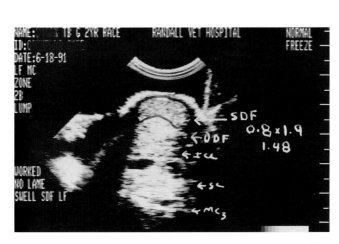

	CSA		
	Abnormal Left Forelimb	Normal Right Forelimb	% CSA increase
Zone 1A	106 mm^2	88 mm^2	17
Zone 1B	120 mm^2	101 mm^2	16
Zone 2A	122 mm^2	107 mm^2	12
Zone 2B	148 mm^2	102 mm^2	45
Zone 3A	123 mm^2	109 mm^2	13
Zone 3B	135 mm^2	104 mm^2	30
Total (1A–3B)	877 mm^2	611 mm^2	% Change 44% T-CSA increase
MIZ(2B)	148 mm^2	102 mm^2	% Change 45% T-CSA increase

MIZ = maximum injury zone

Figure 21.56.

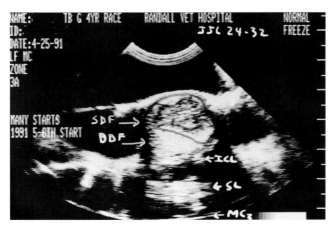

Cross-Sectional Areas of Original Injury	
Zone 1A	132 mm^2
Zone 1B	124 mm^2
Zone 2A	214 mm^2
Zone 2B	243 mm^2
Zone 3A	279 mm^2
Zone 3B	240 mm^2
Total	1232 mm^2
Total hypoechoic areas	650 mm^2
% T-HYP = 53	

Figure 21.57.

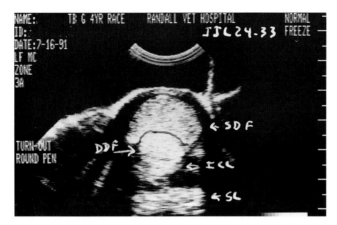

Cross-Sectional Areas 2 Months After Injury

Zone 1A	173 mm²
Zone 1B	264 mm²
Zone 2A	262 mm²
Zone 2B	385 mm²
Zone 3A	350 mm²
Zone 3B	298 mm²
Total	1732 mm²
% Change	500 mm² increase (41% increase of T-CSA)

Figure 21.58.

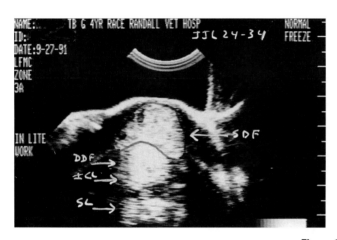

Cross-Sectional Areas 5 Months After Injury

Zone 1A	173 mm²
Zone 1B	182 mm²
Zone 2A	264 mm²
Zone 2B	283 mm²
Zone 3A	323 mm²
Zone 3B	313 mm²
Total	1538 mm²
% Change	25% increase from the tendon volume of the original injury

Figure 21.59.

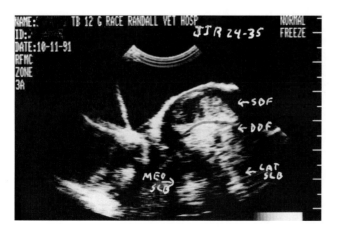

Cross-Sectional Areas of Original Injury

Zone 1A	216 mm²
Zone 1B	203 mm²
Zone 2A	240 mm²
Zone 2B	238 mm²
Zone 3A	244 mm²
Total	1141 mm²

Total Hypoechoic Tendon = 669 mm²
% T-HYP = 59

Figure 21.60.

Figure 21.61 is a cross-sectional right metacarpal zone 3A SDFT sonogram of the same horse shown in Fig. 21.60 made 7 months after injury. The sonogram revealed a marked texture and density improvement with only scattered focal hypoechoic areas comprising a total of 58 mm^2. Although enlarged, the zone 3A shape was slightly crescent.

The T-CSA indicates a stable total volume, which is a favorable finding. On closer inspection, however, all of the decreased CSA occurred in zones 1A and 1B. If the original injury data are further analyzed, the CSA for zones 2A, 2B, 3A, is 721 mm^2. Seven months after the injury, the total CSA for zones 2A, 2B, and 3A is 902 mm^2. This is a 25% CSA increase after 7 months of rehabilitation. In other words, if only the improvement in echogenicity and the maintenance of a reasonable shape are looked at, one would regard this as a favorable SQR. But the CSA increase is a significant enough negative finding to delay an increase in ten-don loading. This was not done, race training resumed and the injury recurred. Obviously, reinjury will not occur in all tendons in which the CSA does not decrease to near original injury level, but an increased CSA can be used as an indicator to prevent premature tendon loading.

Figure 21.62 is a cross-sectional right metacarpal zone 2A SDFT sonogram made from a Thoroughbred race horse that sustained a severe injury. The scan revealed extensive fiber path disruption.

Figure 21.63 is a cross-sectional right metacarpal zone 2A sonogram of the same horse shown in Figure 21.62 made 5 months after injury at EL-2. Echogenicity increased significantly and the shape was more normal. In contrast to the two previous examples, this tendon has made a significant decrease in CSA, which is a favorable finding. The CSA measurements of this tendon at 7 months after injury and EL-7 are given in Figure 21.64.

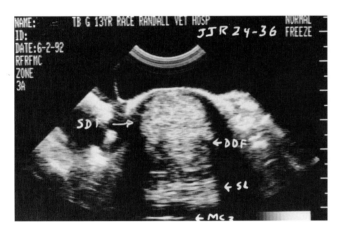

Figure 21.61.

Cross-sectional Areas 7 Months After Injury

Zone 1A	148 mm^2
Zone 1B	142 mm^2
Zone 2A	277 mm^2
Zone 2B	280 mm^2
Zone 3A	345 mm^2
Total	1192 mm^2

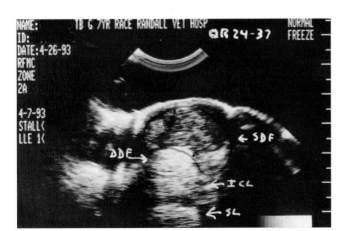

Figure 21.62.

Cross-Sectional Areas of Original Injury

Zone 1A	181 mm^2
Zone 1B	222 mm^2
Zone 2A	435 mm^2
Zone 2B	569 mm^2
Zone 3A	447 mm^2
Zone 3B	192 mm^2
Total	2046 mm^2
Total hypoechoic	1005 mm^2
% T-HYP = 49	

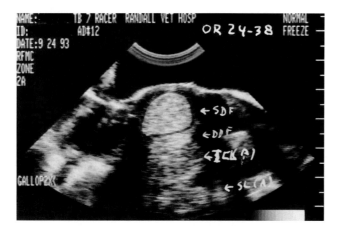

Figure 21.63.

Cross-sectional Areas 5 Months After Injury

Zone 1A	159 mm^2
Zone 1B	179 mm^2
Zone 2A	218 mm^2
Zone 2B	273 mm^2
Zone 3A	255 mm^2
Zone 3B	168 mm^2
Total	1252 mm^2

% Total CSA change = decrease of 794 mm^2
(39% decrease)

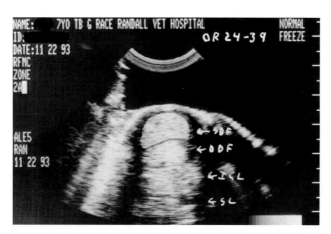

Figure 21.64.

Cross-sectional Areas 7 Months After Injury

Zone 1A	140 mm^2
Zone 1B	173 mm^2
Zone 2A	172 mm^2
Zone 2B	246 mm^2
Zone 3A	263 mm^2
Zone 3B	235 mm^2
Total	1229 mm^2

Figure 21.64 is a cross-sectional right metacarpal sonogram of the same horse shown in Figures 21.62 and 21.63 made 7 months after injury. A few hypoechoic areas were present, and the SDFT shape was more normal, although enlarged. At EL-7, the CSA at 7 months was slightly decreased. Most importantly, the CSA remained stable with increased tendon loading, which is a favorable finding.

The CSA is a practical and sensitive indicator of SDFT abnormality. It is a useful variable to monitor all aspects of tendon healing and rehabilitation, including the SQR and effects of increased tendon loading.

Fiber Alignment

The alignment of collagen bundles in the superficial digital flexor tendon is a difficult variable to influence therapeutically because of inherent physiologic mechanics of tendon fiber injury repair. According to Peacock (25), tendon injury is repaired primarily by the influx of fibroblasts from the paratenon and adjacent vasculature (extrinsic); mature tenocytes contribute little to repair (intrinsic). He believes that tenocytes are mature end-stage cells with little capability to produce collagen. The invading fibroblasts produce collagen fibrils in a random fashion. As healing progresses and the repairing scar matures, the replacement fibrils are remodeled (to varying degrees of efficiency) in a longitudinally oriented pattern consistent with the tension planes of the tendon (25). Buck has shown that slight tension on the injured tendon during the early healing stages of a tendon injury cause fibrin strands to align longitudinally. The practical dilemma, of course, is to apply only enough tension to stimulate the process, not an excessive amount that would result in further damage (26). Goodship suggests that low level exercise in the first 2 months on a graded scale promotes maturation and longitudinal collagen fiber organization, but he also cautions not to exceed the yield strength of the repair tissue (23). Both of these workers imply that longitudinally oriented scar is a more functional physical state for future athletic use. One author (RLG) is currently investigating intralesional BAPTEN as a means to enhance scar remodeling, resulting in a more favorable longitudinal orientation of the repairing scar in SDFT injuries. Therefore, sonographic fiber alignment monitoring is an important aspect of rehabilitation. Fiber alignment is graded as described in the earlier normal sonogram section. The fiber alignment can be graded for the MIZ or any injured SDFT segment. Fiber alignment (FA) is used to: 1) assess the degree of recent tendon injury; 2) assess the SQR at various times; and 3) help contribute to decisions in exercise level management. Fiber alignment is of less concern in low-grade, subtle tendinitis becaue it is not a significant sonographic finding. However, FA has an important roll in evaluating SQR during rehabilitation. One therapy goal is to see longitudinal scar alignment after the remodeling phase.

Figure 21.65 is a cross-sectional right metacarpal zone 1B SDFT sonogram of a normal Thoroughbred in full training. The scan reveals a normal FA. Density comparisons can be made with the DDFT. The FA pattern is completely parallel and, subjectively, the tendon fibers have a "compactness." This tendon would receive a fiber score of 0 (FS-0).

Figure 21.66 is a cross-sectional and sagittal left fore zone 1B normal SDFT sonogram made with a 7.5-MHz linear array transducer. The fiber pattern is compact, parallel, and isoechogenic. The linear array transducer provides excellent sonographic imaging of the sagittal FA. The hypoechoic DDFT density is an artifact caused by sound beam angle.

In SDFT injury, cross-sectional images document the injuries well, and longitudinal views often are not made. However, to be complete, the longitudinal alignment should be documented for every level, not only the MIZ. This baseline information is essential in the repair process. "Healed" tendons with minimal fiber alignment have a more unfavorable prognosis. Because normal tendons have parallel fibers, it is the most desirable endpoint of rehabilitation next to tendon size reduction.

Fiber alignment is useful in confirming subtle, recent SDFT injury. Figure 21.67 is a sagittal left metacarpal zone 2A SDFT sonogram of a Thoroughbred racehorse with a low-grade, diffuse medial swelling. Cross-sectional views of all zones were essentially negative for shape or density abnormalities. There was, however, a slight T-CSA increase and a slight fiber separation seen on the sagittal view. The six zone T-CSA of the normal right SDFT was 526 mm^2. The six zone T-CSA of the suspect left fore SDFT was 686 mm^2. These findings represent a greater than 30% T-CSA increase and highly suggest low-grade tendinitis without identifiable fiber tearing. The obvious question to be asked is "Can I continue training this horse if he responds to symptomatic treatment?" Because there is no obvious tendon fiber tearing, the decision is difficult. Historically, there are racehorses with mild tendonitis that continue racing without mishap. However, some horses suffer further injury that often is career ending. In this case, the sagittal scan may add sonographic information to assist in the clinical decision. Careful examination of the scan reveals a slightly hypoechoic palmar half of the SDFT despite parallel alignment. "Target" fiber bundle "compactness" and separation by echolucent spaces is lacking. This finding supports the slight increase in T-CSA and suspicion of tendonitis. This case

further emphasizes the need to obtain sagittal scans through the "target" area. The ultrasound beam is thin, and lesions may be overlooked in long axis. For example, if there is a small, Type 3 lateral border SDFT lesion seen in cross-section and the sagittal scan is obtained from the normal medial tendon border, erroneous FA data would be obtained.

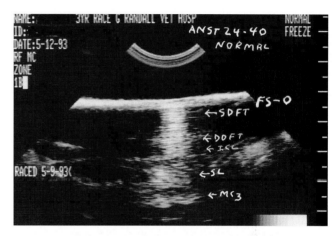

Figure 21.65.

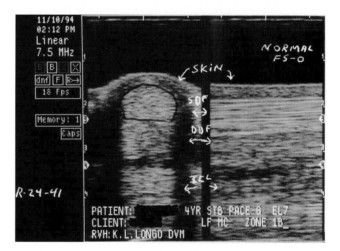

Figure 21.66.

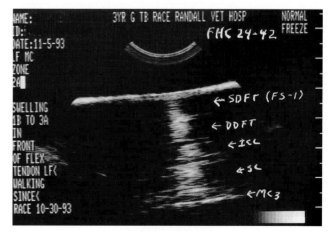

Figure 21.67.

Figure 21.68 is a sagittal left metacarpal zone 2A SDFT sonogram of a Thoroughbred racehorse with low-grade swelling. The cross-sectional sonogram did not indicate any shape, density, or texture abnormalities. There was a significant CSA increase in four of six zones. The sagittal view reveals two hypoechoic tendon fiber tracts that lack parallel alignment. In this tendon, the entire cross-sectional area is the "target" path and fibers are 50 to 75% parallel (FS-1). Based on these parameters, a diagnosis of low-grade tendinitis with focal fiber tearing was made. The trainer was advised that time off from training and long-range treatment were indicated. Because the fiber tearing was low-grade, a favorable prognosis for return to competition was given. Because of unrelated factors, the trainer decided to treat the signs symptomatically, modify the training program, and continue to race. One author (RLG) refers to this as symptomatic treatment and "go on" (S/GO). In this instance, the horse sustained more serious injury, and its racing career was ended. The trainer's decision was not entirely a "bad" one. In this case, it was not favorable, but occasions exist when a

similar decision is the best one for the circumstances. On occasion it can be highly successful. The clinician's role is to discuss management options and the relative chances of success or failure. Furthermore, once the management option is decided on, the clinician can give appropriate treatment and schedule sonographic tendon monitoring schedules. Conversely, long-term rest and treatment offer a favorable prognosis for an injury of this magnitude.

Figure 21.69 is a cross-sectional and sagittal right fore SDFT Zone 2A sonogram of a Thoroughbred racehorse with a focal Type 1 core lesion. The target path for FA assessment is the centrally located fiber bundles only. The target fiber bundles are 25 to 50% axially aligned and are given FS-2.

Figure 21.70 is a normal sagittal left metacarpal zone 2B SDFT sonogram of a Standardbred pacing filly. Texture and axial fiber alignment are normal. In addition, fiber appearance is compact (FS-0).

Figure 21.71 is a sagittal right metacarpal zone 2B SDFT sonogram of the same horse shown in Figure 21.70. Echo-

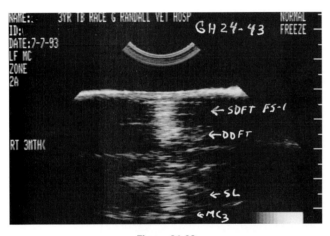

Figure 21.68.

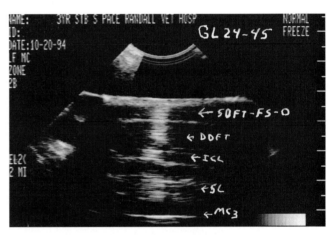

Figure 21.70.

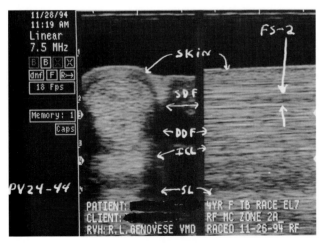

Figure 21.69.

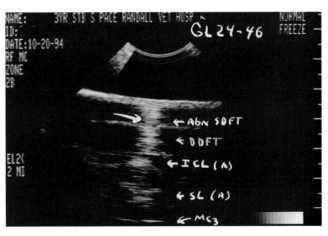

Figure 21.71.

genicity decreased overall, and a fiber tract is in a different plane that is hypoechoic along the dorsal SDFT margin.

Figure 21.72 is a cross-sectional and sagittal right metacarpal zone 3A SDFT sonogram of a Thoroughbred racehorse with a large, Type 2 core lesion. The sagittal scan confirms the lesion and the target core fiber bundles have no significant parallel alignment (FS-3).

Figure 21.73 is a cross-sectional and sagittal left metacarpal zone 1A SDFT sonogram of an 11-year-old Quarterhorse with dorsal border fiber path disruption. The sagittal scan confirms the injury, and the target path has no significant parallel arrangement (FS-3).

Grading of the fiber alignment is based on the estimate of parallel fiber bundles of the target area regardless of whether that target is generalized, as in diffuse tendinitis, or along a

focal, selected path. The target is established by the clinician, who bases it on the pathologic area of interest. This selected path confirms fiber tearing and can be used for evaluating the SQR or the tendon stability or instability if the horse continues to train.

Figure 21.74 is a sagittal left metacarpal zone 1A SDFT sonogram of a Thoroughbred racehorse that has an FS-0. The tendon is normal, and the fiber bundles are compact and parallel in the area of interest. Figure 21.75 is a sagittal left metacarpal zone 3B sonogram of a Thoroughbred racehorse with an FS-1. Figure 21.76 is a sagittal left metacarpal zone 3A sonogram of a Thoroughbred racehorse with FS-2, and Figure 21.77 is a sagittal left metacarpal zone 3B sonogram of a Thoroughbred racehorse with an FS-3.

Parallel fiber alignment in a healing SDFT lesion is eval-

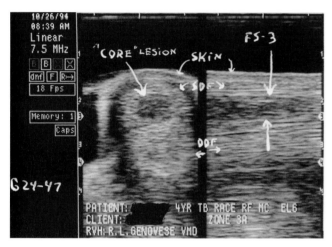

Figure 21.72.

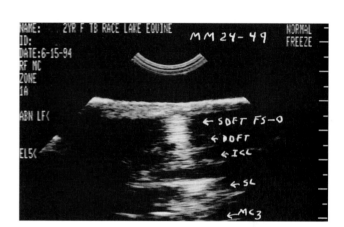

Figure 21.74.

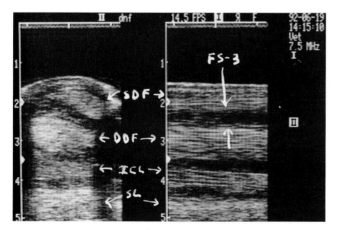

Figure 21.73.

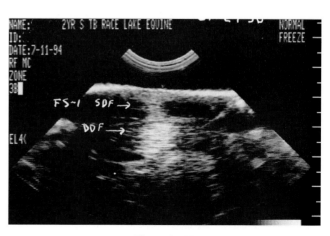

Figure 21.75.

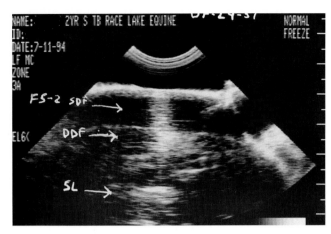

Figure 21.76.

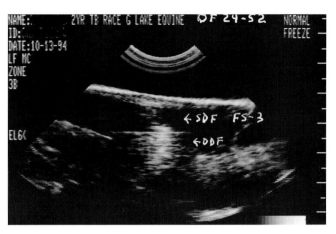

Figure 21.77.

uated in the same manner as recent injuries. Future scores are compared with previous scores and then related to the current EL. Exercise management and prognoses can be based on measurable findings, including the fiber alignment. Scar remodeling is a difficult physiologic process to influence by treatment. Furthermore, collagen realignment is a slow process. If, however, alignment improves, a more favorable prognosis for athletic use would be allowed. A lack of parallel fibers confirms collagen bundle disorientation. This finding indicates an increased chance of mechanical failure. BAPTEN treatment allows scar remodeling to occur more longitudinally when combined with strict exercise control and adequate time off from training.

Figure 21.78 is a sagittal right metacarpal zone 3B SDFT sonogram of a Thoroughbred racehorse with a long history of tendonitis. The tendon was reinjured 1 month before this scan was taken. Since the reinjury, the horse has had stall rest with minimal handwalking (EL-1). A large hypoechoic lesion is present and no significant fiber alignment (FS-3) exists. This sonographic finding at this time with this size lesion is unexpected. It is not physiologically possible to repair an injury with mature collagen and remodel the scar in 30 days. However, 30 days after an acute injury, hematoma resorption and at least partial resolution of the inflammatory infiltrate probably occurs. At this point, the lesion is highly cellular and has immature collagen, causing the hypoechoic appearance. Furthermore, the sonographer can conclude that the hypoechoic paths represent significant tendon fiber damage. This 30-day post-injury sonogram represents the baseline for fiber disruption because the hematoma and inflammatory reaction have had sufficient time to resolve.

Figure 21.79 is a sagittal left metacarpal zone 3B SDFT sonogram made 30 days after injury. This tendon shows reasonably good density and fiber alignment. The dorsal surface has fiber tract disruption; however, there is some evidence of mature, parallel collagen alignment (FS-2). Therefore, a significant number of fiber tracts in the injured area were not disrupted. Even though damage occurred that

requires rehabilitation, it is less severe than in the previous case.

Figure 21.80 is a sagittal left metacarpal zone 2B SDFT sonogram of a Standardbred racehorse injured 3 months earlier and at EL-1 ever since. The scan reveals a large lesion with few isoechogenic fiber bundles and little parallel fiber alignment (FS-3). At 3 months after injury and at EL-1, one would not expect more than a 25% SDFT fiber alignment improvement in a moderate to severe injury.

Figure 21.81 is a cross-sectional and sagittal left metacarpal zone 2B SDFT sonogram of a Thoroughbred racehorse out of training for 8 months because of injury. The scan shows hypoechoic target fiber bundles with slight parallel alignment (FS-2). At this time, based on the minimal alignment and hypoechoic appearance, a guarded prognosis for racing was given. The SDFT size and shape were more favorable. Based on these mixed sonographic parameters, the EL should not be advanced for 1 to 2 months, at which time the tendon should be reevaluated. Traditional tendon injury management in the United States suggests that 8 months is the time to start training; however, the sonographic appearance may show that some horses' tendons are not ready for an EL increase to the training level.

Figure 21.82 is a cross-sectional and sagittal left metacarpal zone 2A SDFT sonogram of a Thoroughbred racehorse currently in pasture (EL-3b) because of an injury 8 months previously. This tendon has similar sonographic parameters as the one shown in Figure 21.81. It was advised to continue the present program and reevaluate in 2 to 3 months.

Figure 21.83 is a sagittal left metacarpal Zone 2A SDFT sonogram of the same horse shown in Figure 21.82 made 12 months after injury. The scan shows hypoechoic and randomly oriented (FS-3) target fiber bundles. Because sonographic improvement was not significant after 4 months, the prognosis for racing is unfavorable.

Figure 21.84 is a sagittal left metacarpal zone 3A SDFT sonogram of a recently injured Thoroughbred racehorse. The scan shows the target fiber bundles as hypoechoic and totally lacking parallel alignment (FS-3).

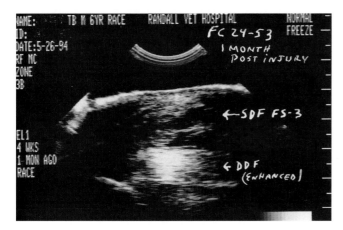

Figure 21.78.

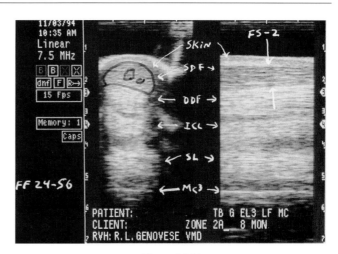

Figure 21.81.

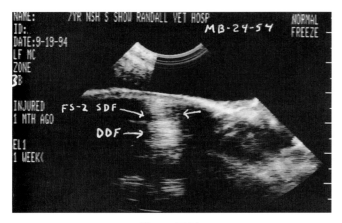

Figure 21.79.

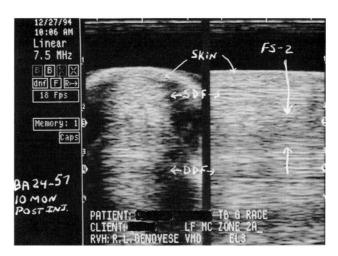

Figure 21.82.

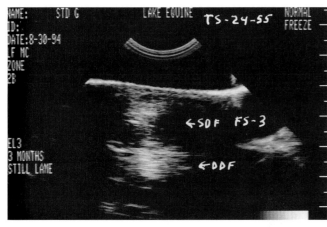

Figure 21.80.

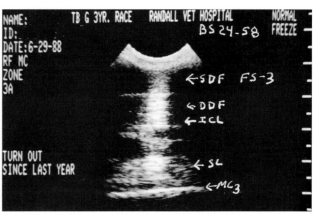

Figure 21.83.

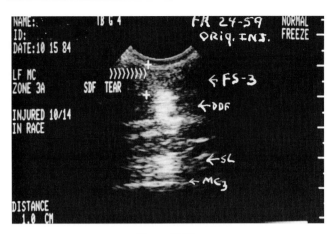

Figure 21.84.

Figure 21.85 is a sagittal left metacarpal Zone 3A SDFT sonogram of the same horse shown in Figure 21.84 7 months after injury and after pasture exercise (EL-3b). Mixed echogenic fiber bundles (Type 2) are present and fiber bundle alignment is less than 25% (FS-3). Based on sonographic parameters, this horse is not ready for exercise (EL-5). However, the trainer felt that enough time was allowed, so the tendon was "set" and training was resumed.

Figure 21.86 is a sagittal left metacarpal zone 3A SDFT sonogram of the same horse shown in Figures 21.84 and 21.85 made 2 months later at EL-5 (galloping). This sonogram indicates obvious reinjury along the palmar half of the SDFT.

Figure 21.87 is a sagittal right metacarpal zone 2A SDFT sonogram of a recently injured Thoroughbred racehorse. Training was stopped and the EL was reduced. The scan shows a large, Type 3 lesion. The target fiber bundles scored an FS-3.

Figure 21.88 is a sagittal right metacarpal Zone 2A SDFT sonogram of the same horse shown in Figure 21.87 made 6½ months after injury. The current exercise level en-

tailed hacking in an arena (EL-4). The scan indicates significant density and FA improvement (FS-1). This sonographic assessment is more favorable. As exercise levels are increased, sonographic monitoring can determine the stability of the healing tendon.

Figure 21.89 is a sagittal right metacarpal zone 2A SDFT sonogram of the same horse shown in Figures 21.87 and 21.88 made 9½ months after injury. The horse had advanced to EL-7; this was a post-race sonogram. The target fiber bundles are isoechogenic and the alignment is FS-1. Subjectively, the fiber bundle lacks compactness. This fiber scoring system used in the BAPTEN SDFT injury management research is being evaluated as a quantitative parameter. The fiber scores of the horse in Figures 21.87 to 21.89 were recorded as follows:

	Initial Injury	6½ Months	9½ Months
zone 1A	2	1	0
zone 1B	3	1	1
zone 2A	3	1	1
zone 2B	3	2	1
zone 3A	3	2	1
zone 3B	1	1	0
Total (T-FS)	15	8 (−47%)	3 (−80%)

In this case, the MIZ (zone 3A) made significant progress at 9 months (greater than 50% FS reduction). The T-FS made a similar favorable reduction at 9 months (greater than 50% reduction).

Currently, a review of BAPTEN and traditionally treated SDFT injuries are being analyzed for FS data that can be used prognostically as an indication of SQR. Our preliminary impression is that at 7 to 9 months at subtraining exercise level, the FS should reduce by 50% before increasing to EL-5. Not all horses satisfying the pre EL-5 FS criteria at the 7 to 9 month period successfully return to competition without reinjury; however, most horses that fail the FS criteria are unsuccessful in their next race and suffer reinjury.

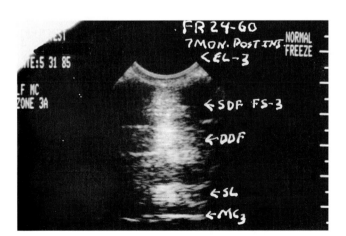

Figure 21.85.

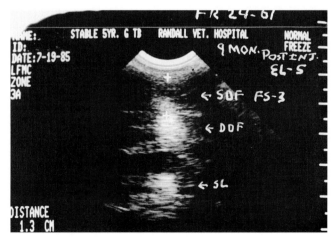

Figure 21.86.

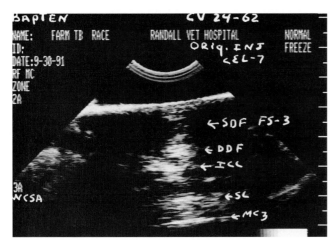

Figure 21.87.

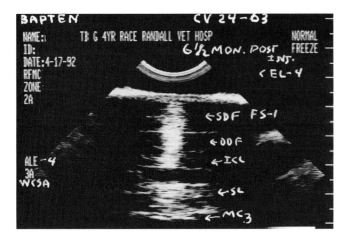

Figure 21.88.

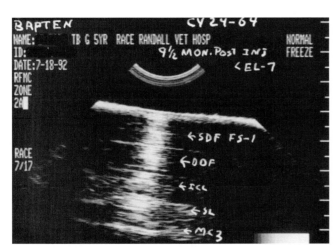

Figure 21.89.

Peritendinous Scar

Sonographic evaluation of the metacarpus/metatarsus should include determining the presence or absence of excessive intratendinous or peritendinous fibrous tissue formation. The most common site for excessive, possibly restrictive, peritendinous scar formation is between the SDFT and DDFT. This finding is most common in chronic, recurring SDFT injuries. Excessive scar formation generally is associated more frequently with tendon lacerations, adverse chemical reactions, and sepsis than with work-related injuries. With work-related SDFT injuries, peritendinous fibrosis is seen mostly in chronic multiple episode injury. Peritendinous fibrosis can impede the SDFT gliding function and can contribute to lameness. Excessive intratendinous fibrosis predisposes the tendon to reinjury.

Figure 21.90 is a cross-sectional right metacarpal Zone 1A SDFT sonogram of an Arab gelding presented for low-grade lameness. SDFT thickness was increased immediately distal to the accessory carpal bone. The scan shows a slightly enlarged tendon with a small, Type 2 core lesion. In Type 2 injuries, lameness is not a common finding. The sonogram shows peritendinous fibrous tissue along the palmarolateral SDFT forming surface adhesions. Furthermore, this fibrous tissue most likely involves the surrounding retinaculum and may be the cause of some tendon gliding restriction, resulting in limb discomfort.

Figure 21.91 is a left metacarpal zone 3B SDFT sonogram of a Thoroughbred racehorse with a more commonly seen low-grade peritendinous fibrosis secondary to a chronic tendonitis. The SDFT has greatly enlarged and fibrous adhesions are present along the medial and lateral border of the DDFT that may result in restricted SDFT gliding.

Figure 21.92 is a cross-sectional left metatarsal Zone 4B SDFT sonogram of a Thoroughbred mare with a markedly thickened tendon sheath on the plantar tendon. Firm adhesions to the tendon have caused restriction of normal gliding movement. There was lameness accompanying this fibrosis, as well as chronic tenosynovitis.

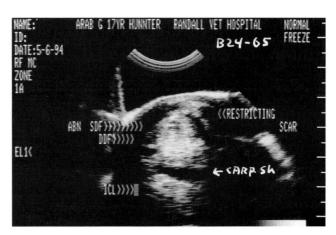

Figure 21.90.

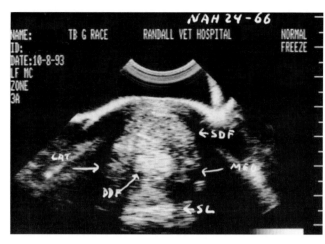

Figure 21.91.

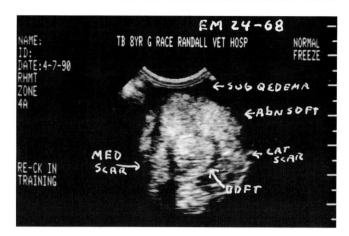

Figure 21.93.

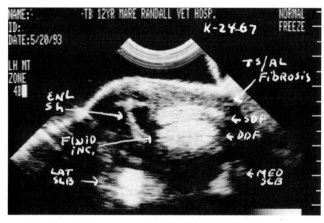

Figure 21.92.

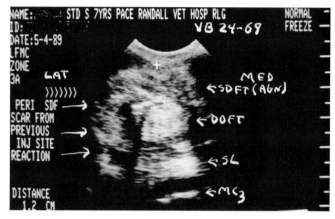

Figure 21.94.

Lacerations and adverse reaction to local chemical injections usually cause the most reactive peritendinous fibrous tissue production. Figure 21.93 is a cross-sectional right metatarsal zone 4A SDFT sonogram of a Thoroughbred racehorse with an abnormal tendon and medial and lateral peritendinous fibrosis. In this case, the interface between the SDFT and the DDFT is visibly distinct. This finding implies that the gliding movement is less restricted and that a more favorable prognosis can be given.

Figure 21.94 is a cross-sectional left metacarpal zone 3A SDFT sonogram of a Standardbred racehorse with excessive lateral border fibrosis. This reaction was in response to medication injected subcutaneously to "treat" the injured tendon. The significance of peritendinous fibrosis must be evaluated from both a clinical and sonographic aspect. It has been our experience that, in chronic tendonitis, fibrous adhesions to the DDFT or the inferior check ligament (ICL) are not common proximal to Zones 3B or 4B. Work-related, painful fibrosis is more common in the distal sheathed

SDFT. In these zones, painful adhesions between the SDFT and the DDFT can be found.

SDFT PATHOLOGY

Introduction

Multiple sonographic variations of SDFT injury exist. In some circumstances, moderate to severe tendon injury is unequivocally diagnosed. Sonographically, the cross-sectional shape changes, various degrees of density and textural fiber bundle abnormalities exist, focal and overall cross-sectional area enlarges, and the normal parallel fiber pattern is disrupted. Sonographically, confirmation of the clinical suspicion of an SDFT injury is more difficult when the degree is slight. In these instances, quantitative assessment is essential to substantiate the injury. The sonographer must identify variation from normal parameters to confirm the injury. From these data, the diagnosis, management program, treatment regimens, and prognoses can be decided. Most of the time, sonographic evaluation is not a diagnostic challenge. In some instances, the presenting problem and the clinical findings do not correlate. Several practical questions are raised when one evaluates the SDFT sonographically, whether for diagnosis or for evaluating the status of a healing injury. Some of the basic questions are as follows:

1. What morphologic abnormality represents an "active" lesion?
2. How does this structural abnormality relate to continued or future athletic use?
3. What method or methods of treatment and case management are indicated?
4. What is the prognosis for return to the present level of athletic use?
5. What constitutes a sonographically "healed" injury?
6. What exercise level should be advised for the present sonographic evaluation?

In other words, after the SDFT status is determined, how does this affect the well being of the horse, and how can it be used to help direct rehabilitation? What advice do we give to the client? Answers to these questions are the essence of SDFT sonography.

Many variations exist in terms of Type, severity, and the response to treatment. Sonography is used to document the SDFT injury, to guide case management, and to evaluate the SQR. Each case has clinical goals, and the endpoint varies from horse to horse, which influences management and treatment suggestions. There are interrelated factors, some of which are based directly on the diagnosis, and other factors that involve stable management and economics. For instance, one may diagnose a new, work-related, moderate SDFT injury in a Thoroughbred racehorse that, at best, has questionable racing talent. This injury will not likely be treated with long-term rehabilitation and surgery because economics most often preclude this option.

These pertinent questions have been addressed for over a decade of clinical information accumulation. Through our experiences, good and bad, we have begun to develop a clinical understanding of SDFT injury management based on sonographic data. The physiologic and economic impact that SDFT injury has on future athletic use of horses is indisputable; there is no question over the tendon's physiologic limitations of repair. Progress of managing tendon injuries has been made over the past decade and continues to improve. Diagnostic ultrasound is credited for allowing earlier diagnosis of tendon injury, determining the severity, and providing valuable data for case management and treatment evaluation.

SDFT Injury Cases

The majority of horses presented for sonographic evaluation have metacarpal or metatarsal swelling with or without lameness. Several of these horses do not have SDFT injury. This group is amenable to symptomatic therapy and cautious, continued use. Horses with SDFT injuries must be separated from those without because the advice and recommended treatment differs. Furthermore, continued training could result in more serious injury. The clinician must determine the cause of the swelling. It is seldom appropriate to advise the client that no abnormalities exist. There is always a reason for the swelling. If the tendon is within normal limits, other causes, such as peritendinous injury or damage to other tissues, should be ruled out. Peritendinous injuries have more favorable prognoses and most often do not significantly prolong athletic use. However, continued training may exacerbate tendon injury that was not detected when the limb was swollen. Careful sonographic examination of the limb is essential. Evaluating all known sonographic parameters greatly assist in this determination. Re-examination within 7 to 10 days after the injury or before re-entering training often shows a lesion.

To emphasize this point, one author (RLG) shares the following case, which was misdiagnosed and mismanaged. Figure 21.95 is a cross-sectional left metacarpal zone 3A SDFT sonogram of a Thoroughbred racehorse with swelling that was detected 1 hour after a 1-mile gallop. The trainer stated that the horse had galloped in elastic support bandages and he wondered if the bandage "pinched" the skin, thus causing the swelling. The horse was scanned within 2 hours after the swelling was noticed. Subcutaneous edema was diagnosed with no tendon injury. The client was advised to apply furacin sweats with double thickness wraps and to continue normal training. Seven days post-examination, the trainer asked for reexamination because the swelling had increased.

Figure 21.96 is a cross-sectional left metacarpal Zone 3A SDFT sonogram of the same horse shown in Figure 21.95. The scan reveals subcutaneous edema and a focal Type 3 palmar midline SDFT lesion. Multiple errors were made in assessing and managing this tendon:

1. The hard copy was too bright for accurate interpretation. This error could easily have masked a small, focal, hypoechoic lesion.

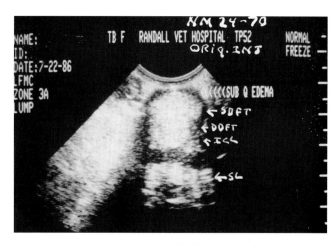

Figure 21.95.

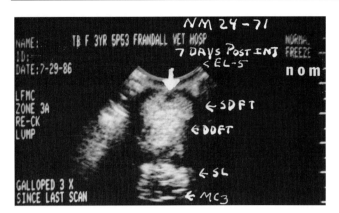

Figure 21.96.

2. The tendon was scanned within 2 hours after injury and the inflammatory response was minimal. Because the early examination was negative for fiber tract disruption or diffuse tendinitis, a repeat examination should have been done 24 to 72 hours later after the post-injury inflammatory response developed.
3. The CSA of at least six levels was not measured.
4. The sonographer failed to compare the contralateral limb CSA. (At that time, however, CSA was not a commonly measured parameter.)
5. The sonographer did not take sagittal scans.
6. The physician did not advise handwalking exercise only and repeating the sonographic examination several days later when the swelling did not totally resolve. A bandage "pinch" is a legitimate syndrome, but within 72 hours, the remaining swelling should have been focal in zone 3A and limited to the skin and subcutis.
7. After fiber damage was diagnosed, the injury was considered slight; therefore, continued training and racing was assumed to be a good prognosis.

Figure 21.97 is a cross-sectional left metacarpal Zone 3B SDFT sonogram of the same horse shown in Figures 21.95 and 21.96 made 3 months later with increased fiber tract tearing. The horse had performed ineffectively since the first

examination and incurred further tendon damage. This case emphasizes the need to follow a **standard sonographic evaluation**, considering all parameters and reserving final judgment until hard copies have been reviewed and the expected clinical response to treatment has been achieved. The value of repeat examinations to confirm that response cannot be overemphasized. Finally, the exercise level should be increased cautiously to ensure that the inflammatory response is under control. Following these principles greatly reduces diagnostic errors and prevents unexpected, more serious, injury.

Figure 21.98 is a cross-sectional and sagittal right metacarpal Zone 2A SDFT sonogram of a horse with recent, diffuse swelling. There was no history of topical medication, nor was any lameness observed. The scan reveals significant anechoic fluid accumulation surrounding the tendon. No significant position, texture, size, shape, or fiber alignment abnormalities of six levels were present. Subcutaneous edema was diagnosed. Sonographically, it is not possible to distinguish edema from recent hemorrhage. In this horse, the extensive swelling and lack of evidence of trauma suggests that hemorrhage is unlikely. A low probability of diffuse, subtle SDFT inflammation exists, even though all parameters are within normal limits. The client was given a good prognosis, symptomatic therapy was advised, and exercise was reduced to walking/trotting under saddle or lunge. Furthermore, if the size of the limb was not normal within 72 hours, the leg should be reexamined before normal activity is resumed.

Figure 21.99 is a cross-sectional right metacarpal Zone 2A SDFT of a racehorse with signs similar to those in Figure 21.98. This scan reveals similar subcutaneous fluid surrounding the SDFT; however, low amplitude echoes existed in the fluid. This finding suggests hemorrhage. In addition, a Type 3 lateral border tendon lesion is present. In horses with subcutaneous fluid accumulation, careful examination of the SDFT is indicated.

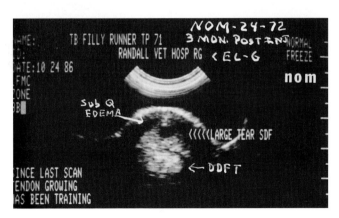

Figure 21.97.

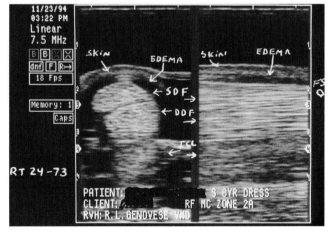

Figure 21.98.

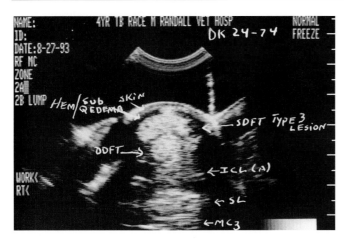

Figure 21.99.

Figure 21.100 is a cross-sectional left metacarpal Zone 3A SDFT sonogram of a Standardbred trotter. The trotter generally exercised in tendon boots. A firm swelling was confined to the middle, plantar metatarsus. The scan reveals no abnormalities of the size, shape, and texture of the tendon, and fiber alignment was normal. Echogenic subcutaneous plantar swelling is present. A clearly visible anechoic interface exists between the tissue and the tendon. Subcutaneous fibrosis or fibrosis resulting from an organizing hematoma was diagnosed. This reaction most likely stems from the use of the tendon boots. Interference while in motion was ruled out because of the plantar location of the fibrous tissue.

One of the most common causes of diffuse peritendinous swelling is application of liniments and paints. Clinically, skin irritation is a salient, but not always accurate, feature. Sonographic evaluation is often requested to rule out low-grade tendinitis, which usually presents as one of two sonographic patterns: 1) dilated vessels without subcutaneous edema; and 2) dilated vessels with subcutaneous edema.

Figure 21.101 is a cross-sectional left metacarpal Zone 2B SDFT sonogram. The scan did not reveal any tendon

abnormalities, and the swelling in this case is caused by marked medial metacarpal and deep metacarpal vessel distention.

Figure 21.102 is a cross-sectional right metacarpal Zone 2A SDFT sonogram of a 2-year-old Standardbred. The SDFT is normal, and medial metacarpal vessel dilatation and subcutaneous edema surrounding the tendon is present. This reaction was caused by leg liniment application.

Figure 21.103 is a cross-sectional right metacarpal Zone 2B sonogram of a Thoroughbred racehorse with a large medial metacarpal vessel distention not caused by liniments. This case is unique because a vascular anomaly is present that results in one large distended vessel as opposed to the usual separate vessels. This filly was scanned repeatedly throughout her racing career, and the vascular anomaly never changed. No tendonitis developed even though persistent, palpable medial metacarpal vascular distention was present.

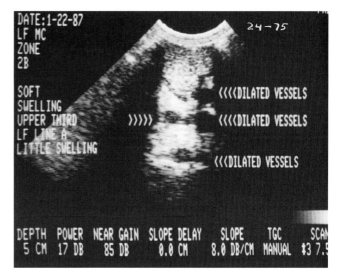

Figure 21.101.

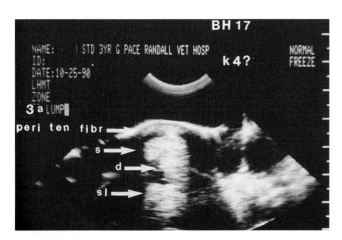

Figure 21.100.

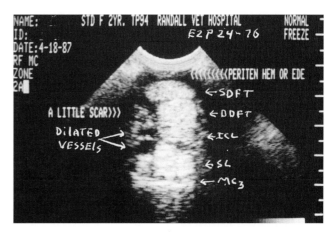

Figure 21.102.

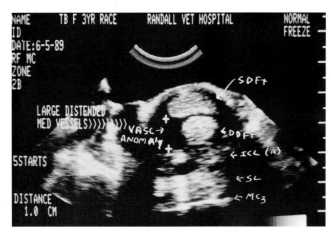

Figure 21.103.

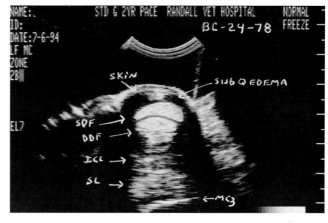

Figure 21.105.

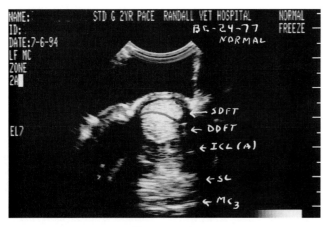

Figure 21.104.

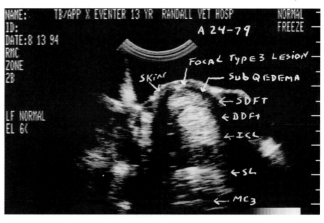

Figure 21.106.

Palmar midmetacarpal focal swelling is a common finding in racehorses. It is common practice after a training exercise to apply a liniment and wrap the leg with a quilt or similar padding covered by a standing bandage. The bandage usually is applied shortly after exercise, and, with slight tendon injuries, swelling is not detectable. The next morning, after the bandage is removed, a focal, palmar metacarpal swelling can be found. This is referred to as the horse being "corded." Physical examination reveals Zone 2B swelling that is sensitive to digital pressure. The differential diagnosis is tendonitis or swelling secondary to a tight bandage. In this instance, a tight bandage was erroneously thought to cause tendonitis. Most trainers do not correlate the injury with the previous day's exercise because the initial inflammatory response was not detected before bandaging. In our opinion, it is impossible to injure tendon fibers with a bandage, but we certainly believe that edema can be caused by improper bandaging. This result most likely stems from a thin and pliable bandage rather than the manner in which it is applied. Veterinarians should explain that it is highly unlikely that a horse with a tendon injury was "bowed" by the bandage. One may save a good groom their job.

Figure 21.104 is a cross-sectional left metacarpal Zone 2A SDFT sonogram of a Standardbred that raced the previous day and was bandaged after the race. The next morning, when the bandage was removed, the trainer noted midmetacarpal swelling. The tendon was normal in Zone 2A.

Figure 21.105 is a cross-sectional left metacarpal Zone 2B SDFT sonogram of the same horse shown in Figure 21.104. There is a large, palmar, hypoechoic fluid accumulation between the SDFT and the skin with some low amplitude echoes. The tendon was within normal limits. This sonogram shows a typical appearance of a "bandage pinched" or "corded" horse. However, as previously noted, a cautious approach is advised. This swelling should abate within 3 to 4 days.

Figure 21.106 is a cross-sectional right metacarpal Zone 2B SDFT sonogram of a racehorse with a similar presentation as the horse in Figures 21.104 and 21.105, except that the lesion was present for a few more days. Subcutaneous edema is present; however, the SDFT sonographic parameters are not normal. There is a focal, mid-palmar, Type 3 fiber disruption. There is a slight shape change and subtle tendon enlargement in two zones. A sagittal scan of this zone revealed a FS-2.

Treatment of SDFT disease is variable. Most of the treatments have inconsistent therapeutic results. None of them have been accepted as the treatment of choice, for many reasons. Tendonitis treatment is be covered in Chapter 27. As far as this chapter is concerned, some potential adverse treatment effects are reviewed to assist in lesion interpretation. Often, previous treatment history is incomplete or unavailable. The sonographer should always be aware that some unusual sonographic presentations may result from previous intratendinous or peritendinous treatment.

Figure 21.107 is a cross-sectional right metacarpal Zone 1A SDFT sonogram of a Quarterhorse with swelling and lameness. This horse had a history of a subcutaneous internal blister injection. The scan reveals no SDFT abnormalities. A 9.0-mm subcutaneous swelling is present, characterized by hyperechoic fibrous tissue reaction and peritendinous edema.

Figure 21.108 is a cross-sectional right metacarpal Zone 2B SDFT sonogram of a Thoroughbred racehorse that had competed two days earlier. In addition, the attending veterinarian had injected the tendon area with subcutaneous ammonium chloride 48 hours before the race. The scan did not reveal any SDFT abnormalities. A large, subcutaneous, anechoic fluid accumulation is present; this was interpreted as an adverse drug reaction.

Figure 21.109 is a cross-sectional left metacarpal Zone 2B SDFT sonogram of a Standardbred trotter that had several peritendinous hyaluronic acid injections over the previous 3 weeks. The limb was progressively swelling. There were no SDFT texture, size, positioning, or fiber alignment abnormalities. The shape changed noticeably from crescent to horizontally shaped. This fluid distribution is unusual because it is around the dorsal SDFT surface on the medial and lateral DDFT borders. The fluid was anechoic and, based on the swelling duration, the lack of echoes would lessen the probability of sepsis but would not rule it out completely. An aspirate was obtained, and culture was negative. Cytology indicated an excessive synovial fluid production and an older hemorrhage. This finding was interpreted as an adverse drug reaction.

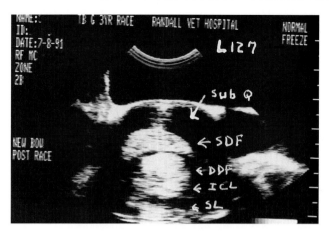

Figure 21.108.

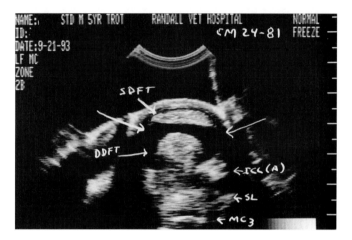

Figure 21.109.

Trauma is another common cause of peritendinous fibrosis. Figure 21.110 is a cross-sectional left metatarsal Zone 4B SDFT sonogram of a Thoroughbred colt that had sustained blunt trauma. There were no lacerations. The scan reveals a subcutaneous fibrosis apparently adherent to the plantar SDFT surface. Most likely, this is an organizing hematoma. The SDFT was within normal limits. Figure 21.111 is a sagittal scan of the same horse shown in Figure 21.110. The scan shows an apparently adherent fibrosis on the plantar SDFT surface and a Zone of subcutaneous hypoechoic fluid or immature fibrous tissue. Low amplitude echoes are present in this area. The mixed level of echogenicity is characteristic of organizing hematomas. Because it is not absolutely possible to distinguish older hematomas from septic reactions, an aspirate for culture is indicated. In this horse, the FS is 0 and there was no lameness or indication of tendon gliding impairment function. This lesion decreased in size and there was no functional impairment. The horse raced successfully throughout the following season.

Figure 21.112 is a cross-sectional right metacarpal Zone 1B SDFT sonogram of a hunter presented for hindlimb lameness evaluation. A focal right metacarpal Zone 1B/2A swelling was found. The swelling was somewhat firm and

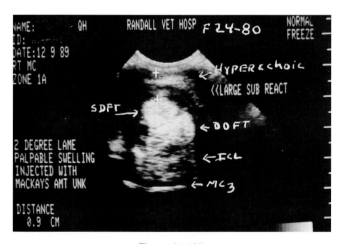

Figure 21.107.

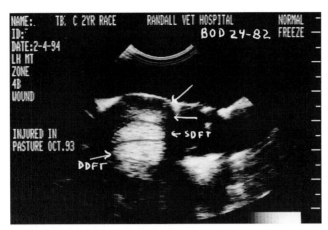

Figure 21.110.

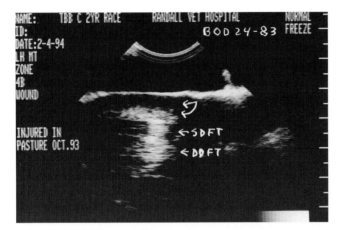

Figure 21.111.

was located along the palmar-lateral SDFT border. The client reported no lameness and had not noticed this swelling. The horse was worked regularly in tendon boots. The scan shows a subcutaneous hypoechoic fibrous tissue reaction along the palmar-lateral SDFT border. This reaction most likely is an organizing hematoma in response to direct trauma (interfering) or secondary to tendon boot placement. It is peculiar that the SDFT CSA was increased only in this Zone and that there is a Type 1, focal, hypoechoic fiber tract along the lateral border only. This injury was diagnosed as the result of direct trauma because: 1) there is a significant peritendinous fibrous reaction; 2) the horse is asymptomatic; 3) the size increase is limited to a 1-cm segment whereas most work-related, active tendonitis lesions are usually longer; and 4) the texture abnormality is slight and the lesion is focal. This would imply a reasonably safe indication to continue normal exercise. We strongly advise monitoring the area; if any gross change is seen, a repeat sonogram is indicated. This lesion is not an incidental finding because several sonographic abnormalities are present. The tendon would be monitored to be certain it is stable and not inflamed. If this were a racehorse, it would be risky to race. A period of galloping (EL-5) is preferred with an additional ultrasound scan. If the tendon was stable, the horse could be allowed to breeze (EL-6) and rescanned before racing.

Persistent peritendinous edema is rare in horses. Figure 21.113 is a cross-sectional left metacarpal Zone 1A SDFT sonogram of a Standardbred pacing filly presented for generalized, low-grade swelling. The scan did not reveal any abnormal tendon parameters. There were several small areas of anechoic fluid accumulation around the SDFT. This was diagnosed as liniment-induced subcutaneous edema. Symptomatic therapy was advised and the horse was kept in normal race training.

Figure 21.114 is a cross-sectional left metacarpal Zone 1A SDFT sonogram of the same horse shown in Figure 21.113 made 2½ months later. The horse was training at EL-6. No gait abnormalities were detected at racing speeds, but the low-grade swelling persisted despite leg liniment changes. The repeat scan did not reveal any abnormalities of shape, texture, or SDFT fiber alignment. Anechoic subcutaneous fluid has accumulated slightly around the tendon, similar to the previous scan. Of interest is a CSA increase from the first scan. In March, the T-CSA of the suspect leg was the same as the contralateral limb. Presently, the six-level CSA was 547 mm^2, a 13% increase. This percent change, in itself, does not confirm tendinitis; however, coupled with the persistent subcutaneous edema, caution is indicated. A subtle tendon strain was diagnosed.

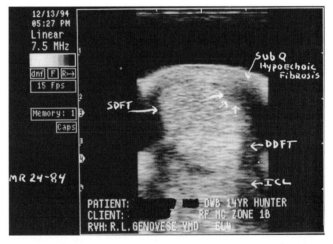

Figure 21.112.

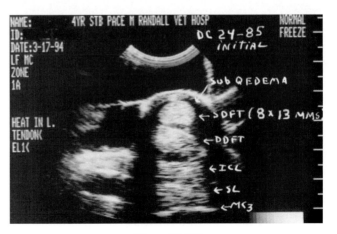

Figure 21.113.

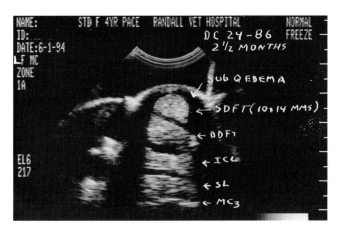

Figure 21.114.

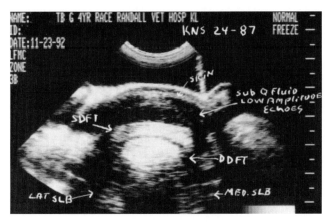

Figure 21.115.

Subcutaneous fluid accumulation can be caused by sepsis, and it is difficult to differentiate the low level amplitude echoes produced by pus from those of early, organizing hematomas. Generally, the clinical signs help differentiate the two. Infection usually results from an open wound or recent drug injection. Skin temperature increases and sensitivity to palpation and lameness is marked. Fluid aspiration for cytology and culture is indicated.

Figure 21.115 is a cross-sectional left metacarpal Zone 3B sonogram with a large, subcutaneous, hypoechoic palmar fluid accumulation. Low level amplitude echoes are scattered throughout the fluid. This swelling had an acute onset 3 days after injection. Fluid was aspirated, and a positive culture was obtained.

INTRATENDINOUS MORPHOLOGIC ABNORMALITIES

SDFT injury appears clinically and sonographically in a variety of ways. There are as many combinations of clinical, economical, intended work use, and sonographic factors that influence diagnosis, treatment, and prognosis. All of these factors must be considered, and each case must be managed accordingly. Each has different priorities to consider. The sonographer will soon discover the clinical and sonographic challenges that tendon disease management can present. When evaluating SDFT injury, always consider

the athletic significance of an injury, and always remember the basic physiologic limits of tendon repair.

Tendon injuries can be secondary to direct trauma, such as laceration, or to the more common work-related fiber damage caused when the elastic limit of SDFT is exceeded. Most use-related injuries are slowly progressive and result from overextension of the limb. This finding is supported by the fact that most SDFT injuries are seen in the racehorses. Many potential contributing factors to fiber tearing exist, such as abnormal collagen turnover, genetic predisposition, track surfaces, improper shoeing, poor training methods, thermal injury increase during exercise, and the role of polysulfated aminoglycans physiology (23).

Work-related SDFT injury is a recent, new injury or a recurring tendonitis. Sonographic abnormalities of recent injury can be slight, moderate, or severe. Sonographic abnormalities can be judged "stable" or "unstable" with serial examinations. When sonographically evaluating repair, the sonographer can view architectural changes as timely, slow, or incomplete. The SQR can be judged favorable or unfavorable. Serial sonographic monitoring of a healing tendon can guide the escalation or de-escalation of exercise levels. Sonography is effective in overall case management.

Sonographic abnormalities can be focal or diffuse in any one cross-sectional plane. The severity of fiber bundle compromise can be determined by doing the following: 1) measuring the percentage of abnormal tendon fibers seen in cross-section; 2) grading the severity of the lesion; and 3) summing the lesion CSA at the predetermined levels and calculating the percent total hypoechoic (% T-HYP) tendon fibers.

We believe that the MIZ is the weakest point in the injured tendon and that more hypoechoic lesions correlate with more fiber strength loss. It follows that a greater volume of fiber loss produces more scar tissue. The more random the scar that is produced, the more likely tendon function will be limited.

Clinical questions that are raised are: Are there times when an incidental, nonclinical sonographic abnormality is present in a normal tendon? Can any abnormal SDFT morphologic feature be considered incidental? Are all identifiable architectural changes from normal signs of tendon disease? (Color changes are seen in otherwise perfectly normal tendons at post mortem [27].) Does this finding represent an early stage of tendon injury, or is it a normal physiologic finding? (Sonographically, color change cannot be detected.) Can normal horses have a few damaged fiber paths and still be considered normal? Does one advise 8 months out of training for a tiny focal lesion? (We think not in some instances. However, in other horses with small focal lesions, one must continue the present exercise level with caution and use serial sonography to monitor the tendon. Small lesions can progress to more severe injuries with continued use.)

Figure 21.116 is a cross-sectional left metacarpal Zone 3A SDFT sonogram of a Thoroughbred racehorse that had been competing regularly for several years. No clinical evi-

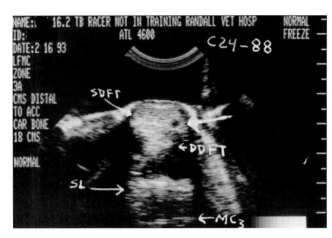

Figure 21.116.

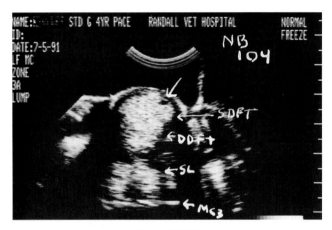

Figure 21.117.

dence of tendonitis was present. This scan was done to test a newly repaired transducer. No abnormalities were found in six of seven levels. The CSA, shape, and fiber alignment were within normal limits in all seven zones. In Zone 3A, however, a focal, Type 4 anechoic area was found on the dorsal lateral tendon. Because this focal defect was only about 5 mm long and because no clinical signs were present, it was considered to be an incidental finding of questionable significance.

Figure 21.117 is a cross-sectional left metacarpal Zone 3A SDFT sonogram of a pacing Standardbred with no clinical evidence of tendonitis. A small defect of the palmar-medial SDFT was found and was considered to be an incidental finding.

Figure 21.118A is a cross-sectional right metacarpal Zone 2A SDFT sonogram of an actively competing jumper with no history of tendonitis. This history presents a slightly different consideration when determining the significance of a small, focal hypoechoic tendon lesion. Palpable, subcutaneous scar tissue was secondary to trauma along the lateral aspect of the tendon. Subcutaneous, hypoechoic fibrous tissue was found along the palmar-lateral SDFT. In addition, a 5-mm, round, Type 2 lateral border tendon defect was present. Also, CSA increased slightly at this level only. This finding appears to be more than incidental. Three sonographic parameters were abnormal: 1) peritendinous fibro-

sis; 2) increased MIZ-CSA; 3) a focal hypoechoic fiber path. The lesion length did not exceed 1 cm and was limited to the fibers adjacent to the subcutaneous scar. Two basic interpretations are possible: 1) this could be a small, subclinical, focal tendon fiber injury with a secondary organizing hematoma; or 2) this could be the result of interference or tendon boot stricture, causing focal tendon inflammation. It was considered to be secondary to direct trauma because no other abnormalities were found. Most focal fiber tearing is, however, caused by strain. Therefore, extreme caution with continued training was advised. If the trainer decides to continue normal training, the tendon should be watched for swelling, heat, or palpable tenderness. The sonogram should be repeated after several weeks of training. When lesions are equivocal, repeat examinations are always indicated. If sonographic parameters remain stable or improve with submaximal stress, one can suspect that the SDFT lesion was secondary to blunt trauma. If abnormal sonographic parameters increase, then primary tendon disease is confirmed. Serial sonography can be used to monitor tendons like radiography can be used to monitor bony lesions. In this instance, the client was surprised that tendonitis was diagnosed. The limb was swollen for a few weeks and there was no other clinical indication that the horse had sustained a tendon injury. The horse continued to be used for flat work and light jumping (EL-5).

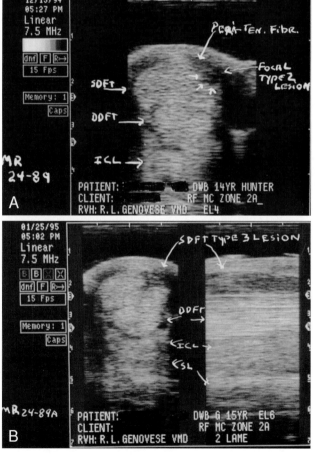

Figure 21.118.

Figure 21.118**B** is a cross-sectional and sagittal right metacarpal Zone 2A SDFT sonogram of the same horse shown in Figure 21.118A made 6 weeks later. The horse had proximal right metacarpal swelling and was slightly lame. The scan shows additional Type 3 fiber path disruption along the palmar-lateral SDFT margin. This lesion had increased in severity, and training was stopped.

Most of the time, an abnormal fiber pattern is evidence of active tendonitis, although small lesion management is often by trial and error. Figure 21.119 is a cross-sectional and sagittal left metacarpal Zone 2B SDFT sonogram of a Thoroughbred racing filly that had been performing well and had a slight mid-tendon swelling. No lameness or heat was associated with the swelling. There is a focal, Type 1, lateral border SDFT lesion. The tendon is enlarged along the palmar-lateral border, and the CSA was increased. The fiber alignment of the target area was FS-2. Furthermore, the lesion was present to a lesser degree in zones 2A and 3A. This focal abnormality is more than incidental because three zones (8 cm) are involved. Continued racing was discouraged even though the damage was slight. Six months rest, a graded exercise regimen, and serial sonographic monitoring would allow a favorable prognosis for return to racing (RTR).

Figure 21.120 is a cross-sectional right metacarpal Zone 3B SDFT sonogram of a Thoroughbred racehorse examined for slight distal tendon swelling. The scan reveals a focal, Type 2 dorsal border lesion. Zone 3A was also damaged, and a 6-cm lesion comprising about 4% of the CSA in Zone 3B (MIZ) was found. The sum of the six-level CSA was 812 mm^2. The six-level CSA of the contralateral normal limb was 583 mm^2, indicating a 39% increase in T-CSA. A significant generalized tendinitis with a small focal tear was diagnosed. An unfavorable prognosis to continue was given.

Focal fiber tearing of any level can be seen with or without significant surrounding tendonitis. A core location is the most common Type of tendon injury described. However, there is a wide variation in lesion location. Lesion distribution and surrounding tendinitis dictates the prognoses and treatment regimens.

Figure 21.121 is a cross-sectional left metacarpal Zone 3A SDFT sonogram of a Standardbred pacer with a focal, Type 4 anechoic dorsolateral border lesion. SDFT did not change shape, and no abnormal fiber pattern was found adjacent to the lesion.

Figure 21.122 is a cross-sectional right metacarpal Zone 3B SDFT sonogram of a Standardbred pacer with an oval, focal Type 4 anechoic mid-dorsal border lesion. There is no obvious adjacent fiber abnormality.

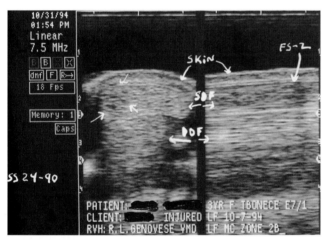

Figure 21.119.

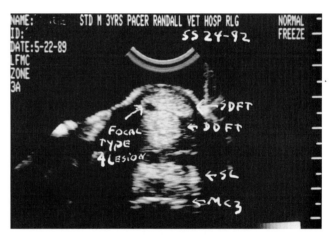

Figure 21.121.

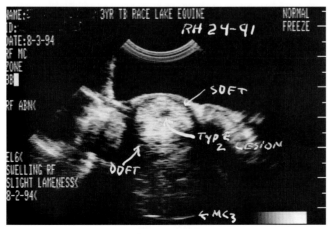

Figure 21.120.

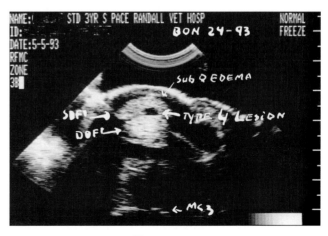

Figure 21.122.

Figure 21.123 is a cross-sectional right metacarpal Zone 3A SDFT sonogram of a Standardbred pacer with a thin horizontal Type 4 anechoic lesion along the dorsal tendon border. Dorsal lesions can be confused with fluid between the SDFT and DDFT. In this tendon, however, a portion of the dorsal margin is damaged, allowing an accurate evaluation. If the lesion extends across the entire tendon width and a small number of surface fibers are damaged, it could be misinterpreted as peritendinous fluid. This horse was pasture rested for 4 months, and the lesion was still present after that time.

Figure 21.124 is a cross-sectional left metacarpal Zone 3A SDFT sonogram of a Standardbred pacer with a large Type 3 dorsal-lateral border lesion.

Figure 21.125 is a cross-sectional right metacarpal Zone 1A SDFT sonogram of a Standardbred pacer with a full width, Type 3 dorsal border lesion. Although this location of SDFT lesions can be seen in any working breed, in our experience, it is more common in the Standardbred.

Because focal fiber tearing can occur at any peripheral tendon location, small, focal, nonreactive lesions are difficult to diagnose. Diagnosing extreme medial and lateral focal lesions requires knowing the shape of the normal tendon borders. Figure 21.126 is a cross-section and sagittal left metacarpal Zone 2B SDFT sonogram of a Standardbred pacer with slight subcutaneous edema and a focal, Type 3 palmar medial tendon border lesion. This finding is confirmed on the sagittal scan (FS-3). Figure 21.127 is a cross-sectional left metacarpal Zone 2B SDFT sonogram with a lesion similar to the one shown in Figure 21.126, but here it is in the palmar lateral border.

Figure 21.128 is a cross-sectional right metacarpal Zone 3A SDFT sonogram of a Thoroughbred racehorse with lateral swelling. Significant shape change occurred caused by a focal Type 3 fiber tearing with peritendonous fluid. If confusion exists, a recheck after inflammation subsides can be helpful. If the lesion is peritendinous, additional sonograms will confirm a normal border. Small, mid-palmar focal lesions can be equally as difficult to identify because most transducers produce an artifactual "specular" reflection because the beam strikes the curved surface at 90°. This focal, bright subcutaneous shadow can mask a small mid-palmar lesion.

Figure 21.129 is a cross-sectional left metacarpal Zone 3A SDFT sonogram of a Thoroughbred racehorse with a focal Type 2 midpalmar lesion. A bright echo is seen at the 12 o'clock position. This artifact can be "moved" by slightly rotating the transducer medially and laterally. The lesion extends across two levels and the CSA is 25% larger than the normal tendon.

Figure 21.130 is a cross-sectional and sagittal left metacarpal Zone 3A SDFT sonogram with a focal Type 3 mid-palmar lesion. The sagittal scan confirms the focal fiber tearing.

Focal fiber disruption can be accompanied by surrounding fiber bundle tendinitis. Figure 21.131 is a cross-sectional

left metacarpal Zone 3B SDFT sonogram of a quarter horse pony with a palmar lateral focal Type 4 anechoic lesion. In addition, a diffuse Type 1 tendinitis surrounds the focal lesion. A low-grade focal fiber tearing with tendinitis was diagnosed.

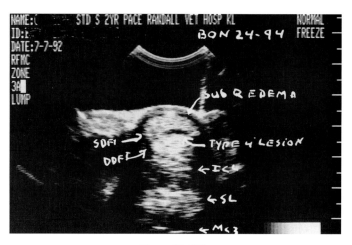

Figure 21.123.

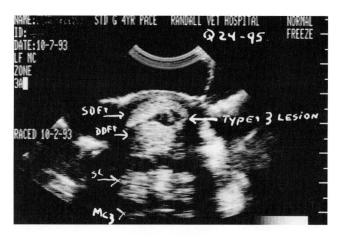

Figure 21.124.

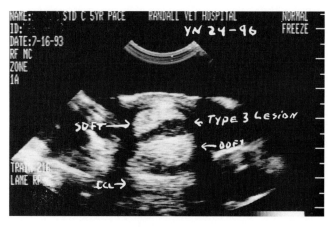

Figure 21.125.

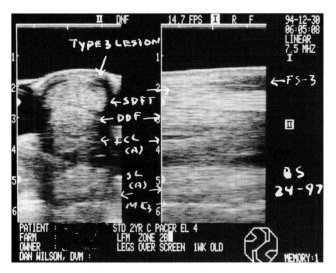

Figure 21.126.

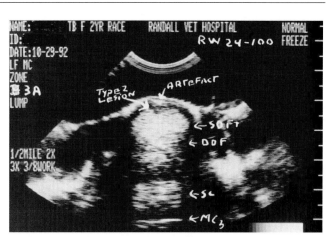

Figure 21.129.

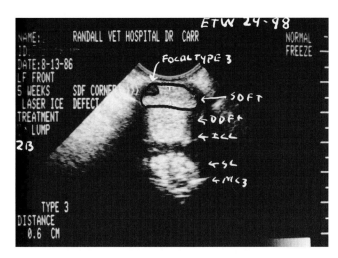

Figure 21.127.

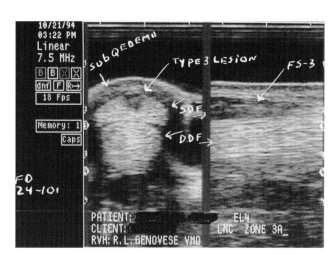

Figure 21.130.

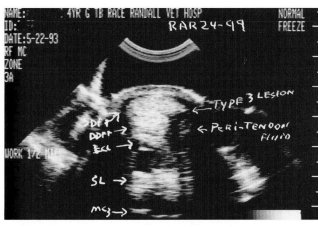

Figure 21.128.

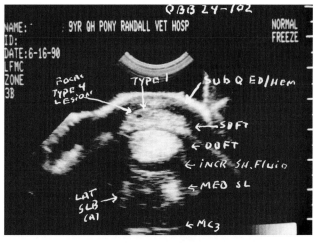

Figure 21.131.

Core lesions are more commonly seen in the racing Thoroughbred. Like peripheral lesions, they can vary in severity and size. Tendinitis may be adjacent to the lesions. Figure 21.132 is a cross-sectional and sagittal right metacarpal Zone 3A SDFT sonogram of a Thoroughbred racehorse with a focal Type 3 core lesion without overt surrounding tendinitis. The sagittal scan confirms the lesion, and the target central fiber path has some axial alignment (FS-2).

Figure 21.133 is a cross-sectional left metacarpal Zone 2B SDFT sonogram of a Thoroughbred racehorse with a moderate-sized focal Type 3 core lesion with no significant adjacent tendinitis. The sagittal scan confirms the lesion. The target fiber bundles lack parallel alignment (FS-3).

Figure 21.134 is a cross-sectional right metacarpal Zone 3B SDFT sonogram of a Thoroughbred racehorse with a focal Type 3 core lesion. A large, diffuse, Type 1 fiber density surrounds the core lesion. A focal core fiber tearing with significant tendinitis was diagnosed.

Figure 21.135 is a cross-sectional left metacarpal Zone 2B SDFT sonogram of a Thoroughbred racehorse with a small, Type 4 anechoic core lesion with adjacent Type 2 tendon fiber bundles. In this tendon, fiber path disruption is greater than the focal lesion suggests. In Type 2 areas, dif-

fuse fiber path disruption is present as is interstitial inflammatory swelling. The larger textural lesion defines the percent HYP fibers, not the smaller focal lesion. Measuring the small focal lesion would underestimate the true severity of the tendon damage.

Besides core and peripheral lesions, a third fiber disruption pattern has been recognized. It may just represent a more severe core lesion Type. This pattern has been seen enough times to warrant a separate discussion. Figure 21.136 is a cross-sectional and sagittal left metacarpal Zone 2B SDFT sonogram demonstrating a large wedge-shaped, triangular, or trough Type 3 central lesion.

Figure 21.137 is a cross-sectional right metacarpal Zone 3B SDFT sonogram of a Thoroughbred racehorse with a large trough lesion. This fiber disruption pattern is along the midline, giving the impression of dividing the tendon into medial and lateral components.

Focal fiber tearing can also occur in multiple unconnected sites within the same tendon. Figure 21.138 is a cross-sectional and sagittal left metacarpal Zone 3B SDFT sonogram of a Standardbred pacer with two separate areas of fiber tearing. One is dorsolateral and the other is palmar medial in location.

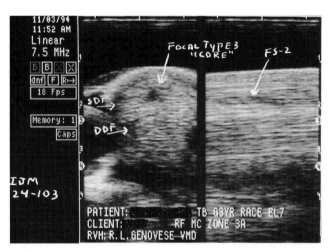

Figure 21.132.

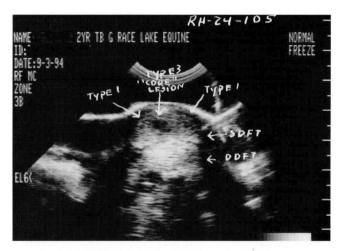

Figure 21.134.

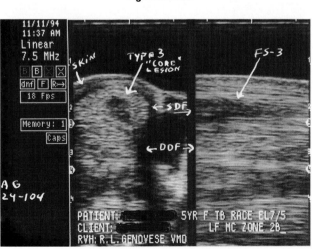

Figure 21.133.

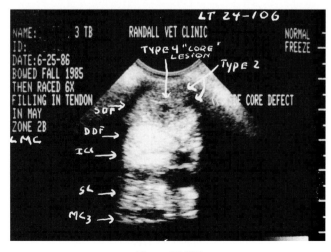

Figure 21.135.

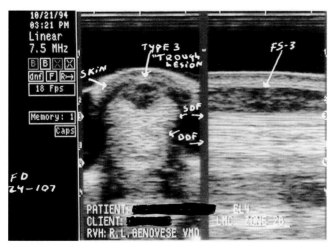

Figure 21.136.

Figure 21.139 is a cross-sectional left metacarpal Zone 3A SDFT sonogram of a Standardbred pacer with two areas of fiber tearing. One is dorsal and the other is located dorsomedially.

Figure 21.140 is a cross-sectional left metacarpal Zone 3A SDFT sonogram of a Standardbred pacer with fiber tearing of the medial and lateral tendon borders.

With the exception of the rare, focal, incidental lesion, textural and density changes usually indicate SDFT injury. When healing is complete, however, there may be persistent hypoechoic foci within the tendon. These foci can be caused by nonparallel fiber alignment, and their presence does not necessarily indicate that the tendon will be unstable when training resumes. Interpretation of hypoechoic fiber bundles seen during the healing process requires serial quantitative sonographic assessments to help determine their significance. This topic is discussed later in this chapter. The present discussion is limited to recent or suspected SDFT injuries.

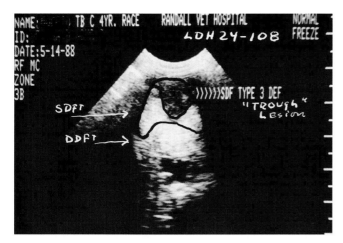

Figure 21.137.

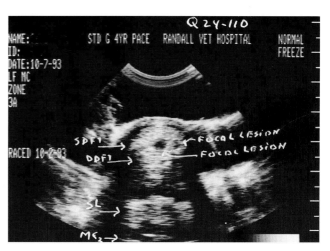

Figure 21.139.

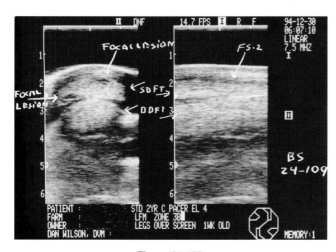

Figure 21.138.

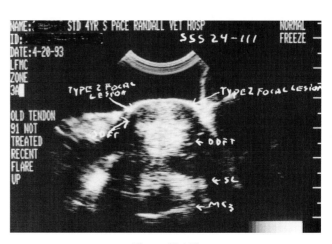

Figure 21.140.

Occasionally, in recent mild injuries, only one sonographic abnormality may be detected. Most recent SDFT injuries, however, have multiple sonographic abnormalities. As a rule, the more extensive the injury, the greater number of abnormal sonographic parameters are found. Although rare, a recent injury can be diagnosed solely on a focal textural change. However, in our experience, a significant CSA increase from normal is the most sensitive indication of early injury. It follows that recently injured tendons with only CSA increases have the best prognosis. Therefore, as expected, early detection of CSA increase vastly improves the chances for return to athletic use. This increase is referred to as subtle tendon enlargement but could be called a tendon strain or a low-grade tendinitis without detectable fiber path disruption. In one author's practice (RLG), this is a category 2 SDFT injury, which means slight injury. It has proven helpful to create categories of SDFT injury, not only for interprofessional communication, but for simplification of injury management. Four basic categories have been created to evaluate the SDFT. Only horses with SDFT injuries are included in the following categorization.

Category 1 are horses with metacarpal or metatarsal swelling with no lameness. On physical examination, the clinician does not suspect that the swelling is caused by tendon or ligament injury. Sonographic examination of the SDFT does not reveal demonstrable position, shape, or fiber alignment abnormalities. The T-CSA does not vary over 15% from the normal contralateral tendon. The potential MIZ-CSA does not vary over 20% from the normal contralateral limb, and the T-HYP (if present) does not exceed 8%. When the quantitative and qualitative sonographic parameters are in this range and there is no evidence of injury to other structures (DDFT, suspensory), the probability is high that the SDFT is not injured significantly. Caution and common sense must be used; however, most of these horses respond to symptomatic treatment and continue athletic use.

Category 2 are horses with metacarpal or metatarsal swelling, and an SDFT injury is suspected on physical examination. Sonographic evaluation does not reveal significant shape and position abnormalities. The quantitative sonographic assessments reveal a T-CSA larger than 15 to 20% of normal, an MIZ-CSA is greater than 25 to 30% larger than normal and T-HYP fiber bundles of 1 to 15%. A high probability exists of a slight SDFT injury in these horses. Often, these horses are kept in training.

Category 3 are horses that have obvious swelling and show physical evidence of SDFT injury. In this category, multiple sonographic abnormalities usually are present. The severity is based on 16 to 25% T-HYP fiber bundles, and these are considered moderate SDFT injuries.

Category 4 are horses that have obvious SDFT injury; many are lame. Multiple sonographic abnormalities are present, and the severity is based on 26% or greater T-HYP fiber bundles. These are considered severe SDFT injuries.

For example, in 1 year (predominately racehorse practice), one author (RLG) examined 42 horses in Category 1. Among these were 22 Thoroughbred racehorses and 3 Standardbred racehorses. Twenty seven (64%) of these horses were treated symptomatically and continued training. Twenty three (85%) did so without sustaining a significant SDFT injury. One horse did well for a short while, then developed significant SDFT injury. Three (11%) sustained SDFT injuries shortly after examination. Fifteen of the 42 were taken out of training. Horses in category 1 have a low probability of further SDFT injury. A favorable prognosis exists for continued use with symptomatic treatment combined with close physical and sonographic monitoring.

In the same year, 63 Thoroughbred and Standardbred racehorses were placed in category 2. Twenty seven (46%) of the trainers elected symptomatic treatment and continued training. Of these 63 horses, 9 (31%) successfully competed without further injury; 3 (10%) raced for a short while before further injury; and 17 (59%) had further injury shortly after continuing training. Therefore, a practical distinction seems to exist between a category 1 and a category 2 classification. Category 1 horses that continue to compete have an 85% chance to do so without further injury. Category 2 horses that continue have only a 31% chance of success. In the same study, only 18% of category 3 racehorses could continue, and none of the category 4 horses successfully continued in training.

Figure 21.141 is a cross-sectional right metacarpal Zone 2A SDFT sonogram of a Thoroughbred racehorse with low-grade swelling. No abnormalities of shape, position, texture or fiber alignment were found in any zone. CSA increased in six zones compared with the normal limb, with a 38% increase in Zone 2A (MIZ-CSA 148 mm²). The six-level T-CSA was 825 mm² compared with 509 mm² for the normal limb, or a 62% increase. This horse has a category 2 SDFT injury and, with symptomatic treatment and continued training, there is a good chance that fiber path disruption will occur. Time off was recommended with a favorable prognosis based upon the findings. The trainer did heed the advice, and the horse was given 3 months off training.

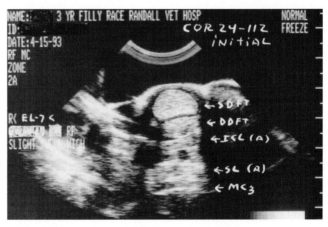

Figure 21.141.

Figure 21.142 is a cross-sectional right metacarpal Zone 2A SDFT sonogram of the same horse shown in Figure 21.141 made after the rest period and before EL-5. There are no sonographic shape, texture, position, or fiber alignment abnormalities. The MIZ-CSA is now 116 mm². Although slightly larger than normal, MIZ-CSA decreased by 22% during the rest period. This finding confirms the original diagnosis and establishes pretraining level baseline data for serial monitoring as the tendon is loaded. With increases in tendon loading, the CSA must remain stable. Exercise level 5 was recommended for 3 to 4 weeks with repeat sonographic examination after that time, or sooner if any new swelling occurs. Before advancing to EL-6, a recheck should be performed.

Figure 21.143 is a cross-sectional and sagittal right metacarpal Zone 2B SDFT sonogram of a Standardbred pacer with slight subcutaneous edema along the palmar aspect. There is a diffuse Type 1 density of the lateral aspect of the tendon. The sagittal scan reveals the "target" fiber path to be slightly less parallel than normal (FS-1) and hypoechoic. In

this tendon, focal tendinitis and low-grade fiber disruption are present. The MIZ-CSA was 140 mm². This is a category 2 injury, but is more advanced than the previous example. This horse would require more time out of training than the previous one.

Figure 21.144 is a cross-sectional right metacarpal Zone 3B SDFT sonogram of a Standardbred trotter with diffuse, Type 1 fiber bundles along the palmar one-half. The sagittal sonogram reveals the target fiber path to be hypoechoic with some loss of normal axial alignment (FS-1). These findings indicate tendinitis with minor fiber bundle disruption.

Figure 21.145 is a cross-sectional left metacarpal Zone 2B SDFT sonogram of a Thoroughbred racehorse presented for slight swelling but no lameness. The horse had been training with an enlarged tendon for several weeks before the examination. The SDFT has an abnormal shape, is enlarged, and has a diffuse Type 2 fiber pattern. Tendinitis is obvious, but fiber disruption is greater than in the previous tendons. This sonogram shows a more serious compromise of tendon strength.

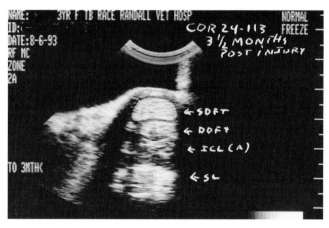

Figure 21.142.

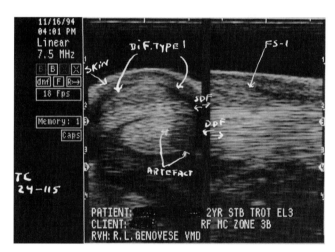

Figure 21.144.

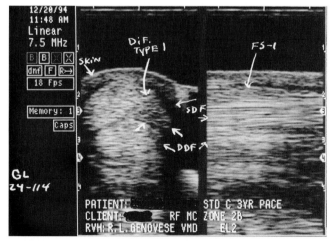

Figure 21.143.

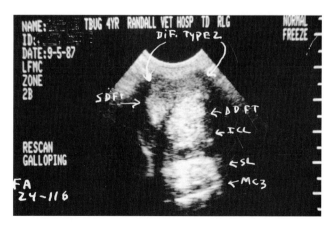

Figure 21.145.

Figure 21.146 is a sagittal left metacarpal Zone 2B sonogram of the same horse shown in Figure 21.145 confirming the fiber path tearing and poor fiber alignment (FS-3). As the severity of fiber path disruption increases, the prognosis for continuing training with symptomatic treatment in racehorses decreases. Similarly, the prognosis for successfully returning to the same training and racing level after rehabilitation decreases as the percentage of fiber damage increases.

Figure 21.147 is a cross-sectional left metacarpal Zone 3A SDFT sonogram of a Thoroughbred racehorse with a recent reinjury. All sonographic parameters are abnormal. CSA and shape have increased. There is an extensive, Type 3 lesion, and the fiber alignment is FS-3. Finally, there is extensive peritendinous fibrosis along the medial DDFT.

Figure 21.148 is a cross-sectional right metacarpal Zone 3B SDFT sonogram of a Standardbred trotter with extensive fiber disruption.

Figure 21.149 is a cross-sectional left metacarpal Zone 3A SDFT sonogram of a Standardbred pacer that had multiple episodes of previous tendon injury. All sonographic parameters are abnormal.

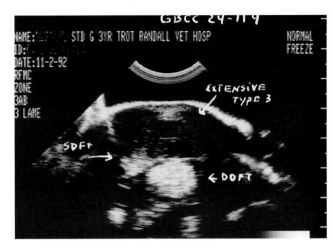

Figure 21.148.

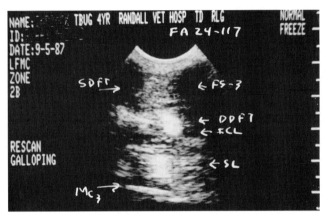

Figure 21.146.

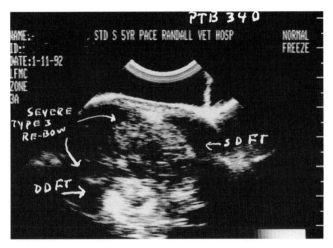

Figure 21.149.

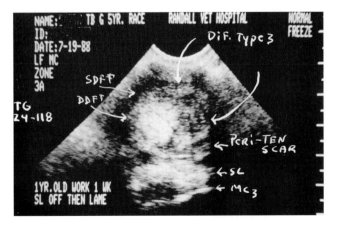

Figure 21.147.

Figure 21.150 is a cross-sectional right metacarpal Zone 3A SDFT sonogram of a tendon that had multiple episodes of injury. All sonographic parameters are abnormal, and this tendon has the most severe tendon injury short of complete division into two parts.

Sonographic evaluation of an acute or recent reinjury is straightforward if done systematically. However, interpretation of more chronic, nonclinical SDFT swelling can be more difficult. Differentiating a stable (set) healing tendon from an early recurring injury can be extremely difficult. Clinical history and physical examination are more important when evaluating enlarged, previously injured tendons. It is not always possible to decide if a fiber abnormality is chronic and stable, inferior SQR, or is a recurring injury at any given EL. This raises questions like: How is sonographic repair determined? Can ultrasound be used to determine whether an SDFT injury is stable (inactive) or unstable (active)?

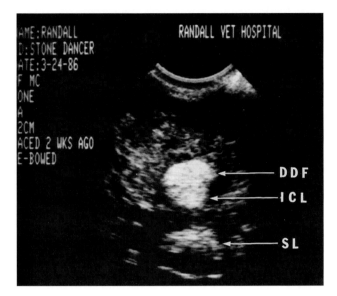

Figure 21.150.

amount of time off and the exercise level. The best that one can do in this situation is give an assessment of the present repair quality and advise an exercise level. If an increase in exercise level was advised after evaluating the tendon, a repeat sonogram after 1 month helps to determine the SDFT stability or instability. Only through serial sonography can one determine the repair status relative to the intended athletic use. If the horse was not going to enter race training, this repair quality may be more than adequate. A poor SQR definitely makes it easier to advise against advancing the exercise level.

Figure 21.153 is a cross-sectional left metacarpal Zone 2B SDFT sonogram of a Thoroughbred racehorse injured 9 months earlier. The highest level of exercise the horse had attained during this time was lunging (EL-2). Once again, the sonographer did not have access to the initial injury scan. The present sonographic evaluation reveals an increased CSA and a reasonably normal shape. Widespread Type 2 fiber paths are present.

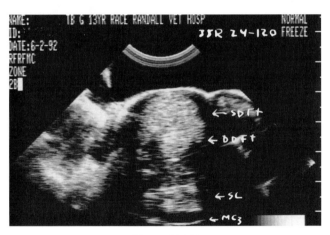

Figure 21.151.

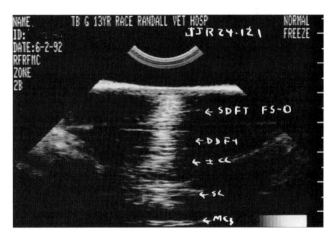

Figure 21.152.

Figure 21.151 is a cross-sectional right metacarpal Zone 2B SDFT sonogram of a Thoroughbred racehorse examined for tendon healing evaluation. The horse had injured the tendon 6 months earlier and had large pasture exercise since the injury (EL-3B). The scan shows an enlarged CSA, a reasonably crescent shape, no significant peritendinous fibrosis, and a partly isoechogenic and partly slightly hypoechoic fiber density.

Figure 21.152 is a sagittal right metacarpal Zone 2B sonogram of the same horse shown in Fig. 21.151. There is near normal fiber alignment (FS-0). Because no baseline sonographic data of the initial injury exists, it is not possible to accurately measure the sonographic parameters. One can provide a qualitative assessment for the present EL. Had the original injury been subtle SDFT enlargement, this would be an inferior SQR. Had the original injury been a large, Type 3 core lesion, this may be a favorable SQR for the

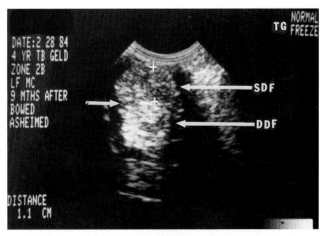

Figure 21.153.

Figure 21.154 is a sagittal left metacarpal Zone 2B sonogram of the same horse shown in Figure 21.153. The tendon fibers are hypoechoic and no significant axial fiber bundle alignment (FS-3) is present. Even without baseline sonographic data, certain conclusions can be derived from the history and sonogram. At 9 months into rehabilitation and at EL-2, the injury is not likely to recur. Therefore, quality of repair is poor and an prognosis for an increase to EL-5 unfavorable. Additional time off is indicated, and sonographic evaluation should be repeated in a month or two. This approach uses the sonographic information to manage SDFT injuries.

Figure 21.155 is a cross-sectional left metacarpal Zone 2A SDFT sonogram of a Thoroughbred racehorse with a chronic injury. The CSA is increased, the shape is oval, and a large Type 3 tendon lesion is present. In this horse, an active recurring injury is likely. Clinical evidence of tendinitis was also present.

Figure 21.156 is a cross-sectional right metacarpal Zone 2A SDFT sonogram of a Thoroughbred racehorse that had multiple injuries. At the time of the scan, the horse was racing (EL-7). The scan shows increased CSA, a reasonable crescent shape, and a mostly isoechogenic density with a few small focal hypoechoic areas and no peritendinous fibrosis.

Figure 21.157 is a sagittal Zone 2A SDFT sonogram of the same horse shown in Figure 21.156. The fibers are 50 to 75% parallel and they scored FS-1. From these parameters and from the EL-7, one can determine this injury to be inactive (stable) at this time. This finding does not indicate, however, that reinjury could not occur. Serial sonographic tendon monitoring during training and racing would be indicated for effective management.

Figure 21.158 is a cross-sectional right metacarpal Zone 3A SDFT sonogram of a Thoroughbred racehorse that had an extensive recovery period. The sonogram was performed before race training. The SDFT is enlarged and has a reasonably normal shape. A typical mixed echogenic texture of a repairing tendon is also present. The CSA of this Zone is 138 mm^2. The six-level T-CSA is 860 mm^2.

Figure 21.159 is the sagittal Zone 3A SDFT sonogram of the same horse shown in Figure 21.158 showing FS-1 fiber alignment.

Figure 21.160 is a cross-sectional right metacarpal Zone 3A scan of the same tendon shown in Figures 21.158 and 21.159 made 2 months after resuming training. The maximum level attained at the time of this scan was EL-5. The scan shows an increased CSA and an oval shape. Both the size and the number of the focal hypoechoic areas increased.

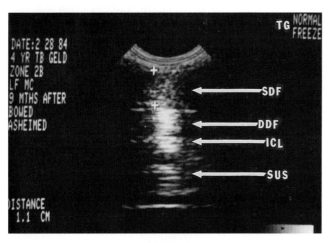

Figure 21.154.

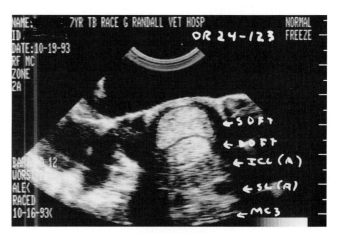

Figure 21.156.

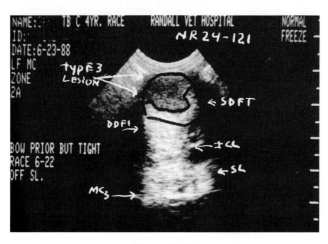

Figure 21.155.

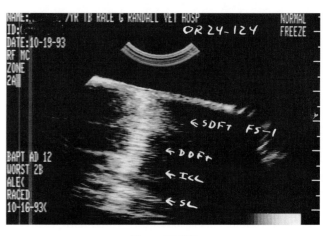

Figure 21.157.

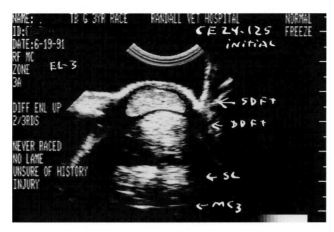

Figure 21.158.

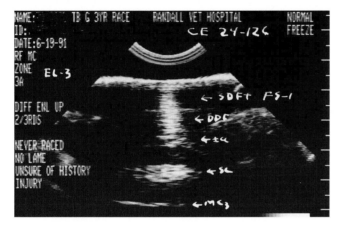

Figure 21.159.

Zone 2B sonogram of the same horse shown in Figure 21.162. The fiber alignment reveals less than 25% parallel fibers and scored FS-3. The horse entered into training with a graded exercise program against advice that said it was too soon.

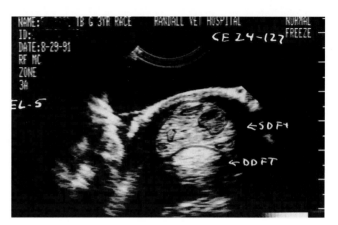

Figure 21.160.

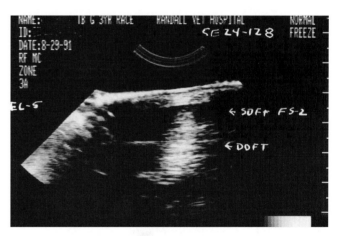

Figure 21.161.

Figure 21.161 is the sagittal Zone 3A SDFT sonogram of the same horse shown in Figures 21.158 through 21.160. The scan reveals a decreased parallel fiber pattern deteriorated to an FS-2. The CSA is 454 mm^2 and the hypoechoic areas represent 25% of the CSA. The six-level T-CSA is 2116 mm^2. Tendon "volume" increased by 146%. This horse started training with what was considered to be an inactive (stable) lesion. As soon as there was a significant upgrade in the exercise level, the SDFT changed from inactive (stable) to reinjured. Sonographic parameters should be considered in terms of SQR and stability or instability with increased loading. This has practical, clinical applications in addressing the client's inquiry: "How is my injured tendon doing?" Sonographic interpretation should be discussed in morphologic terms relative to the current exercise level.

Figure 21.162 is a cross-sectional right metacarpal Zone 2B SDFT sonogram of a Thoroughbred racehorse that had multiple tendon injuries. This scan was taken 4 months after the recent injury. This lesion is considered inactive (stable) at an EL-3. The scan shows an enlarged CSA with an oval tendon shape. The texture reveals scattered, focal hypoechoic areas. The CSA is 299 mm^2 and the six-level T-CSA is 1433 mm^2. Figure 21.163 is the sagittal right metacarpal

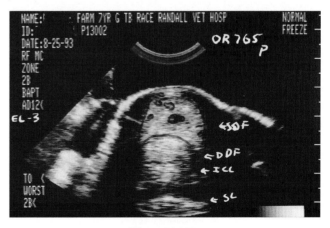

Figure 21.162.

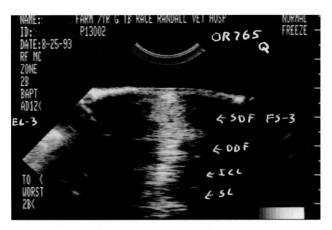

Figure 21.163.

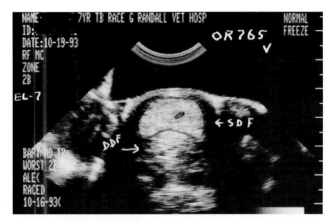

Figure 21.164.

Figure 21.164 is a cross-sectional right metacarpal Zone 2B sonogram of the same horse shown in Figures 21.162 and 21.163 made 2 months later with the training level at EL-7. This scan reveals marked improvement of sonographic parameters. The size is decreased, the shape is more crescent, and the texture is isoechogenic. The MIZ-CSA is 273 mm^2. The six-level T-CSA is 1265 mm^2—a 13% decrease. Figure 21.165 is the sagittal right metacarpal Zone 2B sonogram of the same horse as in Figures 21.162 to 21.164. There is greater than 75% parallel fiber alignment (FS-0). In this case, with increased tendon loading, there is an improved SQR. Although this favorable outcome can occur despite an unfavorable pre-EL-5 SQR, it is rare.

Hindlimb SDFT Injuries

The hind SDFT is susceptible to the same injuries as the fore tendon although the occurrence is less frequent. All principles of forelimb sonography apply to the hindlimb. There is one unique difference on the plantar talus surface (Zones 1A and 1B). Often, horses are presented for plantar hock swelling evaluation, or so-called "curb," with or without lameness. The curb is not a specific clinical entity that applies only to plantar ligament (PL) abnormalities. Rather, it simply refers to plantar talus swelling. One cause of curb is SDF tendonitis, but the swelling is caused more often by subcutaneous, peritendinous fluid or fibrosis. The sonographer should not assume that subcutaneous fibrosis is a primary entity; a combination of abnormalities in the plantar talus is common, and careful sonographic assessment is indicated. Subtle SDFT enlargement can occur here as in any other location; however, peritendinous swelling is the most common cause of curb in all breeds. This swelling may be caused by "sickle" hock conformation or by direct trauma from kicking a solid surface. Subcutaneous fibrosis can result from treatments such as pin firing or external blistering. Also, peritendinous fibrosis can be secondary to SDFT injury or sepsis.

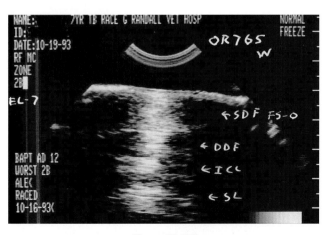

Figure 21.165.

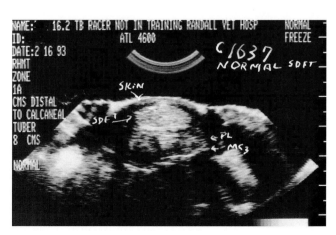

Figure 21.166.

Figure 21.166 is a normal cross-sectional right plantar distal Zone 1A sonogram. The SDFT is on the midline, and the skin and subcutaneous tissue are in direct contact with their plantar surface. The PL contacts the dorsal SDFT surface. The tendon is oval shaped and has an isoechogenic texture.

Figure 21.167 is a normal cross-sectional right plantar Zone 1B sonogram. In this normal scan, the SDFT is on the midline, contacting skin and subcutaneous tissue on its plantar surface and contacting the PL and DDFT dorsally. The DDFT is dorsomedial and the PL is dorsolateral. There is a narrow, horizontal anechoic interface between the SDFT and the DDFT/PL and a vertical, narrow anechoic PL and DDFT interface.

Abnormal SDFT position is rare, but it can luxate or subluxate from its location on the tuber calcaneous. This finding is obviously clinical, but ultrasound can be used to rule out tendon or ligament fiber damage. Figure 21.168 is a cross-sectional and sagittal left plantar Zone 1A sonogram made 6 cm distal to the tuber calcaneous (DTC). Normally, at this level, the PL ligament is on the dorsal SDFT surface and the DDFT is medial and not present on a midline sonogram. In these views, only the PL can be identified. An enthesis is rising from the plantar talus on the sagittal scan, which helps to identify the PL. The SDFT is displaced and not seen on these views.

Figure 21.169 is a cross-sectional left plantar Zone 1B sonogram of a Thoroughbred racehorse with a sudden onset swelling and no lameness after a night of stall rest. The scan was obtained 1 week after injury and shows a hypoechoic subcutaneous fluid accumulation on the plantar SDFT surface. Low amplitude echoes are scattered throughout the fluid, and a distinct fibrous band courses superficially on the plantar medial SDFT surface. The sonographic appearance is compatible with a hematoma or sepsis. A septic lesion most likely has heat and pain; however, an aspirate can be obtained for culture and cytology. The site was surgically drained and a hematoma was confirmed. The SDFT, PL, and DDFT were within normal limits. The hematoma was most likely caused by trauma from kicking the stall walls.

Figure 21.170 is a cross-sectional right plantar Zone 1B sonogram of a Thoroughbred hunter with a history similar to the horse shown in Figure 21.169. Here, however, PL fiber disruption is present. In this horse, the subcutaneous fluid accumulation was partly secondary to the PL inflammatory reaction. Obviously, the treatment differs from that given the horse shown in Figure 21.170.

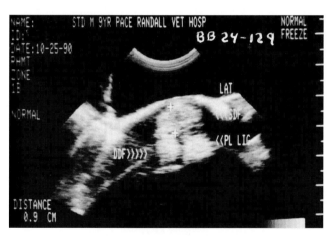

Figure 21.167.

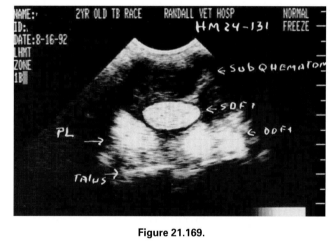

Figure 21.169.

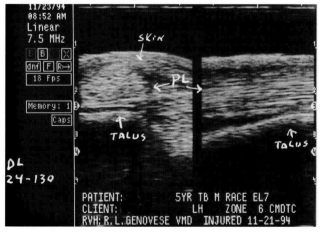

Figure 21.168.

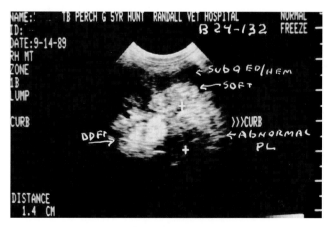

Figure 21.170.

Figure 21.171 is a cross-sectional left plantar Zone 1B sonogram of a Thoroughbred racehorse with a normal SDFT. Uniformly distributed low amplitude echoes were present in the peritendinous fluid. Fluid aspiration yielded purulent exudate and bacterial culture was positive.

Figure 21.172 is a cross-sectional right plantar proximal Zone 1A sonogram of a quarter horse barrel racer. This scan was made proximal to the PL origin. Fluid accumulation is present on the plantar SDFT surface, as is an isoechogenic, 2 mm, horizontal fibrous band on the SDFT plantar surface. This fibrous structure is a thickened bursal wall of a "capped" hock (bursal effusion).

Figure 21.173 is a cross-sectional left plantar Zone 1B sonogram of a horse with a more chronic curb caused by subcutaneous fibrosis. Echogenic fibrous tissue is present on the SDFT plantar surface. Fibrous adhesions to the SDFT margin are apparent. The SDFT was within normal limits.

Figure 21.174 is a sagittal plantar Zone 1B sonogram of same horse shown in Fig. 21.173 confirming the peritendinous fibrosis. The SDFT has normal fiber alignment (FS-0).

Figure 21.175 is a cross-sectional left plantar Zone 1B sonogram of a show jumper with peritendinous fibrosis. This reaction is different from the one in Fig. 21.174, and a fibrous tissue reaction and fluid accumulation are present. The fibrosis is not restricted to the plantar SDFT surface, but extends along the dorsal tendon surface. The SDFT was within normal limits despite the extensive fibrosis.

Figure 21.176 is a cross-sectional right plantar Zone 1B sonogram of a Standardbred pacer with dense, mature scar formation on the SDFT plantar surface and obvious fibrous tendon margin adhesions. There are no reports of extensive palmar fibrosis causing significant SDFT restriction, which is consistent with the authors' findings.

SDFT injury in horses with plantar tarsal swelling must be ruled out because of the greater clinical significance. Figure 21.177 is a cross-sectional left plantar Zone 1A sonogram of Standardbred pacer with nonadhering fibrous tissue adjacent to the SDFT plantar surface. In addition, the SDFT CSA is enlarged, and a Type 3 core lesion is present. Figure 21.178 is a sagittal Zone 1A scan of the same horse shown in Figure 21.177. This scan shows hypoechoic SDFT fibers with 25 to 50% alignment (FS-2).

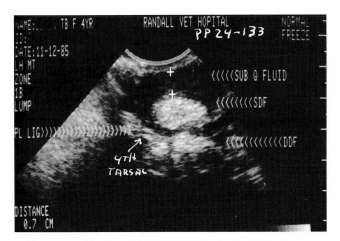

Figure 21.171.

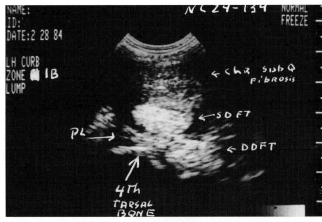

Figure 21.173.

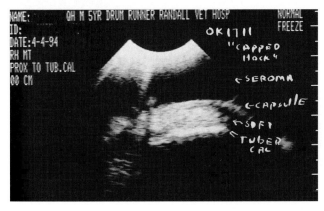

Figure 21.172.

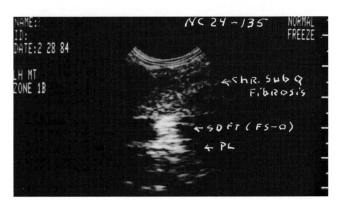

Figure 21.174.

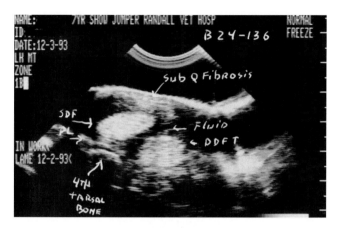

Figure 21.175.

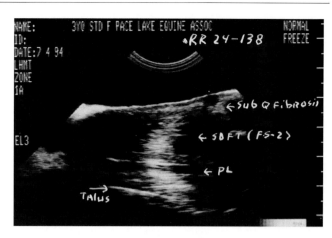

Figure 21.178.

Figure 21.179 is a cross-sectional left plantar Zone 1B sonogram of a Standardbred pacer with subcutaneous, non-adhering fibrous tissue and an abnormal SDFT. The CSA was increased, and a diffuse Type 1 lesion was present.

Figure 21.180 is a cross-sectional left plantar Zone 1B sonogram of a Standardbred racehorse with a history of chronic, intermittent lameness of the affected limb. The trainer identified the curb as the cause. Over the past year, the curb had been symptomatically treated in a variety of ways, including pin-firing, cryotherapy, and several perilesional corticosteroid injections. The scan reveals foci of hyperechoic intratendinous mineral deposition casting acoustic shadows.

Figure 21.181 is a cross-sectional right metatarsal Zone 3B (mid-plantar) sonogram of a Thoroughbred racehorse with anechoic subcutaneous fluid and a focal, Type 3 plantar-medial SDFT lesion.

Figure 21.182 is a cross-sectional right metatarsal Zone 2B (proximal third) sonogram of the same horse shown in Figure 21.181. A rounded, focal Type 4 anechoic medial border SDFT lesion is present.

Figure 21.183 is a cross-sectional right metatarsal Zone 2A sonogram of a Standardbred racehorse made 2 months after the initial injury. A large, diffuse, Type 3 central SDFT lesion is present.

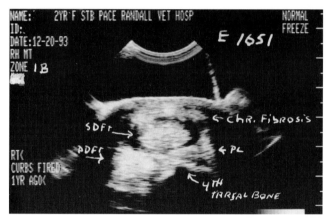

Figure 21.176.

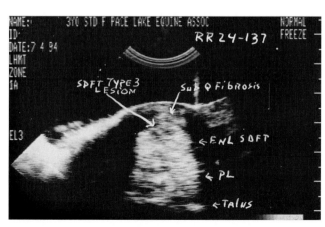

Figure 21.177.

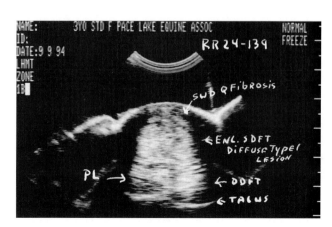

Figure 21.179.

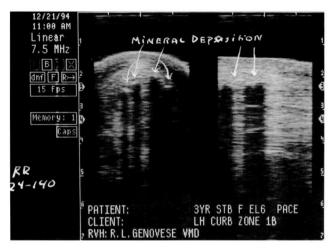

Figure 21.180.

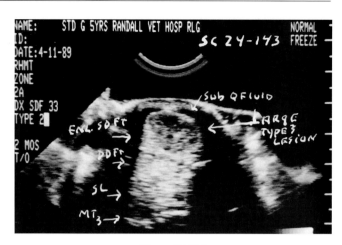

Figure 21.183.

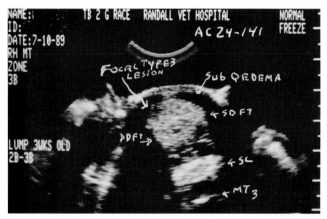

Figure 21.181.

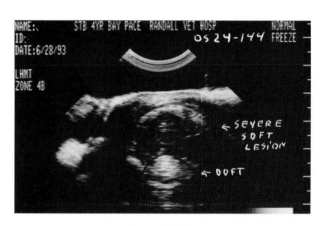

Figure 21.184.

Figure 21.184 is a cross-sectional left metatarsal Zone 4B (distal third) sonogram of a Standardbred pacer with a severe, Type 3 SDFT lesion.

Distal Metacarpal (Zone 3B)/ Metatarsal (Zone 4B) SDFT

The distal metacarpus/metatarsus and palmar/plantar metacarpophalangeal/metatarsophalangeal SDFT is unique because of its anatomic features. The SDFT is narrowed from palmar/plantar to dorsal and is widened medially and laterally. In addition, the tendons have a sheath (TS). At the metacarpo/metatarsophalangeal joint level, the tendons are covered by the palmar digital annular ligament (AL). Injuries and disease can also affect the fibrous tissue structures overlying the SDFT. Redding has published the normal and abnormal ultrasonographic appearance of this zone (28).

Horses usually are referred for clinical evaluation of swelling with or without lameness. Figure 21.185 is a normal cross-sectional and sagittal left metacarpal Zone 3B

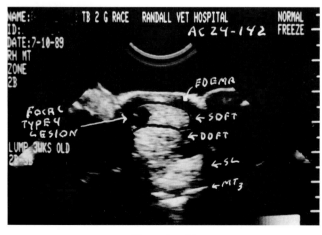

Figure 21.182.

sonogram of a 16.1-hand Thoroughbred. At this level, the SDFT is crescent-shaped and intimately contacts the oval-shaped DDFT palmar surface. The normal tendon sheath (TS) usually is not apparent sonographically. The SDFT is about 4 mm thick and 34 mm wide. The DDFT is about 10 mm thick and 20 mm wide. In a study of Warmbloods, Dik proposed using a ratio of SDFT and DDFT thickness to detect subtle SDFT disease and to categorize palmar/plantar fetlock swellings (22). An increasing ratio suggests SDFT disease while a decreasing ratio indicates DDFT disease. In his report, the normal ratio was 0.4 to 0.6. In our normal example, the SDFT is 4.0 mm thick and the DDFT is 10 mm thick, giving a ratio of 0.4. Measuring this ratio is encouraged to fully evaluate the tendons in this area because tendonitis is often low-grade and subtle. Objective measurements, like thickness ratios and CSA, can help detect these subtle changes. The palmar/plantar fetlock is a common level for DDFT injury.

Figure 21.186 is a normal cross-sectional and sagittal left metacarpal Zone 3C sonogram of a 15.2-hand Standardbred. The scan shows a 3-mm, isoechogenic tissue on the palmar SDFT surface comprising the skin and AL. It often is difficult to recognize the normally thin AL. Because the fluid seldom extends between the annular ligament and SDFT, tendon sheath effusion does not allow better visualization of the ligament. The shape of the DDFT has changed from oval to elliptical with noticeable flattening along the proximal sesamoid bone apices. The SDFT is about 4 mm thick and 27 mm wide and the DDFT is 11 mm by 25 mm.

Figure 21.187 is a cross-sectional right metacarpal Zone 3B sonogram of a horse presented for TS distention. Two anatomic features of the ensheathed tendons are present. First, the TS encloses both the SDFT and DDFT and is referred to as the "outer sheath" with the fluid space as the "outer ring." Practically speaking, the fluid outer ring distention is seen medial, lateral, and dorsal to the DDFT borders. Secondly, there is an "inner sheath" which is the DDFT invagination by the SDFT (macula flexoris). The fluid around the DDFT can be referred to as the "inner ring." No SDFT or DDFT abnormalities were seen on this scan. Amount of fluid increased in both the "inner" and "outer" rings. The inner and outer rings are normally about 2 mm thick. The mesotendon can be seen on the medial and lateral DDFT borders.

Figure 21.188 is a cross-sectional right metacarpal Zone 3B sonogram of a Thoroughbred racehorse with acute onset lameness after a night of stall rest. The filly had been galloped the day before, and the fetlock was routinely bandaged. Physical examination revealed acute palmar distal metacarpal swelling. There were minimal tendon abnormalities and subcutaneous, anechoic fluid accumulation, but no TS distention. The horse was treated symptomatically. The exercise level was decreased, and the swelling resolved within 48 hours. This swelling was most likely caused by a tight bandage.

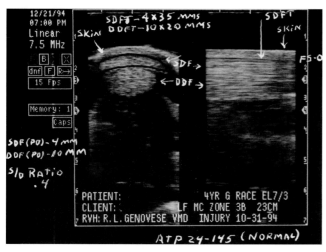

Figure 21.185.

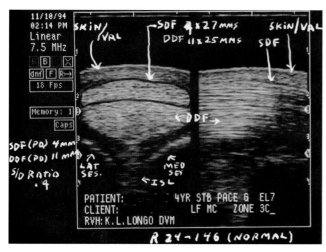

Figure 21.186.

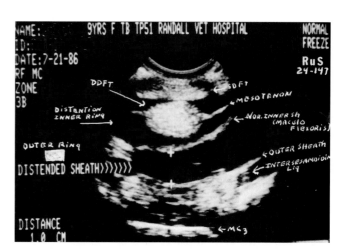

Figure 21.187.

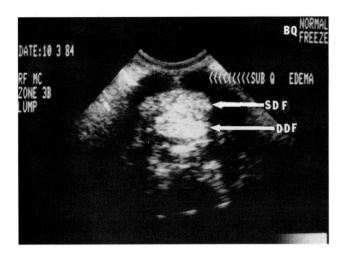

Figure 21.188.

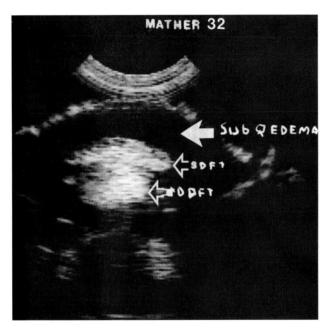

Figure 21.189.

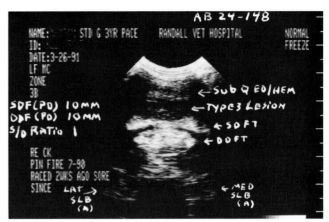

Figure 21.190.

SDFT lesion is present. The SDFT CSA is enlarged to 163 mm². The SDFT and DDFT are 10 mm thick. The SDFT/DDFT ratio is increased to 1, indicating SDFT abnormality. These three horses had the same subcutaneous (not sheath) palmar fetlock swelling, yet all had distinctly different etiologies.

Tendon sheath distention can present in a variety of stages, with and without AL or tendon involvement. Careful assessment is required to determine the presence of tendon injury. Benign TS distention ("windpuffs") is commonly seen in the sport horse. In horses that do not race, low-grade, nonprogressive TS distention seldom affects performance. Occasionally, the more chronic "active" TS disease can cause lameness. In the racehorse, one must always be more cautious of a benign sheath disease diagnosis because this distention can be followed by acute tendon injury with subsequent racing. This finding indicates subthreshold or misdiagnosed tendonitis.

Figure 21.191 is a cross-sectional left metacarpal Zone 3B sonogram of a Thoroughbred racehorse with anechoic fluid distention of the tendon sheath. The SDFT is normal and is 4.0 mm thick. The DDFT is 11 mm and the SDFT/DDFT

Figure 21.189 is a cross-sectional Zone 3B left metacarpal sonogram of an acutely lame Thoroughbred racehorse with post-race palmar fetlock swelling. The scan shows acute, subcutaneous fluid and no apparent tendonitis. Radiographs revealed a proximal sesamoid bone fracture. This case had a similar sonographic presentation as the horse in Figure 21.188, but with significantly different etiologies. It points out the necessity to evaluate each injury completely. In this horse, radiography was a valuable adjunctive diagnostic modality.

Figure 21.190 is a cross-sectional left metacarpal Zone 3B sonogram of a Standardbred presented with a similar, diffuse, palmar fetlock swelling as in Figure 21.189. This scan shows an increase in subcutaneous fluid along the palmar SDFT aspect. In addition, a large, Type 3 palmar

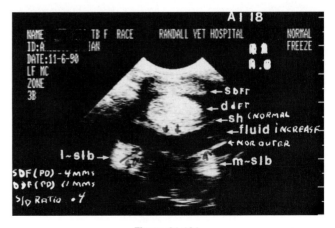

Figure 21.191.

ratio is 0.4. In this case, the palmar swelling was limited to TS distention without concomitant AL or tendon injury. Therefore, the tendon gliding movement should be normal.

Figure 21.192 is a cross-sectional and sagittal left metacarpal Zone 3B sonogram showing TS distention along the palmar SDFT. The TS is thickened and there is a firm fibrous palmar SDFT surface adhesion. If this were extensive, it could result in tendon gliding movement restriction and possible lameness. The normal SDFT is 4 mm thick, the DDFT is 11 mm, and the ratio is 0.4.

Figure 21.193 is a cross-sectional left metacarpophalangeal Zone 3C sonogram showing a fluid accumulation along the palmar SDFT with a small fibrous communication between the tendon surface and the TS. Intimate AL and SDFT contact usually occurs at this site. The fibrous structure most likely represents the normal fibrous connection between the AL/TS/SDFT interface. Mild thickening of the skin and AL are present, but no significant tendon abnormalities were found. The slight thickening of the AL might indicate a strain rather than a benign TS distention.

Because this is a racehorse, training modification, shoeing changes, or support bandaging should be considered to help alleviate strain.

Figure 21.194A is a cross-sectional right metacarpal Zone 3B sonogram of a Standardbred pacing horse with chronic palmar fetlock swelling and decreasing performance level. The scan reveals dense, fibrous, palmar TS thickening with minimal fluid distention. The inner ring is thickened to 4 mm. The SDFT is 6 mm thick, the DDFT is more round than normal and 13 mm thick, and the ratio is normal at 0.5. These findings illustrate a fallacy of ratios if both structures have the same degree of abnormal enlargement.

Figure 21.194B is a cross-sectional Zone 3C sonogram of the same horse shown in Fig. 21.194A showing a thickened dermis and AL. These findings indicate AL constriction because the SDFT, proximal to the AL, is 2 mm thicker. In summary, several abnormalities are present, including a chronic tenosynovitis, low-grade SDF and DDF tendinitis, and AL desmitis with constriction. This horse is a candidate for AL desmotomy.

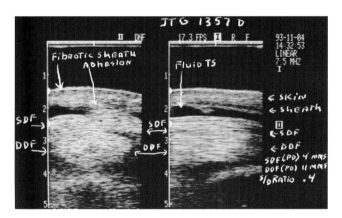

Figure 21.192.

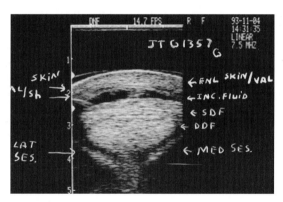

Figure 21.193.

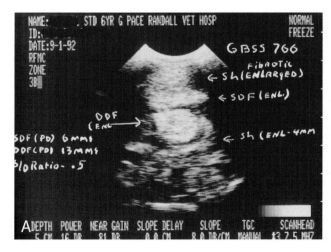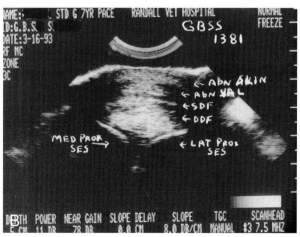

Figure 21.194.

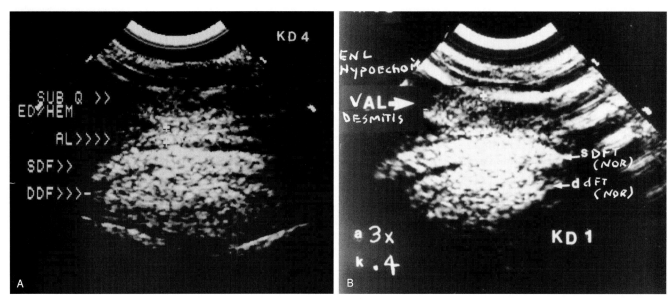

Figure 21.195.

Figure 21.195A is a cross-sectional left metatarsopha-langeal Zone 4C sonogram of an appaloosa showing subcu-taneous hypoechoic fluid accumulation. The fluid has en-hanced AL visualization. The AL, SDFT, and DDFT were within normal limits and the swelling was most likely of traumatic origin ("running down"), allowing a favorable prognosis.

Figure 21.195**B** is a cross-sectional right metacarpo-phalangeal Zone 3C sonogram of a Peruvian Paso (PP) with similar palmar swelling as the horse in Figure 21.195**A**. In this horse, the AL appears to be enlarged and diffusely hypo-echoic. This appearance is compatible with a primary AL desmitis. The SDFT and the DDFT are normal.

Figure 21.196 is a cross-sectional left metatarsal Zone 4B sonogram of an Arab horse showing markedly thickened

"inner and outer" rings (6.0 mm) and TS effusion. The SDFT and DDFT are normal. A diagnosis of chronic, fibri-nous tenosynovitis without tendon involvement was made.

Figure 21.197 is a cross-sectional left metacarpal Zone 3B sonogram of a Standardbred pacer with chronic fibrous palmar TS thickening. There is minimal sheath fluid and the tendons were normal.

Figure 21.198 is a cross-sectional left metacarpopha-langeal Zone 3C sonogram of a quarter horse with fibrous AL thickening. The tendons were normal. There are appar-ent adhesions to the palmar SDFT. A diagnosis of AL desmitis was made.

Figure 21.199 is a gross photograph of a Standardbred pacer with chronic, distal palmar metacarpal swelling. Grossly, differential diagnoses include SDF and/or DDF

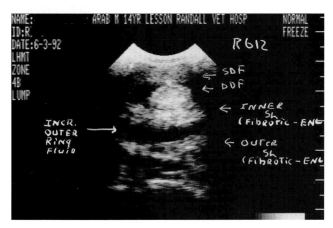

Figure 21.196.

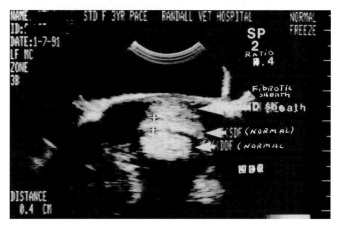

Figure 21.197.

tendonitis with secondary AL constriction, AL desmitis causing constriction with normal tendons, tenosynovitis with or without tendonitis with secondary AL constriction or subcutaneous swelling with normal tendons, sheath and AL. Annular ligament desmotomy may be indicated in the above situations; however, diagnostic ultrasound must be used to accurately diagnose, prognose, and treat this horse.

Figure 21.200 is a cross-sectional left metacarpal Zone 3B sonogram of the same horse shown in Figure 21.199. The scan shows a large, Type 3 SDFT "trough" lesion. The DDFT is normal and the ratio is increased to 1.5. In this case, the surgeon may decide not only to transect the AL, but possibly to split the tendon. This decision could not be made accurately without ultrasonography.

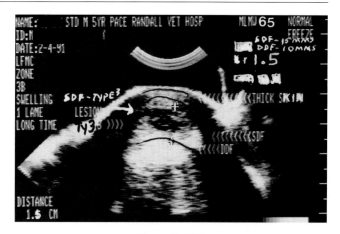

Figure 21.200.

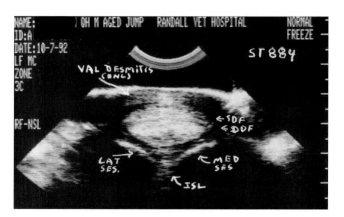

Figure 21.198.

Figure 21.201 is a cross-sectional left metacarpal Zone 3B sonogram of a Standardbred pacer with chronic, palmar fetlock swelling and lameness. The TS had been a clinical problem in the past and was injected on several occasions. Marked hypoechoic TS distention is present with fluid between the tendons. In addition, low amplitude echoes are present in the fluid. Aspiration yielded a positive bacterial culture.

Figure 21.202 is a cross-sectional left metacarpal Zone 3B sonogram of a Standardbred with several chronic abnormalities. The SDFT is enlarged (low-grade tendinitis), the TS is distended, and chronic fibrous thickening of the inner and outer rings is present.

Superficial digital flexor tendonitis in the palmar fetlock (Zones 3B and C) presents clinically similar to more proximal locations. Lesion distribution and severity varies; however, moderate to severe injuries usually are not confined to the distal zones. Slight injuries may be confined to one to three levels, but more extensive injuries usually extend to four or more levels. In a recent review of 114 horses with

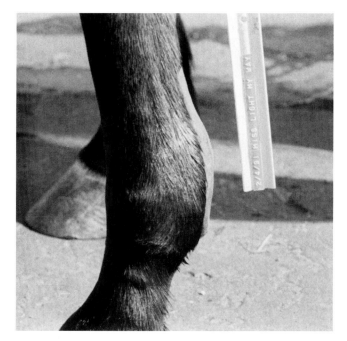

Figure 21.199.

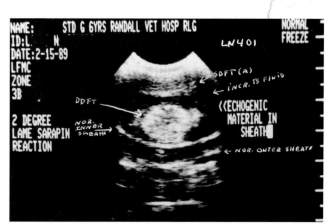

Figure 21.201.

acute or recurrent SDFT tendonitis, the number of affected zones (hypoechoic fibers) were determined for slight, moderate, and severe injuries. Twenty-seven percent of slightly injured tendons (category 2) had one or two affected levels, 39% had three or four levels, 24% had five levels, and only 8% had six or seven abnormal levels. Slight tendon injuries were limited to one to three zones 33% of the time. Moderate injuries (category 3),were limited to one to three zones only 5% of the time. Severe tendon injuries (category 4) were limited one to three zones only 3% of the time, and no moderate or severe injuries were limited to one zone (from unpublished data of R.L. Genovese).

Figure 21.203 is a cross-sectional and sagittal right metacarpal Zone 3B sonogram of a Thoroughbred pleasure horse with a thickened TS with apparent palmar SDFT fibrous adhesions. In addition, there is a focal Type 3 palmar tendon lesion. The SDFT is 7.0 mm and the DDFT is 10, making a ratio of 0.7.

Figure 21.204 is a cross-sectional left metacarpal Zone 3B sonogram of a Standardbred pacer with a focal Type 3 SDFT core lesion.

When examining the distal zones, especially in large horses, medial and lateral border SDFT artifacts are com-

mon when the transducer is positioned midline because of the wide tendon. With wide tendons, it is necessary to move the transducer slightly medially and laterally to image the borders. Focal Type 4 anechoic lesions on the extreme medial and lateral SDFT margins can be overlooked if the borders are not examined carefully.

Figure 21.205 is a cross-sectional right metacarpal Zone 3B sonogram showing a slightly fibrotic tenosynovitis with increased fluid and a focal Type 4 lateral border SDFT lesion. The tendon is 5 mm thick, the DDFT is 11 mm, and the SDFT/DDFT ratio is a normal 0.5. In this case, the SDFT CSA is decreased and a diagnosis of focal fiber tearing was made.

Figure 21.206 is a cross-sectional left metacarpal Zone 3B sonogram of a show pleasure horse with a thickened, fibrotic TS with no appreciable effusion. There are two areas of suspected palmar SDFT adhesions and an enlarged palmar-lateral tendon margin with a Type 1 lesion. The SDFT is 8 mm thick and the DDFT is 10 mm with an increased ration of 0.8. Chronic tenosynovitis with low-grade SDF tendinitis was diagnosed.

Figure 21.207 is a cross-sectional right metatarsal Zone 4B sonogram of a quarter horse with plantar fetlock swelling

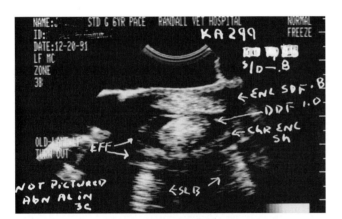

Figure 21.202.

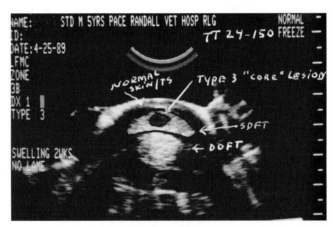

Figure 21.204.

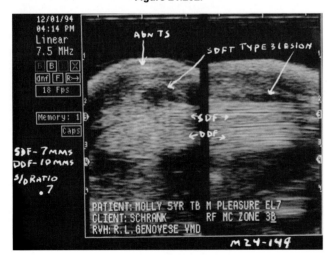

Figure 21.203.

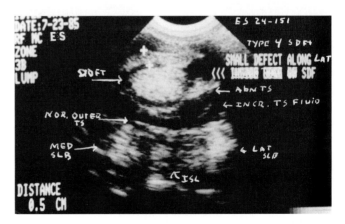

Figure 21.205.

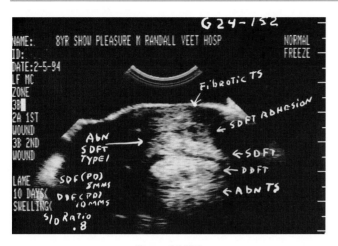

Figure 21.206.

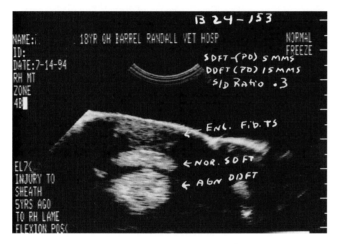

Figure 21.207.

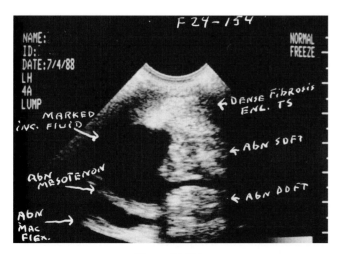

Figure 21.208.

and low-grade lameness. The scan shows a thickened, fibrotic TS and a normal SDFT. There is however, an increased DDFT CSA. The SDFT is 5 mm thick and the DDFT is 15 mm. The SDFT/DDFT ratio is decreased to 0.3, suggesting DDFT enlargement. A chronic tenosynovitis with DDF tendinitis was diagnosed.

Figure 21.208 is a cross-sectional left metatarsal Zone 4A sonogram of a chronically lame horse with a markedly swollen plantar fetlock. This scan shows all soft tissue structures to be abnormal. There is a marked increase in TS fluid, plantar SDFT surface fibrosis, and DDFT mesotendon fibrosis. Both tendons are enlarged and have abnormal fiber patterns. The SDFT is 14 mm thick, the DDFT is 16 mm, and the ratio is increased to 0.8.

SDFT Abnormalities of the Pastern

The SDFT is located on the palmar/plantar medial and lateral aspect of the distal pastern. Distal to the fetlock AL, the SDFT bifurcates into medial and lateral branches approximately at mid P1. The medial and lateral branches course distally and insert on the abaxial surfaces of the distal first phalanx and the proximal second phalanx. The medial and lateral SDFT branches are oval at their origin and become larger and more elliptical near the insertions. Because the SDFT is thin in the upper pastern, it is often difficult to image. In mid P1, the branches course abaxially. Therefore, midline sonography often does not adequately image the SDFT margins. The transducer must be moved laterally and medially just as in imaging the margins of the SDFT in zones 3B and 3C. Midline scans can be used to evaluate the DDFT and the distal sesamoidean ligaments. The SDFT branches intimately contact the medial and lateral DDFT borders. The proximal third of P1 is designated Zone P1A. In this zone (the most difficult pastern Zone to image because of the fetlock angle change and the ergot), the SDFT has not branched. The DDFT lies dorsal to the SDFT and the superficial distal sesamoidean ligament (SDSL) is dorsal to the DDFT. The middle distal, or oblique, sesamoidean ligaments (OSL) are dorsal to the SDSL and adjacent to the bone. The P1 midbody is the second pastern zone (P1B). The SDFT bifurcates in this zone. The distal third of P1 is designated Zone P1C. In this zone, the SDFT branches are abaxial, the DDFT is subcutaneous, and the SDSL is on its dorsal surface. This Zone begins slightly distal to the OSL insertions. The SDFT insertion is seen in P2A, the final pastern zone. This Zone includes the proximal interphalangeal joint. The SDFT branches are located abaxially, and the midline image shows the subcutaneous DDFT and the scutum medium of P2 opposing the dorsal DDFT surface.

The SDFT branches are the most commonly injured palmar/plantar pastern structures, but multiple structures are occasionally involved. Injury to one or both SDFT branches can be primary or secondary to proximal SDFT injury. Usually, these horses have palmar/plantar pastern swelling, and lameness is seen more frequently than with proximal injuries. Because of the variable fiber angle direction of the various structures, ultrasound scans of the pastern are wrought with artifacts. Because of the unique multiplicity of fiber direction, it is not possible at times to obtain a diagnostic image with a given transducer on some horses. Comparison of medial and lateral paired structures and those of the contralateral limb greatly assist the diagnosis. With practice and with proper skin preparation, diagnostic quality images can be obtained. The reader is referred to work by Denoix and Redding (29, 30).

Sonographic evaluation of pastern SDFT injury is the same for injuries proximal to the fetlock. SDFT CSA measurement is difficult in Zone P1A, where branching is incomplete. The SDFT CSA is seldom obtained from a single image. In the branches, however, CSA can be measured accurately. Sagittal scanning is also more difficult because the fetlock is close to the bulbs of the heel. If the scanhead is too long, sagittal images may be impossible. Superficial digital flexor branch injuries have an unfavorable prognosis in racehorses. Lesions must be detected at an early stage and aggressive therapy must be given to remove inflammation and reduce adhesions, or success will be limited.

Figure 21.209 is a normal midline, cross-sectional left palmar pastern Zone P1A sonogram at about 2 cm distal to the ergot base. The SDFT is about 3 mm thick. The skin and proximal digital annular ligament (PDAL) are palmar to the SDFT. The elliptical DDFT opposes the SDFT dorsal border. The SDFT has an isoechogenic texture and, at this level, the medial and lateral borders have the same thickness as the midbody.

Figure 21.210 is a composite cross-sectional oblique right palmar pastern Zone P1A sonogram of a normal Thoroughbred racehorse. The left image was obtained at about a 35 to 45° medial oblique transducer placement. This projection is referred to as the medial offset or oblique view (MO). The image on the right is the same angle from the lateral direction and is referred to as the lateral offset or oblique view (LO). These projections allow visualization of the SDFT margins in the proximal half of P1 and of the me-

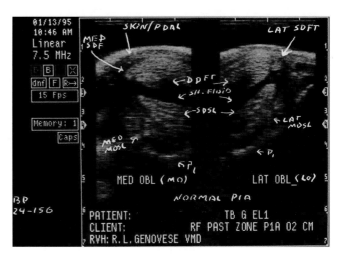

Figure 21.210.

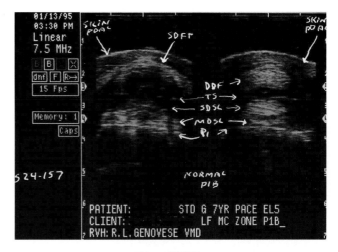

Figure 21.211.

dial and lateral SDFT branches in the distal half of P1 and the proximal third of P2. In this normal horse, the SDFT borders are 2-mm thick and isoechogenic.

Figure 21.211 is a dual cross-sectional left palmar pastern Zone P1B sonogram of a normal Standardbred pacer. This scan is about 4 cm distal to the ergot base and includes the mid P1 area. The skin/PDAL is palmar to the SDFT surface and the artifactually hypoechoic DDFT is dorsal. The midline SDFT is 2 mm thick and the margins are 4 mm thick. The left image is "targeted" at the SDFT, which creates a hypoechoic scanning DDFT and SDSL artifact. The image on the right is "targeted" at the DDFT and the SDFT is artifactually hypoechoic.

Figure 21.212 is a composite cross-sectional oblique left palmar pastern Zone P1B sonogram of a Standardbred pacer with a normal SDFT. The left (LO) image shows the normal lateral SDFT branch border. The skin/PDAL is located on the palmar SDFT surface and the DDFT is dorsal. The lateral border is 5 mm thick. The right image shows the medial SDFT branch border.

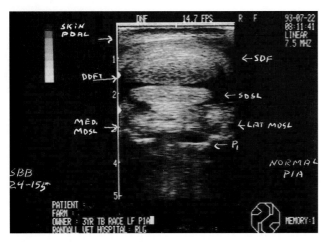

Figure 21.209.

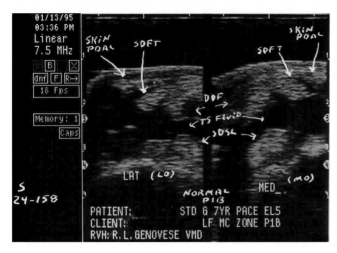

Figure 21.212.

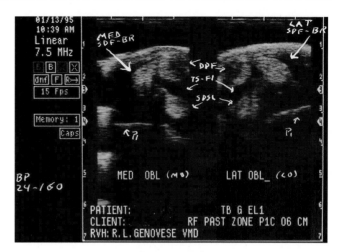

Figure 21.214.

Figure 21.213 is a cross-sectional and sagittal, midline right palmar pastern Zone P1C sonogram of a normal Standardbred 6.0 cm distal to the ergot base. The midline view is distal to the SDFT bifurcation; therefore, the DDFT is subcutaneous. The SDFT branches are poorly and partially seen medial and lateral to the DDFT. The sagittal scan shows the OSL insertions on the palmar surface of P1.

Figure 21.214 is a composite, cross-sectional oblique, right palmar pastern Zone P1C sonogram of a normal Thoroughbred. The left oblique (MO) image shows the medial SDFT branch. The right oblique (LO) image shows the lateral SDFT branch. The branches have enlarged to eight mm thick and have become ovoid, or teardrop shaped.

Figure 21.215 is a midline, cross-sectional and sagittal left palmar pastern Zone P2A sonogram of a normal Standardbred made 9.0 cm distal to the ergot base. This scan does reveal increased thecal fluid; however, this scan is an example of a normal DDFT because of the enhancement of the image by the anechoic fluid. The SDFT is not visible on the midline view at this level.

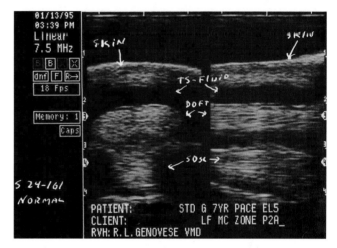

Figure 21.215.

Figure 21.216 is a cross-sectional lateral oblique (LO) and sagittal right palmar pastern Zone P2A sonogram of a clinically normal Thoroughbred. The left image is a cross-section where the SDFT is ovoid and 10 mm thick. The sagittal scan shows the SDFT enthesis (insertion) onto the abaxial proximal P2 surface.

Figure 21.217 is a cross-sectional medial oblique (MO) and sagittal left palmar pastern Zone P2A sonogram of a clinically normal Standardbred pacer. The left image shows the cross-sectional SDFT branch medial view. The right image shows the sagittal image.

One of the most common causes of palmar/plantar pastern swelling is TS effusion. In these horses, there usually is TS distention proximal to the fetlock joint. With benign TS effusion, a soft fluctuant swelling can be detected grossly in the axial pastern at zones P1C and P2A (distal to the PDAL).

Figure 21.218 is a cross-sectional midline right palmar pastern Zone P1B sonogram of a Thoroughbred racehorse The scan reveals increased thecal effusion dorsal to the DDFT. There are no tendon or ligament abnormalities.

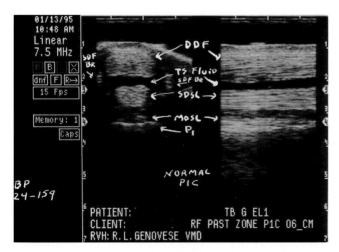

Figure 21.213.

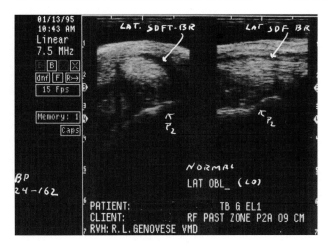

Figure 21.216.

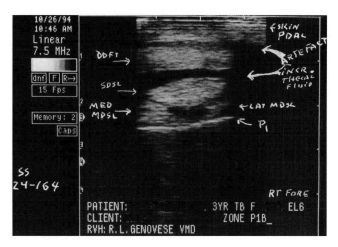

Figure 21.218.

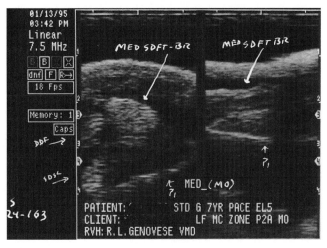

Figure 21.217.

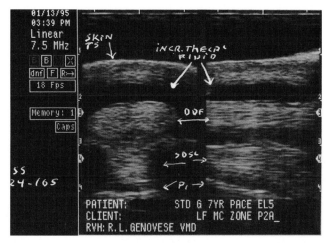

Figure 21.219.

Figure 21.219 is a cross-sectional midline, and sagittal left palmar pastern Zone P2A sonogram of a Standardbred pacer. At this level, the PDAL is not normally seen. The scan reveals an increased thecal effusion and a thickened TS (benign tenosynovitis). The DDFT and the SDSL are normal.

Figure 21.220 is a cross-sectional midline and sagittal left palmar pastern Zone P1C sonogram of a Standardbred pacer. There is TS thickening and fibrosis on the palmar DDFT surface. However, because of the PDAL, increased thecal effusion is seen on the dorsal DDFT aspect. Chronic tenosynovitis was diagnosed.

Figure 21.221 is a cross-sectional midline, right palmar pastern Zone P1B sonogram of a Thoroughbred hunter. This scan reveals subcutaneous, hypoechoic fluid infiltration and low-grade, early fibrosis on the palmar DDFT. This fluid accumulation is not intrathecal. Subcutaneous fluid infiltration of this area could result from dermal infection, sepsis from a penetrating wound, blunt trauma, or could be secondary to SDFT or DDFT injury. Clinical his-

tory and physical examination helps to differentiate. In this case, the fibrosis and inflammatory reaction was attributed to a DDFT injury.

Figure 21.222 is a cross-sectional MO right plantar pastern Zone P1B sonogram of a Thoroughbred racehorse. There is anechoic fluid infiltrate along the medial and dorsal SDFT borders. The medial SDFT border is within normal limits. Aspiration of the fluid pocket yielded serum and some blood. The diagnosis of focal hemorrhage secondary to trauma was made. The horse was treated symptomatically and recovered uneventfully.

Figure 21.223 is a dual, cross-sectional oblique right palmar pastern Zone P1C sonogram of a Thoroughbred with a recent puncture wound. The left scan shows the normal medial SDFT branch with slight peritendinous fibrosis on the palmar tendon surface. The right image shows the normal lateral SDFT. It would be reasonable to continue athletic use with a favorable response to symptomatic therapy because there is no evidence of SDFT injury.

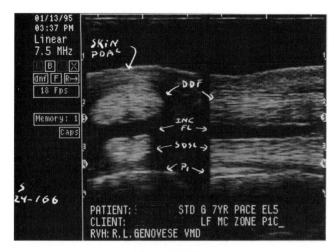

Figure 21.220.

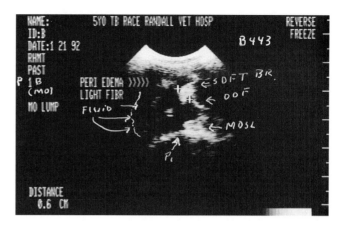

Figure 21.222.

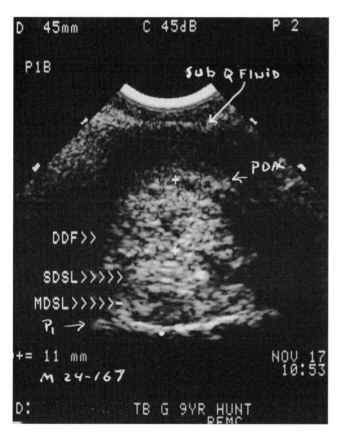

Figure 21.221.

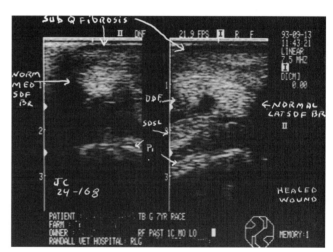

Figure 21.223.

Figure 21.224 is a cross-sectional LO right palmar pastern Zone P1B sonogram of a Thoroughbred racehorse. The scan shows a fibrous tissue reaction on the palmar SDFT surface. The tendon was normal. This Zone includes the PDAL and a possible primary desmitis. Primary PDAL desmitis has been suggested (31). Pastern tendon injury, however, often evokes a significant peritendinous fibrous tissue response, and PDAL involvement is likely. In this case, there was no evidence of pastern trauma. Further clinical investigation and perhaps biopsy of the tissues may establish primary PDAL desmitis as a separate entity.

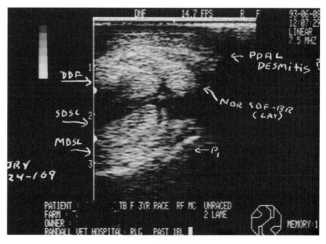

Figure 21.224.

Figure 21.225 is a cross-sectional midline, right palmar pastern Zone P1B sonogram of a Standardbred pacer that had a traumatic pastern injury. It was being assessed for clearance to start training and the palmar pastern has moderate, firm swelling. There is subcutaneous fibrous tissue reaction on the palmar SDFT surface. Unlike the previous horse in Fig. 21.223, however, the SDFT is abnormal. The lateral half is hypoechoic with a poorly defined border. The SDFT was most likely lacerated during the original traumatic injury and has an unfavorable SQR at present. Advancing to EL-5 was advised against until the tendon improved sonographically.

Subtle SDFT enlargement at the pastern level is more difficult to diagnose because the entire cross-section cannot be seen in a single image. Attempts are made to consistently determine the size of the SDFT, however. There are flaws in this approach, but significant CSA increases are significant. Each sonographer is encouraged to develop his or her own technique of CSA measurement data for SDFT branches. In these zones, thickness measurements may be more practical, but attempts should be made to measure CSA. Subtle tendon enlargement has the most favorable prognosis and early diagnosis leads to the best clinical outcome.

Figure 21.226 is an cross-sectional MO left palmar pastern Zone P1B sonogram of a Thoroughbred racehorse with slight medial palmar pastern swelling and no lameness. The scan revealed a 2-mm thick medial SDFT branch enlargement. In addition, three levels were larger compared with both the ipsilateral lateral branch and the contralateral medial branch. Total CSA was 209 mm^2 compared with the lateral branch, which was 135 mm^2. The contralateral medial branch was 139 mm^2. This is a 55% increase in T-CSA, which is compatible with diffuse tendinitis.

Acute, focal SDFT branch lesions can be central or peripheral with varying degrees of severity. Figure 21.227 is a dual cross-sectional MO right palmar pastern Zone P1C sonogram of a Thoroughbred racehorse with post-exercise medial, palmar pastern swelling and low-grade lameness. The scan reveals a medial branch enlargement of 11 mm and a Type 3 core lesion.

Figure 21.228 is a cross-sectional MO right palmar pastern Zone P1B sonogram of a Thoroughbred racing filly with similar signs as the horse in Figure 21.227. The medial SDFT branch was 10 mm thick and two Type 4 peripheral focal fiber tears are present. Both of these injuries were moderate. Severe branch injuries are more commonly seen as distal extensions of more proximal SDFT injury and the pastern should be examined to be complete. There are, however, severe SDFT injuries confined to the pastern.

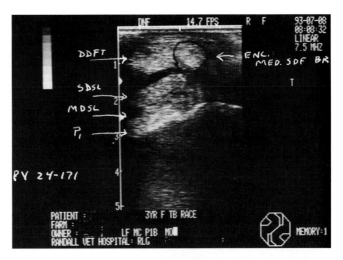

Figure 21.226.

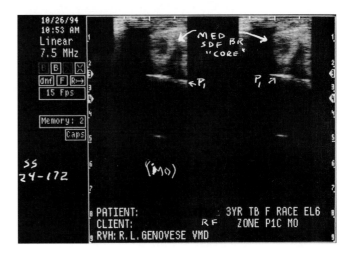

Figure 21.225.   **Figure 21.227.**

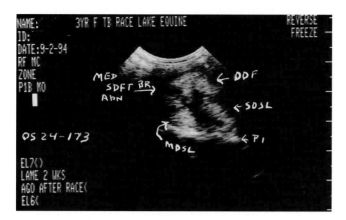

Figure 21.228.

Figure 21.229 is a cross-sectional LO left palmar pastern Zone P1B sonogram of a Standardbred pacer with lateral swelling. The lateral SDFT branch is 11 mm thick and the entire branch is anechoic. Whenever severe distortion of a tendon or ligament is present, the interpretation can be confusing. Several hints can help prevent overlooking this lesion. First, knowledge of the sonographic anatomy is imperative. Secondly, increasing the power or gain may help to visualize low amplitude echoes that would identify the branch. Thirdly, and most importantly, is scanning the tendon proximally and carefully following it distally to the transition Zone from normal echogenic to anechoic lesion. Finally, one can rescan the area 10 to 20 days after injury when the hemorrhage and acute inflammatory response are reduced. At that time, fiber bundles and the tendon outline are easier to identify. This a severe tendon injury. Interestingly, this pacing Standardbred was given 5 months off from training and made a good recovery. The horse returned to racing and after 1 year and injured the contralateral lateral SDFT branch. Superficial digital flexor tendon branch injuries can occur in multiple branches. This finding presents some difficulty when comparing CSA data.

Figure 21.230 is a cross-sectional MO right palmar pastern Zone P1B sonogram of a Thoroughbred racehorse with pastern swelling. The medial SDFT branch is slightly thicker (9.0 mm) and a focal Type 1 palmar abaxial surface lesion is present. Figure 21.231 is a cross-sectional LO P1B sonogram of the same horse shown in Figure 21.230. The scan shows an enlarged lateral SDFT branch with a central core Type 3 lesion.

Acute, focal SDFT branch fiber tearing and peritendonous fibrosis are rare findings. The swelling results mostly from the inflammatory infiltrate and tendon hemorrhage. More chronic findings exist in which palpable swelling is a combination of subcutaneous fibrous tissue response and intratendonous inflammation. The peritendonous fibrosis plus the injury may adversely affect the prognosis for RTR. The horse in Figure 21.229 was evaluated immediately and aggressive therapy was given based on sonographic findings. The horse made a good recovery and raced successfully over 25 times. The healed branch was thickened and isoechogenic, and no appreciable subcutaneous peritendinous fibrosis were present to suggest extensive adhesions.

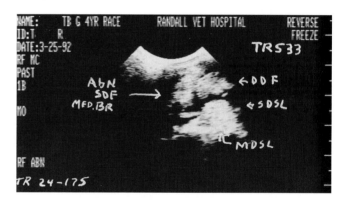

Figure 21.230.

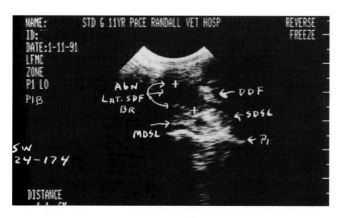

Figure 21.229.

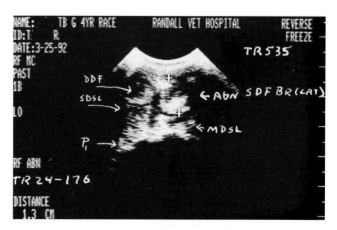

Figure 21.231.

In contrast, a similar Standardbred pacer with a primary lateral branch injury was handled differently by another trainer. Several races before the examination, the trainer noticed palmar pastern swelling and decided to treat symptomatically, and the horse continued racing without sonographic evaluation. The horse raced with intermittent lameness, and performances were deteriorating. Finally, the horse was examined sonographically. Figure 21.232 is a cross-sectional MO left palmar pastern Zone P1A sonogram of a Standardbred pacer revealing chronic, subcutaneous fibrous tissue apparently adhering to the palmar medial SDFT. Some restrictive fibrotic process involving the PDAL most likely occurred. The SDFT has normal texture and size and the medial branch origin is lesion-free. Figure 21.233 is a cross-sectional LO left palmar pastern Zone P1A sonogram of same horse shown in Fig. 21.232. This scan reveals subcutaneous fibrous tissue on the palmar-lateral SDFT surface. The lateral aspect of the tendon and the lateral branch origin are markedly enlarged and a generalized Type 3 density is present; this is significant SDFT fiber disruption. A more unfavorable prognosis was given because of the subcutaneous fibrosis. This Type of reaction may have been responsible for the low number of horses that RTR in the past.

Figure 21.234 is a cross-sectional LO left, palmar pastern Zone P1A sonogram of a pacing Standardbred presented for lameness evaluation and lateral-palmar pastern swelling. The scan reveals a markedly enlarged lateral SDFT branch with a diffuse Type 3 fiber texture; this represents a chronic branch tendinitis with fiber path disruption. In this case, unlike in the previous example, there is no significant PDAL area fibrosis despite the severity and chronicity, which may allow a more favorable prognosis.

Up to this point, we have addressed the normal horse and those horses with obvious clinical pastern SDFT and/or branch injury. However, the sonographer is presented with other situations in which palmar pastern swelling is present. These situations can include during a pre-purchase examination, when new caretakers have assumed the care of the horse and are unfamiliar with the history, or when a client states that an old swelling is present that does not bother the horse. The trainer may ask the clinician to determine the cause of this firm inactive swelling.

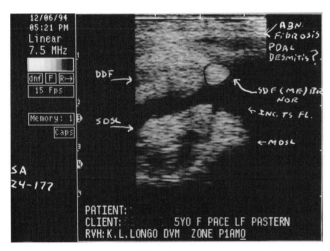

Figure 21.232.

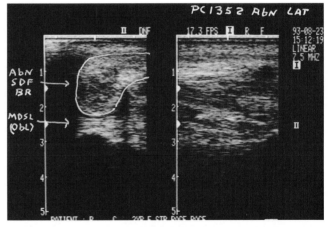

Figure 21.234.

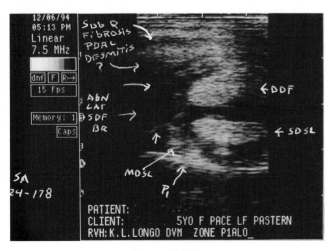

Figure 21.233.

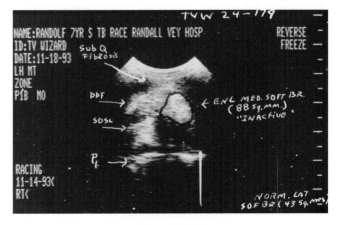

Figure 21.235.

Figure 21.235 is a cross-sectional MO left plantar pastern Zone P1B sonogram of a Thoroughbred racehorse competing without obvious lameness. The trainer was grasping for a poor performance cause. He had been aware of the swelling for a long time, but only recently thought that the horse did not race well because of it. Is this swelling the answer to his dilemma or has the horse just seen better days as a racehorse? This Type of client request is an indication for ultrasonographic examination, and the sonographer must be prepared to offer an evaluation. The scan reveals medial SDFT branch enlargement compared with the normal lateral branch at the same level (9.0 mm). The normal branch CSA was 43 mm^2 compared with 88 mm^2 for the injured branch. The shape and the texture, however, is near normal. Two interpretations are possible: 1) abnormal enlargement that may predispose to fiber tearing with continued training; and 2) abnormal enlargement that has healed and is "stable." Other factors need to be considered in this evaluation. First, this swelling is chronic and the horse has had many races without reinjury, significantly influencing our appraisal. Without earlier scans, it is impossible to sonographically distinguish active subtle branch enlargement from a "stable" repaired lesion. One option is to remove the horse from training for a month and rescan. This decision is risk-free, and if no significant change in CSA or fiber texture occurs, the lesion is most likely chronic and "stable." If there is a reduction in CSA, active tendonitis is present and the horse needs to be rehabilitated gradually.

Secondly, another option is to proceed with training and racing and rescan periodically to see if further changes develop. The risk here is obvious; however, if no changes are seen, the same conclusion can be drawn. If the CSA increases or fiber tearing is seen, training should stop.

Later in the chapter, sonographic assessments are discussed as they relate to tendon repair and the eventual outcome of SDFT injuries. To be complete, several cases are reviewed to illustrate sonographic changes that occur with SDFT branch injuries. It becomes obvious that sonographic repair findings must relate to exercise levels. This information is essential for proper case evaluation. Multiple patient management options are available to trainers and decisions may be based on veterinary advice, past experiences (one failure and they may never try again), and and the economics of each and every situation. From these past experiences, a sonographic criteria data bank can be established to help contribute better advice. In the racetrack community, change is slow to take place and clinicians must relate to the pressures and responsibilities that trainers must face. There always is that one horse who defied all odds and showed up in the winner's circle when veterinary medicine said it could not be done. However, one who stakes his or her career on the chance occurrence that this will happen is foolish. We must approach the assessment of sonographic changes based on the most likely outcome.

The first SDFT branch injury, evaluated over time, is a Thoroughbred racehorse that had successfully returned to

racing after recovery from a metacarpal SDFT injury. This colt was lightly raced, was very speedy, and had an upright conformation. After a winter break from racing in the north, he was trained and raced. Figure 21.236 is a cross-sectional MO left palmar pastern Zone P1A sonogram of the Thoroughbred colt with mild post race lameness and medial, palmar pastern swelling. The scan shows an enlarged medial SDFT branch with a central core Type 2 lesion. The CSA was 94 mm^2 and the lesion affected 41%. Three levels were abnormal and their T-CSA was 288 mm^2. Superficial digital flexor branch tendinitis with 26% focal fiber tearing was diagnosed. Because this horse had been through a previous long-term rehabilitation and because his earnings after recovery were less than optimal, the trainer chose to decrease the exercise level to swimming, apply an external blister, and try a short-term recovery.

Figure 21.237 is a cross-sectional MO left palmar pastern Zone P1A sonogram of the same horse shown in Fig. 21.236 6 weeks into recovery. At this point, swimming and mechanical machine walking was the only exercise (EL-2). The scan reveals an enlarged SDFT medial branch with a Type 1 central core lesion. Sonographic interpretation, at this point, was an immature fibrous tissue response to explain the hypoechoic texture. Inflammatory infiltrate should have

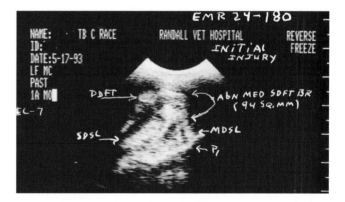

Figure 21.236.

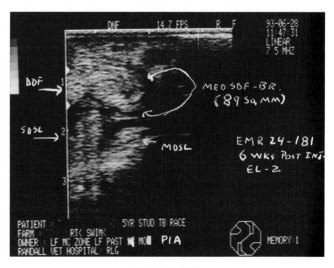

Figure 21.237.

been reabsorbed by six weeks at this EL. This was considered an inadequate sonographic repair at this stage to allow increasing the EL. The lesion comprised a reduced 30% of the cross-sectional area. The CSA of this level decreased to 89 mm². This scan indicates that the improvement was attributed to resolving the acute inflammation. The sonographic improvements are: 1. An 11% reduction in lesion size. 2. A one grade improvement of the texture. 3. Five mm² CSA reduction. 4. The T-CSA of the three abnormal levels was 280 mm² with an average of 20% sonographically abnormal fibers. The trainer decided against advice to stay at EL-2 and progressed up to EL-7 in 21 days.

Figure 21.238 is a cross-sectional MO left palmar pastern Zone P1A sonogram of the same horse shown in Figures 21.236 and 21.237 obtained after the race. The scan reveals an enlarged SDFT medial branch (102 mm²) with a Type 3 lateral lesion involving 48% of the cross-sectional area. The T-CSA for three levels was 275 mm². Even though disaster did not strike in the form of complete breakdown, there was additional injury and acute inflammation. The horse's exercise program was down-scaled again and a short term therapy program instituted. This included 30 days of walking, then a slow return to EL-6.

Figure 21.239 is a dual, LO left and MO right, cross-sectional left palmar pastern Zone P1A sonogram of the same horse as in Figures 21.236 to 21.238 made eight weeks from the last scan with the horse now back to EL-6. The scan reveals an enlarged medial SDFT branch (89 mm²) with a Type 3 lesion comprising 48% of the cross-sectional area. With EL-6, it is not possible to sonographically determine if the hypoechoic texture is due to inadequate collagen fiber repair or partly due to inflammatory infiltration from recurring injury. Based on the CSA the EL should be reduced. The T-CSA for 3 levels was increased to 301 mm² and the average abnormal fibers was reduced to 16%. At this stage, there have been two sonographic evaluations that are inadequate for the present level of exercise and one

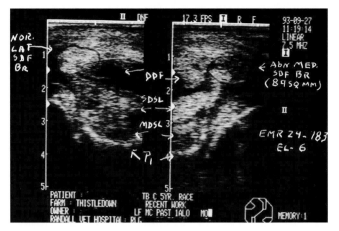

Figure 21.239.

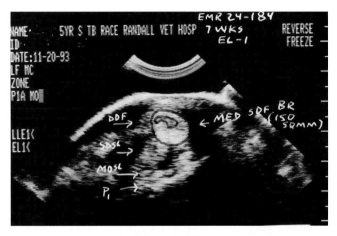

Figure 21.240.

sonographic parameter that is improving. Less severe lesions distal to this Zone are repairing at a favorable rate; but, the MIZ is not. The trainer decided to drastically decrease the EL and remove the horse from race training for an extended period.

Figure 21.240 is a cross-sectional MO left palmar pastern Zone P1A sonogram of the same horse shown in Figures 21.236 to 21.239 made 7 weeks after the previous scan with the horse at machine walking exercise (EL-1). The scan shows a more normal tendon shape and a marked improvement to a Type 1 lesion. The CSA was increased to 150 mm². Cross-sectional involvement decreased to 12%. The three level T-CSA was 437 mm² and the abnormal fiber paths are markedly improved, yet the CSA is increasing. Continued time off was recommended.

Figure 21.241 is a cross-sectional MO left palmar pastern Zone P1A sonogram of the same horse shown in Figures 21.236 to 21.240 made 5 months from the cessation of training. The horse was being given free choice pasture exercise (EL-3). The scan shows a marked improvement of texture, and only 14% abnormal fiber paths was identified

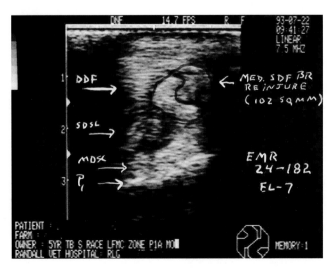

Figure 21.238.

in all three levels. The MIZ had 9.0% hypoechoic fiber bundles. In chronic, multiple injuries, focal Type 1 areas commonly persist as the tendon repairs. These areas indicate immature or inadequate fiber collagen production or, most likely, aggregates of random oriented fibers. The MIZ CSA was reduced to 92 mm² and the total of the three levels was 283 mm². At this stage, all parameters are improved and adequate time has been allowed to suggest an increase in the EL. However, the sonographer cannot be assured that these parameters will remain stable until serial sonographic monitoring is done as the EL increases.

Figure 21.242 is a cross-sectional MO left palmar pastern Zone P1A sonogram of the same horse shown in Figures 21.236 to 21.241 made 10 months after the start of long-term therapy (the horse was out of training for the first 6 months). At the time of this scan, the horse was at EL-6. The scan shows improvement of all parameters. No textural or density abnormalities of any level were present. The CSA of the MIZ was 69 mm². This example shows stability of parameters with increasing tendon loading; from a sonographic evaluation, this is favorable. This horse did not return to racing because of another injury, but this injury did make a favorable recovery.

Figure 21.243 is a cross-sectional MO right palmar pastern Zone P1C sonogram of a Thoroughbred event horse with medial palmar swelling. The scan reveals a peripheral, Type 3 focal medial SDFT branch lesion. Two of three levels were involved. The MIZ had 30% abnormal fiber paths. The MIZ CSA was 48 mm² and the three Zone total was 178 mm². The CSA for the normal lateral branch at the MIZ was 38 mm² and the total of the three comparable zones was 148 mm². The MIZ Zone of the medial SDFT branch was 26% larger and the total of three levels was 20% larger. From these data, one can appreciate the decreased severity of this injury when compared with the last horse. This injury is not as severe and would logically have a more favorable prognosis with remedial therapy and adequate time off. The owner reduced exercise to EL-1 and the horse was returned for re-evaluation of repair.

Figure 21.244 is a cross-sectional MO right palmar pastern Zone P1C sonogram of the same horse in Fig. 21.243 made 2 months after injury. The horse was in EL-2 (ride at the walk). The scan shows resolution of the focal lesion. At the time of this scan, the lesion is isoechogenic and slightly enlarged. This horse's injury is making favorable sonographic progress. Additional time at lower levels of exercise were advised and the suggested total time off was 5 months. After 5 months, a gradual increase in EL stages was recommended, preferably at 1-month intervals, with sonographic monitoring before each EL increase.

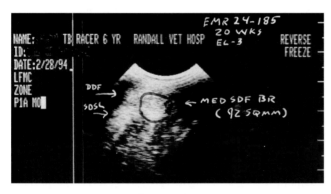

Figure 21.241.

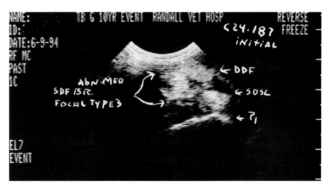

Figure 21.243.

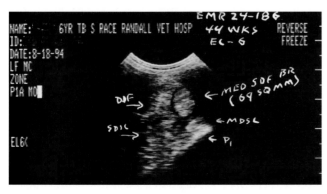

Figure 21.242.

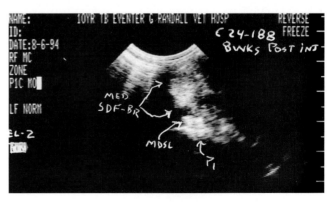

Figure 21.244.

Figure 21.245 is a cross-sectional MO left palmar pastern Zone P1B sonogram of a Thoroughbred racehorse at EL-6 with pastern swelling and lameness. The scan reveals a markedly enlarged SDFT medial branch with a Type 3 lesion. The exercise program was reduced to EL-1 and two external blisters were 1 one month apart.

Figure 21.246 is a cross-sectional MO Zone P1B sonogram of the same horse as in Fig. 21.245 made 2½ months after injury. The horse was still at EL-1. The scan shows the enlarged medial SDFT now with a Type 2 area involving 24% of the cross-sectional area. Based on the persistent enlargement and 24% Type 2 fiber density, exercise should have remained at EL-1. The trainer, however, thought that the horse was doing great and put the horse back into training.

Figure 21.247 is a cross-sectional MO left palmar pastern Zone P1B sonogram of the same horse shown in Figures 21.245 and 21.246 made 2 months after resuming training at EL-6. There is marked medial SDFT branch enlargement with a diffuse, disrupted fiber pattern and Type 3 density. These findings represent retorn tendon fibers and an intense inflammatory reaction. Because of mismanagement, this horse lost 4½ months of rehabilitation, and now has a more serious lesion and a more unfavorable prognosis.

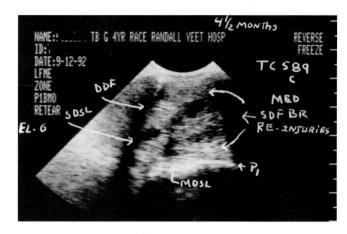

Figure 21.247.

SONOGRAPHIC EVALUATION OF SDFT INJURY REPAIR

Introduction

This section introduces the reader to SDFT sonography in the context of clinical application for maximum utilization of morphologic data. The purpose is to improve technical skills, improve sonographic interpretation, and explore new methods of quantitative assessment that improve case management. The first step towards these goals was to identify sonographic abnormalities through sound use of assessment parameters. Once the SDFT abnormality has been identified and categorized, the clinician must proceed with a management and treatment plan upon which a prognosis for future intended use can be offered. At times, this phase of clinical case management is not a challenge. Regardless of the diagnosis or the extent of the injury, some horses are not used for future athletic use. The owner may use the horse for breeding purposes or maybe the injury is so severe that euthanasia is the option. If the horse has been in the family for years, the trainer may handle it in a manner that does not include veterinary assistance. In these instances, complex treatment, exercise control, and sonographic monitoring techniques are not required. However, this clinical scenario is not common. The more common client request is for restoration of the injured tendon to a functional state so that the horse may continue to perform in its present athletic use without compromise of the quality of that capability. These cases challenge veterinary medicine's expertise of fulfilling the clients goals. Part of that veterinary effort uses periodic sonographic monitoring along with normal physical examinations to evaluate the repairing process. Sonography is used to determine the SQR at various stages of rehabilitation. From these evaluations, the practitioners advise further treatment and appropriate exercise levels.

Considerable variation of morphologic states of repair is seen with SDFT injuries. Some repair states are excellent and lend an optimistic outlook for return to future competition. Other repair states are inferior and are not compatible with athletic use. Yet most of these injured tendons ex-

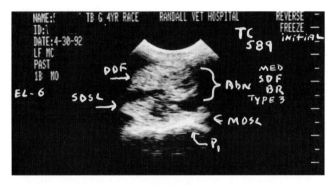

Figure 21.245.

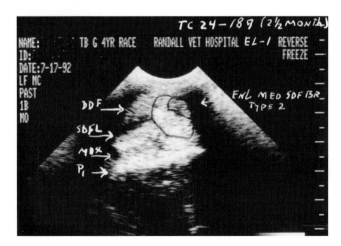

Figure 21.246.

ternally appear clinically stable. Identification of these extremes and all of the combinations in between will be based upon physical examinations and sonographic interpretations. One must also consider that many factors influence the eventual outcome towards the return to competition (RTC) goal. Basic factors include conformation, genetics, shoeing techniques, training skills, work surfaces, other coexisting injuries, and the extent of the present SDFT injury, just to name a few. All of these factors influence the eventual outcome over and above the medical and surgical treatments used. The outcome is complicated further by the physiologic limitations of repairing an injured tendon. Despite these obstacles to a successful end result, veterinary medicine has recently shown significant progress in its ability to improve the RTC. Sonography has been the primary tool responsible for this progress.

Interpretation of the SQR at any given point in the repair process goes beyond indicating to a client at a stall side sonographic assessment that the "black hole" is gone. Meaningful sonographic evaluations are being developed to add a quantitative approach to enhance qualitative sonographic assessments to interpret the SQR more accurately. Earlier diagnosis, better case management, and improved treatment has gradually improved athletic return of bowed horses.

Sonography is a diagnostic tool that compliments clinical evaluation. This modality provides sub gross data to be considered in case management. It does not penetrate the cellular, biochemical, or molecular level for clinical information. However, sonography is a practical means for everyday application that provides morphologic information obtainable by no other practical means. One must also always be aware of the basic principle that tendon fibers and elastic components of normal tendon are not replicated after injury to the SDFT. This limitation of repair sets the tendinous tissue apart from osseous tissue. Functional repair by replacement does occur, however. Over the years, since the introduction of diagnostic ultrasound, we have been addressed by trainers with the misconception that sonography "cures" tendon injuries. The simple fact that one can obtain an image of the SDFT was translated into instant cure for tendon disease. As inappropriate as this may seem, this concept has been perceived by trainers and veterinarians alike. Sonography is not a treatment modality. As a diagnostic tool, however, it can improve case management and favorably influence the outcome of the injury. From that perspective, sonography can help to "cure" a tendon injury. Client education to withhold EL advances until the appropriate time based upon sonographic data is a major step forward in SDFT disease management and the restoration of athletic use. Finally, one should bear in mind that for moderate to severe SDFT athletic use-related injuries, there is seldom a therapeutic short cut to necessary time from training. Beyond sonographic improvement, time is required for remodeling of the scar and vital cross linking.

There are two practical goals of SDFT repair. One is the client's most pressing goal: return to athletic function. In racing, this end result is the return to racing (RTR). This goal is often used by clients and researchers as the end point as a measure of success. However, many factors that influence that end result go beyond treatment. Failure to RTR often is attributed to treatment failure, when in fact case mismanagement was the culprit. This simple principle, which can be so difficult to control and identify, has muddied the waters of clinical research.

The second goal of SDFT repair is clinician related more than trainer related. Because recovery from a SDFT injury takes many months, it is important to recognize that during repair, stages of sonographic evaluation exist that can be used to determine healing quality. Long before the end point of RTR, the repair process can be judged as progressing favorably or unfavorably. Not only do clinicians desire to restore the injured SDFT to athletic function; they also must set sub goals of morphologic progress (SQRs) during rehabilitation. In this manner, clinicians can intervene and possibly change the course of repair in a more favorable direction. The SQR is based on physical evaluation and strongly on qualitative and quantitative sonographic assessments at given time intervals. The clinician can have a significant affect on case management to a point. However, client and horse compliance is essential if the sub goals and ultimate goals of treatment are attained.

To comprehend case management strategy with reference to SDFT injury and recovery, past case experiences and research experiences are the building blocks upon which we can constantly improve the SQR, which (theoretically at least) should improve the ultimate goal—return to competition—more consistently.

Texture and Lesion Density in Rehabilitation

Tendon texture and density are important in identifying SDFT lesions, estimating the injury severity, and evaluating repair quality for prognosis. However, interpretation of a focal or diffuse fiber textural abnormality and of changes over time are relative; interpretation at any given time can be difficult. Formulating a concept of the significance of textural abnormalities can reduce interpretive errors.

Figure 21.248 is a cross-sectional right metacarpal Zone 2B SDFT sonogram of a trotting Standardbred with declining performances and a recent lateral swelling. A Type 3 lesion is present along the lateral SDFT margin. The anatomic structures in the region of this lesion are the lateral SDFT border, the adjacent paratenon, and the subcutaneous tissue. The lesion could be caused by either: 1) tendon fiber disruption; 2) intra or peritendinous hemorrhage/edema; or 3) both 1 and 2. In a recent injury (1 to 14 days), the relative extent of fiber tearing and inflammatory reaction is difficult to determine in this focal hypoechoic area. Even though one can only speculate, the interpretation is of major significance to the diagnosis and treatment. If this lesion was hypoechoic because of 100% fiber, then a significant tendon strength compromise is present. If this hypoechoic lesion in a racing Standardbred is 90% hemorrhage and

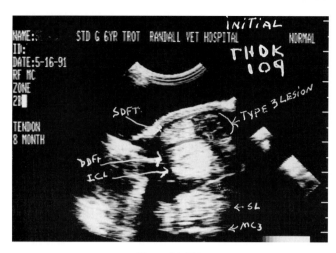

Figure 21.248.

edema and only 10 % fiber damage, the tendon strength compromise might not be as significant as it appears. However, the decision to continue use or institute an expensive, long-term rehabilitation program depends on the sonographer's interpretation of this lesion's severity. It is unrealistic to assume that one can advise long-term rest in all injured horses. In this case, one can assume that there is some fiber damage along this lateral border but concede that part of the hypoechoic texture is caused by recent hemorrhage or edema. For an accurate assessment of fiber loss, a decrease in the EL for 2 to 4 weeks, symptomatic treatment, and repeat sonographic examination is necessary. At the follow-up examination at EL 1 or 2, there should be resolution of the inflammatory process and hematoma resorption, at which point a more accurate fiber evaluation can be made. This approach often is unnecessary simply because either the trainer will not risk any further injury and will automatically rest the horse or the damage is so extensive that it is unequivocal. In certain economic situations, with marginally valued horses, one may be required to compromise. In this case, the horse's value required that an accurate assessment be made. From the trainer's perspective, the option of symptomatic treatment, a reduced EL for a short period, and continued racing was critical to this horse's future. The owner did not choose long-term rehabilitation for this horse. Other alternatives were to sell the horse either to another trainer or for alternative use. The trainer was not receptive and wanted to continue racing if at all possible. Based on these nonmedical influences, a compromise program was designed. The tendon was treated symptomatically and the exercise was decreased to EL-4. A subsequent comparative sonographic examination in 2 to 4 weeks was advised.

Figure 21.249 is a cross-sectional right metacarpal Zone 2B sonogram of the same horse shown in Fig. 21.248 made 4 weeks later. The horse had been treated with perilesional corticorsteroid and sodium hyaluronate when the initial sonogram was made. This treatment was combined with hydrotherapy (ice) and daily leg liniment application. This scan reveals marked improvement of the lesion texture and density. The lateral SDFT border was now Type 1 which is

a two grade improvement in 4 weeks. Therefore, a large part of the Type 3 lesion was caused by hemorrhage and inflammatory infiltrate, and fiber path damage was less than originally suspected. With a Standardbred racehorse it may be possible to continue racing with a training modification. However, further damaging the tendon fibers is still a risk. Because of the trainer's decision to continue racing, the following suggestions were made: 1) repeat the sonographic evaluation after racing to monitor fiber damage; 2) if the tendon seemed clinically stable, but the horse was not performing well, racing should be abandoned, and; 3) even if the horse is economically successful but sustains a significantly more severe tendon injury, racing should be stopped. If this had been a racing Thoroughbred, the chance of success would be lower because of higher tendon loads.

Figure 21.250 is a cross-sectional left metacarpal Zone 3A sonogram of a pacing Standardbred with recent swelling. The scan shows a Type 2 dorsomedial SDFT surface lesion and a small Type 3 midpalmar lesion. The owner decided to treat symptomatically and continue to race. The tendon was treated with a perilesional corticosteroid injection, similar to the horse in Fig 21.249, as well as a reduced EL.

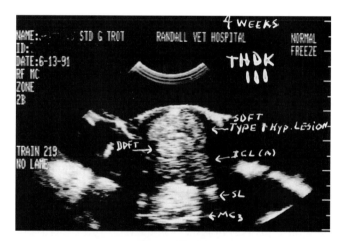

Figure 21.249.

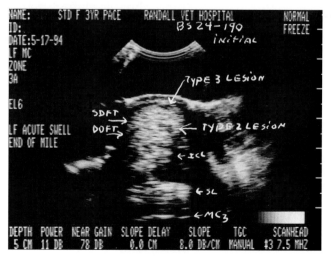

Figure 21.250.

Figure 21.251 is a cross-sectional left metacarpal Zone 3A sonogram of the same horse shown in Fig. 21.250 made 4 weeks after treatment. The scan shows enlargement of the midpalmar SDFT lesion. Unlike the previous horse, texture did not improve and, with a reduced EL, the lesion enlarged, indicating continued fiber damage. The hypoechoic SDFT area is primarily due to tendon fiber disruption. In this case, a long-range treatment program was recommended to avoid more serious injury and to allow repair of the present injury. These two cases contrast textural differences over time with similar injuries treated in exactly the same manner. They illustrate the importance of repeat sonography before increasing the EL. The repeat sonogram confirmed the fiber path damage after resolving the inflammatory reaction.

Figure 21.252 is a cross-sectional left metacarpal Zone 3A SDFT sonogram of a Thoroughbred racehorse that sustained a recent reinjury on the day of the scan. The sonogram shows a diffuse Type 2 lesion.

Figure 21.253 is a cross-sectional left metacarpal Zone 3A sonogram of the same horse shown in Fig. 21.252 made 7 days after injury. The scan reveals a diffuse Type 3 lesion. This tendon lesion degenerated one grade in a 7-day period.

This degradation is probably caused by pressure necrosis and the inflammatory process.

Figure 21.254 is a cross-sectional right metacarpals Zone 3A SDFT sonogram of a Thoroughbred racehorse that sustained a new injury on the previous day. The scan shows a Type 3 core lesion. Figure 21.255 is a cross-sectional right metacarpal Zone 3A sonogram of the same horse as in Fig. 21.254 made 6 weeks after injury at EL-1. The scan shows a remarkable improvement of the lesion texture and density; however, healing in 6 weeks is not possible. There are three likely reasons for what the scan shows. First, this horse was treated with intralesional BAPTEN® and had multiple small gauge needle punctures during intralesional drug injections. These punctures most likely decompressed the tendon causing some degree of hematoma release. Secondly, a favorable drug effect occurred. Thirdly, a significant number of fiber bundles most likely were not injured as was originally suspected. This injury should not be underestimated, however, and long-term treatment is still necessary.

Figure 21.256 is a cross-sectional left metacarpal Zone 3A SDFT sonogram of a Thoroughbred racehorse that sustained a new injury. The scan shows a palmar Type 2 trough lesion.

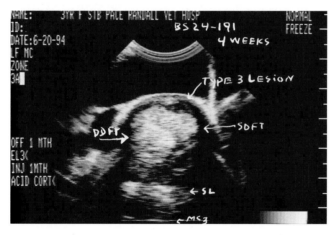

Figure 21.251.

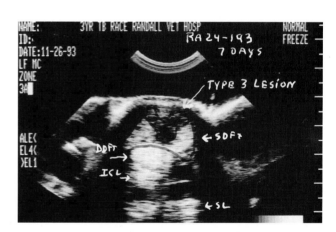

Figure 21.253.

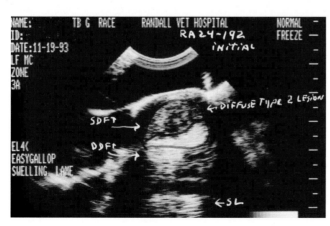

Figure 21.252.

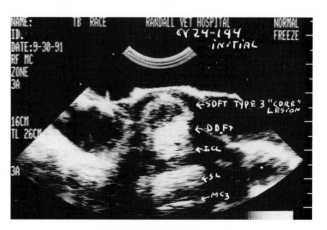

Figure 21.254.

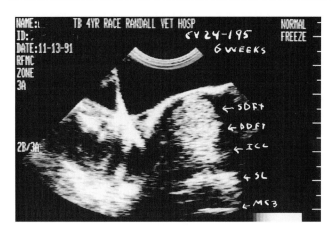

Figure 21.255.

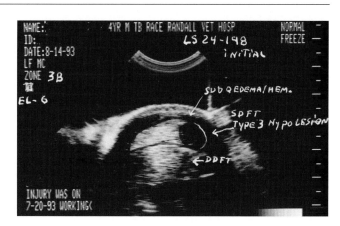

Figure 21.258.

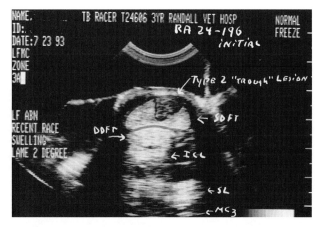

Figure 21.256.

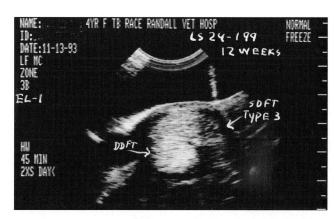

Figure 21.259.

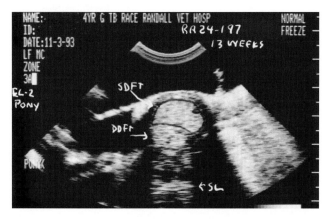

Figure 21.257.

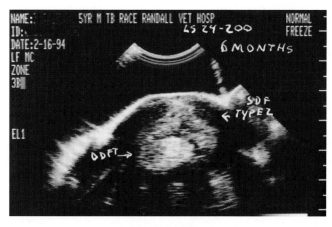

Figure 21.260.

Figure 21.257 is a cross-sectional left metacarpal Zone 3A sonogram of the same horse shown in Fig. 21.256 made 13 weeks after injury. The horse was at EL-2 (pony). The lesion returned to a normal echogenicity. This repair is slightly accelerated, but is compatible for this time period and EL (at 16 weeks, a 70% reduction in hypoechoic fiber bundle volume can be expected). The original Type 2 injury is the main reason why this horse's tendon is ahead of schedule. Type 3 or 4 lesions improve one grade in 12 weeks and two grades in 16 weeks at acceptable exercise levels. Reinjured tendons and severe lesions may resolve at a slower rate.

Figure 21.258 is a cross-sectional left metacarpal Zone 3B SDFT sonogram of a Thoroughbred racehorse that sustained a recent injury. The scan shows a focal Type 3 medial tendon border lesion.

Figure 21.259 is a cross-sectional left metacarpal Zone 3B sonogram of same horse shown in Fig. 21.258 made 3 months after injury. The horse was at EL-1. The scan shows only slight textural improvement; however, the lesion is still a Type 3.

Figure 21.260 is a cross-sectional left metacarpal Zone 3B sonogram of the same horse shown in Figures 21.258 and 21.259 at 6 months and EL-3. The scan reveals a Type 2 lesion. Two possibilities are offered: 1) the repair is basically inferior, consisting of a persistent weaker Type III collagen; or 2) there is continuing injury at EL-3. In this case, there was no history of excessive paddock exercise. Therefore, one can conclude that, at a sub-EL-3 at 12 weeks, resolution of the hypoechoic fiber paths is delayed. This persistent hypoechoic fibrous repair is common in traditionally treated tendon injuries. This sonographic appearance indicates a reduction of the EL and reevaluation of the tendon in 2 to 3 months. The horse should not be put in training just because he has been off for 6 months and the tendon "feels great."

Figure 21.261 is a cross-sectional left metacarpal Zone 3B sonogram of the same horse shown in Figures 21.258 to 21.260 made 11 months after injury. Since the 6 month scan, the horse was not advanced above EL-4. Focal Type 1

fiber bundles are still present. The sonographic appearance has improved, but the horse is not ready to advance to EL-5. This case illustrates the variable textural improvement that can exist in the repair process.

Figure 21.262 is a cross-sectional left metacarpal Zone 3B SDFT sonogram of a Thoroughbred racehorse that sustained a new injury. The scan shows a large, Type 3 SDFT lesion.

Figure 21.263 is a cross-sectional left metacarpal sonogram of the same horse shown in Fig. 21.262 made 13 months after injury. During the time off, the horse never exceeded EL-4. The scan reveals a diffuse Type 1 SDFT texture. With the extended time off and at moderate exercise levels, this tendon did not attain isoechogenic fiber bundles. This is an unfavorable sonographic finding, and a reduced prognosis for RTR would be given. Furthermore, this horse should not advance to EL-5. This horse did advance to EL-5 because the owner said "I have waited a year and I am going to take my chances." The horse reinjured the tendon at EL-6.

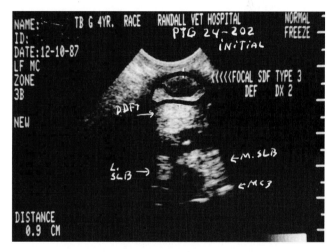

Figure 21.262.

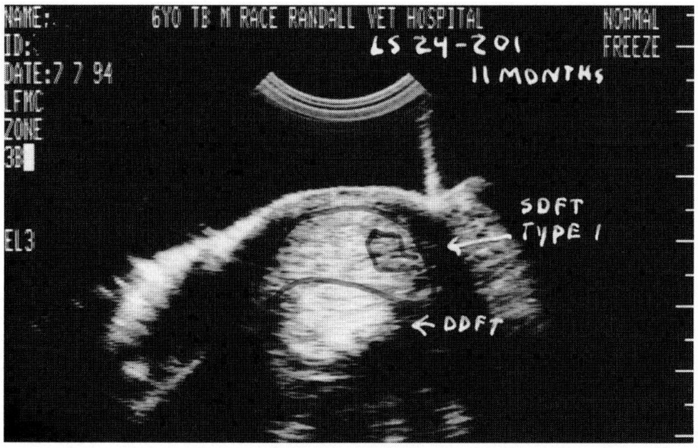

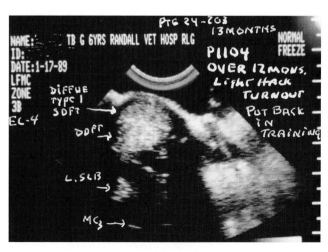

Figure 21.261.

Figure 21.263.

As a tendon injury repairs, it is important to find improving echogenicity at timely intervals, and exercise levels should be adjusted accordingly. Small, focal, Type 1 fiber bundles scattered throughout the length of a repairing tendon may allow increasing the EL, but persistent diffuse hypoechoic fibers past 7 to 9 months after injury are unfavorable findings for RTR. Once a horse is advanced to training levels of exercise, the sonographic monitoring should be done at EL increases to detect regressions of SDFT integrity.

Cross-sectional Area in Rehabilitation

From clinical data gained from the BAPTEN field trials, it became evident that CSA (cross-sectional area), MIZ (maximum injury zone), and T-CSA (total cross-sectional area) were not only sensitive for early injury detection but useful for SQR (sonographic quality of repair) evaluation. We believe this parameter is as important in monitoring repair as are tendon texture and lesion density. The CSA evaluation can be used in the following ways: 1) the CSA of all zones, normal or abnormal. For the metacarpal SDFT, six or seven levels; in the pastern, three levels for each SDFT branch; and for the hind limb, seven to nine levels. When performing serial examinations, repeating the same levels provides meaningful CSA data. Each case has an MIZ-CSA and a T-CSA for that horse's tendon. 2) obtaining the "volume of hypoechoic fiber bundles" for each cross-sectional level. A true mathematic volume is not being determined; however, the sum of the cross-sectional areas of the abnormal zones is meaningful data when serially determined. From these data, the maximum injury zone (MIZ-HYP) is identified and the total "volume" of hypoechoic fiber bundles (T-HYP) can be calculated. Once the total tendon "volume" (T-CSA) and the total hypoechoic fiber bundle "volume" (T-HYP) are determined, the % hypoechoic fiber bundles (%T-HYP) can be calculated. The Zone or level with the largest percentage of compromised fiber bundles is designated the MIZ (the weak link). Moderate to severe injuries usually have five to seven abnormal levels.

For example, if a metacarpal SDFT injury measured at six levels had a T-CSA of 600 mm^2, and all levels had 50% hypoechoic fiber bundles, the total hypoechoic volume would be 300 mm^2. The injury would be 50%T-HYP (severe). The %T-HYP is useful in itself to indicate the injury severity and can be used to monitor the SQR. These same values can be used in the management phase of S/GO (symptomatic treatment and go on) to determine the injury's stability or instability. The CSA is a sensitive indicator of lesion regression once tendon loads increase. The successful BAPTEN project horses are those that have stable CSA with increasing tendon loading. Conversely, unstable CSA indicate impending failure and signal a need for an EL decrease. As seen with textural abnormalities, acute inflammation and hemorrhage can mask the true severity evaluation of an acute injury (1 to 21 days). Therefore, CSA measurements obtained 2 to 4 weeks after injury more accurately represent SDFT fiber compromise and injury severity. The CSA is an important evaluation during rehabilitation to guide EL management. Bypassing CSA evaluations before adjusting the EL can lead to case mismanagement and failure to RTR. Managing exercise levels based on the tendon's measurable sonographic parameters improves the end results.

All significant, work-related tendon injuries result in tendon enlargement. The greater the increase from normal CSA, the more serious the injury. The greater the %T-HYP, the more scar tissue produced. The greater the fibrous tissue volume, the more difficult it is to achieve an athletically functional tendon. A direct relationship exists between increase of tendon volume during repair and the amount of randomly oriented scar tissue. This random scar formation is evident sonographically as inferior texture and/or an increasing CSA. It may also be seen as a failure to see CSA decreases during rehabilitation. We believe that as repair takes place and as longitudinal scar tissue alignment occurs, T-CSA decreases; this is considered a more athletically functional repair. The initial injury CSA data serves as a baseline from which comparison is made throughout rehabilitation. As stated before, the tendon should be rescanned 2 to 4 weeks after injury. Moderately to severely injured tendons seldom return to normal tendon volume. However, CSA decrease is anticipated as repair takes place. Additionally, the CSA should be stable as tendon loading increases.

Figure 21.264 is a cross-sectional left metacarpal Zone 3B normal SDFT sonogram of a Thoroughbred racehorse made at 23 cm DACB. The horse sustained a recent right fore SDFT reinjury and the MIZ was in Zone 3B. Table 21.1 summarizes the six-level CSA data from the initial reinjury through 11 months after injury.

The normal left fore Zone 3B CSA varied from 97 mm^2 to 120 mm^2. This variation reflects the influence of training, transducer positioning, and measurement error. Gillis has reported SDFT hypertrophy as a normal training response (32). In our experience, based on serial sonography of many normal tendons throughout training stages and racing and

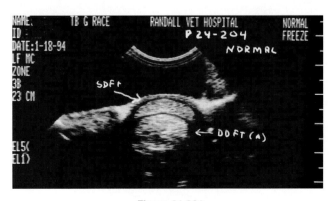

Figure 21.264.

Table 21.1
Normal SDFT (P)*

Date	(MIZ-3B)				(Number of Levels—6)	
	Elapse	EL	MIZ-SA	% Cha.	Total-SA	% Cha.
1/18/94	0	5	112		605	
5/14/94	4 m	2	97	−13	610	+<1
8/16/94	7 m	4	86	−11	583	−04
9/15/94	8 m	5	105	+22	636	+09
9/21/94	8 m	6	107	+02	620	−03
9/29/94	8 m	6	117	+09	621	0
10/13/94	9 m	6	120	+03	624	+<01
10/24/94	9 m	7	99	−18	603	−03
11/14/94	10 m	7	116	+17	652	+08
12/12/94	11 m	7	103	−11	652	0

*Case courtesy of Bapten research—Alaco Corp.

on using the computer CSA quantitation, there is a variation from scan to scan for a given zone. The CSA variation of a normal single Zone can approach 20 to 25%. In this case, the normal SDFT Zone 3B CSA was the lowest after a 7-month period below EL-5 (86 mm^2). Once training started, the CSA increased and varied from 99 mm^2 to 120 mm^2. This same normal technique variation for the sum or total of six or seven levels of the metacarpal tendon is 10 to 15%. In this case, the normal six-level T-CSA varied from 583 mm^2 to 652 mm^2. The largest normal SDFT CSA variation is seen when a horse increases from EL-3 to EL-6. We would support research that indicates a slight CSA increase with conditioning. Furthermore, once racing fitness has been attained, the CSA variations are more stable. At the initial examination, the normal CSA for Zone 3B was 112 mm^2. The maximum CSA attained was 120 mm^2 at 9 months. This is <10% variation over 11 months. These low level CSA variations can be thought of as normal "vibration" indicating minor changes in size, transducer placement and measurement error. The T-CSA in this case had a similar "vibration" or variation at a baseline of 605 mm^2 to a maximum of 652 mm^2 at EL-7. There was never greater than a nine percent

difference between any of the evaluations. This would be considered a stable tendon injury.

Figure 21.265 is a cross-sectional right metacarpal Zone 3B SDFT sonogram of the injured tendon of the same horse shown in Figure 21.264 made at 20 cm DACB. The scan reveals a Type 3 palmar SDFT lesion. Table 21.2 contains the CSA data for this SDFT over an 11-month period. The MIZ-CSA of the initial examination (baseline) was 159 mm^2. The initial T-CSA was 690 mm^2. Three zones had a textural abnormality and three zones had an abnormal CSA increase. Our overall injury evaluation would place it in Category 2 (slight) (10%T-HYP). The MIZ had 29% hypoechoic fiber bundles and an abnormal volume of 70 mm^2. The CSA data indicate progressive MIZ-CSA improvement. The subsequent MIZ-CSA values were always less than the baseline. As exercise levels increased, neither the MIZ-CSA nor the T-CSA exceeded a 20% increase from the previous value. It is interesting that the largest MIZ-CSA increase occurred when this horse went from EL-2 to EL-3b. In the BAPTEN research project, EL-3b can result in low-grade reinjury at the critical 4- to 6-month post-injury period. In the later stages of this project, smaller paddocks were recommended (EL-3a) to prevent these slight reinjuries. Clinically, throughout the 11-month period, there was never any indication of SDFT reinjury. Sonographically, the CSA of the MIZ and T were stable throughout training and racing. On two occasions, the T-CSA was either slightly larger or the same size as the baseline, which caused some concern. The MIZ-CSA, however, always remained smaller than the baseline of 159 mm^2. This variation implies slight strain in Zone 3A, proximal to the MIZ. Texturally, the abnormal SDFT never exceeded 3% T-HYP throughout advances from EL-3 through 3 races. Figure 21.266 is a cross-sectional right metacarpal Zone 3B sonogram of the same horse shown in Figures 21.264 and 21.265 made 11 months after reinjury at EL-7.

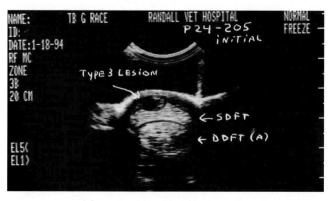

Figure 21.265.

Table 21.2
Abnormal SDFT (P)*

Date	(MIZ-3B)				(Number of Levels—6)	
	Elapse	EL	MIZ-SA	% Cha.	Total-SA	% Cha.
1/18/94	0	5	159		690	
5/14/94	4 m	2	100	−37	608	−12
7/16/94	6 m	3	120	+20	664	+09
9/15/94	8 m	5	115	−04	639	−04
9/21/94	8 m	6	125	+09	638	0
9/29/94	8 m	6	135	+08	703	+10
10/13/94	9 m	6	112	−17	661	−06
10/24/94	9 m	7	117	+04	641	−03
11/14/94	10 m	7	105	−10	655	+02
12/12/94	11 m	7	110	+05	689	+05

*Case courtesy of Bapten research—Alaco Corp.

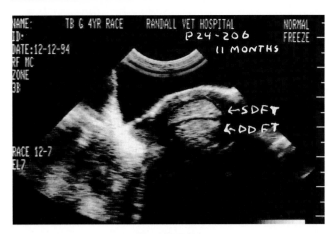

Figure 21.266.

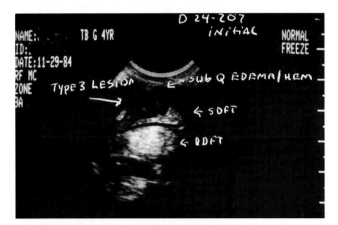

Figure 21.267.

Figure 21.267 is a cross-sectional right metacarpal Zone 3A SDFT sonogram of a Thoroughbred racehorse that sustained a recent injury at EL-7. The scan shows a large Type 3 palmar SDFT lesion. Hypoechoic fiber bundles could be identified in five zones. The MIZ-CSA was 213 mm². The five-level T-CSA was 1138 mm². The overall hypoechoic fiber bundle volume was 451 mm² (40%T-HYP severe injury). Table 21.3 summarizes the CSA data over a 10-month post-injury period. The SDFT injury was treated by percutaneous tendon splitting and traditional pasture rest. At the end of 3 months after injury, the horse was at EL-3b. The MIZ-CSA has increased to 450 mm² (111% increase). The

Table 21.3
Abnormal SDFT (DC)

		(MIZ-3A)			(Number of Levels—5)	
Date	Elapse	EL	MIZ-SA	% Cha.	Total-SA	% Cha.
11/29/84	0	7	213		1138	
02/20/85	3 m	3	450	+111	1351	+19
08/08/85	8 m	3	364	−19	1360	<01
10/08/85	10 m	5	353	−03	1477	+09

T-CSA has increased by 19%. This finding indicates that the MIZ has an unfavorable response at this time and the EL-3b is excessive exercise or that excessive randomly oriented fibrosis is present. At 8 months after injury and the horse still at EL-3b, the MIZ-CSA has improved from the previous examination by 19% yet is still 71% larger than baseline. The T-CSA has shown no decrease since the last scan and is 20% larger than baseline. These CSA data at 8 months after injury at EL-3 are not compatible with a functional repair. Furthermore, the repairing scar is most likely reasonably mature and randomly oriented. The trainer decided to attempt an RTR despite this information for several reasons. Firstly, he had given the horse 8 months off. Secondly, the tendon was grossly tight and cold. Thirdly, the horse was pasture sound.

Figure 21.268 is a cross-sectional right metacarpal Zone 3A sonogram of the same horse as in Fig. 21.267 made at 8 months after injury with the horse at EL-3. After this sonogram, the horse was advanced to EL-5 and suffered a reinjury 2 months later at EL-6.

Figure 21.269 is a cross-sectional left metacarpal Zone 3B sonogram of a pacing Standardbred that recently injured the SDFT. The scan shows several tracts of Type 3 fiber bundles. There were three zones with hypoechoic fiber bundles and six zones that had an abnormal CSA. Table 21.4 summarizes the CSA data obtained over a 19-month period. At initial examination (baseline), the MIZ-CSA was 274 mm². The six-level T-CSA was 1138 mm². The total hypoechoic fiber bundle volume was 180 mm² (15% T-HYP-slight injury). The diagnosis was diffuse tendinitis with focal fiber tearing. At 2 months after injury and at EL-3a, the MIZ-CSA has reduced from baseline by 15%, and the T-CSA has decreased by 7%. This response is favorable. At 6 months after injury and the horse at EL-3b, there is a 37% decrease in MIZ-CSA and an 18% decrease in T-CSA. This is an additional favorable response. These data support two conclusions: First, the EL is not causing low-grade recurrent injury. Second, there is no excessive, nonparallel fiber align-

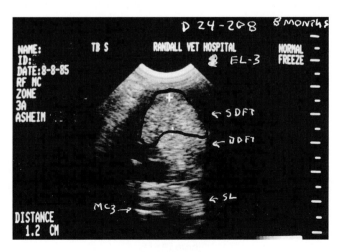

Figure 21.268.

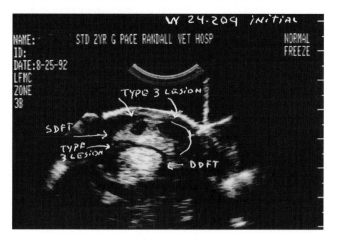

Figure 21.269.

Table 21.4
Abnormal SDFT (W)*

	(MIZ-3B)			(Number of Levels—6)		
Date	Elapse	EL	MIZ-SA	% Cha.	Total-SA	% Cha.
8/25/92	0	7	274		1138	
11/12/92	2 m	3	234	−15	1061	−07
1/22/93	6 m	3	147	−37	867	−18
7/07/93	10 m	6	169	+15	788	−09
2/07/94	17 m	7	154	−09	758	−04
2/18/94	17 m	7	146	−05	703	−07
4/12/94	19 m	7	111	−24	625	−11

*Case courtesy of Bapten research—Alaco Corp.

ment of the repairing scar . This is a more favorably functional repair for RTR. In SDFT injuries, attaining this Type of SQR is the first major step. The second major hurdle is achieving a stable scar when training and racing resumes.

Figure 21.270 is a cross-sectional left metacarpal Zone 3B sonogram of the same horse shown in Figure 21.269 10 months after injury at EL-6. There is a slight palmar decrease in SDFT echogenicity. The MIZ-CSA has increased by 15% (acceptable) and remains below the baseline value. The T-CSA continued to decrease in spite of EL increases. These CSA data would indicate the MIZ is slightly less stable than the overall tendon. With this evaluation in mind as a precautionary measure a one month reduction to EL-5 was advised to allow the MIZ to stabilize.

Figure 21.271 is a cross-sectional left metacarpal Zone 3B sonogram of the same horse as in Figures 21.269 and 21.270 made 17 months post injury at EL-7. The horse has been racing regularly and was clinically asymptomatic. There are a few small focal hypoechoic areas seen on this cross-section. The MIZ-CSA and T-CSA are stable, smaller than baseline and the horse has reached maximum loading.

Figure 21.272 is a cross-sectional right metacarpal Zone 3A SDFT sonogram of a Thoroughbred racehorse with a recent injury. The scan reveals a large, Type 2 core lesion. Table 21.5 summarizes the CSA data over a 16 month pe-

riod. At the initial injury evaluation (baseline), the MIZ-CSA was 258 mm^2 and the six Zone T-CSA was 1147 mm^2. There were six zones that had hypoechoic fiber bundles. The T-HYP was 369 mm^2 and the %T-HYP was 32% (severe injury). The horse was treated with superior check ligament desmotomy (SCLD) and percutaneous surgical tendon splitting (STS) and traditional pasture rest.

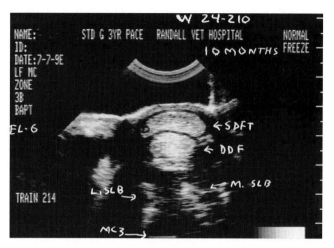

Figure 21.270.

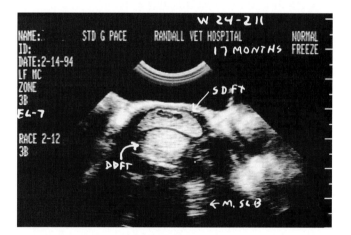

Figure 21.271.

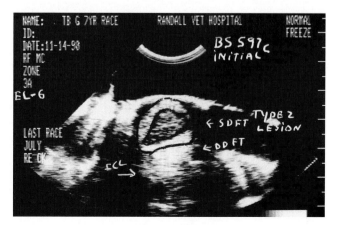

Figure 21.272.

Table 21.5
Abnormal SDFT (B)

| Date | (MIZ-2B) | | | (Number of Levels—6) | | |
	Elapse	EL	MIZ-SA	% Cha.	Total-SA	% Cha.
11/14/90	0	7	258		1147	
3/29/91	4 m	3	240	− 07	1139	− <1
5/16/91	6 m	2	250	+ 04	1254	+ 10
6/13/91	7 m	5	281	+ 12	1647	+ 31
7/20/91	8 m	2	325	+ 16	1595	− 03
8/28/91	9 m	5	330	+ 02	1799	+ 13
3/02/92	16 m	3	201	− 39	1192	− 34

Figure 21.273 is a cross-sectional right metacarpal Zone 3A sonogram of the same horse as in Fig. 21.272 made 6 months post injury at EL-2 (ride at the walk/trot). The SDFT is enlarged with scattered Type 1 fiber bundle foci. Textural abnormalities were identified in five zones. The MIZ-CSA is slightly reduced from baseline but not significantly. As a general guideline at six months and EL-2, at least a 10% reduction is desired. The T-CSA increased by 10% which suggests that zones other than the MIZ have a less favorable repair at this time. Based on the CSA, this horse should not advance beyond EL-2 at this time. However, traditional training (EL-5) was started.

Figure 21.274 is a cross-sectional right metacarpal Zone 3B SDFT sonogram of the same horse as in Figures 21.272 and 21.273 made 7 months post injury with a Type 3 lesion. This reinjury at EL-5 is one Zone distal to the MIZ. The MIZ-CSA has increased only 12% but the T-CSA has an undesirable 31% increase. At this time, the EL was reduced for six weeks to EL-1.

Figure 21.275 is a cross-sectional right metacarpal Zone 3A sonogram of the same horse as in Figures 21.272 to 21.274 made nine months post injury. Since the previous scan, the horse was at EL-1 for six weeks and EL-5 for two weeks. There is a larger Type 2 palmar SDFT lesion. The MIZ-CSA has increased and is significantly larger than base-

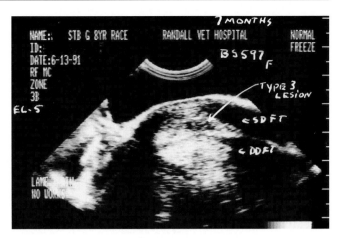

Figure 21.274.

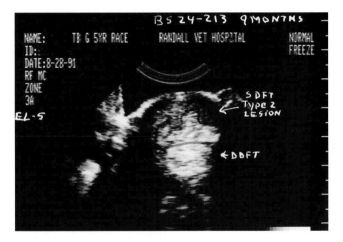

Figure 21.275.

line. The T-CSA has increased to 1799 mm^2 which is 57% larger than the baseline. The T-HYP is 647 mm^2. The reinjury is severe (36%T-HYP). This horse failed to RTR and reinjured the tendon twice at EL-5.

Figure 21.276 is a cross-sectional left metacarpal Zone 3B SDFT sonogram of a Thoroughbred racehorse that was severely injured and was treated for 4 months (EL-3b). The scan shows an enlarged SDFT with Type 3 lesions along the medial and lateral margins. Table 21.6 summarizes the CSA data over a nine month period. Initially, the MIZ-CSA was 395 mm^2 and the 4 level T-CSA was 934 mm^2. The horse was sent back to pasture for an additional month.

Figure 21.277 is a cross-sectional left metacarpal Zone 3B sonogram of the same horse as in Fig. 21.276 made 5 months post injury at EL-6. The scans reveal Type 2 fiber bundles, however, there has been significant textural improvement. The MIZ-CSA made a 12% decrease in spite of the increased EL. These are favorable sonographic data however, the EL is high for this SQR and only five months post injury. Economics and the prospect that it was spring and she could still be used as this year's broodmare, influenced a decision to continue training.

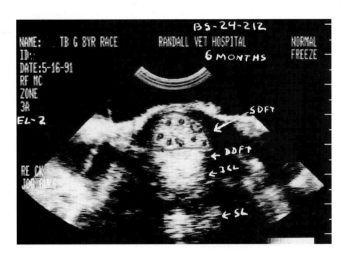

Figure 21.273.

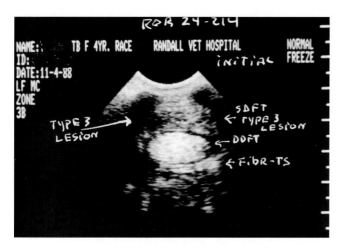

Figure 21.276.

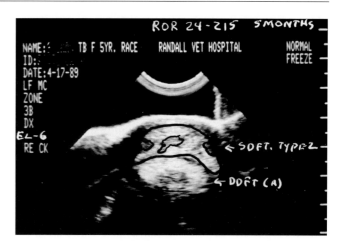

Figure 21.277.

Table 21.6
Abnormal SDFT (ROR)

	(MIZ-3B)			(Number of Levels—4)		
Date	Elapse	EL	MIZ-SA	% CHA.	Total-SA	% CHA.
11/04/88	0	3	395		934	
3/16/89	4 m	5	387	− 01	950	+ 02
4/16/89	5 m	6	339	− 12	749	− 21
5/26/89	6 m	7	255	− 24	766	+ <1
9/12/89	9 m	7	235	− 08	707	− 08

1989—10 starts 5 wins

Figure 21.278 is a cross-sectional left metacarpal Zone 3B sonogram of the same horse as in Figures 21.276 and 21.277 made after her second race. There is a Type 2 medial border SDFT texture. This indicates fiber path weakness. The MIZ-CSA is significantly reduced to 255 mm². The 4 level T-CSA is reduced to 766 mm². This T-CSA reduction is 18% from the baseline and the horse is at EL-7. We believe the reason this filly did so well with this apparently sonographically inferior repair was that the scar fiber alignment was more longitudinal. The reducing CSA with increased loading indicates lesion stability. There was obviously sufficient Zone 3B tensile strength to permit racing. Her performances were credible with five wins in 10 races that year with a class drop. She raced 3 times the following season and reinjured the tendon in the 13th start. The training management, careful sonographic evaluation and a stable MIZ-CSA and T-CSA were responsible for her partial success in RTR.

Figure 21.279 is a cross-sectional left Zone 3B metacarpal SDFT sonogram of a Thoroughbred racehorse that had multiple high value races before injury. The horse had been rested externally blistered and had reinjured the tendon several times prior to this scan and had never exceeded EL-6. This scan was made of the fourth reinjury and serves as baseline. The scan reveals a Type 3 SDFT core lesion. This was the only Zone that had a detectable textural abnormality. Table 21.7 summarizes the CSA data over a 16

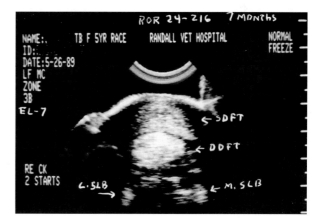

Figure 21.278.

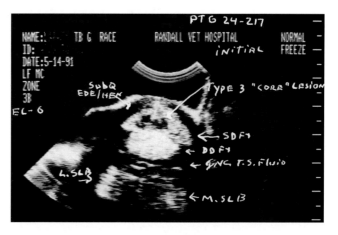

Figure 21.279.

Table 21.7
Abnormal SDFT (PTG)*

| Date | (MIZ-3B) | | | (Numbers of Levels—6) | | |
	Elapse	EL	MIZ-SA	% CHA.	Total-SA	% CHA.
5/14/91	0	6	233		922	
2/01/92	9 m	3	192	−18	702	−24
5/22/92	13 m	7	250	+30	981	+40
7/3/92	14 m	7	289	+15	910	−08
8/25/92	16 m	7	502	+73	1419	+56

*Case courtesy of Bapten research—Alaco Corp.

month period. At the baseline evaluation the MIZ-CSA was 233 mm² and the six-level T-CSA was 922 mm².

Figure 21.280 is a cross-sectional left metacarpal Zone 3B sonogram of the same horse as in Fig. 21.279 made at 9 months post baseline examination at EL-3b. The MIZ-CSA and the T-CSA have significantly reduced by 18% and 24% respectively. There are no significant textural abnormalities found.

Figure 21.281 is a cross-sectional left metacarpal Zone 3B sonogram of the same horse as in Figures 21.279 and 21.280 made at 13 months at EL-7. The scan shows a diffuse Type 1 textural SDFT abnormality. The MIZ-CSA has increased by 30% from the previous scan indicating tendinitis. The T-CSA has also increased by 40% indicating zones proximal to the MIZ are enlarged. At this time, exercise should be reduced to EL-1. The trainer decided against this advise and selected S/GO management with wider race spacing.

Figure 21.282 is a cross-sectional left metacarpal Zone 3B sonogram of the same horse as in Figures 21.279 to 21.281 after three races (EL-7). The scan shows no further texture decrease, however, the MIZ-CSA is increased an additional 15% and there is a slight reduction in the T-CSA from the previous scan. The MIZ-CSA is larger than the baseline. The trainer was advised that the CSA was unstable and there was a high risk of fiber tearing if racing continued. The same management phase was selected, but he decided not to race the horse for a month.

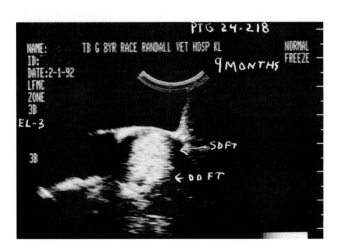

Figure 21.280.

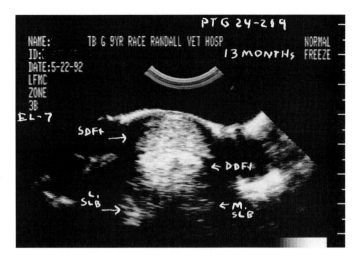

Figure 21.281.

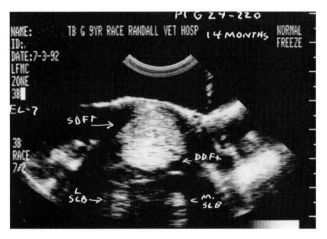

Figure 21.282.

Figure 21.283 is a cross-sectional left metacarpal Zone 3B sonogram of the same horse as in Figures 21.279 to 21.282 made 2 months and one race later. The scan reveals a large, Type 3 SDFT lesion. In this case, the CSA increase was more indicative of impending tendon failure than was the textural evaluation.

An SDFT that has a focal hypoechoic fiber Zone or two and is completely asymptomatic creates a dilemma for the clinician. One may have been asked to examine the horse for TS swelling or a slight thickening of the metacarpus. These horses can be training and/or racing asymptomatically. Most Standardbred practitioners have seen at least one horse with a "black hole" in the tendon that was racing well. As in the last case, the Thoroughbred racehorse had a significant hypoechoic lesion limited to one zone. It did well for a while, but in spite of very careful management and spaced races, the SDFT was reinjured. There were four or five successful races, but the end result was a tendon reinjury more severe than any of the previous episodes. The practitioner was correct in predicting the likelihood of poor performances, most likely lameness, and more severe tendon injury. It is perplexing that other horses with hypoechoic fiber

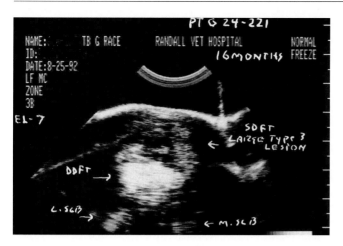

Figure 21.283.

bundles in one or two zones can compete at the same EL and *not* experience tendon failure. This is less likely to happen with Thoroughbred racehorses than with Standardbred racehorses. Horses in less demanding competition have an even a higher success rate with the "symptomatic treatment and go on" (S/GO) management. The authors do not have documented research based explanations for this difference but do have some observations, speculations and experiences that may be informative. Based on our present knowledge, only suggestions can be offered on how to approach this problem relative to the doctor/client relationship. The reason this is important is that the success or failure of a horse returning to its intended use influences client perception and acceptance of the diagnoses, prognoses and medical advice we offer. It should be obvious to any practitioner that client compliance is one the most vital aspects of any therapeutic regimen. Client compliance is based upon their past experiences following the advice of veterinarians as it affected their horses. For instance, one may examine a horse for lameness and diagnose a slight proximal sesamoid bone fracture. The veterinarian recommends six months complete rest to allow fracture healing and at the same time warns the trainer that continued racing may cause breakdown. This would seem to be sound medical advice for a racing Thoroughbred, but in real life, decisions are not always this straight forward. Lets assume, in our hypothetical case, that the trainer thinks this situation over for a few days and explores the options. He decides that the last one of these horses he laid up "never did any good" and the owner lost a lot of money. So the trainer decides to use symptomatic treatment and enters the horse in a claiming race with all intentions to sell the horse. This happens and the horse wins because of the class drop and the new owner, without any medical history, thinks he/she has made the buy of the year. The horse continues to race successfully and a catastrophic breakdown never occurs. The original owner and trainer now question the original diagnosis, prognosis and medical advice. At this point the original veterinarian, who did his best, has lost credibility with the client and it

will take a long time, if ever, to regain it. With talented racehorses and under certain situations this scenario occurs. It is important, however, that a diagnosis or prognosis not be guaranteed and that we continue to predict the most likely outcome and to accept the exception to the rule. Unfortunately, it is often the exception that clients remember.

Some horses can successfully continue to compete with a compromised SDFT fiber pattern. In every subtotal SDFT injury there are medical and nonmedical management decisions. The control of the horse and its athletic future is the responsibility of the trainer on the owner's behalf. The trainer, an integral part of the decision making process, may not agree with the veterinarian's diagnosis, prognosis, and treatment of a SDFT injury. The veterinarians recommendations should be based on the most recent statistical data and past experiences with similar injuries. However, the final disposition rests in the hands of the trainer and/or the owner.

If every injured tendon could be "cured" and if every horse followed the veterinarian's predictions, there would be no dilemma. However, in an imperfect world this is not the case. Trainers that have had past experiences with injured tendons that have been through long term, expensive treatment and repeatedly failed are seldom receptive to long term treatment recommendations. Trainers that have unwittingly gone along successfully racing an injured horse are most likely to select that option again. As veterinarians become more adept at tendon injury diagnosis and treatment regimens prove successful, there will be more trainer and owner compliance.

There are some factors that should be identified in the exceptional horse that races or performs at a highly competitive level with a compromised SDFT. The horse's athletic use is one consideration. For instance, a Thoroughbred racehorse with an asymptomatic Category 2 injury may be at risk with S/GO management for racing; but, would be at a very low risk for weekend trail riding. Continued racing with a Category 2 injury would pose several risks: 1. Performance level may decrease, especially if dropping the racing class is not an option. This horse may already be racing at the bottom of its class or it may be valuable as a breeding animal. 2. Continued use may result in further injury. A Category 2 injury may become a Category 3 or Category 4. 3. The horse may compensate for an painful SDFT injury and cause another musculoskeletal injury. For instance, it is common for a racing Standardbred, to injury the contralateral tendon. 4. There is always the chance of acute breakdown during a race and potential rider injury. Other factors to consider are the current statistical chances of successful RTR after long term treatment the cost of treatment and the length of rehabilitation.

The racing Standardbred is more likely to be able to be successful with S/GO management than Thoroughbred. This is due to the reduced speed of competition and the racing gaits compared to Thoroughbred. Alternative athletic use at times will seldom require long term treatment, for example, racehorses used for breeding or light jumping. A Category 2 SDFT injury in a racehorse may have a guarded prognosis for S/GO management but the prognosis would greatly improve if the intended use was light trail riding.

If the horse is intended for racing and the trainer elects to continue racing, then one should discuss the risks involved. The trainer must also consider the horse's athletic ability and the class level that is intended. It is difficult to continue racing with an SDFT injury and maintain a stakes performance level, but a $10,000.00 claiming horse may do very well with a class drop to $5,000.00. The tendon injury may remain stable, at least for a while. The sonographer's problem with a slight injury is that we cannot determine the elastic limit of the injury. We cannot state with accuracy that a given tendon can sustain loading forces not to exceed "x" number of pounds per square inch and further injury cannot be predicted. Once a horse has raced and a repeat sonographic examination is performed, then we can determine if more injury had occurred. We believe that a small percentage of Thoroughbred racehorses with SDFT injury can effectively continue and most will significantly cause more injury within three or four races. The racing Standardbred is more likely to continue racing and it seems that the rate of deterioration may be slower. It appears that they can complete about eight to ten races before there is clinical discomfort. Another factor that must be considered is the conditioning of the horse for a modified training program after the injury. For example, a very physically fit Thoroughbred racehorse may be reduced to swimming and ponying between races. This would reduce the "in between" races cyclic loading forces. This option is more available to the claiming horse than it would be for the stake class horse. The response to treatment also influences the ability to continue racing. There are many symptomatic treatment options available, but these must be combined with a modified conditioning program. It is interesting that symptomatic treatment programs are more successful with the racing Standardbred than the racing Thoroughbred. Obviously, this difference is due to decreased tendon loading rather than a response to treatment.

Finally, and most importantly, the major factor involved in the decision to select the S/GO management option is the severity of the injury. In a recent analysis of SDFT injuries of Thoroughbred and Standardbred racehorses, the following observations were made: In one year, 29 horses were diagnosed with a Category 2 injuries and in all cases the trainers selected the S/GO management option. Of these 29 horses, nine (31%) continued to race without clinical tendonitis; an additional 3 (10%) raced but were unable to continue in the same year, and 17 (59%) did not reach racing level in that same year. Based on these data, the client can be offered a 30%-40% chance to compete successfully with a slight injury. Conversely, there is a 60%-70% chance to experience tendon failure prior to racing. In a group of 22 horses with a Category 3 (moderate) SDFT injury, there were only 4 horses that attempted to continue racing and two were successful and two failed prior to racing. Both suc-

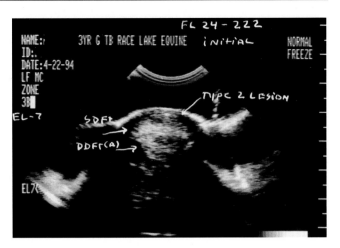

Figure 21.284.

cessful horses were Standardbred racehorses. In a group of 29 Category 4 horses (severe), there were 4 horses that selected S/GO management and all failed to start. As injuries are categorized and large groups are subjected to statistical analysis, more accurate prognoses for the various categories can be given.

Figure 21.284 is a cross-sectional left metacarpal Zone 3B sonogram of a Thoroughbred racehorse with slight distal SDFT thickening. It had recently been purchased for a large sum and was not lame at EL-7. The scan shows a Type 2 palmar SDFT texture involving 29% of the CSA. The T-HYP was 82 mm^2 (13%T-HYP) (slight injury). Table 21.8 summarizes the CSA data over a three and one-half month period. The MIZ-CSA at the baseline evaluation was 123 mm^2 and the T-CSA was 627 mm^2. Hypoechoic fiber paths were detected in five levels.

Three different management options were offered. The first was to rehabilitate the horse for six to eight months (Phase II management), or treat for two to three months to attempt salvaging the racing season, (Phase I management), or finally to treat symptomatically, reduce the training level, and increase time between races (S/GO management). It was carefully pointed out that Phase II was the most protective and offered the best prognosis for RTR, but did offer that, the statistical chance of RTR without recurrent injury was about 25% to 50% depending on treatment success (SQR). It was noted that Phase I management had a 90% failure rate for racing Thoroughbred. And finally, it was explained that the S/GO management option was possible and that it could be successful if managed properly. The risk of converting a Category 2 injury to a Category 3 or 4 with the possibility of acute breakdown was discussed. The trainer had never had any luck "laying up a bowed horse" and it was not an option. It was decided to frequently scan the tendon to monitor the stability of the lesion. It was also decided if the S/GO option wasn't working that it would be abandoned to preclude further more serious injury. The trainer did reduce the training level and was very selective in choosing races. He did agree to allow sonographic examination after each race. All of the advantages and disadvantages were

Table 21.8
Abnormal SDFT (FL)

Date	(MIZ-3B)			(Numbers of Levels—6)		
	Elapse	EL	MIZ-SA	% CHA.	Total-SA	% CHA.
4/22/94	0	7	123		627	
5/04/94	1 w	7	128	+ 04	702	+ 12
5/23/94	1 m	7	156	+ 22	812	+ 16
6/20/94	2 m	7	169	+ 08	914	+ 13
6/29/94	2 m	7	165	− 02	882	− 04
7/16/94	3 m	7	156	− 05	839	− 05
8/10/94	3½ m	7	129	− 17	757	− 10

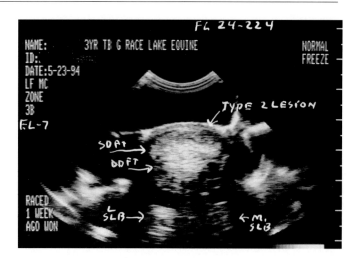

Figure 21.286.

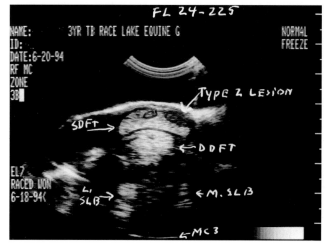

Figure 21.287.

discussed, and everyone involved knew the risks that were being taken.

Figure 21.285 is a cross-sectional left metacarpal Zone 3B sonogram of the same horse as in Fig. 21.284 made 48 hours post race. The scan shows a Type 2 lesion involving 32% of the CSA. Hypoechoic fibers were only found at this level. There was 55 mm^2 of hypoechoic fiber bundles (8% T-HYP). The MIZ-CSA increased by 4% and the T-CSA increased 12%. These increases would not be considered excessive. The post race assessment from qualitative and quantitative points of view would be that there was no additional significant SDFT insult. The horse won the race easily and a maximum effort was not required.

Figure 21.286 is a cross-sectional left metacarpal Zone 3B sonogram of the same horse as in Figures 21.284 and 21.285 1 week post race. The trainer had spaced races by 2 weeks and reduced training to swimming and light gallops. This scan shows the Type 2 lesion involving 26% of the CSA. The MIZ-CSA increased to 156 mm^2 or 22% and the T-CSA increased 16%. These increases are slightly more than technique variation. The total hypoechoic fiber paths was 59 mm^2 (7% T-HYP). An additional strain and an increased low-grade tendinitis was diagnosed. It is noteworthy that this horse is winning, but the overall tendon size is increasing and is larger than the baseline measurements which supports further injury. After two races and a one month,

the MIZ-CSA has increased 27% and the T-CSA has increase 30% from baseline. The trainer was advised to allow one month before the next race and to continue the reduced training program.

Figure 21.287 is a post race, cross-sectional left metacarpal Zone 3B sonogram of the same horse as in Figures 21.284 to 21.286. The scan shows improved echogenicity and only 17% of the CSA was a Type 2. However, more proximal zones had hypoechoic fibers and the T-HYP increased to 105 mm^2 (11%T-HYP). Even though this horse won his race easily, there was slight progression of the tendon injury. Figure 21.288 is a cross-sectional left metacarpal Zone 3B sonogram of the same horse as in Figures 21.284 to 21.287 made after six races and three and one-half months from the baseline evaluation. The horse had been highly successful winning almost all of the races. This scan reveals the Type 2 lesion involving 28% of the CSA. The MIZ-CSA is 129 mm^2 and the six-level T-CSA 757 mm^2. Compared to the initial evaluation the MIZ-CSA has increased 5% and the T-CSA has increased 21%.

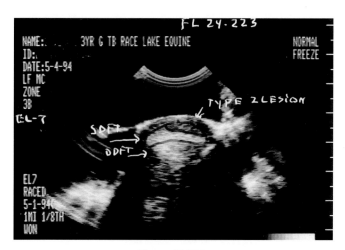

Figure 21.285.

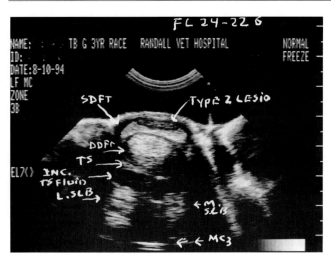

Figure 21.288.

In this case, the S/GO management option was highly successful, but there was acute awareness of the potentially hazardous situation and a proper veterinary/client relationship was established. This horse was exceptional because the tendon injury remained stable at EL-7.

Fiber Alignment Evaluation During Repair

Fiber alignment is a useful parameter to evaluate the SQR. When tendon fiber bundle disruption occurs, there are a physiologic sequence of events that occur. Initially, there is hemorrhage, collagen fiber necrosis, and inflammatory cell infiltration of the lesion. Over the next 3–4 weeks, with proper treatment, the hemorrhage, inflammatory infiltrate, and necrotic tendon fibers will be reabsorbed and removed from the injured area. Simultaneously, fibroblasts infiltrate, produce collagen and fill in the damaged fiber paths. These cells are not tenocytes, but, cells that will eventually function as replacement tendon cells. In the early stages (1–4 months), the collagen produced is smaller in diameter and proliferates randomly in all directions. As these fibers form they cross link in varied directions. This pattern can be monitored sonographically and at two to three months when these immature fibers that are formed have a hypoechoic texture. This should not persist in any significant amount beyond five to six months post injury. Persistent hypoechoic fiber patterns offer 3 possible explanations: 1) The collagen production is abundant and is made up of small diameter, short fibers which are weakly echogenic. 2) The collagen bundles are randomly distributed and are not oriented 90° to the sound beam. 3) Continual or repeated low-grade reinjury is occurring at the present EL.

Persistent hypoechoic fiber patterns beyond six months post injury below EL-4, in any significant amount, is considered an inferior SQR for RTR. A return to isoechogenicity at six months is a favorable parameter of SQR. In moderate to severe lesions, scattered foci of Type 1 fibers will have to be accepted. As the scar tissue matures, evidence of axially aligned fiber bundles is a favorable finding. Poorly aligned, isoechogenic or slightly hypoechoic fibers, indicates an increased reinjury risk with increasing tendon loading. If the scar tissue fibers are "balled up" and "glued together" in a random fashion, there is less chance they will yield to stretching. The chances of successful loading will be more favorable with parallel aligned fibers. Fibrous tissue alignment is a slow process and can be seen about the sixth to eighth month of rehabilitation. Obviously, maintaining the alignment with gradual loading is also a favorable sonographic parameter. In the BAPTEN® research program, fiber alignment is quantitated and the degree of parallelism is correlated with successful RTR. When evaluating sonographic parameters relative to repair, the tissue texture or density and the cross-sectional area changes are seen in the early stages (3-6 months) of repair. Fiber alignment, excessive intratendinous and peritendinous fibrosis are seen in the later stages (four-eight months). In a favorable repair, all parameters remain relatively stable with increased work levels.

Figure 21.289 is a sagittal left metacarpal Zone 3A SDFT sonogram of a racing Thoroughbred that sustained a recent re-injury. There were two zones with Type 1 textural abnormality. Multiple zones had an enlarged CSA. This scan shows the predominately hypoechoic, nonparallel SDFT fiber tracts (FS-3). The total FS for six zones was T-FS 8. The horse was treated with long term rest and SCLD.

Figure 21.290 is a left metacarpal Zone 3A SDFT sonogram of the same horse as in Fig. 21.289 made 7 months post injury at EL-4. There was improvement of texture and a reduction of the MIZ-CSA and the T-CSA, however, the MIZ-FS was 3 and the T-FS still scored 8. Basically, no significant improvement of fiber alignment occurred in seven months. This horse suffered a reinjury during training. This is an interesting case because the only parameter that failed to show progress was the fiber alignment (FA).

Figure 21.291 is a sagittal left metacarpal Zone 3B SDFT sonogram of a pacing Standardbred that recently suffered a re-injury. This horse, as in the previous case, had Type 3 textural lesions of two zones. The FS was 3 for the MIZ. The T-FS for six zones was seven.

Figure 21.292 is a left metacarpal Zone 3B SDFT sonogram of the same horse as in Fig. 21.291 made 6 months post injury at EL-7. The MIZ-FS was 1 and the T-FS was 4. The CSA and textural parameters were also stable. There were many similarities of the last two cases since both had recurrent injuries, limited textural abnormalities and favorable CSA and textural improvement. There was, however, a significant difference in the fiber alignment score.

Figure 21.293 is a sagittal right metacarpal Zone 2B SDFT sonogram of a pacing Standardbred that had a recent injury. The initial MIZ-FS was 3 and the six-level total was FS-9 (maximum is 18 for six levels).

Figure 21.294 is a sagittal right metacarpal Zone 2B SDFT sonogram of the same horse in Fig. 21.293 made at 6 months at EL-3. The scan reveals about half of the fibers to be parallel and the MIZ-FS was 2. The total was FS-10. Other parameters were more favorable and the horse was elevated to EL-5.

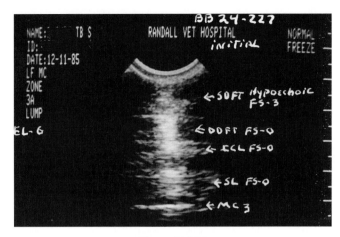

Figure 21.289.

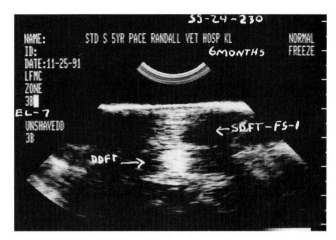

Figure 21.292.

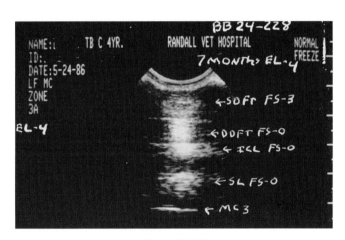

Figure 21.290.

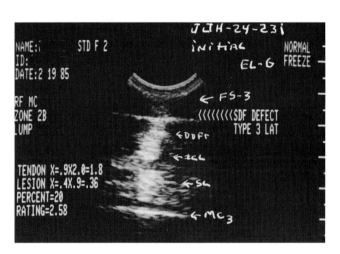

Figure 21.293.

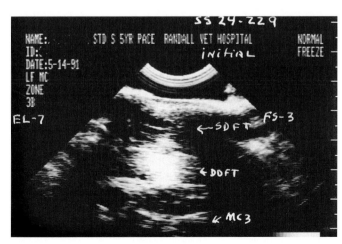

Figure 21.291.

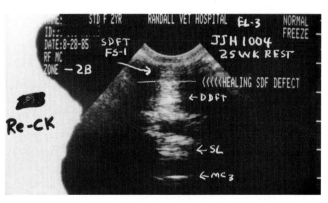

Figure 21.294.

Figure 21.295 is a sagittal right metacarpal Zone 2B SDFT sonogram of the same horse as in Figures 21.293 and 21.294 made at nine months post injury with the horse jogging multiple miles. The fiber MIZ alignment has regressed to FS-3. The total FS was increased to 13. At this point, there were other sonographic abnormal parameters.

Figure 21.296 is a sagittal right metacarpal Zone 2B SDFT sonogram of the same horse made at 11 months post injury at EL-3. The scan shows slight improvement of the FA, but, it is still less than 25% axial and was scored FS-3. The total FS was 10. The later improvement from 13 to 10 was most likely the result of inflammation resolution and the FS was the same as the initial scan. This is an unfavorable parameter for RTR. This filly was given additional time off and was tried again in training only to sustain a third tendon injury.

Figure 21.297 is a sagittal right metacarpal Zone 3A SDFT sonogram of a racing Thoroughbred that sustained a large, core lesion. The scan shows no parallel fiber alignment of the MIZ and is FS-3. The total FS for six zones was 15.

Figure 21.298 is a sagittal right metacarpal Zone 3A SDFT sonogram of the same horse as in Fig. 21.297 made

7 months after injury at EL-2. The scan reveals over 50% parallel fibers of the MIZ and was FS-1. The total FS was 5.

Figure 21.299 is a sagittal right metacarpal Zone 3A SDFT sonogram of the same horse as in Figures 21.298 and 21.299 made 10 months after injury at EL-7. The MIZ-FS was 0 and the total FS was 1. This horse made an excellent recovery, illustrating that parallel fiber alignment can be reestablished and remain stable with increasing tendon loading to EL-7.

Intratendinous/peritendinous Fibrosis in Repair

Excessive, rigid, intratendinous or peritendinous scar is an undesirable response of tendon lesion healing. The reasons are obvious: 1) there is restriction of tendon gliding movement with peritendonous scars, especially in the proximal metacarpus and in the distal sheathed tendon zones; 2) dense intratendinous scar increases the chance of reinjury because scar tissue is weak and inelastic. Excessive, restricting SDFT peritendinous fibrosis is most commonly secondary to lacerations. Work related, excessive scar formation can also be caused by multiple tendon injuries.

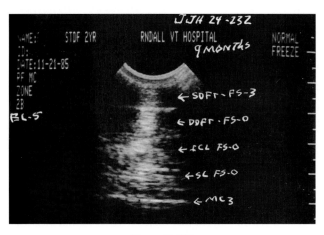

Figure 21.295.

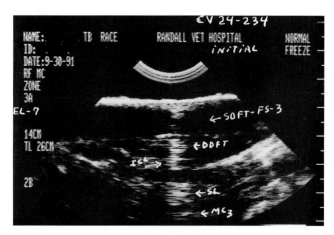

Figure 21.297.

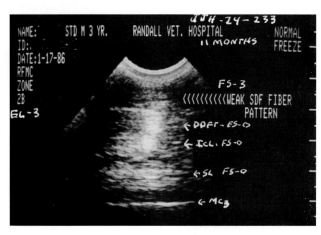

Figure 21.296.

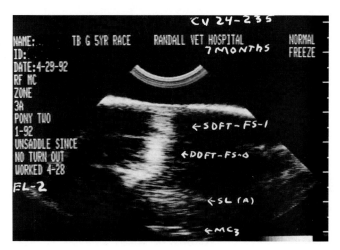

Figure 21.298.

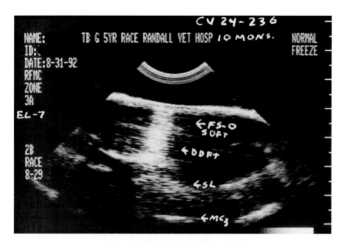

Figure 21.299.

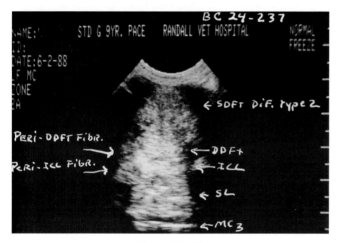

Figure 21.300.

Figure 21.300 is a cross-sectional left metacarpal Zone 2A SDFT sonogram of a Standardbred pacer with a swollen metacarpus. A diffuse Type 2 fiber texture was present in addition to chronic fibrosis along the lateral DDFT and ICL. This is an undesirable fibrous tissue response because adhesions are likely, which may impede the SDFT gliding movement.

Figure 21.301 is a cross-sectional left metacarpal Zone 3A sonogram of a Standardbred with an enlarged SDFT and a markedly thickened tendon sheath (TS). There are potentially restricting palmar tendon surface adhesions.

Figure 21.302 is a cross-sectional left metacarpal Zone 3A SDFT sonogram of a Thoroughbred racehorse with a large diffuse Type 3 lesion (reinjury).

Figure 21.303 is a cross-sectional left metacarpal Zone 3A SDFT sonogram of the same horse shown in Figure 21.302 made 8 months after reinjury. During the recovery period, the horse has not exceeded EL-2. The scan reveals two areas of persistent, Type 3 fibrosis. Additionally, significant peritendinous fibrosis is present along the medial and lateral DDFT borders. Regardless of the deficient textural repair, the peritendinous fibrosis could significantly decrease the functional tendon movement and affect future racing performance. Grossly, this horse had a more upright

fetlock posture because of the scar formation. If this horse returned to racing, increased speeds and tendon stretching will most likely result in recurrent fiber and scar tissue tearing. For occupations other than racing, the prognosis is more favorable because the demand for elasticity is less.

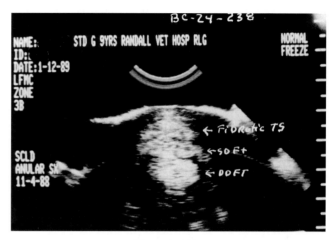

Figure 21.301.

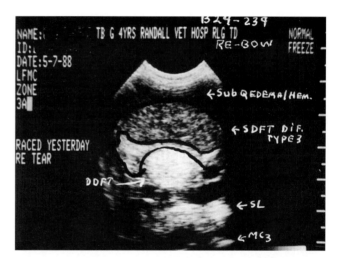

Figure 21.302.

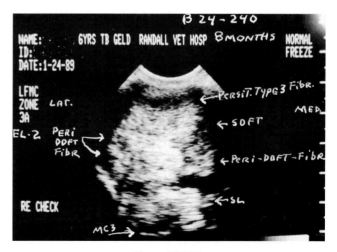

Figure 21.303.

Figure 21.304 is a cross-sectional left metacarpal Zone 3B SDFT sonogram of a Thoroughbred racehorse with a similar reinjury as the horse in Figure 21.303. The scan reveals a large Type 3 tendon enlargement.

Figure 21.305 is a cross-sectional left metacarpal Zone 3B SDFT sonogram of the same horse shown in Fig. 21.304 made 16 months after reinjury at EL-3. This scan reveals a marked palmar digital tendon sheath fibrosis and thickened AL with no apparent DDFT adhesions. The SDFT gliding movement may be restricted. A significant persistent Type 3 lateral SDFT border is present despite 16 months of pasture rest.

Figure 21.306 is a cross-sectional left metacarpal Zone 3B sonogram of a trotting Standardbred that has been competing successfully (EL-7) for over a year with a healed SDF tendonitis. This scan reveals a diffusely enlarged Type 1 tendon; however, there is no significant peritendinous fibrosis or TS thickening. The lack of peritendinous fibrosis is a favorable sonographic finding.

Figure 21.307 is a sagittal left metacarpal Zone 3B sonogram of the same horse shown in Figure 21.306. The scan shows that most of the tendon fibers are axially aligned

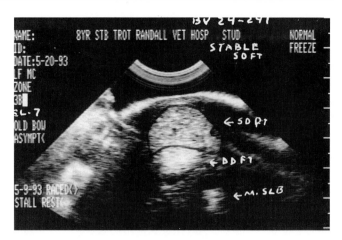

Figure 21.306.

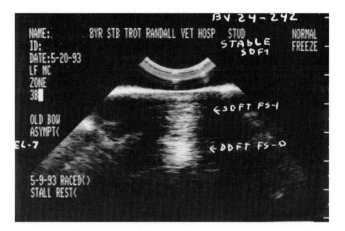

Figure 21.307.

(FS-1). The favorable qualitative and quantitative sonographic assessments correlate with the successful racing for the past year.

Applied SDFT Sonography

Throughout this chapter, we have stressed several techniques of quantitative and qualitative sonographic evaluation to aid in tendon injury diagnosis, prognosis, and treatment. These data can be used to evaluate the healing tendon as well. The quantitative assessments were generated from the intralesional BAPTEN field trial protocol. For the clinician dealing with the injured horse, these concepts can be applied routinely to improve patient care. In this section, "applied" means to relate past experiences when application or lack of application of these principles affected the outcome. A series of cases follows that serve as models, good and bad, that helped establish a sonographic approach to tendon injuries. Hopefully, from these successes and failures, more sophisticated ultrasonographic applications can be developed towards the ultimate goal of improved SQR and RTR.

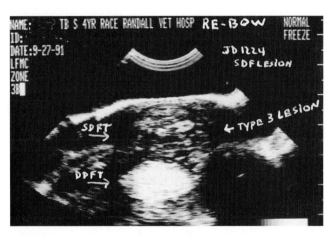

Figure 21.304.

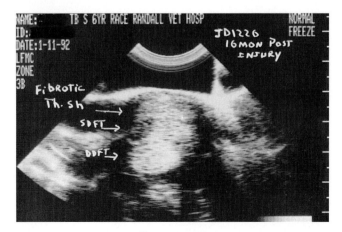

Figure 21.305.

Our training in veterinary medicine has ingrained in us the concept of active or inactive disease processes. We prefer to address a client with a definite opinion that a given abnormality is active or inactive. When we consider SDFT injury, however, we prefer to go beyond this concept. The starting point is to consider any abnormality of the SDFT, regardless of the severity, as a lesion. From this point, we must ascertain whether the lesion is progressive or nonprogressive. Sometimes this requires continued training to answer that question. Continued training obviously imposes additional injury risk, but the decision to stop or continue rests with the owners and trainers. At times, continued training or racing proves to be successful, but more often than not, the opposite occurs. The final sonographic principle of tendon injury evaluation addresses whether the repaired lesion remains stable with increased or continued use. If an injured tendon is grossly enlarged but tight, cold, and nonpainful; and if there is no sonographic evidence of reinjury with increased loading, then it is a stable injury for that EL. The ultimate goal is to attain maximum EL with a favorable SQR that remains stable with loading. Sonographic evaluations are used to detect early instability, and catastrophic recurrence can usually be avoided if appropriate action is taken. Decision-making is less frustrating and more accurate, and SDFT injury management is vastly improved. Regardless of therapy, certain principles need to be applied in the quest for successful return to function.

Figure 21.308 is a cross-sectional left metacarpal Zone 3B sonogram of a racing Thoroughbred that sustained an SDFT injury at EL-7. The filly was a maiden and had made 4 starts earning $498.00. She had normal conformation. There was a Type 3 palmar tendon lesion found. The MIZ-CSA was 198 mm^2 and the lesion comprised 48% of the tendon's cross-sectional area with a FS-3. The T-CSA was 1105 mm^2 and the T-HYP was 17% (moderate injury). The average Type was 1.8 and the T-FS was 16. The lesion was regarded as moderate (15 to 25% T-HYP).

Figure 21.309 is a cross-sectional left metacarpal Zone 3B sonogram of the same horse shown in Figure 21.308

made at 4 months after injury. During that time, the horse had not exceeded EL-2 (pony). The scan reveals a slightly enlarged tendon with a few scattered Type 1 fiber bundles. The MIZ-CSA had decreased by 27% and the T-CSA decreased by 29%. The MIZ-FS was still 3 and the T-FS was 10. This scan shows the expected response of this moderate lesion 4 months after injury at EL 2. The density improved two grades, the CSA reduced significantly with resolution of inflammation, and the FS remained elevated. There are no positioning abnormalities and there is no apparent peritendinous fibrous tissue reaction. At this stage, this horse is being well managed. Exercise is very controlled, as advised. At this point, the SQR is favorable. The next phase was 2 months at EL-3b.

Figure 21.310 is a cross-sectional left metacarpal Zone 3B sonogram of the same horse shown in Figures 21.308 and 21.309 made at 9 months after injury and at EL-5. The texture was similar and the MIZ and T-CSA decreased slightly and are apparently stable. The FS has reduced in the MIZ to 1 and the T-FS to 2. All parameters were stable at this point and the horse was advanced to EL-6 and later to EL-7.

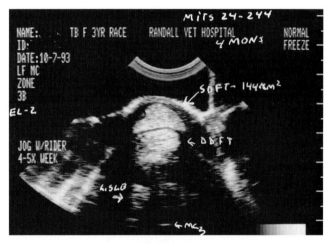

Figure 21.309.

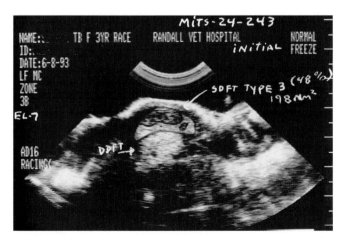

Figure 21.308.

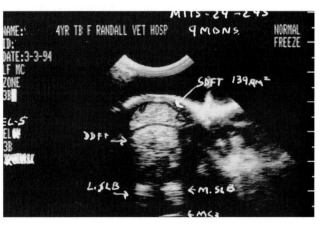

Figure 21.310.

Figure 21.311 is a cross-sectional left metacarpal Zone 3B sonogram of the same horse as in Figures 21.308 to 21.310 made after two races. The scan shows a diffuse palmar SDFT Type 1 texture. The MIZ and T-CSA are stable and are well below the initial injury level. The FS of the MIZ has increased to 2 and the T-FS to 5. The latter two parameters definitely indicate that this lesion is not stable at EL-7. Grossly, no palpable or visible abnormality was present, and the trainer did not complain of decreased performance. At this point, the EL should be reduced until the tendon density improves and remains stable. In this case, economics entered into the decision-making, and the trainer was pressed to accept this advice. This filly had only two races, she was a maiden with little earning capacity, and there had been close to a year's rehabilitation. This filly's injury had done as well as could be expected and she was perfectly managed to this point. From the trainer's viewpoint, the tendon appeared stable and the filly had a chance to win a race. The management decision was to decrease the training level, increase the time between races, and attempt to continue racing (S/GO).

Figure 21.312 is a cross-sectional left metacarpal Zone 3B sonogram of the same filly as in Figures 21.308 to 21.311 made 14 months after injury after 5 races. She raced 3 times from the last scan, earning one second place at the bottom class. She was not lame. The scan reveals a Type 3 palmar SDFT lesion. The MIZ-CSA and T-CSA have increased, but not to the original injury size. The lesion involved 25% of the MIZ cross-sectional area and extended proximally one level. The MIZ-FS was 3 and the T-FS was 7. At this point, reinjury has occurred and three sonographic parameters are unstable. This case exemplifies excellent repair and good case management. The fact is that her SDFT could not remain stable at EL-7. The SDFT instability was predominately related to focal fiber tearing and not tendinitis, hence no significant gross recurrent injury up to this point.

Figure 21.313 is a cross-sectional left metacarpal Zone 3B SDFT sonogram of a racing Thoroughbred with a focal Type 3 core lesion. Similarities to the last case are present, and the damage is limited to the distal metacarpal. The MIZ-CSA was 156 mm^2 and the T-CSA was 801 mm^2. The MIZ-FS was 3 and the T-FS was 8. This was regarded as a slight (7% T-HYP) injury. This horse was managed in the same manner as the previous case. The horse was treated and placed on a graduated exercise program. The EL was increased based on favorable sonographic parameters.

Figure 21.314 is a cross-sectional left metacarpal Zone 3B sonogram of the same horse shown in Figure 21.313 made 4 months after injury at EL-2 (swimming). The scan shows significant textural improvement. The MIZ-CSA and T-CSA have decreased by 11% and 2% respectively. The MIZ-FS has decreased to 2 and the T-FS to 4. This accelerated improvement rate indicates that the initial fiber damage was less than the original estimate. At this stage, three sonographic parameters are improved, indicating a favorable SQR.

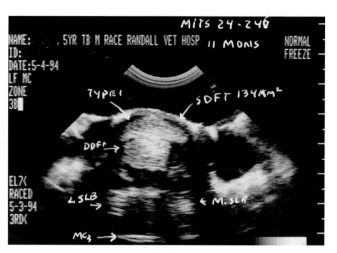

Figure 21.311.

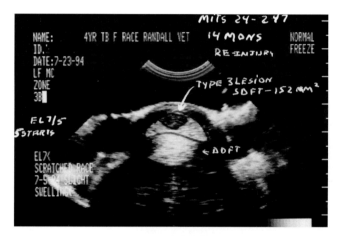

Figure 21.312.

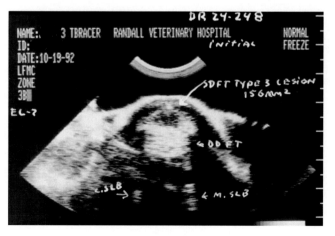

Figure 21.313.

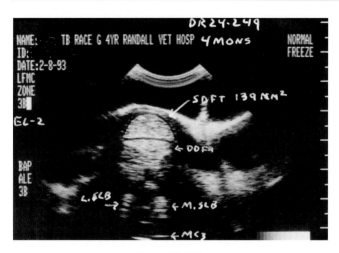

Figure 21.314.

Figure 21.315 is a cross-sectional left metacarpal sonogram of the same horse shown in Figures 21.313 and 21.314 made 7 months after injury at EL-5. The scan shows no textural regressions with the increased work load. The MIZ-CSA is increased by 9% and the T-CSA is increased by 1.5%. This rate of increase suggests more than a physiologic response to training. The MIZ is being slightly overstressed at this EL. The fiber score continues to decrease. Two parameters are stable or improving and only one is slightly questionable. Caution was advised and heeded by the trainer, and the horse remained at EL-5 longer than planned (1 month).

Figure 21.316 is a cross-sectional left metacarpal Zone 3B sonogram of the same horse shown in Figures 21.313 to 21.315 made after the first race (EL-7). The scan shows a stable texture. The MIZ-CSA and T-CSA show significant reductions. The MIZ-CSA reduced by 24% and the T-CSA reduced by 23%. The FS of the MIZ was 0 and total was FS-2. The slight delay in increasing loads was rewarded with

significant improvement and, at this point, all parameters are stable.

Figure 21.317 is a cross-sectional left metacarpal Zone 3B sonogram of the same horse shown in Figures 21.313 to 21.316 made 13 months after injury after 10 races. No textural changes occurred. The MIZ-CSA was stable at 112 mm^2 and the T-CSA at 526 mm^2. The FS was stable at both the MIZ and T at 1 and 2 respectively.

Figure 21.318 is a cross-sectional left metacarpal Zone 3B sonogram of the same horse shown in Figures 21.313 to 21.317 made 18 months after injury. The horse had raced regularly and was completely asymptomatic. The scan shows no textural changes. The MIZ-CSA was 118 mm^2 and the T-CSA was 665 mm^2. The FS for the MIZ and total remained stable at 1 and 2 respectively. This horse competed at an upper-class level and, 2 years after injury, earned in excess of $70,000.00. In this case, the repaired lesion could withstand EL-7 as exemplified by the stable sonographic parameters.

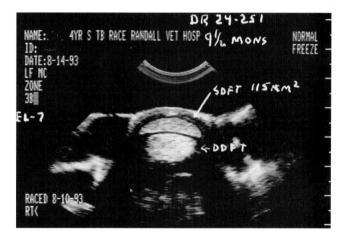

Figure 21.316.

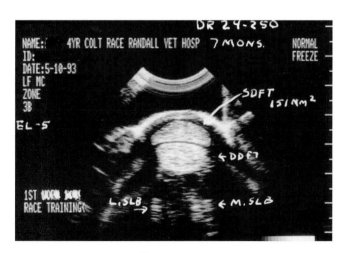

Figure 21.315.

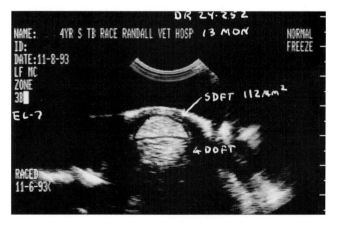

Figure 21.317.

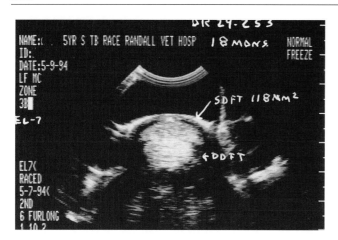

Figure 21.318.

Figure 21.319 is a cross-sectional left metacarpal Zone 3A SDFT sonogram of a pacing Standardbred that was recently injured. The scan shows a Type 3 palmar-medial SDFT lesion. The lesion comprised 43% of the CSA. The MIZ-CSA was 155 mm^2 and the T-CSA was 645 mm^2. Hypoechoic tracts could be identified in four zones. The total hypo-echoic volume was 136 mm^2, which represented 21% of the six-level total volume (21% T-HYP) (moderate injury). The MIZ had a FS-3 and the T-FS was 6.

Figure 21.320 is a cross-sectional left metacarpal Zone 3A sonogram of the same horse shown in Fig. 21.319 made 4 months after injury at EL-3. The scan shows a significant improvement of echogenicity. The MIZ hypoechoic fibers was down to 4% and the T-HYP reduced from 136 mm^2 to 68 mm^2. The MIZ-CSA increased to 192 mm^2 (24%). The T-CSA increased to 954 mm^2 (47%). The FS of the MIZ reduced to 1, but the T-FS increased to 7. This is not a favorable SQR, and it demonstrates a management mistake. The sonographer (RLG) only viewed the texture and advised an exercise level increase (we all learn in time). Had all of the parameters been evaluated properly, this horse should have been reduced to a lower EL for 30 to 60 days then re-evaluated.

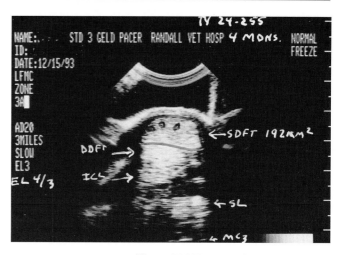

Figure 21.320.

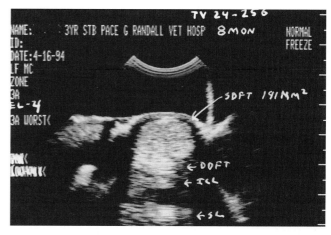

Figure 21.321.

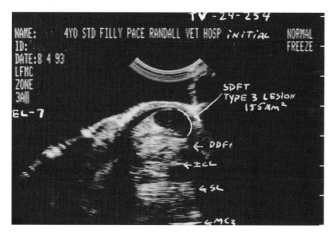

Figure 21.319.

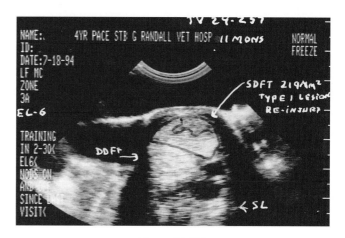

Figure 21.322.

Figure 21.321 is a cross-sectional left metacarpal Zone 3A sonogram of the same horse shown in Figures 21.319 and 21.320 made 8 months after injury at EL-4 (1 mile slow jog). The scan shows a regression of the overall texture. The MIZ-CSA has maintained at 191 mm², but the T-CSA increased further to 1014 mm². It is an unfavorable sonographic evaluation to see the MIZ-CSA or T-CSA significantly increase above the baseline value. The MIZ-FS and T-FS were the same; no improvement in 8 months. At this point, three parameters are unfavorable and indicate tendon instability at the current EL.

Figure 21.322 is a cross-sectional left metacarpal Zone 3A sonogram of the same horse shown in Figures 21.319 to 21.321 made 11 months after injury at EL-6. The scan shows diffuse Type 1 fibers. The MIZ-CSA is increased to 219 mm² and the T-CSA has increased to 1056 mm². The MIZ-FS is 2 and the T-FS is 8.

Figure 21.323 is a cross-sectional left metacarpal Zone 3B sonogram of the same horse shown in Figures 21.319 to 21.322. There is a large, Type 3 SDFT core lesion in the Zone distal to the MIZ. As is often the case, the reinjury appears worse than the original. It is difficult to say whether this reinjury would have occurred had this horse been managed differently. Our impression is that the outcome may have been different if exercise levels would have been reduced when sonographic parameters indicated that an EL increase was not justified. Twenty-five percent plus increases in CSA seldom, if ever, justify increasing exercise levels.

Figure 21.324 is a cross-sectional right metacarpal Zone 3A SDFT sonogram of a pacing Standardbred which sustained a severe reinjury at EL-7. The horse had multiple episodes of previous tendon injury. This was an extremely talented racehorse and the owners decided to attempt another RTR. The scan shows an enlarged tendon with an extensive, Type 3 lesion. The lesion represented 95% of the cross-sectional area. The MIZ-CSA was 776 mm² and the T-CSA was 3335 mm². The MIZ-FS was 3 and the total-FS was 13.

Figure 21.325 is a cross-sectional right metacarpal Zone

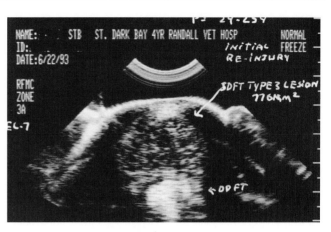

Figure 21.324.

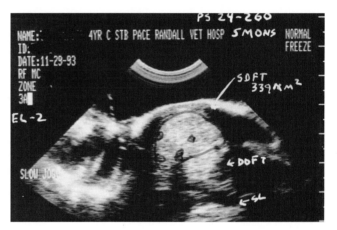

Figure 21.325.

3A sonogram of the same horse shown in Figure 21.324 made 5 months after injury at EL-2 (no turn-out). An extensive textural improvement is present, especially in a lesion of this magnitude. The only treatment to this point was rest, systemic anti-inflammatory drugs and two external blisters. The MIZ-CSA has reduced 56% to 339 mm² and the T-CSA has reduced 54% to 1534 mm². The FS has improved at both the MIZ and T to 1 and 6, respectively. At this point and at this EL, all parameters are favorable.

Figure 21.326 is a cross-sectional right metacarpal Zone 3A sonogram of the same horse shown in Figures 21.324 and 21.325 made 7 months after injury at EL-3. The scan shows a reasonably stable texture for the severity of the injury. The MIZ-CSA and T-CSA have risen slightly (4% and 2%, respectively). This finding indicates that, even after 5 months of hand controlled exercise, paddock exercise (EL-3b) has created some slight fiber compromise. The T-CSA increased from 49 mm² to 260 mm². The parameter change indicating some instability was the FS. The MIZ-FS regressed to 3 and the T-FS regressed to 13. Although not unexpected, these parameter regressions indicate the relative inelasticity of this chronically enlarged tendon. The horse was kept in pasture for 2 additional months before resuming jogging.

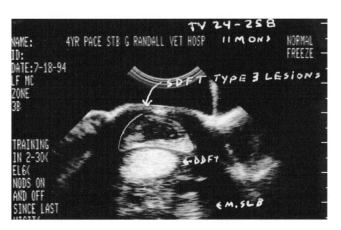

Figure 21.323.

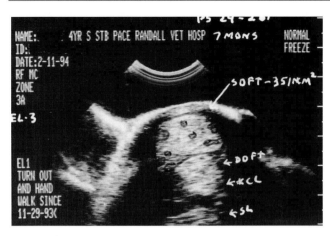

Figure 21.326.

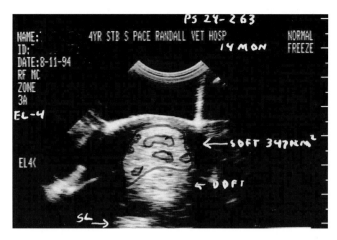

Figure 21.328.

Figure 21.327 is a cross-sectional right metacarpal Zone 3A sonogram of the same horse shown in Figures 21.324 to 21.326 made 12 months after injury. The scan shows focal, hypoechoic areas in the tendon. The MIZ-FS and T-FS was 3 and 15, respectively. A favorable reduction of the MIZ and T-CSA occurred by 23% and 14%, respectively. The horse had completed its first race. The horse was given 1 month rest to recover from a respiratory problem.

Figure 21.328 is a cross-sectional right metacarpal Zone 3A sonogram of the same horse as in Figures 21.324 to 21.327 made at 14 months after injury at EL-4. The scan shows a 20% hypoechoic fiber increase in the MIZ and a 12% increase in the total tendon. The CSA slightly improved. The FS remained elevated at 2 for the MIZ and 13 for the total. These data indicate the instability of two parameters even at this EL. These findings indicate that the EL should not be increased. The horse was reinjured in the next start and was retired. Overall, this lesion did well and the horse was managed properly. The injury and its repair were just not compatible with racing. In this case, the texture and FS were the unstable parameters, indicating fibrous scar weakness.

Figure 21.329 is a cross-sectional left metacarpal Zone

3B SDFT sonogram of a racing Thoroughbred that reinjured its tendon the previous day. The scan reveals a Type 3 lesion of the lateral half of the tendon. The lesion involved 43% of the CSA. Three other levels with a lesser degree of hypoechoic fibers were present. The MIZ-CSA was 310 mm^2 and the six-level total was 1248 mm^2. The MIZ was FS-3 and the T-FS was 9. The horse was rested and treated.

Figure 21.330 is a cross-sectional left metacarpal Zone 3B sonogram of the same horse shown in Figure 21.329 made 4 months after injury at EL-4 (light hacking). The scan shows a diffuse, Type 1 texture. The MIZ-CSA has reduced 17% to 257 mm^2 and the T-CSA has reduced 22% to 910 mm^2. The MIZ-FS is still 3 and the T-FS is 5.

At this point in many tendon injuries, crucial decisions need to be made. The trainer has a horse doing extremely well, grossly. The tendon is cold and tight, and the trainer perceives it to be "set." To complicate matters, the horse is generally very alert and plays and prances when walked in the shed row. It is not easy to report favorable sonographic findings and restrain the trainer at the same time. If you leave this chapter with one principle only, let it be this one: at 4 to 6 months, most moderate injuries should display good sonographic progress, some even perfect progress. However, this does not mean that the repair has reached maximum cross-linking and strength. At least an additional 2 to 3 months of restrained activity is necessary for strengthening and remodeling. In our present program of structured exercise in the BAPTEN trials, most horses are favorable sonographically at 4 to 6 months. Up to that time, all exercise is controlled in hand. We then advise 2 months of paddock exercise in most cases. Many of these horses show slight regression of parameters with just this exercise level increase. Most horses are most likely not going to remain stable at a training level at 5 months. This is a very critical point. Once the horses in the BAPTEN study have completed pasture time, they only advance to EL-4 for 1 month before gradually increasing to EL-5. Furthermore, there is no increase to EL-5 unless the parameters at the 30-day EL-4 level are stable. **Most horses prematurely trained (EL-5), even lightly, from 4 to 7 months after injury reinjure their**

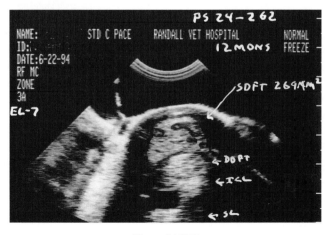

Figure 21.327.

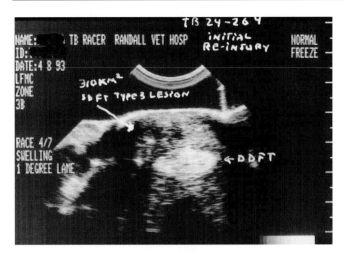

Figure 21.329.

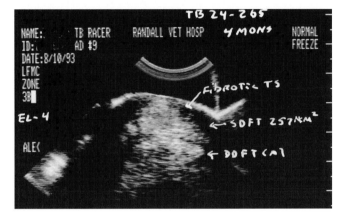

Figure 21.330.

tendons. The time for restraint is mandatory during this period. It is easy to restrain trainers early on when the horse is injured, but 5 to 7 months later the horse's behavior leads the trainer to believe that the tendon is ready to train. The sonographer in part contributes to this impression because parameters should be improving. It is not recommended to advance from EL-2/3 to EL-5 in one step, especially at 5 to 6 months after injury (phase I management). In this case, the trainer was determined to train this horse despite less than ideal sonographic parameters, and he refused to advance the exercise levels in sequence. Instead of remaining at EL-3 for 2 months and then to EL-4 for at least 1 month, he went directly to EL-6 in 2 weeks.

Figure 21.331 is a cross-sectional left metacarpal Zone 3B sonogram of the same horse shown in Figures 21.329 and 21.330 at 5 months after reinjury. The scan reveals a large Type 3 lesion involving 67% of the cross-sectional area. This lesion was present in five other levels to a lesser degree. The MIZ-CSA was 420 mm^2 and the T-CSA was 1608 mm^2. As we have seen previously, more fiber damage has occurred here than in the original injury. This horse was simply advanced too high in EL too rapidly for the stage of repair. This horse was not well managed.

There is a repair phase from 0 to 5–6 months followed by a strengthening phase from 6 months onward. Nothing known today can alter this timetable. We sincerely doubt that many moderate lesions can return to full training before 8 to 9 months after injury. Furthermore, if an unfavorable SQR or CSA instability exists with increased tendon loading, a longer time is required.

Figure 21.332 is a cross-sectional right metacarpal Zone 3B sonogram of a 2-year-old racing Thoroughbred filly at EL-5 with slight sheath filling. The scan did not reveal any textural changes or fiber alignment abnormalities. There was slight TS distention. CSA measurement revealed that the proximal half of the tendon was the same as the opposite limb. The CSA of the proximal three left fore zones was 340 mm^2. The CSA of the right fore proximal three zones was 325 mm^2. Variation in the distal half was greater than expected. The left (normal) distal three zones had a CSA of 254 mm^2 and the right fore was 299 mm^2. This is an 18% variation. Although not alarming, the CSA difference and the TS distention indicated subtle strain of the distal half of the right fore SDFT at EL-5. A 1 month reduced EL was allowed, but rescans before and during EL increases were not done. The exercise levels were increased as part of a normal training schedule.

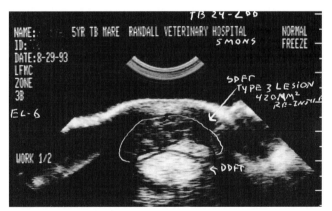

Figure 21.331.

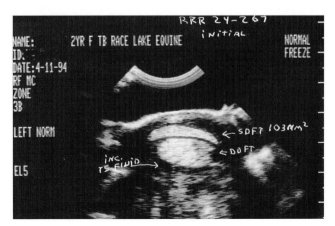

Figure 21.332.

Figure 21.333 is a cross-sectional right metacarpal Zone 3B sonogram of the same horse as in Fig. 21.332 made 5 months later at EL-6. The scan reveals a large Type 2 central SDFT lesion. This injury involved six levels, with the more serious injury occurring in the distal half of the tendon. Some important points to this case include the following: 1) subtle enlargement deserves the clinician's attention, especially in a 2 year old that is only at EL-5; 2) despite the lack of fiber tearing at the time of the initial scan, a short term layoff was obviously inadequate for this horse.

Figure 21.334 is a cross-sectional left metacarpal Zone 3B SDFT sonogram of a seasoned racing Thoroughbred that developed a slight post-race swelling. The scan reveals a small Type 3 focal lesion palmar tendon lesion. CSA data revealed only enlarged zones 3A and 3B. The horse was given 45 days off training and was reduced to EL-1.

Figure 21.335 is a cross-sectional left metacarpal Zone 3B sonogram of the same horse shown in Figure 21.334 made after 6 weeks at EL-1. The scan shows only slight evidence of the focal lesion. In addition, the MIZ-CSA has returned to normal. The horse raced two more times that year without incident.

Figure 21.336 is a cross-sectional right metacarpal Zone

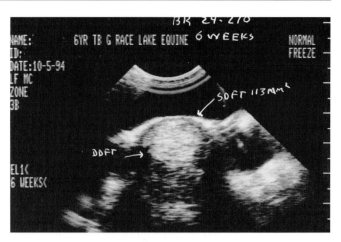

Figure 21.335.

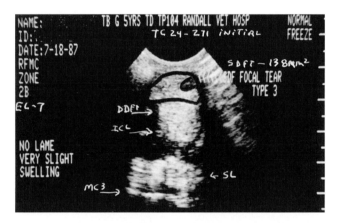

Figure 21.336.

2B sonogram of a regularly competing Thoroughbred racehorse with a focal Type 3 palmar-lateral SDFT lesion. MIZ and T-CSA increased only slightly. The lesion could be identified in three levels. The horse was given 1 month off training and the leg was treated symptomatically.

Figure 21.337 is a cross-sectional right metacarpal Zone 2B sonogram of the same horse shown in Figure 21.336 made 1 month after injury at EL-1. Favorable lesion resolution is present. The horse was returned to training and raced three times.

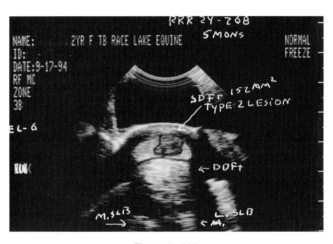

Figure 21.333.

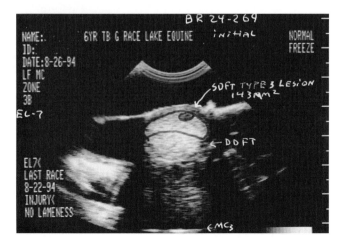

Figure 21.334.

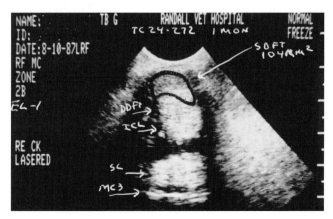

Figure 21.337.

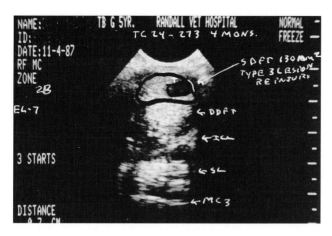

Figure 21.338.

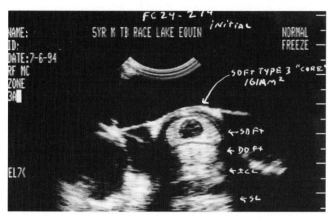

Figure 21.339.

Figure 21.338 is a cross-sectional right metacarpal Zone 2B sonogram of the same horse as in Figures 21.336 and 21.337 made after 3 races and 4 months post injury. The scan shows a focal Type 3 SDFT lesion in the original area. The MIZ-CSA was significantly increased.

These cases demonstrate that it is possible to treat small lesions with small CSA increases and with short time periods away from training. However, if the MIZ CSA or T-CSA approaches a 20 to 30% increase from normal, the client is told that short-term therapy is unsuccessful. Furthermore, short-term lay off is not really a proper choice for horses that have not competed at a maximum EL before SDFT injury. The decision to short-cut the time off is usually an economic one; therefore, each situation must be reviewed carefully and judged on its own merits. In any case, close sonographic monitoring is indicated. In a racing Thoroughbred with moderate SDFT injuries involving over four levels, an attempt at short-term recovery usually is futile.

Figure 21.339 is a cross-sectional left metacarpal Zone 3A sonogram of a regularly raced Thoroughbred stakes filly with a Type 3 SDFT core lesion. The MIZ-CSA was 161 mm^2 and the six-level total was 769 mm^2. The lesion comprised 24% of the CSA. The T-HYP was 126 mm^2 or 16% T-HYP (moderate injury). The MIZ-FS was 3 and the T-FS was 12. A short time-off program, 1 month at EL-1, with diligent leg care was chosen by the trainer.

Figure 21.340 is a cross-sectional left metacarpal Zone 3A sonogram of the same horse shown in Figure 21.339 made 1 month after injury at EL-1. The core lesion texture improved significantly. This finding raises an interesting point. Most likely, the two grade improvement and the shrinking of the black hole is caused by inflammatory fluid and hemorrhage absorption. This horse did not have surgery. There is a diffuse, Type 1 tendon fiber texture. The MIZ-CSA decreased to 136 mm^2, the T-CSA decreased to 712 mm^2, and the T-HYP decreased to 96 mm^2 or 13% T-HYP. The MIZ-FS was reduced to 2 and the T-FS to 7. We have basically seen the effects of a decreased exercise level and resolution of inflammation. The fiber damage is not as severe as the original scan indicated; yet, there is significant injury.

Figure 21.341 is a cross-sectional left metacarpal Zone 3A sonogram of the same horse shown in Figures 21.339 and 21.340 made 2 months after injury and now at EL-5. The scan reveals a Type 1 core lesion involving 30% of the CSA. The MIZ-CSA is increased to 161 mm^2 and the T-CSA is stable at 705 mm^2. The MIZ-FS is still at 2 and the T-FS has increased to 9. Therefore, this increase in EL has caused sonographic parameter regression, and the lesion is considered unstable.

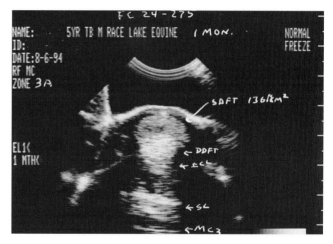

Figure 21.340.

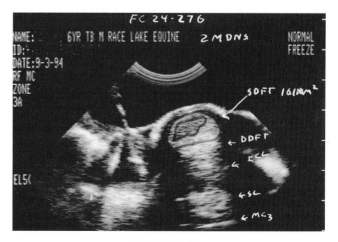

Figure 21.341.

Figure 21.342 is a cross-sectional left metacarpal Zone 3A sonogram of the same horse shown in Figures 21.339 to 21.341 made 2½ months after injury. The trainer has proceeded to EL-6. The scan shows a 52% increase in the MIZ hypoechoic fiber bundles. The MIZ-CSA is slightly reduced to 151 mm². The T-CSA is 752 mm² and the T-HYP is 272 mm² or 36%T-HYP (severe injury). The trainer is controlling the inflammation with systemic and local therapy; however, fiber path disruption is increasing with increased EL. The MIZ-FS is still 2 and the T-FS is up to 11.

Figure 21.343 is a cross-sectional left metacarpal Zone 3A sonogram of the same horse shown in Figures 21.339 to 21.342 made 3 months after injury. The scan shows diffuse, Type 1 fiber texture. The MIZ-CSA is 143 mm² and the T-CSA is 760 mm². The T-HYP is 328 mm² or 43% T-HYP. The MIZ-FS was up to 3 again and the T-FS was at 10. At this point, the trainer was convinced to retire the mare. In this case, the percent of hypoechoic fiber bundles and the FA were the most revealing sonographic parameters. As tendon loading increased, progressive fiber bundle disruption continued despite diligent symptomatic therapy.

No discussion of continuing training with SDFT injury would be complete without an example of the ultimate in tendon injury mismanagement. This case emphasizes that great progress in tendon injury diagnosis and management has been made in the past decade.

Figure 21.344 is a cross-sectional right metacarpal Zone 2B SDFT sonogram of a Thoroughbred racing filly examined for a "bandage pinch". The scan shows a small, focal, Type 3 palmar tendon surface lesion with slight subcutaneous edema. The filly had raced 5 days previously. This lesion involved 11% of the CSA, and the MIZ-CSA was 80 mm². The trainer was advised that this was not a bandage pinch and that he should treat the lesion as a slight bowed tendon. The advice was ignored and the trainer treated it symptomatically and forged onward.

Figure 21.345 is a cross-sectional right metacarpal Zone 3A SDFT sonogram of the same horse shown in Figure 21.344 made 5 months and 2 races after injury. The scan reveals an enlarged tendon with a diffuse Type 2 pattern. The MIZ-CSA was 245 mm². At this time, the trainer decided to rest the horse and treat the tendon injury. This is an extreme example of case mismanagement and stresses the importance of serial sonography.

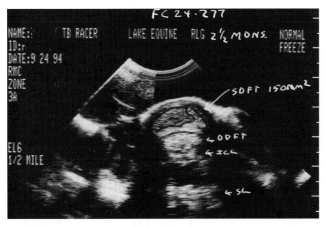

Figure 21.342.

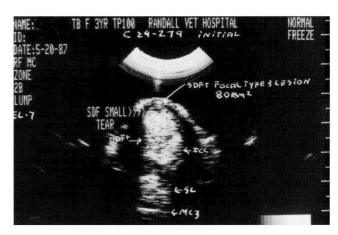

Figure 21.344.

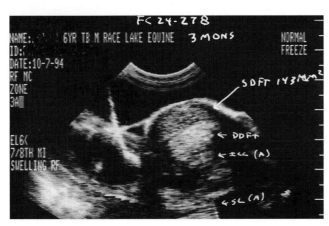

Figure 21.343.

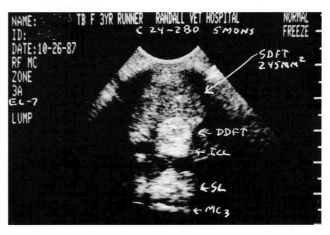

Figure 21.345.

Figure 21.346 is a cross-sectional right metacarpal Zone 3A SDFT sonogram of the same horse shown in Figures 21.344 and 21.345 made 8 months after injury and 3 months at EL-3. The scan reveals a marked improvement of the echogenicity; however, the SQR is unfavorable for RTR because of randomly oriented intratendinous and peritendinous fibrosis. Had the original lesion been managed differently, this tendon would not have progressed to this extent and the prognosis to RTR would most likely have been more favorable.

Figure 21.347 is a cross-sectional left metacarpal Zone 3A SDFT sonogram of a Thoroughbred that was unraced and at EL-6. The scan shows a focal, Type 3 midpalmar tendon margin lesion. The lesion comprised 21% of the CSA. The MIZ-CSA was 142 mm^2 and the six-level T-CSA was 730 mm^2. The T-HYP was 94 mm^2 or 13%T-HYP. The MIZ-FS was 3 and the T-FS was 10. The horse was removed from training and followed a conventional treatment of 6 months' pasture confinement with pin-firing and a series of three external blisters.

Figure 21.348 is a cross-sectional left metacarpal Zone 3B SDFT sonogram of the same horse shown in Figure 21.347 made 6 months after injury at EL-3. The scan shows a Type 2 fibrous lesion repair with some palmar peritendinous fibrosis. This is considered a delayed or poor quality fibrous tissue response consisting of immature small diameter collagen (weak) or randomly arranged collagen fibers (weak) or continuing low-grade tendonitis. The hypoechoic fiber bundles comprised 15% of the CSA at this level. The T-HYP for five of the six levels was 118 mm^2, or 17% T-HYP. This percent is higher than the original injury. The MIZ-CSA (Zone 3A) was increased to 155 mm^2 and the T-CSA was 696 mm^2, which is lower than the initial calculation. The MIZ-FS was decreased to 1 and the T-FS was 9. For the elapsed time and EL, the SQR is poor for almost all parameters. This finding dictates a reduction or maintenance of the same EL and additional time. Most certainly, these data *do not* justify an EL increase. The trainer entered the horse in training against advice.

Figure 21.349 is a cross-sectional left metacarpal SDFT Zone 3B sonogram of the same horse shown in Figures 21.347 and 21.348 made 7 months after injury at EL-5 for only 3 days. The scan shows a large Type 3 midpalmar tendon lesion in exactly the same area of the previously noted weak fiber repair. The lesion comprised 44% of the CSA. The five-level T-HYP was 309 mm^2, or 35%T-HYP. The MIZ-CSA was 230 mm^2 and the T-CSA was 887 mm^2. The MIZ-FS was 3 and the T-FS was 13.

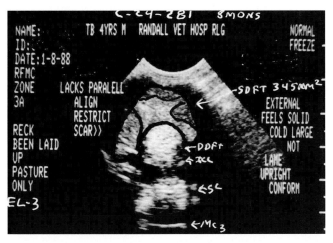

Figure 21.346.

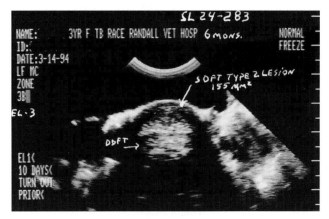

Figure 21.348.

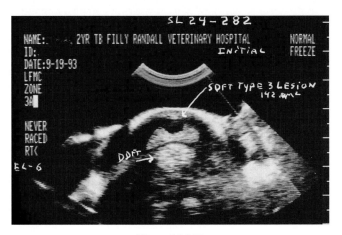

Figure 21.347.

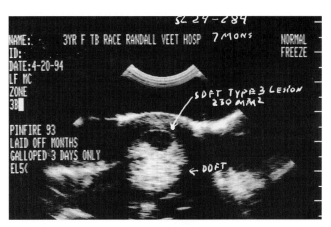

Figure 21.349.

Figure 21.350 is a cross-sectional left metacarpal Zone 3B SDFT sonogram of a racing Thoroughbred with focal palmar distal swelling. The filly was purchased recently and had been racing regularly. The scan shows a focal Type 3 palmar-medial tendon lesion with surrounding, diffuse, Type 1 tendinitis and subcutaneous edema/hemorrhage. Focal fiber tearing and diffuse tendinitis were diagnosed. The lesion was present in three other zones to a lesser degree. The MIZ-CSA (3B) was 121 mm^2 and the five-level T-CSA was 493 mm^2. The T-HYP was 37 mm^2. The trainer was given options of long-range treatment and rehabilitation or symptomatic treatment and continuedracing. The trainer decided to allow a short time off in an attempt to salvage the racing year for new owners. The horse was allowed EL-1 for 6 weeks and an external blister was applied.

Figure 21.351 is a cross-sectional left metacarpal Zone 3B sonogram of the same horse shown in Figure 21.350 made after 2 races 2 weeks apart. Both performances were poor. The scan shows that the focal lesion is slightly more echogenic (Type 2), but more diffusely distributed along the palmar medial tendon. The MIZ-CSA had increased to 171 mm^2 and the five-level T-CSA has increased to 728 mm^2. The T-HYP was increased to 146 mm^2. The trainer decided

against continuing to race because, even with a modified training program and better race selection, the horse was nonproductive and tendon injury was increasing. The trainer decided to enter long-range therapy. The horse was pin-fired and eventually turned out (EL-3). The horse was given 5 months at EL-3 and 2 weeks at EL-4.

Figure 21.352 is a cross-sectional left metacarpal Zone 3B sonogram of the same horse shown in Figures 21.350 and 21.351. The scan shows a smaller, persistent, focal Type 2 lesion. The MIZ-CSA was reduced significantly to 133 mm^2. The five-level T-CSA decreased to 526 mm^2. The T-HYP was 114 mm^2.

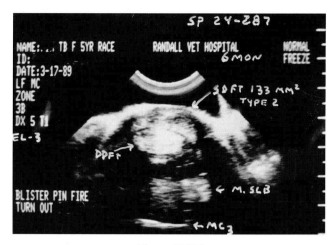

Figure 21.352.

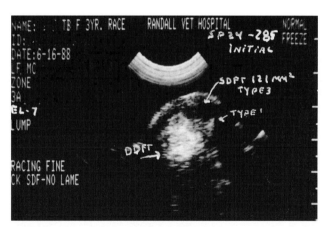

Figure 21.350.

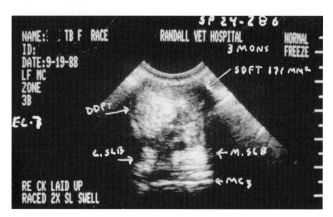

Figure 21.351.

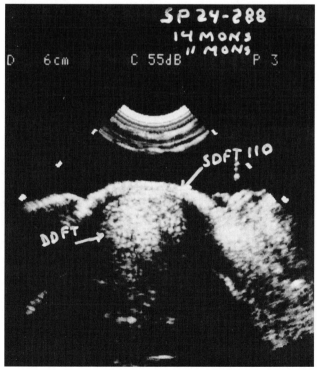

Figure 21.353.

Figure 21.353 is a cross-sectional left metacarpal Zone 3B sonogram of the same horse shown in Figures 21.350 to 21.352 made 14 months after the initial sonographic examination. The horse had raced over 20 times since the 5½-month lay-off. The scan shows a slight, medial, SDFT margin enlargement with a slight decrease in texture quality. The MIZ-CSA was decreased to 110 mm² at EL-7.

Figure 21.354 is a cross-sectional left metacarpal Zone 3B sonogram of the same horse shown in Figures 21.350 to 21.353 made 24 months after the original examination. The horse had raced 40 times before this scan and 20 times after this scan. The scan shows persistent, palmar-medial Type 2 fibers. The MIZ-CSA has remained stable 2 years after injury even though this lesion never attained isoechogenicity. The most significant parameter, in this case, was the CSA stability attained once the EL was reduced. This horse was well managed and the trainer was extremely compliant once his initial efforts to continue racing failed.

Figure 21.355 is a cross-sectional right metacarpal Zone 3A SDFT sonogram of a racing Thoroughbred that had competed on a regular basis for the past 3 years. The horse

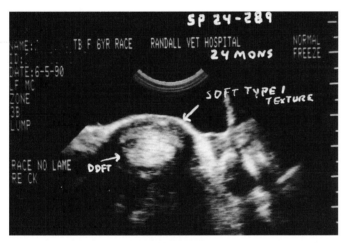

Figure 21.354.

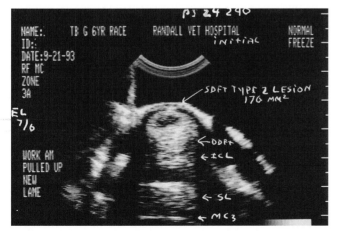

Figure 21.355.

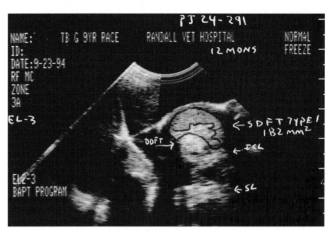

Figure 21.356.

was examined for a post-EL-6 lameness and swelling. The scan shows a Type 3 SDFT core lesion that was identified at 3 levels. The MIZ-CSA was 176 mm² and the six-level T-CSA was 722 mm². The T-HYP was 51 mm² or 7% T-HYP for the 6 levels. The MIZ-FS was 3 and the T-FS was 5. The acute inflammation was treated symptomatically for 2 weeks. After this period, the horse was externally blistered and turned out (EL-3) for 1 year.

Figure 21.356 is a cross-sectional right metacarpal Zone 3A sonogram of the same horse shown in Fig. 21.355 made 12 months after injury at EL-3. The scan reveals SDFT enlargement with a diffuse, 61% Type 1 fiber texture of the cross-sectional area. Type 1 tendon fibers could be identified in four zones. The six-level T-HYP was 181 mm² or 24%T-HYP. The MIZ-CSA was 182 mm², increased from 176 mm². The T-CSA was also slightly increased from 722 mm² to 770 mm². The MIZ-FS was 2 and the T-FS was 7. In this case, all sonographic parameters are basically inferior to 1 year post-injury evaluations at EL-3 that successfully RTR. The FS is elevated, the CSA has not decreased below the original injury values, and the percent hypoechoic fibers (weak or random distribution) has significantly increased. Sonography has truly advanced tendon management to a more sophisticated level. This client chose not to risk reinjury in a potentially futile attempt to race. The trainer decided to use this horse for an alternate, less stressful, occupation.

CONCLUSION

Fiber disruption can occur in several patterns; however, these patterns have some consistency. The core lesion is an example of this. Injury patterns that occur may eventually correlate to the athletic use of the horse. This might suggest a specific physiologic process that is associated with a given athletic function. Goodship has addressed the core lesion and suggests that temperature changes within the center of the SDFT may play a role in this injury in racehorses (23). Correlating common lesion locations with a specific athletic function can ultimately result in a better understanding of tendon injury pathogenesis. Prevention programs might reduce the injury rate. For instance, anecdotally, at least, it seems that central core lesions are more common in Thoroughbred racehorses, whereas peripheral lesions seem more common in Standardbred racehorses. The next decade will see great advances in scar manipulation during rehabilitation and will hopefully return more horses to performance. At present, early diagnosis and treatment of tendon injuries are the keys to a successful return to performance. Serial ultrasonographic monitoring of tendon injuries allows more accurate decisions regarding increasing or decreasing exercise levels during rehabilitation. The fairly predictable stages of tendon healing discussed in this chapter should preclude returning horses to training and racing too soon. Finally, in our opinion, it is no longer valid to assess tendon injuries by inspection and palpation only.

REFERENCES

1. Rantanen NW. The use of diagnostic ultrasound in limb disorders of the horse: a preliminary report. J Equine Vet Sci 1982;2:62–64.
2. Hauser ML, Rantanen NW, Modransky PD. Ultrasound examination of the distal interphalangeal joint, navicular bursa, navicular bone and deep digital tendon. J Equine Vet Sci 1982;2:95–97.
3. Hauser ML, Rantanen NW. Ultrasound appearance of the palmar metacarpal soft tissues of the horse. J Equine Vet Sci 1983; 3:19–22.
4. Modransky PD, Rantanen NW, Hauser ML, et al. Diagnostic ultrasound examination of the dorsal aspect of the equine metacarpophalangeal joint. J Equine Vet Sci 1983;3:56–58.
5. Rantanen NW, Genovese R L, Gaines RD. The use of diagnostic ultrasound to detect structural damage to the soft tissues of the extremities of horses. J Equine Vet Sci 1983;3:134–135.
6. Hauser ML, Rantanen NW. Ultrasound appearance of the palmar metacarpal soft tissues of the horse. J Equine Vet Sci 1983; 3:19–22.
7. Lamb CL, Stowater JL, Pipers FS. The first twenty-one years of veterinary diagnostic ultrasound. Vet Radiol 1988;29:37–45.
8. Reef VB, Martin BB, Elser A. types of tendon and ligament injuries detected with diagnostic ultrasound: description and follow-up. Proceedings 34th Annual Meeting. American Association of Equine Practitioners, 1988; 245–248.
9. Spurlock GH, Spurlock SL, Parker GA. Ultrasonographic, gross and histologic evaluation of a tendinitis disease model in a horse. Vet Radiol 1989;30:184–188.
10. Genovese RL, Rantanen NW, Hauser ML, et al. The use of ultrasonography in the diagnosis and management of injuries to the equine limb. Compend Contin Educ Pract Vet 1987; 9:945–957.
11. Reef VB, Martin BB, Stebbins K. Comparison of ultrasonographic, gross and histologic appearance of tendon injuries in performance horses. Proceedings 35th Annual Meeting. American Association of Equine Practitioners, 1989;279.
12. Genovese RL, Rantanen NW, Simpson BS. Clinical experience with quantitative analysis of superficial digital flexor tendon injuries in thoroughbred and standardbred racehorses. Vet Clin North Am Equine Pract 1990;6:129–145.
13. Genovese RL. Prognosis of superficial flexor tendon and suspensory ligament injuries. Proceedings 39th Annual Meeting. American Association of Equine Practitioners 1993;17–19.
14. Reef VB. Evaluation of tendon and ligaments. In: Robinson NE, ed. Current therapy in equine medicine 3. Philadelphia: WB Saunders, 1991;796–798.
15. Chvapil M. Present status of the pharmacology of fibrosis and scar contractures. First Annual Dubai International Equine Symposium. Dubai, UAE. 395–406, 1996
16. Davis, WM. The clinical application of scar remodeling in disease states. Proceedings First Annual Dubai International Equine Symposium, Dubai, UAE, 1996;407–416.
17. Reef VB, Genovese RL, Byrd JW, et al. Treatment of superficial digital flexor tendon injuries with beta-aminoproprionitrile fumarate (BAPN-F): sonographic evaluation of early tendon healing and remodeling. Proceedings First Annual Dubai International Equine Symposium, Dubai, UAE, 1996;423–30.
18. Genovese RL, Reef VB, Longo KL, et al. Superficial digital flexor tendinitis—long term sonographic and clinical study of racehorses. Proceedings First Annual Dubai International Equine Symposium, Dubai, UAE, 1996;187–205.
19. Gillis C. Tendon and ligament rehabilitation. Proceedings First Annual Dubai International Equine Symposium, Dubai, UAE 1996;417–421.
20. Genovese RL, Rantanen NW, Hauser ML, et al. Diagnostic ultrasonography of equine limbs. Vet Clin North Am Equine Pract 1986;2:145–226.
21. Denoix JM. Functional anatomy of tendons and ligaments in the distal limbs (manus and pes). Vet Clin North Am Equine Pract 1994;10:323–349.
22. Dik K, van den Belt AJM, Keg PR. Ultrasonographic evaluation of fetlock annular ligament constriction in the horse. Eq Vet Jour 1991;23:285–288.
23. Goodship AE, Birch HL, Wilson AM. The pathobiology and repair of tendon and ligament injury. Vet Clin North Am Equine Pract 1994;10:323–349.
24. Goodship AE. 33rd BEVA Congress. 1994.
25. Peacock EE, Van Winkle W. In: Surgery and biology of wound repair. WB Saunders, 1970;331–348.
26. Buck RC. J Pathol Bacteriol 1953.
27. Silver IA, Goodship AE, et al. A clinical and experimental study of tendon injury healing and treatment in the horse. Eq Vet Jour (Suppl) 1. Section A, 1983.
28. Redding WR. Evaluation of the equine digital flexor tendon sheath using diagnostic ultrasound and contrast radiography. Vet Radiol Ultrasound 1994;35:42–48.
29. Denoix JM, Crevier N, Azevedo C. Ultrasound examination of the pastern. Proceedings 37th Annual Meeting. American Association of Equine Practitioners, 1991;363–380.
30. Redding WR. Sonographic examination of the structures of the digital sheath. Proceedings 39th Annual Meeting. American Association of Equine Practitioners, 1993;11–15.
31. Dik KJ, Boroffka S, Stolk P. Ultrasonographic assessment of the proximal annular ligament in the equine forelimb. Eq Vet Jour 1994;26:59–64.
32. Gillis C, Meagher D. Tendon response to training. Equine Athlete 1991;4:26–27.

22. The Deep Digital Flexor Tendon, Carpal Sheath, and Accessory Ligament of the Deep Digital Flexor Tendon (Inferior Check Ligament)

RONALD L. GENOVESE AND NORMAN W. RANTANEN

INTRODUCTION

Deep digital flexor tendon (DDFT) injuries are less common than superficial digital flexor (SDFT) injuries or suspensory ligament (third interosseous muscle or TIOM) injuries. Accessory ligament of the deep digital flexor tendon (ALDDFT) injuries are rarely found except in older sport horses. Because the carpal sheath is intimately associated with all of the above, it deserves discussion as a structure secondarily involved in a variety of injuries. All of the basic principles developed for the SDFT in Chapter 21 certainly are valid for the DDFT and ALDDFT. The theme emphasizing initial accurate sonographic and clinical diagnoses, short-term follow-up examinations to ascertain more accurate prognoses, well-planned rehabilitation programs, and serial sonographic and clinical monitoring schedules must be followed with any soft tissue support structure injury. Arbitrary treatment and management decisions based on history and physical examination alone are fortunately becoming a thing of the past.

THE NORMAL DEEP DIGITAL FLEXOR TENDON

The normal, sonographically accessible fore deep digital flexor tendon (DDFT) can be scanned from the accessory carpal bone level to the distal one third of the pastern. The DDFT insertion onto the distal phalanx is inaccessible to sonographic evaluation. Unlike the superficial digital flexor tendon (SDFT), textural abnormalities secondary to scanning artifact are more commonly seen during DDFT sonographic examination. Therefore, one should become familiar with these common artifactual echolucent areas when evaluating DDFT textural abnormalities. The DDFT is bounded on its palmar surface by the SDFT in the metacarpus and at the metacarpophalangeal joint level. In the pastern, the SDFT is adjacent to the DDFT palmar surface only in the proximal fourth (2 to 3 cm distal to the ergot). Distally in the pastern, the palmar DDFT surface is subcutaneous. In the proximal half to two-thirds of the metacarpus, the DDFT is bounded dorsally by the carpal sheath and the accessory ligament of the DDFT (ALDDFT). In Zone 1A (0 to 4 cm distal to the accessory carpal bone (DACB), the DDFT is triangular to round-shaped.

Figure 22.1 is a cross-sectional and sagittal Zone 1A (3 cm DACB) sonogram of a normal 15.3-hand Thoroughbred (TB) racehorse. The DDFT is slightly triangular shaped and

no textural artifacts are seen. The computer determined cross-sectional area (CSA) to be 80 mm^2. The SDFT is seen on the palmar surface and a slightly, but considered normal, distended carpal sheath is seen dorsally. Dorsal to the carpal sheath is the rectangular shaped ALDDFT. The ALDDFT CSA is 73 mm^2. Both the DDFT and the ALDDFT have 100% parallel fiber alignment. Closer cross-sectional view inspection reveals a thin, horizontal, focal hypoechoic dorsal medial border artifact not to be confused with a lesion.

Figure 22.2 is a normal cross-sectional and sagittal left metacarpal Zone 1B (6 cm DCAB) sonogram. The DDFT is rounder with a uniform texture. The palmar border is bounded by the SDFT and the dorsal surface bounded by the ALDDFT CSA is 81 mm^2. The ALDDFT is rectangular shaped and has a 52 mm^2 CSA.

Figure 22.3 is a normal cross-sectional and sagittal left metacarpal Zone 2A (9 cm DCAB) sonogram. The DDFT is oval shaped and the ALDDFT is rectangular. The DDFT and the ALDDFT have a uniform texture. The DDFT CSA is 87 mm^2 and the ALDDFT is 69 mm^2. At this level, there is a distinct DDFT/ALDDFT interface.

Figure 22.4 is a normal cross-sectional and sagittal left metacarpal Zone 2B (13 cm DCAB) sonogram. The DDFT is slightly oval and there is intimate contact between it and the ALDDFT, however, a distinct sonographic interface is still appreciated. The DDFT CSA is 75 mm^2 and the ALDDFT is 59 mm^2.

Figure 22.5 is a normal cross-sectional and sagittal left metacarpal Zone 3A (16 cm DCAB) sonogram. The DDFT is oval and the ALDDFT is crescent shaped. The DDFT CSA is 92 mm^2 and the ALDDFT is 47 mm^2. The DDFT/ALDDFT interface may or may not be visible. At the suspensory ligament (interosseous muscle, TIOM) bifurcation in Zone 3A, the ALDDFT inserts into the DDFT. This insertion can cause some error in normal CSA measurement. In this case, the DDFT and ALDDFT borders are visible and separate CSA measurements were made. The DDFT CSA is 92 mm^2 and the ALDDFT is 47 mm^2. DDFT CSA increased at this level. In some normal horses, however, the ALDDFT is not separate from the DDFT, and the CSA is larger.

Figure 22.6 is a normal cross-sectional and sagittal left metacarpal Zone 3B (21 cm DCAB) sonogram. The DDFT is distinctly oval and the ALDDFT is no longer seen as a separate structure. The DDFT CSA is 122 mm^2.

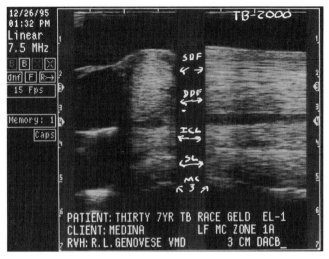

Figure 22.1.

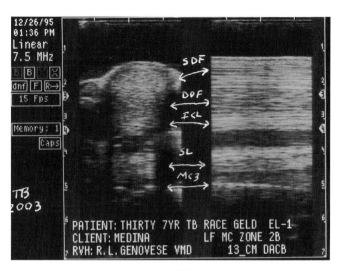

Figure 22.4.

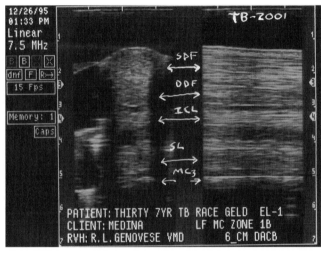

Figure 22.2.

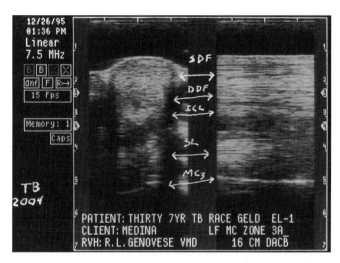

Figure 22.5.

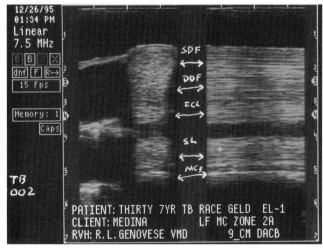

Figure 22.3.

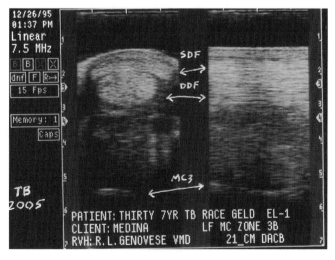

Figure 22.6.

Figure 22.7 is a normal cross-sectional and sagittal left metacarpophalangeal joint Zone 3C (24 cm DCAB) sonogram. The DDFT is oval, the SDFT is on its palmar surface, and the DDFT dorsal surface is bounded by the proximal sesamoid bone apices and the sesamoidian ligament. In this figure, there is a central-dorsal DDFT echolucent scanning artifact. During the real time sonographic examination, this reduced echogenicity is commonly produced. It is caused by the tendon fiber curvature as it passes over the palmar fetlock. In real time, sections are viewed independently for textural evaluation, but it may not be possible to produce one image that accurately displays the density of all the structures. Multiple cross-sectional views may be required at this and more distal levels to present the true textural evaluation. The CSA of the DDFT at this level is 148 mm².

As with the SDFT, the CSA of the levels can be summed to estimate a "volume" of sonographically accessible DDFT and ALDDFT. When this is done, it consistently provides information relative to a decrease or increase in size of the tendon. It is referred to as total cross-sectional area, or T-CSA. In the normal example, the 7 level DDFT T-CSA is 685 mm². The 5 level T-CSA of the ALDDFT is 300 mm². The reader is referred to Chapter 21 for an in-depth discussion of basic CSA, texture, position, and fiber alignment concepts derived for the superficial digital flexor that apply to the DDFT in most instances.

The ability to obtain single-view, accurate textural information of the DDFT in the palmar/plantar pastern is even more difficult than in the metacarpus/metatarsus. Multiple cross-sectional views are often required. At times, because of fiber angulation, pastern conformation, and transducer configuration, it is not possible to obtain an artifact-free cross-sectional DDFT sonogram. This problem can cause interpretation error; however, clinical evaluation, CSA values, and sagittal views help to assess the DDFT accurately.

Figure 22.8 is a cross-sectional and sagittal left pastern Zone P1A sonogram of a Thoroughbred (2 cm distal to the ergot) in which the DDFT is elliptical. Its palmar surface is

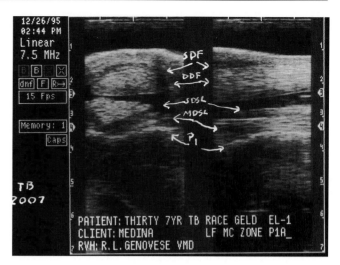

Figure 22.8.

bordered by the SDFT and the dorsal surface is bordered by the superficial distal or straight sesamoidian ligament (SDSL). In this figure, slight distal tendon sheath distention is visible between the DDFT and the SDSL. Commonly, there is artifactual echolucency of the DDFT mid-dorsally and medially. However, the shape and size of the DDFT is normal. The DDFT CSA is 108 mm².

Figure 22.9 is a cross-sectional and sagittal left palmar Zone P1B pastern sonogram (4 cm distal to the ergot in mid P1). The DDFT is elliptical and the CSA is 110 mm². Figure 22.10 is a cross-sectional and sagittal left palmar pastern Zone P1C sonogram (6 cm distal to the ergot). At this level, the DDFT is subcutaneous between the abaxial SDFT branches. The SDSL borders its dorsal surface. The DDFT has a bilobed shape and the CSA is 98 mm². Figure 22.11 is a cross-sectional and sagittal left pastern Zone P2A sonogram (8 cm distal to the ergot) in which the DDFT is enlarged but the appearance is bilobed. The DDFT is bordered on its dorsal surface by the scutum medium of the second phalanx. The DDFT CSA is 157 mm² and the 4 level T-CSA is 473 mm².

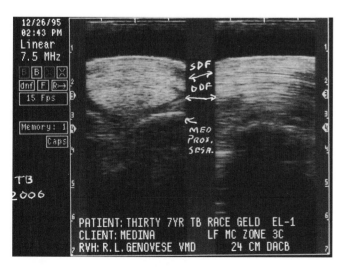

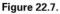
Figure 22.7.

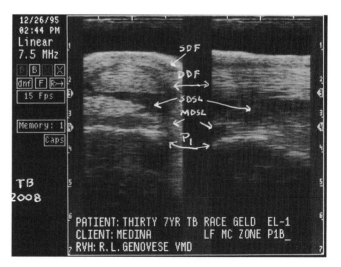

Figure 22.9.

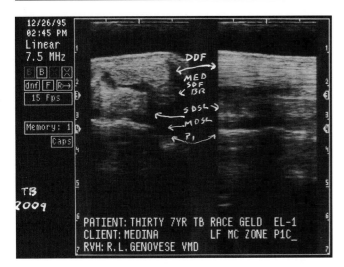

Figure 22.10.

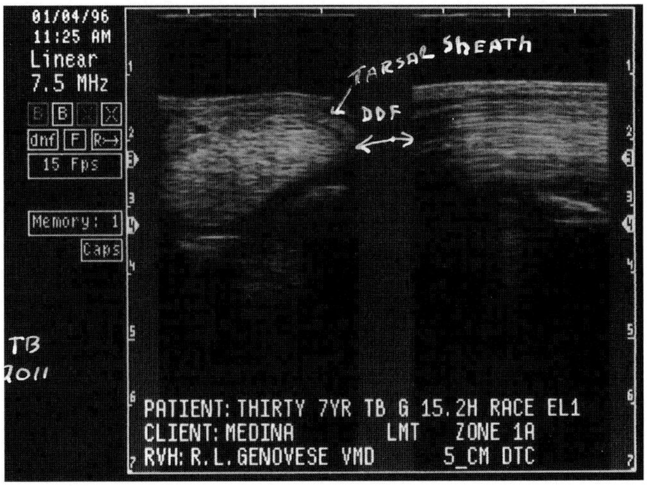

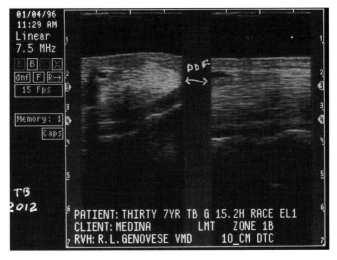

Figure 22.12.

These normal DDFT and ALDDFT CSA data are from a single, clinically normal horse obtained by a specific method. These values may vary between horses, and the reader is referred to Chapter 21 for a discussion of CSA measurement techniques for the SDFT. In this instance, the CSA information is valid for this normal horse.

In the hindlimb, the DDFT is derived from a group of muscles that join at various levels near the hock. The DDFT is mostly intact in the crus about 4 to 8 cm proximal to the tuber calcaneous. However, some muscle fibers extend distally into the proximal metatarsus. The sonographic importance of this is that hypoechoic muscle bundles may be seen when examining the DDFT in the plantar talus and may cause confusion. Usually, the DDFT cannot be imaged on a midline scan of the upper half of the plantar talus because of its medial location. The transducer must be rotated medially to obtain an image as it courses laterally to its plantar midmetatarsus position.

Figure 22.12 is a normal cross-sectional and sagittal left talus Zone 1A sonogram (5 cm distal to the tuber calcaneous [DTC]). The transducer was rotated medially to obtain the image. At this level, the DDFT is subcutaneous and is surrounded by the tarsal sheath. The DDFT is oval and the CSA is 248 mm². Artifactual echolucency of the dorsal axial border is present. Figure 22.13 is a normal cross-sectional and sagittal left talus Zone 1B sonogram (10 cm DTC). The transducer is positioned medially over the DDFT. The tendon is oval and the CSA is 229 mm². There is a dorsal, axial margin Type 3 area in the DDFT most likely caused by hypoechoic muscle bundles.

Figure 22.14 is a normal cross-sectional and sagittal left metatarsal Zone 2A sonogram (18 cm DTC). The DDFT is round in this midline sonogram and positioned towards the medial aspect. The SDFT is on its plantar border and the rudimentary ALDDFT is on its dorsal border. The DDFT CSA is 138 mm². Figure 22.15 is a normal cross-sectional

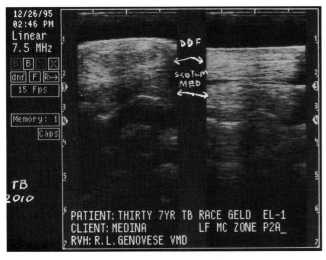

Figure 22.11.

Figure 22.13.

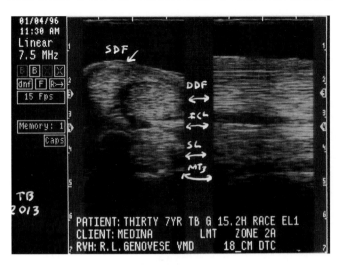

Figure 22.14.

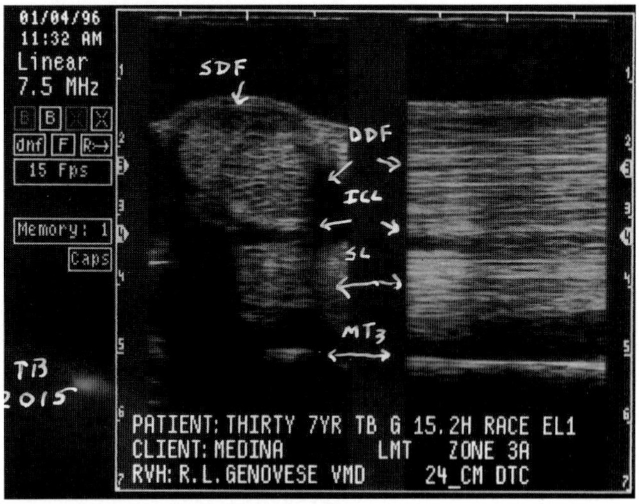

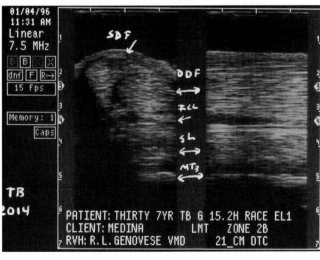

Figure 22.15.

and sagittal left metatarsal Zone 2B sonogram (21 cm DTC). The DDFT is round and the CSA is 129 mm^2. Figure 22.16 is a normal cross-sectional and sagittal left metatarsal Zone 3A sonogram (24 cm DTC). The DDFT is round and has a 107 mm^2 CSA. Figure 22.17 is a normal cross-sectional and sagittal left metatarsal Zone 3B sonogram (27 cm DTC). The DDFT is round and the CSA is 125 mm^2. The small ALDDFT is still present and distinct from the DDFT. Figure 22.18 is a normal cross-sectional and sagittal left metatarsal Zone 4A sonogram (30 cm DTC). This sonogram shows the level of the suspensory ligament bifurcation and the point at which the ALDDFT and the DDFT join. The DDFT CSA is 122 mm^2. In this horse, the ALDDFT is still a sonographically distinct structure. Figure 22.19 is a cross-sectional and sagittal left metatarsal Zone 4B sonogram (36 cm DTC). The DDFT is oval and the CSA is 164 mm^2. As in the forelimb, at this level, an artifactually produced, slight echolucency of the mid-dorsal

DDFT surface is present. Figure 22.20 is a normal cross-sectional and sagittal left plantar metatarsophalangeal joint sonogram. The DDFT is elliptical and has a CSA of 182 mm^2. Artifactual echolucency of the mid-dorsal DDFT aspect is present. The 9-level DDFT T-CSA is 144 mm^2. More commonly, however, seven metatarsal levels are measured which, in this horse, is 967 mm^2.

DDFT Abnormalities

Figure 22.21 is a normal dual cross-sectional right metacarpal Zone 3B sonogram. The SDFT is normally crescent shaped and the palmar tendon sheath is not clearly visible. The DDFT has a normal elliptical shape and is located dorsal to the SDFT. The mid-dorsal DDFT aspect has an artifactual hypoechoic texture. The tendon sheath dorsal to the DDFT surface is not visible. There is no increased tendon sheath fluid. The palmar to dorsal (PD) SDFT mea-

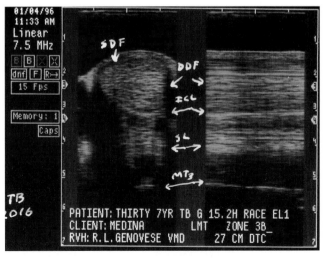

Figure 22.16.

Figure 22.17.

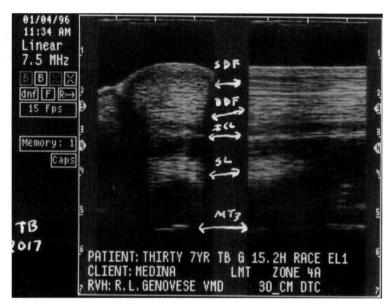

Figure 22.18.

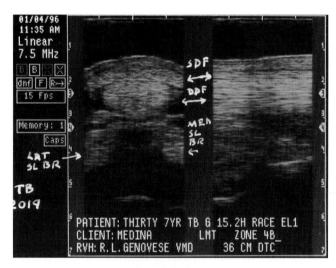

Figure 22.19.

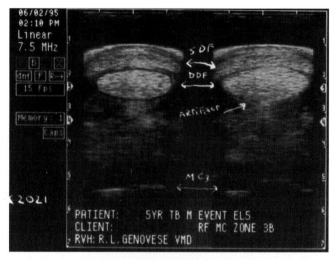

Figure 22.21.

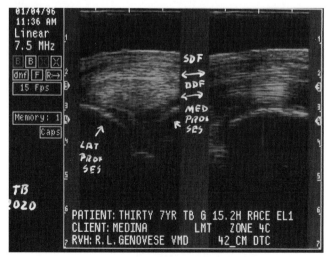

Figure 22.20.

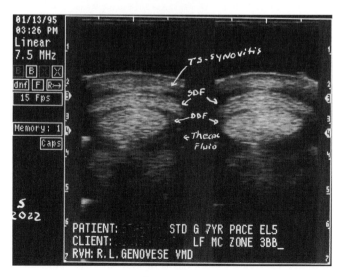

Figure 22.22.

surement is 5 mm. The PD DDFT measurement is 11 mm. The SDFT to DDFT ratio is five, which is normal according to a study of Warmblood horses reported by Dik (1). There are no sonographic tendon or tendon sheath abnormalities. Figure 22.22 is a dual cross-sectional left metacarpal Zone 3B sonogram. In this scan, there are no tendon abnormalities. The SDFT is 5 mm and the DDFT is 10 mm thick. The SDFT/DDFT ratio is a normal 0.5. There is an increased palmar TS thickness and a slight increase in thecal fluid. Fluid is visible on the dorsal DDFT surface. The diagnosis was a low-grade benign tenosynovitis without tendonitis.

Figure 22.23 is a dual cross-sectional right metacarpal Zone 3B sonogram. In this horse, no tendon abnormalities are present. The SDFT is 0.6 mm and the DDFT is 10 mm thick. The SDFT/DDFT ratio is a normal 0.6. There is no noticeable thickness of the palmar TS; however, slight TS thickening on the dorsal DDFT aspect is present. This sonogram shows an example of a slightly more chronic tenosynovitis.

Figure 22.24 is a cross-sectional left metacarpal Zone 3B sonogram. The SDFT is normal, but the DDFT is more round than normal with a central echolucency. Thecal fluid has increased significantly and TS thickening is apparent. The SDFT/DDFT ratio is a low 0.3, which indicates an increased DDFT CSA. In this horse, there is chronic tenosynovitis with DDFT tendinitis.

Figure 22.25 is a cross-sectional left metacarpal Zone 3B sonogram of a 4-year-old Thoroughbred racehorse with a thickened palmar TS. The SDFT was normal; however, the DDFT is oval and is enlarged with a slight dorsomedial echolucency. The SDFT is 4 mm, the DDFT is 13 mm thick, and the ratio is 0.3, confirming DDF tendonitis.

DDFT injury is rare in Thoroughbred (TB) and Standardbred (STD) racehorses. In our experience, work-related DDFT injuries are more commonly seen in sport horses such as polo ponies or eventing horses. Figure 22.26 is a dual

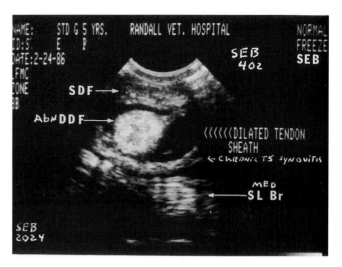

Figure 22.24.

cross-sectional Zone 3B sonogram of the left and right metacarpals of a Thoroughbred racehorse with left fore tendon swelling at the junction of the middle and distal thirds. The horse was not lame but was slightly sensitive to direct tendon palpation. The right fore cross-sectional sonogram is normal. The SDFT CSA is 77 mm^2 and the DDFT is 122 mm^2. The SDFT/DDFT ratio is 0.7. No definitive shape or textural abnormalities of the left fore SDFT or DDFT are present. The SDFT CSA is similar to the right leg at about 80 mm^2 (4% CSA increase). The DDFT CSA is 136 mm^2, which is increased by 9%. The SDFT/DDFT ratio is 0.6. The CSA difference between the right and left DDF tendons seems equivocal; however, DDFT strain can be a subtle finding. As in SDFT injury, there may be only a DDFT CSA increase with low-grade tendinitis. This finding is especially true of low grade DDFT injury around the metacarpo/metatarsophalangeal joints. In this horse, slight swelling was noted by the trainer. A diagnosis of mild DDFT strain was made. The horse was treated with anti-in-

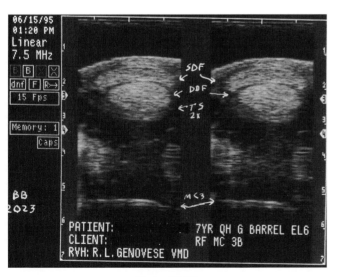

Figure 22.23.

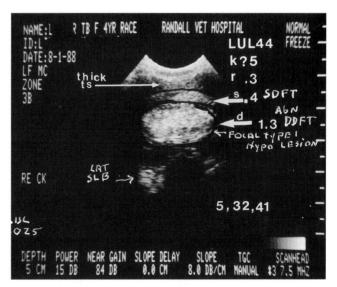

Figure 22.25.

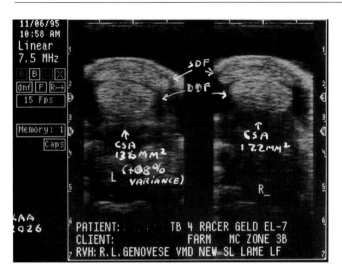

Figure 22.26.

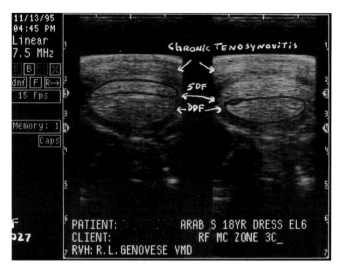

Figure 22.27.

flammatory medication, corrective shoeing, and several weeks rest from work. It made an uneventful recovery.

Distal metacarpal/metatarsal swelling is caused most frequently by TS filling. An associated lameness may or may not be present, and careful sonographic assessment of the TS, SDFT, and DDFT is indicated. Because of the high probability of DDFT scanning artifact in these zones, textural abnormalities may be difficult to assess. One can rely heavily on CSA measurement. Careful consideration should be given to both the absolute DDFT values and the SDFT/DDFT ratio. Because the DDFT size and shape changes from Zone 3A to the first pastern zone, exact level CSA comparisons to the opposite normal limb need to be made. In these evaluations, careful measurements from the base of the accessory carpal bone (DACB) help provide accurate level location for comparison.

For example, consider this clinical presentation. An 18-year-old Arab school horse was presented with the complaint of low-grade right fore leg lameness. The horse had chronic bilateral forelimb tenosynovitis for the past several years and had never been lame. Right fore digital tendon sheath anesthesia relieved the discomfort. Figure 22.27 is a dual cross-sectional right palmar metacarpophalangeal joint sonogram. There was no apparent DDFT textural or shape abnormality. Chronic TS thickening is present. Cross-sectional areas of both fore limbs were obtained.

	Left	Abn. Right	Variance
SDFT T-CSA (7 levels)	438 mm²	480 mm²	+10%
SDFT (3B, 3C)	160 mm²	160 mm²	0
SDFT (3C)	80 mm²	78 mm²	−2%
DDFT T-CSA (7 levels)	630 mm²	635 mm²	+ <1%
DDFT (3B, 3C)	223 mm²	252 mm²	+13%
DDFT(3C)	112 mm²	151 mm²	+35%

Using the measurements, this horse has a significant 35% CSA Zone 3C DDFT increase compatible with low grade

tendinitis. Because the DDFT is firmly bound dorsally by the proximal sesamoid bones and the SDFT and annular ligament (AL) palmarly, discomfort secondary to tendon swelling is likely.

When gross DDFT enlargement or an unequivocal textural abnormality occurs, the diagnosis of injury becomes more obvious. Figure 22.28 is a normal cross-sectional right metacarpal Zone 3B sonogram of an 11-year-old quarter horse event horse. The horse had left fore metacarpal tendon swelling and lameness. The right fore DDFT was normal and the CSA is 159 mm². Figure 22.29 is a cross-sectional left metacarpal Zone 3B sonogram of the same horse shown in Figure 22.28. The TS was thickened, and the DDFT was enlarged and slightly oval to round with a Type 2 lateral lesion. The hypoechoic fiber bundles involve 37% of the CSA. The CSA is 271 mm², a 70% increase over the opposite limb. Figure 22.30 is a cross-sectional left metacarpal Zone 3C sonogram of the same horse shown in Figure 22.29. The DDFT fiber injury extended distally. In addition, focal mineralization of the medial cen-

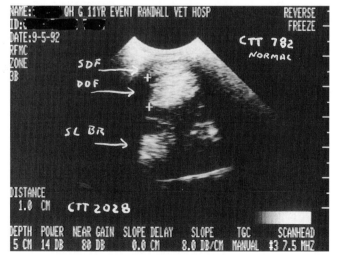

Figure 22.28.

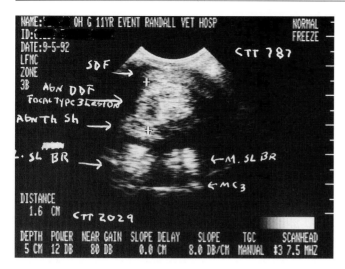

Figure 22.29.

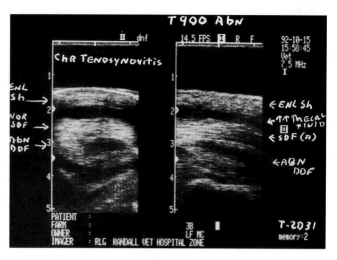

Figure 22.31.

tral aspect of the tendon is present. The mineralization indicates chronicity. This case demonstrates an athletic, use-related focal DDFT injury.

Figure 22.31 is a cross-sectional and sagittal left metacarpophalangeal joint Zone 3C sonogram of a horse presented for chronic tenosynovitis evaluation. Chronic swelling of the distal TS was present, and the owner noted recent lameness. The TS is thickened, and an increase in thecal fluid of the outer sheath compartment was present. The SDFT was normal; however, a large, Type 3 DDFT core lesion is present and loss of palmar border definition has occurred.

Figure 22.32 is a cross-sectional palmar metacarpophalangeal joint Zone 3C sonogram of a Standardbred racehorse with a recent low grade lameness. The horse had previously been rested for an SDFT injury and had been racing well. The SDFT was clinically and sonographically stable. There was a thickened AL, an enlarged SDFT, and an abnormal DDFT with a focal Type 3 mid-dorsal border DDFT lesion. In the area of the lesion, the tendon border

was ill-defined and peritendinous fibrosis was apparent between the DDFT and the intersesamoidean ligament.

Figure 22.33 is a dual cross-sectional left and right metacarpophalangeal joint Zone 3C sonogram of a Thoroughbred hunter with SDFT and DDFT textural abnormalities. The left fore SDFT is enlarged compared with the right and focal hypoechoic fiber bundles are present centrodorsally. Closer inspection reveals a left fore DDFT size increase and a slight shape change from elliptical to oval compared with the normal right tendon. SDFT dorsal and DDFT palmar border definition are decreased. Figure 22.34 is a dual cross-sectional left and right metacarpophalangeal joint Zone 3C sonogram of the same horse shown in Figure 22.33. Diffuse, Type 1 hypoechoic DDFT fiber bundles are present on the central-palmar aspect. The acoustic interface between the SDFT and the DDFT is reduced. The palmar DDFT border is nondistinct and poorly defined. At this level, the right fore DDFT CSA is 164 mm^2 and the left fore CSA is 210 mm^2 (28% increase). In this case, SDFT

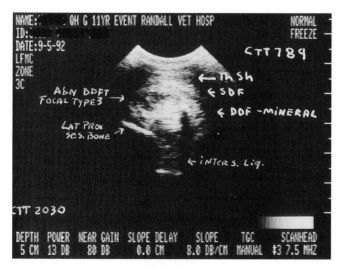

Figure 22.30.

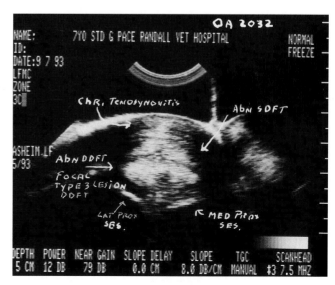

Figure 22.32.

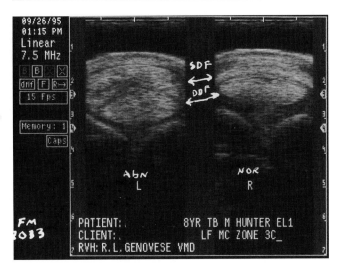

Figure 22.33.

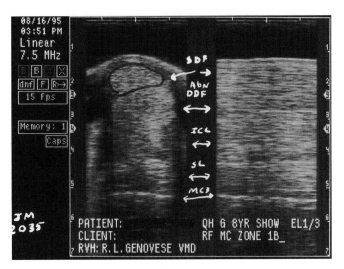

Figure 22.35.

and DDFT injuries are present. In our experience, DDFT work related injury is seen more commonly at the level of the fetlock and pastern than in the metacarpus. However, a primary DDFT injury can occasionally be found in the metacarpus. As a rule, metacarpal injury is more commonly seen in the ALDDFT than in the DDFT. In the hind limb, work related DDFT injury is more common in the metatarsus compared with ALDDFT injuries. This finding suggests that the well developed ALDDFT has a protective role in the forelimb.

Figure 22.35 is a cross-sectional and sagittal right metacarpal Zone 1B sonogram of an 8-year-old quarter horse used for English pleasure. The DDFT was enlarged and had diffuse, Type 1 fiber bundles along the medial aspect. The normal left fore DDFT CSA for this level is 125 mm² and the right fore is 218 mm² (74% increase). The hypoechoic fibers are 22% of this CSA. This is the maximum injury zone (MIZ). The left fore five level T-CSA is 592 mm² and the right fore five level T-CSA is 794 mm² (34% increase).

Distal DDFT injury commonly has poor repair with traditional treatment regimens. Moderate to severe lesion fiber repair commonly produces a scar that cannot withstand athletic use. Figure 22.36 is a cross-sectional left metacarpal Zone 3B sonogram of a 5-year-old quarter horse used for English pleasure that had a painful palmar fetlock injury. The horse had a noticeable contracted DDFT conformation of the affected limb. The horse had a sudden onset of lameness. A large, Type 3 central DDFT lesion was present in zones 3B and 3C. The maximum injury zone (MIZ) was 3B, which had 16% compromised fibers. The normal right fore DDFT CSA was 128 mm² and the left DDFT was 250 mm² (95% increase). The horse was given stall rest and had corrective shoeing. Figure 22.37 is a cross-sectional left metacarpal Zone 3B sonogram of the same horse shown in Figure 22.36 made 2 months after the original injury. Since the previous sonographic evaluation, the horse had been stall rested and hand walked (EL-1). This scan reveals a persistent, Type 3 DDFT lesion involving 20% of the CSA in

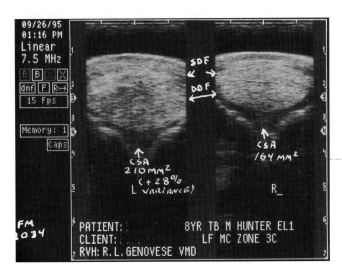

Figure 22.34.

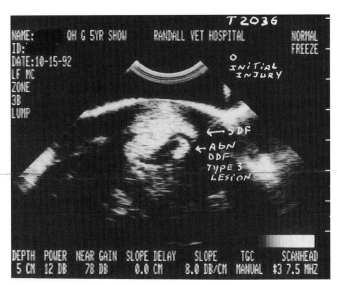

Figure 22.36.

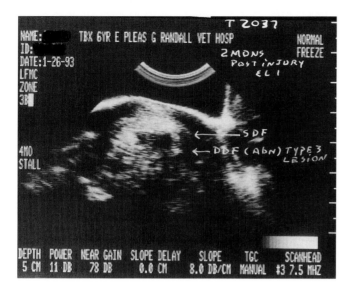

Figure 22.37.

both levels. The MIZ CSA decreased from 250 mm^2 to 200 mm^2 (20% improvement). Figure 22.38 is a cross-sectional left metacarpal Zone 3B sonogram of the same horse shown in Figure 22.37 made 7 months after injury. During the 7 months of rehabilitation, the horse had only been hand walked (EL-1). The sonogram revealed persistent hypoechoic centromedial DDFT tendon fibers. Hypoechoic fibers comprised 20% of the CSA, but the texture improved one grade from Type 3 to Type 2. The CSA is 236 mm^2. Despite 7 months of strictly controlled exercise, this lesion has a poor quality of repair. This horse was eventually used for light trail riding, but had occasional lameness until retirement.

DDFT Pastern Abnormalities

Deep digital flexor tendon pastern abnormalities can be primary or can be a distal extension of more proximal injury.

DDFT injuries can be work related or secondary to traumatic injury. Injury can be isolated to the DDFT or can involve other ligament or tendon injuries. The most commonly injured pastern structure is the SDFT branch(s). However, DDFT injuries do occur, and one of the most common is secondary to palmar digital neurectomy. This injury can be seen as an insidious onset or as acute fiber tearing. As a rule, palmar pastern swelling with some degree of lameness occurs. The low grade swelling and slight lameness can be secondary to neuroma formation, failure of the neurectomy to resolve the pain, and DDF tendinitis. Sonography should be done to detect early DDFT tendinitis and to prevent acute tendon rupture.

Figure 22.39 is a dual cross-sectional left palmar pastern Zone P2A sonogram of a mixed breed gelding. There is a mature subcutaneous fibrous tissue reaction on the palmar DDFT surface. Loss of palmar DDFT border definition is present. In addition, the tendon is enlarged and the shape has changed significantly from bilobed to elliptical. This 10-year-old trail horse had been nerved 2 years previously and had not demonstrated any lameness or significant swelling until recently. These sonographs can be interpreted in two ways: subcutaneous tissue fibrosis with firm adhesions to the palmar DDFT surface, or low-grade DDF tendinitis. Anti-inflammatory medication and corrective shoeing were instituted and this horse made clinical improvement.

Figure 22.40 is a cross-sectional and sagittal left fore palmar pastern Zone P2A sonogram of a quarter horse used for barrel racing. The horse had a palmar digital neurectomy several months previously for chronic palmar foot disease. The horse had marked lameness, pastern swelling, and foot instability. There was sonographic evidence of marked DDFT fiber disruption.

Athletic injury of the distal DDFT can occur without concurrent SDFT injury. This Type of injury may be isolated or may be complicated by TS/AL injury. Figure 22.41 is a cross-sectional left palmar metacarpophalangeal joint Zone 3C sonogram of a 5-year-old quarter horse presented

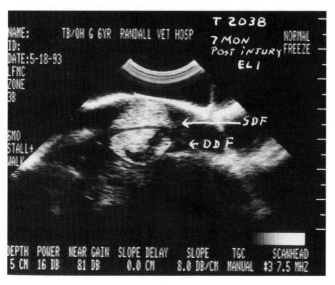

Figure 22.38.

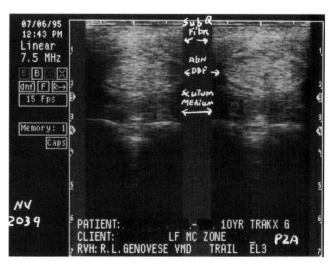

Figure 22.39.

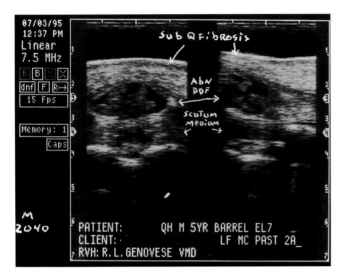

Figure 22.40.

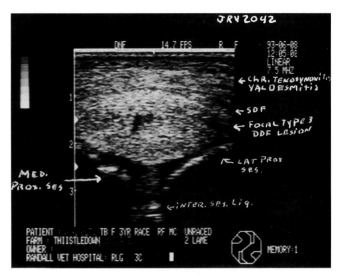

Figure 22.42.

for palmar fetlock swelling. The horse had low-grade lameness. The sonogram indicates a large Type 3 DDFT core defect. There is no sonographic evidence of TS or AL abnormality.

Figure 22.42 is a cross-sectional right palmar metacarpophalangeal joint Zone 3C sonogram of a Thoroughbred racehorse with a similar presentation as the horse shown in Figure 22.41. A Type 3 midpalmar DDFT lesion was present. The SDFT was normal. The TS and AL have thickened significantly. Figure 22.43 is a cross-sectional right palmar Zone P1A pastern sonogram of the same horse shown in Figure 22.42. A focal, Type 3 midpalmar DDFT lesion is present. The SDFT was normal. There is marked palmar TS and AL thickening on the SDFT and what appears to be firm fibrous tissue adhesions to the palmar SDFT border. Echolucent DDFT lesions are common secondary findings to annular ligament constriction. Figure 22.44 is a cross-

sectional right palmar pastern Zone P1B sonogram of the same horse shown in Figure 22.43. The sonogram reveals extension of this lesion into this zone. Palmar border DDFT definition loss is present. In addition, proximal digital annular ligament (PDAL) fibrosis is adjacent to the palmar SDFT surface. The SDFT was normal at this level. In this horse, not only DDFT injury, but concomitant AL and PDAL injury, are present. This finding may affect the treatment decisions in this case as opposed to the previous case.

More subtle swelling and lameness caused by DDFT injury, as seen in the fetlock, can be seen in the pastern. Figure 22.45 is a normal dual cross-sectional left fore palmar pastern Zone P1C sonogram of a quarter horse used for trail riding. The DDFT is a normal, slightly bilobed shape. The borders are distinct and the homogeneous echogenicity is normal. Figure 22.46 is a dual cross-sectional right fore palmar pastern Zone P1C sonogram of the same horse shown

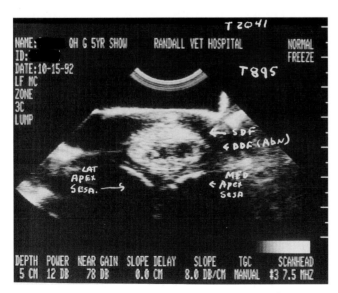

Figure 22.41.

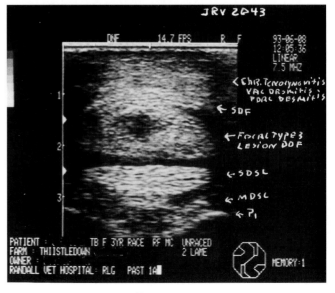

Figure 22.43.

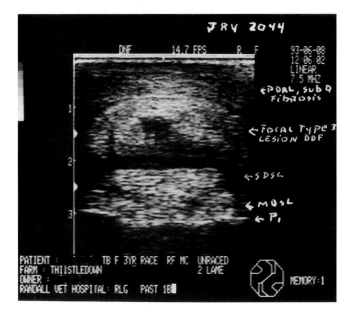

Figure 22.44.

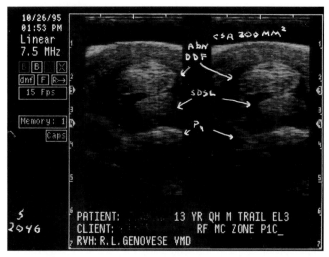

Figure 22.46.

in Figure 22.45. This palmar TS was thickened and thecal fluid was increased. In addition, the DDFT has a more rounded shape and is distinctly, abnormally curved along the palmar border. Slight medial and lateral dorsal border echolucency is present. The normal left DDFT CSA is 144 mm^2 and the right DDFT CSA is 200 mm^2 (38% increase). A diagnosis of chronic tenosynovitis with low grade DDFT tendinitis was made.

Figure 22.47 is a dual cross-sectional left palmar pastern Zone P1A sonogram of a Thoroughbred racehorse. There are no DDFT textural, shape, or CSA abnormalities; however, the tendon is malpositioned relative to the SDSL.

Figure 22.48 is a cross-sectional right palmar Zone P1C pastern sonogram of an 8-year-old Thoroughbred hunter presented for moderate lameness and palmar pastern swelling. This leg had a palmar digital neurectomy 1 year

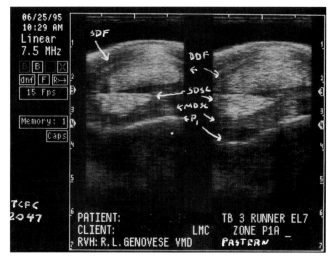

Figure 22.47.

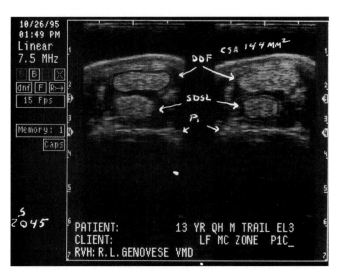

Figure 22.45.

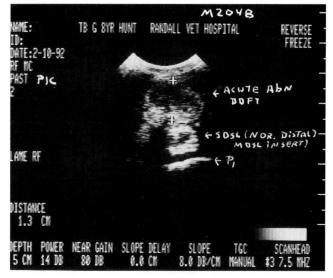

Figure 22.48.

before admission. The DDFT was enlarged with a large Type 3 lesion of the palmar one-half. Along with this DDFT injury, the SDSL has a focal hypoechoic center. The finding of the center at this level, distal to the middle distal or oblique sesamoidean ligament insertions, is normal in many horses. The echolucency is reported to be the fibro-cartilagenous scutum of the second phalanx.

Figure 22.49 is a dual cross-sectional left palmar pastern Zone P2A sonogram of a 10-year-old jumper that had a palmar digital neurectomy 2 years earlier. The horse was markedly lame and had left fore palmar pastern swelling. The DDFT was enlarged with generalized echolucency, and the tendon borders were poorly defined.

Palmar pastern lacerations can result in severe DDFT disease. Figure 22.50 is a cross-sectional and sagittal left metacarpal Zone 3B sonogram of a 2-year-old Arab colt with a palmar fetlock laceration. DDFT enlargement with palmar border definition loss is present, as is diffuse echolucency. The sagittal scan had no significant parallel tendon fiber alignment. Interestingly, with such an extensive DDFT injury, the SDFT was spared.

Figure 22.51 is a dual cross-sectional left metacarpal Zone 3B sonogram of a 15-year-old quarter horse that was lacerated several years previously. The mare had a slight flexural deformity and was lame in the pasture. The DDFT was enlarged with loss of normal shape and with nondistinct palmar and dorsal borders. A mixed echogenic texture and firm restrictive adhesions between the DDFT and SDFT are present. Despite the years since the injury, hypoechoic fibers were still present. The lameness was apparently secondary to extensive scar contraction and restriction of SDFT and DDFT gliding movement.

Tendon sheath infection usually causes severe palmar metacarpophalangeal joint and pastern swelling and lameness. Figure 22.52 is a cross-sectional pastern Zone P1C sonogram of a Standardbred racehorse that had the TS injected with corticosteroids 1 week before admission. The pastern was markedly swollen and there was 3/5 degree

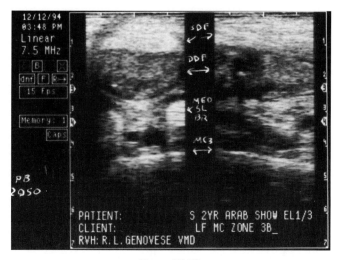
Figure 22.50.

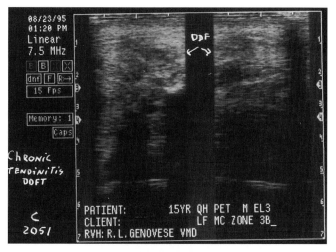
Figure 22.51.

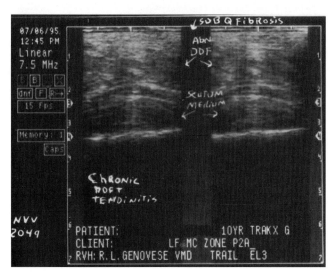
Figure 22.49.

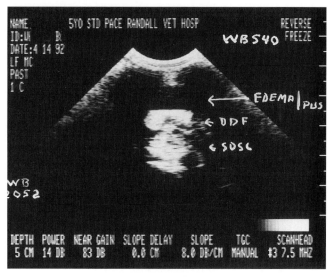
Figure 22.52.

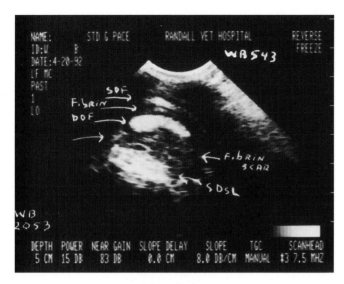

Figure 22.53.

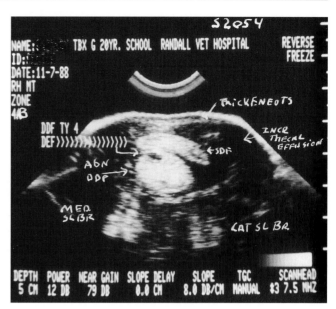

Figure 22.54.

lameness. A large subcutaneous fluid deposition was present. At this point, the fluid could not be identified as pus because fluid texture can be nonspecific. Purulent exudate, however, usually has an echogenic, composite fluid appearance. The instrument gain may have to be increased to visualize the low amplitude echoes. To confirm infection, an aspirate was obtained and submitted for culture. The DDFT has a normal shape and size. There is, however, a focal echolucent dorsal medial border defect and a slight dorsal medial peritendinous fibrous tissue reaction. A focal echolucent palmar medial SDSL border defect is also present. These focal hypoechoic areas are not specific for infection.

Figure 22.53 is a cross-sectional left fore palmar pastern Zone P1A sonogram of the same horse shown in Figure 22.52. An enlarged thecal compartment surrounded the DDFT. The TS fluid compartment has diffuse increased echogenicity, indicating the presence of an organizing hematoma, fibrin deposition, or inflammatory exudate. An aspirate is indicated for culture and cytology to classify the fluid. In this case, the cytologic examination was positive for fibrin and inflammatory exudate and the culture was positive for a bacterial pathogen. The DDFT is normal in size and shape; but the focal hypoechoic lesions seen in Zone P1C were apparent in this zone.

Hindlimb DDFT Abnormalities

Hindlimb DDFT injuries are more commonly associated with lacerations. However, sport related injuries do occur. Sport horses have a greater injury incidence than racehorses. In our experience, hindlimb DDFT injuries are more common in Standardbred than in Thoroughbred racehorses. Although DDFT injuries are rare compared to SDFT injuries, a variety of clinical and sonographic presentations exist.

Figure 22.54 is a cross-sectional right metatarsal Zone 4B sonogram of a 20-year-old Thoroughbred cross. Slight TS thickening with an increased thecal fluid is present. The

SDFT was normal. The DDFT has a focal Type 4 plantar medial border lesion.

Figure 22.55 is a cross-sectional right metatarsal Zone 4B sonogram of a Thoroughbred polo horse presented for metatarsal swelling and a work-related lameness. The DDFT shape is abnormally round and there is a Type 4 central lesion. The amount of thecal fluid has increased.

Figure 22.56 is a cross-sectional right metatarsal Zone 3B sonogram of a Thoroughbred racehorse presented for acute onset lameness and swelling after a race. A Type 3 plantar border DDFT lesion is present.

Figure 22.57 is a cross-sectional left metatarsal Zone 4B sonogram of a 17-year-old quarter horse presented for left hind metatarsal swelling and lameness. A large, Type 3 DDFT lesion is present.

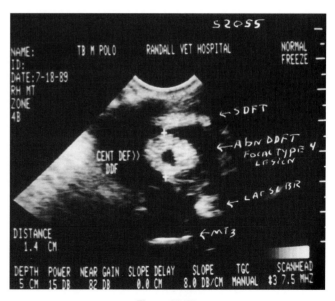

Figure 22.55.

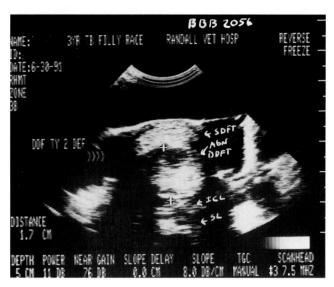

Figure 22.56.

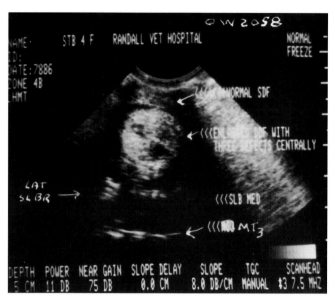

Figure 22.58.

Figure 22.58 is a cross-sectional left metatarsal Zone 4B sonogram of a 4-year-old Standardbred presented for poor performances and metatarsal swelling. The DDFT was enlarged and rounded with several Type 3 lesions. The texture abnormality is more diffuse, suggesting widespread tendinitis and focal fiber tearing.

The DDFT status is of utmost importance when evaluating horses with painful chronic tenosynovitis. It is common practice to treat the chronic tenosynovitis with intrathecal corticosteroid or corticosteroid/hyaluronic acid combinations and allow continued athletic use. Arthroscopic surgery has been used to excise adhesions to restore tendon gliding movement. Postoperative rest periods are generally short. It is clinically important to rule out SDFT/DDFT injury in these cases. Failure to identify ten-

don injury can result in case mismanagement and treatment failure.

Figure 22.59 is a cross-sectional left metatarsal Zone 4B sonogram of a 17-year-old Dutch Warmblood hunter with over a 1-year history of chronic tenosynovitis. Occasional lameness was associated with plantar fetlock swelling. The horse was injected on several occasions with corticosteroid/hyaluronic acid combination without consistent lameness improvement. The horse was recently presented for arthroscopic surgery without preoperative sonographic evaluation. After surgery, the horse was rested for 1 month and returned to light work. The lameness intensified postoperatively and, over a 1-month period of light exercise, the plantar fetlock continued to enlarge, necessitating a cessation of exercise. Just before this evaluation, the horse would

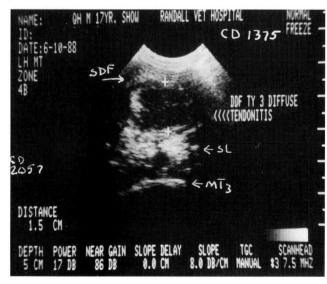

Figure 22.57.

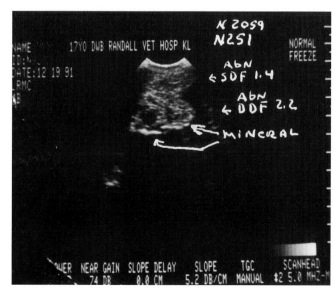

Figure 22.59.

stand without the heel of the affected foot touching the ground. There was an enlarged DDFT with scattered, focal Type 3 lesions of the dorsal, medial, and lateral regions. The entire cross-section had a generalized echolucency. In addition, extensive dorsal border mineral deposition is present, casting a large acoustic shadow. This is an extensive DDFT injury with gliding restriction and mineralization. The SDFT was also enlarged and diffusely hypoechoic. Figure 22.60 is a sagittal left metatarsal Zone 4B sonogram of the same horse shown in Figure 22.59. Both the SDFT and DDFT have little parallel scar alignment and the dorsal border mineralization is also seen in this plane.

Deep digital flexor tendon injury can have an insidious onset in the working horse. Figure 22.61 is a dual cross-sectional left and right metatarsal Zone 4B sonogram of a Standardbred racehorse presented for poor performances and bilateral distal tendon sheath swelling. The trainer noted that the right hind seemed "to bother the horse." The left hind SDFT and DDFT are normal, however, there is an increase in thecal fluid volume. The right hind SDFT is slightly enlarged without evidence of fiber tearing. When the CSA of zones 4A, 4B, and 4C were compared with the left hind, the right SDFT was 15% larger. This increase is equivocal but certainly suspect. It may indicate a low grade SDFT tendinitis. In the right hind, the DDFT is more rounded than normal and has a definite focal Type 2 plantar medial border lesion. In addition, DDFT border definition loss has occurred laterally and dorsally. The left distal Zone 3 CSA is 514 mm^2 and the right is 893 mm^2 (73% increase). Figure 22.62 is a dual cross-sectional left and right metatarsal Zone 4C sonogram of the same horse shown in Figure 22.61. The DDFT is enlarged with several echolucent areas and an indistinct dorsal border.

Figure 22.63 is a cross-sectional right plantar talus Zone 1B sonogram of a 5-year-old Standardbred presented for lameness and a possible left hind curb. The right hind is

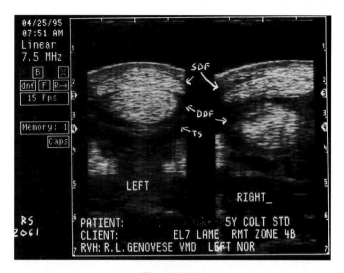

Figure 22.61.

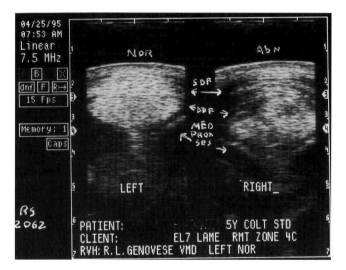

Figure 22.62.

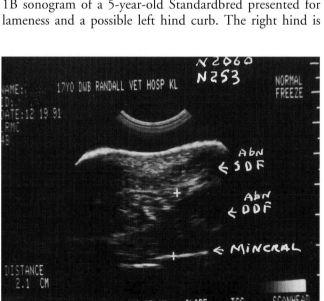

Figure 22.60.

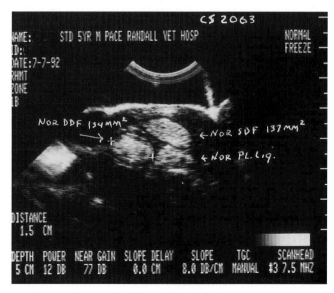

Figure 22.63.

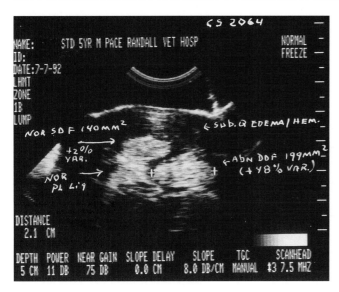

Figure 22.64.

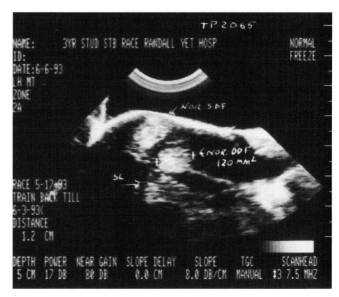

Figure 22.65.

normal and the SDFT CSA is 137 mm². The left hind SDFT CSA is 140 mm² (2% increase). The right DDFT CSA is 134 mm² and the left DDFT is 199 mm² (48% increase). Figure 22.64 is a cross-sectional left plantar talus Zone 1B in sonogram of the same horse shown in Figure 22.63. Marked subcutaneous plantar swelling is present on the SDFT surface. There are no SDFT, DDFT, or PL textural or shape abnormalities; however, the DDFT CSA is increased. No significant increase in SDFT CSA has occurred, which indicates that the subcutaneous swelling is not from a generalized CSA increase of all ligamentous and tendinous structures. The left hind DDFT CSA is increased 48% greater than the right. This finding is compatible with DDFT tendinitis. In this case, the curb was more than subcutaneous edema or hemorrhage.

Figure 22.65 is a normal cross-sectional left metatarsal Zone 2A sonogram of a 3-year-old Standardbred racehorse right hind limb lameness. There was a right hind low curb that concerned the trainer. Figure 22.66 is a cross-sectional right metatarsal Zone 2A sonogram of the same horse. A large, Type 3 SDFT lesion of the medial half and DDFT enlargement are present. The left DDFT CSA is 120 mm² and the right CSA is 228 mm² (90% increase). In this case, SDF and DDF tendinitis are present.

Low grade hind limb lameness secondary to subtle DDF tendinitis in athletic horses is rare. Figure 22.67 is a normal cross-sectional right metatarsal Zone 2B sonogram of a 10-year-old Canadian hunter presented for low grade, sudden onset, left hind lameness. The proximal third of the left DDFT/ALDDFT had slight, diffused thickening. The lameness was relieved with regional anesthesia of this area. The right DDFT CSA is 115 mm². Figure 22.68 is a cross-sectional left metatarsal Zone 2B sonogram of the same horse shown in Figure 22.67. There is a slight increase in tarsal sheath fluid. The DDFT has a normal shape and texture, but the size has increased. The left DDFT CSA is

201 mm² (75% increase). This finding indicates low grade DDFT tendinitis.

Athletic hind pastern DDFT injury can be seen clinically. Figure 22.69 is a dual cross-sectional left and right hind plantar pastern Zone P1C sonogram of a 16-year-old trail horse with low grade right hind lameness. There is marked right hind DDFT swelling with echolucency of the dorsal half. The shape is distinct and abnormal and the borders are nondistinct. This case illustrates a chronic DDF tendinitis causing lameness not associated with previous neurectomy.

It is not uncommon to see hind limb lacerations that cause isolated DDFT injury or a combination injury with other tendons or ligaments. Figure 22.70 is a cross-sectional right metatarsal Zone 4B sonogram of a 3-year-old Standardbred that had sustained a wound the previous year; healing appeared complete externally. However, with train-

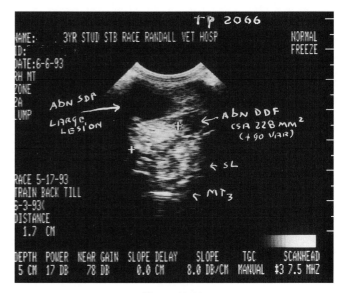

Figure 22.66.

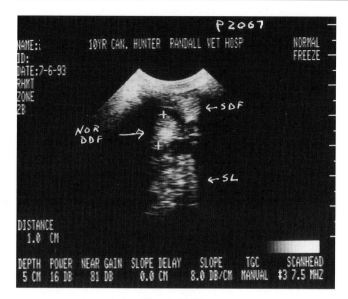

Figure 22.67.

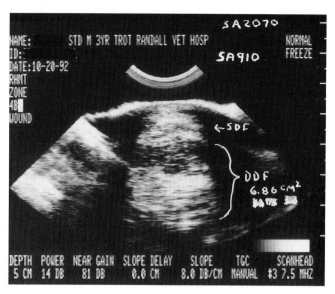

Figure 22.70.

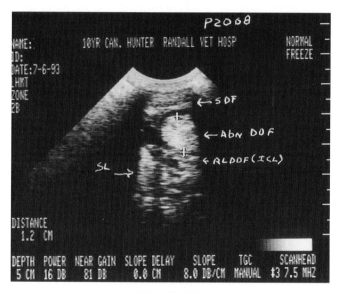

Figure 22.68.

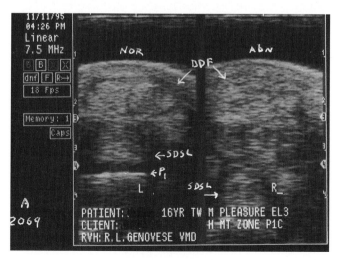

Figure 22.69.

ing, the horse had right hind lameness. DDFT is markedly enlarged with a large plantar Type 3 lesion. The repaired DDFT failed to withstand race training (EL5/6; see Chapter 27). This is a common complication of repaired tendon injuries secondary to lacerations.

THE CARPAL SHEATH

Introduction

According to Budras, the carpal sheath is a double layered synovial structure used to protect the SDFT and the DDFT as they pass through the carpal canal (2). The normal carpal sheath extends from 8 to 10 cm proximal to the palmar antebrachiocarpal joint to approximately the mid-metacarpus. The carpal sheath completely envelops the DDFT and the SDFT partially. For sonographic purposes, carpal sheath fluid can be seen on the dorsal DDFT surface and the medial and lateral SDFT/DDFT surfaces. Dyson reports that in a study of 350 clinically normal horses, there were varying amounts of detectable fluid in the proximal metacarpal extension of the carpal sheath (3). She pointed out that SDFT and DDFT evaluation within the carpal canal is difficult because there is only a small sonographic "window" on the medial surface. Furthermore, in her experience, increased carpal sheath fluid can be associated with SDFT injury.

Sonographic carpal sheath evaluation should routinely begin with caudal antebrachial evaluation commencing approximately 10 cm proximal to the accessory carpal bone. The architecture of the digital flexor muscle groups, the developing tendons, the carpal sheath cranial to the deep digital muscle bundle, and the caudal radial contour should be evaluated. In the 10 cm proximal to the accessory carpal bone, the digital flexor muscles gradually give rise to the SDF and the DDF tendons. The smaller superficial digital muscle and tendon are located caudomedially to the larger deep digital flexor muscle and tendon. One can sonographically follow the transition of muscle to tendon through the carpal canal by rotating the transducer medially. In the carpal canal, the SDFT is superficial to and more rounded than the DDFT. The DDFT is larger, opposes the dorsal lateral SDFT surface, and has a triangular shape. Figure 22.71 is a normal cross-sectional and sagittal caudal antebrachial sonogram 10 cm proximal to the accessory carpal bone of a Thoroughbred racehorse. In cross-section, the digital flexor muscles and early tendon formation are centrally located. The septate architecture is distinct and a distinct fibrous capsule is present on the caudal superficial digital flexor muscle surface. The SDFT and DDFT origins can be appreciated medially. The normal carpal sheath is seen as a 5 mm anechoic space between the caudal radius and the cranial deep flexor muscle and tendon fiber border. The sagittal scan shows the musculotendinous SDFT and DDFT junctions. On the cranial DDFT and DDF muscle lies the anechoic fluid carpal sheath compartment. Figure 22.72 is a normal cross-sectional and sagittal antebrachial sonogram of the same horse shown in Figure 22.71 made 7 cm proximal to the accessory carpal bone. The SDF and DDFT tendons are more prominent at this level of the musculotendinous junction.

Figure 22.73 is a normal cross-sectional right metacarpal Zone 1A sonogram of a 6-year-old Standardbred pacer. The SDFT CSA of this level is 120 mm^2. There is no detectable carpal sheath fluid increase. Figure 22.74 is a normal cross-sectional caudal right antebrachial sonogram made 6 cm proximal to the accessory carpal bone of the same horse shown in Figure 22.73. The digital flexor muscle group CSA is 9 cm^2 and the carpal sheath (CS), cranial to the DDF muscle group surface, is 10 mm thick. Figure 22.75 is a cross-sectional left metacarpal Zone 1A sonogram of the same horse shown in Figure 22.74. The left SDFT is more rounded than the right and focal, hypoechoic lateral margin fiber bundles are present. The SDFT CSA is 242 mm^2 (102% increase). There is no noticeable CS fluid increase.

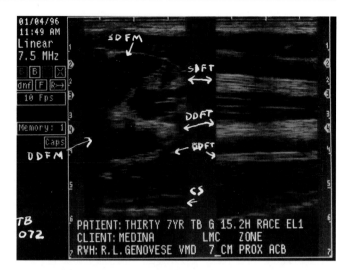

Figure 22.72.

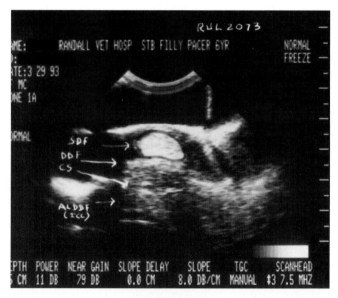

Figure 22.73.

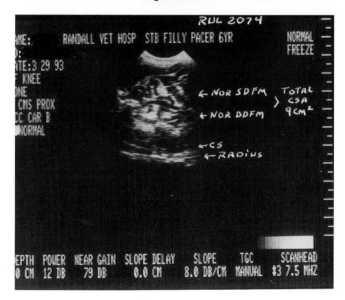

Figure 22.74.

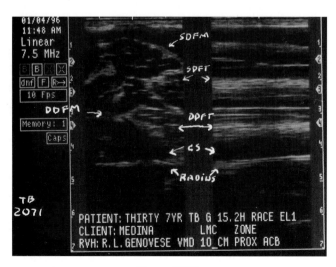

Figure 22.71.

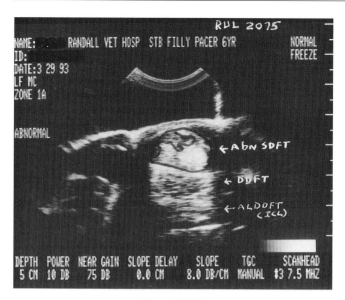

Figure 22.75.

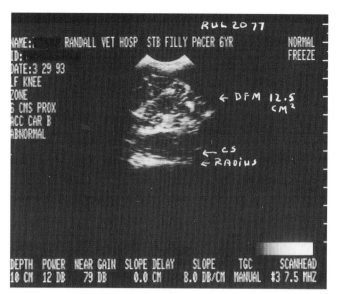

Figure 22.77.

Figure 22.76 is a cross-sectional left metacarpal Zone 2A sonogram of the same horse shown in Figure 22.75. A large Type 3 lateral border SDFT lesion is present. Figure 22.77 is a cross-sectional left caudal antebrachial sonogram made 6 cm proximal to the accessory carpal bone. There are no detectable morphologic or textural digital flexor muscle group abnormalities. However, the muscle group CSA is increased over the normal leg at the same level. The CSA is 12.5 cm². In addition, the CS is increased to 17 mm. This racehorse was presented for left fore lameness, a palpable metacarpal SDFT abnormality, and thickening of the antebrachial flexor muscle group. There is increased pressure in the carpal sheath at and proximal to the carpal canal level but not *distal* to the carpal canal.

Figure 22.78 is a cross-sectional left caudal antebrachial sonogram made 6 cm proximal to the accessory carpal bone

of a 6-year-Standardbred presented for left fore leg lameness and palpable swelling proximal and distal to the palmar carpus. The shape, architecture, and flexor muscle group CSA (9 cm²) are within normal limits. There is an increased CS fluid adjacent cranial to the muscle group. Figure 22.79 is a cross-sectional left metacarpal Zone 1A sonogram of the same horse shown in Figure 22.78. The tendons and ligaments were within normal limits. In this case, the lameness was caused by a primary CS effusion without tendon or ligament abnormalities (benign CS synovitis). This sonographic evaluation influences the treatment program and the advised time from training as opposed to the previous case. In this instance, symptomatic intrathecal treatment and a short rest period are indicated. However, the limb should be monitored clinically and sonographically after treatment.

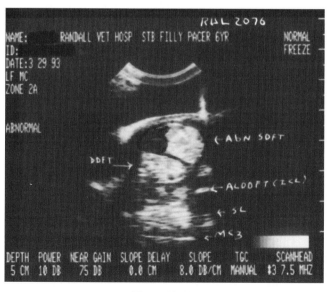

Figure 22.76.

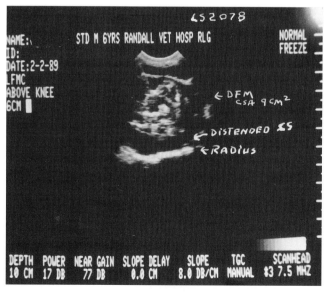

Figure 22.78.

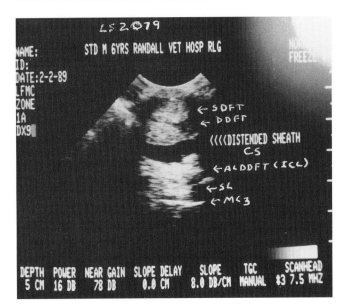

Figure 22.79.

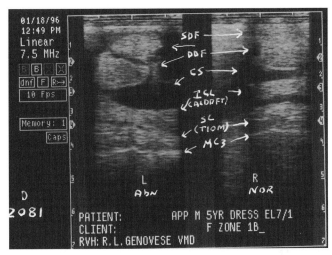

Figure 22.81.

Figure 22.80 is a dual cross-sectional right and left caudal antebrachial sonogram of a 5-year-old dressage horse presented for sudden onset left fore leg lameness and distal, caudal antebrachial, and proximal metacarpal swelling. The right fore limb was normal and the CSA is 12.9 cm². The CS is 5 mm thick. The left antebrachium had a slight textural deep flexor muscle abnormality characterized by a diffuse central echogenicity increase. The CSA is 14.4 cm². The CS is 10 mm thick. These findings indicate not only a CS synovitis, but also sonographic evidence of deep flexor muscle strain and inflammation.

Figure 22.81 is a dual cross-sectional right and left metacarpal Zone 1B sonogram of the same horse shown in Figure 22.80. The left and right SDFT and DDFT were within normal limits. The amount of left CS fluid has increased. The left fore ALDDFT had a slight shape abnormality most likely caused by increased CS fluid pressure. Figure 22.82 is

a dual cross-sectional right and left metacarpal Zone 2A sonogram of the same horse shown in Figure 22.81. The left and right SDFT and DDFT were normal. The left CS fluid increase is significant, causing an apparent left ALDDFT shape abnormality. The ALDDFT appears elongated in a medial to lateral dimension and the palmar to dorsal size has decreased. This case requires a slightly different treatment approach because there is sonographic evidence of flexor muscle strain near the musculotendinous junction.

Figure 22.83 is a normal cross-sectional left caudal antebrachial sonogram made 7 cm proximal to the accessory carpal bone of a 2-year-old Standardbred presented for right fore lameness that occurred after a training mile. The CSA is 9 cm². The trainer indicated that right caudal antebrachial swelling was present. Figure 22.84 is a cross-sectional right caudal antebrachial sonogram made 7 cm proximal to the accessory carpal bone of the same horse shown in Figure 22.83. There was a hypoechoic caudal lateral margin superficial digital flexor muscle lesion. A distinct fascial plane loss

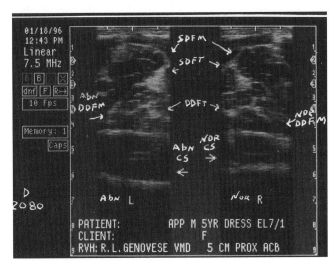

Figure 22.80.

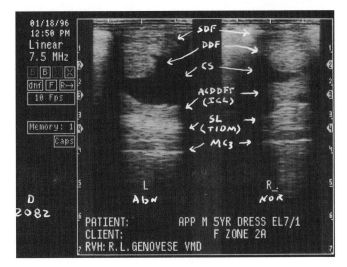

Figure 22.82.

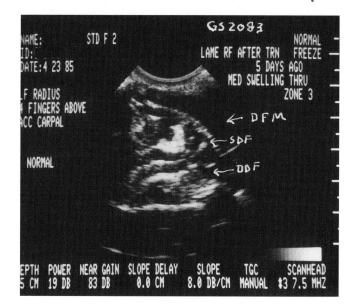

Figure 22.83.

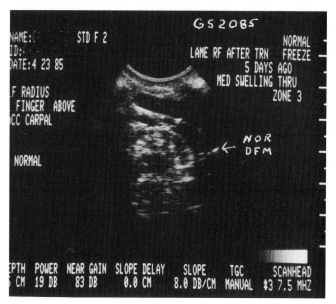

Figure 22.85.

is present as well as enlargement of the border. In addition, there is a central fascial architecture loss of both muscles. The CSA is 14.7 cm². Figure 22.85 is a normal cross-sectional left caudal antebrachial sonogram made 2 cm proximal to the accessory carpal bone of the same horse shown in Figure 22.84. The CSA is 4.8 cm². Figure 22.86 is a cross-sectional right caudal antebrachial sonogram made 2 cm proximal to the accessory carpal bone of the same horse shown in Figure 22.85. An abnormal digital flexor muscle architecture is present characterized by a loss of distinct fascial borders and an increased medial superficial and deep flexor muscle echogenicity. The CSA is slightly larger than the left (6.3 cm²). In this case, the antebrachial swelling was not caused by CS synovitis but rather by a digital flexor muscle injury at the musculotendinous junction.

Figure 22.87 is a cross-sectional right caudal antebrachial sonogram made 8 cm proximal to the accessory carpal bone of an 8-year-old quarter horse presented for lameness and CS distention. The muscles are within normal limits; however, CS fluid has increased. Figure 22.88 is a cross-sectional right caudal antebrachial sonogram made 2 cm proximal to the accessory carpal bone of the same horse shown in Figure 22.87. The muscles are normal and the increased CS fluid is present at this level. Figure 22.89 is a cross-sectional right metacarpal Zone 1B sonogram of the same horse shown in Figure 22.88. The tendons and ligament are normal, but the CS fluid increase is present and has low amplitude echoes. This finding indicates either hemorrhage or septic inflammatory exudate. A fluid aspirate is needed to confirm the diagnosis.

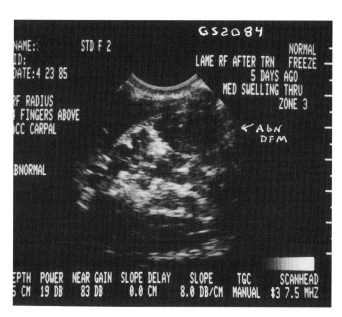

Figure 22.84.

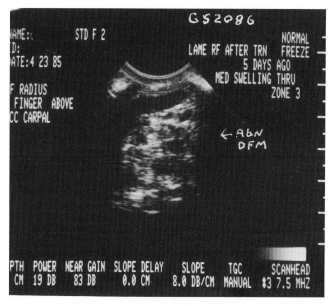

Figure 22.86.

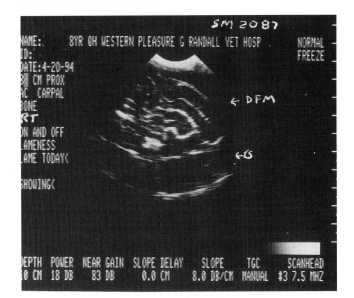

Figure 22.87.

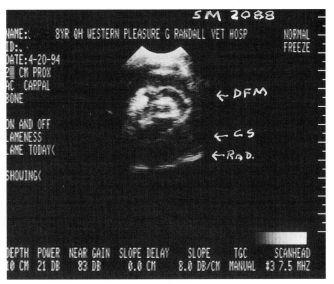

Figure 22.88.

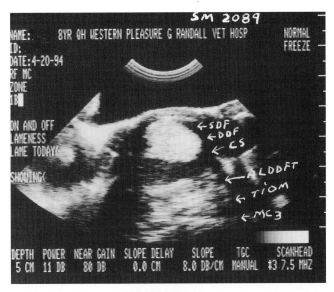

Figure 22.89.

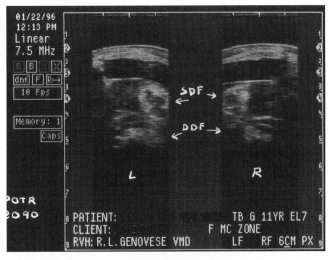

Figure 22.90.

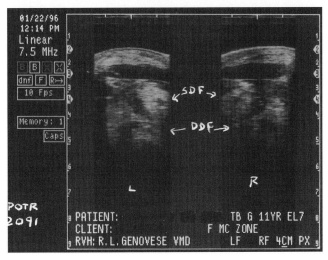

Figure 22.91.

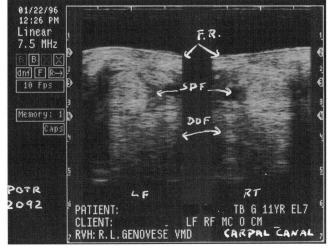

Figure 22.92.

Carpal canal SDFT injury is rare, but the cases that we have seen usually involve carpal tunnel syndrome, even though proximal metacarpal tendon swelling can be subtle. Horses with this SDFT strain usually are lame, and only with careful palpation and contralateral limb comparison is slight SDFT swelling recognized. In colder climates, a winter hair coat can obscure swelling recognition. Figure 22.90 is a dual cross-sectional right and left fore antebrachial sonogram made 6 cm proximal to the accessory carpal bone of an 11-year-old Thoroughbred gelding jumper with a sudden onset lameness after a jumping round. The horse was 2/5 degree lame at the trot. Physical examination revealed slight swelling and increased upper third metacarpal skin temperature. At this level, the SDFT is oval and located centromedially, and central echolucent muscle fibers are visible. There is no significant CSA difference. Figure 22.91 is a dual cross-sectional right and left caudal antebrachial sonogram made 4 cm proximal to the accessory carpal bone of

the same horse shown in Figure 22.90. The right and left fore SDFT had normal texture; however, there is a CSA difference. The right is 99 mm^2 and the left is 120 mm^2 (21% increase). Figure 22.92 is a dual cross-sectional medial oblique right and left carpal canal sonogram. At this level, muscle bundles are not seen. There are no significant SDFT textural or shape abnormalities; however, the CSA has increased. The normal right SDFT CSA is 160 mm^2 and the left fore is 191 mm^2 (19% increase). Figure 22.93A is a dual cross-sectional left and right metacarpal Zone 1A sonogram of the same horse shown in Figure 22.92. There are no textural abnormalities detected in either SDFT, however the normal right SDFT is round and the abnormal left is oval. The right SDFT CSA is 118 mm^2 and the abnormal left SDFT CSA is 144 mm^2 (22% increase). Superficial digital flexor tendon swelling of this magnitude at this level most likely causes lameness. In this example, there was lameness, carpal sheath distention, and a first episode SDFT strain.

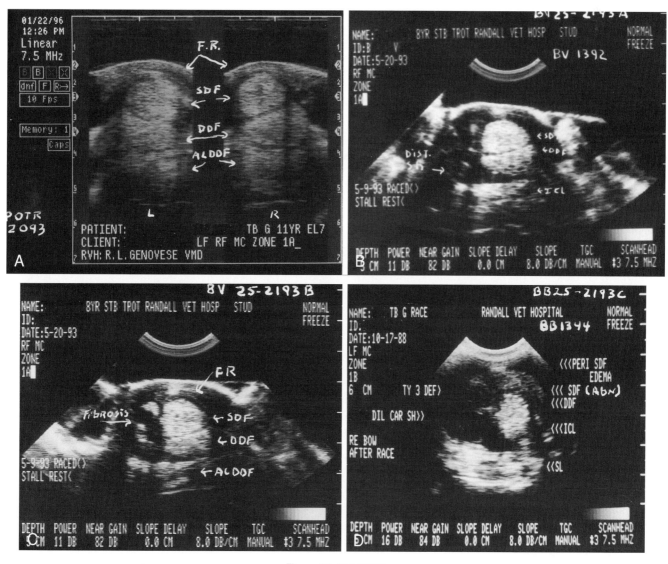

Figure 22.93 A,B,C,D.

In some circumstances, the SDFT status and its contribution to lameness presentation is not as clearly defined. Figure 22.93**B** is a cross-sectional right metacarpal Zone 1A sonogram of a recently raced 8-year-old Standardbred trotter with right fore lameness. The trainer noted carpal sheath distention proximal and distal to the carpus. The horse had been racing with a clinically stable tendonitis for several months. Carpal sheath fluid has increased. No SDFT textural abnormalities are present at this level. The trainer reported that no external changes were seen in the tendon since the onset of lameness. Figure 22.93**C** is a cross-sectional right medial oblique metacarpal Zone 1A sonogram of the same horse shown in Figure 22.93B. This scan shows increased carpal sheath fluid and evidence of flexor retinaculum fibrosis. Based on the reported SDFT stability by the trainer and the lameness onset coincidental to the carpal sheath distention, the carpal sheath effusion was treated as the primary injury. The sheath was injected with corticosteroid/hyaluronate combination. The aspirate was hemorrhagic, and the trainer was cautioned about continuing racing. Instructions were given to monitor the tendon.

At other times, SDFT injury associated with acute CS distention is not a difficult finding. Figure 22.93**D** is a cross-sectional left metacarpal Zone 1B sonogram of a Thoroughbred racehorse with acute onset lameness and metacarpal swelling after a race. Extensive SDFT injury and marked CS distention were present.

Figure 22.94 is a normal cross-sectional and sagittal left caudal antebrachial sonogram made 10 cm proximal to the accessory carpal bone of a 20-year-old Warmblood event horse that had been presented 1 month previously for SDFT reinjury. Since that visit, the horse was stall rested and hand-walked. Three days before this examination, the horse was found acutely lame in the right fore with right caudal antebrachial swelling. The left caudal antebrachial sonogram was normal. The CSA is a normal 9 cm^2. Figure 22.95 is a cross-sectional and sagittal right caudal antebrachial sonogram made 9 cm proximal to the accessory carpal bone of the

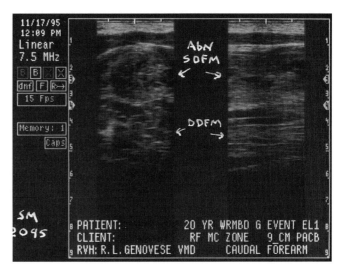

Figure 22.95.

same horse shown in Figure 22.94. There was a loss of fascial planes in the superficial digital muscle and a diffuse increased echogenicity. The deep digital flexor muscle group is normal. The combined digital flexor muscle group CSA is 12 cm^2. Figure 22.96 is a dual cross-sectional left and right caudal antebrachial sonogram made 16 cm proximal to the accessory carpal bone of the same horse shown in Figure 22.95. There is complete loss of normal fascial planes of the right fore with a generalized increase in echogenicity. Myositis was diagnosed as the cause of the lameness and swelling.

Figure 22.97 is a cross-sectional and sagittal left metacarpal Zone 1B sonogram of a 4-year-old Hackney pony presented for mild persistent lameness and CS distention. The SDFT and DDFT are normal. Moderate CS fluid distention is present. The ALDDFT does not have any textural abnormalities but slight shape abnormality exists because of increased CS fluid pressure. Figure 22.98 is a cross-sectional and sagittal left caudal antebrachial sonogram made 5 cm

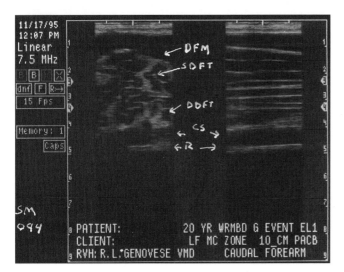

Figure 22.94.

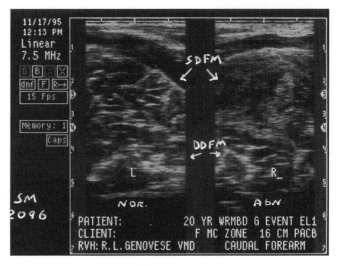

Figure 22.96.

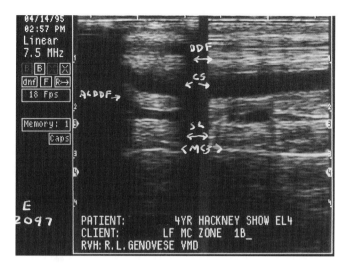

Figure 22.97.

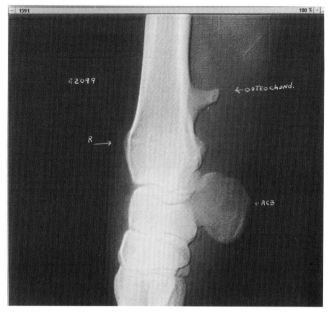

Figure 22.99.

proximal to the accessory carpal bone of the same horse shown in Figure 22.97. Mineral deposition is apparent in the cranial deep flexor muscle group. This mineral deposition can be seen on both the cross-sectional scan and the sagittal scan. Figure 22.99 is a left carpal radiograph of the same horse shown in Figure 22.98. A large osteochondroma is protruding from the caudal radial surface. It traumatizes the deep flexor muscle and causes a hemorrhagic tenosynovitis. Osteochondromas can occur in any age horse and can occasionally have confusing clinical signs. The most reliable signs are lameness and CS distension, when present. Some horses do not fully extend the affected limb but are not noticeably lame. Not all horses with carpal tunnel syndrome secondary to osteochondromas have CS distension. Radiographs are reliable only if the bony projection(s) can be seen unequivocally. A complete series should be taken depending on the degree of suspicion; however, dorsopalmar projections often show the roughened bone as a radiodense focal area(s) while they may be obscured on other views. The normal caudolateral bone surface irregularity at the rudimentary ulnar at-

tachment on the radius should not be confused with osteochondromas, which occur more toward the midline or medial aspect. Horses with lesions similar to the one in Figures 22.98 and 22.99 are straightforward. Osteochondroma should not, however, be ruled out because radiographs are negative and CS distension is minimal or absent.

Slight CS distension generally does not result in lameness and may be within normal range. Many normal horses may have some degree of CS fluid increase. Figure 22.100 is a cross-sectional and sagittal left metacarpal Zone 1B sonogram of a 4-year-old Standardbred pacer with a slight increase in CS fluid. There are no SDFT, DDFT, or ALDDFT sonographic abnormalities.

Figure 22.101 is a cross-sectional left metacarpal Zone 1B sonogram of a 3-year-old Standardbred pacer with slight to moderate CS fluid increase. The SDFT, DDFT, and ALDDFT were normal.

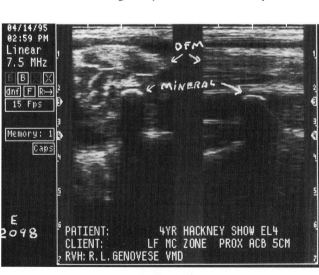

Figure 22.98.

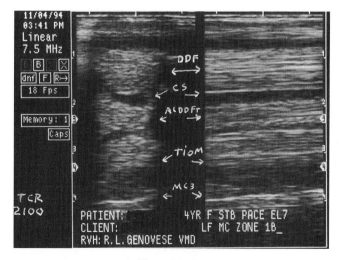

Figure 22.100.

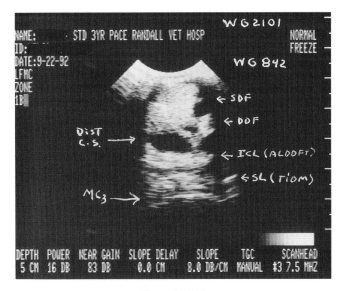

Figure 22.101.

Figure 22.102.

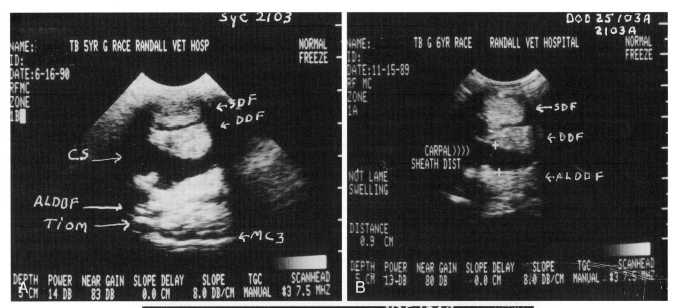

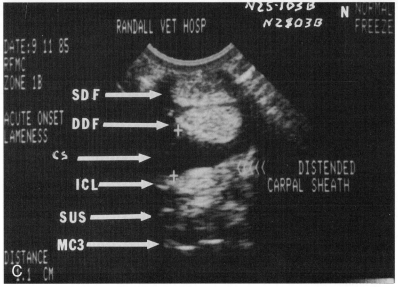

Figure 22.103 A,B,C.

Figure 22.102 is a dual cross-sectional left and right metacarpal Zone 1B sonogram of a 2-year-old Standardbred pacer with slight bilateral CS fluid increase. None of the horses in Figures 22.100 to 22.102 were lame or had performance compromise.

Figure 22.103A is a cross-sectional right metacarpal Zone 1B sonogram of a Thoroughbred racehorse with moderate to severe CS fluid increase. The SDFT, DDFT, and ALDDFT were normal. This horse, however, was clinically lame because of the increased CS fluid pressure.

Figure 22.103B is cross-sectional right metacarpal Zone 1A sonogram of a Thoroughbred racehorse presented for proximal metacarpal swelling evaluation. No lameness was evident at any gait even though there was marked CS distention. The SDFT, DDFT, and the ALDDFT were normal.

Figure 22.103C is a cross-sectional right metacarpal Zone 1B sonogram of a horse presented with proximal metacarpal swelling similar to the horse in Figure 22.103B; however, there was lameness. CS distention was significant without any identifiable SDFT, DDFT, or ALDDFT injury.

Figure 22.104 is a cross-sectional left and right metacarpal Zone 1B sonogram of a 3-year-old mixed breed dressage horse with slight left CS distention and moderate right CS distention. No SDFT or DDFT abnormalities were present; however, the right ALDDFT was enlarged. When summed for 4 levels, the right had a 21% CSA increase compared with the left. In this case, there is evidence of CS distention and slight right ALDDFT strain.

Figure 22.105 is a dual cross-sectional left and right caudal antebrachial sonogram of the same horse shown in Figure 22.104 made 7 cm proximal to the accessory carpal bone. There was increased CS fluid on the dorsum of the deep digital flexor muscle group; however, no muscle abnormalities are present.

Figure 22.106 is a cross-sectional left metacarpal Zone

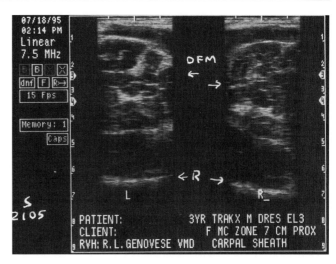

Figure 22.105.

2A sonogram of a Thoroughbred racehorse with chronic CS swelling that had been injected on several occasions. Recently, the horse was severely lame, and the owner reported that the CS swelling was greater than usual. Severe CS swelling was present and, because of the lameness degree and the recent injection history, sepsis was strongly suspected. An aspirate of pus was obtained, which was positive for a bacterial pathogen, and the horse was humanely destroyed.

Carpal sheath distention can occur as a nonclinical benign synovitis; however, it can be associated with a variety of soft tissue and bony abnormalities. The sonographer should always examine the distal antebrachium in all horses with CS distention associated with performance decline or lameness. Radiographic evaluation of the carpus for osteochondroma or accessory carpal bone fracture should be a standard procedure. One author (RLG) includes at least a lateral projection radiograph of all horses that present with palpable CS distention proximal to the carpus.

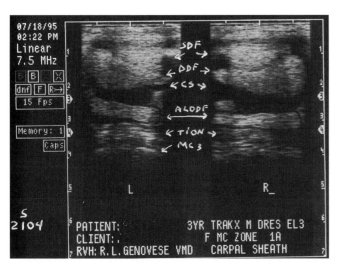

Figure 22.104.

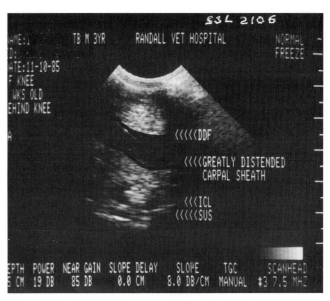

Figure 22.106.

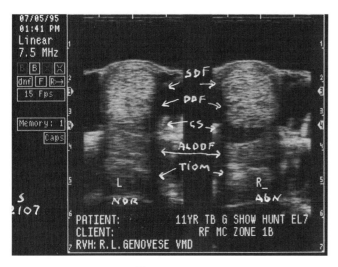

Figure 22.107.

Figure 22.107 is a dual cross-sectional right and left metacarpal Zone 1B sonogram of an 11-year-old jumper presented for a sudden onset lameness after a jumping round. The trainer noted fluctuant swelling along the SDFT below the carpus and thought the horse had injured the tendon. This scan reveals an increase CS fluid. The fluid had low amplitude echoes, suggesting hemorrhage. Figure 22.108 is a lateral-medial right carpal radiograph confirming an accessory carpal bone fracture. A careful evaluation of the SDFT, DDFT, and ALDDFT is always indicated, however. As seen in other areas of soft tissue evaluation, examining both the normal and injured limb assists one in detecting subtle tendon, ligament, or muscle injury by comparing CSA measurements.

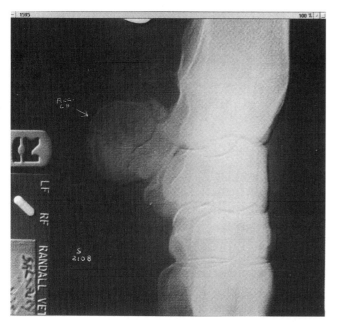

Figure 22.108.

THE ACCESSORY LIGAMENT OF THE DEEP DIGITAL FLEXOR TENDON (ALDDFT) (INFERIOR CHECK LIGAMENT)

According to Getty, the ALDDFT of the forelimb is a direct continuation of the broad palmar carpal ligament. It has the dorsal carpal sheath extension on its palmar surface and the third interosseous muscle (TIOM) on its dorsal surface (4). It has a palmar attachment to the distal row of carpal bones as well. The ALDDFT joins the DDFT in the middle to distal third of the metacarpus. Sonographically, the ALDDFT can be distinguished as a separate structure to Zone 3A. In the hindlimb, the ALDDFT originates from the plantar distal tarsal fascia and is a less developed ligamentous structure than it is in the forelimb. It has been reported that it is not present in mules and some horses.

There are few references in the literature relative to clinical ALDDFT disease. An in-depth report by Dyson described 27 cases of ALDDFT injury (5). She reported ALDDFT injury occurrence more frequently in horses used for athletics other than racing. She also indicated that injury was more common in the older equine athlete. The range of injury spanned the usual focal fiber tearing to diffuse desmitis with a predominance of diffuse injury. It was a primary finding or was in combination with SDFT or DDFT injury. In her experience, the return to athletic function was fair when an SDFT injury was not involved. Our experiences are similar with injury more common in older horses, which can be bilateral. Clinical ALDDFT injury is usually sudden in onset with metacarpal or metatarsal swelling, and lameness is common. In recently injured horses, the ALDDFT injury diagnosis is confirmed by physical examination and ultrasonographic confirmation. Sonographic evaluation allows determining the extent of the injury and whether concomitant SDFT, DDFT, or third interosseous muscle (TIOM) injury is present. In some instances, subtle acute ALDDFT origin injury or lameness secondary to chronic ALDDFT fibrosis is not clinically apparent. Furthermore, the rate and quality of recovery is variable. Therefore, as with other ligament and tendon injuries, a thorough sonographic examination of both limbs is often indicated. In Dyson's report, the prognosis was greatly decreased in horses with concomitant SDFT injury (5).

The ALDDFT origin can partially be examined sonographically in Zone 1A. The ligament enthesis on the palmar third carpal bone surface can be seen in most horses. This area is slightly difficult to examine because of the accessory carpal bone contour and some transducer configurations. Scanning artifact can be seen; however, basic understanding of the causes of sonographic artifacts can reduce error (see Chapter 8).

In Zone 1A, there are several anatomic and sonographic pitfalls to consider that may cause focal or diffuse hypoechoic scanning artifacts in the equine forelimb. At the skin level, in the area of transducer contact, the flexor retinaculum is coursing obliquely from the accessory carpal bone to the metacarpal bone. The palmar third carpal bone contour is sloped and the palmar proximal third metacarpal surface is vertical. The ALDDFT origin from the palmar carpal fascia and palmar third carpal bone is vertical. Therefore, it may not be possible to obtain an artifact-free complete ALDDFT origin image because it is difficult to achieve parallel skin/transducer contact. Transducer rotation can allow parallel alignment of a portion of the ALDDFT. Images along the sloping palmar metacarpal are easier to obtain because in that segment, the slope of the flexor retinaculum and the palmar third carpal bone are parallel. In addition, there are two synovial compartments of the carpus. The more proximal synovial compartment is the middle carpal joint and the more distal is the carpometacarpal joint. If these joints are distended adequately with synovial fluid, rounded, focal, anechoic structures will be present on the dorsal ALDDFT surface. These structures should not be interpreted as a focal ALDDFT origin fiber rupture.

Figure 22.109 is a normal dual sagittal left palmar carpal Zone 1A sonogram of a Thoroughbred racehorse. The image on the left is the normal ALDDFT insertion onto the palmar distal third carpal bone surface. At the level of the proximal metacarpus, the carpometacarpal joint is seen as a normal, several millimeters long, anechoic structure between the dorsal ALDDFT surface and the third metacarpal bone. The figure on the right is a sagittal sonogram of the ALDDFT origin on the palmar third carpal bone, proximal to the left image. The rounded anechoic structure is the middle carpal joint and does not represent fiber tearing of the origin of the ALDDFT.

Figure 22.110 is a sagittal left palmar carpal Zone 1A sonogram of a Thoroughbred show hunter. In this image, there is normal ALDDFT fiber attachment onto the palmar third carpal bone that does not show the hypoechoic carpometacarpal joint. ALDDFT fibers originating more proximally from the palmar carpal fascia can be seen. It is ad-

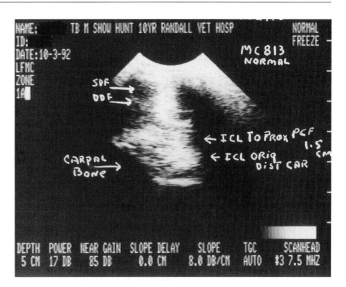

Figure 22.110.

vantageous and less confusing to begin the sonographic examination in Zone 1B and proceed proximally after identification of the TIOM (suspensory ligament) origin. This process enables identification of the transition of the slight proximal metacarpal slope from the more sloping palmar third carpal bone contour.

Figure 22.111 is a normal sagittal right metacarpal Zone 1B sonogram of a Thoroughbred racehorse. The scan shows the origin of the TIOM from the palmar third metacarpal surface. Note that, in this area, the proximal palmar metacarpal bone has a gentle sloping contour. This slope is less than the palmar third carpal bone. If the TIOM origin is identified as the starting point and the ALDDFT is followed proximally, sonographic orientation and interpretation is easier. ALDDFT injury limited to the origin at the palmar third carpal bone is rare.

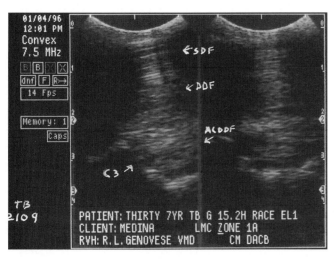

Figure 22.109.

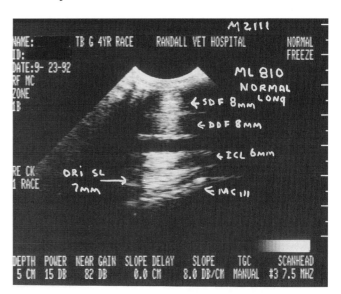

Figure 22.111.

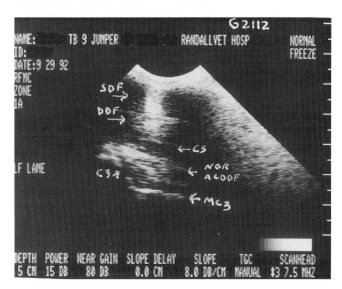

Figure 22.112.

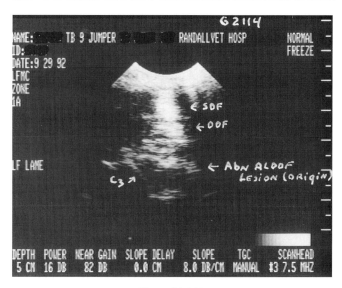

Figure 22.114.

Figure 22.112 is a normal sagittal right palmar carpal Zone 1A sonogram of a 9-year-old jumper that was examined for a sudden onset left fore lameness. Palpation did not reveal any palpable carpal or metacarpal abnormalities. Diagnostic anesthesia confirmed pain in the left proximal palmar metacarpus. Figure 22.113 is a sagittal left palmar carpal Zone 1A sonogram of the same horse shown in Figure 22.112. A palmar third carpal bone avulsion fracture was present, as was an echolucent ALDDFT origin distal to the cartilaginous or bony fragment. In addition, the palmar to dorsal right fore ALDDFT is 10 mm thick and the left is 15 mm.

Figure 22.114 is a sagittal left palmar carpal Zone 1A sonogram of the same horse shown in Figure 22.113 showing a hypoechoic ALDDFT origin lesion.

Figure 22.115 is a cross-sectional right palmar carpal

Zone 1A sonogram of a Thoroughbred racehorse presented for sudden onset lameness. No palpable carpal or metacarpal abnormalities were present. Diagnostic anesthesia confirmed the palmar carpus as the source pain, and carpal radiographs were unremarkable. A focal avulsion fracture is seen arising from the palmar third carpal bone along the lateral ALDDFT border.

Figure 22.116 is a cross-sectional right palmar carpal Zone 1A sonogram of the same horse shown in Figure 22.115. A rounded Type 3 dorsal lateral border ALDDFT lesion is present. In both of these cases, the onset of lameness was sudden without palpable swelling. Regional anesthesia confirmed the location of the lameness cause. In both instances, carpal radiographs were unremarkable and no TIOM injury could be identified.

Figure 22.117 is a cross-sectional left palmar carpal Zone

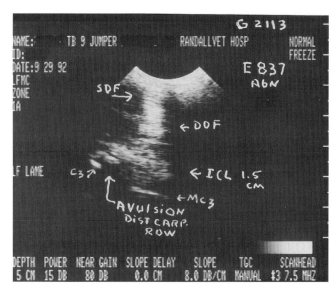

Figure 22.113.

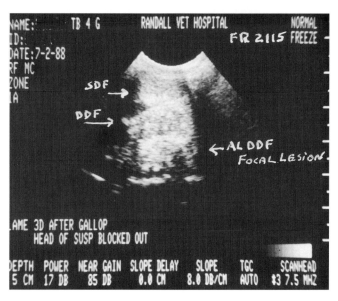

Figure 22.115.

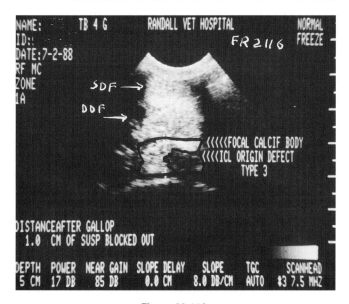

Figure 22.116.

1A sonogram of a Standardbred racehorse presented for right fore lameness. Palpation revealed nonpainful, low grade ALDDFT swelling. The ALDDFT was enlarged with minimal texture abnormality. The enlargement decreased distally and no focal fiber tearing was seen. The sonographic dilemma in this case is determining whether the ALDDFT enlargement represents an older repaired injury or a more acute, strain-related desmitis. In this instance, it is not possible to make this determination from a single sonographic examination. The clinical history indicated that this was a recent onset lameness and the palpable swelling was only recently observed. This trainer had been training this horse for an extended period and had not detected any swelling before this episode, nor did any previous lameness or swelling indicate a past injury. Therefore, our interpretation was

ALDDFT desmitis. The horse was treated symptomatically and given a 2-week rest period. The trainer was instructed to submit the horse for repeat examination if the lameness persisted. The horse made an uneventful recovery and continued its athletic career. It is worth speculating in this case and similar injuries in the Standardbred racehorse that ALDDFT is predominantly seen in trotters. It is common practice in the United States to shoe trotters with a long toe (4+ inches) and a low heel for possible gait enhancement. It has been recognized by one author (RLG) that ALDDFT injury in other athletic horses that this longer toe—lower heel foot conformation is generally seen. It is our opinion that this Type of foot conformation increases the chance of ALDDFT injury.

Figure 22.118 is a normal cross-sectional right metacarpal Zone 2A sonogram of a Standardbred trotter presented for left fore lameness and metacarpal swelling. The right fore ALDDFT is normal for this level and the CSA is 85 mm^2. Even though no textural right metacarpal SDFT abnormalities were present, the six level T-CSA was 16% larger than the left tendon.

Figure 22.119**A** is a cross-sectional left metacarpal Zone 2A sonogram of the same horse shown in Figure 22.118. The ALDDFT is enlarged with a nondistinct generalized echolucency and loss of the distinct palmar and dorsal borders. The ALDDFT CSA is 143 mm^2 (68% increase) and, unlike the previous horse, there is textural abnormality. An interesting question to be asked is "Is the ALDDFT a primary problem resulting in low grade contralateral SDFT strain, or is the ALDDFT desmitis the result of compensation for the contralateral SDFT strain?" No direct association may exist. However, this illustrates that bilateral evaluation of all structures should be done to rule out multiple soft tissue injuries.

Rarely, one may encounter what the authors believe to be an incidental finding of mineral deposition in the palmar

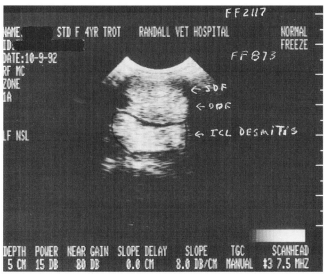

Figure 22.117.

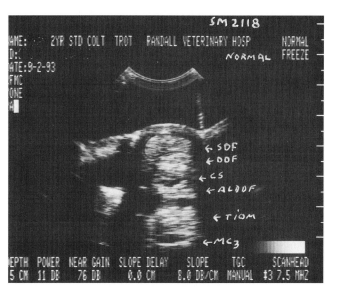

Figure 22.118.

carpometacarpal region. Figure 22.119**B** is a cross-sectional and sagittal palmar carpal Zone 1A sonogram of a Thoroughbred event horse being evaluated for a medial suspensory ligament branch injury. There was no clinical evidence of palmar carpal abnormality. This scan shows focal mineral deposition on the dorsomedial DDFT/carpal sheath junction. This ectopic mineralization creates an acoustic shadow of the ALDDFT. Both authors have seen this focal mineralization on several occasions. On most of these occasions, there was no history of clinical signs referable to this area or any medical history indicating treatment of this area. Occasionally, one author (NWR) has found it in horses with pain on palpation and proximal suspensory ligament desmitis. We regard this ectopic mineralization as an incidental finding if there are no other structural abnormalities or clinical evidence that this lesion is causing lameness. The main differential diagnosis is the introduction of air from regional anesthesia injections. Occasionally, ultrasonographic examination of this area has to be delayed for several days if recent injections have been made.

It is unusual to find peri-ligamentous fibrous tissue reaction around the ALDDFT. Figure 22.120 is a cross-sectional right metacarpal Zone 2A sonogram of a quarter

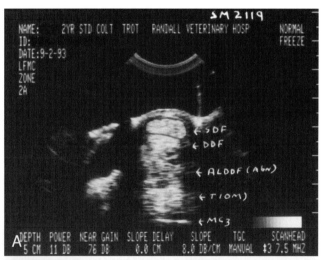

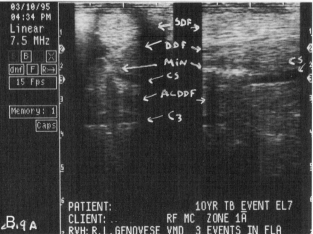

Figure 22.119.

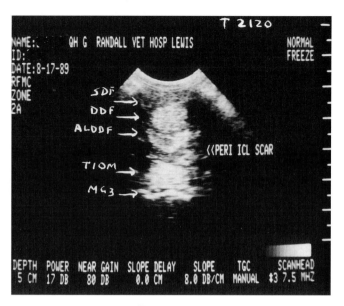

Figure 22.120.

horse gelding presented for swelling. The ALDDFT is within normal limits. A peri-ligamentous fibrous tissue reaction is present between the ALDDFT and the TIOM.

Sonographic ALDDFT lesions range from subtle enlargement, suggesting low grade strain, to focal areas of fiber tearing, to severe fiber pattern disruption and extensive desmitis. Figure 22.121 is a cross-sectional and sagittal right metacarpal Zone 1A sonogram of a quarter horse hunter with a focal Type 3 centrolateral ALDDFT lesion. This finding is confirmed on the sagittal sonogram.

Figure 22.122 is a cross-sectional left metacarpal Zone 1A sonogram of mixed breed event horse with a focal Type 2 dorsolateral ALDDFT lesion.

Figure 22.123 is a cross-sectional left metacarpal Zone 2B sonogram of Standardbred pacer with a large Type 3 central ALDDFT lesion. The ALDDFT is enlarged and the shape is more rounded than normal.

Figure 22.124 is a cross-sectional left metacarpal Zone 1B sonogram of a Thoroughbred hunter with an enlarged echolucent ALDDFT consistent with a diffuse desmitis.

Figure 22.125 is a cross-sectional and sagittal right metacarpal Zone 1B sonogram of a Morgan trail horse with an enlarged generalized echolucent ALDDFT. The ALDDFT CSA is 134 mm^2.

Figure 22.126 is a normal cross-sectional right Zone 3A sonogram of a Thoroughbred racehorse. In this zone, an indistinct interface between the DDFT and the ALDDFT can still be seen. The TIOM is just beginning to bifurcate.

Figure 22.127 is a cross-sectional and sagittal right metacarpal Zone 3A sonogram of the same horse shown in Figure 22.125. This is the sonographic level of "insertion" of the normal ALDDFT. However, in this case, the ligament is enlarged and there is a diffuse Type 2 texture. In addition, a Type 3 dorsolateral DDFT lesion is present.

Figure 22.128 is a cross-sectional right metacarpal Zone 2B sonogram of a Thoroughbred racehorse that became

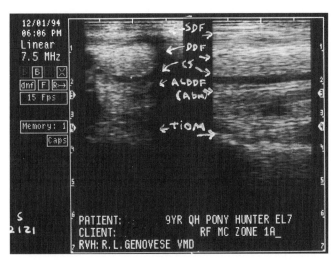

Figure 22.121.

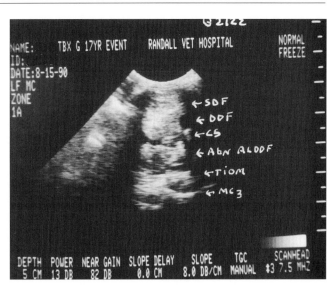

Figure 22.122.

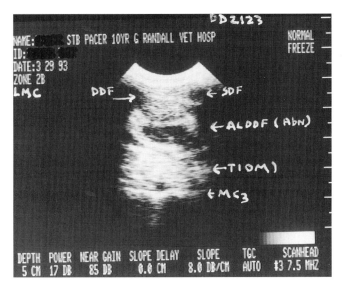

Figure 22.123.

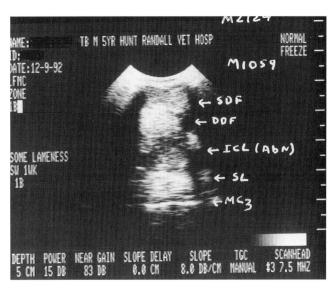

Figure 22.124.

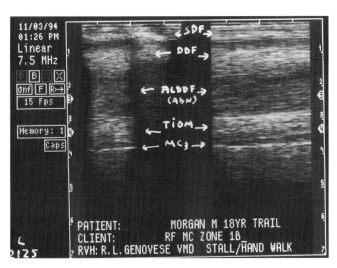

Figure 22.125.

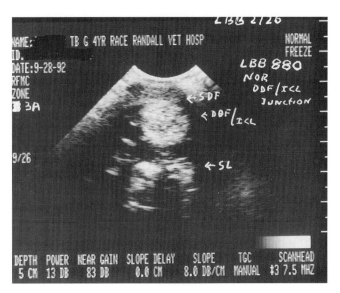

Figure 22.126.

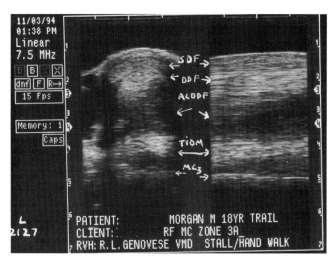

Figure 22.127.

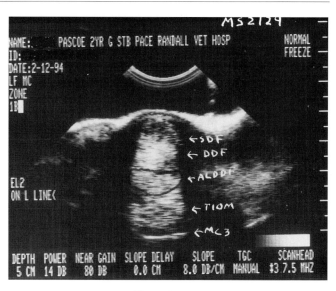

Figure 22.129.

acutely lame after a race 1 month earlier. The metacarpus was swollen, and scans revealed an enlarged and almost totally anechoic ALDDFT compatible with severe injury.

More subtle ALDDFT injury can be difficult to diagnose if careful attention is not given to all sonographic assessment parameters. Figure 22.129 is a normal cross-sectional left metacarpal Zone 1B sonogram of a 2-year-old Standardbred pacer presented for "recently being on the right line." There was slight palpable swelling of the right proximal metacarpus. The normal left ALDDFT CSA is 128 mm^2.

Figure 22.130 is a cross-sectional right metacarpal Zone 1B sonogram of the same horse shown in Figure 22.129. The ALDDFT is enlarged and has a focal echolucency along the medial border. The ALDDFT CSA is 161 mm^2 (26% increase). The three level normal left fore ALDDFT CSA is 402 mm^2. The three level abnormal right fore ALDDFT CSA is 485 mm^2 (21% increase). The CSA data combined with the slight textural and shape abnormalities confirms the ALDDFT desmitis diagnosis.

Figure 22.131 is a dual cross-sectional left and right metacarpal Zone 2A sonogram of a mixed breed jumper presented for slight mid-metacarpal swelling and no reported lameness. The owner was concerned that this recent slight "thickening" was not resolving. The scan on the left is the clinically normal limb. The right ALDDFT had a slightly rounded lateral border compared with the left. The left CSA obtained from zones 2A and 2B is 125 mm^2 and the right is 168 mm^2 (34% increase). The right SDFT CSA is 3% less than the left. The right DDFT CSA is 14% less than the left. There is significant subtle right ALDDFT enlargement without textural change. This finding explains the slight palpable midmetacarpal swelling and is consistent with a slight ALDDFT strain. Since this early diagnosis was made, the horse was given a short rest period and made an unremarkable recovery.

Care must be taken to place linear array scanheads in ex-

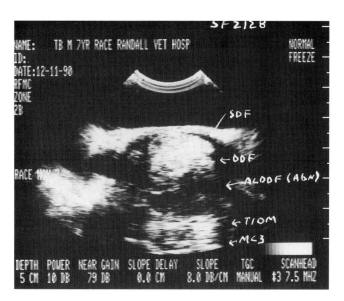

Figure 22.128.

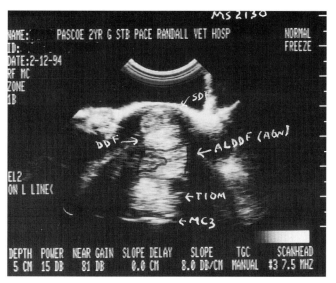

Figure 22.130.

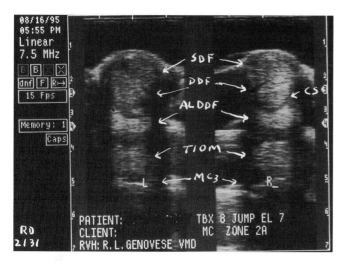

Figure 22.131.

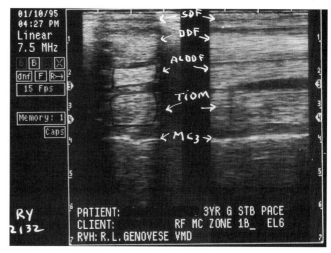

Figure 22.132.

actly the same cross-sectional plane on both limbs because the medial and lateral ALDDFT and TIOM image borders are determined by the ultrasound transducer contact area created by the flat transducer contacting the rounded palmar/plantar metacarpal/metatarsal surfaces. If the scanning plane is slightly oblique, left and right comparisons are invalid. Sector or convex array scanheads are less of a problem because their beams diverge and the medial and lateral borders of the ALDDFT are more likely to be included in the image. This is especially true of the TIOM. The lateral and medial suspensory ligament margins are not imaged with rectangular beams and and are sometimes not imaged with divergent beams. The reason for this is that skin indentations usually are present palmar to the ligament margins and the sound beams often encounter the air/skin interface in the indentation. The beam is then "cut off," missing the true ligament margins. Lateral or medial TIOM body and branch lesions often are missed unless the scanhead (and standoff pad) is placed directly medial or lateral over the ligament margin. It is nearly impossible to image the TIOM branches from the palmar aspect effectively with a linear array transducer. Cross-sectional area measurements made with linear array (rectangular beams) are less than those measured with sector or convex arrays (divergent beams). Therefore, it is important to use the same Type of scanhead configuration for serial examinations of the ALDDFT and TIOM. The problem is not as great with the SDFT and DDFT because the standoff pads create more ultrasound beam contact width. Compare the TIOM width in Figure 22.129 and Figure 22.131 for comparison of divergent (pie-wedge) versus rectangular beams. The divergent sector image in Figure 22.129 includes more TIOM width than the rectangular linear array image of Figure 22.131.

Figure 22.132 is a normal cross-sectional and sagittal right metacarpal Zone 1B sonogram of a Standardbred pacer presented for "recently being on the left line." Figure 22.133 is a cross-sectional and sagittal left metacarpal sonogram Zone 1B of the same horse shown in Figure 22.132. There is ALDDFT enlargement with a diffuse echolucency.

There is slight TIOM enlargement and a focal hypoechoic medial border lesion. The three level right ALDDFT CSA is 198 mm^2 and the left is 278 mm^2 (40% increase). The four level right TIOM CSA data is 469 mm^2 and left is 543 mm^2 (16% increase). In this limb, there is a slight TIOM and ALDDFT desmitis.

Incidentally found hypoechoic lesions always create a dilemma for the clinician. Figure 22.134 is a dual cross-sectional right metacarpal Zone 2A sonogram of a Welsh Pony presented for low grade, bilateral carpal sheath distention evaluation. There is a focal Type 2 central ALDDFT lesion, but no change in shape of the ligament. The CSA of this level and the five level total did not reveal any significant difference between the left and the right ligaments. Furthermore, there was no proximal or distal extension of this hypoechoic lesion. In this rare instance, inflammatory response has no sonographic support. Even though this finding may be incidental, as clinicians, we advise continued athletic use with careful observation and repeat sonography to determine whether or not the ALDDFT is stable.

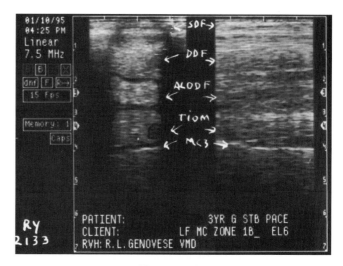

Figure 22.133.

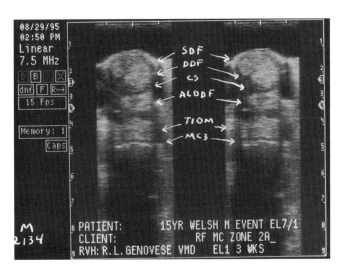

Figure 22.134.

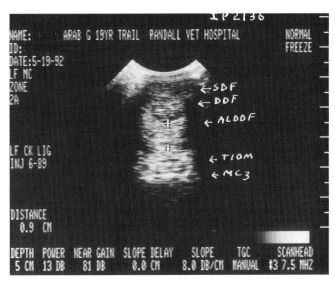

Figure 22.136.

Bilateral ALDDFT lesions are common clinical findings in older horses. Because CSA measurements are currently a routine part of our sonographic evaluation, diagnosing bilateral injuries is more common. Examining the apparently normal contralateral limb should be a standard procedure.

Figure 22.135 is a dual cross-sectional left and right metacarpal Zone 2A sonogram of a 21-year-old dressage horse. The left ALDDFT is enlarged and diffusely echolucent with adhesions to the dorsal DDFT and the palmar TIOM. The right fore ALDDFT is enlarged and had a focal Type 2 medial border lesion.

At times, assessing the significance of a chronically enlarged ALDDFT is difficult. Clinical history is pertinent because it is not always possible to differentiate recent from nonclinical poorly repaired lesions. As with tendon injuries, repair often is accompanied by hypoechoic, randomly oriented fibrosis.

Figure 22.136 is a cross-sectional left metacarpal Zone 2A sonogram of an Arab trail horse. The enlarged ALDDFT had been present for several years after an acute injury, and the horse had not experienced any clinical signs related to the thickening. The horse was in full work. The ALDDFT CSA is 136 mm^2, but the texture and shape are reasonable and there are no apparent adhesions to the DDFT. This repair is favorable and clinically has not resulted in reinjury or discomfort.

Figure 22.137 is a cross-sectional left metacarpal Zone 2A sonogram of a 14-year-old American Saddlebred presented for sonographic evaluation of a chronic nonclinical ALDDFT enlargement. The horse was in full work and no gait abnormalities were observed. The ALDDFT is enlarged and there is apparent slight adhesion between the ALDDFT and DDFT. As reported by Dyson, the DDFT seems to be smaller than normal (5). The authors have observed similar

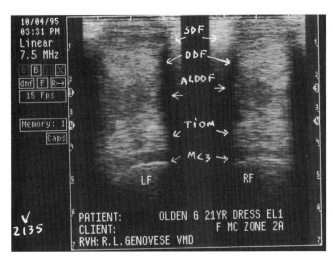

Figure 22.135.

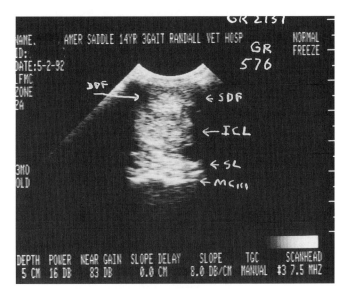

Figure 22.137.

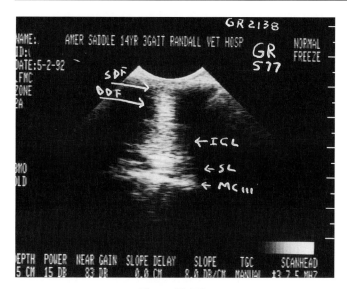

Figure 22.138.

findings in some horses with chronic ALDDFT enlargement. The texture has slight, randomly distributed, Type 1 areas. Figure 22.138 is a sagittal left metacarpal Zone 2A scan of the same horse shown in Figure 22.137. Parallel ALDDFT fiber alignment is reasonably normal.

Figure 22.139 is an actively competing Standardbred racehorse. This amazing horse has an enlarged, stable ALDDFT. There are no apparent significant TIOM or DDFT adhesions. In addition, the DDFT and SDFT are enlarged. All three of these sonographically abnormal structures were presently stable and no lameness was present.

Repair of an injured ALDDFT follows the general pattern of tendinous and ligamentous injury healing. The repair quality depends, in part, on the extent of the injury. Injuries with fiber tearing heal with randomly oriented fibrosis as opposed to injuries that are predominantly inflammatory with little fiber tearing. The functional end result is based on

the quality of the collagenation and fiber alignment and on the lack of restrictive adhesions surrounding tendinous and ligamentous structures. The overall prognosis for return to athletic use reported by Dyson is more favorable than for horses with SDFT injury (5). She reported that 10 of 13 horses returned to full work with primary ALDDFT injury within 3 to 9 months after injury; however, the study covered a variety of occupations. Intended future use after any tendon or ligament injury greatly influences prognosis.

The second most important factor is injury severity. In all cases, the same quality of repair principles apply. All tendon and ligament injury repair is inferior to normal tendon and ligament. The importance is how inferior the repair is relative to the intended athletic use. The ALDDFT seems to be a more protected and forgiving structure in consideration of future athletic use. Further research on ALDDFT injury and return to racing or high level evening is needed to provide a more accurate assessment. In our experience, most horses with ALDDFT injuries 1) are not racehorses; 2) are older; 3) have some degree of correctable feet abnormalities; or 4) perform on manageable working surfaces (not race tracks) that help prevent reinjury.

Figure 22.140 is a 12-year-old jumper presented for sudden onset lameness and swelling. A focal Type 3 lateral ALDDFT lesion is present. Treatment consisted of anti-inflammatory medication, locally applied hydrotherapy, and regular bandaging. Exercise was limited to handwalking.

Figure 22.141 is a cross-sectional right metacarpal Zone 2A sonogram of the same horse shown in Figure 22.140 3½ months after injury. The echogenicity returned to normal. The CSA increased and there is slight adhesion formation dorsal to the palmar TIOM. The DDFT is of normal size and shape. Figure 22.142 is a sagittal right metacarpal Zone 2A sonogram of the same horse shown in Figure 22.141. There is near normal parallel scar alignment. The traditional therapy program of rest, leg work, and controlled exercise has resulted in a favorable, but not ideal, sonographic qual-

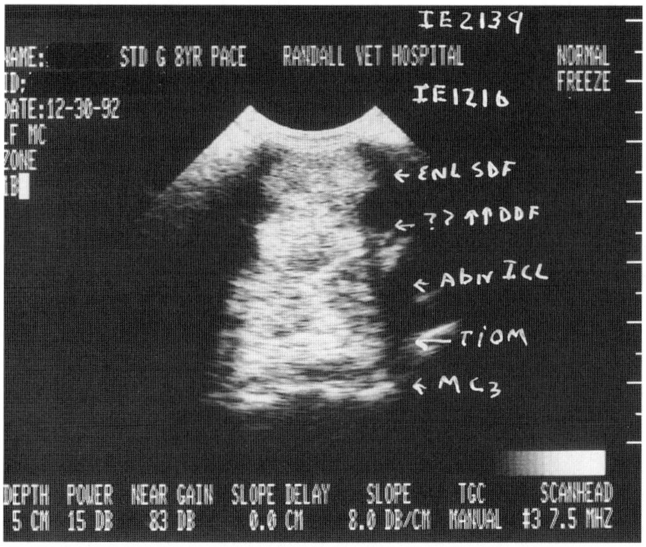

Figure 22.139.

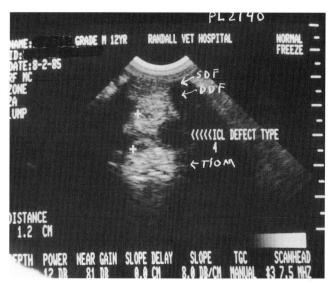

Figure 22.140.

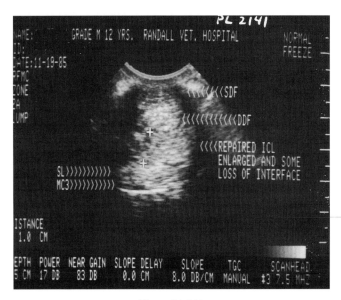

Figure 22.141.

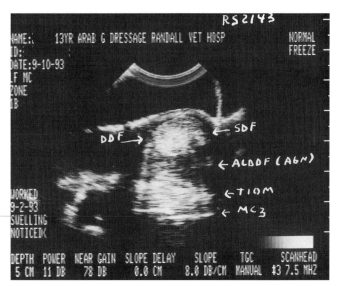

Figure 22.143.

ity of repair (SQR). Texture and fiber alignment are favorable; however, the CSA is increased and there is slight adhesion formation. This horse's intended use was low level jumping and was returned to work without injury recurrence.

Figure 22.143 is a cross-sectional left metacarpal Zone 1B sonogram of a 13-year-old Arab dressage horse presented for sudden onset swelling and no lameness. A diffuse ALDDFT injury is characterized by an echolucent lateral half, suggesting inflammation, and a mostly anechoic medial half, suggesting inflammation and fiber disruption. The left CSA is 178 mm^2 and the right is 88 mm^2 (102% increase). The contralateral limb was normal. This horse was treated in the same manner as the previous case.

Figure 22.144 is a cross-sectional left metacarpal Zone

1B sonogram of the same horse shown in Figure 22.143 made 2 months after injury. The lateral half texture is now isoechoic and there is a two-grade textural medial half improvement. There appears to be adhesion formation to the dorsal DDFT surface and the palmar TIOM surface. The CSA increased to 210 mm^2. This horse was returned to a gradual increase in work and resumed normal dressage work the next year. During the subsequent year, the horse's athletic use was advanced from flat work to flat work accompanied with low level jumping. One and one half years after the original injury, the horse was presented for left metacarpal swelling. Figure 22.145 is a dual cross-sectional right and left metacarpal Zone 2A sonogram. There is a generalized echolucency of the enlarged left ALDDFT as well as a focal Type 2 central contralateral right fore ALDDFT

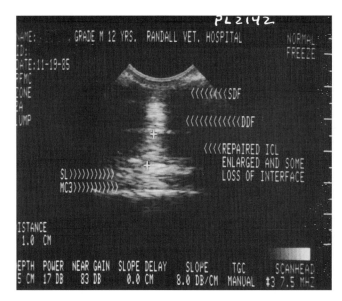

Figure 22.142.

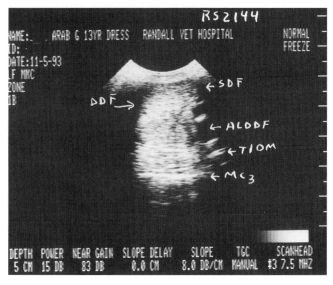

Figure 22.144.

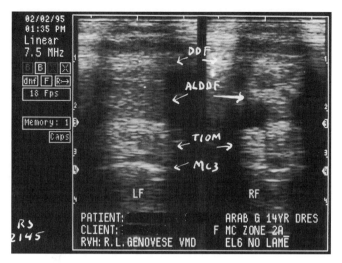

Figure 22.145.

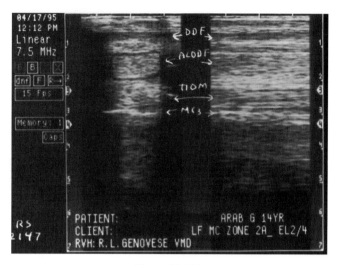

Figure 22.147.

lesion. A recurrent left ALDDFT desmitis and a focal fiber disruption of the right were diagnosed. The left GSA is 121 mm² and the right is 52 mm². The left fore ALDDFT was injected peri-ligamentously with triamcinolone and legend, and the horse was given 6 weeks at a reduced exercise program and then returned to normal walk, trot, and canter exercise. The CSA values are considerably decreased from the 2-month post injury measurements. This decrease may be caused partially by the difference in the sector scanner used in the earlier studies and the linear array used for this study based on the previous discussion.

Figure 22.146 is a dual cross-sectional left and right metacarpal Zone 2A sonogram of the same horse shown in Figure 22.145. There was a marked left ALDDFT echogenicity improvement, but the right fore focal lesion is unchanged. The left CSA is 121 mm² and the right is slightly smaller at 50 mm². A repeat peri-ligamentous triamcinolone/legend combination injection was done, and the horse was sent back to normal walk, trot, and canter exercise. In this selected case, the decision to medicate the left

fore ALDDFT locally was based on several factors, of which the owner was fully informed. First, the reinjury was not accompanied by lameness despite the elevated work level. There was no sonographic evidence of fiber tearing. Because of the horse's age, the owner was not prepared to give this horse an extensive time off for a reinjury. Finally, it was clearly stated that periodic sonographic monitoring would be done.

Figure 22.147 is a cross-sectional and sagittal left metacarpal Zone 2A sonogram of the same horse shown in Figure 22.146 made approximately 1 month after a return to full walk, trot, and canter exercise. The left ALDDFT remained enlarged but apparently stable with this increased work load.

Figure 22.148 is a cross-sectional and sagittal left metacarpal Zone 2B sonogram of a 5-year-old barrel racing quarter horse that had a previous palmar digital neurectomy. This horse suffered a recent metacarpal and pastern injury during a race. The horse was acutely lame and had palmar metacarpal and pastern swelling. At the walk, the toe of the

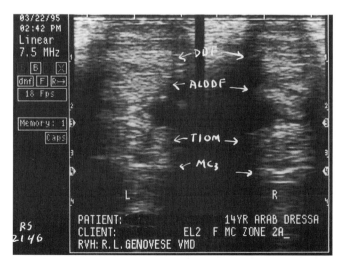

Figure 22.146.

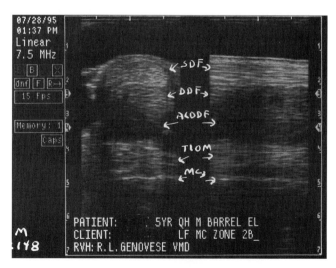

Figure 22.148.

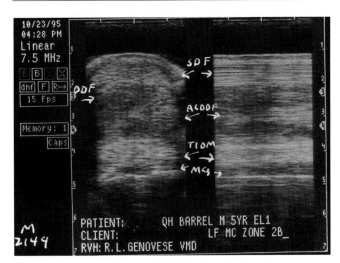

Figure 22.149.

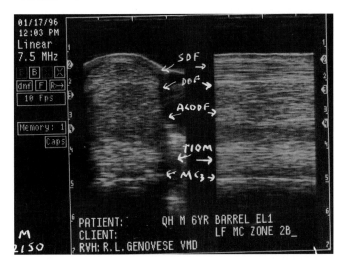

Figure 22.150.

foot was not stable. The left ALDDFT is totally hypoechoic with indistinct margins. There is total lack of fiber alignment. This was the acute injury phase or baseline sonographic information examination. There was also extensive DDFT injury extending from Zone 3A and through the palmar pastern.

Figure 22.149 is a dual cross-sectional and sagittal left metacarpal Zone 2B sonogram of the same horse shown in Figure 22.148 made 3 months after baseline. During the past 3 months, the horse has been confined to a stall. Local leg treatment was being done and the horse had corrective shoeing to improve the stability of the toe of the foot. The DDFT is slightly enlarged and has a generalized echolucency. The ALDDFT is enlarged and the texture has improved significantly. Shape is reasonably normal, with the medial, lateral and dorsal borders more clearly visible. There is, however, apparent adhesion formation between the ALDDFT and DDFT. The horse is still slightly unstable and, without the bar shoe, the toe was still slightly unstable and would elevate upon foot placement. However, 12 weeks later, a significant return of echogenicity was evident. The sagittal sonogram indicates some parallel fiber alignment centrally.

Figure 22.150 is a cross-sectional and sagittal left metacarpal Zone 2B sonogram of the same horse shown in Figure 22.149 made 6 months after baseline. Since the previous sonogram, the horse was only allowed to hand walk (EL-1). The DDFT is enlarged and the central core is echolucent. The ALDDFT is enlarged and hypoechoic fiber bundles are present along the dorsomedial aspect. There is firm adhesion between the DDFT and the ALDDFT. The sagittal sonogram reveals some attempt at parallel alignment of both the DDFT and ALDDFT. The sagittal sonogram reveals some attempt at parallel alignment of both the DDFT and ALDDFT. There has been reasonable fibrous repair of this severe DDFT and ALDDFT injury; however, because of apparent extensive adhesion formation, DDFT gliding movement may be limited. Clinically, the horse is

slightly more upright as healing has progressed. The future athletic use of this horse for barrel racing with this SQR is in jeopardy.

Bilateral injury should always be considered, especially in older horses. Figure 22.151 is a cross-sectional and sagittal left metacarpal Zone 2A sonogram of an aged dressage horse. There is a Type 3 ALDDFT injury involving 79% of the 252 mm^2 CSA with no visible parallel fiber alignment.

Figure 22.152 is a cross-sectional and sagittal right metacarpal Zone 2A sonogram of the same horse shown in Figure 22.151. There is a slightly enlarged ALDDFT with a Type 3 centrally located lesion. The CSA is 115 mm^2. The left fore had the more severe injury with 5 levels of injury; the right had 4 levels.

Figure 22.153 is a cross-sectional and sagittal left metacarpal Zone 2A sonogram of the same horse shown in Figure 22.152 made 2 months after injury. During the 2 months, the horse was allowed hand walking only. Repair was favorable for 2 months after injury considering the mag-

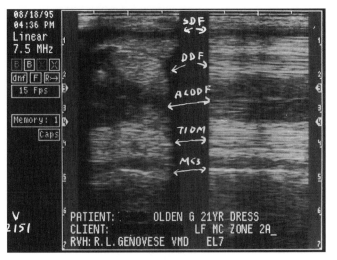

Figure 22.151.

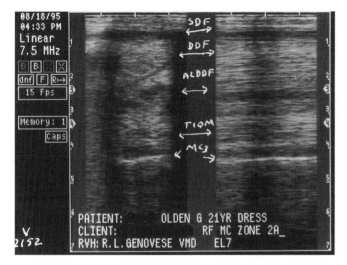

Figure 22.152.

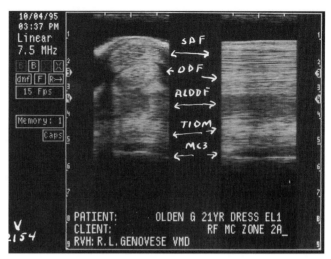

Figure 22.154.

nitude of the lesion. The ALDDFT is enlarged but has normal echogenicity. All the borders are distinct with no evidence of DDFT or TIOM adhesions. The sagittal scan reveals slightly reduced parallel fiber alignment. The CSA decreased to 228 mm^2.

Figure 22.154 is a cross-sectional and sagittal right metacarpal Zone 2A sonogram of the same horse shown in Figure 22.153 made 2 months after injury. The ALDDFT still has a diffuse echolucency and is enlarged. There is a significant lack of parallel fiber alignment. Although this was the less severely injured ligament, this injury has not repaired to the sonographic quality of the contralateral limb. The CSA increased to 171 mm^2.

Figure 22.155 is a cross-sectional and sagittal left metacarpal Zone 2A sonogram of the same horse shown in Figure 22.154 made 3 months after injury. Since the previous scan, the horse has slightly increased the exercise level to EL-2 (ride at the walk only). The ALDDFT remains enlarged,

but there is normal echogenicity, parallel fiber alignment, and no significant DDFT or the TIOM adhesions. The CSA is reduced to 142 mm^2.

Figure 22.156 is a cross-sectional and sagittal right metacarpal Zone 2A sonogram of the same horse shown in Figure 22.155 made 12 weeks after injury. The ALDDFT remains enlarged and has a slightly echolucent palmar aspect. There is near normal parallel fiber alignment. The CSA is further reduced to 128 mm^2. This case illustrates the expected favorable repair with traditional therapy consisting of complete exercise control through the early months. In the clinical management of this horse, even though there is a near ideal sonographic repair, we would not recommend the start of normal work. It is our opinion that additional time is required for scar remodeling and strengthening. The exercise level would be increased gradually over a 2 to 3 month period and sonographic monitoring as loading increases would be recommended.

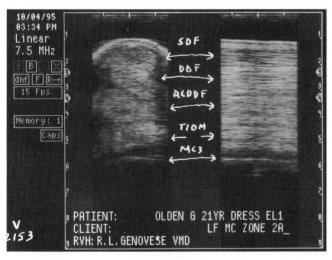

Figure 22.153.

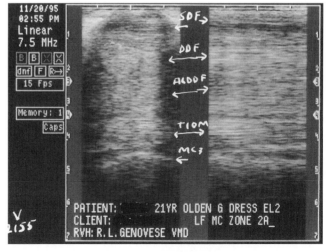

Figure 22.155.

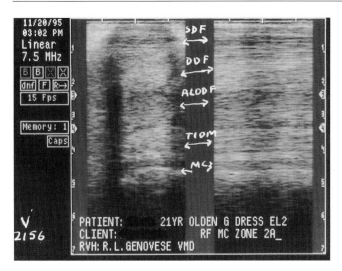

Figure 22.156.

Hind Limb ALDDFT Injuries

Hind limb ALDDFT injuries are rare in our experience. There can be sonographic abnormalities of the metatarsal ALDDFT, but the clinical significance and the definitive metatarsal ALDDFT injury diagnosis is equivocal. At times, it is difficult to establish injury of this rudimentary structure.

Figure 22.157 is a normal cross-sectional right metatarsal Zone 3A sonogram of a Standardbred. The ALDDFT is a thin, crescent shaped, 3-mm thick ligamentous structure seen on the DDFT dorsal surface. An anechoic interface exists between it and the DDFT. Dorsal to the ligament, a several millimeter long anechoic space represents loose connective tissue containing neurovascular structures separating it from the TIOM. The dorsal ALDDFT and the plantar TIOM borders are distinct.

Figure 22.158 is a cross-sectional right metatarsal Zone 3A sonogram of an aged field hunter presented for firm, low grade, metatarsal swelling evaluation. The SDFT and

DDFT tendons are normal. The ALDDFT is 7 mm thick. The neurovascular/loose connective tissue dorsal to the ALDDFT surface is compressed and displaced, and a visible interface exists between the dorsal ALDDFT and the plantar TIOM. No TIOM abnormalities are present at this level. This sonogram is presented to demonstrate that previous ALDDFT injury can result in a thickened stable structure, causing palpable metatarsal enlargement.

Figure 22.159 is a cross-sectional right metatarsal Zone 2B sonogram of a 3-year-old Standardbred presented for evaluation of firm metatarsal swelling. Previously, this horse had sustained a traumatic injury to this area. As in the previous case example, the ALDDFT is enlarged and is in intimate, yet separate, contact with the DDFT on its plantar surface and the TIOM dorsally. Both of these cases demonstrate the sonographic appearance of a healed, clinically stable, primary metatarsal ALDDFT injury. At this point, one can appreciate a healed injury resulting in an enlarged ALDDFT. However, it is more difficult to sonographically confirm an acute primary injury.

Figure 22.160 is a cross-sectional right metatarsal Zone 2B sonogram of a 4-year-old quarter horse presented for sudden onset metatarsal swelling. The SDFT was normal. To determine whether the DDFT is normal, CSA and texture comparison to the contralateral limb is essential. When this horse was examined in 1986, this step was not commonly done. Comparison is made for two reasons: first, to establish normal CSA data and secondly, to confirm that this individual has a sonographically detectable hind ALDDFT because it may be absent. This was not done, and information is missing. Based on the images, there is an absence of identifiable ALDDFT tissue. The hypoechoic structures on the dorsal DDFT may represent acute injury with a loss of identifiable morphology or edema and hemorrhage of the loose connective tissue. It was assumed that images represented an injury to the ligament, and it was decided to treat with a 1-month rest period and a follow-up

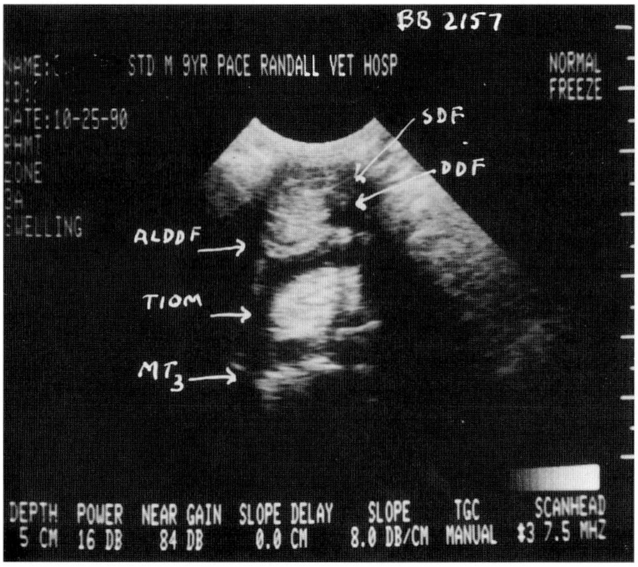

Figure 22.157.

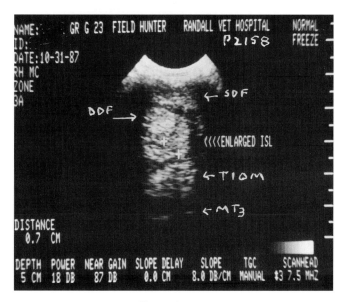

Figure 22.158.

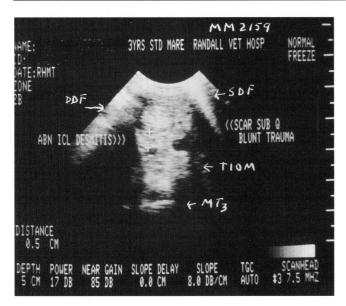

Figure 22.159.

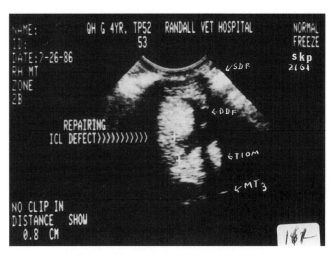

Figure 22.161.

examination. We believe that prevention of further injury is a clinically sound judgment. Therefore, we assumed the worst case scenario and used repeat sonography as a tool to confirm the diagnosis. There are many times when the diagnosis is equivocal, and repeat sonography adds pertinent data to help establish a diagnosis and prognosis.

Figure 22.161 is a cross-sectional right metatarsal Zone 2B sonogram of the same horse shown in Figure 22.160 made 1 month later. This scan reveals a return of ALDDFT echogenicity, which is enlarged (8 mm thick). In this case, there was a primary ALDDFT injury, but this was not established firmly until the 1-month repeat sonogram was done.

Figure 22.162 is a cross-sectional right metatarsal Zone 3A sonogram of a Standardbred trotter presented for low grade swelling that was nonresponsive to symptomatic treatment. The trainer reported that the horse's performances in the last two starts were suboptimal. It was his opinion that this leg "bothered the horse at high speeds." The DDFT and

ALDDFT have a normal shape and near normal size. An equivocal, focal hypoechoic area is present on the dorsomedial-medial DDFT border. The dorsal ALDDFT margin is distinct and no textural abnormalities are present. As has been shown previously in the section on the normal DDFT, normal artifactual hypoechoic fiber bundles can be present on the dorsal surface. However, the question is: "Is this hypoechoic area more than one would expect and is there an abnormality of the ALDDFT/DDFT junction?"

Figure 22.163 is a cross-sectional right metatarsal Zone 4A sonogram of the same horse shown in Figure 22.162 at the time of the initial examination. At this level, a more distinct hypoechoic area is present on the dorsomedial DDFT border; however, unlike Zone 3A, it appears to be located at the interface between the tendon and ligament instead of within the DDFT tendon fibers. It was recommended that this horse be taken out of training, treated symptomatically, and re-examined.

Figure 22.164 is a cross-sectional right metatarsal Zone 3A sonogram of the same horse shown in Figure 22.163

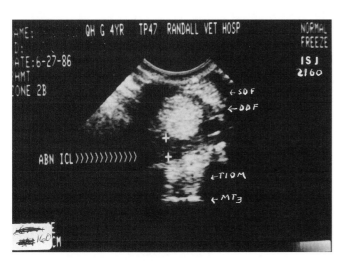

Figure 22.160.

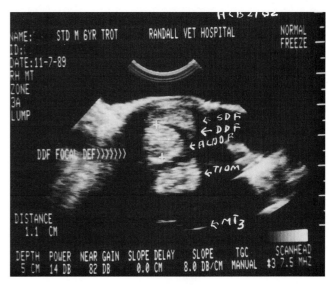

Figure 22.162.

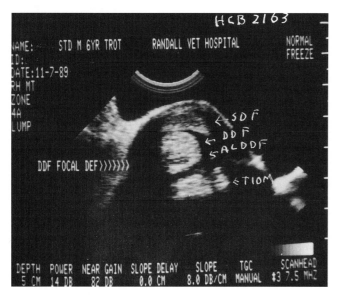

Figure 22.163.

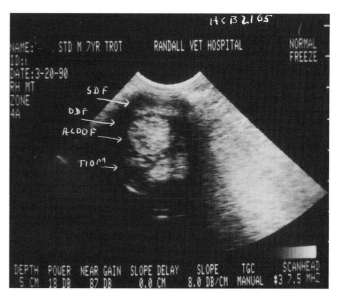

Figure 22.165.

made 4½ months after injury with the horse turned out in a paddock for exercise (EL-3). The ALDDFT has an abnormal shape and a slight size increase. Furthermore, there is a loss of the sharp dorsal border and slight periligamentous fibrosis. A focal hypoechoic segment is still present in the dorsomedial DDFT. This finding may represent a healing lesion or it could be a scanning artifact.

Figure 22.165 is a cross-sectional right metatarsal Zone 4A sonogram of the same horse shown in Figure 22.164 made during the repeat examination. An apparent fibrosis appeared between the DDFT and the ALDDFT as did significant periligamentous fibrosis. A persistent and more dorsally located focal hypoechoic DDFT lesion is still present. Taking all of the clinical and sonographic information into consideration, it is our opinion that a DDFT and ALDDFT injury occurred near the insertion.

Figure 22.166 is a cross-sectional and sagittal left metatarsal Zone 3A sonogram of a Standardbred racehorse that had an on and off racing career because of a left hind TIOM desmitis. Currently, the horse had been racing and the TIOM seemed clinically stable. After the most recent race, generalized metatarsal swelling was present. The owner was concerned that a TIOM reinjury had occurred. The scan DDFT was normal, and ALDDFT appears normal, with increased echogenicity of the neurovascular-loose connective tissue dorsally. The plantar TIOM margin appears normal.

Figure 22.167 is a cross-sectional and sagittal left metatarsal Zone 4A sonogram obtained at the same examination. The DDFT and the TIOM are normal. The ALDDFT is distinct and has an increased echogenicity connective tissue on the dorsal margin. Diffuse metacarpal swelling is present, yet there is no firm evidence of tendon

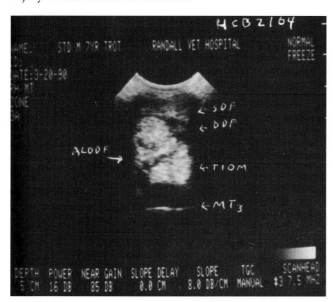

Figure 22.164.

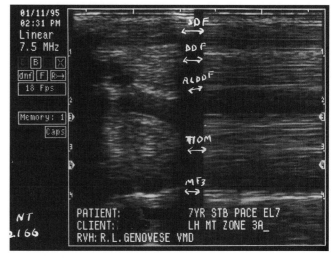

Figure 22.166.

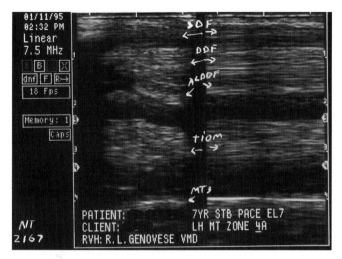

Figure 22.167.

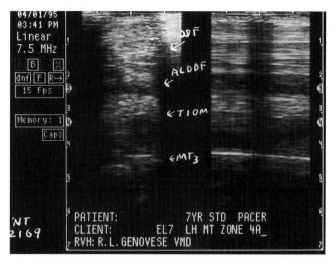

Figure 22.169.

or ligament injury. This finding raises questions about the etiology of this persistent swelling. The increased metatarsal thickness is apparently caused by edema, hemorrhage, or active inflammation of the connective tissue between the ALDDFT and the TIOM. A conservative approach was taken because of the previous TIOM injury. The owner decided to reduce the exercise level and treat the leg symptomatically. However, over the next 3 months, despite EL reduction to EL-5, there was no significant gross improvement of the metacarpal swelling.

Figure 22.168 is a cross-sectional left metatarsal Zone 3A sonogram of the same horse shown in Figure 22.167 made 3 months after injury. There was a distinct ALDDFT enlargement and a near normal echogenicity. There is a detectable interface between the ALDDFT and the TIOM. The important sonographic question is: "Does this thickened fibrous tissue represent a healing and enlarged ALDDFT, or is it a healing injury of the plantar TIOM surface?" In this case, the interface appears to separate the

ALDDFT from the plantar TIOM. Figure 22.169 is a cross-sectional and sagittal left metatarsal Zone 4A sonogram of the same horse shown in Figure 22.168 made during the 3 month post-injury sonographic evaluation. ALDDFT was clearly enlarged with near normal echogenicity and a distinct interface between the ALDDFT and the plantar TIOM surface. ALDDFT fiber alignment in the sagittal scan was poor. Therefore, a primary ALDDFT injury was diagnosed.

The systematic sonographic and clinical evaluation of equine extremity soft tissue injuries are valid concepts for the commonly injured SDFT. The preceding case studies indicate that the DDFT and ALDDFT benefit from a similar program. Certain tissue responses are somewhat predictable for the majority of cases, but individual variation in injury types and repair processes dictate that absolute recommendations cannot be made. The major difference in the last decade in soft tissue injury diagnosis and management in the horse can be directly attributable to diagnostic ultrasound. Without the ability to image the injured structures, intelligent decisions regarding treatment and management cannot be made.

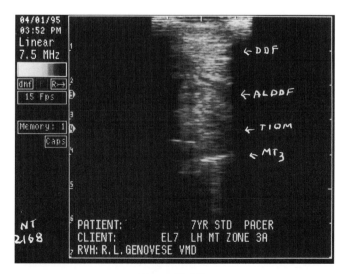

Figure 22.168.

REFERENCES

1. Dik KJ, Van Den Belt AJM, Keg PR. Ultrasonographic evaluation of fetlock annular ligament constriction in the horse. Equine Vet J 1991;23:285–288.
2. Budras KD, Sack W0. Anatomy of the horse. 2nd ed. Philadelphia: Mosby-Wolfe, 1994:12.
3. Dyson SJ, Dik KJ. Miscellaneous conditions of tendons, tendon sheaths and ligaments. Vet Clin North Am Equine Pract 1995; 2:315–337.
4. Getty R. In: Sisson, Grossman, eds. The anatomy of the domestic animals. 5th ed. Philadelphia: WB Saunders, 1975:1:431.
5. Dyson SJ. Desmitis of the accessory ligament of the deep digital flexor tendon: 27 cases (1986–1990). Equine Vet J 1991;23: 438–444.

23. Suspensory Apparatus

SUE DYSON

ANATOMY

The interosseous (medius) has been so much modified in the horse that it is termed the superior sesamoidean or suspensory ligament. It is predominantly a strong tendinous band containing variable amounts of muscular tissue (1). Sisson (1) inferred that the amount of striated muscle tissue was greater in younger horses; however, a survey of forelimb suspensory ligaments found no such variations with age (2), although differences were noted among Thoroughbreds, sexes, and state of training. This finding was confirmed (3), although the total content of muscle in the body of the suspensory ligament ranged from 2.1 to 11%.

The number and size of muscle bundles vary among individuals, but they are consistent between left and right forelimbs (3). The muscle bundles are scattered throughout the middle third of the body of the suspensory ligament, but they divide into two distinct bundles distally. Some horses have little muscle tissue proximally, whereas distally they have large muscle bundles. The muscle bundles are usually adjacent to or within sheets of loose connective tissue that run the length of the ligament. The quantity of loose connective tissue increases distally. A sheet often continues proximally from the division of the ligament deep into the structure.

The forelimb suspensory ligament originates from the palmar carpal ligament and the proximal aspect of the third metacarpal bone, whereas the hind limb suspensory ligament originates principally from the plantar proximal aspect of the third metatarsal bone. A close relationship exists between the combined joint capsule of the middle and carpometacarpal joints and the proximal suspensory ligament in the forelimb (4) and between the tarsometatarsal joint capsule and the proximal suspensory ligament in the hind limb (5). The body of the suspensory ligament descends between the second and fourth metacarpal (metatarsal) bones and in the distal metacarpus divides into two branches that insert on the proximal sesamoid bones. Extensor branches pass obliquely forward to join the common digital extensor tendon on the dorsoproximal aspect of the proximal phalanx. The suspensory apparatus is continued distally as the short, cruciate, oblique, and straight distal sesamoidean ligaments.

ULTRASONOGRAPHY OF THE NORMAL SUSPENSORY APPARATUS

For ease of reference, the suspensory apparatus can be divided into four areas: the proximal suspensory ligament (referring to the proximal one third of the metacarpus or metatarsus); the body of the suspensory ligament; the me-dial and lateral branches of the suspensory ligament; and the distal sesamoidean ligaments. The suspensory ligament may be imaged ultrasonographically using either a linear-array transducer or a sector transducer (6–8). Transverse images are easy to obtain and to interpret with either transducer, whereas the greater contact length of a linear-array transducer produces longitudinal images that are easier to assess, because a greater length of the ligament can be seen at any one time. The shape and size of the transducer head influence the ease of obtaining images of the distal sesamoidean ligaments in the pastern region.

The horse should be bearing full weight on the limb, if possible, with the limb positioned vertically, or even slightly caudal to the vertical axis. This position is particularly useful when imaging the pastern region. In general, a 7.5-Mhz transducer is ideal, or a transducer of variable frequency can be used. However, some 7.5-Mhz transducers have poor image resolution in the far field, and this may impair assessment of the proximal suspensory ligament, especially in the hind limbs of large horses. A 5-Mhz transducer is therefore preferable.

The proximal suspensory ligament and the body are best evaluated from the palmar (plantar) aspect of the limb, using a 7.5-Mhz transducer *without* a stand-off (offset). If the transducer has a built-in stand-off, this may result in an artifact partially superimposed over the suspensory ligament. In small ponies only (less than 250 kg body weight), the use of a stand-off may enhance image quality. When interpreting longitudinal images, the most proximal palmar (plantar) aspect of the third metacarpal (metatarsal) bone is not vertical, but slopes slightly palmad.

The medial and lateral branches of the suspensory ligament are best imaged from the palmar (plantar) medial and palmar (plantar) lateral aspects of the limb, and because they are positioned superficially, a stand-off is generally required. It may also be useful to assess the area between the two branches, usually filled by loose areolar connective tissue, from the palmar (plantar) aspect of the limb.

The distal sesamoidean ligaments are usually best evaluated using a stand-off. This alters the position of the focal zone of the transducer and also aids in obtaining a larger area of contact. The pastern should be examined from palmar (plantar), palmar medial, and palmar lateral aspects.

The ultrasonographic appearance of the proximal part of the forelimb suspensory ligament and its body is variable (3) (Figs. 23.1 and 23.2). The suspensory ligaments of 350 clinically normal horses and ponies were examined ultrasonographically; 22 horses were reexamined 3 to 8 months after initial examination. These comprised a random selection of horses that had either a central poorly defined or well-de-

447

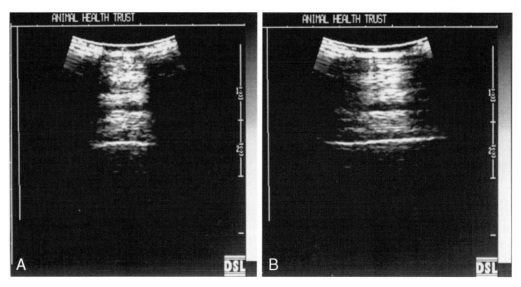

Figure 23.1. Transverse **A,** and longitudinal **B,** ultrasonograms of the proximal metacarpus of a normal horse.

fined hypoechoic area in the proximal part or body of the suspensory ligament, or in which variability in the appearance of the accessory ligament of the deep digital flexor tendon had been noted.

No significant difference in size of the suspensory ligament exists between left and right forelimbs of an individual horse at any level in the limb. The ligament is approximately rectangular in cross-section and may arise from two heads, separated by a less echogenic band. The echogenicity of the suspensory ligament is usually bilaterally symmetric, but it varies among horses. The suspensory ligament may be of uniform echogenicity to the deep digital flexor tendon, but in the proximal suspensory ligament in 13% of limbs studied, a well-defined or poorly defined central hypoechoic area was identified extending a variable distance proximodistally (see Fig. 23.2). At and immediately proximal to its bifurcation, the central area of the ligament may be less echogenic than the periphery (Figs. 23.3 and 23.4). The suspensory ligament was of patchy echogenicity in 4% of limbs studied. The palmar medial and lateral borders were usually well defined, but the dorsal margin of the suspensory ligament in

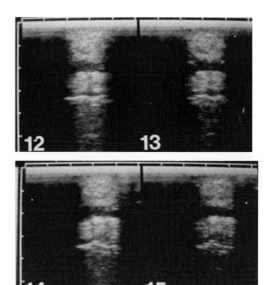

Figure 23.3. Transverse ultrasonograms of the mid-metacarpal region of a normal horse in the region of the bifurcation of the suspensory ligament, obtained at 12, 13, 14, and 15 cm distal to the accessory carpal bone.

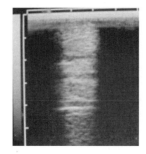

Figure 23.2. Transverse ultrasonogram of the palmar metacarpal soft tissues of a normal horse obtained 6 cm distal to the accessory carpal bone. Note the central hypoechoic area in the suspensory ligament.

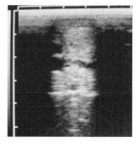

Figure 23.4. Transverse ultrasonogram of a normal horse at 11 cm distal to the accessory carpal bone. Note the hypoechoic area on the dorsal margin of the suspensory ligament, a normal feature.

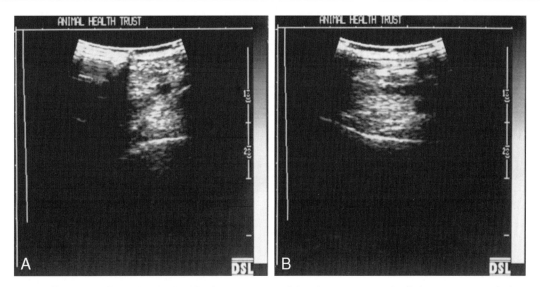

Figure 23.5. Transverse **A,** and longitudinal **B,** ultrasonograms of the plantar metatarsal soft tissue structures in the proximal metatarsus.

the region 2 to 3 cm distal to the accessory carpal bone was poorly defined or hypoechoic in 9% of limbs.

The proximal part of the suspensory ligament in the hind limb is rounder in cross-section but of more uniform echogenicity among horses than in the forelimb (Fig. 23.5). Shadowing artifacts frequently complicate interpretation proximally.

The medial and lateral branches of the suspensory ligament are usually of similar size, tending to be larger in hind limbs than in forelimbs, and are of uniform echogenicity. The branches are approximately circular in cross-section (Fig. 23.6) and lie immediately below the skin, not separated by any echodense material. Each ligament blends with

a smoothly outlined curved, proximal sesamoid bone. When viewed from the palmar (plantar) aspect of the limb, the medial and lateral branches are separated by echogenic, loose areolar connective tissue. From this view, the intersesamoidean ligament can also be clearly seen.

The short, cruciate (deep), oblique (middle), and straight (superficial) distal sesamoidean ligaments are well-defined structures in the pastern region, clearly demarcated from adjacent structures and of uniform echogenicity (Figs. 23.7 and 23.8). The straight sesamoidean ligament inserts by a cartilaginous scutum onto the proximopalmar (plantar) aspect of the middle phalanx. This results in a large central hypoechoic region that should not be confused with a lesion.

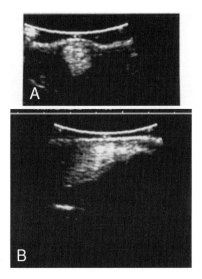

Figure 23.6. Transverse **A,** and longitudinal **B,** ultrasonograms of the lateral branch of the suspensory ligament of a normal horse.

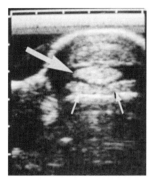

Figure 23.7. Transverse ultrasonogram of the proximal pastern of a normal horse. Note the straight sesamoid ligaments (*large arrow*) and the oblique sesamoidean ligaments (*small arrows*).

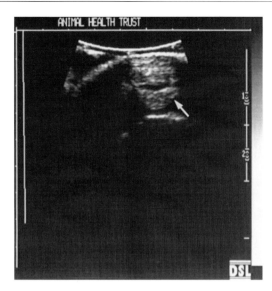

Figure 23.8. Transverse ultrasonogram of the mid-pastern region. Note the straight sesamoidean ligament (*arrow*).

INDICATIONS FOR ULTRASONOGRAPHIC EXAMINATION

Active lesions involving the body or branches of the suspensory ligament or the distal sesamoidean ligaments are usually associated with the development of localized heat, swelling, and pain, although the correlation with the presence or absence of lameness is poor. Swelling may be subtle and confined to slight rounding of the medial and lateral margins of the ligament. Localized heat, pain, and swelling are all indications for ultrasonographic appraisal. The most proximal part of the suspensory ligament lies between the bases (heads) of the second and fourth metacarpal (metatarsal) bones and is therefore virtually inaccessible to direct palpation, although indirect pressure can be applied over the palmar (plantar) aspect. Localized heat or pain detectable by palpation and pain isolated to this area using local analgesic techniques are indications for ultrasonographic examination. Extensive, diffuse soft tissue swelling in the metacarpal (metatarsal) region may make it impossible to determine which structures are involved. This is another indication for ultrasonographic evaluation.

The close relationship among the suspensory ligament, the second, third, and fourth metacarpal bones, and the proximal sesamoid bones must also be borne in mind. Radiographic and scintigraphic examinations may yield vital additional information.

PROXIMAL SUSPENSORY DESMITIS

The term *proximal suspensory desmitis* is restricted to lesions confined to the proximal one third of the metacarpus (metatarsus) and is a common condition affecting both forelimbs and hind limbs of horses of all ages in a broad cross-section of disciplines (9–17). In contrast to lesions involving the body or branches of the suspensory ligament, the horse usually has associated lameness or "poor performance" or "poor action." The condition may occur unilaterally or, less commonly, bilaterally. It sometimes occurs in association with more distal limb pain, such as in navicular disease, and is frequently seen in horses with poor mediolateral or dorsopalmar foot balance. Straight hock conformation or hyperextension (excessive dorsiflexion) of the metatarsophalangeal joints may predispose to injury in the hind limb (17). Palmar cortical fatigue fractures of the third metacarpal bone and avulsion fractures of the proximal suspensory ligament are considered separately.

Clinical Signs

Lameness can vary from mild to severe and in early cases is generally exacerbated by work, especially fast work, and improved by rest. Low-grade hind limb lameness frequently goes unrecognized until it deteriorates. No pathognomonic gait abnormalities have been detected. In horses with low-grade early forelimb cases, lameness may only be detectable on a circle with the lame limb on the outside, especially on a soft surface. In both forelimbs and hind limbs, lameness may be more readily detected by an astute rider than by an observer.

Forelimb lameness may be accentuated by flexion of the fetlock and interphalangeal joints, but it is generally unaffected by carpal flexion, whereas hind limb lameness may be increased by flexion of the fetlock and interphalangeal joints or by flexion of the hock and stifle joints.

Horses with acute-onset cases may have localized heat in the proximal metacarpal (metatarsal) region, with or without periligamentous soft tissue swelling, but those with more chronic cases frequently have no detectable palpable abnormality. Occasionally, the margins of the most proximal part of the suspensory ligament that can be palpated are rounded. Pressure applied over the proximal palmar (plantar) aspect of the suspensory ligament may elicit pain.

Local Analgesic Techniques

Even in animals with detectable clinical abnormalities in the proximal metacarpal (metatarsal) region, it is useful to employ local analgesic techniques to confirm the source or sources of pain, although interpretation is not always straightforward. The clinician must identify any concurrent cause of lameness, and distal limb nerve blocks should be performed to eliminate a more distal source of pain. Occasionally, slight improvement may be seen after perineural analgesia of the palmar (plantar) and palmar metacarpal nerves in the middle or distal third of the metacarpus (18), probably because of slight proximal diffusion of local anesthetic solution. Perineural analgesia of the palmar metacarpal (plantar metatarsal) nerves (2 × 2.5 mL), 4 to 6 cm distal to the carpometacarpal (tarsometatarsal) joint, should substantially improve or alleviate lameness associated with proximal suspensory desmitis, although in a small proportion, perineural analgesia of the ulnar (2%) (unpublished data) or tibial (12%) (16) nerves may be necessary. Nonetheless, when performing subcarpal or subtarsal analgesia, the clinician must recognize, first, that local anesthetic solution may diffuse proximally and, second, that a close relationship exists between the proximal suspensory ligament and the carpometacarpal and tarsometatarsal joint capsules in the forelimbs and hind limbs (4, 5). Therefore, subcarpal or subtarsal analgesia may inadvertently alleviate pain associated with the middle carpal or carpometacarpal joints or the tarsometatarsal joint. Intra-articular analgesia of the middle carpal or tarsometatarsal joints should ideally be performed on a separate occasion. Leakage from the joint capsule should also be considered, especially if a palmar approach to the middle carpal joint is used, rather than a dorsal approach. Thus, intra-articular analgesia may improve or alleviate pain associated with the proximal metacarpal (metatarsal) region. False-negative results of subtarsal analgesia of the plantar metatarsal nerves may result from inadvertent placement of the local anesthetic into the tarsal sheath.

Ultrasonographic Features

Ultrasonography is invaluable for the definitive diagnosis of proximal suspensory desmitis. It is easier to obtain consistent transverse images of the proximal suspensory ligament in both the forelimb and the hind limb than to obtain longitudinal images. This is in part related to the orientation of the fibers, given their origin on the third metacarpal (metatarsal) bone. Lesions may be focal and often extend only 1 to 2 cm proximodistally. Careful comparison with the contralateral limb is invaluable, particularly in view of the variability among normal horses in the ultrasonographic appearance of the forelimb suspensory ligament. Accurate measurements of the dimensions of the right and left suspensory ligaments in transverse and median planes at sites equidistant to the accessory carpal bone or to the tarsometatarsal joint are useful.

Ultrasonographic abnormalities associated with proximal suspensory desmitis include one or more of the following (Figs. 23.9 through 23.16):

1. Enlargement of the suspensory ligament in median or transverse planes (see Figs. 23.9, 23.11, and 23.13 through 23.15).

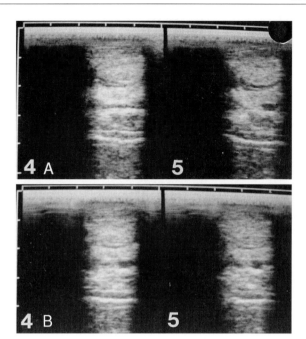

Figure 23.10. A, Transverse ultrasonogram of the palmar metacarpal soft tissues of a 6-year-old novice event horse, obtained 4 and 5 cm distal to the accessory carpal bone. Moderate lameness of 4 days' duration was alleviated by perineural analgesia of the palmar metacarpal (subcarpal) nerves. Poorly defined hypoechoic areas in the suspensory ligament extended approximately 1 cm proximodistally. **B,** The same horse 5 weeks later. The suspensory ligament is of much more uniform echogenicity. The horse resumed walking and trotting exercise, was in full work 5 weeks later, and has had no recurrent injury.

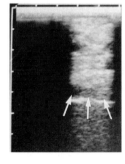

Figure 23.9. Transverse ultrasonogram of the palmar metacarpal soft tissues of the left forelimb of a 7-year-old novice event horse, obtained 5 cm distal to the accessory carpal bone. The horse had been purchased recently and been intermittently lame. Lameness was alleviated by perineural analgesia of the palmar metacarpal (subcarpal) nerves. The suspensory ligament is enlarged and its dorsal border (*arrows*) is poorly defined.

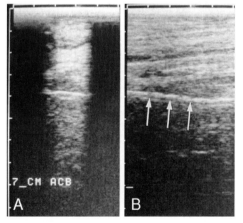

Figure 23.11. A, Transverse ultrasonogram of the palmar metacarpal soft tissues of the right forelimb, obtained 7 cm distal to the accessory carpal bone, of a 13-year-old Anglo-Arab endurance horse with intermittent lameness of nearly 9 months' duration. The lameness had recently deteriorated and become more consistent. The dorsal two thirds of the enlarged suspensory ligament is diffusely hypoechoic. **B,** Longitudinal ultrasonogram. The rather irregular outline of the palmar cortex of the third metacarpal bone (*arrows*) is indicative of enthesophyte formation and the diffuse reduction of echogenicity of the suspensory ligament.

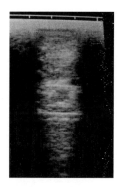

Figure 23.12. Transverse ultrasonogram of the palmar metacarpal soft tissues of an 8-year-old Prix St. Georges dressage horse, obtained 6 cm distal to the accessory carpal bone. The horse had shown transient lameness of 2 days' duration associated with heat in the proximal metacarpus. A well defined central hypoechoic area was present in the suspensory ligament and extended approximately 1.5 cm proximodistally. The lesion was no longer detectable 6 weeks later, at which time the horse resumed full work without recurrent injury.

2. Poor definition of one or more margins of the suspensory ligament, usually the dorsal margin (see Fig. 23.9).
3. A diffuse hypoechoic area involving part or all of the cross-sectional area of the suspensory ligament (see Figs. 23.11, 23.13, and 23.14**B**).
4. A well-defined central hypoechoic (or anechoic) area (see Figs. 23.12 and 23.16).
5. One or more poorly defined central hypoechoic areas (see Fig. 23.10).
6. Hyperechogenic foci; this feature has generally only been seen in chronic cases and has been identified more commonly in hind limbs than forelimbs, associated with fibrosis or mineralization.
7. An irregular palmar (plantar) contour of the third metacarpal (metatarsal) bone associated with enthesophyte formation (see Fig. 23.11**B**); this feature has been identified more frequently in hind limbs than in forelimbs.

At the time of an acute injury, detectable ultrasonographic abnormalities may be subtle and may become more obvious with time (7 to 14 days), despite rest. A change in a suspected lesion with time (increased or decreased echogenicity) is a good indicator of its potential significance.

Radiography

Radiographic examination is useful to identify or to confirm the presence of any concurrent lesion that may contribute to pain (e.g., an avulsion fracture of the origin of the suspensory ligament) and to identify any secondary bony abnormalities (14, 15, 19–22), including the following:

1. Sclerosis of the proximal third metacarpal (metatarsal) bone seen in a dorsopalmar (dorsoplantar) view.
2. Alteration of the trabecular pattern of the palmar (plantar) subcortical bone seen in a lateromedial view (see Fig. 23.15**B**).

3. Enthesophyte formation (see Fig. 23.15**B**); in my experience, ultrasonography is a more sensitive indicator of enthesophyte formation than radiography.

Radiographic abnormalities have been seen more commonly in hind limbs (66%) than in forelimbs (<5%) (15, 16); this may reflect the chronicity of the injury. Diagnosis of proximal suspensory desmitis is not based on radio-

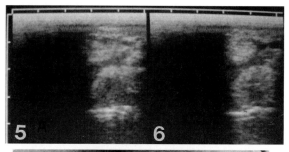

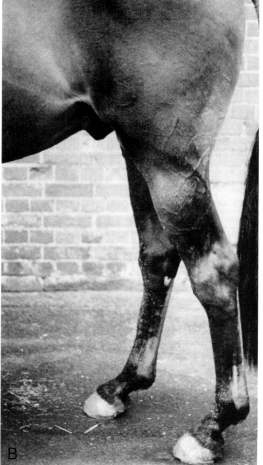

Figure 23.13. A, Transverse ultrasonograms of the plantar metatarsal soft tissues of a 12-year-old dressage horse, obtained 5 and 6 cm distal to the tarsometatarsal joint. The suspensory ligament is enlarged and has diffuse areas of reduced echogenicity. The horse had been intermittently lame for approximately 3 months and has had persistent lameness, repeatedly alleviated by subtarsal analgesia. **B,** Note the relatively straight conformation of the hocks and tendency towards hyperextension of the metatarsophalangeal joints.

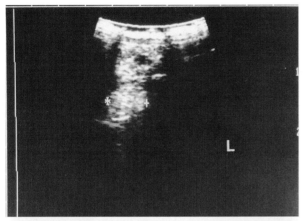

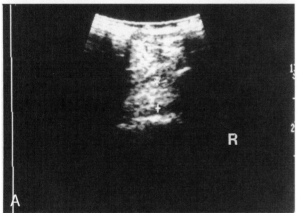

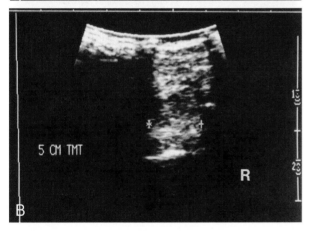

Figure 23.14. A, Transverse ultrasonograms of the plantar metatarsal soft tissues of the left (L) and right (R) hind limbs of a 9-year-old Thoroughbred endurance horse that had developed right hind limb lameness 8 weeks previously after a 50-mile ride. Lameness was alleviated by subtarsal analgesia. The suspensory ligament of the right hind limb is enlarged (10.1 × 18.9 mm) compared with that of the left hind limb (10.3 × 14.5 mm) and has less uniform echogenicity. **B,** Transverse ultrasonogram of the right hind limb 3 months later. The lameness had persisted despite rest, and the margins of the suspensory ligament body felt rounded. The suspensory ligament at 5 cm distal to the tarsometatarsal joint is further enlarged (17.1 × 16 mm) and is diffusely hypoechoic.

graphic abnormalities. Similar radiographic abnormalities may be seen in the hind limbs of some sound horses (Dyson, unpublished data). However, postmortem examination has shown a good correlation between the presence of radiographic abnormalities and subclinical pathologic changes of the proximal suspensory ligament.

Nuclear Scintigraphy

Nuclear scintigraphy has been described as a sensitive means of diagnosis of proximal suspensory desmitis (19, 20, 23), but no reliable reports have correlated nuclear scintigraphic with clinical and ultrasonographic findings. I routinely employ local analgesic techniques and ultrasonography to diagnose proximal suspensory desmitis. I have examined a few horses with nuclear scintigraphy; these animals had forelimb (4) or hind limb (3) lameness in which pain was localized to the proximal palmar (plantar) metacarpus (metatarsus) but in which no ultrasonographic or radiographic lesion was identified. One horse had a slightly increased uptake of radionucleotide in the proximal palmar metacarpus, but in the remainder, the results were negative. This disappointing result may have been improved by using more sophisticated techniques of analysis.

Treatment and Follow-Up

In my experience, horses are all treated by box rest and a controlled ascending exercise program, combined with correction of foot imbalance and application of shoes set long and wide at the heels or egg bar shoes. Concurrent treatment with local or systemic administration of a glycosaminoglycan polysulfate (Adequan), local injection of sodium hyaluronate, or local injection of an internal iodine blister does not appear to influence the outcome. Local corticosteroid treatment produces only transient improvement in clinical signs. Horses are serially reassessed clinically and ultrasonographically usually at 6- to 12-week intervals, depending on the likely duration of the injury at the time of diagnosis. Acute forelimb injuries (less than 4 weeks' duration) are associated with a rapid improvement in or alleviation of lameness within 7 to 21 days and progressive increase in echogenicity of the lesion (see Figs. 23.10 and 23.16A and B). Decrease in size of an enlarged suspensory ligament has been documented less frequently. A close-to-normal echogenicity of the lesion has been restored within 12 weeks of acute injuries. Horses have successfully resumed full work at this stage. An attempt to return horses to full work in less than 6 weeks despite partial or almost total resolution of the lesion has resulted in re-injury (see Fig. 23.16B and C). More chronic injuries usually "heal" less completely; a hypoechoic area may have persisted on a long-term basis. There is a higher rate of re-injury in this group of horses, although the period of rest and controlled exercise is often longer (6 to 9 months). A decision to return a horse to work in this situation is generally based on no further change in the ultrasonographic appearance over

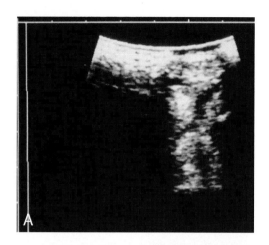

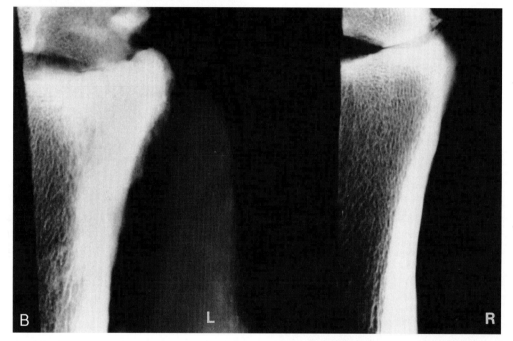

Figure 23.15. A, Transverse ultrasonogram of the plantar metatarsal soft tissues of the left hind limb of a 14-year-old hunter (former steeplechaser), obtained 5 cm distal to the tarsometatarsal joint. The suspensory ligament is enlarged and has a central hypoechoic area. The lesion extended approximately 6 cm proximodistally. The horse had been intermittently lame for more than 6 months with associated progressive hyperextension of the fetlock. The horse was humanely destroyed. **B,** Lateromedial radiographs of post mortem sagittal slices of the left (L) and right (R) hind proximal metatarsi. The plantar cortex of the third metatarsal bone of the left hind limb is markedly thickened; subcortical sclerosis and enthesophyte formation are present. *(continued on next page)*

a 3-month period. In my experience, the overall success rate of treatment of forelimb proximal suspensory desmitis is approximately 90%.

Experience with hind limb proximal suspensory desmitis has been far less favorable (16). Only 6 of 27 (22%) of horses studied had resolution of detectable lameness and were able to resume full work without recurrent injury in the period of follow-up (up to 3 years). All these horses had been lame for 4 weeks or less, whereas most of the rest had a more chronic history. There was generally a slow progressive improvement in the ultrasonographic appearance of the suspensory ligament, but in 75% of horses, persistent hy-

poechoic areas were still present up to 12 months after rest was initiated, associated with persistent lameness or recurrence of lameness if work was resumed. These poor results may be improved by recognizing lesions earlier, but riders and trainers are often less aware of (or ignore) subtle hind limb gait abnormalities than they are of mild forelimb lameness. Possibly, results are biased because my experience is in a second-opinion practice. However, the success rate of treatment in 10 of 17 (58%) of a series of horses similarly treated in a first-opinion practice is still disappointingly low (Leitch, M., personal communication). In a small proportion of horses, lesions deteriorate despite rest (see Fig.

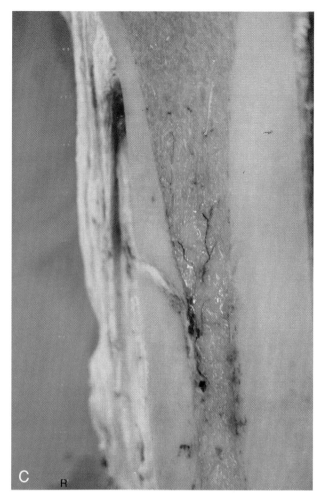 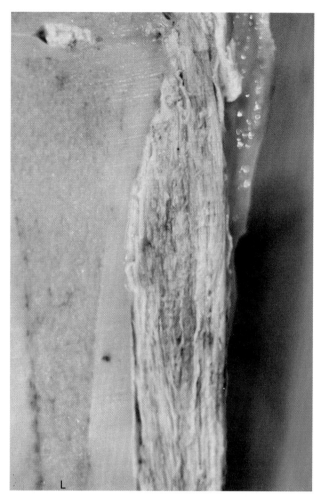

Figure 23.15. C, Sagittal sections of the proximal metatarsus of the left and right hind limbs (the flexor tendons have been removed). Note the very marked enlargement of the left hind suspensory ligament.

23.14). Some horses with forelimb or hind limb proximal suspensory desmitis have worked satisfactorily while being treated with phenylbutazone, without apparent deterioration of clinical signs.

AVULSION FRACTURES OF THE PROXIMAL SUSPENSORY LIGAMENT

Avulsion fractures of the proximal suspensory ligament occur in both the forelimb and the hind limb (22–25). They have been documented to occur most commonly in racehorses (Standardbreds more than Thoroughbreds) and my experience supports this finding. Young horses are particularly at risk. In my experience, the classification as an avulsion fracture is sometimes open to question, because some documented examples appear to have occurred immediately distal to the area of attachment of the suspensory ligament.

Clinical Signs

The horse usually has an acute onset of moderate to severe lameness. In the acute stage, the animal generally resents pressure applied over the palmar (plantar) proximal metacarpus (metatarsus), and pain is more severe than that associated with proximal suspensory desmitis. In horses with chronic cases, it may be more difficult to elicit pain. Lameness generally improves with, but may not be alleviated by, box rest.

Diagnosis

In acute cases, diagnosis can usually be based on the clinical signs and ultrasonographic or radiographic demonstration of the fracture. In more chronic cases, local analgesic techniques may be required. Perineural analgesia of the palmar metacarpal (plantar metatarsal) nerves immediately distal to

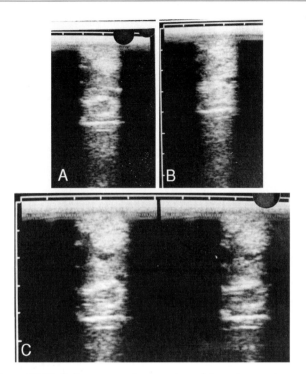

Figure 23.16. A, Transverse ultrasonogram of the palmar metacarpal soft tissues of the right forelimb of a 12-year-old advanced event horse with mild lameness of 2 days' duration. There was slight heat in the proximal metacarpus. Lameness was alleviated by perineural analgesia of the palmar metacarpal (subcarpal) nerves. There is a central hypoechoic area in the suspensory ligament at 8 cm distal to the accessory carpal bone, extending less than 1 cm proximodistally. **B,** Sonogram of the same animal 3 weeks later. The horse was in a slow, controlled exercise program and clinical signs had resolved. The lesion has a central echogenic core but is still detectable. The horse resumed full work, but lameness recurred 2 weeks later. **C,** Seven days after recurrence of lameness. The central hypoechoic area is now more obvious, occupies a larger proportion of the cross-sectional area, and extends further (2 cm) proximodistally. The horse was rested for 2 months and made a complete recovery, competing successfully at championship level for 2 more years.

the carpus (tarsus) or local infiltration of local anesthetic usually improves lameness substantially. Intra-articular analgesia of the middle carpal joint (6 mL mepivacaine) by the palmar approach has also been followed by rapid improvement in forelimb lameness.

Ultrasonography

In my experience, fractures are usually more readily detectable in longitudinal than in transverse images. An acute displaced fracture is seen as a complete discontinuity of the palmar (plantar) cortex (Fig. 23.17A). An incomplete fracture may be much more difficult to detect. Examining the limb during both weight bearing and non–weight bearing can be helpful. In a more chronic fracture, slight periosteal callus may be seen.

I generally note ultrasonographic evidence of localized suspensory desmitis (Fig. 23.17B). An insufficient number

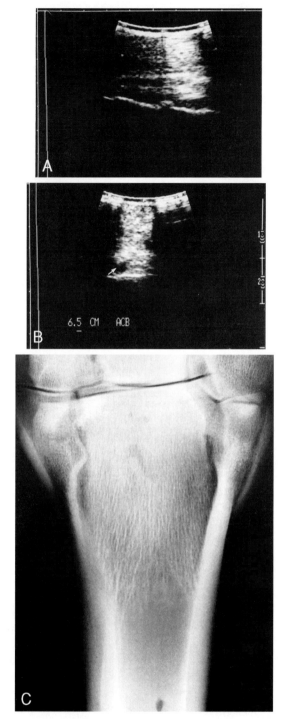

Figure 23.17. A, Longitudinal ultrasonogram of the palmar metacarpal soft tissues of the proximal left metacarpus of a 3-year-old Thoroughbred flat racehorse with recurrent lameness of 6 weeks' duration. There were no detectable localizing signs, but moderate lameness was alleviated by perineural analgesia of the palmar metacarpal (subcarpal) nerves. Note the discontinuity of the palmar cortex of the third metacarpal bone, indicative of a fracture. **B,** Transverse ultrasonogram at 6.5 cm distal to the accessory carpal bone. The dorsomedial border of the suspensory ligament (*arrow*) is almost anechoic. **C,** Dorsopalmar radiographic view of the metacarpus. Curved lucent line and discrete opacity represent an avulsion fracture of the palmar cortex of the third metacarpal bone.

of cases has been followed on a long term basis to determine whether the extent of suspensory damage influences the long-term prognosis.

Radiography

Avulsion fractures of the suspensory ligament are best detected in dorsopalmar (dorsoplantar) or slightly oblique dorsopalmar views and in lateromedial or flexed lateromedial projections. They may be seen as almost straight or saucer-shaped lucent lines (with the base proximal or distal) (Fig. 23.17C) or as a "punched out" lesion. An insufficient number of cases of each type of lesion has been examined both radiographically and ultrasonographically to know whether any good correlation exists between radiographic and ultrasonographic appearance.

Nuclear Scintigraphy

Nuclear scintigraphy may be a more sensitive means of detecting an acute, incomplete fracture than either ultrasonography or radiography.

Treatment and Prognosis

Horses are treated by box rest for 6 weeks, followed by box rest and controlled exercise for at least another 6 weeks. Horses are monitored clinically, ultrasonographically, and radiographically. In my experience, lameness generally takes longer to resolve than that associated only with proximal suspensory desmitis, sometimes up to 2 months. Fractures have remained detectable radiographically for 2 to 4 months; periosteal callus has been recognized ultrasonographically at 4 to 6 weeks after injury in a few horses. The total convalescence period has ranged from 4 to 6 months. Most horses have ultimately made a complete recovery and returned to full athletic function without associated recurrent injury; one horse with forelimb lameness developed a sequestrum (I.M. Wright, personal communication); a second horse developed progressive suspensory desmitis despite healing of the fracture. Recurrent lameness associated with a fracture was successfully treated by forage of the bone (26). It remains open to debate whether this was a true avulsion fracture or a fatigue or stress fracture of the palmar cortex of the third metacarpal bone.

PALMAR CORTICAL FATIGUE FRACTURES

Proximal palmar cortical fatigue fractures of the third metacarpal bone were previously confused with both proximal suspensory desmitis and avulsion fractures of the proximal suspensory ligament (23, 25), but I believe that they should probably be regarded as a separate clinical entity probably unrelated to disorders of the suspensory ligament. They are included because they are important in a differential diagnosis of proximal palmar metacarpal pain and to highlight them as a distinct clinical condition.

The condition occurs in young horses, generally associated with an increase in work intensity. Although these injuries occur most commonly in racehorses (flat and jumpers) (25, 27), they have been seen in horses in other disciplines including dressage, showjumping, and long-distance riding (25, 28). Fractures may occur unilaterally or bilaterally. Although many horses have a history of acute-onset lameness, a small proportion have a longer-standing mild gait abnormality.

In the acute stage, the horse may have pain on palpation of the proximal palmar metacarpus. Lameness varies from mild to severe and is usually worse on hard ground and is rapidly accentuated by work. Diagnosis is confirmed by localization of pain, by perineural analgesia of the palmar metacarpal nerves immediately distal to the carpus, and by radiographic demonstration of the fracture. Some fractures have apparently extended to the carpometacarpal joint, and lameness has been improved by intra-articular analgesia of the middle carpal joint (27).

Fractures are most readily detectable radiographically in a dorsopalmar (or slightly oblique) dorsopalmar view, and they extend longitudinally a variable distance proximodistally almost exclusively in the *medial* proximal metaphyseal–diaphyseal region. Surrounding sclerosis is generally present even in the acute stage, suggestive of preexisting subclinical bone modeling.

I previously questioned the relationship between palmar cortical fatigue fractures and proximal suspensory desmitis (25). Since then, 25 horses with radiographic evidence of a palmar cortical fatigue fracture have been examined radiographically and ultrasonographically. No abnormality of the suspensory ligament has been detected.

Treatment has been box rest (6 weeks), followed by a further 6 weeks of box rest and controlled walking before resumption of work. In my series, all horses returned to full athletic function without recurrent injury. In those horses that were reexamined radiographically, the fracture had disappeared and sclerosis had become less obvious.

DESMITIS OF THE BODY OF THE SUSPENSORY LIGAMENT

Desmitis of the body of the suspensory ligament is principally an injury of horses that race, both Thoroughbreds (flat racehorses and jumpers) and Standardbreds (12, 13, 9, 30). Injuries are generally restricted to the forelimb in Thoroughbreds, whereas they occur in both forelimbs and hind limbs in Standardbreds, and several limbs may be affected concurrently. Standardbreds appear to be able to tolerate a much greater amount of damage while still being maintained in work compared with Thoroughbreds. Overall, a poor correlation exists between the extent of lesions and the degree of lameness. Nonetheless, performance may be compromised even in the absence of overt lameness. Although proximal suspensory desmitis and desmitis of the medial or lateral branches of the suspensory ligament are common injuries in event horses, showjumpers, and endurance horses, body lesions are recognized less frequently and are often a sequel to a previous branch injury.

Soreness on palpation of the forelimb suspensory ligament is a common finding in horses with lameness associated with a more distal limb problem, but only rarely is any structural abnormality of the ligaments identifiable ultrasonographically. Event horses frequently have sore suspensory ligaments for one to several days after competing cross country, but rarely does this appear to be related to a significant problem. In these horses, it does not appear to be a warning sign of impending desmitis.

Clinical Signs

The clinical signs associated with suspensory body desmitis are variable in presence and degree and may include the following:

1. Rounding of the margins of the body of the suspensory ligament.
2. Enlargement of the body of the suspensory ligament.
3. Periligamentous edema; severe periligamentous soft tissue swelling can make accurate assessment of the suspensory ligament per se impossible by palpation.
4. Localized heat.
5. Pain on palpation of the margins of the suspensory ligament (and the second or fourth metacarpal or metatarsal bones).
6. Lameness; the absence of lameness does not preclude significant desmitis.

Diagnosis of desmitis of the body of the suspensory ligament is usually based on clinical signs and can be confirmed ultrasonographically. Only rarely are local analgesic techniques required. Analgesia may be necessary if more than one cause of lameness is suspected or if recurrence of previous desmitis is suspected. In this case, a previously enlarged suspensory ligament may have no detectable change in size, shape, or reaction to palpation. Although blockade of the palmar metacarpal nerves proximal to the site of the lesion may improve lameness, it may be necessary also to block the palmar nerves.

Ultrasonographic Features

Identification and interpretation of suspected lesions of the body of the suspensory ligament are not always easy, given the variable ultrasonographic appearances among normal horses. The precise level of the bifurcation is also variable among horses of similar size. Comparison with the contralateral limb can be invaluable in a horse with unilateral clinical signs.

Ultrasonographic abnormalities include (Fig. 23.18) the following:

1. Enlargement of the body of the suspensory ligament in median or transverse planes.
2. Loss of definition of one or more of the margins of the suspensory ligament.
3. A diffuse reduction in echogenicity of a large proportion of the cross-sectional area of the ligament.

4. Focal hypoechoic areas, central or peripheral, extending a variable distance proximodistally.
5. Focal hyperechoic lesions in horses with chronic cases.

The extent of ultrasonographic abnormalities is not always correlated with the severity of clinical signs.

Unlike lesions identified ultrasonographically in the superficial digital flexor tendon, many lesions in the suspensory ligament persist on a long term basis (more than 12 months) regardless of the method of management, although focal lesions in Standardbreds may "fill in." Although the area of the lesion and its proximodistal extent may reduce slightly, and there may be some increase in echogenicity, a readily detectable defect often remains in Thoroughbreds. This finding limits the value of serial ultrasonographic evaluations for determining when a horse may be able to withstand a return to work. We have no objective method of determining the extent of healing and the "strength" of the repair tissue. This may explain the high rate of recurrence of body lesions in both Thoroughbreds and Standardbreds. Standardbreds can frequently be managed (31), with a useful extension to their competitive lives, whereas management is more difficult in Thoroughbreds (32).

Management

Treatment is aimed at reducing inflammation by systemic nonsteroidal anti-inflammatory drugs, hydrotherapy, and controlled exercise (31). Progress is monitored both clinically and by serial ultrasonographic examinations. In Standardbreds, hand-walking exercise is advocated for the first 4 weeks (31). Provided some improvement is noted in the ultrasonographic appearance of the ligament and the horse is sound when jogged in hand, the horse is harnessed and walked in the bike for a further 4 weeks. Flat shoes are preferred. The horse is reassessed ultrasonographically 8 weeks after surgery, and if some further filling in of the defect has occurred, short slow jogging is reintroduced and gradually increased. A third ultrasonographic examination is performed after 8 weeks of jogging, and provided the lesion is of uniform echogenicity to the remainder of the suspensory ligament and has a linear arrangement of fibers, normal jogging and speed work are resumed.

PERIOSTITIS OF THE SECOND OR FOURTH METACARPAL (METATARSAL) BONE AND SUSPENSORY LIGAMENT DESMITIS

Periostitis of the second or fourth metacarpal (or less commonly, metatarsal) bone (a splint) is frequently seen in association with localized or more diffuse suspensory ligament desmitis (20). It is often difficult to determine the sequence of events: does periostitis lead to localized inflammation and irritation of the suspensory ligament and result in adhesion formation? Alternatively, can suspensory ligament desmitis induce periostitis? The pair of conditions is seen in all types of horses. Clinical signs include localized heat and pain on pressure over the affected bone, usually with a variable de-

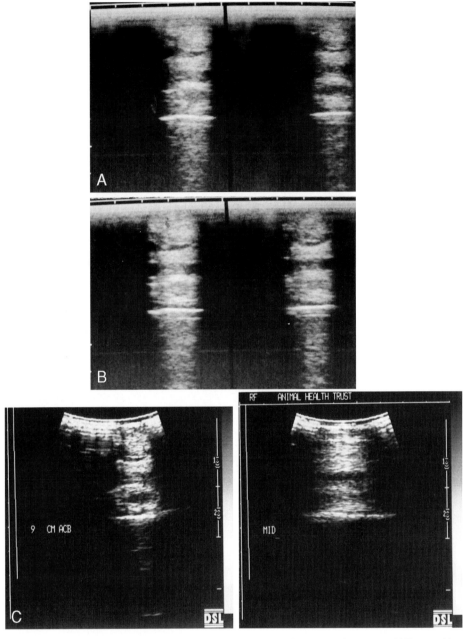

Figure 23.18. A, Transverse ultrasonogram of the palmar metacarpal soft tissues of a 6-year-old Thoroughbred flat race-horse with "filling" in the right forelimb since racing 6 weeks previously but no lameness. The body of the suspensory ligament was enlarged throughout its length and felt stiffer than that of the contralateral limb. The medial palmar vein was enlarged. The suspensory ligament has a large central hypoechoic area at 7 and 9 cm distal to the accessory carpal bone, which extended approximately 8 cm proximodistally. **B,** The same horse 5 months later. There is considerable increase in echogenicity of the suspensory ligament. The horse resumed slow cantering at this stage and when reevaluated 3 months later, the suspensory ligament was of almost uniform echogenicity. **C,** Transverse (*left*) and longitudinal (*right*) ultrasonograms from the mid-metacarpal region of the same horse 14 months after the original injury. The horse had raced twice with recurrence of clinical signs of heat and pain but no detectable lameness. A large central hypoechoic lesion extended throughout the body of the suspensory ligament.

gree of localized enlargement of the diaphysis. There may be surrounding soft tissue swelling. Palpation of the margin of the suspensory ligament on that side may be difficult. Palpable enlargement of the suspensory ligament is a variable feature. There is usually mild to moderate lameness, worst on a hard surface. Diagnosis is based on clinical signs and radiographic and ultrasonographic abnormalities.

Radiology

The extent of radiographic abnormalities and the ease of their detection depend on the duration of clinical signs. Periosteal new bone formation takes approximately 10 days before it is sufficiently radiodense to be detected, and it may be detectable more accurately by ultrasonography. Precise orientation of the x-ray beam and the use of "soft" exposures is essential if this active new bone is to be detected (Fig. 23.19A). It can be difficult to determine accurately the axial extent of this new bone. Later, the new bone becomes progressively more radiopaque, although radiolucent "pillars" may persist because of incorporation of fibrous tissue. The new bone gradually models and becomes more smoothly outlined, although it may still have an irregular contour. These changes take place over 6 to 8 weeks.

Ultrasonography

Associated ultrasonographic abnormalities are usually localized and include the following:

1. Focal enlargement of the suspensory ligament.
2. A focal reduction of echogenicity, medially (associated with periostitis of the second metacarpal bone), laterally (associated with periostitis of the fourth metacarpal bone), or, less commonly, centrally.
3. Loss of definition of the medial or lateral border of the suspensory ligament (Fig. 23.19B).
4. Echogenic material abaxial to the suspensory ligament. This may represent adhesion formation between the suspensory ligament and the second or fourth metacarpal bone.

Treatment

Generally, box rest for 6 to 8 weeks results in total resolution of the problem with or without topical application of antiinflammatory agents such as dimethylsulfoxide. Local injection of corticosteroids subjectively may be beneficial. In some horses, adhesions do develop between the suspensory ligament and the enlarged metacarpal bone, resulting in recurrent desmitis. Surgical transection of these adhesions once the active bony reaction has subsided, usually with osteotomy of the exostosis or amputation of the distal splint bone, has been beneficial.

FRACTURE OF THE SECOND OR FOURTH METACARPAL (METATARSAL) BONE AT THE JUNCTION OF THE PROXIMAL TWO THIRDS AND DISTAL ONE THIRD AND SUSPENSORY DESMITIS

A close anatomic relationship exists between the suspensory apparatus and the second and fourth metacarpal (metatarsal) bones. The distal ends of both the second and fourth metacarpal (metatarsal) bones are connected by fibrous bands to the abaxial surface of the medial and lateral proximal sesamoid bones. Fracture of the second or fourth metacarpal (metatarsal) bone is frequently seen either in association with desmitis of the body of the suspensory ligaments or with desmitis of the medial or lateral branch of the suspensory ligament (20, 33, 34), and it may be the result of hyperextension of the fetlock and stretching of the aforementioned fibrous bands. The fracture consistently occurs at the junction between the proximal two thirds and the distal one third of the bone (Figs. 23.20 and 23.22), in conjunction with either body or branch suspensory lesions. In

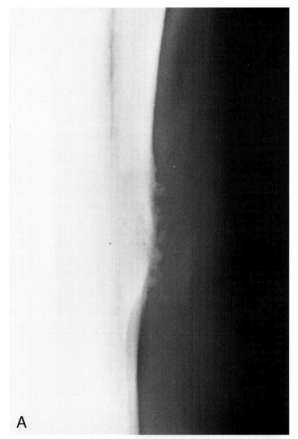

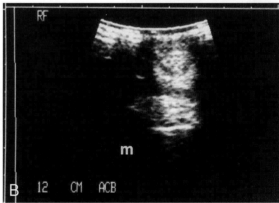

Figure 23.19. A, Dorsomedial-palmarolateral oblique view of the left metacarpus of a 7-year-old hunter with mild lameness. There was pain on palpation of the mid-diaphysis of the second metacarpal bone and the adjacent suspensory ligament. There is an active appearing periosteal proliferative reaction on the diaphysis of the second metacarpal bone. **B,** Transverse ultrasonogram of the palmar metacarpal soft tissues obtained at the same level as the "splint." The medial margin (m) of the suspensory ligament is hypoechoic and poorly defined.

association with desmitis of the body of the suspensory ligament or of one of the branches, one frequently sees a deformation in shape or modeling of the distal aspect of the second or fourth metacarpal bones (Fig. 23.21). Whether this is mechanical deformation resulting from pressure or from the presence of adhesions is difficult to determine. Adhesions are often identified surgically. Preexisting suspensory desmitis is one major factor, but some fractures occur acutely and the cause of these fractures remains poorly understood. Two horses were examined with a recent fracture and localized desmitis while confined to box rest for another cause of lameness.

Concurrent splint bone fractures and suspensory desmitis (branch or body lesions) are seen in many types of horses including Thoroughbred racehorses (especially jumpers), Standardbreds, Hunters, and, less commonly, event horses and pleasure horses. One generally notes diffuse or localized soft tissue swelling, the extent of which may prohibit accurate palpation of both the suspensory ligament and the affected metacarpal bone. The horse has localized heat and pain on palpation, and lameness may be mild to moderate. Diagnosis is based on clinical signs, radiography, and ultrasonography.

Radiography

Both the metacarpal bone and the proximal sesamoid bone should be evaluated, because lesions at both sites may occur concurrently. Preexisting abnormalities of either the medial or lateral proximal sesamoid bone suggest long-term sus-

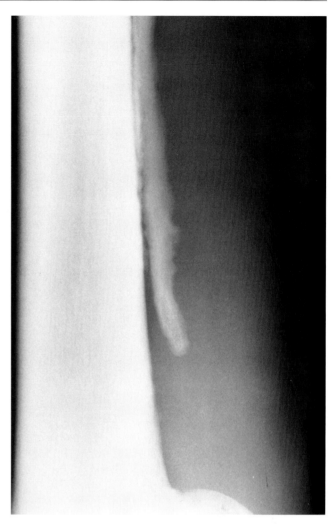

Figure 23.21. Dorsolateral-palmaromedial oblique view of the left metacarpus of a 6-year-old Thoroughbred steeplechaser with suspensory ligament desmitis. The distal third of the fourth metacarpal bone is considerably modeled.

pensory desmitis. The fracture should be evaluated to determine (see Figs. 23.20 and 23.22) the following:

1. The site of the fracture (most occur at the same location).
2. The degree of displacement.
3. The presence of comminution; comminution may indicate external trauma as the underlying cause.
4. The presence of callus formation and its extent. Fractures may also be detected ultrasonographically.

Ultrasonography

Ultrasonography is used to identify the extent of suspensory ligament desmitis; the clinician must bear in mind that the degree of suspensory ligament disorder is likely to influence the long-term prognosis, unless the fracture was due to external trauma (see Fig. 23.22).

Ultrasonographic abnormalities include those already discussed under suspensory ligament desmitis. In addition, depending on the chronicity of the lesion, there may be poorly defined or well-defined echogenic material between

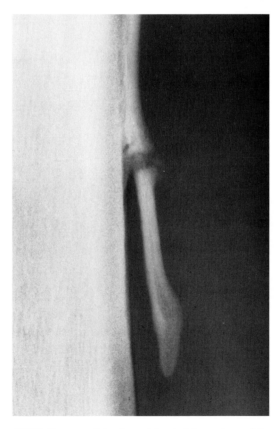

Figure 23.20. Dorsomedial-palmarolateral oblique view of the right metacarpus of an 11-year-old hunter with severe recurrent suspensory desmitis. A healing fracture is at the junction of the proximal two thirds and distal third of the second metacarpal bone. There was a similar fracture of the fourth metacarpal bone. When explored surgically, both the second and fourth metacarpal bones were completely shrouded in thick fibrous tissue.

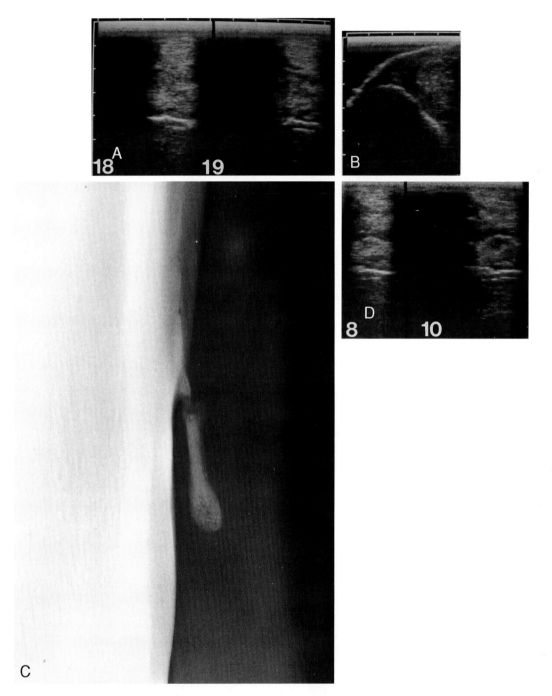

Figure 23.22. A, Transverse ultrasonogram of the palmar metacarpal soft tissues of an 8-year-old Grand Prix show jumper that had shown intermittent right forelimb lameness for approximately 8 weeks but had been "managed" in order to be kept in competition. The distal aspect only of the suspensory ligament was sore on palpation. The suspensory ligament at 18 and 19 cm distal to the accessory carpal bone is enlarged and has central hypoechoic areas. **B,** Transverse ultrasonogram of the medial branch of the suspensory ligament, which was enlarged but not painful. The medial branch is enlarged and its margins poorly defined and surrounded by moderate echoes. Poorly defined hypoechoic areas are within the branch. **C,** Dorsomedial-palmarolateral oblique radiographic view of the metacarpus. There is a slightly displaced fracture of the distal end of the second metacarpal bone with some callus formation. The fracture fragment was removed surgically. **D,** Transverse ultrasonograms of the palmar metacarpal soft tissues 7 months postoperatively obtained at 8 and 10 cm distal to the accessory carpal bone. The horse had resumed work 2 months earlier but suffered recurrent lameness associated with enlargement of the suspensory ligament and localized pain at this level, i.e., significantly further proximally than the previous lesion. The horse has been managed by aggressive local therapy and judicious selection of competitions.

the fractured metacarpal bone and the suspensory ligament. Nonetheless, not all fractures of the distal second or fourth metacarpal bones are associated with detectable ultrasonographic abnormalities of the suspensory ligament at the time of the initial injury.

Management

Some controversy exists concerning the optimal treatment for fractures of the distal one third of the second or fourth metacarpal bones. Some clinicians advocate surgical removal of the fracture fragment, and others infer that most fractures can be treated conservatively (33–36). In my opinion, there is a place for surgical removal of selected fracture fragments, but despite surgical treatment, suspensory ligament desmitis may recur. To my knowledge, although retrospective studies have compared the results of surgical and conservative treatment, no prospective studies have been conducted. The prognosis is better in Standardbreds than in Thoroughbreds (33, 37).

With conservative treatment, nondisplaced or slightly displaced fractures usually heal satisfactorily within 4 to 6 weeks if the horse is confined to box rest. Only a small amount of callus develops, and it subsequently remodels. Small radiolucent defects may persist because of incorporation of fibrous tissue. If the fracture is moderately displaced, a larger amount of callus may develop, or a thick layer of fibrous tissue may be laid down that envelops the entire distal metacarpal bone. A large exostosis may impinge on the suspensory ligament and may cause recurrent lameness.

Several questions remain unanswered satisfactorily:

1. Can adhesions develop between callus and a normal suspensory ligament, thus predisposing to subsequent suspensory desmitis?
2. Is a displaced fracture seen in association with suspensory desmitis more likely to be associated with adhesion formation?
3. Does a correlation exist between the degree of displacement of the fracture and the severity of suspensory desmitis?

The prognosis ultimately depends on the degree of suspensory desmitis and the extent of adhesion formation. Standardbreds therefore have a more favorable prognosis than Thoroughbreds.

INFECTIOUS OSTEITIS OR OSTEOMYELITIS OF THE SECOND OR FOURTH METACARPAL (METATARSAL) BONES

Infectious osteitis or osteomyelitis usually is a sequel to direct trauma to the limb, which may also result in concurrent localized inflammation of the suspensory ligament. Diagnosis can be by radiography or ultrasonography. Infectious osteitis is characterized ultrasonographically by an anechoic area immediately adjacent to the diaphysis. Ultrasonographic abnormalities are usually detectable before the development of any radiographic changes. Some horses do respond adequately to aggressive systemic antimicrobial therapy if treated in the acute stage. The localized suspensory inflammation generally resolves satisfactorily. In longer-standing cases with sequestrum formation, surgical curettage is indicated. The radiographs should be inspected carefully to assess the integrity of the bone, because the initiating trauma may result in a fracture. Amputation of part of the splint bone may have to be considered.

DESMITIS OF THE MEDIAL OR LATERAL BRANCH OF THE SUSPENSORY LIGAMENT

Desmitis of the medial or lateral branch of the suspensory ligament is a common injury, occurring in all types of horses, in both forelimbs and hind limbs (13, 29, 30). Usually, only a single branch is affected, in a single limb, although both branches may be affected, especially in hind limbs. Foot imbalance is often recognized in affected horses, and this may be a predisposing factor. Detection of radiographic abnormalities (modeling of the distal second or fourth metacarpal bones or a proximal sesamoid bone) in some horses at the time of an acute, first-time injury suggests a subclinical preexisting problem. I have also seen many event horses that have presented with concurrent suspensory branch desmitis and ipsilateral metacarpophalangeal joint pain associated with degenerative joint disease.

Clinical Signs

The clinical signs depend on the degree of damage and on the chronicity of the lesions and include localized heat and swelling. Swelling is often due to enlargement of the branch per se and periligamentous edema or periligamentous fibrous material. One may see associated distention of the metacarpophalangeal (metatarsophalangeal) joint capsule. I have seen cases in hind limbs with massive distention and enlargement of the digital flexor tendon sheath making accurate appraisal of the suspensory branches difficult by palpation. Pain is usually elicited either by direct pressure applied to the injured branch or by passive flexion of the fetlock. Lameness is variable and may be absent, but it is usually proportional to the degree of damage and is inversely related to the duration of the injury.

Diagnosis

Diagnosis is based on clinical signs and ultrasonographic examination. Only rarely are local analgesic techniques required. Analgesia may be necessary when more than one lesion is suspected or in horses with more chronic or recurrent cases that have no reaction to palpation of the branch and no localized heat. In my experience, it is usually necessary to block both the palmar (plantar) and palmar metacarpal (palmar metatarsal) nerves to alleviate lameness fully. Perineural analgesia of the palmar metacarpal or palmar nerves alone usually does not alleviate lameness. If the blocks are performed ipsilateral to the affected branch, there is usually significant improvement in lameness, although bilateral blocks may be necessary to alleviate it fully. In acute cases with concurrent distention of the metacarpophalangeal joint and severe pain on passive flexion of the joint, I generally reassess the horse 2 to 3 weeks later, when the acute inflammatory reaction has subsided. If joint capsule distention and pain on manipulation persist, then the joint is blocked intra-articularly. In a few horses, joint pain is a long-term limiting factor, rather than suspensory desmitis, so medication of the joint or arthroscopic evaluation may be indicated.

Ultrasonography

The entire suspensory ligament should be examined ultrasonographically because lesions may extend further proximal or distal than detectable clinical signs.

Ultrasonographic abnormalities may include the following (Figs. 23.23 through 23.28):

1. Abnormalities of the body of the suspensory ligament (see the discussion of desmitis of the body of the suspensory ligament).
2. Enlargement of the branch (see Figs. 23.23, 23.24, 23.27, and 23.28**A**).
3. Change in shape of the branch (see Fig. 23.25).
4. Loss of definition of one or more margins of the branch (see Figs. 23.24, 23.25, and 23.28).
5. Well-defined or poorly defined hypoechoic areas, central or marginal (see Figs. 23.24, 23.26, 23.27, and 23.28).
6. A diffuse reduction in echogenicity involving all or most of the cross-sectional area of the branch (see Fig. 23.23).
7. Echodense material subcutaneously (see Figs. 23.23, 23.25, and 23.27).
8. Echodense material between the medial and lateral branches (Fig. 23.28**B**).
9. Hyperechoic foci or larger masses within the branch; this finding tends to imply a chronic lesion (see Fig. 23.23).

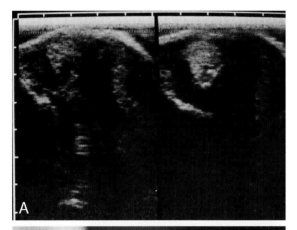

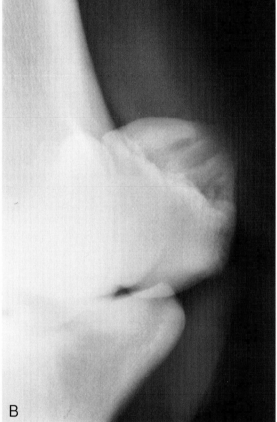

Figure 23.24. A, Transverse ultrasonogram of the lateral branch of the suspensory ligament of the right forelimb of an advanced event horse with acute onset desmitis. The branch is enlarged and has a large hypoechoic area axially. **B,** Dorsolateral-palmaromedial oblique view of the lateral proximal sesamoid bone. Broad radiating lucent lines and irregular palmar border of the bone are indicative of entheseophyte formation. The horse experienced recurrent desmitis when finally returned to compete at championship level 3-day events but is able to compete successfully at 1-day level.

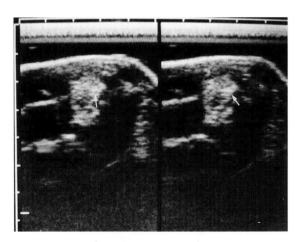

Figure 23.23. Transverse ultrasonogram of the lateral branch of the suspensory ligament of a 12-year-old hunter with recurrent right forelimb lameness associated with heat and enlargement of the branch. The enlarged branch has a diffuse decrease in echogenicity. Focal hyperechoic areas (*arrows*) are indicative of fibrosis or dystrophic mineralization. There is some periligamentous echodense material. The horse had recurrent lameness.

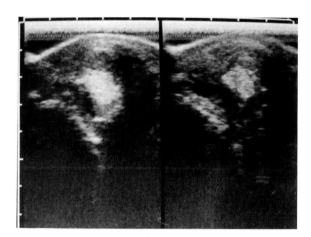

Figure 23.25. Transverse ultrasonogram of the lateral branch of the suspensory ligament of an 11-year-old hunter. The branch is abnormally shaped and is surrounded by considerable echodense material, especially subcutaneously. The distal part of the body of the suspensory ligament has a central hypoechoic area.

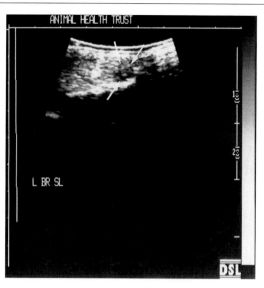

Figure 23.26. Longitudinal ultrasonogram of the lateral branch of the suspensory ligament of the right forelimb of a 10-year-old advanced event horse. There was lameness associated with focal pain on pressure in the region of the insertion of the branch on the lateral proximal sesamoid bone. A focal hypoechoic area is at the site of insertion (*arrows*).

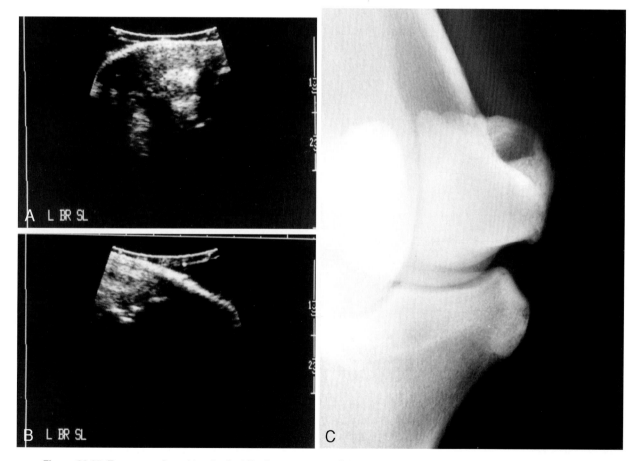

Figure 23.27. Transverse **A,** and longitudinal **B,** ultrasonograms of the lateral branch of the suspensory ligament of the right hind limb of a 13-year-old pleasure horse. The horse had moderate lameness of 2 months' duration associated with enlargement and periligamentous thickening of the lateral branch. **A,** The lateral branch of the suspensory ligament is enlarged; its margins are poorly demarcated and there is a central hypoechoic area. Considerable echodense material is present subcutaneously. **B,** Note the lack of linearity of most of the echoes and the irregular outline of the lateral proximal sesamoid bone. **C,** Dorsolateral-plantaromedial oblique view of the lateral proximal sesamoid bone. There is modeling of the plantar and distal aspects of the bone and a large well-circumscribed radiolucent zone in the proximal plantar aspect of the bone.

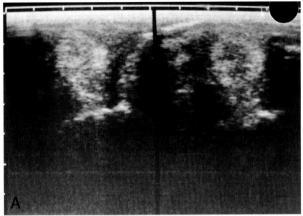

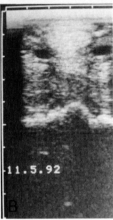

Figure 23.28. A, Transverse ultrasonograms of the lateral branch of the suspensory ligament of the right hind limb of an 11-year-old Grand Prix dressage horse with intermittent moderate right hind limb lameness. Both hind fetlocks were moderately hyperextended, both the medial and lateral branches of the suspensory ligament of the right hind limb were enlarged, and localized heat and pain were present. The lateral branch of the suspensory ligament is massively enlarged, its margins are poorly demarcated, and there are poorly defined hypoechoic areas. **B,** Transverse ultrasonogram of the plantar metatarsal soft tissues in the distal quarter of the metatarsus. The branches of the suspensory ligament cannot be seen, but extensive echodense material is dorsal to the deep digital flexor tendon and represents fibrous material between the branches.

10. An irregular contour or fracture of the ipsilateral proximal sesamoid bone.
11. An abnormal amount of fluid in the digital flexor tendon sheath.

The branches should be examined in both transverse and longitudinal planes; lesions restricted to the insertion per se may only be detectable in longitudinal images.

I have seen several horses that presented with slight localized swelling and heat in the region of a suspensory ligament branch and a subtle alteration in gait in which no detectable ultrasonographic abnormalities were identified. The swelling appeared to be principally periligamentous. Although, in some horses, continued work did not unduly exacerbate clinical signs, in others, the clinical signs deteriorated and ultrasonographic abnormalities of the suspensory ligament became evident.

Radiography

It is prudent to examine radiographically both the ipsilateral splint bone and the proximal sesamoid bone. However, the presence of radiographic abnormalities consistent with so-called sesamoiditis (38) secondary to suspensory desmitis does not necessarily appear to be well correlated with the outcome of the horse (3, 39). Primary sesamoiditis, unassociated with suspensory desmitis, has caused recurrent lameness in Standardbreds (39). Radiographic abnormalities may include the following (see Figs. 23.24, 23.27, and 23.29):

1. Dystrophic mineralization of the soft tissues (see Fig.23. 29).
2. An avulsion fracture of the proximal sesamoid bone.
3. Radiating lucent lines of variable size in the proximal sesamoid bone (see Fig. 23.24).
4. A large, well-defined lucent zone in the proximal sesamoid bone (see Fig. 23.27).
5. Modeling of the palmar (plantar) aspect of the proximal sesamoid bone; enthesophyte formation (see Fig. 23.24).
6. Distortion in shape of the ipsilateral splint bone.
7. A fracture of the ipsilateral splint bone.

Management

Management depends on the severity of both the clinical signs and of the ultrasonographic abnormalities, and the breed and occupation of the horse. Some dressage horses with minor ultrasonographic abnormalities have been shod with egg bar shoes; the training program has been modified for 6 to 8 weeks, and the horses have then successfully re-

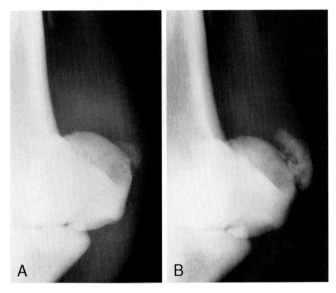

Figure 23.29. A, Dorsolateral-palmaromedial oblique radiographic view of a right forelimb 6 weeks after the onset of lameness associated with desmitis of the lateral branch of the suspensory ligament in a 7-year-old dressage horse. A poorly defined opacity is palmar to the lateral proximal sesamoid bone. Note also the lucent zone in the sesamoid bone. **B,** Six months later, the horse was still lame. The radiopacity is considerably larger and more opaque. The horse remained lame.

sumed full work. A few horses with large, well-defined central core lesions have been treated by a method analogous to tendon splitting with apparently good results, and they have returned to work within 6 to 9 months. Many horses, however, present with poorly demarcated lesions, many of which are marginal or restricted to the region of the insertion of the ligament branch. These have been treated conservatively by corrective trimming and shoeing, box rest, and a controlled ascending exercise program.

Ultrasonographic lesions appear to be slow to resolve, taking longer than comparable lesions in the superficial digital flexor tendon. Some appear to persist on a long-term basis (or at least as long as the period of follow up, up to 18 months). Nonetheless, some horses do successfully resume work despite the persistence of a lesion readily detectable ultrasonographically, although with a significant incidence of re-injury despite convalescent periods of up to 12 months. In the face of persistent ultrasonographic lesions, in my experience, it is difficult to predict accurately when a horse may be able to return to work successfully. I usually recommend return to full work either when the lesion has "healed" or when no appreciable change is seen in the ultrasonographic appearance between two examinations 3 months apart and the horse has been rested for at least 6 months.

Some horses can successfully be "managed" and maintained in work by using aggressive local therapy (e.g., cold, sweats, laser or ultrasound therapy, use of whirlpool boots), provided that the limb is monitored carefully. No good studies have considered the efficacy of other methods of medical therapy, such as intralesional sodium hyaluronate, nor have any comprehensive studies determined whether the type of ultrasonographic abnormality influences progress. The presence of dystrophic mineralization warrants a more guarded prognosis in non–Standardbreds for return to full athletic function without recurrent injury. However, the presence or absence of radiographic abnormalities consistent with "sesamoiditis" does not seem to influence the outcome. To my knowledge, the value of nuclear scintigraphic evaluation has not been properly appraised. Fractured or misshapen distal splint bones or apical sesamoid fractures are treated surgically.

In horses with a hind limb suspensory branch lesion, with echodense material extending between the medial and lateral branches, the prognosis is uniformly poor, regardless of the method of management. Lameness is persistent. The echodense material represents firm adhesion formation between the branches.

APICAL AND ABAXIAL PROXIMAL SESAMOID FRACTURES

Apical sesamoid fractures are defined as those fractures involving not more than the proximal one third of the bone. They occur in either young foals or mature horses. In young foals, frequently both medial and lateral proximal sesamoid bones are fractured, and more than one limb may be affected (40). The predominant clinical sign is localized heat and soft tissue swelling; lameness may be minimal or not detectable. Rarely is there significant damage to the suspensory ligament. Treatment is by box rest, and the prognosis is favorable, although the healed bone does remain persistently enlarged with an abnormal shape. Apical sesamoid fractures in mature horses occur most commonly in racehorses, although they can occur in any type of horse, with a higher incidence in forelimbs than hind limbs. Bramlage and associates (41) demonstrated that conditioning work enhanced the strength of the suspensory ligament. In vitro studies with limbs tested to failure in a limb jig showed that rupture of the suspensory ligament occurred in limbs from unfit horses, whereas failure occurred in the proximal sesamoid bone in trained horses (42).

Clinical signs of an acute fracture include localized heat, a variable degree of soft tissue swelling, pain on pressure over the proximal sesamoid bone, and lameness. There may be associated distention of the fetlock joint capsule. The amount of soft tissue swelling depends to an extent on the degree of associated suspensory desmitis. Ultrasonographic examination is important to verify the presence or absence of suspensory desmitis and its degree, because this factor has an important influence on prognosis (43). In horses with minimal evidence of suspensory desmitis, the prognosis after surgical removal of the fracture fragment is favorable (44–46) provided that the fracture does not involve a large amount of the articular surface and can be removed with minimal damage to the suspensory ligament and the intersesamoidean ligament. Convalescent time depends the extent of compromise of the attachment of the suspensory ligament. Involvement of the intersesamoidean ligament warrants a more guarded prognosis. Ultrasonography can also be used to identify the fracture, but it is not a substitute for radiographic examination.

Abaxial sesamoid fractures occur much less frequently and tend to involve a larger amount of the insertion of the suspensory ligament. Atraumatic removal of the fracture fragment is more difficult; thus, the prognosis is generally more guarded.

Transverse mid-body proximal sesamoid fractures occur most commonly in the forelimbs of racehorses. Lameness is usually acute in onset and severe, associated with localized soft tissue swelling and pain. The incidence of concurrent suspensory branch desmitis is poorly documented. Conservative management usually results in persistent lameness associated with a fibrous union. Surgical management by lag screwing, use of a cancellous bone graft, and wiring techniques have yielded better results (47–50).

BASILAR PROXIMAL SESAMOID FRACTURES

Basilar sesamoid fractures occur in all types of horses, especially Thoroughbreds (51), in both forelimbs and hind limbs, forelimbs predominating. Fractures are usually transverse, but they may be comminuted. Although in the acute stage, pain may be induced by pressure over the base of the sesamoid or by passive manipulation of the fetlock, these signs may be absent in horses with more chronic cases. Lameness ranges from mild to severe and may be improved by palmar (plantar) nerve blocks at the level of the proximal sesamoid bones or palmar (junction of proximal two thirds and distal one third of metacarpus) and palmar metacarpal nerve blocks. The fractures are usually readily identified radiographically and may also be visualized ultrasonographically. The incidence of concurrent distal sesamoidean ligament desmitis is poorly documented. Conservative management usually results in either fibrous union or nonunion and persistent low-grade lameness (43). Small fragments do not lend themselves to internal fixation. Favorable results have been achieved by surgical removal of the fragments by arthrotomy (51) or by arthroscopy (51) (Wright, I., personal communication). Some fracture fragments are amenable to internal fixation using a wiring technique (49). The prognosis is best for noncomminuted, small fractures with no or minimal displacement (51).

SAGITTAL PROXIMAL SESAMOID FRACTURES

Sagittal proximal sesamoid fractures have only been described in conjunction with lateral condylar fractures of the third metacarpal bone. No reports of the ultrasonographic appearance of these fractures have been published, nor do reports describe whether there are detectable abnormalities of either the intersesamoidean ligament or the suspensory branches. The prognosis for return to athletic function is guarded.

OSTEOMYELITIS OF THE PROXIMAL SESAMOID BONES

Osteomyelitis of the proximal sesamoid bones and associated abnormalities of the intersesamoidean ligament have been described in both forelimbs and hind limbs, characterized by radiolucent zones involving the axial margin of either or both the medial and lateral proximal sesamoid bones (52). Distention of the fetlock joint capsule or the distal flexor tendon sheath is a variable feature. Lameness ranges from moderate to severe. Associated ultrasonographic abnormalities have not been described. Medical therapy has been unsuccessful. I have seen two cases of osteomyelitis of both medial and lateral proximal sesamoid bones associated

with marked abnormalities of the digital flexor tendon sheath in young Thoroughbreds in training. The first, of unknown duration, had irregularly demarcated radiolucent zones on the abaxial aspect of the left fore lateral proximal sesamoid bone and in the axial aspect of the medial proximal sesamoid bone. Ultrasonographically, the abaxial surface of the lateral proximal sesamoid bone was irregular, and echolucent areas were present between the bone and the suspensory ligament attachment. There was loss of echogenicity of the intersesamoidean ligament proximally. The horse had an abnormal amount of synovial fluid in the digital flexor tendon sheath and echodense material. Surgical treatment was unsuccessful.

The second case, of 6 weeks' duration, had massive swelling of the distal left metatarsus, fetlock, and pastern and severe lameness. Poorly defined radiolucent zones involved the proximal half of the axial borders of both proximal sesamoid bones, and poorly demarcated new bone was noted on the abaxial surfaces. Ultrasonographically, the axial borders of the proximal sesamoid bones were irregular (Fig. 23.30); there was a diffuse reduction in echogenicity of the proximal half of the intersesamoidean ligament. The horse had considerable echodense material in the digital flexor tendon sheath proximal to the fetlock and an abnormal amount of fluid distally. In the region of the fetlock, both the superficial and deep digital flexor tendons were enlarged but of normal echogenicity. In the pastern, the deep digital flexor tendon was of abnormal shape and had focal areas of reduced echogenicity with some adhesion formation.

A third horse, with a history of a penetrating wound on the palmar aspect of the right fore pastern 5 months previously, had diffuse thickening around the fetlock and palmar pastern and severe lameness. Radiographically, diffuse mineralization was visible on the abaxial aspect of the proximal sesamoid bones. Ultrasonographically, a thick layer of subcutaneous echodense material on the palmar aspect of the fetlock and pastern, thickening of the wall of the digital flexor tendon sheath, and extensive echodense material palmar to the proximal sesamoid bones were noted. There was loss of definition between the superficial and deep digital flexor tendons in the pastern and on the palmar aspect of the

Figure 23.30. A, Transverse ultrasonogram of the plantar metatarsal soft tissues of a 3-year-old Thoroughbred flat racehorse with sudden onset of severe left hind limb lameness 6 weeks earlier. Diffuse hot swelling of the left hind metatarsus and pastern was present: the horse would bear weight only on the toe. Note the considerable amount of echodense material within the digital flexor tendon sheath (*small arrows*) and the thickened sheath wall (*large arrow*). **B,** Transverse ultrasonogram slightly further distally. Considerable echodense material is present subcutaneously. Note the irregular outline of the axial aspect of the medial proximal sesamoid bones (*arrow*). **C,** Transverse ultrasonogram of the plantar aspect of the pastern at the distal end of the proximal phalanx. A thick layer of subcutaneous echodense material is present. An abnormal amount of fluid is within the digital flexor tendon sheath, with faint echoes within. In the central dorsal aspect of the deep digital flexor tendon is a hypoechoic area (*arrows*) that correlated with degenerative change post mortem, which extended to the level of the fetlock. **D,** Dorsoplantar view of the metatarsophalangeal joint. The axial margins of the proximal sesamoid bones are irregular in outline. **E,** Dorsolateral-plantaromedial oblique view of the metatarsophalangeal joint. Poorly defined new bone is on the plantar and distal aspects of the lateral proximal sesamoid bone (*arrows*). **F,** Post mortem dorsoplantar radiographic view of the proximal sesamoid bones. Note the extensive lytic areas along the proximal axial margins of the bones and the new bone on the abaxial aspect of the lateral (L) proximal sesamoid bone.

(continued on next page)

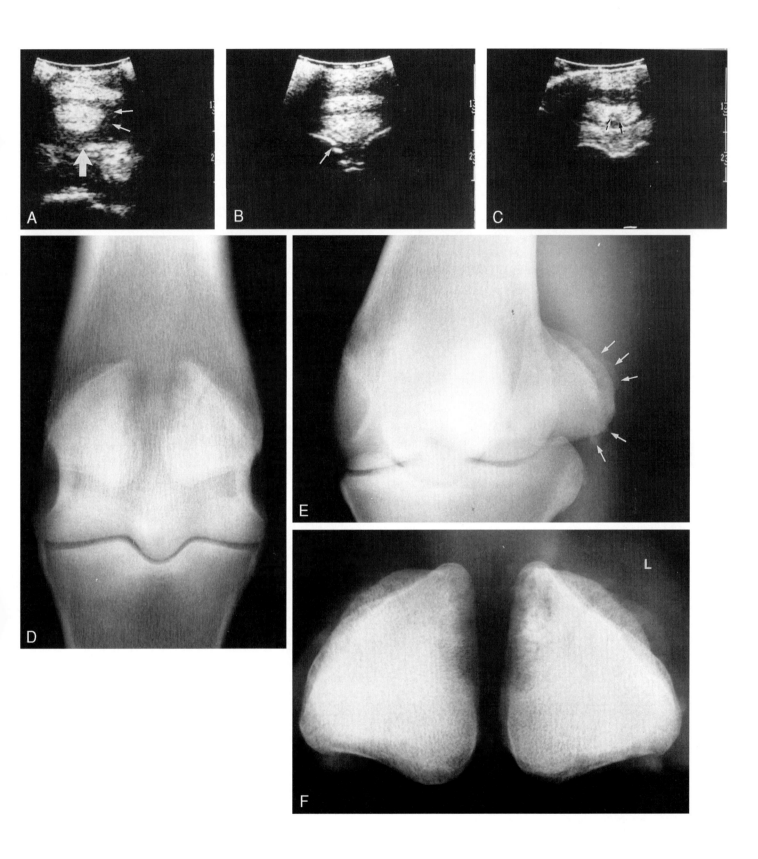

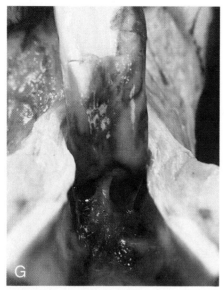

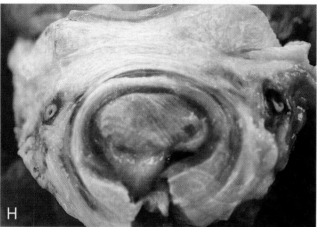

Figure 23.30. *(Continued)* **G,** Post mortem examination of the enlarged deep digital flexor tendon in the pastern showed multiple adhesions. **H,** Post mortem transverse section of the distal metacarpus. Note the extensive subcutaneous fibrosis and the enlarged deep digital flexor tendon.

fetlock and loss of mobility between these structures. Postmortem examination confirmed extensive adhesion formation and a thick layer of fibrous material on the palmar aspect of the proximal sesamoid bones, each of which had new bone formation on their palmar aspects.

BREAKDOWN OF THE SUSPENSORY APPARATUS

Traumatic disruption of the suspensory apparatus occasionally occurs in foals (40, 53), but it is generally an injury of the forelimbs of Thoroughbred racehorses (54, 55). The horse has acute-onset, severe lameness, with dropping of the fetlock, pain, and swelling. The most common injury is fracture of both proximal sesamoid bones. Less commonly, complete avulsion of the distal sesamoidean ligaments occurs, with proximal displacement of the proximal sesamoid bones. Rarely, complete disruption of the body or branches of the suspensory ligament occurs. In any type of injury,

there may be concurrent damage to either or both the superficial and deep digital flexor tendons.

All the palmar metacarpal soft tissue structures should be evaluated ultrasonographically. If there is either a transverse fracture of both proximal sesamoid bones or avulsion of the distal sesamoidean ligaments, tension in the suspensory ligament is lost, so reduction in echogenicity and loss of its normal fiber pattern are noted. Complete tearing of the suspensory ligament produces complete loss of continuity of the ligament.

Treatment is aimed only at salvaging the horse and is prolonged and expensive. Although long-term splinting has been successful (54, 55), potential complications include severe laminitis in the contralateral limb resulting from excessive weight bearing. Surgical management by fetlock arthrodesis has better long-term results (56, 57).

BREAKDOWN OF THE HIND LIMB SUSPENSORY APPARATUS

Progressive "degenerative" changes in hind limb suspensory ligaments have been seen in a few horses that originally presented with proximal suspensory desmitis, which had straight hock conformation, with or without hyperextension (excessive dorsiflexion) of the fetlocks. This condition has been characterized by a diffuse decrease in echogenicity of the proximal suspensory ligaments that becomes progressively more extensive distally. A similar clinical condition has also been recognized in brood mares. Progressive hyperextension of the hind fetlocks may result in abrasions on their plantar aspects. There is a diffuse reduction in echogenicity of most of the body of the suspensory ligament. The incidence in brood mares seems to be higher than in breeding stallions of a similar age. Flat shoes with caudal extensions may be helpful.

DESMITIS OF THE DISTAL SESAMOIDEAN LIGAMENTS

The cruciate and short distal sesamoidean ligaments insert on the proximal aspect of the proximal phalanx. The cruciate ligaments are easiest to identify ultrasonographically in longitudinal images; in transverse images, they are closely applied to the dorsal aspect of the straight sesamoidean ligament. The short sesamoidean ligaments are difficult to differentiate from the oblique sesamoidean ligaments. The oblique (middle) sesamoidean ligaments lie to the left and right of the palmar mid-line proximally and become smaller and closer together toward the middle of the proximal phalanx. Proximally, the medial and lateral oblique sesamoidean ligaments are seen ultrasonographically as well-defined, uniformly echogenic structures, approximately triangular in transverse images (Fig. 23.31). They lie adjacent to the palmar (plantar) cortex of the proximal phalanx. Each ligament is separated from the superficial digital tendon by an anechoic space. It is easiest to identify the oblique sesamoidean ligaments in a longitudinal plane by identifying the base of one of the proximal sesamoid bones and following the ipsi-

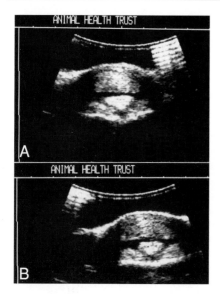

Figure 23.31. **A,** Transverse ultrasonogram and diagram of the proximal palmar pastern region. 1 = superficial digital flexor tendon; 2 = deep digital flexor tendon; 3 = straight sesamoidean ligament; 4 = oblique sesamoidean ligament; 5 = palmar cortex of proximal phalanx. **B,** Transverse ultrasonogram of the palmar pastern region obtained approximately 1 cm distal to the ultrasonogram in **A.** The oblique sesamoidean ligaments are closer together.

lateral ligament distally, bearing in mind its oblique orientation. The straight (superficial) distal sesamoidean ligament lies between the deep digital flexor tendon and the cruciate sesamoidean ligaments proximally, between the deep digital flexor tendon and the oblique sesamoidean ligaments in the middle of the proximal phalanx, and then between the deep digital flexor tendon and the palmar cortex of the middle phalanx as well as the palmar recess of the proximal interphalangeal joint, before inserting by the scutum medium on the proximal aspect of the middle phalanx. The straight sesamoidean ligament is the most echodense of the soft tissue structures on the palmar (plantar) aspect of the pastern. It changes from trapezoidal proximally, through oval, to square distally in transverse section. Distally, a central hypoechoic area is seen in normal horses that should not be confused with a lesion (Fig. 23.32). The ease with which the soft tissue structures on the palmar (plantar) aspect of the pastern can be imaged depends on the shape of the pastern and the position of the limb. Horses with an upright pastern conformation are easiest to examine, especially if the bulbs of the heel are well separated. In horses with a less favorable conformation, for example, in those with a short pastern and marked palmar (plantar) concavity, it can be helpful to place the limb to be examined behind the contralateral limb, with the fetlock hyperextended. Sometimes, elevating the horse's foot on a block facilitates the examination. Although transverse images are readily obtained using a linear-array transducer, it is generally easier to achieve good-quality longitudinal images using a sector scanner, unless the horse has long pastern conformation.

Although the clinical features of distal sesamoidean desmitis have been described (58), the diagnosis was not substantiated by ultrasonography. Since then, it has become clear that superficial digital flexor tendon branch lesions were previously misdiagnosed as oblique sesamoidean ligament damage (59). Periosteal new bone on the palmar (plantar) medial or lateral aspects of the proximal phalanges is a common incidental radiological abnormality, especially in non–Thoroughbred horses. Generally, it is not possible to identify ultrasonographically any structural abnormality of the oblique sesamoidean ligaments, which insert in these areas, and usually no associated clinical signs are present.

Injury to one or both oblique distal sesamoidean ligaments most commonly is associated with sudden-onset lameness and swelling on the palmar (plantar) medial or lateral aspect of the proximal half of the proximal phalanx. The swelling may be difficult to differentiate from that associated with a branch lesion of the superficial digital flexor tendon. The injury has been seen in horses from various sports disciplines. Ultrasonographic abnormalities (Fig 23.33) may include one or more of the following:

1. Enlargement.
2. Diffuse reduction of echogenicity.
3. Focal hypoechoic areas.
4. Poor demarcation of the margins of the ligament.
5. Reduction in the space between the ligament and the superficial digital flexor tendon.
6. Periosteal new bone on the palmar/plantar aspect of the proximal phalanx.
7. Concurrent basilar fracture of the ipsilateral proximal sesamoid bone.

Horses managed conservatively have had a high incidence of recurrent lameness; however, an enlarged oblique

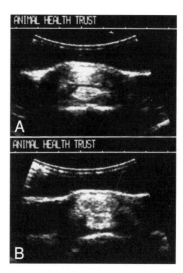

Figure 23.32. **A,** Transverse ultrasonogram and diagram of the mid-palmar pastern region. 1 = deep digital flexor tendon; 2 = straight sesamoidean ligament. **B,** Transverse ultrasonogram of the palmar pastern obtained approximately 1 cm distal to the ultrasonogram in **A.** Note the central hypoechoic area in the straight sesamoidean ligament. This is a normal feature.

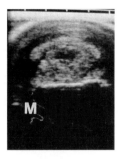

Figure 23.33. Transverse ultrasonogram of the palmar soft tissues of the proximal pastern of the left forelimb of a 10-year-old steeplechaser with slight intermittent lameness of 3 months' duration, accentuated after a race 3 weeks previously. Diffuse soft tissue swelling on the palmar pastern made it difficult to palpate individual structures. Some subcutaneous echodense material (thickening of the proximal digital annular ligament) is present. The medial (M) oblique distal sesamoidean ligament is enlarged and diffusely hypoechoic. The hypoechoic area in the deep digital flexor tendon is an artifact.

distal sesamoidean ligament of uniform, normal echogenicity is an incidental finding in some horses with lameness from another cause.

Desmitis of the straight sesamoidean ligament is uncommon and has only been seen in forelimbs. This condition is characterized ultrasonographically by the following:

1. Enlargement.
2. Focal hypoechoic areas.
3. Increased fluid in the digital flexor tendon sheath.

Care should be taken not to misinterpret the normal central hypoechoic area on the most distal aspect of the ligament at its insertion. Occasionally, concurrent lesions of the straight and oblique sesamoidean ligaments occur. The prognosis for return to full athletic function for a horse with any injury of the straight sesamoidean ligament appears to be guarded.

Loss of tension (relaxation) of the straight sesamoidean ligament may occur if the suspensory ligament is ruptured, resulting in instability or subluxation of the proximal interphalangeal joint. Ultrasonographic abnormalities include the following:

1. Apparent enlargement of the cross-sectional area.
2. Loss of "fiber" alignment.
3. Focal hypoechoic areas resulting from lack of tension.

REFERENCES

1. Sisson S. Equine syndesmology. In: Getty R, ed. Sisson and Grossman's anatomy of domestic animals. 5th ed. Philadelphia: WB Saunders, 1975;1:349–375.
2. Wilson D, Baker G, Pijanowski G, et al. Morphology and maturation of the proximal sesamoidean ligament in the horse. Abstract Vet Surg 1988;17:47.
3. Dyson S, Vatistas N, Thorp P. Ultrasonographic appearance of the equine forelimb suspensory ligament. In: Proceedings of the Dubai International Equine Symposium, 1996: 207–225.
4. Ford T, Ross M, Orsini P. A comparison of methods for proximal metacarpal anaesthesia in horses. Vet Surg 1988;18:146–150.
5. Dyson S, Romero J. An investigation of injection techniques for local analgesia of the equine distal tarsus and proximal metatarsus. Equine Vet J 1993;25:30–35.
6. Hauser M, Rantanen N. Ultrasound appearance of the palmar metacarpal soft tissues of the horse. Equine Vet Sci 1983;3:19–22.
7. Pharr J, Nyland T. Sonography of the equine palmar metacarpal soft tissues. Vet Radiol 1984;25:265–273.
8. Hauser M. Ultrasonographic and correlative anatomy of the horse. Vet Clin North Am Equine Pract 1986;2:127–144.
9. Marks D, Mackay-Smith M, Leslie A, et al. Lameness resulting from high suspensory disease (HSD) in the horse. Proc Am Assoc Equine Pract 1981;24:493–497.
10. Personett L, McAllister S, Mansmann R. Proximal suspensory desmitis. Mod Vet Pract 1983;64:541–545.
11. Rantanen N, Gaines R, Genovese R. The use of diagnostic ultrasound to detect structural damage to the soft tissues of the extremities of horses. Equine Vet Sci 1983;3:134–135.
12. Hauser M, Rantanen N, Genovese R. Suspensory desmitis: diagnosis using real time ultrasound imaging. Equine Vet Sci 1984; 4:258–262.
13. Genovese R, Rantanen N, Hauser M, et al. Diagnostic ultrasonography of equine limbs. Vet Clin North Am Equine Pract 1986; 2:145–226.
14. Huskamp B, Nowak M. Insertion desmopathies in the horse. Pferdheilkunde 1988;4:3–12.
15. Dyson S. Proximal suspensory desmitis: clinical, ultrasonographic and radiographic features. Equine Vet J 1991;23:25–31.
16. Dyson S. Proximal suspensory desmitis of the hind limb. In: Proceedings of the Fifteenth Bain-Fallon Memorial Lectures. Artarmon, Australia: Australian Equine Veterinary Association, 1993: 55–62.
17. Dyson S. Proximal suspensory desmitis in the hind limb: 42 cases. Br Vet J 1994;150:279–291.
18. Dyson S. Nerve blocks and lameness diagnosis in the horse. In Pract 1984;6:102–107.
19. Ueltschi G. Zur Diagnose von Interosseuslasionen an der Ursprungsstelle. Pferdeheilkunde 1989;5:65–69.
20. Young R, O'Brien T, Craychee T. Examination procedures for the diagnosis of suspensory desmitis in the horse. Proc Am Assoc Equine Pract 1989;35:233–241.
21. Dik K, Gunsser I. Atlas of diagnostic radiology of the horse. Part 2. Diseases of the hind limb. London: Wolfe, 1989:74–75.
22. Butler J, Colles C, Dyson S, et al. Clinical radiology of the horse. Oxford: Blackwell Scientific, 1993.
23. Pleasant R, Baker G, Muhlbauer M, et al. Stress reactions and stress fractures of the proximal palmar aspect of the third metacarpal bone in horses: 58 cases (1980–1990). J Am Vet Med Assoc 1992; 201:1918–1923.
24. Bramlage L, Gabel A, Hackett R. Avulsion fractures of the origin of the suspensory ligament in the horse. J Am Vet Med Assoc 1980; 176:1004–1010.
25. Dyson S. Some observation on lameness associated with pain in the proximal metacarpal region. Equine Vet J 1988; (Suppl 6):43–52.
26. Wright I, Platt D, Houlton J, et al. Management of intracortical fractures of the palmaroproximal third metacarpal bone in a horse by surgical forage. Equine Vet J 1990;22:142–144.
27. Ross M, Ford T, Orsini P. Incomplete longitudinal fracture of the proximal palmar cortex of the third metacarpal bone in horses. Vet Surg 1988;17:82–86.
28. Lloyd K, Kobluk P, Ragle C, et al. Incomplete palmar fracture of

the proximal extremity of the third metacarpal bone in horses: ten cases (1981–1986). J Am Vet Med Assoc 1988;192:798–803.

29. Genovese R, Rantanen N, Hauser M, et al. The use of ultrasonography in the diagnosis and management of injuries to the equine limb. Compend Contin Educ Pract Vet 1987;9:945–955.

30. Dyson S, Arthur R, Palmer S, et al. Suspensory ligament desmitis. Vet Clin North Am Equine Pract 1995;11:177–215.

31. Palmer S. Management of suspensory ligament desmitis in Standardbred racehorses. In: Suspensory ligament desmitis. Vet Clin North Am Equine Pract 1995;11:199–206.

32. Arthur R. Management of suspensory ligament desmitis in Thoroughbred racehorses. In: Suspensory ligament desmitis. Vet Clin North Am Equine Pract 1995;11:197–199.

33. Bowman K, Evans L, Herring M. Evaluation of surgical removal of fractured distal splint bones in the horse. Vet Surg 1982;11:116–120.

34. Verschooten F, Gasthuys F, De Moor A. Distal splint bone fractures in the horse: an experimental and clinical study. Equine Vet J 1984;16:532–536.

35. Allen D, White N. Management of fractures and exostoses of the metacarpals and metatarsals II & IV in 25 horses. Equine Vet J 1987;19:326–330.

36. Harrison L, May S, Edwards G. Surgical treatment of open splint bone fractures in 26 horses. Vet Rec 1991;128:606–610.

37. Jones R, Fessler J. Observations on small metacarpal and metatarsal fractures with or without associated suspensory desmitis in Standardbred horses. Can. Vet J 1977;18:29–32.

38. O'Brien T, Morgan J, Wheat J, et al. Sesamoiditis in the Thoroughbred: a radiographic study. J Am Vet Radiol Soc 1971;12:75–87.

39. Hardy J, Maroux M, Breton L. Clinical relevance of radiographic findings in proximal sesamoid bones of 2 year old Standardbreds in their first year of training. J Am Vet Med Assoc 1991;198:2089–2094.

40. Ellis D. Fractures of the proximal sesamoid bones in Thoroughbred foals. Equine Vet J 1979;11:48–52.

41. Bramlage L, Bukowiecki C, Gabel A. The effect of training on the suspensory apparatus of the horse. Proc Am Assoc Equine Pract 1989;35:245–247.

42. Bukowiecki C, Bramlage L, Gabel A. In vitro strength of the suspensory apparatus in training and resting horses. Vet Surg 1987;16:126–130.

43. Bukowiecki C, Bramlage L, Gabel A. Proximal sesamoid bone fractures in horses; current treatments and prognosis. Compend Contin Educ Pract Vet 1985;7:S684–S698.

44. Spurlock G, Gabel A. Apical fractures of the proximal sesamoid bones in 109 Standardbred horses. J Am Vet Med Assoc 1983;183:76–79.

45. Fretz P, Barker S, Bailey J, et al. Management of proximal sesamoid fractures in the horse. J Am Vet Med Assoc 1984;185:282–284.

46. Palmer S. Arthroscopic removal of apical and abaxial sesamoid fracture fragments in five horses. Vet Surg 1989;18:347–352.

47. Fackelmann G. Compression screw fixation of proximal sesamoid fractures. J Equine Med Surg 1978;2:32–39.

48. Medina L, Wheat J, Morgan J, et al. Treatment of basal fractures of the proximal sesamoid bone in the horse using an autologous bone graft. Proc Am Assoc Equine Pract 1980;26:345–380.

49. Martin B, Nunamaker D, Evans L, et al. Circumferential wiring of mid-body and large basilar fractures of the proximal sesamoid bones in 15 horses. Vet Surg 1991;20:9–14.

50. Henninger R, Bramlage L, Schneider R, et al. Lag screw and cancellous bone graft fixation of transverse proximal sesamoid fractures in horses: 25 cases (1983–1989). J Am Vet Med Assoc 1991;199:606–612.

51. Parente E, Richardson D, Spencer P. Basal sesamoidean fractures in horses: 57 cases (1980–1991). J Am Vet Med Assoc 1993;202:1293–1297.

52. Wisner E, O'Brien T, Pool R, et al. Osteomyelitis of the axial border of the proximal sesamoid bones in seven horses. Equine Vet J 1991;23:383–389.

53. Honnas C, Snyder J, Meagher D, et al. Traumatic disruption of the suspensory apparatus in foals. Cornell Vet 1990;80:123–133.

54. Wheat J, Pascoe J. A technique for management of traumatic rupture of the equine suspensory apparatus. J Am Vet Med Assoc 1980;176:205–210.

55. Bowman K, Leitch M, Nunamaker D, et al. Complications during treatment of traumatic disruption of the suspensory apparatus in Thoroughbred horses. J Am Vet Med Assoc 1984;184:706–715.

56. Bramlage L. Arthrodesis of the metacarpophalangeal joint: results in 43 horses. Vet Surg 1985;14:49.

57. Richardson D, Nunamaker D, Sigafous R. Use of an external skeletal fixation device and bone graft for arthrodesis of the metacarpophalangeal joint in horses. J Am Vet Med Assoc 1987;191:316–321.

58. Moyer W. Distal sesamoidean desmitis. Proc Am Assoc Equine Pract 1982;28:245–251.

59. Dyson S, Denoix J-M. Tendon, tendon sheath and ligament injuries in the pastern. Vet Clin North Am Equine Pract 1995;11:217–234.

24. Joints and Miscellaneous Tendons (Miscellaneous Tendons and Ligaments)

JEAN-MARIE DENOIX

INTRODUCTION

In the last few years, much effort has been directed toward the diagnosis and treatment of equine locomotor disorders resulting in acute or chronic lameness.

Ultrasonography has significantly improved the diagnosis of soft-tissue injuries of the equine limbs. With conventional diagnostic procedures such as palpation, gait evaluation, regional or articular anesthesia, and radiology, it is difficult to accurately diagnose soft-tissue joint injuries. The use of ultrasonography has expanded considerably during the last few years, and this technique has become a very useful tool for the identification of injuries of tendons, ligaments, and associated structures in the horse distal limbs.

It is presently used for the evaluation and documentation of every soft-tissue deformation and in a large number of clinical cases to determine soft-tissue–associated injuries with osteoarticular abnormalities identified with radiology. When abnormal radiographic findings are present in joints, ultrasonography allows the veterinarian to determine whether associated soft-tissue lesions are present as well. Therefore, evaluation of lesions is improved, and prognosis and treatment of joint injuries take advantage of this combination of complementary imaging procedures. Moreover, as a safe noninvasive method, ultrasonography has advantages over advanced radiographic procedures such as contrast arthrography and fistulography, or diagnostic arthroscopy. Ultrasonography has become important in the diagnosis of lameness in horses, and a detailed knowledge of the ultrasonographic anatomy is an essential part of this diagnosis.

GENERAL APPROACH FOR DIAGNOSIS

Tendons and Ligaments

For each tendon and ligament injury, the ultrasonographic signs are quite consistent. They include modifications of size, shape, and position, as well as modifications of echogenicity and architecture.

Modifications of Size and Shape

One of the most reliable criteria in the identification of tendon and ligament injuries is the evaluation of the size of the anatomic structure considered. Because of the large number of tendons and ligaments in the horse limbs, as well as individual variations, size evaluation can require comparison with the same structure in the opposite limb.

Generally, tendinopathies and desmopathies are accompanied by an increase in size. In recent injuries this enlargement is due to edema, hemorrhage, and an increasing content in fibroblastic tissue. When the hypoechoic injury is located on the margins of the structure involved, the shape of the echogenic part of the tendon or ligament is changed; the apparent size of the structure can decrease, and the real size can be underestimated. Thus size of tendons and ligaments must be evaluated very cautiously, and every shape modification suggests marginal injuries.

A true reduction in size of a structure may indicate disuse atrophy. In older injuries the apparent size of the structure usually increases; nevertheless, when peripheral fibroblastic metaplasia is present, the shape of the echogenic part of the structure is altered and its size can actually decrease.

Modifications of Echogenicity and Architecture

Injuries of tendon and ligament induce modifications of echogenicity. For each structure, hypoechogenicity can be due to an inflammatory process, fluid accumulation, or fibroplasia. Hyperechoic images are induced by fibrous tissue and cartilage or bone metaplasia. Chronic injuries are often accompanied by hyperechoic, thickened, peritendinous tissue.

Insertion-Site Abnormalities

Insertion sites of tendons and ligaments on bone surfaces (called entheses) must be examined carefully when tendon or ligament insertion injuries are suspected.

In recent injuries, if hypoechoic images extend all the way to the bony surface of attachment, an insertion desmopathy or tendinopathy, also called *enthesopathy*, must be considered. Hyperechoic images casting acoustic shadows are indicative of bony fragment avulsion (or previous undiagnosed calcification).

In old or chronic enthesopathies, several ultrasonographic findings can be observed:

1. Subterminal thickening, which induces bending of the collagen fibers bundles
2. Irregular patterns of echogenicity with hypoechoic (fibroblastic tissue) and hyperechoic (fibrosis, cartilaginous metaplasia) spots
3. Irregular contour of the insertion surfaces, which is indicative of bone remodeling (osteolysis and osteoproliferation). In some anatomic locations, chronic enthesopathies induce a deepening of the insertion fossa (metacarpal insertion of the collateral ligaments of the fetlock, femoral insertion of the medial collateral ligament of the stifle)

475

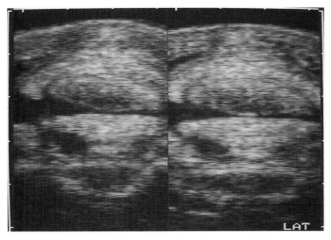

Figure 24.1. Transverse ultrasound scan of the palmar aspect of the pastern just distal to the proximal sesamoid bones. The proximal digital annular ligament is thickened, and localized hypoechoic images are present within this ligament. A synovial effusion within the digital sheath is also present.

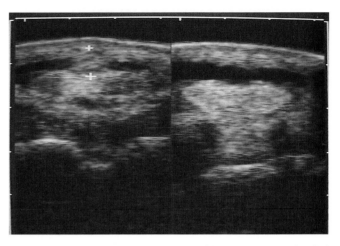

Figure 24.3. Transverse ultrasound scan of the pastern at the level of the distal P1. An anechoic space is present between the digital annular ligaments and the DDFT, indicative of synovial effusion within the digital sheath. *Left scan,* Thickening of the mesotendon (*crosses*) is also seen.

4. Hyperechoic spots casting acoustic shadows, which are indicative of bony fragment avulsion, calcification, or bone metaplasia

Complementary Imaging

As indicated previously, tendon and ligament injuries may involve the corresponding bony surface of insertion. Because of the respective indications and limitations of radiography and ultrasonography, when enthesopathies are suspected, it is always recommended to combine both procedures to get a better evaluation of bone, as well as soft-tissue involvement.

Associated Structures

Canal syndromes can be observed in any location where tendons are surrounded by synovitis and fibrous sheaths.

Recent injuries (tenosynovitis) are usually accompanied by a degree of synovitis. In old or chronic injuries abnormal findings include synovial distention, synovial membrane hyperplasia (membrane plicas, mesotendons), and thickening of the fibrous wall (annular ligament or retinaculum). Chronic distention generally induces bony proliferation at the insertion sites of the fibrous part of the canal wall. When the synovial fluid is echogenic, a septic tenosynovitis

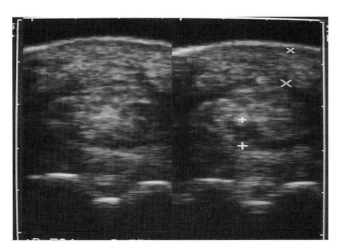

Figure 24.2. Transverse ultrasound scan of the palmar aspect of the pastern at the level of the proximal interphalangeal joint. The deep hyperechoic line represents the palmar profile of the distal condyles of P1. The distal digital annular ligament is thickened (*oblique crosses*), and a hypoechoic image is present within the DDFT (*crosses*).

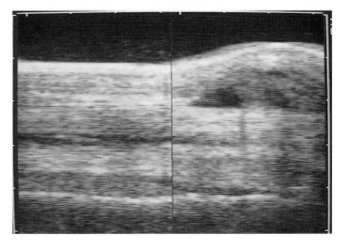

Figure 24.4. Longitudinal ultrasound scan of the pastern at the palmar aspect of P1. An echogenic mass (with a hypoechoic center) is present between the DDFT and the superficial wall of the synovial sheath, and a synovial effusion is present within the synovial cavity. These findings are compatible with chronic proliferative synovitis of the DDF mesotendon.

or hemorrhage within the synovial sheath should be suspected.

SPECIFIC INJURIES

Pastern

Abnormal findings can be found in every anatomic structure of the pastern area, including the digital sheath (annular ligaments and synovial sheath), the flexor tendons, the distal sesamoid ligaments, and the ligaments of the proximal and distal interphalangeal joints.

Annular Ligaments and Digital Sheath

Desmopathy of the *proximal and distal digital annular ligaments* (PDAL and DDAL) is common and can be imaged and documented on transverse and longitudinal ultrasound scans. The thickness of these structures can increase up to 3 to 15 mm, and the echogenicity varies according to the evolution stage of the disease process; it can be decreased, normal, or heterogenous.

When desmopathy of the PDAL is observed (Fig. 24.1), injuries of the superficial digital flexor tendon (SDFT) are often also detected at the same level. In some horses, lesions of the SDFT in the distal metacarpus can also be recorded.

Desmopathy of the DDAL (Fig. 24.2) is often accompanied with distal lesions of the deep digital flexor tendon (DDFT), particularly those that are sequelae of podotrochlear syndrome (navicular disease) and/or digital neurectomy.

Effusion of synovial fluid within the *digital sheath* is commonly identified in clinical cases (Fig. 24.3). In many horses no other abnormal findings can be detected within the tendons and ligaments of the pastern and distal metacarpus. The most common simultaneous lesions are found within

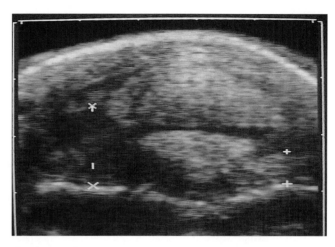

Figure 24.6. Transverse ultrasound scan of the palmar aspect of the pastern at the level of the proximal P1. The medial oblique sesamoid ligament (*left side*) is thickened and hypoechoic compared with the lateral sesamoid ligament (*right side*). These findings are consistent with a recent injury of this ligament.

the DDFT. It can also be a sequela of septic tenosynovitis. Synovial effusion within the digital sheath can accompany tendon injuries above the proximal sesamoid bones.

Hypoechoic to echogenic masses are occasionally identified in the distal recess of the digital sheath, usually in the sagittal plane (Fig. 24.4). This injury can be found as a sequel of a septic tenosynovitis. In most horses an aseptic effusion is also present, and on longitudinal and transverse sonograms, long synovial folds can be easily identified in a totally anechoic synovial fluid. These ultrasound findings are consistent with a chronic proliferative synovitis affecting the palmar mesotendon of the DDFT.

Superficial and Deep Digital Flexor Tendon Injuries (see Chapters 21 and 22)

Distal Sesamoid Ligament Injuries

Distal sesamoid ligament injuries are observed mainly in sport and race-horses and most commonly identified in the oblique sesamoid ligaments.

Straight sesamoid ligament (SSL) injuries were found only in forelimbs (Fig. 24.5). They include relaxation and desmopathy.

- *Relaxation* of the SSL (Fig. 24.5) occurs when the third interosseus muscle (suspensory ligament) is ruptured and this injury is accompanied by various degrees of proximal interphalangeal joint instability or subluxation. Ultrasonographic findings include lack of alignment of the ligament fibers, hypoechoic spots due to fiber relaxation and waves, and thickening of the cross-sectional area of the SSL.
- *Desmopathy* of the SSL has also been documented. Abnormal findings include thickening of the SSL, hypoechoic images identified in various locations (abaxial, central, dorsal, palmar), and synovial fluid effusion within the digital sheath (inconsistent).

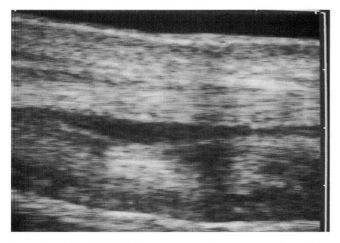

Figure 24.5. Longitudinal ultrasound scan of the palmar aspect of the pastern. The straight sesamoid ligament is relaxed, wavy, and thickened. The ligament appears hypoechoic where the fiber bundles are not perpendicular to the ultrasound beam. This horse had a rupture of the third interosseus muscle and a subluxation of the proximal interphalangeal joint.

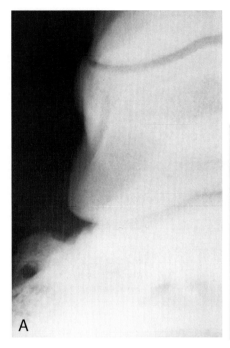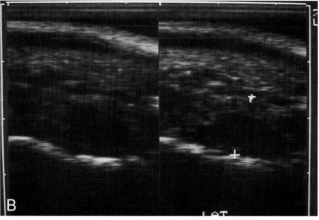

Figure 24.7. A. Dorsopalmar radiograph of the lateral aspect of the pastern and coronary areas of the right forelimb. Bony avulsion is present in the distal insertion fossa of the lateral collateral ligament (*LCL*) of the distal interphalangeal joint (*DIPJ*). This sport horse was injured 5 days previously. **B.** Transverse ultrasound scan of the lateral aspect of the coronary band shows thickening of the LCL of the DIPJ (*between the two crosses*); the deep layer of this ligament is hypoechoic. Superficially lie the coronary band and the echogenic periople, which represents the junction between the skin and the hoof. Complementary imaging demonstrated strain and distal avulsion fracture of the LCL of the DIPJ.

Oblique sesamoid ligament (OSL) injuries were found in forelimbs (Fig. 24.6) and in hind limbs. Only one (lateral or medial) or both of the OSL may be involved. Ultrasonographically, the lesions of the OSL were characterized by a moderate, but usually extensive, thickening; hypoechoic spots or diffuse and strong hypoechogenicity in recent injuries; thickening and moderate but diffuse hypoechogenicity in old or chronic injuries; and bone remodeling at the distal insertion of the OSL on the triangular palmar surface of insertion on the proximal phalanx (P1).

In a number of horses a chronic lesion of the distal branch of the suspensory ligament can also be found on the same aspect of the limb. Osteochondral fragmentation of the proximopalmar aspect of P1 can sometimes be identified on the same clinical cases. On the hind limbs chronic OSL desmopathy is sometimes accompanied by degenerative joint disease of the metatarsophalangeal joint and proximal interphalangeal joint subluxation.

Palmar Ligament of the Proximal Interphalangeal Joint

Because of its orientation, lesions of this ligament are difficult to establish ultrasonographically. It was suspected in a small number of horses presenting a mild swelling of the pastern, a positive proximal digital nerve block (with ambiguous response to the distal digital nerve block), but no evidence of osteoarticular damage, nor any other abnormal ultrasound findings in the other soft tissues of the pastern. Ultrasonographic diagnosis is based on the identification of a thickened hypoechoic space between the distal branch of

the SDFT and the SSL, especially on transverse sonograms with a lack of visualization of the normal structure. These findings are consistent with an injury of the axial palmar ligament of the proximal interphalangeal joint.

Collateral ligaments of the Distal Interphalangeal Joint

Acute strain with avulsion fracture of the lateral collateral ligament of the distal interphalangeal joint (DIPJ) has been identified radiographically and ultrasonographically in the forelimb (Fig. 24.7) and hind limb (Fig. 24.8). Radiographs demonstrated an avulsion fracture at the distal insertion fossa of the distal phalanx. Ultrasound findings were as follows:

1. Thickening of the collateral ligament (compared with the opposite one)
2. Hypoechoic images, especially located in the deep part of the ligament (Fig. 24.7*B*)
3. Hyperechoic spots casting acoustic shadows, indicating bony fragments (Fig. 24.8*B*)
4. Periarticular edema
5. Pain when too much pressure was applied with the probe

Fetlock

Dorsal Aspect

Ultrasonography is an interesting tool for the differential diagnosis of swelling or thickening at the dorsal aspect of the

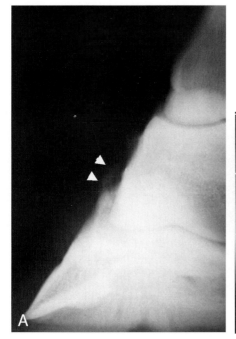
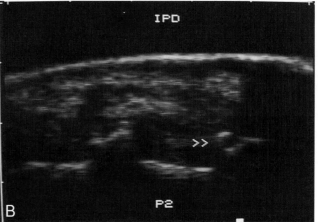

Figure 24.8. A. Dorsomedial-lateroplantar oblique radiograph of the pastern and coronary areas of the right hind limb. A bony avulsion (*arrowheads*) is present in the distal insertion fossa of the lateral collateral ligament (*LCL*) of the distal interphalangeal joint (*DIPJ*). This sport horse was injured 40 days ago. **B.** Longitudinal ultrasound scan of the lateral aspect of the coronary area. This scan shows bony irregularities and hyperechoic spots within the LCL of the DIPJ at the lateral aspect of P2. This ligament is thickened and moderately hypoechoic. Comparative imaging shows subacute strain, bony avulsion, and bony proliferation (enthesopathy) at the insertion sites of the LCL of the DIPJ. On the right side of the scan the hoof wall creates an acoustic shadow.

fetlock. It allows us to pinpoint specific involvements of the different anatomic layers.

Subcutaneous Connective Tissue. Abscesses are seen as large hypoechoic or anechoic images between the skin and the underlying structures (dorsal articular capsule and extensor tendons). Pressure on the transducer makes the abnormal space thinner; this finding is indicative of fluid distention.

Tendinopathy. Fibrosis and thickening of the dorsal (thoracic limb) or long (pelvic limb) digital extensor tendon (DDET or LDET) due to trauma can be documented (Fig. 24.9). This finding is most common on the hind limbs and is usually associated with subcutaneous fibrosis of the dorsal digital fascia. These injuries induce the same ultrasonographic abnormalities as those described for the flexor tendons.

Subtendinous Bursitis. The subtendinous bursa of the digital extensor tendons is difficult to image in a clinically normal limb. A mild to moderate amount of synovial fluid makes the extensor tendon appear clearly separated from the dorsal articular capsule. The increased volume of synovial content can induce out-pouching at the medial aspect of the digital extensor tendon. The pressure within the bursa may elevate the extensor tendon (Fig. 24.10), which becomes apparent in the distal metacarpus (metatarsus).

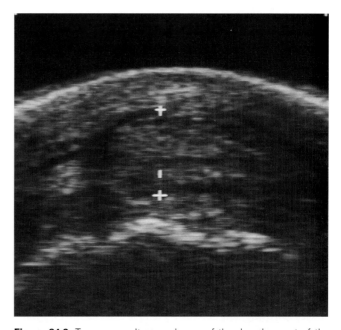

Figure 24.9. Transverse ultrasound scan of the dorsal aspect of the fetlock. This scan was obtained at the proximal border of the metatarsal condyle on the right hind limb of a 3-day-event horse who had a previous traumatic injury. The long digital extensor tendon is thickened (*crosses*); a moderate hypoechogenicity and peritendinous fibrosis are present within this tendon. At the deep aspect of the scan, the hyperechoic profile of the metarsal condyle is imaged.

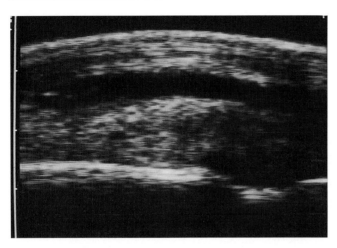

Figure 24.10. Longitudinal ultrasound scan of the dorsal aspect of the fetlock. The echogenic deep line represents the dorsal profile of the distal third metacarpal bone. A totally anechoic fluid-filled space is present between the dorsal digital extensor tendon and the dorsal articular capsule. Transverse ultrasound images also showed that this abnormal finding was the result of a subtendinous bursitis.

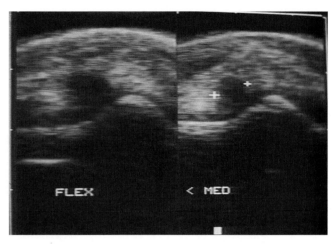

Figure 24.12. Transverse ultrasound scans of the dorsal aspect of the fetlock. These scans are focused on the medial aspect of the intermediate sagittal ridge of the metacarpal condyle. A hypoechoic area is present within the dorsal articular capsule adjacent to the medial aspect of the metacarpal sagittal ridge and is also demonstrated when the fetlock is flexed (*left*). This finding is consistent with a focal capsulitis.

Capsulopathies

- *Hypoechoic images* and thickening can be identified within the thick, dorsal, articular capsule of the fetlock (Figs. 24.11 and 24.12). They are usually asymmetrical (lateral or medial) and located at the dorsal aspect of the metacarpal condyle. Only the deep layer of the capsule or the totality of this structure can be involved. When a capsulopathy is suspected in a limb in a weight-bearing position, it must be confirmed when the fetlock is flexed, in a non–weight-bearing position, to avoid relaxation artifacts. These hypoechoic images can represent either inflammatory processes (capsulitis) or fibroblastic tissue in old lesions.

- *Localized hyperechoic images* with acoustic shadowing can be found in several locations: proximally, near the dorsal border of the metacarpal condyle (usually sagittal or parasagittal); distally, near the capsule attachment on the proximal phalanx, in a parasagittal position; and laterally or medially, at the level of the dorsoabaxial border of the metacarpal condyle.

- *Proximal hyperechoic images* represent calcification of either the dorsal capsule or the proximodorsal synovial fold; abaxial hyperechoic images correspond to calcification, as well as bony osteochondral fragments within the dorsal capsule. Distal hyperechoic images could be due to calcification, osteochondral fragments, or acquired chip fractures.

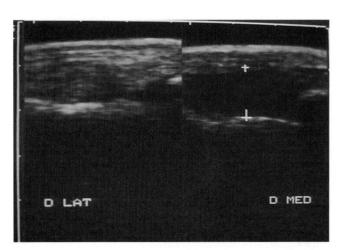

Figure 24.11. Longitudinal ultrasound scans of the dorsal aspect of the fetlock. On each scan the proximal border of the proximal phalanx appears on the right. Compared with the dorsolateral approach (*left*), the dorsomedial approach (*right*) showed thickening and a decrease in echogenicity of the dorsal articular capsule. These findings indicate extensive dorsal capsulitis.

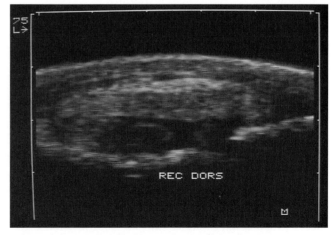

Figure 24.13. Longitudinal ultrasound scan of the dorsal aspect of the fetlock. Between the echogenic dorsal articular capsule and the dorsal profile of the third metacarpal bone (*on the left*) and proximal phalanx (*on the right*), synovial fluid distention and moderate thickening of the dorsoproximal synovial fold are present. Hyperechoic osteophytes appear at the proximal border of P1. These findings are indicative of proliferative synovitis with degenerative joint disease.

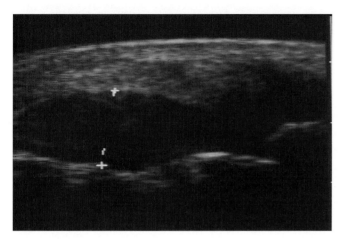

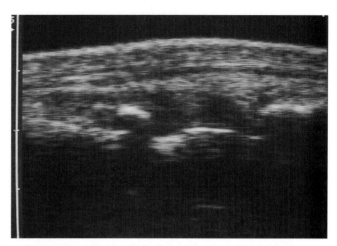

Figure 24.14. Longitudinal ultrasound scan of the dorsal aspect of the fetlock. Between the echogenic dorsal articular capsule and the dorsal aspect of the distal metacarpal bone, extensive thickening of the dorsoproximal synovial fold is present. Bone remodeling (osteolysis) of the dorsal metacarpus is also seen. These imaging findings indicate that chronic proliferative synovitis is present.

Figure 24.15. Longitudinal ultrasound scan of the dorsal aspect of the fetlock. A hyperechoic spot is present at the proximal aspect of the metacarpal condyle, indicating a calcification of the dorsoproximal synovial fold. The dorsal digital extensor tendon runs between the skin and the dorsal capsule.

- *Diffuse hyperechoic images* without acoustic shadowing are found when fibrosis of the dorsal capsule is present. It is usually associated with limited passive flexion of the fetlock joint.

Synovial Membrane

- Thickening of the synovial membrane is common in inflammatory processes (arthritis), but the membrane can barely be differentiated from the anechoic or poorly echogenic synovial fluid.
- Longitudinal and transverse sections at the dorsal aspect of the fetlock allow imaging of the *synovial fold* of the proximal recess and a precise evaluation of its size and architecture (Figs. 24.13 and 24.14).

Abnormal findings include the following:

1. Thickening of the proximal synovial fold (thickness >2 mm) and elevation of the dorsal articular capsule
2. Diffuse hypoechoic images within the fold
3. Synovial fluid effusion between the articular surfaces and the dorsal articular capsule
4. Fibrosis of this fold
5. Osteolysis on the proximal border of the metacarpal condyle
6. Diffuse hyperechoic images, indicating fibrosis of the synovial fold
7. Hyperechoic images with acoustic shadows demonstrating calcification (Fig. 24.15)

These lesions represent a synovial hyperplasia and/or metaplasia.

Articular Margins of the Proximal Phalanx

- Ultrasonography is more sensitive than radiology in detecting irregularities, remodeling, or osteophytes of the proximal bor-

der of P1 (Fig. 24.16). It is also more thorough as the entire contour of the dorsoabaxial border of P1 can be examined by moving the probe.

- Hyperechoic images casting acoustic shadows are indicative of bony fragments (Fig. 24.17). These fragments could be chip fractures, osteochondral fragments, or areas of calcification within the distal insertion of the dorsal capsule. On transverse sections, ultrasonography allows location of these bony fragments with accuracy (Fig. 24.17*B*), even when they are small and difficult to see on dorsopalmar radiographs. Moreover, it is possible to calculate the depth of the fragments without distortion. During the ultrasound examination, flexion and extension movements allow determination of the degree of mobility of the fragments (Fig. 24.17*C*). When surgical removal is considered, ultrasonography, as a preoperative examination,

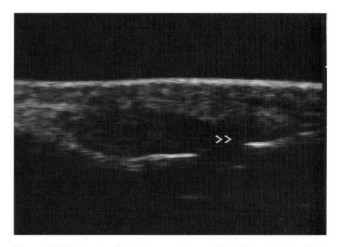

Figure 24.16. Longitudinal ultrasound scan of the dorsal aspect of the fetlock. Hyperechoic extension of the proximal border of the proximal phalanx indicates formation of a periarticular osteophyte. The dorsal articular capsule and the dorsoproximal synovial fold look hypoechoic.

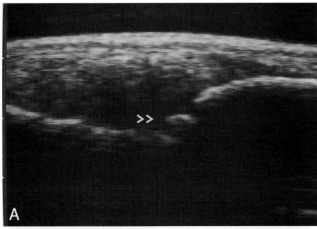

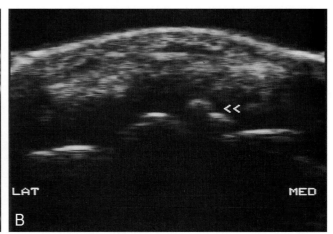

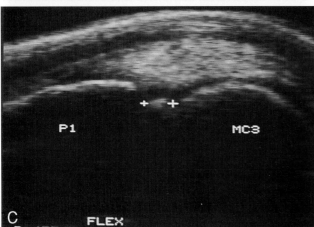

Figure 24.17. A. Longitudinal ultrasound scan of the dorsal aspect of the fetlock. Thickening of the dorsal articular capsule is seen and a hyperechoic spot is present at the dorsal aspect of the metacarpophalangeal space. This image corresponds to an osteochondral fragment. **B.** Transverse ultrasound scan of the dorsal aspect of the fetlock of the same horse. This complementary scan shows that there are two bone nodules adjacent to the medial aspect of the sagittal ridge of the metacarpal condyle. **C.** Longitudinal ultrasound scan of the dorsal aspect of the fetlock of the same horse in a flexed (*FLEX*) position. This scan shows that the bony fragments fit into the articular space during flexion. *MC3*, metacarpal condyle.

gives precise landmarks for the surgical approach. The position of the limb during the surgery must be taken into consideration to make ultrasonographic images in the same attitude, because of the relative proximal displacement of the skin during metacarpophalangeal flexion.

Metacarpal Condyle

- Longitudinal sections can demonstrate irregularities of the contour of the metacarpal condyle sagittal ridge (osteochondritis dissecans or defects). They also highlight abnormal contours of the lateral or medial parts of the distal condyle, which may be inapparent on lateromedial radiographic views because of superimposition.
- Transverse sections easily reveal parasagittal osteochondral defects of the metacarpal condyle, which require proximodistal, skyline, radiographic projection to be identified.

Abaxial (Lateral or Medial) Aspects

With ultrasonography several structures on the abaxial aspect of the fetlock can be evaluated.

Dorsoabaxial Aspect

- *Collateral ligament* (lateral or medial). This ligament does not have a homogenous echogenicity because of the different orientation of its fibers. On most longitudinal and transverse sec-

tions, its deep layer looks hypoechoic because of the obliquity of the fibers near the bone insertion in the abaxial fossa.

Nevertheless, the evaluation of the size and echogenicity of each part of the collateral ligaments of the fetlock allows identification and documentation of injuries (Figs. 24.18 and 24.19).

Usually *desmitis* of the collateral ligament of the fetlock induces thickening and hypoechogenicity of the deep part of this structure.

Chronic proximal *insertion desmopathies* (enthesopathies) are characterized by a deepening of the insertion fossa of the collateral ligament at the abaxial aspect of the metacarpal condyle (Fig. 24.20).

Other common findings include thickening and obliquity of the fibers at the attachment of the ligament; hypoechoic images within the ligament; and remodeling, bony avulsion, or calcification at the insertion site.

- *Hyperechoic images* can be identified within the collateral ligament, usually at the most distal part of the metacarpal condyle near the metacarpophalangeal joint space (Fig. 24.21).

These images casting acoustic shadows are either areas of calcification after an injury or osteochondral fragments, which can also be demonstrated on oblique radiographs.

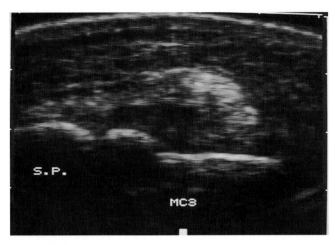

Figure 24.18. Transverse ultrasound scan of the lateral aspect of the fetlock. This 10-year-old mare had a total luxation of the metacarpophalangeal joint. The lateral proximal sesamoid bone (*SP*) is on the left, and the lateral aspect of the metacarpal condyle (*MC3*) is on the right. The deep layer of the lateral collateral ligament is thickened and hypoechoic. These findings are compatible with rupture. Extensive periarticular thickening compatible with edema and hemorrhage is also seen.

These findings were often found with both a thickening and a heterogenous pattern of echogenicity within the collateral ligament indicating chronic desmitis (Fig. 24.21).

- *Articular margins.* The abaxial articular margins of the proximal phalanx and metacarpal condyle can present abnormal sharp borders. This finding is indicative of periarticular osteophytes.

Palmoabaxial Aspect
Proximopalmar (plantar) recess of the metacarpo-(metatarso)phalangeal joint. Distention of this synovial recess is a common (but not consistent) finding when degenerative

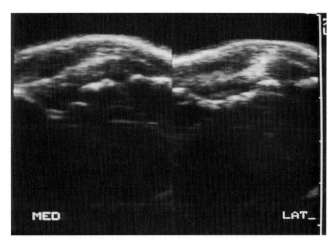

Figure 24.20 Longitudinal ultrasound scans of the medial (*left*) and lateral (*right*) aspects of the fetlock. On the medial aspect, the insertion fossa of the lateral collateral ligament (*LCL*) is deeper than normal and the bone surface is irregular. These findings indicate that chronic proximal enthesopathy of the LCL is present.

joint disease of the fetlock is present (Fig. 24.22). It is also observed when acute trauma to the joint has occurred.

When the synovial fluid is echogenic, hemorrhage or sepsis within the metacarpophalangeal articular cavity should be considered (Figs. 24.23 and 24.24).

Distal insertion of the third interosseus muscle (suspensory ligament) (see also Chapter 23). Thickening of the distal portion of the third interosseus muscle (TIOM) branches and hypoechoic images within it are indicative of desmitis. In chronic desmopathy these findings are usually accompanied by the presence of a thick peritendinous echogenic area indicative of peritendinous fibrosis. When the distal insertion

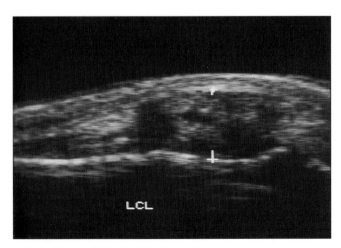

Figure 24.19. Longitudinal ultrasound scan of the lateral aspect of the fetlock. The metacarpophalangeal space appears on the right. The lateral collateral ligament (*LCL*) is thickened, and the superficial layer of this structure is hypoechoic. These findings are consistent with desmopathy of the LCL.

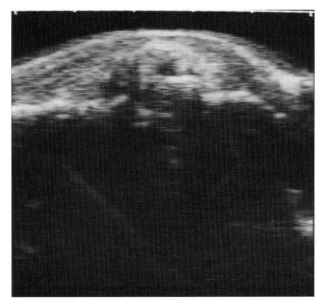

Figure 24.21. Longitudinal ultrasound scan of the lateral aspect of the fetlock. Thickening and an irregular pattern of echogenicity of the lateral collateral ligament (*LCL*) are seen. A hyperechoic spot casts an acoustic shadow. These findings are compatible with a chronic desmopathy and calcification or bone fragments within the LCL.

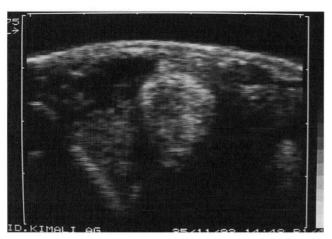

Figure 24.22. Transverse ultrasound scan of the lateral aspect of the fetlock. The palmar aspect of the third metacarpal bone is on the left, and the palmar aspect of the area is on the right. The distal branch of the third interosseus muscle looks thickened and slightly hypoechoic. An anechoic synovial fluid effusion is present with chronic proliferative synovitis within the proximopalmar recess of the metacarpophalangeal joint.

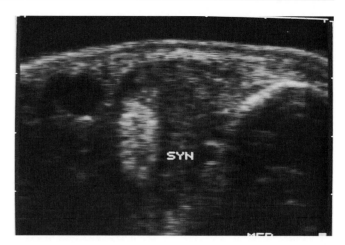

Figure 24.23. Transverse ultrasound scan of the lateral aspect of the fetlock. Same mare shown in Figure 24.18 (metacarpophalangeal joint luxation). The palmar aspect of the third metacarpal bone is on the right and the palmar aspect of the area is on the left. The synovial recess (*SYN*) content is echogenic, and because of the history and physical examination, hemorrhage was suspected within the articular cavity. Notice the dilatation of the digital vein at the palmar aspect of the interosseus branch.

of the suspensory branch is involved (enthesopathy), the abaxial surface of insertion (interosseus face) of the corresponding proximal sesamoid bone looks irregular. Hyperechoic images casting acoustic shadows in the distal insertion of the suspensory ligament are indicative of avulsion fracture or calcification.

Proximal Sesamoid Bones. As mentioned previously, the abaxial surface of insertion for the TIOM distal branch (interosseus face) may present an irregular contour or avulsion fractures. Fractures of the proximal sesamoid bones are better documented by radiology. Nevertheless, ultrasonographic images can help in assessing topographic relationships between the bony fragments and the surrounding soft tissues, especially the suspensory ligament. This information is useful in determining the best surgical approach when removal of the bony fragments is considered, especially at the apex or at the base of the proximal sesamoid bones.

Palmar Aspect. At the palmar aspect of the fetlock, several ligaments must be considered. The flexor tendons are described elsewhere (Chapters 21 and 22).

- Partial rupture or desmitis of the palmar (or intersesamoid) ligament was suspected but never established definitely in this retrospective study, although they were described at necropsy and reproduced experimentally.

Adhesions between the palmar ligament and the DDFT were observed in chronic injury with fibroplasia and calcification of this tendon. During the dynamic examination on the flexed limb, decreased mobility between these two structures was demonstrated. These findings were confirmed at necropsy.

- Proximal desmitis of the distal sesamoid ligaments most often occurred within the oblique sesamoid ligaments (OSL). In-

juries of the straight sesamoid ligament (SSL) were observed at their proximal insertion in some instances.

Desmopathies of the OSL usually involved their proximal part. They were characterized by a thickening and, depending on their stage of evolution, a hypoechogenicity or an heterogenous pattern of echogenecity. They were located on one side of the limb (medially or laterally) or on both sides, and were frequently accompanied by injuries of the TIOM branches.

- Hyperechoic images casting acoustic shadows within the sesamoidophalangeal space at the palmar aspect of the fetlock may represent osteochondral fragments (Fig. 24.25), avulsion

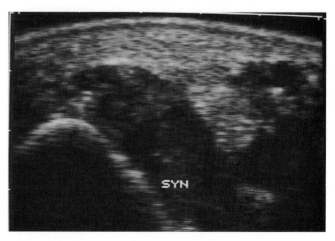

Figure 24.24. Transverse ultrasound scan of the lateral aspect of the fetlock. The palmar aspect of the third metacarpal bone is on the left and the palmar aspect of the area is on the right. The synovial recess (*SYN*) content is markedly distended and echogenic. History and clinical examination indicated that the horse had septic arthritis.

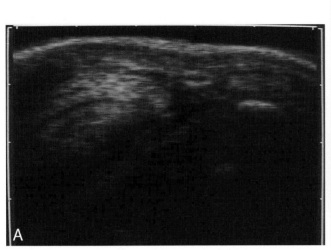
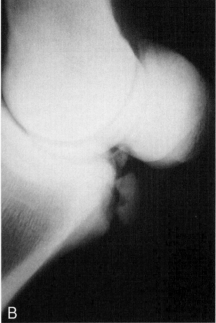

Figure 24.25. A. Transverse ultrasound scan of the plantarolateral aspect of the fetlock distally to the lateral proximal sesamoid bone. At the plantarolateral aspect of the proximal P1 a hyperechoic bony fragment is within the lateral oblique sesamoid ligament. On the left side of the ultrasound scan the deep and superficial digital flexor tendons are imaged. **B.** Lateromedial radiograph of the same fetlock. There are two osteochondral bony fragments within the sesamoidophalangeal space.

fracture of the palmo(planto)proximal border of the proximal phalanx or of the base of the proximal sesamoid bones, or calcification within the oblique or short sesamoid ligaments. The intraarticular or extraarticular position of the fragment can be assessed with radiography and ultrasonography to decide which technique (arthroscopy or extraarticular approach) should be used if surgical removal is considered. In the extraarticular approach, ultrasonography is of primary importance for determining the exact location, depth, and size of the fragment.

The ultrasonographic examination of the palmar annular ligament (PAL) is easy and gives precise information about injuries of this ligament, as well as associated lesions of the flexor tendons and digital sheath. The normal PAL is less than 2 mm thick (Fig. 24.26). Thickening of the PAL may be the result of recent or chronic desmopathy (Figs. 24.27 and 24.28) and is usually accompanied by a digital-sheath tenosynovitis with synovial effusion (Figs. 24.28 and 24.29)

- The dynamic examination on the flexed limbs allows assessing of the functional relationships between the flexor tendons and

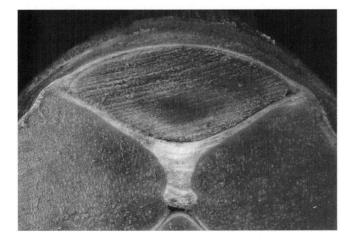

Figure 24.26. Transverse anatomic section of the palmar aspect of the fetlock. In a dorsopalmar direction the following structures can be identified: the two proximal sesamoid bones, the palmar (or interesamoid) ligament, the DDFT, the SDFT, and the thin palmar annular ligament.

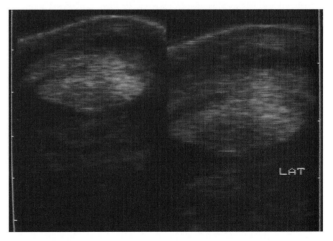

Figure 24.27. Transverse ultrasound scans of the palmar aspect of the fetlock above the proximal sesamoid bones. Superficial to the SDFT, the palmar annular ligament is thickened and hypoechoic. These findings indicate desmitis of this structure. Dorsal to the DDFT, the proximal part of the palmar ligament has a normal hypoechoic representation.

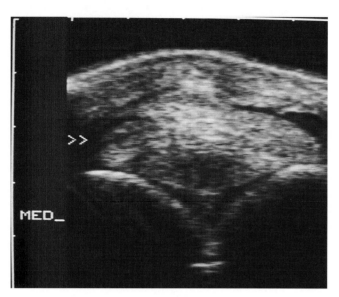

Figure 24.28. Transverse ultrasound scan of the palmar aspect of the fetlock at the level of the proximal sesamoid bones. The palmar annular ligament is thickened, but has normal echogenicity. Synovial fluid is between the SDFT and the palmar annular ligament. This finding shows that chronic injury of this ligament is not accompanied by stenosis of the flexor tendons.

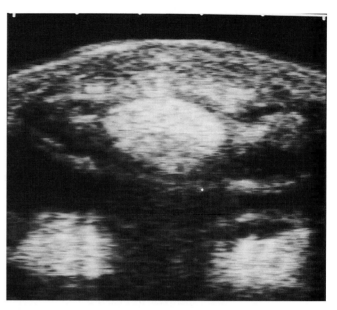

Figure 24.29. Transverse ultrasound scan of the palmar aspect of the fetlock proximal to the proximal sesamoid bones. The thickening of the palmar annular ligament is accompanied by an extensive synovial fluid effusion within the proximal recess of the digital sheath. The synovial membrane and the mesotendons are also thickened, showing the chronicity of the injuries. Because of the synovial effusion, the distal branches of the third interosseus muscle are very clearly imaged.

the palmar annular ligament. During the flexion and extension of the metacarpophalangeal joint of clinically normal horses, both flexor tendons slide at the same speed except at the end of each movement. When the superficial and deep flexor tendons do not synchronize in a proximal direction during flexion and in a distal direction during extension, adhesions must be suspected. These adhesions usually take place between the SDFT and the palmar annular ligament.

Metacarpus/Metatarsus

Long Digital Extensor Tendon

Traumatic injuries of extensor tendons at the dorsal aspect of the metacarpus or metatarsus are common. They include accidental sectioning/rupture, most common on the hind limbs, and bruising, most common on the front limbs.

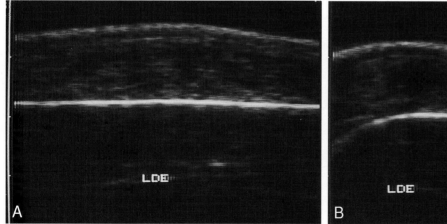
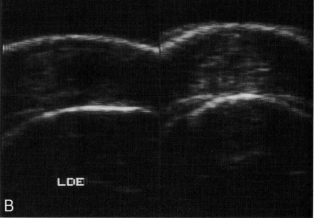

Figure 24.30. A. Longitudinal ultrasound scan at the dorsal aspect of the metatarsus. The long digital extensor tendon is thickened and has abnormal, irregular hypoechogenicity. These findings are compatible with a traumatic injury or elongation of this tendon. The dorsal aspect of the third metacarpal bone cortex looks regular and hyperechoic. **B.** Transverse ultrasound scans at the dorsal aspect of the metatarsus of the same horse. Ultrasound findings were the same. The long digital extensor tendon is thickened and has an abnormal, irregular hypoechogenicity. These findings are compatible with a traumatic injury or elongation of this tendon. The dorsal aspect of the third metacarpal bone cortex looks regular and hyperechoic. *LDE,* long digital extensor.

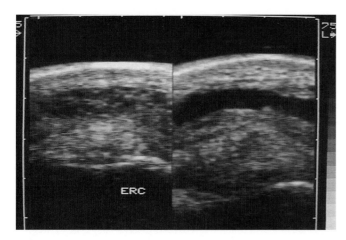

Figure 24.31. Transverse ultrasound scans of the dorsal aspect of the carpus at the level of the distal radius. Between the extensor retinaculum and the subcutaneous tissue, there is a hypoechoic (*left*) and an anechoic (*right*) space. The extensor carpi radialis (*ECR*) has normal shape, size, and echogenicity. These findings indicate that the dorsal swelling of the carpus is caused by a subcutaneous hygroma.

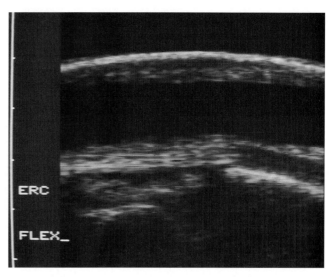

Figure 24.32. Longitudinal ultrasound scan of the dorsal aspect of the carpus in flexion. An extensive synovial effusion is present within the extensor carpi radialis (*ECR*)[9] synovial sheath. Between the distal aspect of the radius (*on the left*) and the radial carpal extensor tendon, the dorsal articular capsule of the carpus is imaged.

- When the tendon has been recently ruptured, a very hypoechoic gap due to hemorrhage can be observed between the proximal and distal stumps. During the healing process, the echogenicity gradually improves because of fibrous scar-tissue formation and hemorrhage resorption. In old injuries the tendon appears thickened with an irregular pattern of echogenicity and fiber alignment over several centimeters. Functional sequelae may include tendon and fetlock laxity, or tendon adhesion to the metatarsus and partial deficit of digital extension.

- Bruising induces a thickening of the dorsal or long digital extensor tendon, anechoic or hypoechoic areas of hemorrhage, and a very hypoechoic peritendinous (subcutaneous) space of fluid accumulation (Fig. 24.30). Evolution of these abnormal ultrasonographic findings does not differ from other traumatic injuries of tendons resulting in an increase in size and a diffuse, irregular pattern of echogenicity with smaller and disoriented fiber bundles.

Carpus

Dorsal Aspect

When a swelling is present at the dorsal aspect of the carpus, extensor tendon injuries or tenosynovitis should be differentiated from subcutaneous lesions (Fig. 24.31).

Extensor Carpi Radialis Tendinopathy. Injuries of the distal tendon of the extensor carpi radialis muscle were documented in several horses. Abnormal findings included thickening of the tendon, hypoechoic images within the tendon, and in most cases tenosynovitis of the tendon sheath at the dorsal aspect of the distal radius and carpus (Fig. 24.32). In most horses the flexion range of the carpus was reduced because of the thickening of the tendon and possibly adhesion to the radius periosteum, as well as to the tendon sheath wall. Rupture of the retinaculum extensorum with synovial

fluid effusion in the subcutaneous tissue was also observed (Fig. 24.33).

Dorsal Digital Extensor Tenosynovitis. Different amounts of synovial fluid distention were observed within the synovial sheath of the dorsal digital extensor tendon at the dorsolateral aspect of the carpus (Fig. 24.34). The synovial fluid

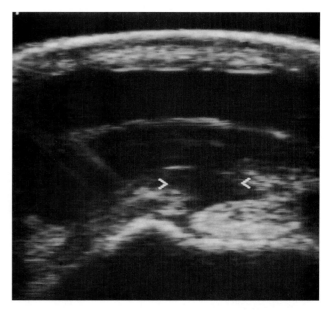

Figure 24.33. Transverse ultrasound scan of the dorsal aspect of the carpus at the level of the distal radius. An extensive fluid effusion (with an oblique echogenic artifact on the left) is between the superficial structures and the extensor carpi radialis tendon. An anechoic gap was identified within the extensor retinaculum in longitudinal and transverse scans (*arrowheads*), indicating a communication between the extensor carpi radialis synovial sheath and the superficial fluid effusion.

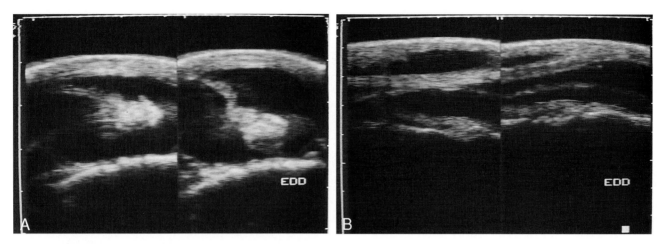

Figure 24.34. A. Transverse ultrasound scan of the dorsal aspect of the carpus. An extensive synovial fluid effusion is present within the dorsal digital extensor tendon (*EDD*) sheath. The mesotendon is thickened and lengthened and is clearly imaged because of the contrast with the surrounding anechoic fluid. **B.** Longitudinal ultrasound scan of the dorsal aspect of the same carpus. The EDD has no contact with the dorsal aspect of the radius and is elevated distally (*on the right*). It is relaxed and its size is reduced. These findings are consistent with atrophy and elongation of this tendon.

was always totally anechoic, and in most cases the thickening of the synovial membrane made the mesotendon very apparent (Fig. 24.34*A*). Old or chronic distention stretched the retinaculum extensorum. In one particular horse, which also suffered from antebrachiocarpal degenerative joint disease, the tendon was lengthened and totally separated from the dorsal articular capsule of the carpus (Fig. 24.34*B*).

Dorsal Articular Capsule

• Rupture of the dorsal articular capsule was imaged (Fig. 24.35). In this case subcutaneous fluid accumulation was present, and communication with the joint cavity was established on flexed joint. Pressure on the dorsal aspect of the joint caused one of the synovial folds to enter the opened articular space.

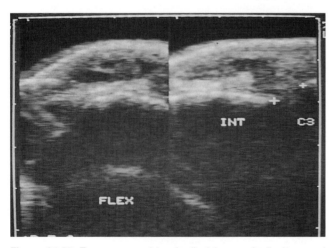

Figure 24.35. Transverse and longitudinal (parasagittal) ultrasound scans of the dorsal aspect of the carpus in flexion. A synovial fluid effusion is around the dorsal digital extensor tendon (*left side*). On the longitudinal scan (*right side*) a hypoechoic pathway (*crosses*) goes between the intermediate (*INT*) and third carpal (*C3*) bones. Dynamic examination and pressure on the tendon sheath showed communication between the articular cavity and the tendon sheath.

• Distention and thickening of the dorsal articular capsule was observed in traumatic injuries to the joint (Fig. 24.36). When fractures occurred, synovial fluid accumulation induced alterations of the dorsal articular capsule.

Lateral Aspect

Proximal to the accessory carpal bone, the synovial fluid distention of the proximal recess of the carpal sheath is easy to identify when carpal canal syndrome exists (Fig. 24.37). This large recess is located cranially to the distal part of the ulnaris lateralis muscle, caudally to the lateral digital extensor tendon, and at the lateral aspect of the digital flexor muscle bodies.

At the lateral aspect of the accessory carpal bone, a tenosynovitis of the long and thin tendon of the lateralis ulnaris muscle was identified in two horses who presented with a partial fracture of the proximodorsal angle of the accessory carpal bone.

Palmaromedial Aspect: Carpal Canal

Tenosynovitis of the carpal canal is a common problem in race horses and sport horses. Distention of the proximal recess is easy to document at the lateral aspect of the distal forearm (Fig. 24.37), proximal to the accessory carpal bone and cranial to the ulnaris lateralis muscle (see above). Distention of the distal recess makes the anechoic space between the deep digital flexor tendon and its accessory ligament wider in the proximal third of the metacarpus. In some cases fluid distention can also be found at the lateral and/or medial aspect of the flexor tendons in this area.

Tenosynovitis of the carpal canal can be found alone (Fig. 24.38) or can be due to other injuries of the canal wall (parietal injuries) or to the content of this canal.

Parietal Injuries of the Carpal Canal Accompanied by Synovial Sheath Distention

1. *Accessory ligament desmopathies.* Injuries of the accessory ligament of the superficial digital flexor tendon (AL-SDFT,

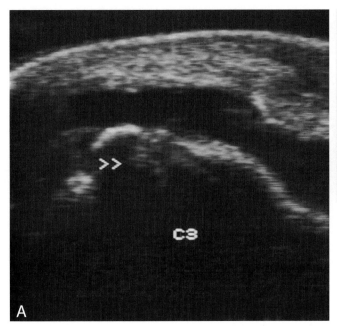
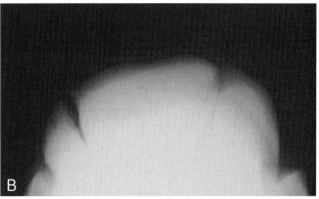

Figure 24.36. A. Transverse ultrasound scan of the dorsal aspect of the distal row of the carpus shows a sagittal slab fracture. The dorsal surface of the third carpal bone (*C3*) is separated from the thickened and elongated dorsal articular capsule by an anechoic synovial fluid distention space. There is an echogenic gap within the dorsal hyperechoic aspect of C3 that is compatible with an enlarged fracture line. **B.** Proximodistal radiograph of the distal row of the same carpus shows a slab fracture line in the medial part of C3. This horse had sudden onset of left forelimb lameness 10 weeks ago.

proximal check ligament) are not unusual in race and sport horses. Evaluation of this ligament is made by placing the probe at the medial aspect of the distal antebrachium, between the chestnut and the styloid process of the radius. In this region the AL-SDFT is located between the palmar aspect of the radius, the distal tendon of the flexor carpi radialis, the median artery, and the flexor tendons and looks echogenoic with irregular borders (Fig. 24.38). Abnormal findings indicative of desmopathy include the following (Fig. 24.39):

- Local or diffuse hypoechogenicity
- Thickening
- Synovial fluid accumulation between the AL-SDFT and the radius
- Decrease of visualization of the deep limit of the tendon sheath of the flexor carpi radialis

Injuries of the accessory ligament of the deep digital flexor tendon (AL-DDFT or distal check ligament) are described elsewhere (Chapter 22), and are often accompanied

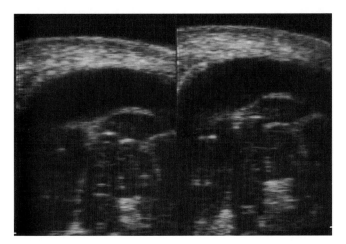

Figure 24.37. Transverse ultrasound scan of the lateral aspect of the distal forearm. Between the digital flexor muscle bodies and the thickened antebrachial fascia and subcutaneous tissue is an anechoic fluid distention space. This image is the result of distention of the proximal lateral recess of the carpal sheath.

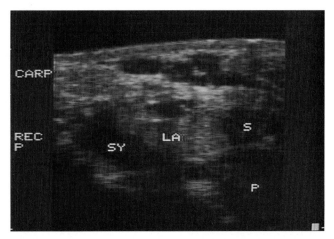

Figure 24.38. Transverse ultrasound scan of the palmaromedial aspect of the distal forearm. Synovial fluid distention (*SY*) is present in the proximal recess (*REC P*) of the carpal sheath. The accessory ligament (*LA*) of the superficial digital flexor tendon has a normal echogenic appearance. The digital flexor muscle bodies still have hypoechogenic muscular fibers. *P*, deep; *S*, superficial.

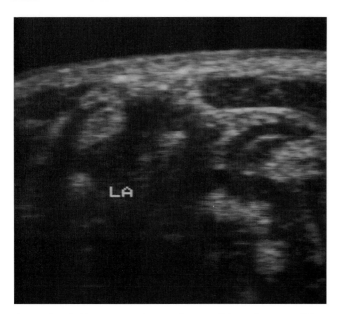

Figure 24.39. Transverse ultrasound scan of the palmaromedial aspect of the distal forearm of the same horse shown in Figure 24.44. An enlarged hypoechoic area is present between the flexor carpi radialis tendon and the SDF and DDF muscle body–tendon junction. The accessory ligament of the SDFT (proximal check ligament) is not apparent; thus the hypoechoic area can be interpreted as an injured accessory ligament (*LA*). Hypoechoic images within the digital flexor components represent muscular fibers.

by a synovial fluid distention of the distal recess of the carpal sheath.

2. *The dorsal wall of the carpal canal* is the common palmar ligament of the carpus. This ligament inserts on the transverse crista radialis and is continued by the AL-DDFT. Lesions of this ligament make it thicker and hypoechoic and are accompanied by proximal desmopathy of the AL-DDFT (Fig. 24.40).

3. *The lateral wall of the carpal canal* is formed by the accessory carpal bone and its ligaments. Fractures of the accessory

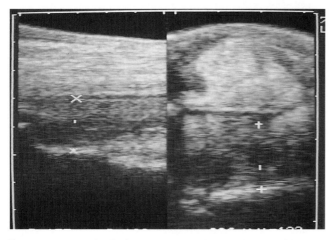

Figure 24.40. Longitudinal and transverse ultrasound scans of the palmar aspect of the distal carpus. The junction between the common palmar carpal ligament and the accessory ligament of the DDFT is thickened and hypoechoic images are within it, indicating desmopathy of the dorsal wall of the carpal canal.

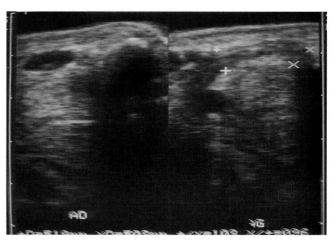

Figure 24.41. Transverse ultrasound scans of the palmar medial aspect of the right and left carpus. On the left carpus (*right scan*) the flexor retinaculum appears thickened and hypoechoic (*crosses*). These findings are compatible with desmopathy of the retinaculum.

carpal bone usually induce carpal canal synovial effusion and in some horses, bony fragments can be found within the carpal sheath.

4. Finally, *carpal canal syndrome* can be accompanied by distention or desmopathy of the fibrous palmaromedial wall of the carpal canal named retinaculum flexorum (RF). Distention of the RF can be caused by either chronic synovial fluid accumulation or thickening of the flexor tendons. The diagnosis of desmopathy of the RF is based on the thickening of this structure and a generally moderate hypoechogenicity (Fig. 24.41).

Injuries of the Carpal Canal Content Causing Synovial Effusion: Tendinopathies and Vascular Lesions. Proximal injuries of the SDFT and DDFT are described elsewhere (Chapters 21 and 22) and usually induce carpal sheath effusion (Fig. 24.42).

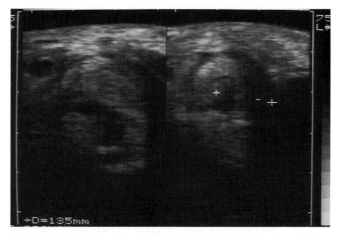

Figure 24.42. Transverse ultrasound scans of the palmaromedial aspect of the carpus. *Left,* An abnormal hypoechoic space is present between the superficial and deep digital flexor tendons, which is compatible with chronic synovitis. *Right,* The lateral part of the SDFT looks hypoechoic. The hyperechoic curve line on the right is the palmar border of the accessory carpal bone. A surgical debridement of the carpal canal showed a laceration of the lateral aspect of the SDFT.

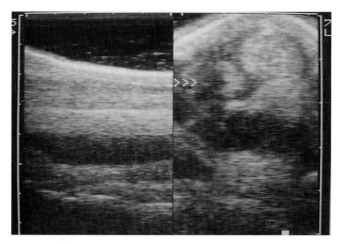

Figure 24.43. Longitudinal and transverse ultrasound scans of the palmar aspect of the carpometacarpal junction. A hypoechoic distended synovial fluid space is present in the distal recess of the carpal sheath. The transverse scan (*right*) shows an abnormal image of the median artery wall (*arrowheads*). Paracentesis revealed blood in the carpal canal synovial sheath.

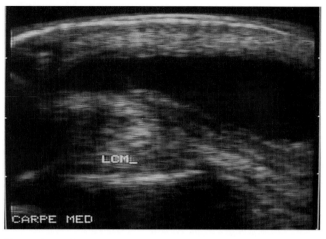

Figure 24.45. Transverse ultrasound scan of the medial aspect of the carpus. The medial collateral ligament (*LCM*) is inserted on the medial aspect of the radial carpal bone. Between the cross-section of this ligament and the subcutaneous tissue is a large anechoic fluid space. History and other clinical investigations showed that this finding was the result of a traumatic hematoma.

Blood effusion within the carpal sheath has been also found in association with wall injuries of the median artery (Fig. 24.43).

Tenosynovitis of the Distal Tendon of the Flexor Carpi Radialis. This can be found in association with desmopathy of the AL-SDFT. Distention of the tendon sheath is easy to identify because of the very echogenic aspect of its fibrous surroundings (antebrachial fascia and retinaculum flexorum) and of the distal tendon of the flexor carpal radialis (Fig. 24.44). Associations between these abnormal findings are easily explained as the AL-SDFT forms the deep wall of the tendon canal.

Medial Aspect

At the medial aspect of the joint, periarticular and ligament injuries were observed.

- Subcutaneous anechoic fluid accumulation observed after recent traumatic interference was due to a hematoma.(Fig. 24.45).
- Thickened echogenic material between the skin and the medial collateral ligament, indicative of subcutaneous fibrosis, was observed as a result of chronic interference (Fig. 24.46).
- Several types of medial collateral ligament (MCL) injuries could be imaged: An irregular profile of the medial styloid

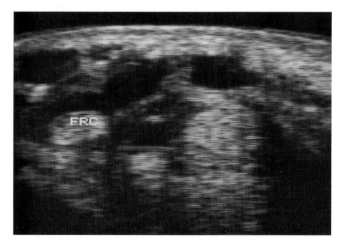

Figure 24.44. Transverse ultrasound scan of the palmaromedial aspect of the distal forearm. An anechoic fluid distention is present around the distal tendon of the flexor carpi radialis (*FRC*), and the corresponding mesotendon is thickened. These findings are indicative of flexor carpi radialis tenosynovitis. The digital flexor tendons and the distal part of the accessory ligament of the SDFT appear normal.

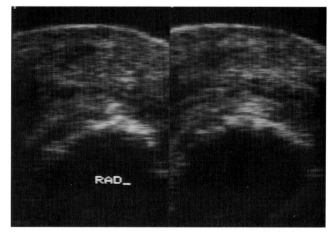

Figure 24.46. Transverse ultrasound scan of the medial aspect of the carpus. The medial collateral ligament is inserted on the styloid process of the radius (*RAD*). Superficially, thickening and fibrosis of the subcutaneous tissue are present as a result of repeated, interfering, traumatic injuries with the other limb. On the left scan, the proximal insertion site of the medial collateral ligament looks irregular, indicating insertion desmopathy (enthesopathy).

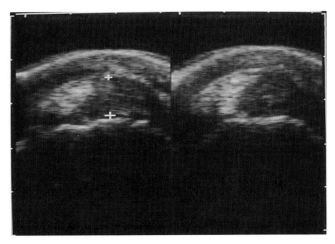 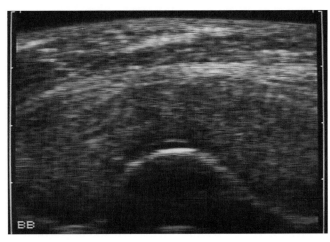

Figure 24.47. Transverse ultrasound scans of the medial aspect of the carpus. The palmar part of the medial collateral ligament looks thickened and hypoechoic. On normal horses, because of the spiral disposition of the fiber bundles, this ligament does not have homogenous echogenicity. Thus, although the findings shown here are compatible with medial collateral ligament desmopathy, they are not indicative of this lesion and should be compared with findings in the opposite limb.

Figure 24.48. Transverse ultrasound scan of the cranial aspect of the shoulder. Normal ultrasound representation of the proximal tendon of the biceps brachii. This tendon has uniform echogenicity. The deep hyperechogenic line represents the bone surface of the intertuberal groove, and the biceps tendon is closely molded to the intermediate ridge of this groove. Normally, the bicipital (intertuberal) bursa lies between the tendon and the groove and is not clearly represented.

process of the radius is consistent with proximal enthesopathy of the MCL. Thickening and abnormal hypoechoic images are indicative of MCL desmopathy (Fig. 24.47).

Shoulder

On sound horses the proximal tendon of the biceps brachii muscle has an homogenous pattern of echogenicity. At the proximal end of the humerus, this tendon is applied on the intertubercular groove (Fig. 24.48); some muscular fibers can produce hypoechoic images in the cranial part of the tendon. Abnormal ultrasonographic images were mainly recorded at the cranial aspect of the point of the shoulder.

Traumatic Tendinopathy of the Brachial Biceps

Lesions of the proximal tendon of the biceps brachii muscle were identified after traumatic injuries of the cranial aspect of the shoulder (Fig. 24.49). In one injured tendon, thickening and hypoechoic images were found (Fig. 24.50).

Fracture of the Supraglenoidal Tubercle

This lesion is best diagnosed with radiology, but ultrasonography can demonstrate the lack of tension within the proximal tendon of the biceps brachii muscle. This structure appears less echogenic with hypoechoic spots (Fig. 24.51). Calcifications and/or bony fragmentations were also observed and appeared as hyperechoic spots casting acoustic shadows.

Bicipital Bursitis (Intertubercular Bursitis)

Normally, no fluid appears at the caudal (deep) aspect of the biceps brachii muscle. In descriptions of bicipital bursitis, synovial fluid distention between the proximal tendon of the biceps and the intertubercular groove has been mentioned. If fluid distention is great enough, the bursa is seen to fill over the cranial aspect of the tendon.

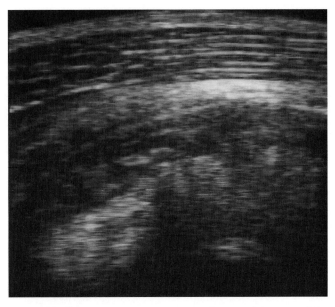

Figure 24.49. Transverse ultrasound scan of the cranial aspect of the shoulder. This mare had a traumatic injury of the cranial aspect of the shoulder 13 days ago. Thickening and diffuse hypoechoic images are present in the superficial part of the bicipital tendon. Hypoechoic images are also found in the intermediate part of the tendon.

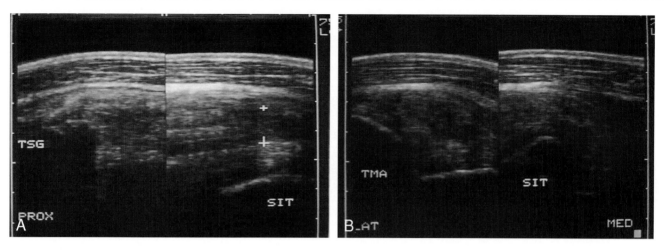

Figure 24.50. A. Longitudinal ultrasound scan of the cranial aspect of the shoulder. Longitudinal hypoechoic images are located within the tendon at the cranial aspect of the intertubercular groove. This mare also had enthesophytes at the proximal insertion of the biceps brachii on the supraglenoid tubercule. Both abnormal imaging findings indicate the presence of enthesopathy and proximal tendinopathy of the biceps. **B.** Transverse ultrasound scan of the cranial aspect of the same shoulder. There are hypoechoic spots within the proximal tendon of the biceps brachii that are compatible with tendinopathy.

Hock

Dorsal Aspect

Tenosynovitis of the *long digital extensor tendon* (LDET): The long digital extensor tendon (LDET) passes through three retinacula (proximal, middle, and distal) at the dorsal aspect of the hock and is surrounded by a vaginal tendon sheath. Tenosynovitis induces distention and swelling of this sheath from the distal crus to the proximal metatarsus. Transverse and longitudinal ultrasonographic images demonstrate fluid accumulation, synovial membrane thickening, and sharpening of the tendon limits (Fig. 24.52).

Differential diagnosis of swelling at the dorsal aspect of the hock includes (a) tenosynovitis of the long digital extensor tendon, (b) tenosynovitis of the tibialis cranialis and peroneus tertius tendons, (c) thickening of the distal part of the peroneus tertius muscle, and (d) distention of the tibial extensor retinaculum.

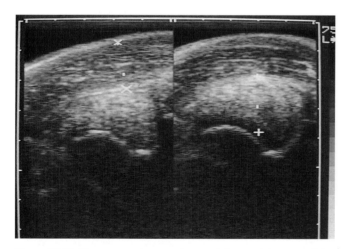

Figure 24.51. Transverse ultrasound scan of the cranial aspect of the shoulder. This 2-year-old horse had a supraglenoid tubercule fracture. The lateral part of the biceps brachii tendon looks hypoechoic (*left image*), and at the proximal aspect of the intertubercular groove (*right image*) an anechoic space is present between the tendon and the bone surface, which is compatible with bicipital bursitis.

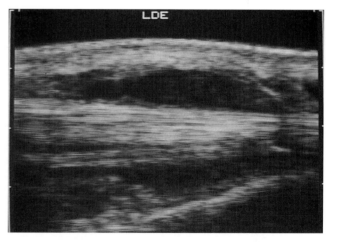

Figure 24.52. Longitudinal ultrasound scan of the dorsal aspect of the hock. The deep, oblique, hyperechoic line represents the dorsal aspect of the tibia. The hypoechoic line within the tendon on the left side of the scan represents muscular fibers of the long digital extensor muscle body. Fluid effusion and synovial membrane proliferation are present on each aspect of the long digital extensor tendon. These abnormal findings are consistent with a long extensor tenosynovitis. *LDE,* long digital extensor.

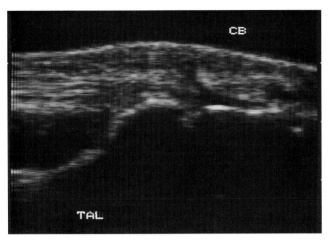

Figure 24.53. Longitudinal ultrasound scan of the medial aspect of the hock. The deep hyperechogenic lines represent the medial profile of the talus (*TAL*) and the central and third tarsal bones. The long medial collateral ligament (on the left side) inserts on the distal tubercule of the talus. The cunean branch (*CB*) of the tibialis cranialis muscle is separated from the underlined structures by an anechoic space representing a subcutaneous bursitis.

Figure 24.54. Transverse ultrasound scan of the dorsomedial aspect of the hock. The cunean branch (*BC*) is located under the cranial branch of the medial saphenous vein (*V*). Dorsally (*CR>*) there is an anechoic space (*crosses*) representing synovial fluid within the cunean bursa; the synovial membrane is thickened. These abnormal signs indicate chronic cunean bursitis. This horse had also a bone spavin.

Medial Aspect

On the medial aspect of the hock, several structures can be imaged, including the long and short medial collateral ligaments, the talometatarsal ligament, and the tarsal (medial) tendon of the tibialis cranialis muscle.

Subtendinous bursitis of the tarsal tendon of the tibialis cranialis muscle was imaged at the dorsomedial aspect of the distal tarsus (Figs. 24.53 and 24.54). Abnormal findings included synovial fluid distention, synovial membrane proliferation, and sometimes thickening of the cunean tendon. These findings were always accompanied by various degrees of degenerative joint disease of the distal tarsus.

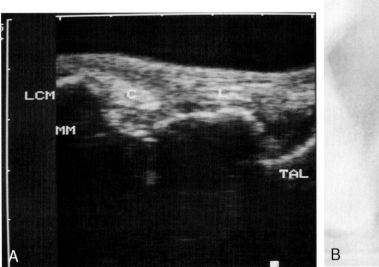

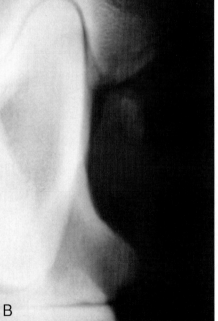

Figure 24.55. A. Longitudinal ultrasound scan of the medial aspect of the distal hock. The long (*L*) and short (*S*) parts of the medial collateral ligament (*LCM*) are clearly imaged. Both of them originate from the medial malleolus (*MM*) of the tibia. The long medial collateral ligament runs to the distal tubercule of the talus (*TAL*) on the right. In the deep portion of this ligament, a hyperechoic curve line casts an acoustic shadow suggestive of calcification or bone material. **B.** Dorsolateral plantaromedial oblique radiograph of the same hock. A large bony fragment is located dorsomedially. Comparative imaging findings showed that this fragment was inserted in the dorsal aspect of the long medial collateral ligament.

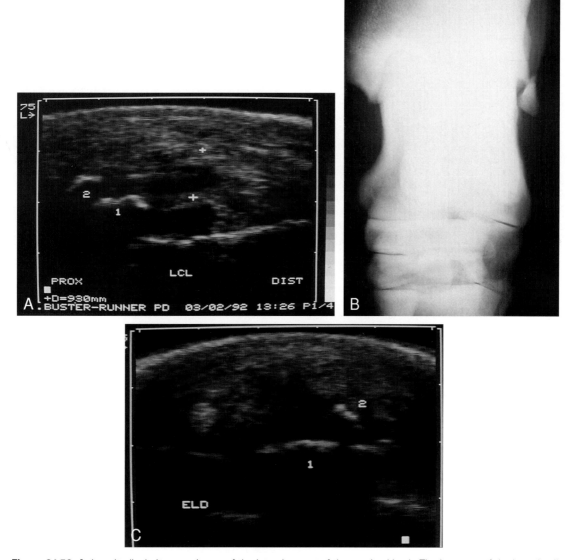

Figure 24.56. A. Longitudinal ultrasound scan of the lateral aspect of the proximal hock. The long part of the lateral collateral ligament (*LCL*) is thickened, and hypoechoic images are present within this ligament at the lateral aspect of the talus. Proximally (*on the left*) are two bony fragments (*1* and *2*) avulsed from the lateral malleolus (distal fibula). Subcutaneous thickening is also present, probably the result of hemorrhage and edema. **B.** Dorsoplantar radiograph of the same hock. An avulsion fracture of the lateral malleolus is present, with mild bony proliferation at the lateral aspect of the talus. **C.** Transverse ultrasound scan of the lateral aspect of the same proximal hock. The dorsal aspect is on the left, the plantar aspect on the right. The echogenic round structure on the left is the lateral digital extensor tendon; plantar to it are the two bony fragments (*1* and *2*). Subcutaneous swelling is also apparent. These findings can be helpful if surgical removal of the fragments is considered.

Distal enthesopathies of the long medial collateral ligament on the distal tubercle of the talus and calcifications within this ligament were easily documented with radiography and ultrasonography (Fig. 24.55).

Lateral Aspect

On the lateral aspect of the hock, the long and short lateral collateral ligaments can be imaged. The short ligament is only stretched when the hock is flexed. Diagnosed injuries include desmopathies and enthesopathies at the proximal at-

tachment on the lateral malleolus and at the distal insertion on the calcaneus, 4th tarsal bone, and 4th metatarsal bone.

When avulsion fractures occur at the *proximal attachment* on the lateral malleolus (Fig. 24.56), ultrasonography helps characterize the size, location, depth, and anatomic relationships of the bony fragments, and this information is particularly valuable when surgical extraction is considered (Fig. 24.56C).

Imaging signs of *distal enthesopathy* of the lateral collateral ligament of the hock include the following:

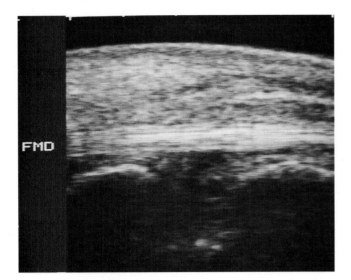

Figure 24.57. Longitudinal ultrasound scan of the plantaromedial aspect of the proximal hock. This image shows the medial digital flexor (*FMD*) tendon, which runs over two underlying bones, the tibia on the left and the talus (sustentaculum tali) on the right. Extensive thickening of the subcutaneous tissue without any other abnormal findings on sonograms and radiographs is caused by trauma.

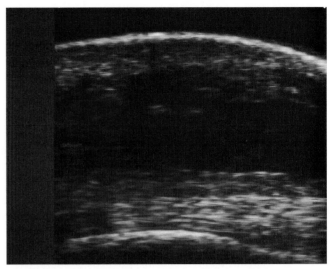

Figure 24.58. Longitudinal ultrasound scan of the plantar aspect of the point of the hock. Superficial to the plantar aspect of the calcaneus and the superficial digital flexor tendon, is a large fluid accumulation in a subcutaneous location at the point of the hock. Because no communications were established with any other synovial component of this region, it was concluded that the fluid distention was the result of a capped hock.

1. Radiographic signs: (a) periosteal proliferation and (b) radiolucent lines within the distal calcaneus.
2. Ultrasound findings: irregular surface of the lateral aspect of the distal calcaneus.

The lack of visualization of the lateral digital extensor tendon at the lateral aspect of the lateral malleolus is indicative of surgical tenectomy for the treatment of stringhalt. Trauma to the lateral hock is common and induces subcutaneous thickening (Fig. 24.57).

Plantar Aspect

At the plantar aspect of the hock, two distinct areas must be considered; these are the point of the hock and the tarsometatarsal junction (versus).

Point of the Hock. Ultrasonographic examination of the capped hock helps in determining the amount of fluid and/or fibrosis (Fig. 24.58) before considering the treatment of the condition.

Instability and luxation of the SIDFT can be documented with ultrasonography.

Lateral luxation of the superficial digital flexor tendon (SDFT) is a well-known pathologic entity. Ultrasonography allows documentation of this injury and evaluation of the tendon itself within the peritendinous swelling or fibrosis and demonstrates the abnormal positioning of the tendon.

Clinical instability of the SDFT on the tuber calcanei is correlated with distention of the medial attachment of the SDFT cap. Abnormal ultrasonographic findings include (a) thickening of the medial attachment, (b) hypoechoic images

within the medial attachment, synovial fluid distention of the subtendinous bursa, and (d) bony irregularities at the medial aspect of the calcaneus.

Medial luxation of the SDFT cap was also documented ultrasonographically.

Subtendinous bursitis of the SDF tendon bursa can occur independently.

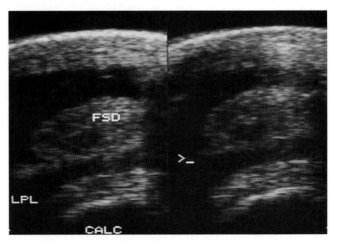

Figure 24.59. Transverse ultrasound scans of the plantar aspect of the point of the hock. Fluid accumulation is present at the plantar and dorsal aspects of the superficial digital flexor tendon (*FSD*). Communication exists between these two locations (*arrow*) on the lateral aspect of the superficial digital flexor tendon; thus the capped hocklike deformation was considered to be the result of synovial herniation of the superficial digital flexor tendon subtendinous bursa. The deep echogenic structure is the long plantar ligament (*LPL*) inserted on the plantar aspect of the calcaneus.

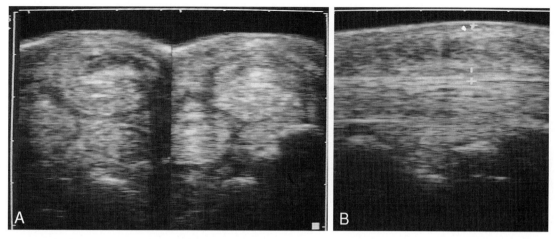

Figure 24.60. A. Transverse ultrasound scans of the plantar aspect of the tarsometatarsal area. These scans, which were performed on a "curb" deformation, show a subcutaneous thickening, partially hypoechoic on the left scan, between the superficial digital flexor tendon (*SDFT*) and the skin. The dorsal aspect of the SDFT is in contact with the lateral digital flexor tendon (*on the left*) and the long plantar ligament, inserted on the proximal fourth metatarsal bone on the right scan. These scans show that the curb deformation was induced by thickening of the plantar tarsal fascia. **B.** Longitudinal ultrasound at the plantar aspect of the tarsometatarsal joint of the same hock. Extensive thickening is also present between the skin and the SDFT and is compatible with desmopathy of the plantar tarsal fascia. Dorsal to the SDFT lies the long plantar ligament. The deep bony structures are the fourth tarsal bone (*on the left*) and the proximal metatarsus (*on the right*).

Usually, the synovial fluid distention causes protrusion at the lateroplantar aspect of the SDF tendon and ultrasonography helps to avoid confusion with a capped hock (Fig. 24.59).

Tarsometatarsal Junction

Curbs. Hard thickening distal to the tuber calcanei was often considered as desmopathy with enlargement of the long plantar ligament (calcaneometatarsal ligament). On clinical cases examined ultrasonographically, longitudinal and transverse images demonstrated a thickening between the SDFT and the skin (Fig. 24.60), whereas the long plantar ligament and the flexor tendons demonstrated normal size, shape, and echogenicity. On these clinical cases, these findings indicated that the "curb" deformation was induced by a desmopathy of the plantar tarsal fascia. Distention of the distal recess of the plantar tarsal sheath may induce a curb-like deformation (Fig. 24.61), as can superficial or deep digital flexor tendinitis and desmitis of the plantar ligament.

Figure 24.61. Transverse ultrasound scan of the plantar aspect of the tarsometatarsal area. Fluid distention is present between the medial and lateral flexor tendons and the accessory ligament of the deep digital flexor tendon. Hypoechoic tissue is present between the superficial (*FSD*) and deep flexor tendons, and the subcutaneous tissue is thickened. The soft curblike deformation of this hock was created by chronic synovial fluid distention of the distal recess of the tarsal sheath.

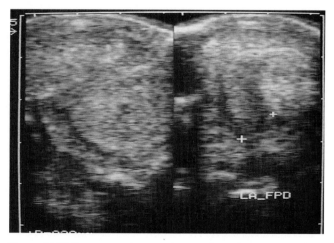

Figure 24.62. Transverse ultrasound scans of the plantar aspect of the proximal metatarsus. The accessory ligament of the deep digital flexor tendon (*AL-FPD*) is thickened (*crosses*) without any significant changes of echogenicity. These findings suggest that chronic desmopathy of the accessory ligament of the deep digital flexor tendon is responsible for the thickening of the area.

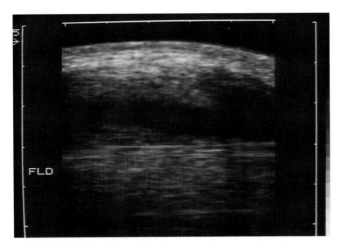

Figure 24.63. Longitudinal ultrasound scan of the caudomedial aspect of the hock proximal to the sustentaculum tali. The thick echogenic tendon is the lateral digital flexor tendon (*FLD*). Synovial fluid effusion is present caudomedially to this structure. Synovial membrane thickening is also imaged. These findings are consistent with tarsal sheath tenosynovitis.

Accessory ligament desmopathy. In the hind limb the deep digital flexor tendon (DDFT) is made by the junction between the strong tendon of the lateral digital flexor muscle and the small medial digital flexor tendon. The accessory ligament of the DDFT is thinner than in the forelimb; it is 2 to 3 mm thick.

Desmopathy of the accessory ligament of the DDFT is an uncommon injury and was found on trotters (there are no

pacers in France), as well as on dressage horses. Abnormal ultrasound findings were similar to other tendon injuries (Fig. 24.62). Ultrasonography helps differentiate this injury from other injuries of the plantar and proximal metatarsus such as proximal suspensory desmitis, deep or superficial digital flexor tendinitis, and desmopathy of the plantar tarsal fascia.

Plantaromedial Aspect

At the plantaromedial aspect of the hock lies the plantar tarsal sheath. The fibrous wall of this sheath is made by the flexor retinaculum, and within the tarsal sheath are located the lateral digital flexor tendon (LDFT) and the plantar nerves and arteries. Tarsal canal syndrome was observed mainly in sport horses and secondly in race horses. In *recent injuries* only the proximal recess of the synovial sheath can be distended at the medial aspect of the common calcanean tendon, proximal to the tuber calcanei (Fig. 24.63). In *old or chronic injuries,* the distention of the distal recess may be ob-

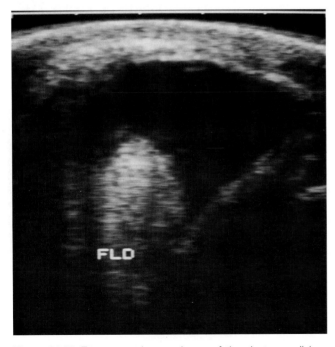

Figure 24.64. Transverse ultrasound scan of the plantaromedial aspect of the proximal hock. Fluid distention is present plantaromedially to the lateral digital flexor tendon (*FLD*) and is in contact with the flexor surface of the sustentaculum tali (*oblique hyperechogenic line on the right*). These findings are consistent with synovial fluid effusion within the tarsal sheath. The synovial fluid pressure induces traction on the flexor retinaculum, which is distended.

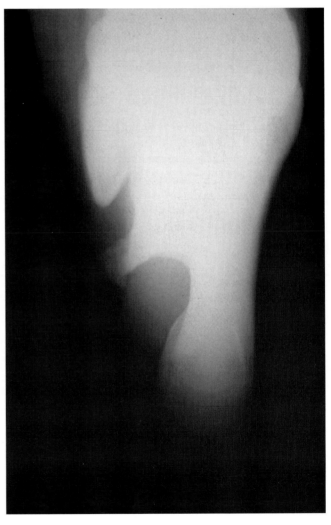

Figure 24.65. Proximodistal skyline view of the hock of a 5-year-old mare afflicted by tarsal canal syndrome. The chronic tension on the medial insertion of the flexor retinaculum induces bony proliferation along the medial border of the sustentaculum tali.

served in the proximal third of the metatarsus. Ultrasonography is a very valuable tool to differentiate tarsal caudal syndrome from other tendon and ligament injuries in this area such as (a) proximal suspensory desmopathy (third interosseus muscle tendinopathy), (b) accessory ligament of the DDFT desmopathy, (c) DDFT or SDFT tendinopathy, and (d) plantar tarsal fascia desmopathy. Older or chronic injuries may induce synovial membrane proliferation and flexor retinaculum elongation at the plantaromedial aspect of the sustentaculum tali (Fig. 24.64). Chronic tension on the retinaculum induces bony proliferation at the medial border of the sustentaculum tali (Fig. 24.65).

Because of the inflexion of the LDFT on the sustentaculum tali inducing nonhomogenous echogenicity in transverse and longitudinal ultrasound sections, it is difficult to clearly demonstrate abnormal echogenicity of this tendon within the tarsal canal. Nevertheless, ultrasonography is adequate to identify some bony irregularities of the gliding surface of the sustenculum tali.

Crus

Cranial Aspect

Peroneus Tertius Muscle Rupture and Healing. In the horse the peroneus tertius (PT) muscle is entirely fibrous and contributes to the joint angles' solidarization (stay apparatus) of the pelvic limb. On normal horses this structure is easy to image with ultrasonography as it is a very echogenic structure surrounded by the hyperechoic muscle bodies of the long digital extensor and tibialis cranialis muscle. Rupture of the PT muscle is a clinical diagnosis. In *recent injuries,* there is a lack of visualization of this structure as it becomes hy-

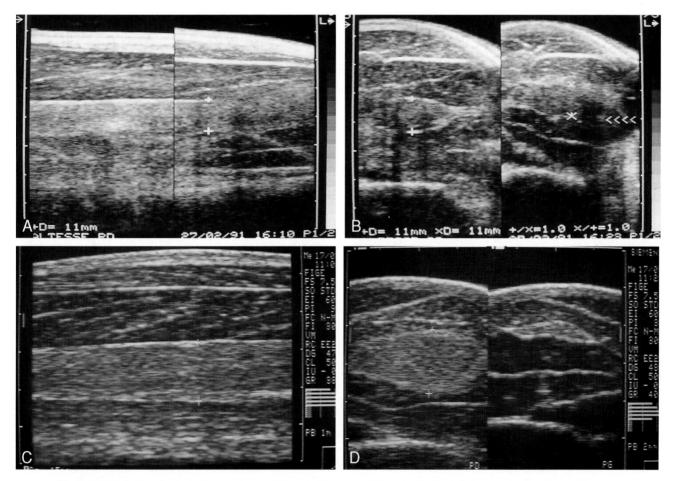

Figure 24.66. A. Longitudinal ultrasound scan of the cranial aspect of the crus. On the left scan, under the skin and the crural fascia, three anatomic structures can be identified: the body of the long digital extensor muscle, the echogenic peroneus tertius muscle, and the cranial tibial muscle body. On the right scan the peroneus tertius muscle is not visualized; it has become hypoechoic (*crosses*). This finding was accompanied clinically by a recent rupture of the peroneus tertius muscle. Ultrasonographic images show that the rupture occurred within the distal third of the crus. **B.** Transverse ultrasound scan of the cranial aspect of the crus. On the left image, which is of the mid-tibia, the peroneus tertius muscle (*crosses*) is thickened and hypoechoic. In the distal third of the crus this structure is more hypoechoic and anechoic. These findings are compatible with rupture. On both longitudinal and transverse scans, the cranial tibial muscle body is hypoechoic, also suggesting a muscle injury. **C.** Longitudinal ultrasound scan of the cranial aspect of the crus of the same horse. The peroneus tertius muscle, which remains slightly hypoechoic with homogenous tenuous architecture, is extensively thickened. **D.** Transverse ultrasound scans of the cranial aspect of the crus of the same horse. On the left scan the peroneus tertius muscle of the right hind limb is markedly thickened, causing compression of the adjacent muscle bodies. The right scan shows the normal peroneus tertius muscle of the opposite limb at the same level of the crus.

poechoic at the level of the rupture (Fig. 24.66A), usually located at the distal third of the tibia. Some anechoic, fluid-filled vesicles are indicative of hemorrhage. During the healing process the PT muscle becomes thicker and more echogenic. Finally, when function returns to normal, the cross-sectional area of the injured PT muscle is four to five times as large as the sound, contralateral one on most of its length.

Muscle Abnormalities

1. General muscle atrophy as documented on horses undergoing stringhalt.
2. Amyotrophy of the lateral digital extensor muscle belly was documented on horses who sustained surgical tenectomy of the corresponding tendon for the treatment of stringhalt-like syndrome.
3. Calcification within the LDE muscle body was documented with radiography and ultrasonography in two horses. Hyperechoic images casting acoustic shadows indicated that calcification can be found in the common proximal tendon of the PT and LDE muscles at the level of the sulcus extensorius.

Caudal Aspect

Injuries of the common calcanean tendon were documented in race horses and sport horses. Tendinopathies of the superficial digital flexor tendon (SDFT) or the gastrocnemius tendon have been described. Ultrasonographic signs do not differ from those described for the flexor tendons of the distal limbs and include modification of size, shape, echogenicity, and architecture (Figs. 24.67 and 24.68).

Stifle

Three distinct topographic areas can be differentiated when ultrasonographic examination of the stifle is considered. The anatomic structures of the femoropatellar joint can be examined mostly at the cranial aspect of the stifle. The soft-tissue structures of the femorotibial joint should be examined within two areas: a medial one to evaluate the femorotibial compartment of the joint, and a lateral one to evaluate the lateral femorotibial component of the joint.

Femoropatellar Joint

Hematoma. Prepatellar hematomas between the skin and the patellar fascia were documented. Anechoic fluid spaces are indicative of recent injuries (Fig. 24.69); in older injuries the distended subcutaneous space has a very heterogenous pattern of echogenicity with anechoic fluid pockets separated by echoic trabecula.

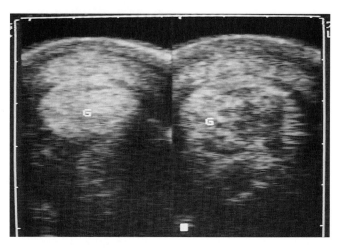

Figure 24.68. Transverse ultrasound scans of the caudal aspect of the crus. These two scans present a cross-section of the common calcanean tendon. On the left scan (representing the sound limb), the gastrocnemius tendon has a normal size and regular echogenicity. On the right scan, the gastrocnemius tendon is markedly thickened and large hypoechoic images can be seen within the tendon. These abnormal findings are consistent with gastrocnemius tendinopathy.

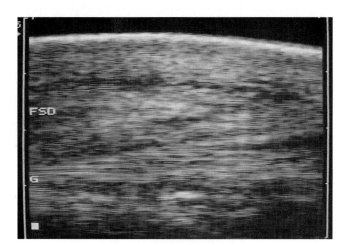

Figure 24.67. Longitudinal ultrasound scan of the caudal aspect of the crus. The caudal profile of the common calcanean tendon is curved; the superficial digital flexor tendon (*FSD*) is thickened and has irregular echogenicity. The deep structures correspond to the gastrocnemius tendon (*G*) and the calcanean tendons of the femoral muscles. The abnormal findings presented here are consistent with an old superficial digital flexor tendinopathy.

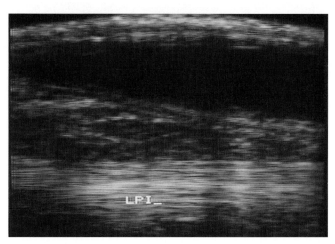

Figure 24.69. Longitudinal ultrasound scan of the cranial aspect of the stifle. An anechoic fluid accumulation is present between the skin and the patellar fascia. The moderately echogenic infrapatellar adipose pad is located between this fascia and the thick intermediate patellar ligament (*LPI*). This superficial fluid pocket was a hematoma.

Patellar Ligaments. Abnormal ultrasonographic findings were documented in each patellar ligament.

Intermediate patellar ligament (IPL). Injuries causing lameness were documented at each insertion site of this ligament. *Proximal* enthesopathy with bony proliferation was documented at the cranial aspect of the patella after traumatic injuries on 3-day-event horses and steeplechasers. Abnormal findings included moderate thickening, irregular pattern of echogenicity, and bony proliferation or irregularities at the cranial aspect of the patella.

Periarticular osteophytes, at the apex of the patella occurring after medial patellar desmotomy, were also documented ultrasonographically as hyperechoic images located at the caudal aspect of the IPL (Fig. 24.70).

Distal IPL desmopathy causing lameness was also identified (Figs. 24.71 and 24.72). Abnormal findings included peripheral or central hypoechoic area ("core lesion") and bony proliferation at the insertion site on the tibial tuberosity.

Medial patellar ligament (MPL). Avulsion fracture of the medial angle of the patella (proximal insertion of the MPL) was documented ultrasonographically and radiographically. Ultrasonography was particularly useful for the surgical removal of the bony fragments.

MPL desmitis was suspected in horses and ponies with chronic upward fixation of the patella (Fig. 24.73*A*). Following MPL desmotomy, ultrasonographic images demonstrated several abnormal findings (Fig. 24.73*B*): thickening of the MPL; hypoechoic and anechoic images indicative of hemorrhage, edema, and ligament relaxation; and subcutaneous hypoechoic space compatible with edema.

It must be mentioned that these findings are not only located at the surgical site but involve the whole length of the

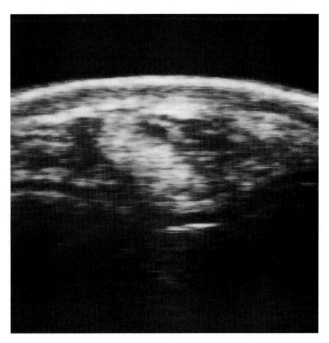

Figure 24.71. Transverse ultrasound scans of the cranial aspect of the stifle. The superficial echogenic line is the skin, and the deep sinuous hyperechogenic line is the subchondral bone surface of the femoral trochlea with the medial ridge on the left and the lateral ridge on the right. The intermediate patellar ligament looks irregular and the craniolateral part of it is irregularly hypoechoic. These findings, also demonstrated on longitudinal scans, are compatible with intermediate patellar ligament desmitis.

MPL, probably due to laxity of this ligament. Ultrasonographic images made several months after surgery demonstrate extensive thickening and architecture remodeling of the MPL (Fig. 24.74).

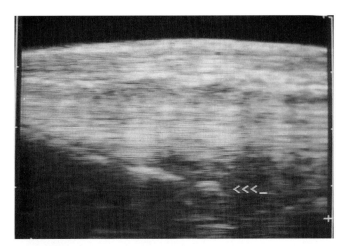

Figure 24.70. Longitudinal ultrasound scan of the cranial aspect of the stifle. The deep oblique hyperechogenic line on the left is the cranial aspect of the patella. The thick intermediate patellar ligament inserts on this bone surface, and when the limb is in a weight-bearing position with the patella locked, the infrapatellar fat pad herniates between the intermediate patellar ligament and the skin. At the deep aspect of the intermediate patellar ligament there is an echogenic spot (*arrowheads*), indicating the presence of a bony fragment at the apex of the patella. This mare had a medial patellar ligament desmotomy 8 months earlier.

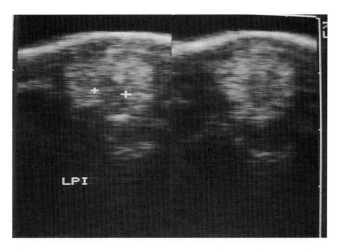

Figure 24.72. Transverse ultrasound scans of the cranial aspect of the stifle at the level of the proximal tibia. The superficial echogenic line is the skin, and the deep line is the tibial tuberosity sulcus. The distal part of the intermediate patellar ligament has a hypoechoic center. This finding was also shown on longitudinal scans with the limb in a weight-bearing position. It is indicative of intermediate patellar ligament desmopathy. The horse's lameness was improved after administration of local analgesia.

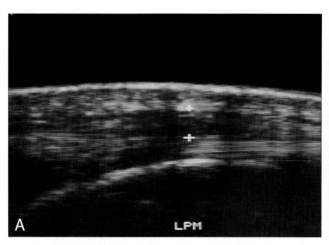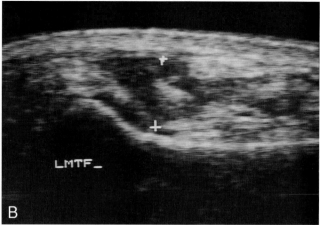

Figure 24.73. A. Longitudinal ultrasound scan of the medial aspect of the stifle of a pony with upward fixation of the patella. The deep hyperechogenic curved line is the rnedial ridge of the femoral trochlea. The medial patellar ligament (*LPM*) runs over this bone surface; its superficial part is thickened and hypoechoic. These findings are consistent with medial patellar ligament desmitis. **B.** Transverse ultrasound scan of the medial aspect of the same stifle after recent medial patellar desmotomy. The deep hyperechoic concave line is the medial aspect of the distal femur (*LMTF*). The medial patellar ligament is thickened with a heterogenous pattern of echogenicity. These abnormal images are caused by injuries induced by the surgery (laceration, retraction, hemorrhage, and edema).

Lateral patellar ligament (LPL). Traumatic LPL desmopathy associated with tibial tuberosity fracture were imaged (Figs. 24.75 and 24.76). Abnormal ultrasound findings included extensive hypoechoic images, fiber disruption, periligamentous edema, and bony-fragment displacement with echogenic fracture site.

Synovial Components. Synovial evaluation is presented in Chapter 26; thus only specific data for the femoropatellar joint will be mentioned. The most common cause of synovial abnormalities is femoral trochlea osteochondrosis (Fig. 24.77).

Synovial membrane thickening can be measured at the deep aspect of the infrapatellar pad. Synovial fold proliferation is easily identified because of the anechoic synovial fluid. Synovial fluid accumulation is a common finding associated with osteochondral lesions of the femoral trochlea and can be very extensive.

Articular Surfaces. Because of its thickness the articular cartilage of the femoral trochlea is easily imaged. It is thicker on the lateral trochlear ridge than on the medial one. The subchondral bone surface is seen as a regular hyperechogenic line.

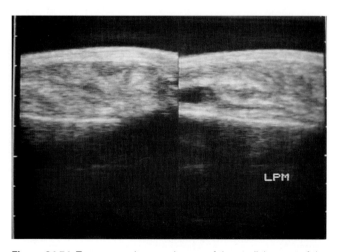

Figure 24.74. Transverse ultrasound scans of the medial aspect of the stifle; medial patellar desmotomy was performed 8 months before the scans were made. The deep hyperechogenic line is the medial aspect of the femoral trochlea. The medial patellar ligament (*LPM*) is thickened and has a heterogeneous pattern of echogenicity. These findings reflect the repair of the ligament after surgery.

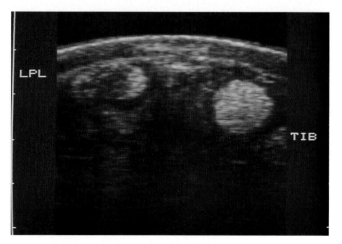

Figure 24.75. Transverse ultrasound scan of the craniolateral aspect of the stifle. The superficial echogenic lines are the skin and the patellar fascia. The rounded echogenic structure on the right is a normal intermediate patellar ligament. On the left the oval structure with a heterogenous pattern of echogenicity is the lateral patellar ligament (*LPL*). This abnormal finding was caused by an injury of the lateral patellar ligament that accompanied a tibial tuberosity fracture. *TIB*, tibia.

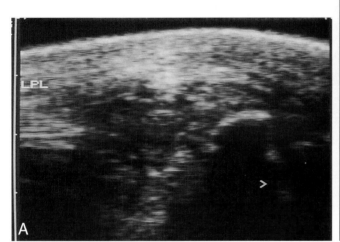
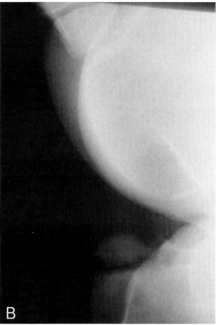

Figure 24.76. A. Longitudinal ultrasound scan of the craniolateral aspect of the stifle. The superficial echogenic structures are the skin and the patellar fascia. The lateral patellar ligament is echogenic (*on the left*), but its distal part (*on the right*) is markedly thickened and hypoechoic. On the right side of the scan is a gap in the hyperechogenic bony surface and an echogenic line within the tibial tuberosity (*arrowhead*). These linked findings are the result of trauma that caused a tibial tuberosity fracture. **B.** Lateromedial radiograph of the cranial aspect of the same stifle. A large separated bony fragment is at the proximal aspect of the tibial tuberosity, and small displaced chip fragments are present more caudally. This case shows why comparative imaging is done for complete documentation of bone and soft-tissue injuries after trauma.

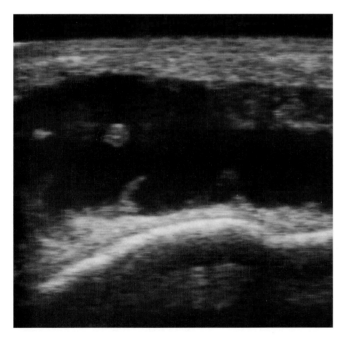

Figure 24.77. Longitudinal ultrasound scan of the cranial aspect of the stifle of a 7-month-old filly. The superficial echogenic structures are the skin and the patellar fascia. The deep hyperechogenic line is the bone surface of the medial ridge of the femoral trochlea. An extensive synovial fluid effusion is present within the femoropatellar joint; synovial membrane thickening and proliferation is also seen. High villous synovial folds are clearly imaged in the anechoic synovial fluid.

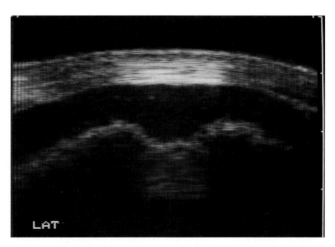

Figure 24.78. Longitudinal ultrasound scan of the craniolateral aspect of the stifle of a 5-month-old colt. The superficial echogenic structures are the skin and the cranial border of the lateral patellar ligament. The deep irregular hyperechoic line is the subchondral bone surface of the lateral ridge of the femoral trochlea. A depression is present in this line, with echogenic material in place of the subchondral bone corresponding to a notch. A subchondral bone defect and radiolucencies were seen on lateromedial radiographs. The large, strongly hypoechoic space between the lateral patellar ligament and the subchondral bone surface corresponds to thickened synovial membrane and articular cartilage.

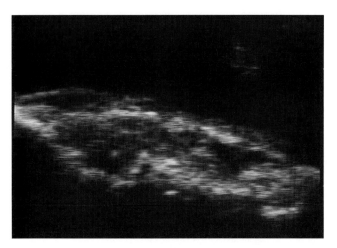

Figure 24.79. Longitudinal ultrasound scan of the craniolateral aspect of the stifle of a 7-month-old filly (the same horse shown in Figure 24.77). An extensive synovial fluid effusion is present within the femoropatellar joint cavity with some high villous synovial folds. The deep hyperechoic subchondral bone surface of the lateral trochlear ridge looks markedly irregular. Radiographs showed a large radiolucent bone defect of the femoral trochlea. On this sonogram this defect is occupied by irregular echogenic material, representing degenerative and partially calcified cartilage or synovial material.

Abnormal findings observed in osteochondrosis lesions of the femoral trochlea included the following:

1. Abnormal thickening of the articular cartilage (Fig. 24.78)
2. Abnormal echogenic images superficial to the subchondral hyperechoic line, compatible with partial ossification of the abnormal cartilage, synovial proliferation, and/or osteochondral avulsion (Figs. 24.79 and 24.80)
3. Abnormal profile of the subchondral bone surface (Fig. 24.81)

Femoral trochlea osteochondrosis usually induces synovial fluid accumulation within the femoropatellar com-

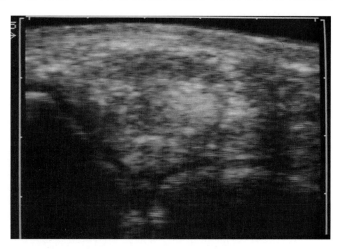

Figure 24.81. Transverse ultrasound scan at the cranial aspect of the femoral trochlea. The superficial structures represent the skin, patellar fascia, infrapatellar fat pad, and intermediate patellar ligament. The deep hyperechoic line is the subchondral bone surface of the femoral trochlea. A sagittal defect of the subchondral bone profile of the trochlear groove is present.

partment but also frequently within the medial and/or lateral femorotibial recesses.

Tibial Tuberosity. Usually, traumatic injuries of the tibial tuberosity can easily be demonstrated on lateromedial radiographs. Sagittal fractures are sometimes difficult to image on caudocranial radiographs. Ultrasonographic examination may give additional documentation of the injury as the fracture site appears as an echogenic line within the bone substance (Fig. 24.82) and soft-tissue–associated injuries can be documented (Fig. 24.76).

Patella. Fractures of the patella were documented with radiography and ultrasonography. Avulsion fracture of the

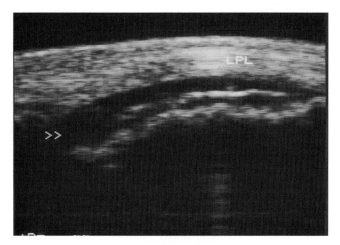

Figure 24.80. Longitudinal ultrasound scan of the craniolateral aspect of the stifle of a 7-month-old colt. The echogenic superficial structures are the skin and the lateral patellar ligament (*LPL*). The deep, irregular hyperechoic line is the subchondral bone surface of the lateral ridge of the femoral trochlea. An additional echogenic line appears in the intermediate anechoic space and corresponds to an osteochondral fragment separated from the underlying bone.

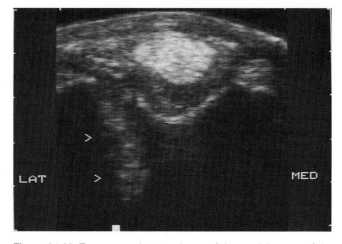

Figure 24.82. Transverse ultrasound scan of the cranial aspect of the stifle. The superficial echogenic line is the skin, and the deep hyperechogenic line is the tibial tuberosity with its sagittal sulcus. The distal intermediate patellar ligament has a homogenous echogenicity within the moderately echogenic infrapatellar pad. On the lateral side, a gap is seen in the bony surface and a large and regular echogenic sagittal line (*arrowheads*) is present within the tibial tuberosity. These findings corresponded to a tibial tuberosity fracture.

medial angle of the patella was demonstrated with both methods, but ultrasonography had advantages over radiography to identify soft-tissue–associated injuries (patellar ligament desmopathies) and to locate the bony fragments accurately for surgical removal.

Enthesopathies at the cranial aspect of the patella are described above.

Medial Femorotibial (MFT) Joint

At the medial aspect of the stifle two distinct areas can be identified: a craniomedial area and a caudomedial area.

Craniomedial Area. Caudal to the medial patellar ligament, longitudinal and transverse sections allow imaging of the following:

1. The proximal recess of the medial femorotibial joint filled with anechoic synovial fluid and the concave medial aspect of the distal femur (Fig. 24.83); it decreases in size when pressure is applied on the transducer. Normally, it was less than 10 mm thick, 15 mm in a proximodistal direction, and 20 mm craniocaudally. Generally, the synovial membrane shows high, villous, synovial folds.
2. The triangular-shaped echogenic cranial part of the medial meniscus, the border of which protrudes inside the synovial cavity (Fig. 24.83) because the synovial membrane inserts its abaxial medial surface.
3. The medial aspect of the tibial plateau is imaged as a hyperechogenic line.

Caudomedial Area. This area extends around the *medial collateral ligament* (MCL).

Longitudinal (frontal) sections demonstrate three layers of anatomic structures (Fig. 24.84):

1. The superficial layer corresponds to the thick echogenic femoral fascia and, proximally, to the heterogenous hypoechoic distal end of the sartorius and gracilis muscles.
2. The intermediate layer is occupied by the echogenic MCL. This ligament is made of parallel fibers and is 4 to 5 mm thick. It becomes hypoechoic when the ultrasound beam is not perpendicular to its fibers.

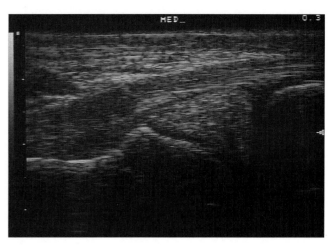

Figure 24.84. Longitudinal (frontal) ultrasound scan of the medial aspect of the femorotibial joint. The medial meniscus is located between the medial condyles of the femur and the tibia. It is covered by the medial collateral ligament.

3. The deep layer is formed by the medial condyle of the femur (imaged as an hyperechoic line), the homogenous echogenic medial meniscus, and the medial condyle of the tibia. The *medial meniscus* (MM) has a typical triangular shape and is separated from the hyperechoic subchondral bone surface of the femur and tibia by a totally anechoic space that represents the articular cartilage. Normal ultrasound images clearly demonstrate that the medial (abaxial) border of the medial meniscus is in contact with the deeper aspect of the MCL.

Abnormal findings include synovial distention of the recess of the MFT joint; modification of size and echogenicity of the MCL; modifications of shape, position, and echogenicity of the MM; and modifications of shape of the articular margins and condyle.

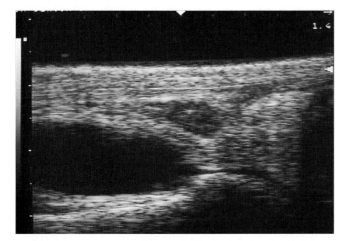

Figure 24.83. Longitudinal (frontal) ultrasound scan of the craniomedial area of the femorotibial joint. This image shows the relationships between the medial meniscus, the medial condyles of the femur and the tibia, and the medial femorotibial recess.

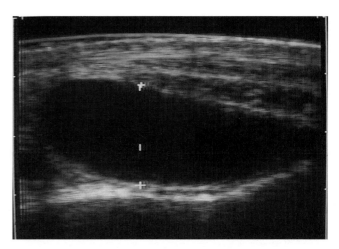

Figure 24.85. Transverse ultrasound scan of the craniomedial aspect of the stifle. The medial recess of the medial femorotibial joint is extensively distended by synovial fluid. The superficial echogenic structures are the skin and the medial femoral fascia; caudally (*on the right*), the hypoechogenic layers correspond to the sartorius muscle. The deep hyperechogenic line is the medial profile of the femoral trochlea (the cranial aspect is on the left; the caudal aspect is on the right).

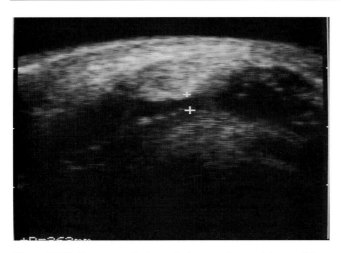

Figure 24.86. Transverse (horizontal) ultrasound scan of the medial aspect of the stifle. Under the skin and the medial femoral fascia, the oval echogenic structure is the medial collateral ligament. The deep semicircular echogenic element is the medial meniscus sectioned horizontally. Between the medial meniscus and the medial collateral ligament is a hypoechoic space, on each side of which synovial fluid distention is present. These findings frequently accompany synovial effusion and synovitis. This horse had a tibial tuberosity fracture.

1. *Synovial distention:* Distention of the synovial recess of the MFT joint (Figs. 24.85 and 24.86) can be found alone as a manifestation of synovitis or can be a consequence of a femorotibial or femoropatellar pathology as there is often communication between the synovial compartments of the joint, at least under pathologic conditions.

Distention of the medial recess of the MFT joint is often accompanied by distention of other recesses of the joint. On transverse imaging, this recess can be larger than 40 mm long, 30 mm high, and 20 mm thick. Pressure on the probe makes the fluid space thinner. When moderate distention is present, ultrasonography can help as a preoperative procedure to perform arthrocentesis of the joint.

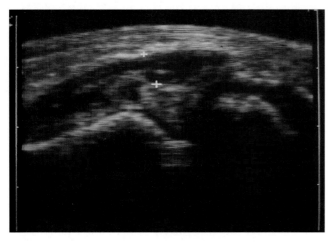

Figure 24.87. Longitudinal (frontal) section at the medial aspect of the femorotibial joint. This 2-month-old filly had stifle trauma. The medial collateral ligament (*crosses*) is thickened and hypoechoic, indicating rupture and inflammation. This filly also had an eminentia intercondylaris avulsion fracture.

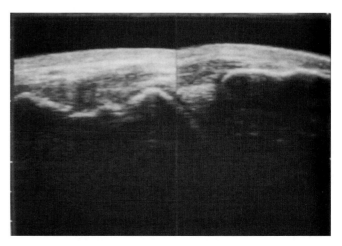

Figure 24.88. Longitudinal (frontal) ultrasound scans of the medial aspect of the stifle. Extensive thickening and hypoechoic areas are present in the medial collateral ligament. Bone remodeling is seen at the proximal attachment of this ligament on the medial femoral condyle. These findings are correlated with chronic desmopathy of the medial collateral ligament. On this image (made in a non–weight-bearing position) the medial meniscus is not displaced.

2. *Medial collateral ligament (MCL):* MCL desmopathy induces the usual ultrasound abnormalities of tendon and ligament injuries such as thickening, heterogenous pattern of echogenicity and architectural remodeling, and insertion desmopathy with deepening of the insertion fossa at the medial aspect of the medial femoral condyle (Figs. 24.87 and 24.88).

Associated lesions of meniscal injuries, synovial fluid effusion, and degenerative disease of the femorotibial joint can be imaged.

3. *Medial meniscus (MM):* Abnormal images of the MM include (a) abnormal positioning and relationships and (b) modification of echogenicity.

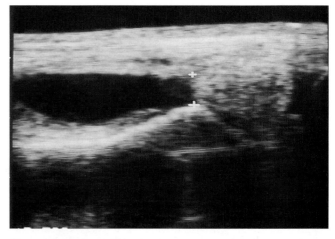

Figure 24.89. Longitudinal (frontal) ultrasound scan of the medial aspect of the stifle. Synovial fluid distention is present in the medial recess of the medial femorotibial joint. On this image (made in a non–weight-bearing position) the medial meniscus appears slightly displaced out of the femorotibial articular space (*crosses*). The medial aspect of the femur is on the left, and the distance between the tibial plateau (*on the right*) and the medial meniscus is enlarged.

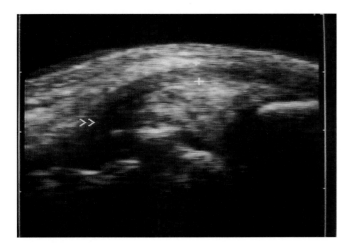

Figure 24.90. Longitudinal (frontal) ultrasound scan of the medial aspect of the stifle. The medial collateral ligament (*crosses*) bends over the medial meniscus, which is displaced out of the femorotibial space. A large osteophyte (*arrowheads*) is present on the medial margin of the femoral condyle.

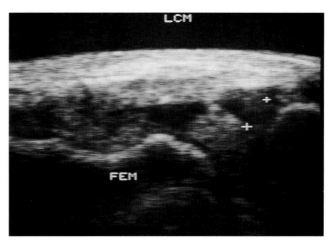

Figure 24.92. Longitudinal (frontal) ultrasound scan of the medial aspect of the stifle. This 1-year-old filly had a fracture of the eminentia intercondylaris of the tibia. At the medial aspect of the femur (*FEM*) ultrasound manifestations of synovitis (fluid effusion and synovial membrane proliferation) are seen. A hypoechoic triangular space (*crosses*) is between the medial collateral ligament (*LCM*) and the medial tibial condyle, compatible with an injury of the distal border of the medial meniscus.

Prolapse of the medial meniscus (Figs. 24.89 and 24.90) is easier to document when the limb is in a weight-bearing position than when it is semiflexed in a resting position. Because of the presence of the medial collateral ligament, it mostly appears in the craniomedial aspect of the stifle.

When synovial distention is extensive and when the synovial membrane is thickened, a hypoechoic space can be identified between the medial meniscus and the superficial structures (femoral fascia and MCL). This hypoechoic gap (Fig. 24.86) between the MM and the MCL is abnormal, since normally these two structures adhere to each other.

Hypoechoic images are mainly located in the intermediate part of the meniscus (Fig. 24.91) and could represent either fibroblastic tissue, tear, or collapse. They are also identified on the proximal or distal borders on horses who

presented tibial tuberosity or eminentia intercondylaris fractures (Fig. 24.92). These variations of the superficial structures should not be confused with lesions (Fig. 24.93).

Hyperechoic images within the MM have also been found (Fig. 24.94). Hyperechoic images casting acoustic shadows were not necessarily imaged as radiopaque material on caudocranial and lateromedial radiographs; thus fibrosis or focal calcification of the MM are to be considered.

Hyperechoic images casting acoustic shadows were observed in a horse with radiopaque material within the femorotibial space (Fig. 24.95). Necropsy examination

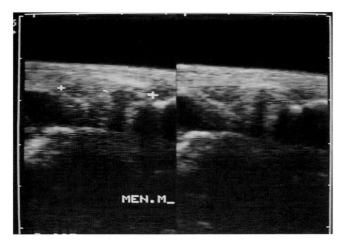

Figure 24.91. Longitudinal (frontal) ultrasound scans of the medial aspect of the stifle. The medial femoral condyle is on the left, and the tibial plateau is on the right. A sharply delineated hypoechoic bundle is within the medial meniscus (*MEN.M*). This finding is compatible with a collapse or tear of the meniscal fibers, as well as an inflammatory process or scar tissue.

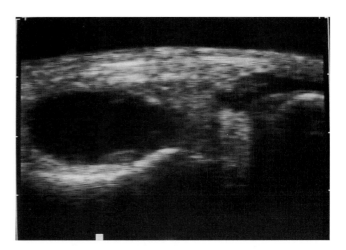

Figure 24.93. Longitudinal (frontal) ultrasound scan of the medial aspect of the stifle of the same horse shown in Figure 24.86. A synovial fluid effusion is within the medial recess of the medial femorotibial joint, and the joint is distended distally to the meniscus at the medial aspect of the tibia (*on the right*). The proximal border of the medial meniscus looks hypoechoic. Although this finding is compatible with an inflammatory process, modification of the echogenic aspect of the medial meniscus induced by the acoustic properties of the superficial strutures should also be considered.

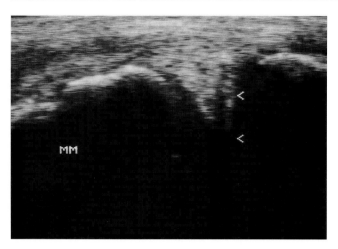

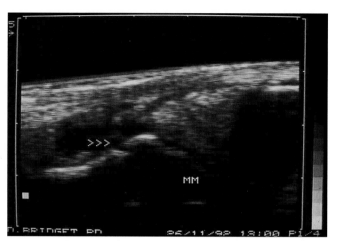

Figure 24.94. Longitudinal (frontal) ultrasound scan of the medial aspect of the stifle. A hyperechoic spot cast an acoustic shadow near the medial border of the medial meniscus (*MM*). Bone remodeling is present at the proximal insertion of the medial collateral ligament on the medial aspect of the medial femoral condyle (*on the left*). This horse had a bone cyst in the medial femoral condyle.

Figure 24.96. Longitudinal (frontal) ultrasound scan of the medial aspect of the stifle. Periarticular bony proliferation is present on the medial margin of the medial femoral condyle (*arrowheads*), and the articular surface is slightly irregular. Moderate synovial membrane thickening is present in the medial recess of the medial femorotibial joint. *MM*, medial meniscus.

demonstrated the presence of bone nodules within the medial meniscus. This horse also has osteochondrodysplasial lesions of the femoral condyles and an extensive synovial distention.

> 4. *Articular surfaces: Femoral or tibial periarticular osteophytes can easily be identified on longitudinal (frontal) ultrasoundscans (Fig. 24.96). In these cases the hyperechoic articular margin looks prominent and irregular.*

An abnormal medial condyle profile and an abnormal

anechoic space between this condyle and the MM or between the MM and the tibial plateau were also identified in horses with medial femoral condyle bone cysts (Fig. 24.97).

Lateral Femorotibial Joint (LFT)

At the lateral aspect of the stifle two distinct areas can be identified: a craniolateral area and a caudolateral area.

Craniolateral Area. A longitudinal section in a sagittofrontal plane and transverse sections demonstrate the echogenic

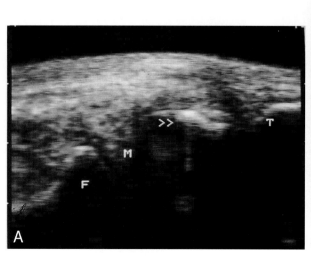

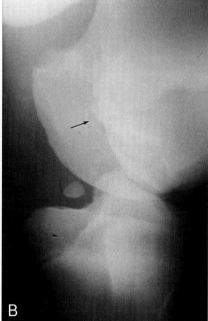

Figure 24.95. A. Longitudinal (frontal) ultrasound scan of the medial aspect of the stifle of a 15-month-old colt. The articular surface of the medial femoral condyle (*F*) lacks convexity, indicating osteochondrodysplasia, and a hyperechoic image cast an acoustic shadow (*arrowheads*) within the medial meniscus (*M*). **B.** Caudolateral-craniomedial oblique view of the same stifle. Radiopaque nodules are within the femorotibial space and femoral condyle dysplasia (*arrow*) is present. *T*, tibia.

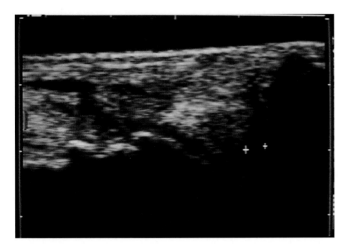

Figure 24.97. Longitudinal (frontal) ultrasound scan of the medial aspect of the stifle. Bone remodeling is present at the medial aspect of the medial femoral condyle, and the space between the medial meniscus and the tibia is thickened (*crosses*). This horse also had a subchondral bone cyst within the medial femoral condyle.

proximal tendon of *long digital extensor* (LDE) and peroneus tertius (PT) muscles (Fig. 24.98). This tendon is 15 to 20 mm thick and inserts obliquely in the extensor fossa of the femur. Its medial aspect is in contact with the moderately echogenic infrapatella fat of the stifle and with the craniolateral aspect of the lateral meniscus. Distally, this tendon slides on the fibrocartilaginous surface of the sulcus extensorius and is prolonged by the echogenic fibrous peroneus tertius muscle and by the hypoechoic long digital extensor muscle belly. The deep aspect of this tendon is underlined by a hypoechoic line that represents the synovial membrane of the lateral femorotibial joint subextensorius recess.

Caudolateral Area. This area is located around the *lateral collateral ligament* (LCL). Longitudinal sections showed this

ligament (Fig. 24.99) as a thick echogenic fibrous structure with oblique fibers.

At the lateral aspect of the lateral condyle of the femur, the LCL inserts obliquely on the lateral epicondyle. It is separated from the fascia lata by the hypoechoic distal end of the biceps femoris muscle.

At the level of the femorotibial space, the LCL is 6 to 9 mm thick and 16 to 20 mm craniocaudally. Deeply, the echogenic *lateral meniscus* is located between the lateral condyle of the femur and the lateral condyle of the tibia. This meniscus looks less triangular than the medial one (its shape is more trapezoidal), and due to the shape of the lateral condyle of the femur, its proximal border is less regularly concave; the thickness of its abaxial (lateral) border is 13 to 18 mm. The LCL is separated from the lateral meniscus by a 3- to 5-mm space. In this space the proximal tendon of the popliteus muscle runs obliquely in a caudodistal direction so that, on longitudinal scans, only oblique sections of this tendon can be imaged.

Distally, the LCL runs over the lateral condyle of the tibia and inserts on the proximal fibula. The fibulotibial space is easily identified.

Identified abnormal findings include synovial distention of the subextensorius recess of the lateral femorotibial joint, modifications of echogenicity of the lateral meniscus, shape modifications of the articular surfaces, and long digital extensor tendon injuries already mentioned as injuries of the cranial aspect of the crus.

1. *Synovial distention:* Distention of the lateral recess of the patellar joint can be documented at the lateral aspect of the femoral trochlea.

Distention of the LFT joint is indicated by a different amount of synovial fluid within the subextensorius recess (Figs. 24.100 and 24.101). This recess is located in the sulcus extensorius of the tibia at the deep aspect of the proxi-

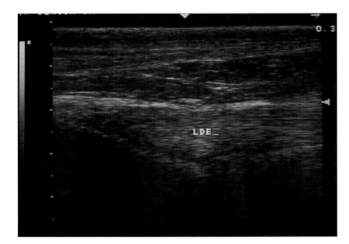

Figure 24.98. Longitudinal (frontal) ultrasound scan of the lateral aspect of the normal stifle. The proximal tendon of the long digital extensor (*LDE*) and peroneus tertius muscles insert on the extensor fossa of the femur (*on the left*). It is covered by the skin, the crural fascia, and the body of the LDE muscle. It apposes the cranial part of the lateral meniscus and, on the right, the sulcus extensorius.

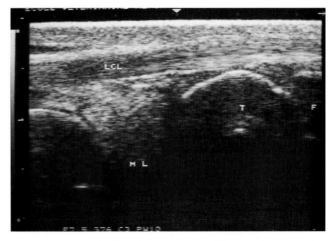

Figure 24.99. Longitudinal ultrasound scan of the lateral aspect of the normal stifle. This scan images the lateral collateral ligament (*LCL*), the lateral meniscus (*ML*), the lateral condyle of the tibia (*T*), and the head of the fibula (*F*). The echogenic structure between the LCL, the lateral femoral condyle (*on the left*), and the lateral meniscus is the proximal tendon of the popliteus muscle.

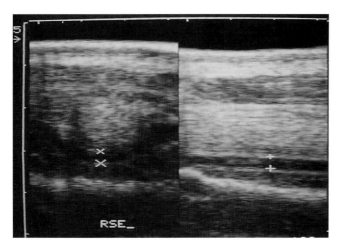

Figure 24.100. Transverse and longitudinal ultrasound scans of the craniolateral aspect of the stifle at the level of the proximal tibia. The echogenic intermediate structure is the proximal common tendon of the long digital extensor and peroneus tertius muscle. Superficially, it is covered by the skin, the crural fascia, and the long digital extensor muscle body. Its deep aspect is separated from the proximal cranial tibial muscle body by a hypoechoic space (*crosses*), indicating synovitis of the subextensorius recess of the lateral femorotibial articular cavity. The deep hyperechogenic line is the sulcus subextensorius of the tibia in transverse (*left*) and longitudinal profile (*right*).

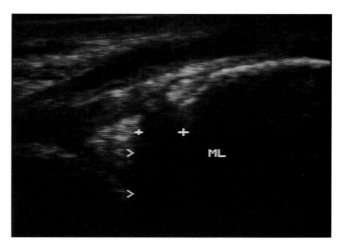

Figure 24.102. Longitudinal (frontal) ultrasound scan of the lateral aspect of the stifle. The distal half of the lateral meniscus (*ML*) appears strongly hypoechoic; only the proximolateral part of this structure has normal echogenicity. The left, regular, curved hyperechogenic line is the medial condyle of the femur; the more superficial hyperechogenic line on the right is the lateral aspect of the tibia. The lateral collateral ligament appears hyperechoic because its fibers are not perpendicular to the ultrasound beam.

mal tendon of the LDE and PT muscles. Distention of the LFT joint is usually accompanied by injuries and distention of the FP joint and/or MET joint. Extensive fluid accumulation in the subextensorius recess is often found in clinical cases with femoral trochlea osteochondritis (Fig. 24.101).

2. *Lateral meniscus:* Hypoechoic images within the distal part of the LM were found in clinical cases afflicted with severe

femoral trochlea osteochondrosis or with bone cyst in the lateral condyles of the tibia or femur (Fig. 24.102). The deep (axial) part of the LM looked hypoechoic in a filly who had also an avulsion of the cranial attachment of this meniscus on the cranial intercondylar area of the tibia (Fig. 24.103).

3. *Articular surfaces (subchondral bone surface):* Irregular contour of the hyperechogenic lateral femoral condyle and thickening of the anechoic space between this surface and the LM were identified in horses presenting subchondral bone cysts.

4. *Long digital extensor tendon (LDET):* Hypoechoic images with thickening of the tendon were found in horses that presented

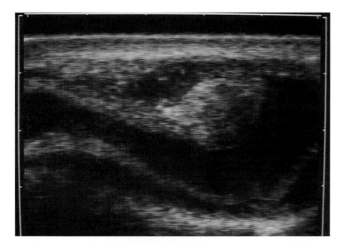

Figure 24.101. Transverse ultrasound scan of the craniolateral aspect of the stifle. An extensive synovial fluid effusion is present within the subextensorius recess of the lateral femorotibial joint. The superficial and deep walls of the synovial membrane are thickened. Superficially, the two echogenic layers are the skin and the crural fascia. The deep hyperechogenic line is the transverse profile of the sulcus subextensorius of the tibia.

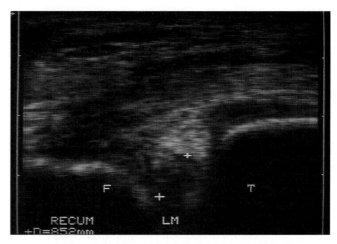

Figure 24.103. Longitudinal (frontal) ultrasound scan of the lateral aspect of the stifle of a 2-month-old filly. Same clinical case shown in Figure 24.87. This scan was made with the filly in lateral recumbency, and the lateral condyles of the femur (*F*) and tibia (*T*), as well as the lateral meniscus (*LM*), are imaged. The deep, axial part of this meniscus is hypoechoic, and radiographs showed avulsion of the cranial attachment of this structure.

with tibial tuberosity fractures. These injuries were accompanied by distention of the subextensorius recess.

Large hyperechoic images casting acoustic shadows were identified within the LDE tendon in horses undergoing proximal hind limb lameness. On lateromedial and caudocranial radiographic views, these horses had radiopaque bony nodules in the proximal long digital extensor tendon.

CONCLUSIONS

Ultrasonography is useful as a complementary procedure for imaging the soft tissue of the equine joints. Interpretation of sonograms requires a precise knowledge of descriptive and topographic anatomy of the horse limb structures to obtain the adequate images and avoid misinterpretation. The use of ultrasonography for the diagnosis of injuries to the tendons, joints, and associated structures needs the support of reference images and a good technique.

ACKNOWLEDGEMENTS

This paper was supported by the Institut National de la Recherche Agronomique, Paris, France, and by the Service des Haras, des Courses et de l'Equitation.

The authors would like to thank Patricia Perrot and Benoît Bousseau for their help in the preparation of the manuscript. Several ultrasound scans were performed at the Equine Clinic of Grosbois. Many thanks to the practitioners, especially Drs. Corde, Delecroix, Desbrosse, Lang, and Pechayre, who referred several clinical cases included in this study.

SUGGESTED READINGS

General

Barone R. Anatomie comparée des mammifères domestiques. Tome 2. Arthrologie et myologie. 2nd ed. Paris: Vigot, 1980.

Dik KJ. Ultrasonography in the diagnosis of equine lameness. Vet Ann 1990;30:162.

Ellenberger W, Baum M. Handbuch der Vergleichenden Anatomie der Haustiere. l3rd ed. Berlin: Verlag Von August Mirschwald, 1912.

Fornage B. Echographie du système musculo-tendineux des membres. Atlas d'anatomie ultrasonore normale. Paris: Vigot, 1987.

Genovese RL, et al. Clinical application of diagnostic ultrasound to the equine limb. Proc 31st Ann AAEP 1985; p. 701.

Getty R. Sisson and Grossman's: The anatomy of domestic animals. 5th ed. Philadelphia, London: WB Saunders, 1975.

International Committee on Veterinary Gross Anatomical Nomenclature. Nomina anatomica veterinaria. 3rd ed. Ithaca, NY: World Association of Veterinary Anatomists, 1983.

Nickel R, Schummer A, Seiferle E. Lehrbuch der Anatomic der haustiere. Band 1. Berlin und Hamburg: Verlag Paul Parey, 1977, pp. 213–215.

O'Keeffe D, Mamtora H. Ultrasound in clinical orthopaedics. J Bone Joint Surg 1992;74–88.

Schmaltz R. Atlas der Anatomie des Pferdes. Teil 2. Berlin: Schoetz, 1909; pp. 36–40.

Stashak TS. Adams' Lameness in horses. 4th ed. Philadelphia: Lea & Febiger, 1987.

Pastern

Boening KJ, von Saldem FC, Leenderste IP, et al. Diagnostic and surgical arthroscopy of the equine coffin joint. Proc 35th Ann AAEP 1989; p. 311.

Denoix JM, et al. L'examen échographique du paturon chez Ic cheval. Pract Vét Equine 1993;25:19.

Denoix JM. Etude biomécanique de la région phalangienne chez le cheval. CEREOPA 1985; pp. 60–75.

Denoix JM, Crevier N, Azevedo C. Ultrasound examination of the pastern in horses. Proc 37th Ann AAEP 1991; p. 363.

Dyson SJ. Lameness due to pain associated with the distal interphalangeal joint: 45 cases. Equine Vet J 1991;23:128.

Edwards GE. Interpreting radiograph 2: the fetlock joint and pastern. Equine Vet J 1984;16:4.

Hago B de, Vaughan C. Use of contrast radiography in the investigation of tendonsynovitis and bursitis in horses. Equine Vet J 1986;18:375.

Hauser ML, Rantanen NW, Genovese RL. Ultrasound anatomy and scanning technic of the distal extremities in the horse. Proc 31st Ann AAEP 1985; pp. 693.

Hauser ML, Rantanen NW. Ultrasound examination of distal interphalaneal joint, navicular bursa, navicular bone and deep digital tendon. III. Equine Vet Sci 1982;2:95.

Hertsch B, Neuberth M. Zur Dislokation der Gleichbeine nach partieller bzw. voliständiger Ruptur der distalen Gleichbeinbänder. (Sesamoid dehiscence after partial and total rupture of the distal sesamoidean ligaments). Pferdeheilkunde 1991;7:335.

McClellan PD, Colby J. Ultrasonic structure of the pastern. J Equine Vet Sci 1986;6:99.

Moyer W. Distal sesamoidean desmitis. Proc 28th Ann AAEP 1982; p. 245.

Moyer W, Raker CW. Diseases of the suspensory apparatus. Vet Clin North Am Equine Pract 1980;2:61.

Nyack B. Treatment of ruptured distal sesamoidean ligaments in a pony. Mod Vet Pract 1983;64:294.

Park RD, Nelson TR, Hoopes PJ. Magnetic resonance imaging of the normal equine digit and metacarpophalangeal joint. Vet Radiol 1987;28:105.

Rantanen N. Assessing tenovaginitis (editorial). J Equine Vet Sci 1983;4:171.

Redding W. Ultrasonic imaging of the structures of the digital flexor tendon sheath. Comp Cont Educ Pract Vet 1991;13:1824.

Van Pelt RW. Diagnosis and treatment of tendosynovitis. J Am Vet Med Assoc 1969;154:1022.

Verschooten F, De Moor A. Tendinitis in the horse: its radiographic diagnosis with airtendograms. J Am Vet Radiol Soc 1978;19:23. Watrous BJ, Dutra FR, Wagner PC, et al. Villonodular synovitis of the palmar and plantar digital flexor tendon sheaths and the calcaneal bursa of the gastrocnemius tendon in the horse. Proc 33rd Ann AAEP 1987; pp. 413–428.

Williams FL, Campbell DY. Tendon radiography in the horse. J Am Vet Med Assoc 1961;139:224.

Fetlock

Adams OR. Constriction of the palmar (volar) or plantar annular ligament of the fetlock in the horse. Proc 23rd Ann AAE 1977; p. 213.

Barclay WP, Foerner JJ, Phillips TN. Lameness attributable to osteochondral fragmentation of the plantar aspect of the proximal phalanx in horses: 19 cases (1981–1985). J Am Vet Med Assoc 1987;191:855.

Bukowiecki CF, Bramlage LR, Gabel AA. Palmar/plantar process fractures of the proximal phalanx in 15 horses. Vet Surg 1986;15:383.

Denoix JM, Bousseau B, Crevier N. Ultrasound examination of the fetlock in the horse. Proc 3rd Cong World Equine Vet Assoc, Swiss Rev Vet Med 1993;11-S:103.

Dik KJ, Van Den Belt AJM, Keg PR. Ultrasonographic evaluation of fetlock annular ligament constriction in the horse. Equine Vet J 1991;23:285.

Foerner J, Barclay WP, Phillips TN, MacHarg MA. Osteochondral fragments of the palmar/plantar aspect of the fetlock joint. Proc 33th Ann AAEP 1987; p. 739.

Gerring EL, Webbon PM. Fetlock annular ligament desmotomy: a report of 24 cases. Equine Vet J 1984;16:113.

Grondahl AM. Incidence and development of ununited proximoplantar tuberosity of the proximal phalanx in Standardbred trotters. Vet Radiol Ultrasound 1992;33:18.

Hago B de, Vaughan LC. Radiographic anatomy of the tendon sheaths and bursae in the horse. Equine Vet J 1986;18:102.

Haynes P. Disease of metacarpophalangeal joint and metacarpus. Vet Clin North Am (Large Anim Pract) 1980;2:33–59.

Kannegieter NJ. Chronic proliferative synovitis of the equine metacarpophalangeal joint. Vet Rec 1990;127:8.

Modransky PD, Rantanen NW. Diagnosic ultrasound examination of the dorsal aspect of the equine metacarpophalangeal joint. Equine Vet Sci 1983;3:56–58.

Nickels FA, Grant BD, Lincoln SD. Villonodular synovitis of the equine metacarpophalangeal joint. J Am Vet Med Assoc 1976;168:1043.

O'Brien TR. Disease of the thoroughbred fetlock joint—a comparison of radiographic signs with gross pathologic lesions. Proc 23rd Ann AAEP 1977; pp. 367–380.

Palmer SC. Radiography of the abaxial surface of the proximal sesamoid bones of the horse. J Am Vet Med Assoc 1982;181:264.

Pettersson H, Ryden G. Avulsion fractures of the caudoproximal extremity of the first phalanx. Equine Vet J 1982;14:333.

Rantanen N. Assessing tenovaginitis (editorial). J Equine Vet Sci 1983;4:171.

Steyn P, Schmitz D. The sonographic diagnosis of chronic proliferative synovitis in the metacarpophalangeal joints of a horse. Vet Radiol 1989;30:125.

Swanstrom OG, Lewis RE. Arthrography of the equine fetlock. Proc AAEP 1969; p. 221.

Vail TB, Stashak TS, Park RD, Powers BE. Desmotomy of the fetlock annular ligament in the horse: clinical ultrasonographic and histopathological findings in 47 patients (abstract 105). 27th Ann Meet Am Col Vet Surg. Vet Surg 1992;21:408.

Versehooten F, Picavet TM. Desmitis of the fetlock annular ligament in the horse. Equine Vet J 1986;18:1386.

Weaver JCB, Stover SM, O'Brien TR. Radiographic anatomy of soft tissue attachments in the equine metacarpophalangeal and proximal phalangeal region. Equine Vet J 1992;24:310.

White NA, Sullins KE, Spurlock SL, Parker GA. Diagnosis and treatment of metacarpophalangeal synovial pad proliferation in the horse. Vet Surg 1988;17:46.

Yovich JV, Turner AS, Stashak T.S, McIlwraith CW. Luxation of the metacarpophalangeal and metatarsophalangeal joints in horses. Equine Vet J 1987;19:295.

Yovich JV, McIlwraith CW, Stashak TS. Osteochondrosis dissecans am sagittalen Rollkamm von Mc III und Mt III beim. Pferd Pferdeheilkunde 1986;2:109.

Metacarpus/Metatarsus

Baxter GM. Retrospective study of the lower limb wounds involving tendons, tendon sheaths or joints in horses. Proc 33rd Ann AAEP 1987; pp. 715–728.

Foland JW, et al. Traumatic injuries involving tendons of the distal limbs in horse: a retrospective study of 55 cases. Equine Vet J 1991;23:422.

Yovich JV, Stashak TS, McIlwraith CW. Rupture of the common digital extensor tendon in foals. Comp Cont Educ Pract Vet 1984;6:S373.

Carpus

Auer J. Diseases of the carpus. Vet Clin North Am (Large Anim Pract) 1980;2:81.

Bailey JV, Barber SM, Fretz PB, Jacobs KA. Subluxation of the carpus in thirteen horses. Can Vet J 1984;25:311.

Dietze AE, Rendano VT. Fat opacities dorsal to the equine antebrachicarpal joint. Vet Radiol 1984;25:205.

Dik KJ. Radiographic and ultrasonographic imaging of soft tissue disorders of the equine carpus. Tijdschr Diergeneesk 1990;115:1168.

Doran RE, Collins LG. Mastocytoma in a horse. Equine Vet J 1986;18:500.

Ford TS, Ross MW, Orsini PG. Communications and boundaries of the middle carpal and carpometacarpal joints in horses. Am J Vet Res 1988;49:2161.

Hurtig MB, Fretz PB, Doige CE, Naylor J. Accuracy of arthroscopic identification of equine carpal lesions. Vet Surg 1985;14:93.

Jann H, Slusher SU, Courtney Q. Treatment of acquired bursitis (hygroma) by en-bloc resection. Equine Pract 1990;12:8.

Kannegieter NJ, Burbridge HM. Correlation between radiographic and arthroscopic findings in the equine carpus. Aust Vet J 1990;67:132.

Kohler L. Rupture de la synoviale articulaire an niveau de l'articulation du carpe chez le cheval, images radiologiques et possibilités de traitement. (Rupture of the carpal joint capsule in horses, radiography and treatment methods). Pract Vet Equine 1984;16:133.

Lingard TR. Strain of the superior check ligament. J Am Vet Med Assoc 1966;148:364.

McIlwraith CW. Tearing of the medial palmar intercarpal ligament in the equine midcarpal joint. Equine Vet J 1992;24:367.

Mackay-Smith MP, et al. Carpal canal syndrome in horses. J Am Vet Med Assoc 1972;160:993.

Martin GS, McIlwraith CW. Arthioscopic anatomy of the intercarpal and radiocarpal joints of the horse. Equine Vet J 1985;17:373.

Mason TA. Chronic tenosynovitis of the extensor tendon sheaths of the carpal region in the horse. Equine Vet J 1977;9:186.

Nemeth F, Dik KJ. Carpal swelling in horses. Prakt Tierärzt 1990;71:12.

Rantanen NW. The use of diagnostic ultrasound in limb disorders of the horse: a preliminary report. Equine Vet Sci 1982;2:62.

Rapin CMJ. Sur certains efforts de la région sus-carpienne chez le cheval—luxation de l'os sus-carpien. Thèse Méd Vét, Ecole Nationale Vétérinaire d'Alfort, no 78, 1929.

Squire KR, et al. Arthroscopic removal of a palmar radial osteochondroma causing carpal canal syndrome in a horse. J Am Vet Med Assoc 1992;201:1216.

Stahre L, Tuffvesson G. Supracarpal exostoses as causes of lameness. Nord Vet Med 1967;19(7–8):356.

Suann CJ, Homey FD. The treatment of transection of the extensor carpi radialis muscle as a result of a lacerating wound in a horse. Can Vet J 1983;24:243.

Turner AS, et al. Acute eosinophilic synovitis in a horse. Equine Vet J 1990;22:215.

Wallace CE. Chronic tendosynovitis of the extensor carpi radialis tendon in the horse. Aust Vet J 1972;48:585.

Shoulder

Adams SB, Blevins WE. Shoulder lameness in horses. I. Compend Cont Educ Pract Vet 1989;11:64.

Adams SB, Blevins WE. Shoulder lameness in horses. II. Compend Cont Educ Pract Vet 1989;11:190.

Adams S. Surgical repair of a supraglenoid tubercule fracture in a horse. J Am Vet Med Assoc 1987;191:332.

Dyson S. Shoulder lameness in horses: diagnosis and differential diagnosis. Proc 32th Ann AAEP 1987; pp. 461–480.

Dyson S. Diagnostic techniques in the investigation of shoulder lameness. Equine Vet J 1986;18:25.

Dyson S. Shoulder lameness in horses: an analysis of 58 suspected cases. Equine Vet J 1986;18:29.

Dyson S. Sixteen fractures of the shoulder region in the horse. Equine Vet J 1985;17:104.

Lucas C, et al. Radiology 1989;32:234.

Meagher DM, Pool RR, Brown MP. Bilateral ossification of the tendon of the biceps brachii muscle in the horse. J Am Vet Med Assoc 1979;174:282.

Nixon AJ, Spencer CP. Arthrography of the equine shoulder joint. Equine Vet J 1990;22:107.

Nixon AJ. Diagnosis and surgical arthroscopy of the equine shoulder joint. Vet Surg 1987;116:44.

Yovich JV, Aanes WA. Fracture of the greater tubercle of the humerus in a filly. S Am Vet Med Assoc 1985;187:74.

Hock

Brcuer D, Becker M. Luxation of the calcaneus cap in the horse. Prakt Tierärzt (Collegium Veterinarium XV) 1985;66(Sondernummer):35–36, 38.

Denoix JM. Le jarret des équidés: eléments d'anatomie topographique, fonctionnelle et appliquée (The equine hock: elements of topographic, functional and applied anatomy). Point Vét 1983;15:21.

Dik KJ. Ultrasonography of the equine tarsus. Vet Radiol Ultrasound 1993;34:36.

Dik KJ, Merkens HW. Unilateral distention of the tarsal sheath in the horse: a report of 11 cases. Equine Vet J 1987;19:307.

Dik KJ, Keg PR. The efficacy of contrast radiography to demonstrate "false thoroughpins" in five horses. Equine Vet J 1990;22:223.

Edwards GB. Changes in the sustentaculum tali associated with distention of the tarsal sheath (Thoroughpin). Equine Vet J 1978;10:97.

Gabel AA. Treatment and prognosis for cunean tendon bursitis-tarsistis of Standardbred horses. J Am Vet Med Assoc 1980;175:1086.

Gabel AA. Diagnosis, relative incidence and probable cause of cunean tendon bursitis-tarsitis of Standardbred horses. J Am Vet Med Assoc 1979;175:1079.

Meagher DM, Aldrete AV. Lateral luxation of the superficial flexor tendon from the calcaneal tuber in two horses. J Am Vet Med Assoc 1989;195:495.

Mettenleiter E, Meier HP, Ueltschi G, Waibl H. Examination of the common tendon sheath of the M. *flexor hallucis* longus and the M. *tibialis caudalis* by ultrasound in the horse. Anat Histol Embryol 1992;21:246.

O'Brien TR. Radiographic interpretation of the equine tarsus. Proc 19th Ann AAEP 1973; pp. 289–300.

Phillips TN. Unusual hock problems. Proc 32th Ann AAEP 1986; pp. 663–667.

Scott EA. Surgical repair of a dislocated superficial digital flexor tendon and fractured fibular tarsal bone in a horse. J Am Vet Med Assoc 1983;182:332.

Scott EA, Breuhaus B. Surgical repair of a dislocated superficial digital flexor tendon in a horse. J Am Vet Med Assoc 1982;181:171.

Shively MJ. Correct anatomic nomenclature for the joints of the equine tarsus. Equine Pract 1982;4:9.

Updike SJ. Functional anatomy of the equine tarsocrural collateral ligaments. Am J Vet Res 1984;45:867.

Updike SJ. Anatomy of the tarsal tendons of the equine tibialis cranialis and peroneus tertius muscles. Am J Vet Res 1984;45:1379.

Van Pelt RW, Riley WF. Treatment of calcaneal bursitis. S Am Vet Med Assoc 1968;153:1176.

Van Pelt RW. Inflammation of the tarsal synovial sheaths. J Am Vet Med Assoc 1969;155:1481.

Watrous BJ, Dutra FR, Wagner PC, et al. Villonodular synovitis of the palmar and plantar digital flexor tendon sheaths and the calcaneal bursa of the gastrocnemius tendon in the horse. Proc Ann AAEP 1987; pp. 413–428.

Welch RD, Auer JA, Watkins JP, Baird AN. Surgical treatment of tarsal sheath effusion associated with an exostosis on the calcaneus of a horse. J Am Vet Med Assoc 1990;196:1992.

Wheat JD, Rhode EA. Luxation and fracture of the hock of the horse. J Am Vet Med Assoc 1964;145:341.

Wilderjans HC. New bone growth on the sustentaculum tali and medial aspect of the calcaneal bone surrounding the deep digital flexor tendon in a pony. Equine Vet Educ 1990;2:184.

Wright IM. Fractures of the lateral malleolus of the tibia in 16 horses. Equine Vet J 1992;24:424.

Crus

Carleton LL, Trout DR. Equine limb anatomy: peroneus tertius muscle relationships. Zbl Vet Med C Anat Histol Embryol 1984;13:313.

Dik KJ. Ultrasonography of the equine crus. Vet Radiol Ultrasound 1993;34:28.

Dyson JS, Kidd L. Five cases of gastrocnemius tendinitis in the horse. Equine Vet J 1992;24:351.

Léveillé R, Lindsay WA, Biller DS. Ultrasonographic appearance of ruptured peroneus tertius in a horse. J Am Vet Med Assoc 1993;202:1981.

Proudman CJ. Common calcaneal tendinitis in a horse. Equine Vet Educ 1992;4:277.

Reimer P, Milbradt H, Wegner U, Braumann KM. The sonographic assessment of acute and chronic achilles pain. J Med Imaging 1989;3:1.

Shoemaker RS, Martin GS, Hillman DJ, Haynes PF, et al. Disruption of the caudal component of the reciprocal apparatus in two horses. J Am Vet Med Assoc 1991;198:120.

Szabuniewiez M, Titus RS. Rupture of the peroneus tertius. VM/SAC 1967;62:993.

Trout DR, Lohse CL. Anatomy and therapeutic resection of the peroneus tertius muscle in a foal. J Am Vet Med Assoc 1981;179:247.

Updike SJ. Fascial compartments of the equine crus. Am J Vet Res 1985;46:692.

Stifle

Aisen AM, McCune WJ, McGuire A, et al. Sonographic evaluation of the cartilage of the knee. Radiology 1984;153:781.

Badoux DM. The geometry of the cruciate ligaments in the canine and equine knee joint, a Tchebychev mechanism. Acta Anat 1984;119:60.

Baker GJ, Moustafa MAI, Boero MJ, Foreman JH, Wilson DA. Caudal cruciate ligament function and injury in the horse. Vet Rec 1987;121:319.

Brown MP, Moon PD, Buergelt CD. The effect of injection of an iodine counter irritant into the patellar ligaments of ponies: application to stifle lameness. J Equine Vet Sci 1984;4:82.

Bukowiecki CF, Sanders-Shamis M, Bramlage LR. Treatment of a ruptured medial collateral ligament of the stifle in a horse. J Am Vet Med Assoc 1988;193:687.

Denoix JM. L'examen radiographique du grasset du cheval. II. Images radiologiques normales. Point Vet 1986;18:109.

Denoix JM. Functional anatomy and biomechanics of the equine stifle and hock. Proc 2nd Cong World Equine Vet Assoc. Swiss Rev Vet Ultrasound Med 1991;11a:48.

Derks WHJ, deHooge P, Van Linge B. Ultrasonographic detection of the patellar plica in the knee. J Clin Ultrasound 1986;14:355.

Dik KJ, Nemeth F. Traumatic patella fracture in the horse. Equine Vet J 1983;15:244.

Dyson S, Wright I, Kold S, Vatistas N. Clinical and radiographic features, treatment and outcome in 15 horses with fracture of the medial aspect of the patella. Equine Vet J 1992;24:264.

Dufour M, et al. Dérangement interne du genou. IRM et corrélation arthroscopique (70 cas). (Internal derangement of the knee. MRI appearances with arthroscopic correlation in 70 cases). Rev Im Med 1993;5:151.

Foland JW, McIlwraith CW, Trotter GW. Equine femoropatellar osteochondritis dissecans: results of arthroscopic surgery in 153 horses. Vet Surg 1991;20:335.

Fornage BD, et al. Diagnostic des calcifications du tendon rotulien. Comparaison échoradiographique. J Radiol 1984;65:355.

Fornage BD, et al. Sonography of the patellar tendon: preliminary observations. Am J Radiol 1987;149:549.

Frija G, et al. Ménisques macroscopiquement normaux: corrélation entre l'IRM et l'histologie. Rev Im Med 1989;1:37.

Gerring EL, Davies JV. Fracture of the tibial tuberosity in a polo pony. Equine Vet J 1982;14:158.

Gibson KT, et al. Production of patellar lesions by medial patellar desmotomy in horses. Proc 35th Ann AAEP 1989; pp. 298–303.

Hendrickson DA, Nixon AJ. A lateral approach for synovial fluid aspiration and joint injection of the femoropatellat joint of the horse. Equine Vet J 1992;24:399.

Jeffcott LB, Kold SE. Stifle lameness in the horse: a survey of 86 referred cases. Equine Vet J 1982;14:31.

Jones C, Schmitz DG. Sonographic anatomy of soft tissue structures of the equine femorotibial joint. Tex Vet Med 1989;51:17.

Laine HR, Harjula A, Peltokaillo P. Ultrasound in the evaluation of the knee and patella regions. J Ultrasound Med 1987;6:33.

McIlwraith CW. Osteochondral fragmentation of the distal aspect of the patella in horses. Equine Vet J 1990;22:157.

Nickels FA, Sande R. Radiographic and arthroscopic findings in the equine stifle. J Am Vet Med Assoc 1982;181:918.

O'Brien TR, Baker TW, Koblik P. Stifle radiology: how to perform an examination and interpret the radiographs. Proc 32th Ann AAEP 1986; pp. 531–552.

Parks AH, Wyn-Jones G. Traumatic injuries of the patella in five horses. Equine Vet J 1988;20:24.

Penninck DG. Ultrasonography of the equine stifle. Vet Radiol 1990;31:293.

Prades M, et al. Injuries to the cranial cruciate ligament and associated structures: summary of clinical, radiographic, arthroscopic and pathological findings from 10 horses. Equine Vet J 1989;21:354.

Reeves MJ, Trotter GW, Kainer RA. Anatomical and functional communications between the synovial sacs of the equine stifle joint. Equine Vet J 1991;23:215.

Sanders-Shamis M, Cabel AA. Surgical reconstruction of a ruptured medial collateral ligament in a foal. J Am Vet Med Assoc 1988;193:80.

Sanders-Shamis M, Bukowiecki CF, Biller DS. Cruciate and collateral ligament failure in the equine stifle: seven cases (1975–1985). J Am Vet Med Assoc 1988;193:573.

Selby B, Richardson ML, Montana MS, Teitz CC, et al. High resolution sonography of the menisci of the knee. Invest Radiol 1986;91:335.

Selby B, Richardson ML, Nelson BD, et al. Sonography in the detection of meniscal injuries of the knee: evaluation in cadavers. Am J Radiol 1987;149:549.

Smith BL, Auer JA, Watkins JP. Surgical repair of tibial tuberosity avulsion fractures in four horses. Vet Surg 1990;19:117.

Squire KRE, Blevins WE, Frederick M, Fessler JF. Radiographic changes in an equine patella following medial patellar desmotomy. Vet Radiol 1990;31:208.

Tegtmeyer CJ, McCue FC, Higgins SM, Ball DW. Arthrography of the knee: a comparative study of the accuracy of single and double contrast techniques. Radiology 1979;132:37.

Vacek JR, Ford TS, Honnas CM. Communication between the femoropatellar and medial and lateral femorotibial joints in horses. Am J Vet Res 1992;53:1431.

25. Muscle Evaluation, Foreign Bodies, and Miscellaneous Swellings

RENÉE LÉVEILLÉ AND DAVID S. BILLER

Improved technology and the development of high-resolution transducers have made ultrasonography of the musculoskeletal system possible. The major advantages over other diagnostic imaging techniques are the ability to evaluate internal architecture of soft tissues, dynamic evaluation of structures, relatively low cost, absence of radiation, and wide availability. Ultrasonography allows differentiation of a firm, solid, or thick-walled cystic lesion, clearly reveals injuries to tendons, muscle, and ligaments, and reveals minor irregularities of the wall and lumen of distended tendon sheaths, and it may demonstrate radiolucent foreign material more clearly than contrast radiography (1). Determining the presence of a lesion may be all that is necessary, or it may lead to a more specific workup. Ultrasonography has the advantage of enabling the examiner to determine whether a lesion is vascular, cystic, or solid, a determination that is valuable in selecting the next diagnostic step (2).

This chapter reviews the application of ultrasonography to the evaluation of musculoskeletal disorders including soft tissue masses, identification of foreign bodies, osteomyelitis, cellulitis, and certain joint abnormalities.

TECHNIQUE

The most common imaging technique, radiography, is capable of identifying soft tissue swelling, but the cause is often not diagnosed.

As with all sonographic imaging, images are obtained in longitudinal, transverse, and, if needed, oblique projections for all structures and entities evaluated. This method contributes the most information, by allowing three-dimensional localization and measurement of lesions. It is frequently useful to scan the contralateral asymptomatic side of paired structures if one questions what is normal for each patient. The lesions should be characterized according to size, pattern of distribution, internal echo characteristics, and relationship with other anatomic structures.

Maximum resolution of the target tissue is obtained using a transducer with a frequency of 5 Mhz or higher (7.5 or 10 Mhz). High-frequency transducers provide optimal spatial and contrast resolution; however, depth of penetration and field of view are limited. Linear transducers of lower frequency (3 Mhz) are advantageous in large muscular areas if the pathologic process is deep (such as the thigh), where the increased penetration and larger field of view are necessary to visualize deep structures. The transducers are usually applied directly onto the skin; however, a stand-off pad is useful for visualizing superficial structures. The stand-off pad allows the superficial structures to be within the focal zone and away from the artifact created at the surface off the transducer, especially with mechanical scanners (2, 3).

NORMAL MUSCLE ANATOMY

The sonographic patterns of normal skeletal muscles are similar for all groups of muscles (4). Muscle is generally less echogenic than subcutaneous fat or tendons. The appearance of normal skeletal muscle imaged longitudinally is that of homogeneous, multiple, fine, parallel echoes (Fig. 25.1). Transverse imaging shows a more disorganized pattern of fine echoes scattered throughout the muscle fibers (Fig. 25.2). This appearance of muscle is due to multiple muscle bundles (fasciculi) surrounded by fibroadipose septa (perimysium). Larger septa may be clearly visualized, giving a thin reticular pattern on transverse scans. Vascular structures situated within the muscles may be imaged (4). A brightly echogenic outer margin of each muscle is formed by connective tissue fascia. The echogenicity of contracted muscle is often less than that of relaxed muscle (2, 4). Muscle tonicity at rest tends to flatten and smooth the area of discontinuity.

SOFT TISSUE MASSES

Ultrasound can differentiate between solid and cystic masses. Doppler imaging (spectral or color) can be used to differentiate cystic from vascular lesions such as arteriovenous fistula, aneurysm, or pseudoaneurysmal structure (2, 5, 6). The appearance of solid lesions depends more on the particular tissue and pathologic characteristics. Although edema may appear sonolucent, fibrosis is usually echogenic (4). Small or thin fluid collections may not show distal acoustic enhancement (4).

In one report, ultrasonography of a prominence at the coronary band in a horse confirmed the diagnosis of a keratoma as a well-delineated hypoechoic soft tissue mass between the hoof wall and the articulation of the distal and middle phalanges (7).

MUSCLE INJURIES

Muscular trauma may result in the formation of hematomas, muscle tears, compartment syndrome, abscess, or myositis ossificans (2). Various abnormal sonographic patterns have been identified. These include 1) fluid-filled

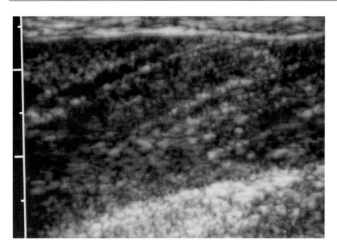

Figure 25.1. A longitudinal scan of normal skeletal muscle demonstrates homogeneous, multiple fine parallel echoes.

collections, 2) small, irregularly shaped lesions with scattered low-level echoes, 3) ill-defined echogenic areas, 4) highly reflective zones with acoustic shadowing, and 5) acoustically mixed lesions with hypoechogenic and echogenic areas (4).

Ultrasonographically typical cavitary lesions have been found in hematomas associated with recent large muscular tears (Fig. 25.3). This pattern has also been found in less recent trauma associated with older hemorrhagic or serous encysted collections. The organizing hematoma can display internal echoes or septations (Fig. 25.4). Small partial ruptures or separations exhibit irregularly shaped anechoic areas, occasionally with poor low-level background echoes (4, 8).

The sonographic characteristics of hematomas depend on the age and status of clot formation and on the frequency of the transducer. Recent hemorrhage and organized clots appear echogenic (9). In general, high-frequency transducers produce increased echogenicity from clotted

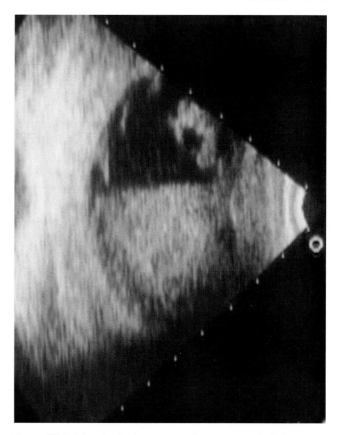

Figure 25.3. A longitudinal sonogram shows an anechoic hematoma with accumulation of echogenic material at its dependent portion.

hematomas. Hematomas may have well-defined or irregular margins with or without internal septa. The incidence of septations within hematomas ranges from 10 to 44% among hematomas in all locations (10). Muscular hemorrhage often results in focal or diffuse muscle enlargement and is usually confined to the compartment of origin. A hematoma may dissect around a muscle or may be associated with muscle tears. In human patients, dynamic exami-

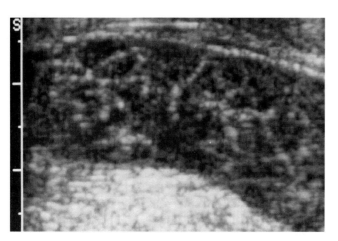

Figure 25.2. A transverse scan of normal skeletal muscle shows fine echoes scattered throughout muscle fibers. Large septa give a thin reticular pattern.

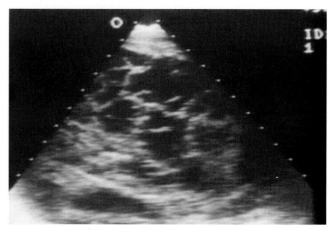

Figure 25.4. A longitudinal scan shows a large hematoma containing internal echoes and septations. Surgical exploration confirmed the presence of an organized hematoma.

nations with muscle contraction and relaxation have been reported and may be valuable in differentiating a hematoma from a muscle tear associated with a hematoma. Contraction shows retraction of muscle with an increased size of the lesion if a tear is present (2). Recurrent or chronic muscle injuries develop fibrosis and scarring characterized by heterogeneous areas of increased echoes that do not increase in size with contraction (2).

Chronic lesions with ossification have demonstrated highly echogenic foci with acoustic shadowing (4, 11). The sonographic appearance of hematomas is not specific; in particular, the overlap with abscesses may be considerable. Because there is no reliable ultrasonographic means of detecting the presence of infection in a hematoma, needle aspiration is necessary in certain clinical situations.

ABSCESS

The ultrasonographic appearance of abscesses varies from a cystlike to a solid echogenic (hyperechoic) pattern, the variable appearance reflecting the physical characteristics of the fluid at the time of examination. In a large percentage of cases, weak echoes are dispersed throughout the fluid, although well-defined fluid–debris levels may be seen (Fig. 25.5). Large amounts of strong echogenic debris may also be encountered, often in the dependent portion of the cavitary lesion, but occasionally creating a complex or solid echo pattern. The abscess is easily distinguishable from the surrounding tissue (5). The presence of internal echoes with higher echogenicity is also a common ultrasonographic abscess pattern that could be in the form of septations (12). Gas-containing abscesses may appear as densely echogenic masses with acoustic shadowing or reverberation.

Intramuscular injection of various drugs into the gluteal musculature has been reported to cause abscess formation at the injection site (12). The appearance of the tissue surrounding the abscess is carefully evaluated for the presence of early fistulous tract formation or a foreign body (12).

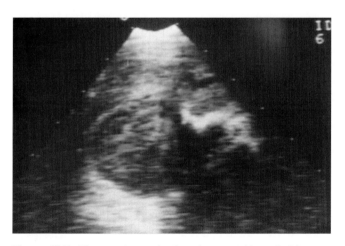

Figure 25.5. Ultrasound examination shows a thin-walled hyperechoic mass. Pus was obtained on fine-needle aspiration.

Cartee and Rumph (13) described the following protocol using ultrasonography in the evaluation of fistulous tracts: 1) locate the tract from its point of drainage and follow its length as far as possible; if the tract does not contain enough fluid to appear anechoic or hypoechoic, the instillation of sterile fluid or antibiotic solution should be considered; 2) If a hyperechoic area is located within the tract, the transducer should be manipulated so the presence or absence of an acoustic shadow can be determined; 3) if an acoustic shadow is seen, its deeper portion should be observed; 4) If hypoechoic areas are present within the acoustic shadow, a tentative diagnosis of fibrous tissue or tendon should be considered; 5) If no echoes are present within the acoustic shadow, bone or wood may be suspected; and 6) If no acoustic shadowing is noted and the echoes within the fistula are of low intensity, cellular debris or material may be suspected (e.g., blood, abscess, fibrin tag).

The difficulties in using ultrasonography in the evaluation of foreign objects within fistulous tracts are as follows: the presence of air or gas in the tract may cause a false-positive diagnosis of a dense object such as bone or wood (13); a large beam width may add to the apparent size of an object; a change in the pressure applied with the probe may help one to differentiate gas from solid foreign body; and the direction of the transducer so the object will be in the focal zone is sometimes difficult to predetermine.

FOREIGN BODIES

Ultrasonography has been reported as a useful adjunct to conventional radiographs in diagnosing the presence and location of radiolucent (glass, wood) foreign bodies that have become embedded in soft tissue (2, 13–15). The shape, size, and location of foreign bodies are best determined by conventional radiographs if the foreign body is radiopaque. Only the nearest surface of the foreign body is evident with ultrasound, so the configuration and size cannot be accurately determined (2).

In all cases of sonographically visualized foreign bodies, an accurate three-dimensional localization should be obtained by using longitudinal and transverse scans. The location of the foreign body can be marked on the skin, and its depth can be measured accurately on the scan to enable the surgeon to retrieve it through the shortest route and with the least damage to the surrounding structures (14).

On ultrasonography, the reflectivity of a foreign body depends on its acoustic impedance, which varies with density. Thus, steel and glass are significantly more reflective than Plexiglas and wood. Low-density nonopaque foreign bodies, however, may reflect ultrasound beams sufficiently well to be detectable sonographically. Hyperechoic foci, particularly when they lack shadowing or reverberating hyperechoic comet tail artifact, are better detected when they are in a homogeneous, slightly hypoechoic area such as subcutaneous fat, muscle, or inflammatory tissue (14). Other factors that must be considered in the discrimination of a foreign object are its width and reflector incidence in

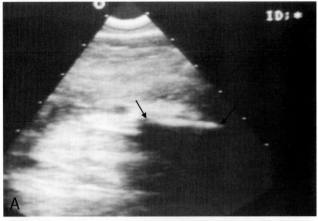

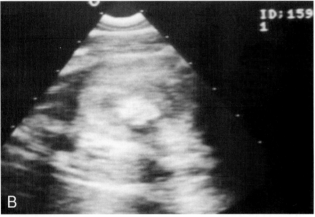

Figure 25.6. Piece of wood in the flank. Hyperechoic linear structure represents the piece of wood surrounded by an anechoic to hypoechoic inflammatory rection. Only a small portion of the piece of wood (*arrows*) creates an acoustic shadowing. **A**, Longitudinal scan. **B**, Transverse scan.

relation to the ultrasound beam width. This "side lobe" phenomenon can result in an image in which the object appears thicker than it really is. The image can also appear to have echoes within a shadow leading to the assumption

that either it is a weak reflector or has not produced a true acoustic shadow (2).

All foreign bodies (glass, metal, vegetable material) produce hyperechoic foci on sonography. Wood usually cannot be seen on plain films, whereas sonography can readily demonstrate the presence of wood (2). The acoustic shadow produced by a piece of wood may be seen only when the transducer is in certain positions (Fig. 25.6) (13). Occasionally, glass shows acoustic shadowing (Fig. 25.7) (2). Lead shot has created focal echogenicities, with strong posterior reverberation echoes. One would expect to find a clean acoustic shadow posteriorly, but we have no explanation for this unusual phenomenon. It should not be mistaken for the presence of gas within a lesion. Comparison with plain films may help one to differentiate lead shot from collections of gas large enough to be visible radiographically (16).

Ultrasonography is sensitive in the diagnosis of foreign bodies, but specificity needs further evaluation. The ultrasonographic differential diagnosis includes calcifications, bone interface, and the presence of gas (14).

OSTEOMYELITIS

Osteomyelitis, soft tissue abscesses, and cellulitis may have overlapping clinical symptoms. Radiographic lesions of osteomyelitis appear 10 to 14 days after the onset of the infection. Ultrasound has been used successfully in the diagnosis of osteomyelitis. When the draining tract can be followed to the bone source, foreign bodies, fracture fragments, and sequestra can be delineated ultrasonographically (17). The location of the fluid with respect to the bone is an important aspect in differentiating osteomyelitis from cellulitis (2, 17, 18).

Acute osteomyelitis is difficult to diagnose. Various modalities, including conventional radiography, bone scintigraphy, gallium-67 scintigraphy, and magnetic resonance imaging, have been used. Radiographic changes are

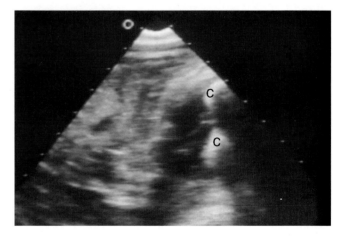

Figure 25.8. Sonogram of osteomyelitis of the proximal radius. A transverse scan reveals a fluid collection in direct contact with bone. Cortical destruction is shown by interruption of the hyperechoic cortical line. C = cortex.

Figure 25.7. Glass fragment at the palmar aspect of the metacarpus. Transverse scan shows bright reflection associated with comet-tail artifact. G = glass fragment.

seen only when significant bone destruction or periosteal production or reaction has occurred. Accumulation of fluid adjacent to the bone, without intervening soft tissue, has been seen sonographically in patients with osteomyelitis before the detection of radiographic abnormalities (Fig. 25.8) (17).

Because of its physical properties, bone is not visualized with ultrasound. It typically appears as a longitudinal or convex echogenic density with acoustic shadowing posterior to it. Focal accumulations of fluid are not normally present in the soft tissues or surrounding the bone. In human patients, the sonographic appearance of fluid around or adjacent to bone suggests acute osteomyelitis and correlates well with the pathophysiologic features of the disease. With hematogenous dissemination of organisms, an acute inflammatory response is initiated in bone. This response results in vascular ischemia, edema, and bone necrosis. As the exudative response continues and as tissue pressure increases in children, one may see the periosteum elevated by subperiosteal fluid or abscess formation. In adults, the periosteum is firmly attached to the bone; therefore, inflammatory debris may erode through the periosteum and may produce extraperiosteal fluid and abscess collections (2, 18, 19).

If soft tissue is demonstrated between the fluid and bone, then a nonosseous origin of fluid should be considered (Fig. 25.9) (17). Pathologic processes that may appear as anechoic fluid collections confined to the soft tissues include abscesses, hematomas, seromas, and lymphedema (18). Care should be taken to avoid misinterpreting joint effusions, which also appear as fluid accumulation adjacent to bone. The ultrasonographic diagnosis of osteomyelitis is also made in humans based on detection of cortical destruction, sequestrum formation, and subperiosteal abscesses (17).

JOINT ABNORMALITIES

Joint effusions can be diagnosed sonographically even when small amounts of fluid are present. Although ultrasound cannot determine the nature or cause of effusions (2), pyogenic arthritis is suggested by the presence of hyperechoic synovial fluid and capsular thickening (20).

Other indications may be the assessment of capsular lesions associated with osteochondrosis, if joint effusion is not associated with bony abnormalities, to differentiate between extra-articular avulsed bone fragments and intra-articular loose bodies, fragments floating, attached to or incorporated into the joint capsule (Figs. 25.10 and 25.11) (21).

Ultrasonographic image differentiates cartilage from subchondral bone, and this finding may be useful to detect early or small cartilage lesions (22, 23). Cartilage appears as a distinct hypoechoic band having sharp anterior and posterior margins, with the cartilage–bone interface usually appearing more echogenic because of the larger impedance mismatch than the synovial space–cartilage interface (24). In human patients, cartilage measurements are less precise or reproducible when the margins are obscured or degraded by disease. In general, clarity and sharpness correlate better with the clinical impression than do the absolute measurements of thickness (24). Perhaps the most striking ultrasonographic finding is "rough" cartilage, which is frequently seen in arthritic patients. Possibly such roughening or irregularity precedes actual thinning of cartilage in many patients (24).

In the carpus, the only articular cartilage that can be evaluated ultrasonographically is located at the distal radius. To achieve this visualization, the carpus has to be held in the fully flexed position, and the transducer is applied in a transverse position The articular cartilage appears as a smooth, anechoic layer surrounded by two echogenic lines representing the soft tissue–cartilage interface and the cartilage–radial bone interface, respectively. In a weight-bearing position, it is not possible to outline any carpal cartilage.

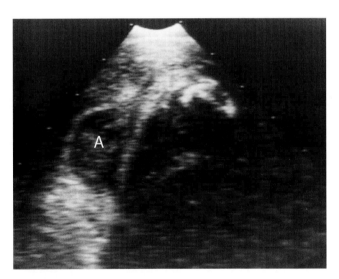

Figure 25.9. A longitudinal scan of the humerus shows a fluid collection separated from the bone by echogenic soft tissue. Surgical exploration confirmed periosseous abscess without osteomyelitis. A = abscess.

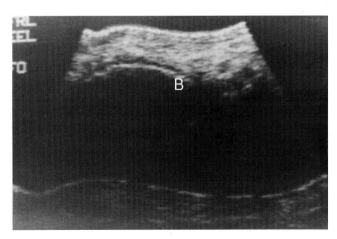

Figure 25.10. Sonogram of a normal joint surface. B = subchondral bone.

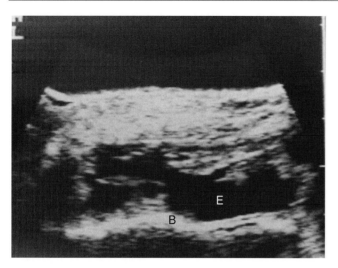

Figure 25.11. Sonogram of joint effusion. B = subchondral bone; E = effusion.

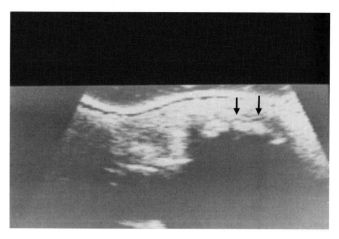

Figure 25.13. Calcinosis circumscripta at the lateral aspect of the hock. The longitudinal scan shows hyperechoic reflectors creating acoustic shadowing (*arrows*).

The carpal joint capsule with its two fat areas at the level of the antebrachiocarpal joint and the proximal row of carpal bones was identified on sonograms (22).

The articular surface is seen as a hypoechoic line surrounded by two hyperechoic interfaces. The cranial interface represents the interface between soft tissue and the hypoechoic cartilage, and the caudal interface represents the interface between the hypoechoic cartilage and subchondral bone. Anechoic lines compatible with synovial fluid are not identified in normal horses. The joint capsule is not identified separately. In the stifle, anatomic structures that can be imaged are the three patellar ligaments, collateral ligaments, articular cartilage of the femoral trocheal ridges, and the medial and lateral menisci. Visualization of the cruciate ligaments is not obtained on standing, weight-bearing horses

(23). In humans, cruciate ligaments are seen ultrasonographically as linear, hypoechoic structures crossing the knee (25). Ultrasonography of the tarsus has also been described by Dik (26).

Whether sonography has sufficient specificity for one to advocate surgery based on an abnormal sonography is not known (27).

FRACTURES

Reef described the diagnosis of pelvic fractures using ultrasound in five horses. Multiple fragments were detected ultrasonographically in each horse, with areas of muscle disruption and hemorrhage surrounding the fractured ilium (28). During ultrasonographic examination, irregular bone contour suggests callus formation (29).

MYOSITIS OSSIFICANS

Sonography has been used in the evaluation of posttraumatic myositis (2, 30). Hyperechoic foci within the musculature represent fibrosis from previous injury (Fig. 25.12).

Calcinosis circumscripta is imaged as a soft tissue mass, distorting the fascial planes. A bright reflector within the mass represents calcification, dating the lesion to at least 3 to 4 weeks. Air or metal within the soft tissue produces a bright reflector with distal acoustic shadowing. Acoustic shadow may obscure the underlying bone; if possible, the transducer should be angled so soft tissue can be imaged between the calcification and the adjacent cortex (Fig. 25.13). If this can be done, the diagnosis of a primary bone tumor with extension can be eliminated (30).

CONCLUSION

The information obtained with ultrasonography may help the veterinarian to make a prognosis and to provide the best management of patients, as follows: 1) surgery may not be indicated if the ultrasonographic examination is normal; 2)

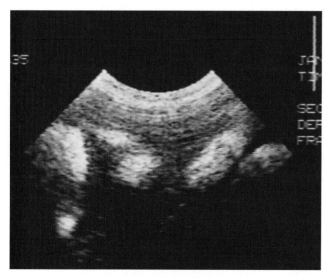

Figure 25.12. Sonographic examination of the semitendinous region of a horse with a history of previous trauma revealed hyperechoic foci scattered throughout the musculature. Sonographic findings are compatible with fibrotic myositis.

minimal ultrasonographic findings may be followed by serial ultrasonographic studies; 3) surgery may be indicated if perfect healing is necessary (4); and 4) the evolution of the lesions can be monitored during therapy. Ultrasonography is a method of evaluation that documents the added diagnostic information often unavailable with conventional radiography.

REFERENCES

1. Dik K. Soft tissue lesions of the equine carpus: roentgenological and echographic studies. Tijdschr Diergeneeskd 1990;115:1168–1174.

2. Kaplan PA, Matamoros A, Anderson JC. Sonography of the musculoskeletal system. AJR Am J Roentgenol 1990;155:237–245.

3. Biller SD, Myer W. Ultrasound scanning of superficial structures using an ultrasound stand off pad. Vet Radiol 1988;29:138–142.

4. Fornage BD, Touche DH, Segal P, et al. Ultrasonography in the evaluation of muscular trauma. J Ultrasound Med 1983;2:549–554.

5. Hager DA. The diagnosis of deep muscle abscesses using two-dimensional real time ultrasound. Proceedings of the Thirtieth Annual Convention of the American Association of Equine Practitioners 1986:523–529.

6. Williams J, Bailey HQ, Schertel ER, et al. Compartment syndrome in a Labrador Retriever. Vet Radiol Ultrasound 1992;34:244–248.

7. Seahorn TL, Sams AE, Honnas CM, et al. Ultrasonographic imaging of a keratoma in a horse. J Am Vet Med Assoc 1992;200:1973–1974.

8. Neuberth M, Stefansson P, Hertsch B. Ultrasonographic diagnosis of hematomas and abscesses in the proximal parts of the equine locomotor system. Pferdeheilkunde 1990;6:237–244.

9. Mittelstaedt CA. Abdominal ultrasound. New York: Churchill Livingstone, 1989.

10. Wicks JD, Silver TM, Bree RL. Gray scale features of hematomas: an ultrasonic spectrum. AJR Am J Roentgenol 1978;131:977.

11. Dik KJ, Belt JM. [Sonography applied to muscles of horse's limb.] Muskelsonographie der Pferdeextremitat. Pferdeheilkunde 1992;8:261–266.

12. Love NE, Nickels F. Ultrasonographic diagnosis of a deep muscle abscess in a horse. Vet Radiol Ultrasound 1993;34:207–209.

13. Cartee RE, Rumph PF. Ultrasonographic detection of fistulous tracts and foreign objects in muscles of horses. J Am Vet Med Assoc 1984;184:1127–1132.

14. Fornage BD, Schernberg FL. Sonographic diagnosis of foreign bodies of the distal extremities. AJR Am J Roentgenol 1986;147:567–569.

15. Little CM, Parker MG, Callowich MC, et al. The ultrasonic detection of soft tissue foreign bodies. Invest Radiol 1986;21:275–277.

16. Wendell BA, Athey PA. Ultrasonic appearance of metallic foreign bodies in parenchymal organs. J Clin Ultrasound 1981;9:133–135.

17. Reef V, Reimer J, Reid C. Ultrasonographic findings in horses with osteomyelitis. Proceedings of the Thirty-seventh Annual Convention of the American Association of Equine Practitioners 1991:381–391.

18. Abiri MM, Kirpekar M, Ablow RC. Osteomyelitis: detection with ultrasound. Radiology 1989;172:509–511.

19. Abiri MM, Kirpekar M, Ablow RC. Osteomyelitis: detection with ultrasound: work in progress. Radiology 1988;169:795–797.

20. Shiv VK, Jain AK, Taneja K, et al. Sonography of hip joint in infective arthritis. J Assoc Can Radiol 1990;41:76–78.

21. Dik KJ. Ultrasonography in the diagnosis of equine lameness. In: Grunsell CSA, Raw ME, eds. The Veterinary Annual 30. London: Wright Butterworth Scientific, 1990: 162–171.

22. Tnibar M, Kaser-Hotz B, Auer JA. Ultrasonography of the dorsal and lateral aspects of the equine carpus: technique and normal appearance. Vet Radiol Ultrasound 1993;34:413–425.

23. Pennick DG, Nyland TG, O'Brien TR, et al. Ultrasonography of the equine stifle. Vet Radiol 1990;31:293–298.

24. Aisen AM, McCune WJ, MacGuire A, et al. Sonographic evaluation of the cartilage of the knee. Radiology 1984;153:781–784.

25. Laine HR, Harjula A, Peltokallio P. Ultrasound in the evaluation of the knee and patella regions. J Ultrasound Med 1987;6:33–36.

26. Dik KJ. Ultrasonography of the equine tarsus. Vet Radiol Ultrasound 1993;34:36–43.

27. Selby B, Richardson ML, Montana MA, et al. High resolution sonography of the menisci of the knee. Invest Radiol 1986;4:332–335.

28. Reef VB. Diagnosis of pelvic fractures in horses using ultrasonography. Vet Radiol Ultrasound 1992;33:121 (abstract).

29. Pilsworth RC, Shepherd MC, Herinckx, et al. Fracture of the wing of the ilium, adjacent to the sacroiliac joint, in Thoroughbred racehorses. Equine Vet J 1994;24:94–99.

30. Kramer FL, Kurt AB, Rubin C, et al. Ultrasound appearance of myositis ossificans. Skeletal Radiol 1979;4:19–20.

26. Sonographic Examination of Synovial Structures in the Horse

W. RICH REDDING

Swellings of the synovial sheaths and bursae of the equine limb occur commonly. The clinical significance of some of these disorders can be difficult to ascertain. Acute effusions of these synovial structures may be due to a primary inflammatory response, or they may be secondary to an injury of one or more of the tendons or ligaments with which they are associated. Effective management of these disorders therefore requires a diagnosis that identifies the structure involved and the specific damage incurred. Diagnostic ultrasound provides an excellent means to image synovial structures and associated tendons and ligaments accurately, as well as to provide insight into the pathophysiologic state at the time of the examination.

Sonographic evaluation of synovial structures requires a detailed knowledge of the anatomy of the equine limb. This chapter reviews the anatomy of the synovial sheaths and bursae and associated tendons and ligaments of the equine limb (1–4). The sonograms of some normal synovial sheaths and the sonographic appearance of some common clinical problems of these structures are reviewed.

GENERAL SYNOVIAL SHEATH ANATOMY

Tendons are bound to the limb by *annular ligaments* or *retinacula*. An annular ligament or retinaculum is a bandlike thickening of the deep fascia that crosses over one or more tendons and begins and ends on close bony prominences. Where there is increased motion or a severe change in direction of the tendon, such as at a joint, it is surrounded by a *synovial sheath* (*vagina synovialis tendinis*). A synovial sheath is composed of inner visceral (pars tendinae) and outer parietal (pars parietalis) layers. Closely surrounding and included in the parietal layer is the fibrous portion of the sheath. Both layers are lined by synovial cells that produce a synovial-like fluid medium that facilitates movement of the tendon by minimizing friction and thereby aiding the gliding action of the tendon. The visceral and parietal layers of a sheath are continuous through the *mesotendon,* which carries the extrinsic blood supply to the tendon. In areas of increased motion, the mesotendon disappears or is replaced by threads of tissue called *vincula*. The proximal aspect of a synovial sheath has a redundant sickle-shaped fold of the parietal and fibrous layer that allows the tendon to travel freely within the sheath. The distal aspect of most sheaths does not have a large range of movement and therefore inserts directly on a distal aspect of the tendon. For simplicity, some anatomists have classified sheaths as bursae that are folded over the tendon. This characterization may be seen more clearly when viewing some tendon sheaths that do not surround the tendon fully at all levels, particularly the sheaths of the extensor surface of the carpus.

The anatomic locations of the most common clinically apparent synovial sheaths in the horse are the digital flexor tendon sheath found on all four limbs, the tarsal sheath found on the plantar aspect of the tarsus, the carpal sheath found on the palmar aspect of the carpus covering the deep digital and superficial digital flexor tendons, the individual sheaths of the digital extensor tendons as they cross the dorsal aspect of the carpus, and the individual sheaths of the extensor digital tendons of the hind limb crossing the dorsal surface of the tarsus.

DIGITAL SHEATH

Anatomic descriptions of the digital flexor tendon sheath apply to both the forelimb and the hind limb; for purposes of this discussion, the term palmar equates with plantar. The digital flexor tendon sheath begins in the distal third of the metacarpus or metatarsus and extends to the distal pastern approximately at the proximal end of the middle phalanx. In the young horse, the digital flexor tendon sheath is generally longer and begins more proximad than in the adult. The digital flexor tendon sheath covers the deep digital flexor tendon and the dorsal border of the superficial digital flexor tendon just before the superficial digital flexor tendon bifurcates to form a ring around the deep digital flexor tendon along the palmar aspect of the fetlock joint. Slightly distal to the proximal aspect of this ring, the tendons are bound to the limb by the annular ligament, which forms the palmar aspect of the fetlock canal. The superficial digital flexor tendon has a natural axial connection to the annular ligament and therefore forms the palmar border of the digital flexor tendon sheath. The deep digital flexor tendon is held more central throughout its course in the digital flexor tendon sheath by the ring formed by the superficial digital flexor tendon termed the *manica flexoria.*

The superficial digital flexor tendon bifurcates in the palmar pastern into two branches that insert on the distal abaxial aspect of the proximal phalanx and the proximal abaxial aspect of the middle phalanx. These branches are contained within the digital flexor tendon sheath. The dorsal border of the digital flexor tendon sheath distal to the proximal sesamoid bones and intersesamoidean ligament is formed by the distal sesamoidean ligaments. The digital flexor tendon sheath extends further distal on the limb on the dorsal aspect than on the palmar aspect. The distal extent of the dorsal component of the digital flexor tendon sheath is the so-called "T ligament," a transverse fibrous band that separates the digital flexor tendon sheath from the proximal palmar pouch of the distal interphalangeal joint and the navicular bursa. In one area of the distal palmar pastern just proximal to the bulbs of the heel, the deep digital flexor tendon is not contained within the digital flexor tendon sheath before it courses over the navicular bone and its associated bursa to insertion on the palmar aspect of the distal phalanx.

CARPUS

Craniolateral Forearm

The muscles on the craniolateral forearm are the extensors of the distal limb (carpus, fetlock, pastern, and coffin joints). All tendons of these muscles cross the dorsal surface of the carpus and have an associated synovial sheath. These synovial sheaths begin at variable distances proximal to the carpus and generally extend distal to the carpus (only the flexor carpi radialis and the ulnaris lateralis tendons with their insertions on the accessory carpal bone have insertions on the bones of the carpus). The deep fascia over the dorsal surface of the carpus is thickened to form a wide fascial band called the *extensor retinaculum.* The extensor retinaculum binds down the tendons of the extensor carpi radialis, the common digital extensor, and the extensor carpi obliquus as they cross the dorsal surface of the radius. The medial groove of the radius is shallow and allows the extensor carpi obliquus to pass obliquely from lateral to medial in its course to insertion on the head of the second metacarpal bone. The middle groove is for the tendon of the extensor carpi radialis. The lateral groove is for the tendon of the common digital extensor. There is a groove in the lateral styloid process, and a canal is formed in the lateral collateral ligament for the lateral digital extensor tendon. The deep surface of the extensor retinaculum serves as the dorsal aspect of the common fibrous joint capsule of the antebrachial, midcarpal, and carpometacarpal joints of the carpus. This retinaculum blends with the medial and lateral collateral ligaments of the carpus.

The extensor carpi obliquus tendon crosses over the tendon of the extensor carpi radialis in its course to insertion on the second metacarpal bone. This tendon is covered by a sheath as it crosses the extensor carpi radialis tendon and distal radius. A bursa is also interposed between the tendon and the medial collateral ligament of the carpus (5). In the adult horse, the tendon sheath and bursa frequently communicate.

The extensor carpi radialis crosses the dorsal surface of the carpus and inserts on the third metacarpal tuberosity. The sheath begins approximately 8 to 10 cm proximal to the carpus and extends to the middle of the carpus. The sheath ends at about the level of the intercarpal joint, wherein the tendon becomes closely associated with the fibrous portion

of the joint capsule befor insertion on the metacarpal tuberosity.

The common digital extensor tendon sheath begins approximately 7 to 8 cm above the carpus and extends to the carpometacarpal articulation and proximal metacarpus. A small tendon that originates from the radial head of the common digital extensor muscle shares the synovial sheath with the larger tendon beginning just proximal to the carpus.

The lateral extensor tendon sheath begins 6 to 8 cm proximal to the carpus and extends to the proximal metacarpus. The lateral digital extensor tendon passes through a canal formed between the superficial and deep parts of the lateral collateral ligament.

The origin of the ulnaris lateralis muscle is the lateral epicondyle of the humerus and the lateral collateral ligament of the elbow joint. As the muscle crosses the elbow, an associated sheath along its deep surface sometimes communicates with the elbow joint. As the ulnaris lateralis courses distad, the tendon bifurcates proximal to the accessory carpal bone into a short and a long tendon branch. The short tendon inserts on the proximal and lateral aspect of the accessory carpal bone and does not have a tendon sheath. The long tendon becomes surrounded by a sheath just distal to the bifurcation passing through a groove on the lateral surface of the accessory carpal bone to insert on the fourth metacarpal bone.

Caudomedial Forearm

The muscles of the caudomedial forearm are associated with flexion of the distal limb. The deep fascia over the palmar surface of the carpus is thickened to form a wide fascial band called the *flexor retinaculum,* similar to the extensor retinaculum of the dorsal carpus. The flexor retinaculum extends from the medial collateral ligament of the carpus to the accessory carpal bone. The carpal canal is thus formed, bounded palmarly by the flexor retinaculum, laterally by the accessory carpal bone, and dorsally by the palmar carpal ligament. Three tendons pass through the carpal canal: the deep digital flexor tendon; the superficial digital flexor tendon; and the flexor carpi radialis tendon. The tendon of the humeral head of the superficial digital flexor is joined by the accessory ligament or radial head of the muscle just under the flexor retinaculum. The tendon of the ulnar head of the deep digital flexor muscle is joined by the tendon of the humeral head of the muscle just before being enclosed by the carpal sheath. The superficial and deep digital flexor tendons are enveloped by a common synovial sheath called the *carpal synovial sheath,* which passes through the carpal canal. This sheath begins approximately 8 to 10 cm proximal to the carpus and extends distad to the middle of the metacarpus. At the medial aspect of the tendons of the superficial and deep digital flexor muscles and the carpal sheath are the large medial palmar artery and the medial palmar nerve. At the junction of the flexor retinaculum and the medial collateral ligament of the carpus a canal is formed to allow the passage of the flexor carpi radialis tendon. The flexor carpi radialis tendon is covered by a synovial sheath just proximal to this canal until just proximal to insertion on the second metacarpal bone. Caudal to the flexor carpi radialis tendon are the medial palmar vein and the radial artery. The palmar carpal ligament is the thickened palmar part of the common fibrous membrane of the joint capsule. This ligament is continued distally as the accessory ligament of the deep digital flexor.

The tendon of insertion of the flexor carpi ulnaris does not have a synovial sheath associated with it before insertion on the accessory carpal bone.

TARSUS

Craniolateral Aspect of Hind Leg

The *long digital extensor tendon* lies on the cranial aspect of the crus and courses over the dorsum of the tarsus just lateral to the medial trochlear ridge of the talus. A proximal, middle, and distal extensor retinaculum cover the long digital extensor tendon at the level of the tarsus. A synovial sheath encompasses this tendon from approximately the level of the lateral tibial malleolus and continues coverage through the distal retinaculum almost to the junction with the lateral digital extensor tendon. At this level, the conjoined tendons of the long digital and lateral digital extensor muscles continue distally similarly to the common digital tendon of the front limb.

In the area of the tarsocrural joint, the *peroneus tertius tendon* lies superficial to the tendon of the cranial tibial muscle. The peroneus tertius tendon forms a sleevelike cleft to allow passage of the cranial tibial tendon and associated synovial sheath. The peroneus tertius tendon divides into a dorsal branch that inserts on the third tarsal and third metatarsal bones and a lateral branch that blends with the middle retinaculum and inserts on the calcaneus and fourth tarsal bone. The *cranial tibial tendon* also divides into dorsal and medial branches. The dorsal branch inserts on the third metatarsal bone. The medial branch or cunean tendon courses over the long medial collateral ligament of the tarsus and inserts on the first tarsal bone. A subtendinous bursa called the *cunean bursa* is present between the medial branch of the cranial tibial tendon and the long medial collateral ligament (see the section of this chapter on bursas).

The lateral digital extensor tendon of the hind limb courses distad across the lateral surface of the hock. The tendon crosses the lateral malleolus in a groove and is bound by two retinacula, a lateral digital extensor retinaculum and a distal extensor retinaculum. A synovial sheath surrounds the tendon, which extends from just proximal to the proximal retinaculum and ends distal to the distal retinaculum to just before the lateral digital extensor tendon joins the long digital extensor tendon.

A small muscle, the *short digital extensor* (*extensor digitorum brevis*), fills the angle between the long digital extensor tendon and the lateral digital extensor tendon just on the distal aspect of the tarsus. This muscle originates from the lateral collateral ligament, the lateral branch of the peroneus tertius tendon, and the middle extensor retinaculum and inserts on the two large extensor tendons on which it acts.

Caudal Aspect of Hind Leg

The *superficial digital flexor muscle* is almost entirely tendinous in the hind limb. It courses distally from the supracondyloid fossa of the caudodistal femur cranial to the lateral and medial gastrocnemius tendons. The *superficial digital flexor tendon* emerges from the medial aspect of the gastrocnemius tendon to lie superficial to the gastrocnemius tendon. The superficial digital flexor tendon is then joined by the flat tarsal tendons of the biceps femoris and semitendinosus muscles. At this point, the superficial digital flexor tendon flattens before inserting on the medial and lateral aspects of the tuber calcis. The calcaneal tendon of the gastrocnemius muscles inserts on the plantar surface of the tuber calcaneus. A small bursa lies between the superficial digital flexor tendon and the tuber calcaneus. A subtendinous calcanean bursa is also present between the superficial digital flexor and gastrocnemius tendons just above the insertion onto the tuber calcaneus. This subtendinous bursa extends 7 to 10 cm above and below the point of the hock. A communication usually exists between these two bursa along the lateral aspect of the gastrocnemius tendon. There is no accessory ligament of the superficial digital flexor muscle in the hind limb because of the primarily tendinous nature of this muscle.

The *deep digital flexor muscle* consists of three heads: a medial head (long digital flexor); a superficial head (caudal tibial); and a deep head (flexor digiti I longus). The caudal tibial muscle is cranial (deep) to the superficial digital flexor and medial to the lateral digital extensor and long digital flexor. The flexor digiti I longus is the largest of the three heads and is cranial to the caudal tibial muscle. These two muscles combine to form one tendon just above the hock. The tendon lies deep to the flexor retinaculum, which runs from the tuber calcaneus to the medial collateral ligament of the tarsus. The tarsal synovial sheath surrounds the deep digital flexor tendon from 4 to 6 cm proximal to the tarsus and extends to about 12 to 16 cm distal to tarsus. The long digital flexor tendon crosses the medial surface of the tarsus and joins the deep digital flexor tendon distal to the tarsus. This tendon is held in position as it crosses the tarsus by two flexor retinacula, which are thickenings of the deep tarsal fascia. A synovial sheath surrounds the long digital flexor tendon, which begins proximal to the proximal retinaculum and extends distal to the distal retinaculum.

The tarsal fascia on the plantar surface of the tarsus thickens to form the *flexor retinaculum*. This retinaculum blends medially with fascia from the plantar aspect of the medial collateral ligament of the tarsal joint. It also attaches to the calcaneus above the sustentaculum tali, to the sustentaculum tali, and to the medial surfaces of the central tarsal bone, the fused first and second tarsal bones, and the second metatarsal bone. Laterally, it is continuous with the long plantar ligament on the plantar surface of the calcaneus. The plantar surface of the sustentaculum tali of the calcaneus has a smooth surface with a groove for the passage of the principal tendon of the deep digital flexor muscle.

The tibial nerve divides in the distal crural region into the medial and lateral plantar nerves, which course through the tarsal canal on the lateral aspect of the deep flexor tendon. The medial plantar nerve and artery cross the plantar surface of the deep digital flexor tendon at the level of the tarsometatarsal articulation. The medial and lateral plantar arteries course through the tarsal canal with the deep digital flexor tendon.

CLINICAL PRESENTATION OF TENOSYNOVITIS

Tenosynovitis by definition is inflammation of a tendon sheath. Tenosynovitis has been reported to present with distention of a tendon sheath with synovial effusion (6–8). The manifestation of tenosynovitis usually depends on the amount and the duration of the inflammation. Classification of tenosynovitis has previously been reported (6). This scheme is based on inflammation and divides tenosynovitis into 1) idiopathic, 2) acute, 3) chronic, and 4) septic. The inflammatory response of the synovial structures is nonspecific, and the difference is more of degree than of type. The inflammatory response can be described much like inflammation of a joint capsule. The term *synovitis* implies that inflammation is limited to the synovial lining of a tendon sheath. *Capsulitis,* generally found in more chronic tenosynovitis, implies that inflammation has extended into the fibrous portion of the tendon sheath. Chronic tenosynovitis can manifest as a proliferative fibrosis that may obliterate the synovial sheath. Tenosynovitis should be further defined by anatomic location.

Examinations of horses with tenosynovitis should include careful palpation of the limb, manipulation of the tendons, ligaments, and joints associated with the sheath, and application of digital pressure to all relevant structures to elicit a painful response and, if possible, to exacerbate or create a lameness. Lameness associated with tenosynovitis varies considerably and probably depends on the degree of inflammation and the amount of effusion present within the sheath. Acute tenosynovitis typically presents with mild to moderate effusion of the synovial sheath without associated lameness. Serious injuries to some of the tendons and ligaments associated with a sheath can have moderate effusion without apparent lameness. The lack of lameness therefore should not preclude the use of diagnostic ultrasound in evaluating synovial effusions of tendon sheaths.

The clinical examination should indicate that the tendon sheath and tendons or ligaments associated with the sheath are the clinical problems. If this is not possible and if lameness is present, then perineural or intrasynovial anesthesia should be used. Synovial fluid analysis may help one to determine the intensity of the inflammatory response if other findings are equivocal. A complete series of high-detail ra-

diographs of the area may also be necessary. Clinical assessment is critical before the significance of the sonographic findings can be interpreted and an accurate treatment and prognosis can be given.

Structural damage or primary injury to tendons or ligaments within or around the synovial sheath resulting in tenosynovitis is discussed in detail elsewhere in this book.

Idiopathic Tenosynovitis

Idiopathic tenosynovitis is present when there is synovial effusion within a tendon sheath without obvious signs of inflammation, pain, or lameness. Clinical examination reveals a nonpainful synovial distention of the tendon sheath and, if a synovial sample is collected, a normal synovial fluid analysis. Usually, the horse has no history of an inciting cause for the tendon sheath distention. Effusion without inflammation is thought to occur insidiously from low-grade chronic trauma. Poor conformation is thought to predispose animals to some forms of tenosynovitis, such as that seen in tarsal sheath effusion (thoroughpin). Tendon sheath effusion may occur because of stretching of the sheath resulting from an increasing workload, obesity, or pregnancy. The most common sites for idiopathic effusion are the digital sheath, tarsal sheath, and extensor tendon sheaths of the carpus. Although most cases of idiopathic tenosynovitis are considered cosmetic blemishes, sonographic evaluation may be necessary to document normal architecture of the sheath and associated structures. Foals born with or that later develop extensor tendon sheath effusion should be carefully evaluated with ultrasound for underlying extensor tendon damage.

Distention of the synovial sheath by an effusion is probably self-perpetuating. Gross distention stretches the synovial cells lining the synovial membrane, with subsequent gap formation between the cells. This allows fluid and protein to leak into the sheath, thereby adding more volume to the effusion. The duration of the effusion may therefore limit a dramatic response to simple drainage. Investigators have reported that idiopathic tenosynovitis may be treated by injection of the synovial sheath with a corticosteroid (8). The underlying cause (e.g., prevailing management practices, workload, abnormal shoeing) should be defined and corrected.

Acute Tenosynovitis

Acute tenosynovitis is present when effusion, inflammation, pain, or lameness rapidly develops within a tendon sheath. Acute tenosynovitis is usually associated with some form of traumatic injury. A known incident such as hitting a jump or a fall during a work or turnout may indicate the origin of the injury. A delayed onset with otherwise rapid development of synovial sheath effusion may occur. This situation may occur when a racehorse returns from a work or race and develops effusion hours to days after the suspected injury. Structural damage to one or more of the tendons or ligaments associated with the tendon sheath may be the underlying cause of the effusion present in the sheath.

Complete sonographic examination is indicated in this form of tenosynovitis, to preclude further damage to injured structures (Fig. 26.1). Documentation of the specific structures involved and classification of the injury are necessary to institute appropriate therapy and to monitor the reparative process. Those horses without sonographic evidence of structural damage to the soft tissues associated with the sheath should have a complete set of high-detail radiographs taken to rule out osseous abnormalities such as fractures. Those horses with tendinitis or desmitis should have therapy aimed at reducing inflammation of the appropriate structure. Treatment of tendinitis or desmitis will be discussed in other chapters of this book.

If no structural damage of the tendons or ligaments can be documented, then rest combined with cold hydrotherapy, anti-inflammatory agents, and support wraps should be employed initially. Aspiration of the effusion and injection of corticosteroid or hyaluronic acid may be used if signs persist longer than a week.

Chronic Tenosynovitis

Chronic tenosynovitis typically is unresolved acute tenosynovitis. Repeated trauma to a specific area may cause multiple episodes of acute tenosynovitis and may subsequently lead to chronic tenosynovitis. Persistent effusion and inflammation present in chronic tenosynovitis frequently leads to a thickening of the fibrous portion of the sheath. Typically, the function of the sheath must be compromised to be classified as chronic; otherwise, idiopathic tenosynovitis would be classified with chronic tenosynovitis. Fibrous adhesions of the parietal and visceral layers of the sheath may form and may restrict the gliding motion of the tendon through the sheath. Structural damage to the sheath, tendon, or related structures without appropriate rest or therapy is frequently the cause of the persistent inflammation. Chronic tenosynovitis may occur after a laceration involving skin, subcutaneous tissue, tendon sheath, and sometimes a portion of or the entire tendon. Attempts to suture the tendon should be made only when lacerations involve the entire tendon. The one-wound, one-scar concept of wound healing leads one to expect adhesions across full-thickness lacerations and prompts strategic measures for prevention (9). Infections of the sheath secondary to lacerations may lead to chronic restrictive tenosynovitis.

An attempt to define the inciting cause of the inflammation should be made before treatment is instituted. Elimination of the cause of any repeated trauma should be the primary goal of therapy. Sonographic examination frequently reveals a diffuse proliferative response of the sheath that complicates accurate identification of underlying structural damage. Villonodular masses do occur within synovial sheaths (10) (Fig. 26.2). Care should be taken to define the location of villonodular masses as intraluminal or extraluminal and to determine that no other masses exist. Adhe-

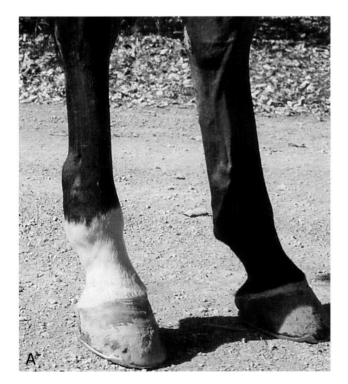
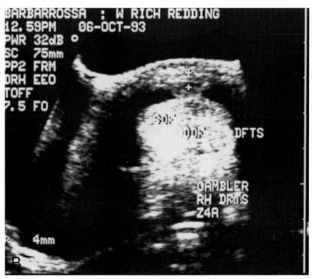

Figure 26.1. A, Clinical appearance of acute tenosynovitis of the digital sheath of the hind limb in a hunter. Notice the digital sheath has a prominent lateral protrusion, which at this stage is primarily effusion. **B,** Sonogram of the same animal with acute tenosynovitis. Notice the anechoic fluid surrounding the superficial and deep digital flexor tendon at zone 3A. The natural axial connection of the annular ligament to the superficial digital flexor tendon is evident at the cursors.

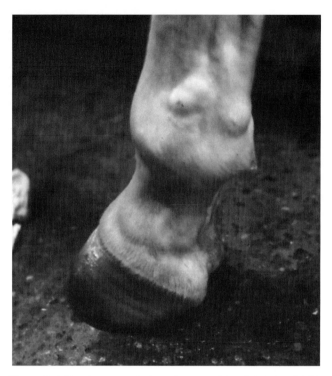

Figure 26.2. Focal mass on the lateral aspect of the digital sheath. This was found to be an intraluminal mass consistent with a villonodular synovitis.

sions between a tendon and the sheath and between a tendon and another tendon or between any of these structures and a villonodular mass or masses may be found on sonographic examination. It may become necessary to inject a contrast or fluid medium to define the synovial membrane and the structures within the sheath. Contrast radiography, which has been previously reported, may also be used and may complement the sonographic examination (10–12). Symptomatic treatment of chronic tenosynovitis includes drainage and injection of a hyaluronic acid product or a corticosteroid. These injections may be repeated at regular intervals. Persistence of lameness after medical therapy may dictate surgical exploration to define and remove the specific problem. Endoscopy with an arthroscope has been reported and allows adequate access to the structures of the digital sheath (13). The same principles of triangulation with an arthroscope and instrumentation can be used in other synovial sheaths. More extensive surgical exploration of the sheath may be warranted in cases of proliferative synovitis because the operator's ability to distend the sheath and to attain adequate exposure with an arthroscope is limited. In some instances, resection of the retinaculum or the annular ligament may be warranted to relieve compression on soft tissue structures within a carpal or fetlock canal, respectively.

Septic Tenosynovitis

Infection of a tendon sheath is typically presented as a severe, non–weight-bearing lameness with heat, pain, and diffuse swelling. Punctures, lacerations, and iatrogenic infections are the most common causes of septic tenosynovitis, although infections of hematogenous origin do occur. The nonspecific action of many of the enzymes of inflammation can destroy the fibrils and matrix of the tendon within the synovial sheath. Fibrin deposition within the synovial sheath may lead to fibrous adhesion formation. Therapy should be aggressive and should follow the same principles as for septic arthritis. Broad-spectrum bactericidal parenteral antibiotics and some form of a sheath drainage procedure typically involving lavage with a balanced electrolyte solution should be instituted immediately. The location of the sheath may dictate the form of drainage procedure. An incision to open the sheath, to remove fibrin and debris, and to lavage the interior of the sheath is frequently necessary. Placement of Penrose drains, closed-suction drains, and irrigation devices may be used at the discretion of the clinician.

Sonographic examination is not necessary to make a diagnosis of septic tenosynovitis, but it is a useful adjunct to subsequent treatment. Sonographic examination may be helpful in finding a pocket of fluid for collection of a synovial fluid sample for culture and sensitivity testing as well as for synovial fluid analysis. The sonographic appearance of the synovial fluid can vary depending on the cellular content and the formation of fibrin. The prognosis can be modified based on the extent of degenerative changes of the tendon or tendons. Placement of a closed-suction drain at the distalmost extent of the sheath may be assisted by the use of ultrasound. Sequential sonographic examinations should be used to assess the response to therapy. This is particularly important to evaluate the effectiveness of a closed-suction apparatus in collecting the accumulating fluid formed within the sheath.

Intrasynovial fistulas can occur between a tendon sheath and a joint. Fistulas are thought to have a traumatic origin. The clinical presentation of a synovial fistula is similar to that of tenosynovitis, with effusion of the involved synovial sheath. Lameness may be present in a horse with a synovial fistula. The effusion can be massaged between the tendon sheath and the joint. Sonographic evidence of the fistula or movement of the fluid from one synovial cavity to the next may be visualized. Contrast radiography may also be used. Fistulas have been reported between the common digital extensor tendon sheath and the intercarpal joint or radiocarpal joint, the extensor carpi radialis tendon sheath and the intercarpal joint, and under the long digital extensor tendon in association with the proximal or distal interphalangeal joint of the digit. Surgical repair of the fistula is necessary to close the fibrous defect in both the sheath and the joint.

Digital Flexor Tendon Sheath

Most current literature on sonographic examination of the palmar metacarpus routinely evaluates the distal carpal sheath and the proximal digital flexor tendon sheath (14,

15). Most of this literature emphasizes examination of the superficial and deep digital flexor tendons, the suspensory ligament, and the inferior check ligament. Sonographic examination of the structures of the fetlock canal and palmar pastern has been reported (16–19). Although "wind puffs" or "wind galls" may be used to describe a swelling of a joint or sheath, these terms are most frequently used to describe idiopathic tenosynovitis of the digital flexor tendon sheath. The digital flexor tendon sheath is also frequently involved in traumatic acute tenosynovitis. Acute tenosynovitis occurring in the digital flexor tendon sheath of a performance horse necessitates close evaluation of the superficial digital flexor and deep digital flexor tendons and the annular ligament. Injury to the distal sesamoidean ligaments, which are outside the digital flexor tendon sheath in the digit, may also cause mild acute tenosynovitis because of the proximity of the inflammatory response.

Chronic tenosynovitis is usually due to unresolved acute tenosynovitis. Injuries involving multiple structures or severe injuries to a single structure that instigate an intense and prolonged inflammatory response are more likely to lead to chronic tenosynovitis of the digital sheath. Clinical and sonographic examinations reveal an inflammatory response characterized by fibrous thickening of the tendon sheath (Fig. 26.3). Lameness is more likely to be present in horses with chronic tenosynovitis of the digital flexor tendon sheath. Chronic tenosynovitis of the digital flexor tendon sheath may cause type 2 annular ligament constriction syndrome within the palmar or plantar fetlock canal (19) (Fig. 26.4). This condition may resemble type 3 annular ligament constriction syndrome, characterized by thickening of the annular ligament and a loss of echogenicity of the superficial digital flexor tendons (Fig. 26.5). Both may appear to have a notched appearance along the palmar or plantar border of the fetlock when viewed from the side. In both syndromes, horses may have a history of chronic lameness not improving with rest and worsening with exercise. Intrasynovial corticosteroid injection may provide temporary relief in the case of chronic tenosynovitis. Repeated injections may be necessary to manage this condition. Typically, animals with type 2 annular ligament constrictions are candidates for annular ligament resection. Type 3 annular ligament constrictions require appropriate therapy for the tendinitis, and, in some instances, annular ligament resection may be beneficial. Villonodular synovitis, discussed earlier, has been reported to occur in the digital flexor tendon sheath and the calcaneal bursa (10). Isolated masses may be found, or the condition may be part of a chronic proliferative tenosynovitis.

The digital flexor tendon sheath is also commonly involved in lacerations and puncture wounds. Close inspection of wounds in this area is essential to rule out involvement of the digital sheath. Lacerations that involve the sheath should be examined sonographically to ascertain whether the tendon is involved. Meticulous debridement of the wound edges with copious lavage ideally allows the

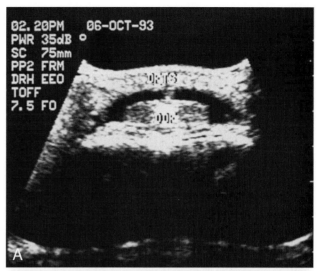

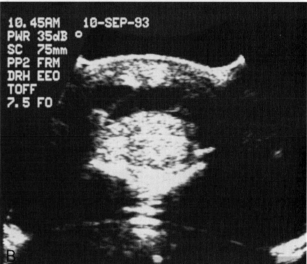

Figure 26.3. A, Chronic tenosynovitis of the distal digital flexor tendon sheath at distal aspect of the pastern. Anechoic fluid surrounds the deep digital flexor tendon, which is of normal size and appearance, but the sheath wall is thickened. **B,** Chronic tenosynovitis of the proximal digital flexor tendon sheath within the fetlock canal. Anechoic fluid fills the sheath while fibrous tags adhere to the sheath wall.

sheath to be sutured primarily. Horses with wounds to the digital flexor tendon sheath should have a sonographic examination after an appropriate period to determine whether adhesions have formed. Intrasynovial hyaluronic acid given early in the repair process may prevent adhesion formation and may therefore be included in the treatment of healing wounds of the digital flexor tendons or of the digital flexor tendon sheath (20).

Extensor Tendon Sheaths that Cross the Carpus

Tenosynovitis of the extensor tendon sheaths of the carpus is frequently due to direct trauma to the dorsal surface of the carpus, particularly in horses that jump fences. Effusions of the extensor tendon sheaths are most commonly as-

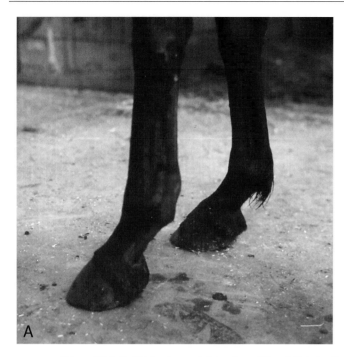

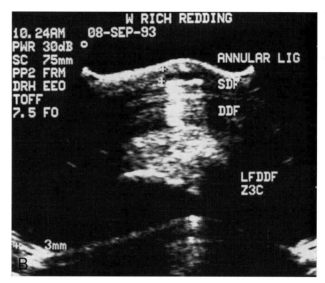

Figure 26.4. A, Thickening and distention of the digital sheath. The notched appearance is caused by palmar protrusion of the distended digital sheath proximal to the annular ligament. **B,** Longitudinal sonogram of the same limb. The proximal aspect is to the right and the distal aspect is to the left. Notice the palmar protrusion of the digital sheath, which is filled with fluid. The skin and annular ligament measure 3 mm, which is considered within normal limits; therefore, this is classified as a type 1 annular ligament constriction.

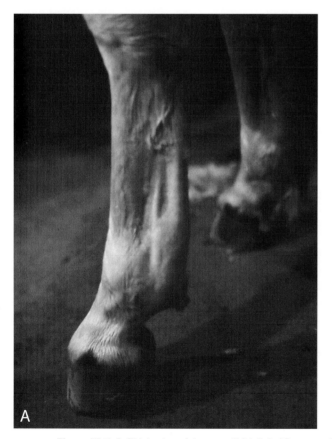

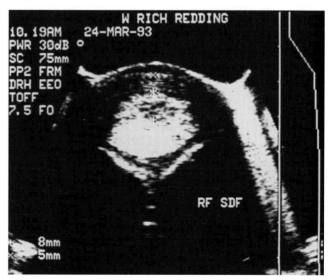

Figure 26.5. A, Thickening of the superficial digital flexor tendon caused by diffuse tendinitis. Although tendinitis is the dominant feature, the digital flexor tendon sheath is also thickened. **B,** Sonogram of the same limb shows a thickened annular ligament with a focal core type of defect of the superficial digital flexor tendon.

sociated with the common digital extensor tendon (Fig. 26.6). The sheath is distended and typically presents as two swellings proximal and distal to the extensor retinaculum. The fluid can be manually pressed from proximal to distal, and this feature may be used to generate more complete images of the borders of the common digital extensor tendon during the ultrasound examination. Sonographic evidence that the fluid is escaping the synovial sheath and entering the underlying joint indicates a synovial fistula. The sonographic appearance of the fluid can vary with the amount of cellular and inflammatory debris. This may suggest the origin and duration of the tenosynovitis. A cellular effusion implies an acute injury, possibly with hemorrhage or intense inflammatory response. Anechoic fluid with fibrous tags may develop in more long-standing synovial sheath effusion.

Foals born with or that later develop extensor tendon sheath effusion may have flexural deformity of the carpus. Whether such common digital extensor tendon damage results from the flexural deformity or is created by the deformity is unknown. Sonographic examination may help to determine whether active tendon damage or tendon rupture has occurred. The prognosis is good even in foals with tendon rupture if the flexural deformity is not severe.

Carpal Canal

The carpal sheath in the proximal palmar metacarpus is seen on routine sonographic examinations as an anechoic space between the deep digital flexor tendon and the inferior check ligament. Mild effusions of the carpal sheath may be seen primarily as an enlargement of this anechoic space in

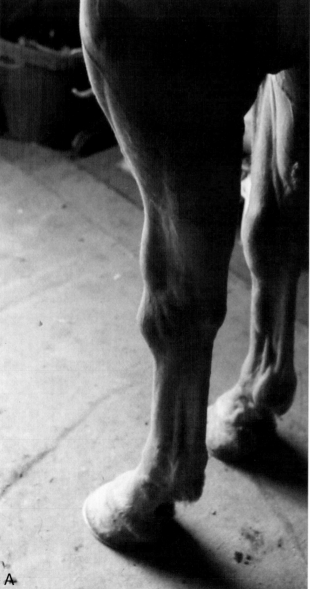

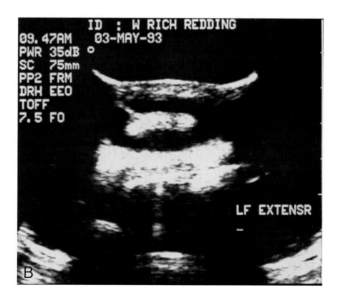

Figure 26.6. A, Acute tenosynovitis of the common digital extensor tendon sheath. The proximal and distal pouches are filled with effusion on either side of the extensor retinaculum. **B,** Sonogram of the common digital extensor sheath. Effusion surrounds the tendon demonstrating a mesotendon attaching to the tendon from the dorsal aspect of the sheath.

the proximal palmar metacarpus. Some effusions may extend to the midmetacarpus or as far as the proximal digital sheath. Larger effusions may extend proximal to the carpus with pronounced swellings laterally between the ulnaris lateralis and lateral digital extensor muscles and medially between the flexor carpi ulnaris and flexor carpi radialis muscles. Although idiopathic tenosynovitis does occasionally occur in the carpal sheath, acute tenosynovitis is probably more typical. Acute tenosynovitis of the carpal sheath may be due to injuries to the deep or superficial digital flexor tendon in the proximal metacarpus (21). Tendinitis of the deep digital flexor and superficial digital flexor tendons should therefore be ruled out before therapy for primary tenosynovitis is instituted. Acute tenosynovitis of the carpal sheath accompanied by severe lameness on flexion of the carpus may be due to fractures within the carpus, particularly fracture of the accessory carpal bone. A complete set of high-detail radiographs should routinely be included in evaluations of horses with acute tenosynovitis with mild to moderate lameness of the forelimb.

Various conditions may create chronic tenosynovitis of the carpal sheath. Direct trauma to the soft tissues of the carpal canal and fractures of the palmar aspect of the carpus (accessory carpal bone) may cause acute synovitis of the carpal sheath. Continued trauma to the soft tissues of the palmar carpus and callus formation resultant from fracture repair may lead to chronic tenosynovitis of the carpal sheath. Osteochondroma or slow-growing exostosis of the distal caudal radius may create chronic tenosynovitis (Fig. 26.7).

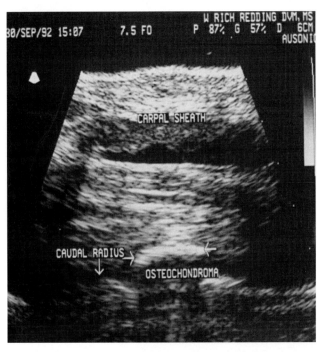

Figure 26.7. Longitudinal sonogram of chronic tenosynovitis of the carpal sheath caused by an osteochondroma of the caudomedial aspect of the distal radius. The proliferative synovial membrane adjacent to the effusion appears less echogenic than the fibrous capsule.

Proliferative fibrous thickening of the carpal sheath characteristic of chronic tenosynovitis of the carpal sheath can result in carpal canal syndrome from compression of the neurovascular structures that course through the carpal canal. Intrasynovial corticosteroid may provide temporary relief, but carpal canal syndrome frequently requires sectioning of the flexor retinaculum for return to soundness. Osteochondromas should be removed, and if this is not successful, sectioning of the flexor retinaculum may be required.

Tarsus

Tarsal Sheath

The normal tarsal sheath is not routinely visualized on sonographic examinations of the plantar tarsus. A moderate amount of effusion is typically present and is apparent as two swellings cranial to the calcaneal tendon on both medial and lateral aspects of the distal crus. In more pronounced effusions of the tarsal sheath, a distal swelling may be seen distal to the hock on the medial aspect of the tarsometatarsal joint. Swellings of the tarsal sheath are called *thoroughpin*. Thoroughpin is a morphologic description and can exist with varying degrees of inflammation. Most cases of thoroughpin, however, are classified as idiopathic tenosynovitis. Idiopathic tenosynovitis can occur bilaterally and in some instances is probably due to conformation.

Acute tenosynovitis of the tarsal sheath, however, can manifest with varying degrees of inflammation and lameness. This necessitates a more accurate definition of the underlying cause of acute tenosynovitis of the tarsal sheath. Acute tarsal sheath effusion usually occurs unilaterally, with sudden onset of moderate to severe lameness. Acute tenosynovitis of the tarsal sheath is thought in most instances to be traumatically induced. Frequently, the horse has a history of a known trauma to the medial aspect of the tarsus. Fractures of the bones of the tarsus, avulsion fracture of the sustentaculum tali (around the attachment of the middle short medial tarsocrural ligament, which attaches to the distomedial aspect of the sustentaculum tali), or overstretching of the sheath may cause aseptic tenosynovitis of the tarsal sheath. Radiographs of the tarsus including the dorsomedial–plantarolateral and dorsplantar (flexed) projections should be included in the diagnostic workup. Previous reports of chronic unilateral tarsal sheath effusion with lameness frequently revealed new bone production on the sustentaculum tali and fibrillation of the deep digital flexor tendon on gross inspection (22, 23). Contrast radiography may assist in further defining both acute and chronic tarsal sheath abnormalities.

Wounds to the tarsus should be evaluated for the possibility of penetration into the tarsal sheath and the closely positioned tibiotarsal joint. Treatment of septic tenosynovitis has been discussed previously in this chapter. Chronic septic tenosynovitis may progress to osteomyelitis of the sustentaculum tali and adhesions of the deep digital flexor tendon and carries an unfavorable prognosis.

Extensor Tendons that Cross the Tarsus

Direct trauma is the most likely cause of tenosynovitis of the extensor tendons of the tarsus. The lateral digital extensor tendon sometimes develops idiopathic or acute tenosynovitis (Fig. 26.8). The swelling within the synovial sheath protrudes proximal and distal to the retinaculum of the lateral digital extensor. Sonographic examination rarely determines associated tendon injury. These effusions often persist in spite of appropriate treatment.

The long digital extensor tendon is rarely affected. I have seen one case of acute tenosynovitis initiated by blunt trauma to the dorsal surface of the tarsus. The distal aspect of the peroneus tertius tendon was damaged as well (Fig. 26.9). The horse remained sound, but a prominent swelling of the dorsal tarsus remained.

GENERAL BURSAL ANATOMY

A *bursa* (*bursa synovialis*) is a closed sac lined with a membrane closely resembling a synovial membrane. A bursa is present on a limb or at specific areas of the body that generally have limited movement but with untoward pressure against a portion of bone, tendon, or ligament. A bursa can also be found in areas to facilitate the gliding action of a tendon, particularly in an area of stress such as in the vicinity of the tendon's attachment. The surface of the bone or the portions of the tendon or ligament contacting the bone may become cartilaginous. Bursae have been classified based on anatomic position (subcutaneous, subfascial, subligamentous, submuscular, and subtendinous) or by the method of formation (congenital and acquired). *Congenital bursae* are located in a predictable position and are termed true or constant bursae. *Acquired bursae* typically develop subcutaneously in response to pressure and friction and are called inconstant bursae. Skin movement causes tearing of the subcutaneous tissue allowing fluid to accumulate that later becomes encapsulated by fibrous tissue. In the later stages of development, bursae develop a synovial-like membrane which has a similar structural appearance to congenital bursae. In general, bursae beneath the deep fascia or among tendon, muscle, and bone are constant, whereas those between the skin and other structures (subcutaneous bursae) are inconstant.

A bursa may communicate with a joint or tendon sheath in close proximity (e.g., bursa beneath the long digital extensor tendon and the lateral femorotibial joint of the stifle, subtendinous bursa with the tendon sheath of the abductor pollicis longus in older horses (5), and bicipital bursa and the scapulohumeral joint). These may become clinically apparent because of effusions from the respective joint or sheath that cause filling of the bursa.

The constant bursae most commonly found of clinical significance are the navicular bursa, the cunean bursa, the bicipital bursa, the trochanteric bursa, and the subtendinous bursae of the common calcaneal tendon. The acquired bursae most commonly found of clinical significance are the

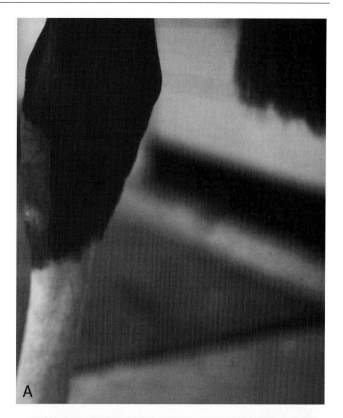

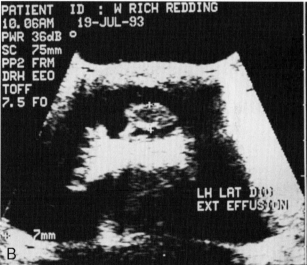

Figure 26.8. A, Dorsal surface of the tarsus with effusion present in the lateral digital extensor synovial sheath. **B,** Sonogram of the lateral digital flexor tendon and sheath of the hind limb. Effusion surrounds the tendon, showing a mesotendon attaching to the tendon from the medial aspect of the sheath. Dorsal is to the right and plantar is to the left.

olecranon bursa, the subcutaneous calcaneal bursae, and carpal hygroma.

SPECIFIC BURSAE

The cunean and calcaneal bursae have been discussed previously in this chapter.

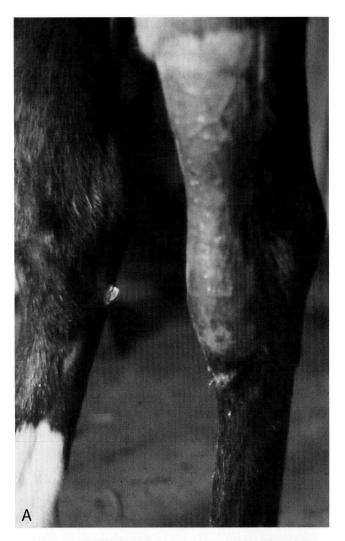

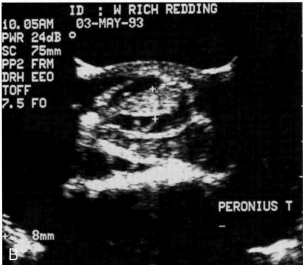

Figure 26.9. A, Soft tissue swelling of the dorsal surface of the tarsus. This swelling is filled with fluid. **B,** Sonogram of the long digital flexor tendon just above the medial trochlea of the talus. Diffuse swelling of the subcutaneous tissues is present as well as effusion within the synovial sheath of the long digital flexor tendon. The increased inflammatory debris present in the fluid appears as echogenic material.

Navicular Bursa (Bursa Podotrochlearis)

The navicular bursa is interposed between the deep digital flexor tendon and the navicular bone before insertion of the tendon on the distal phalanx. The bursa is lined by a synovial membrane, except along the fibrocartilage of the navicular bone and along the surface of the deep digital flexor tendon, which apposes the fibrocartilage.

Bicipital Bursa (Bursa Intertubercularis)

The tendon of origin of the biceps brachii passes from the supraglenoid tubercle of the scapula and occupies the intertubercular groove. The bicipital (intertubercular) bursa lies under the tendon of the biceps brachii in the intertubercular groove and surrounds the tendon. The tendon at this level is partly cartilaginous and is closely molded to the intermediate ridge. This bursa does not typically communicate with the scapulohumeral joint.

Trochanteric Bursa

The trochanteric bursa is large and lies between the flat tendon of the gluteus accessorius muscle and the cartilage of the convexity of the trochanter major as the tendon courses to its insertion on the crest distal to the trochanter.

Bursa of the Common Digital Extensor Tendon at the Fetlock and Pastern Joints

The common digital extensor muscle has a bursa interposed between the tendon of insertion and the dorsal aspect of the fetlock and pastern joint. The common digital extensor tendon often has a bursa near the union with the extensor branches of the suspensory ligament.

Bursae of the Extensor Branches of the Suspensory Ligament

Bursae are present under the extensor branches of the suspensory ligament as they course dorsodistad to joint the common digital extensor tendon. These bursae are so extensive that they may be considered synovial sheaths. Small subcutaneous bursae may occur on the palmar surface of the fetlock joint and on the lateral surface of the fetlock just proximal to the extensor branches of the suspensory ligament.

Other Bursae

Many bursae are not discussed in detail in this chapter primarily because of a lack of clinical significance. Some of these include the bursa of the infraspinatus tendon of insertion, which may communicate with the shoulder joint, a bursa associated with the coracobrachialis tendon of origin, a bursa associated with the tendon of insertion of the subscapularis. A constant bursa is present deep to the flexor tendons at the distal extent of the third metacarpal bone, which lies between the fibrous joint capsule of the palmar fetlock. This bursa may communicate with the fetlock joint.

CLINICAL PRESENTATION OF BURSITIS

Bursitis by definition is inflammation present within a bursa. Constant or acquired bursae may be involved, but they have different clinical presentations. True bursitis involves a constant bursa and is caused by direct trauma, or it may be associated with the stress of racing or performance (use trauma). *Traumatic bursitis,* as this condition is known, is the most common form of bursitis in true bursae. Traumatic bursitis most commonly occurs in the bicipital, trochanteric, and cunean bursae. Varying degrees of lameness are present in horses with bursitis in these areas. Rest is the preferred method of treatment for direct traumatic bursitis such as bicipital bursitis. Use-trauma forms of traumatic bursitis are generally secondary to an underlying primary problem such as tarsitis or bone spavin. Appropriate treatment requires addressing the primary problem.

Acquired bursitis has been defined as the development of a subcutaneous bursa and or inflammation of that bursa (6). Acquired bursae usually develop after direct mechanical trauma with subsequent hemorrhage or fluid accumulation. Acquired bursitis does not typically result in lameness, but with chronicity, it can cause a mechanical limitation to flexion of the corresponding joint. The most common locations of acquired bursitis are over the olecranon (capped elbow), the dorsal carpus (carpal hygroma), and the tuber calcaneus (capped hock). These acquired bursae first and foremost require the prevention of repeated trauma to the area. Acute lesions may resolve spontaneously. Lesions that do not resolve spontaneously may require drainage and injection of corticosteroid followed by pressure bandage. If response to treatment is poor at this time, the placement of drains may be necessary to empty the cavity and to enhance fibrosis across the cavity.

Septic bursitis occurs when a bursa becomes infected. This most often occurs following a puncture wound. Septic bursitis can occur within any constant bursa, but it is more frequent in the navicular and the calcaneal bursae. Aggressive treatment in the form of surgical debridement is necessary. Septic bursitis carries a guarded prognosis.

Traumatic Bursitis

Bicipital Bursa

Bicipital bursitis is commonly due to a traumatic injury to the point of the shoulder. The horse has a characteristic way of traveling if the shoulder is fixed because of pain. Direct pressure and palpation of the bicipital bursa may elicit a painful response in horses with an acute case. Frequently, it becomes necessary to inject a local anesthetic agent into the bursa to prove that the lameness originates in the bicipital bursa. Radiographs of the shoulder may need to be included to rule out other causes of shoulder lameness such as

calcification of the biceps tendon, fractures of the supraglenoid tuberosity or the proximal humerus, and osteochondrosis of the scapulohumeral joint. Injection of corticosteroid into the bursa and rest are the preferred methods of treatment.

Cunean Bursa

The cunean bursa is present under the medial branch of the cranial tibialis tendon of insertion. *Cunean bursitis* usually occurs in conjunction with inflammation of the soft tissues around the distal tarsal joints (cunean bursitis or tarsitis). Usually, one sees no obvious swelling of this bursa, and diagnosis requires resolution of the lameness by placement of a local anesthetic directly into the bursa. The response of the medial tarsus of characteristic of bone spavin (Jack spavin) should not be confused with swelling of the bursa. Sonographic examination may be of value to evaluate effusion if it is present or to document changes within the cranial tibial tendon if it exists.

The injection of corticosteroid into the cunean bursa and the tarsometatarsal and distal intertarsal joints is usually sufficient to treat cunean tarsitis. Treatment should also include shoeing changes, appropriate rehabilitation to strengthen the soft tissues of the tarsus, and rest, if necessary. I have seen several cases of persistent cunean bursa effusion after repeated injection of corticosteroid into the bursa. This effusion did not appear to cause lameness or untoward effect.

Navicular Bursitis

Navicular disease is a degenerative disease involving the navicular bone, navicular bursa, and deep digital flexor tendon. Although the pathogenesis is not completely understood, one typically sees erosion and ulceration of the fibrocartilage on the flexor surface of the navicular bone and tearing of the fibers of the deep digital flexor tendon, with an accompanying chronic synovitis or bursitis of the navicular bursa. Unfortunately, sonographic examination of the navicular area is difficult at best and adds little to defining this problem. The bursa can be seen in part on longitudinal scan of the distal palmar digit, but little information can be gained because of the position of the bursa within the foot. More experience with the use of diagnostic ultrasound in clinical navicular disease may prove useful in determining changes developing within the deep flexor tendon and navicular bursa. At present, clinical examination and radiographic evidence of degenerative changes of the navicular bone are most critical to a diagnosis.

Trochanteric Bursitis

Trochanteric bursitis is a poorly defined inflammation of the trochanteric bursa. This problem is generally secondary to tarsal problems. Sometimes trochanteric bursitis presents with a localized area painful to palpation and lameness can be alleviated when this area is blocked. This area of pain frequently extends cranially into the gluteal muscle. Sonographic examination of the gluteal muscle, tendon and trochanteric bursa has not been routinely performed by the author. Continued use of diagnostic ultrasound in clinical cases of trochanteric bursitis might provide insight as the cause of the lameness and palpable pain.

Acquired Bursitis

Olecranon Bursitis

Olecranon bursitis (*shoe boil, capped elbow*) is an acquired bursitis typically due to trauma from contact of the ipsilateral horseshoe with the elbow. The injury may occur when the animal lies down or, in the gaited horse, during work. Repeated trauma is prevented by wrapping the foot in a boot or cotton bandage. In the acute stages, fluid is usually present within the bursa. Lameness is typically not present unless the bursitis has become septic. Draining tracts suggest infection, which may be iatrogenic or due to a foreign body. As the condition becomes chronic, the fluid is sometimes replaced by fibrous tissue. Sonographic examination reveals a subcutaneous position of the bursa and may be helpful to characterize the bursitis as acute or chronic (fluid filled or fibrous). The presence of a foreign body or bone sequestrum may be seen with diagnostic ultrasound. Drainage and injection with a corticosteroid may be necessary if conservative therapy is not effective. Strict aseptic technique is necessary to prevent infection of the bursa. Once the bursa wall thickens with fibrous tissue, treatment becomes more problematic. Surgical drainage and the placement of drains may become necessary. More extreme measures may be necessary if there is no response. Opening the cavity and applying or packing with Lugol's iodine may be necessary to promote fibrosis between the bursal walls. Repeated sonographic examination can assist the clinician in determining the response to each stage of treatment.

Calcaneal Bursae

Acquired calcaneal bursitis (*capped hock*) is thought to be due to trauma, usually from the horse's kicking the wall or trailer. Sonographic examination typically reveals a subcutaneous position of the bursa and, in the early stages, a primarily fluid-filled pocket (Fig. 26.10). The fluid may have fibrin or the appearance of a large clot within the cavity. A capped hock appearance has been reported in cases of gastrocnemius tendinitis and in some bony abnormalities of the tuber calcis (24). *Plantar ligament desmitis* or *curb* manifests as a swelling along the plantar aspect of the calcaneus. Curb occurs commonly and may be related to conformation. Lameness is typically minimal and of short duration. Horses with persistent lameness with swelling more distal to the plantar ligament should be evaluated more carefully. Superficial digital flexor tendinitis of the proximal metatarsus may have a similar appearance, with swelling distal to the calcaneus. Occasionally, similar swelling exist without lameness.

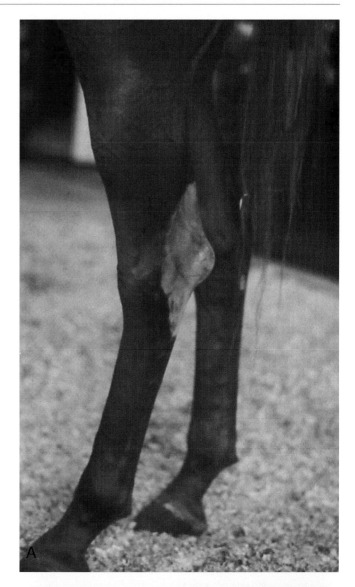

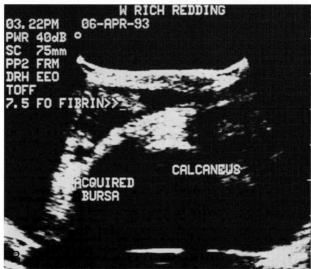

Figure 26.10. A, Acquired calcaneal bursa on the point of the hock (capped hock). **B,** Longitudinal sonogram of the same limb. Subcutaneous fluid is present with a fibrinous mass (considered fibrin because of the acute history).

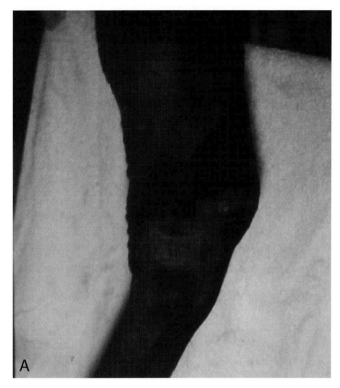 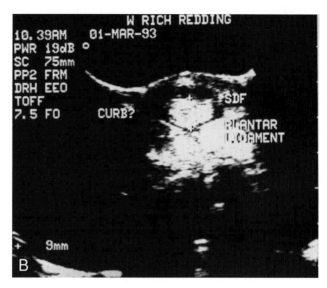

Figure 26.11. A, Plantar swelling of the proximal metatarsus associated with the superficial digital flexor tendon. Fluid is palpable within the swelling. **B,** Sonogram of the same limb with a normal appearing superficial digital flexor tendon. Subcutaneous fluid surrounds the tendon.

This swelling has a fluid consistency and appears sonographically as a fluid pocket surrounding the superficial digital flexor tendon (Fig. 26.11). Drainage may alleviate the problem, but persistence of the fluid may warrant corticosteroid injection.

The constant bursa of the calcaneus can develop effusion in luxation of the superficial digital flexor tendon. The constant bursae can be involved in septic processes, particularly punctures and lacerations around the tarsus. Appropriate treatment includes systemic antibiotics, surgical debridement as necessary, and possibly placement of drains. Radiographs may provide evidence of sequestrum formation or osteomyelitis, which may be the primary problem, with the bursa secondarily infected.

Carpal Hygroma

A carpal hygroma is a subcutaneous swelling that develops after repeated trauma to the dorsal carpus (Fig. 26.12). In the acute stage, a carpal hygroma contains fluid that appears consistent with a hematoma. Sonographically, this fluid can have a range of cellular and inflammatory debris, frequently with an organized clot. Fluid aspiration and pressure bandaging may be sufficient to resolve the problem initially. In the chronic state, loculation of fluid by fibrous bands can occur, but more commonly, a distinct bursal cavity develops. Sonographic evaluation is useful in differentiating swellings of the dorsal aspect of the carpus. Swellings of the dorsal carpus must be differentiated from carpal hygroma.

Synovitis of the extensor carpi radialis tendon sheath, subcutaneous herniation of a carpal joint capsule, ganglion, synovial fistula of the extensor sheaths and carpal joints, and synovitis of the carpal joints all may cause swellings of the dorsal carpus. Once carpal hygroma has been documented, it may be necessary to lance the bursa, to place a Penrose drain in the cavity, and to maintain a pressure wrap on the limb.

CONCLUSION

Sonographic evaluation of the equine limb has become a useful adjunct in the examination of lameness in horses. Sonographic findings in cases of tenosynovitis and bursitis should, however, be interpreted in conjunction with a complete history, physical examination, perineural or intrasynovial anesthesia, and radiologic study. A knowledge of the pathophysiology of disease affecting synovial sheaths and bursae and the relation to sonographic evidence of disease is necessary for accurate interpretation of injuries in this area.

Evaluation of tendon architecture requires the limb to be in extension and under stress; orientation of the transducer 90° to the tendon fibrils is critical. A tendon sheath allows the tendon to have freedom of movement at radical changes in direction. The gliding motion may be difficult to document in the standing or extended position. It may be of interest to scan the tendon while the operator holds the horse's limb off the ground and manually flexes and extends the limb to document range of motion. This procedure

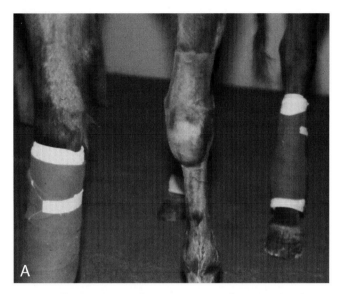
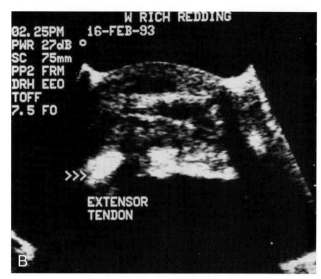

Figure 26.12. A, Fluctuant swelling of the dorsal surface of the carpus consistent with a carpal hygroma. **B,** Sonogram of the same limb shows the subcutaneous nature of the fluid. The fluid surrounds what appears to be a clot.

may be especially important when evidence of an adhesion or fibrous tissue is apparent within a sheath on the initial scan. In horses with proliferative synovitis or capsulitis, it may be difficult to interpret accurately the tendons and ligaments associated with the sheath. A fluid medium may be injected intrasynovially to define the lining of the synovial sheath and to document normal tendon and ligament architecture.

REFERENCES

1. Sack W, Habel R. Rooney's guide to the dissection of the horse. Ithaca, NY: Veterinary Textbooks, 1977.
2. Sisson S. Equine myology. In: Getty R, ed. Sisson and Grossman's the anatomy of the domestic animals. 5th ed. Philadelphia: WB Saunders, 1975.
3. Dyce KM, Sack WO, Wensing CJ. Textbook of veterinary anatomy. Philadelphia: WB Saunders, 1987.
4. Kainer RA. Functional anatomy of the equine locomotor organs. In: Stashak TS, ed. Adams' lameness in horses. 4th ed. Philadelphia: Lea & Febiger, 1987.
5. Sack WO. Subtendinous bursa of the medial aspect of the equine carpus. J Am Vet Med Assoc 1976;167:315–316.
6. McIlwraith CW. Diseases of joints, tendons, ligaments and related structures. In: Stashak TS, ed. Adams' lameness in horses. 4th ed. Philadelphia: Lea & Febiger, 1987.
7. Bowman K. Tenosynovitis. 15th annual Veterinary Surgical Forum, Chicago, October 19–21, 1987.
8. Van Pelt RW. Tenosynovitis in the horse. J Am Vet Med Assoc 1969;154:1022–1032.
9. Peacock EE, Van Winkle W. Repair of tendons and restoration of gliding function. In: Wound repair. 2nd ed. Philadelphia: WB Saunders, 1976.
10. Watrous BJ, Dutra FR, Wagner PC, et al. Villonodular synovitis of the palmar and plantar digital flexor tendon sheaths and the cal-

caneal bursae of the gastrocnemius tendon in the horse. Proc Am Assoc Equine Pract 1987;33:413–428.
11. Hago BED. Radiographic anatomy of tendon sheaths and bursae in the horse. Equine Vet J 1986;18:102–106.
12. Hago BED. Use of contrast radiography in the investigation of tenosynovitis and bursitis in horses, Equine Vet J 1986;18:375–382.
13. Nixon AJ. Endoscopy of the digital flexor tendon sheath in horses. Vet Surg 1990;19:266–271.
14. Rantanen NW. The use of diagnostic ultrasound to detect structural damage to the soft tissues of the extremities of horses. J Equine Vet Sci 1985;3:134–135.
15. Genovese RL, Rantanen NW, Hauser M L, et al. Diagnostic ultrasound of equine limbs. Vet Clin North Am Equine Pract 1986;2:145–225.
16. McClellan PD. Ultrasonic structure of the pastern. Equine Vet Sci 1986;6:99–101.
17. Redding WR. Ultrasound imaging of the structures of the digital flexor tendon sheath. Compend Contin Educ Pract Vet 1991;13:1824–1832.
18. Denoix J, Crevier N, Azevedo C. Ultrasound examination of the pastern in horses. Proc Am Assoc Equine Pract 1991;33:363–380.
19. Dik KJ, Van Den Belt JM, Keg PR. Ultrasonographic evaluation of fetlock annular ligament constriction in the horse. Equine Vet J 1991;23:285–288.
20. Gaughn EM, Nixon AJ, Krook LP. Effects of sodium hyaluronate on tendon healing and adhesion formation in horses. Am J Vet Res 1991;52:764–773.
21. Rantanen NW. Assessing tenosynovitis [editorial]. J Equine Vet Sci 1983;4:171.
22. Dik KJ, Merkens HW. Unilateral distention of the tarsal sheath in the horse: a report of 11 cases. Equine Vet J 1987;19:307–313.
23. Edwards GB. Changes in the sustentaculum tali associated with distention of the tarsal sheath (thoroughpin). Equine Vet J 1978;10:97–102.
24. Dyson S, Kidd L. Five cases of gastrocnemius tendinitis in the horse. Equine Vet J 1992;24:351–356.

27. Section A

The Effects of Polysulfated Glycosaminoglycan on the Healing of Collagenase-Induced Tendinitis of the Equine Superficial Digital Flexor Tendon[1]

W. RICH REDDING, LARRY C. BOOTH, AND ROY R. POOL

SUMMARY

Eight (four thoroughbred and four standardbred) horses had tendinitis induced in the superficial flexor tendon of both forelimbs by the injection of 4000 IU of collagenase. One group of four horses (treatment group) was treated with 500 mg polysulfated glycosaminoglycan IM every 5 days for seven treatments beginning 24 hours after injection of collagenase. The second (control) group of four horses received the same volume of saline on the same schedule. Sonographic examination of each limb was performed on days 1, 3, 5, and 7 post injection and weekly thereafter for 8 weeks. The sonographic images of the superficial digital flexor tendons and collagenase lesions were recorded on thermal print paper at each time period. The outlines of the tendons and the core defects were then traced onto clear unexposed radiograph film for measurement using a computerized image analysis system. Clinical examinations to evaluate pain and lameness were also performed at the same time periods. Horses were euthanized at 8 weeks, and histologic evaluation was performed on longitudinal sections of excised tendons.

The sonographic examinations revealed that tendon core defects from treatment horses developed echogenic patterns earlier than did tendons from saline controls. The core defects also decreased in size significantly more rapidly in the treatment group ($P < .03$). Treatment horses had a subjectively less painful gait than did control horses during the first week of the study after which none of the horses manifested pain. Histologic evaluation of the core defects confirmed what was seen sonographically. The core defects were not obvious in six of the eight treated tendons. Remnants of the core defects in the form of amorphous collagenous tissue was present in all the control tendons.

The same general types of microscopic changes were encountered in both groups, but degenerative collagenous tissue was present in the core defects of all control tendons, while little evidence of degenerative tissue could be found in the treated tendons after 2 months. It would appear that polysulfated glycosaminoglycan encouraged tenocyte proliferation and presumably repair within the original tendon bundles that were damaged by the initial injection of collagenase.

---

[1]This abstract was presented at the 1992 ACVS meeting in Miami.

TREATMENT OF TENDINITIS WITH POLYSULFATED GLYCOSAMINOGLYCAN

Tendinitis is a common and career-threatening injury in horses of all breeds. In the racehorse damage to the superficial digital flexor tendon (SDFT) is thought to occur due to traumatic overstrain and/or may be the result of cyclic loading, which can lead to degeneration of the tendon (1–6). Diagnostic ultrasound has proven very useful in defining the type and extent of injury to the tendinous structures of the palmar metacarpus/metatarsus (7, 8). Probably the most common form of tendinitis present in the racehorse appears sonographically as a core type defect of the SDFT. Experimentally, this core type of SDF tendinitis has been induced by injection of collagenase and has become a model for this type of injury (9). Previous studies have documented sonographic and morphologic similarities between this experimental tendinitis and clinical tendinitis (10–12). This similarity has allowed a somewhat objective comparison of treatment regimens of the SDF tendinitis and was incorporated into our study for this reason.

The exact cause of tendinitis is poorly understood and in fact may be multifactorial. The use of diagnostic ultrasound to confirm the presence of tendinitis should be utilized whenever possible and may lend insight into the most appropriate therapy. In any instance, when tendon tissue has been damaged, the initial therapy should address the inflammatory cascade and may make the difference between success and failure. The incorporation of several modes of therapy is common, and some of the alternative therapies will be discussed in other papers of this chapter. The objective of this paper is to propose that PSGAG be incorporated in the medical treatment of the early stages of tendinitis.

As with any wound, a tendon injury progresses through an initial vascular phase into an inflammatory phase, which is followed later by a fibroproliferative phase. During the vascular phase there is an increase in permeability of the venous endothelial cells allowing an influx of noncellular plasma components into the wound cavity. A wound matrix is produced that is high in fibronectin, a physiologic adhesive produced by fibroblast and endothelial cells that binds fibrin, cells, and other matrix components. Shortly thereafter, the cellular components of the inflammatory phase (polymorphonuclear leucocytes and monocyte-derived macrophages) migrate into the wounded area. The intensity of this inflammatory reaction is thought to be proportional

539

to the amount of trauma associated with the injury. Early in the inflammatory phase, hydrolytic enzymes released from these polymorphonuclear leucocytes and by cells damaged in the traumatic event (tenocytes, fibroblasts, and endothelial cells in the case of tendinitis) begin the debridement of damaged tissue in the wounded area. Later in the inflammatory phase, the monocyte-derived macrophages begin to dominate the cellular reaction at 3 to 5 days post injury. These cells synthesize and release proteases that continue the debridement of the wound, as well as produce mitogenic factors and cytokines that influence healing in the later stages.

During the fibroproliferative phase of tendon healing, the fibrin-fibronectin meshwork is invaded by undifferentiated fibroblasts and blood vessels (endothelial cells). These fibroblasts can originate from the peritendinous tissue (extrinsic component) or from proliferating tenocytes of the epitenon and endotenon (intrinsic component). These fibroblasts surround themselves with elastin, fibronectin, sulfated and nonsulfated glycosaminoglycans, proteases, and fibrillar collagen. Fibroblast proliferation and differentiation, as well as the subsequent neovascularization, appear to be regulated by the macrophage series of cells probably through the production of heparin-binding growth factor. This stimulation of fibroblasts creates a marked increase in the levels of glycosaminoglycans (GAG) at the repair site after tendon injury during this fibroproliferative phase (13). Of the three major glycosaminoglycans found in the tendon (hyaluronate, chondroitin sulfate, and dermatan sulfate), hyaluronate production predominates at this stage. Tissues rich in hyaluronate contain predominantly small-diameter fibrils (<60 nm) and tissues containing predominantly dermatan sulfate have primarily large-diameter fibrils (>150 nm) (14). Secondary remodeling of the scar with removal of these small fibrils and replacement with larger fibrils allows a gradual increase in strength over time.

The goal of medical therapy in tendinitis is to reduce the inflammatory response to the minimum necessary for repair of the tendon and thereby limit the damage (directly or indirectly due to the inflammatory response) to the abnormal tendon tissue. Bramlage (15) has divided tendon healing into stages consisting of an acute (inflammatory) period occurring within the first 48 hours; a subacute period (during fibrous deposition) occurring from 2 days out to 3 to 4 weeks; a remodeling period (with collagen maturation and remodeling) of approximately 21 to 60 days or more; and a period of retraining (with stabilization and reorganization of the injured tendon tissue for use), which begins when the tendon is again stressed.

The most common forms of medical therapy for the acute stage of tendinitis have included an initial period of hypothermia utilizing hydrotherapy and/or ice; nonsteroidal anti-inflammatories (NSAIDs); pressure bandaging; sweats; poultices; and, more recently, intravenous, oral, or topical DMSO during the acute and subacute inflammatory stages. Additional forms of parenteral or local therapy

will be discussed in detail in other papers of this chapter. Polysulfated glycosaminoglycans (Adequan, Luitpold Pharmaceuticals, Shirley, NY) have recently been utilized with some success in experimental, as well as clinical, SDF tendinitis.

Polysulfated glycosaminoglycan is a drug similar in composition to hyaluronate, which is made up of repeating units of hexosamine and hexuronic acid with a molecular weight of approximately 10,000 daltons. While PSGAG has been most extensively reported for its effects on cartilage and in the treatment of osteoarthritis, some recent reports are finding that PSGAG should be considered in the initial therapy of tendinitis. Goodship (16) has suggested that PSGAG be administered at a dose of 1 mg/kg intramuscularly every 4 days for 4 weeks. The manufacturer has maintained that PSGAG be administered as a-500 mg dose (approximately 1 mg/kg) given intramuscularly beginning 24 to 48 hours after injury and continued every 5 days for seven treatments (Dr. Gary White, Luitpold Pharmaceuticals, Shirley, NY, personal communication). More recently it has been suggested that PSGAG should be given locally, if not by intralesional injection, primarily to maintain a higher concentration of the drug at the site of injury (17).

The rationale for the use of PSGAG in tendinitis, like in osteoarthritis, probably lies in the ability of this product to attenuate the inflammatory response to injury, thereby limiting the destruction of normal collagen and reducing the loss of proteoglycans from the tendon matrix. This effect has been demonstrated in in vitro cartilage and chondrocyte studies, as well as in in vivo osteoarthritis models. Given that the structure of tendon and cartilage is similar, modification of the inflammatory response with PSGAG would seemingly be of benefit in tendinitis.

CATABOLIC EFFECT

Polysulfated glycosaminoglycan has been shown to be effective in slowing the degradation of collagen in osteoarthritic cartilage. While the catabolism of collagen occurs through the action of neutral collagenase, it also involves cathepsin B1, elastase, and lysosomal enzymes. Polysulfated glycosaminoglycans have been shown to be a potent competitive inhibitor of the collagenase activity of cathepsin B (18). Polysulfated glycosaminoglycan has also been tested in vitro against a number of enzymes thought to be associated with matrix degradation by intracellular lysosomal enzymes and extracellular neutral proteinases (19–21). One report evaluated the inhibitory effects of PSGAG on lysosomal enzymes prepared and purified from rabbit kidneys. In that report, beta-galactosidase, beta-glucuronidase, beta-N-acetylglucosaminodase, alpha-glucosidase, and alpha-mannosidase were inhibited in descending order by 167 μg/ml PSGAG (19). Another report showed that the actual release of enzymes from polymorphonuclear leukocytes was not influenced by PSGAG, but neutral protease, beta-glucuronidase, and myeloperoxidase were inhibited in a dose-dependent manner (20). By reducing the action of these inflammatory enzymes, PSGAG may decrease degradation of the collagen and ground substance of the normal tendon. Sparing normal tendon fibrils and maintaining as much normal tendon architecture as possible should support the structural reorganization of the repair tissue and increase the mechanical strength of the tendon both initially and during healing.

ANABOLIC EFFECT

While the previous studies evaluated the effect of PSGAG on some of the enzymes of the inflammatory response, there has been some suggestion that the quality of repair tissue may also be positively affected. Elevated amounts of proteoglycans and hyaluronic acid have been produced by chondrocytes harvested from articular cartilage in vitro when PSGAG was added to the culture media. Proteoglycans are also thought to enhance the deposition of large collagen molecules. One in vitro study evaluating the effects of PSGAG on equine fetlock cartilage tissue in organ culture demonstrated a dose-dependent stimulation of net collagen and glycosaminoglycan synthesis (22). Increasing overall synthesis of collagen with production of larger-diameter collagen fibrils would certainly be advantageous in increasing the tensile strength of tendons with tendinitis.

BIOAVAILABILITY

For PSGAG to exert in vivo effects similar to those described in the previous in vitro studies, it is critical that parenteral administration attains sufficient concentration in tendon tissue. Two studies have evaluated ^{3}H-labeled PSGAG administration in laboratory animals and human volunteers, and the distribution was monitored (23, 24). These studies found the fibrous types of connective tissue such as tendon, menisci, and the annulus fibrosus of the intervertebral disc to have a high affinity for PSGAG. It was also suggested that PSGAG had a greater affinity for noncollagenous matrix proteins and proteoglycan than for type 1 collagen (23).

DISCUSSION

As our understanding of tendon injury and repair has increased, the utilization of staged treatments at different times in the inflammatory response (i.e., acute to subacute to chronic) has become increasingly more important than the use of any single treatment. Aggressive therapy aimed at minimizing the inflammatory response and limiting the destruction of normal tendon collagen fibrils should begin immediately. As mentioned previously, the use of hydrotherapy, nonsteroidal anti-inflammatories, and other parenteral medications such as dimethyl sulfoxide should be included in the acute stage of tendinitis because of their effects on reducing the intensity of the inflammatory reaction. At present, PSGAG appears to be beneficial in the treatment of tendinitis when used in the acute stage of the inflammatory response and should be utilized in the medical management of tendinitis.

In our study a significant decrease in lesion size was found in the PSGAG-treated tendons. This effect was thought to be due primarily to an attenuation of the inflammatory response. Treatment with PSGAG appeared to encourage tenocyte proliferation and presumably repair within the original tendon bundles. Whether this tenocyte proliferation was due to a protective effect of this treatment or due to a stimulation of the tenocyte by PSGAG is unknown. There did appear to be less damage to the arterioles of the endotenon in the treated tendons, which should have supported a more normal pattern of blood flow than that found in the control group. This maintenance of blood flow could explain an increased survival rate of the tenocytes, but also may have allowed an accelerated maturation of the tendon lesions over controls. Because the amount of necrosis can be related to the degree of vascular compromise and, given that the control tendons appeared to have more vascular compromise than in the treated tendons, it is certainly possible that there was more necrosis in the control tendons.

More information is needed with regard to the specific content of the tendon matrix and the role glycosaminoglycans (endogenous and exogenous) may play in normal tendon function and tendon healing. It is apparent that the matrix has a regulatory function on the cell. This ground substance is thought to influence ion transport, diffusion of nutrients, and cell-to-cell interaction. It has also been shown that the specific constituents of the matrix influences the type of the collagen that is produced by the fibroblasts (i.e., hyaluronate stimulates the production of smaller fibrils). Tenocytes and fibroblasts certainly produce glycosaminoglycans, but it is unknown whether PSGAG can directly influence these cells to produce these substances. While polysulfated glycosaminoglycans have been shown to stimulate synoviocytes to produce sodium hyaluronate in vitro (25), no information about their effect on fibroblast/tenocyte production of hyaluronate is available. What effect hyaluronate plays in tendon repair or how PSGAG may affect the glycosaminoglycan concentrations in normal tendons or in the injury and repair of tendons needs further evaluation.

The final outcome of the healing process is ultimately determined at a cellular level and is based on a balance of reparation and regeneration coordinated by intercellular communication. This cellular communication is generally through several peptidergic and chemical mediators that influence cell reproduction and growth. These mediators include such catalysts as epidermal growth factor, transforming growth factor, insulin-like growth factor, and heparin-binding growth factor, as well as many more. Heparin-binding growth factors are thought to have a potent impact on proliferation of fibroblasts. It is unknown whether the heparin-like PSGAG may have a similar effect on fibroblasts. Whether PSGAG simulates heparin-like growth factor or influences the production of this mediator or other mediators needs further evaluation.

Mechanical deformation of cell membranes can influence cell shape and pressure, which is thought to activate ion channels. Mobility of a tendon can therefore potentially influence cellular function and/or mediate matrix composition. Early mobility in the repair process may therefore prove to be important in the ultimate outcome of tendon healing. Our study revealed treated animals were lame for a shorter period than the control animals. Increased weight bearing and mobility in the early, post-injection period may have indirectly improved repair tissue organization and maturation by increasing vascular flow and potentially decreasing tissue fluid accumulation. As mentioned earlier, there could also be some form of mechanical stimulation of tenocytes and/or fibroblasts with earlier mobility, and this may account for the tenocyte proliferation and the repair within the original tendon bundles. How exercise and mobility of injured tendons influence tendon repair in the horse certainly needs further evaluation

REFERENCES

1. McCullagh KG, Goodship A E, Silver IA. Tendon injuries and their treatment in the horse. Vet Rec 1979;105:54–57.
2. Williams I F, Heaton A, McCullagh KG. Cell morphology and collagen types in equine tendon scar. Res Vet Sci 1980;28:302–310.
3. Stromberg B, Tufvesson G. Lesions of the superficial flexor tendon in racehorses. A microangiographic and histopathologic study. Clin Orthop 1969;62:113.
4. Selway SJ. Diseases of the tendons. In: Equine medicine and surgery. 3rd ed. Santa Barbara, CA: American Veterinary Publications, 1982;1071–1088.
5. McIllwraith CW. Diseases of joints, tendons, ligaments and related structures. In: Stashak TS, ed. Adams' lameness in horses. 4th ed. Philadelphia: Lea & Febiger, 1987; 463–468.
6. Pool RR, Meagher DM. Pathological findings and pathogenesis of racetrack injuries. Vet Clin North Am Equine Pract 1990; 6(1):1–30.
7. Genovese RL, Rantanen NW, Hauser ML, Simpson BS. Diagnostic ultrasonography of equine limbs. Vet Clin North Am Equine Pract 1986;2:145–226.
8. Genovese RL, Rantanen NW, Simpson BS, Simpson DM. Clinical experience with quantitative analysis of superficial digital flexor tendon injuries in thoroughbred and standardbred racehorses. Vet Clin North Am Equine Pract 1990;6(1):129–145.
9. Silver IF, Brown PN, Goodship AE, Lanyon LE, McCullagh KG, Perry G, Williams IF. Studies on the pathogenesis of equine tendonitis following collagenase injury. Equine Vet J 1983;(Suppl 1):1–43.
10. Spurlock GH, Spurlock SL, Parker GA. Evaluation of Hylartin V therapy for induced tendonitis in the horse. Equine Vet Sci 1989; 9(5):242–246.
11. Gaughan EM, Nixon AJ, Lennart PK, et al. Effects of sodium hyaluronate on tendon healing and adhesion formation in horses. Am Soc Vet Res 1991;52(5):764–773.
12. Henninger R. The effects of tendon splitting on the healing of collagenase induced tendonitis of the superficial digital flexor tendon in the horse. Vet Comp Ortho Traum January 1992; 1:1–19.
13. Reid T, Flynn MH. Changes in glycosaminoglycan content of healing rabbit tendon. J Embryol Exp Morphol 1974;31:489–495.
14. Merrilees MJ, Tiaug KM, Scott L. Changes in collagen fibril diameters across artery walls including a correlation with glycosaminoglycan content. Conn Tiss Res 1987;16:327–357.
15. Bramlage, LR. Medical treatment of tendinitis. In: Robinson NE, ed. Current therapy in equine medicine. Philadelphia: WB Saunders, 1992; pp.146–149.
16. Goodship AE, Birch HL, Wilson AM. The pathobiology and repair of tendon and ligament injury. Vet Clin North Am Equine Pract 1994;10(2):323–349.
17. Smith RKW. A case of superficial flexor tendinitis: ultrasonographic examination and treatment with intralesional polysulfated glycosamnioglycans. Equine Vet Educ 1992;4:280–303.
18. Trnavsky K. Action of arteparon on collagenolytic activity of cathepsin B1. Proceedings of the 9th European Congress on Rheumatology. Basle: Eular Publishing, 1979; 27–29.
19. Greiling H, Kanreko M. The inhibition of lysosomal enzymes by a glycosaminoglycan polysulfate. Drug Res 1973;23:593–597.
20. Biaci A, Fehr K. Inhibition of human lysosomal elastase by arteparon. Proceedings of the 9th European Congress on Rheumatolgy. Basle: Eular Publishing, 1979; 19–26.
21. Mikul-Ikov AD, Trnavsky K. Influence of a glycosaminoglycan polysulfate (arteparon) on lysosomal enzyme release from human polymorphonuclear leukocytes. Z Rheumatol 1982;41(2):50–53.
22. Glade MJ. Polysulfated glycosaminoglycan accelerates net synthesis of collagen and glycosaminoglycans by arthritic equine cartilage tissues and chondrocytes. Am J Vet Res 1990;51:779–785.
23. Andrews JL, Sutherland J, Ghosh P. Distribution and binding of glycosaminoglycan polysulfate to intervertebral disc, knee joint cartilage and meniscus. Arzneim-Forsch Drug Res 1985;42:355.
24. Muller W, Panse P, Brand S, Staubli A. In vivo study of the distribution, affinity to cartilage and metabolism of glycosaminoglycan polysulfate (GAGPS [arteparon]). Z Rheumatol 1983; 42:144.
25. Burkhardt F, Ghosh P. Laboratory evaluation of glycosaminoglycan polysulfate ester for chondroprotective activity: a review. Curr Ther Res 1986;40:1034-1053.

27. Section B

Treatment of Superficial Digital Flexor Tendinitis—An Opinion

RONALD L. GENOVESE

HISTORY

Prior to the use of diagnostic ultrasonography, evaluation of a tendon injury was based on clinical examination and gait evaluation. Often the results of treatment were judged successful by the return to athletic use. The prognosis for return to high-level equine athletic activities such as racing was regarded as unfavorable. This was evidenced by the high recurrence of injury rate once horses were returned to maximum exercise. Adams (1) reported a 20% chance to return to high-level exercise such as racing. During the late 1950s treatments consisted of extensive rest, external and internal blistering, and pin and line firing. Since many racehorses failed to return to racing, the so-called "bowed" tendon was regarded as one of the most career compromising injuries that could happen to a racehorse. In spite of this unfavorable prognosis, there were horses that successfully returned to racing, but the majority did so at a significantly lower class level. The low success rate stimulated little incentive for long-term treatment programs. Most clinicians were apt to choose treatment programs that were the most recently successful in their hands. There was little research directed toward the so-called "bowed" tendon for many reasons. Among those reasons was the inability to assess the injury morphologically and the inescapable physiologic fact that one could not recreate new tendon fibers. In the 1960s Asheim et al. (2) reported an improved return to athleticism using a surgical tendon splitting technique. This surgical approach renewed interest in the injured tendon. Carbon implants were tried to improve tendon injury repair, but results were not consistently favorable. In the 1980s further progress was made when Silver et al. (3) reported that beneficial results from firing could not be established. Bramlage (4) reported a significantly improved athletic return following superior check ligament desmotomy with or without tendon splitting. In the 1990s Goodship (5) reported the use of polysulfated glycosaminoglycans (PSGAG) in the early injury stages accompanied by strict exercise control as possibly improving tendon lesion repair.

The introduction of diagnostic ultrasonography, allowing a morphologic tendon architectural evaluation, has greatly enhanced research and clinical interest. This has enhanced not only tendon injury diagnosis but also so-called "bowed" tendon treatment evaluation. In spite of the more recent surgical and medical approaches to so-called "bowed" tendons, successful return to high-level competition has been inconsistent in many veterinarians' hands. From this point on the term "bow," which is a colloquial term for a change in tendon profile, will not be used whenever possible.

In the 1990s I became involved in a clinical field trial evaluating the therapeutic benefit of intralesional β-amino-proprionitrile-fumarate (BAPTEN®, Alaco Corp., Tucson, AZ) for superficial digital flexor tendon (SDFT) injury treatment. As of July 1997, this drug had not received FDA approval for use in horses in the United States. From this experience I developed my present injured-tendon treatment concepts. The project design utilized objective sonographic data to evaluate tendon repair. Many of the previously reported therapies lacked measurable objective parameters to evaluate the treatment success, except for return to racing (RTR). Although return to high-level competition is a practical end point, it is questionable to use RTR as the single parameter to evaluate specific tendon injury treatment success. Valid questions are as follows: Even if a horse has returned to racing, is it reinjury free? How is repair evaluated and morphologically documented? Were the horses in the Asheim study all slightly or severely injured? What type of athletic activity did study horses perform? Is there a severity of injury definition? Are all lesions in the same location? Lameness is a poor criteria since many injured horses are not lame. Furthermore, it became apparent that previous studies lacked categorization of injury severity or even documentation that a tendon was injured. These are the questions that have clouded the issue of treatment success. I am convinced that all tendon injuries are not the same.

From the BAPTEN® clinical studies, an approach was developed to quantitate tendon injury and treatment response. I believe that tendon injuries vary, that different therapeutic approaches are necessary, and that only through serial sonographic examinations can the response be evaluated. The bases of my tendon treatment are as follows:

1. Establish the type and injury extent.
2. Select an exercise management phase based on objective measurements and nonmedical considerations.
3. Institute an appropriate treatment regimen for each individual case.
4. Sonographically monitor the response to increasing exercise levels and adjust accordingly.
5. Sonographically monitor the effects of maximum exercise.

INTRODUCTION

The discussion of my treatment and management approach to SDFT injury should start with a disclaimer. The following discussion will not include total tendon ruptures, lacerations, or septic tendinitis. It is beyond the scope of this section to include these unique situations. My discussion is directed toward varying degrees of subtotal, athletic-use–related injury with the primary emphasis on racehorses.

It is also acknowledged that tendon repair physiology dictates that healing occurs not by replication of normal tenocytes but by damaged tendon fiber replacement with modified fibroblasts. In other words, all tendon injury repairs are inferior to normal tendon fibers. It is a question of the repair quality relative to the intended loading level that most likely determines the return to training and racing. It is the goal of therapy to affect the best quality repair. In my efforts to restore a horse to high-level competition, I keep in mind that the faster the horse will have to go, the better the repair has to be. Furthermore, I constantly remind myself that the reason I am treating my patient is because, at its athletic level, an injury occurred to a *normal* tendon. I am trying to make a less than normal tendon do the same or more work. To that end, I direct all of the rehabilitation steps to the most structurally functional repair possible. I refer to sonographic evaluations during rehabilitation as the sonographic quality of repair (SQR). As obvious as this concept may seem, it is basic to clinical management and the eventual athletic return. I also realize that the higher the competitive level, the more difficult it is to achieve with a repaired tendon. I believe the success rate for return to athletic use allows a lesser SQR when there is a decrease in the competitive level. For instance, if an injured racehorse is used for weekend trail riding, the SQR can be inferior. Conversely, return to stakes-class racing requires the best-quality, most-functional repair. This type of repair is difficult if not impossible to achieve. This most functional SDFT repair is the challenge that clinicians must face when the future intended use is racing .

There are many variables to consider in tendon injury treatment. Each case will emphasize its unique set of variables. At times, economics is the prevailing consideration, and the horse's value may be the primary concern. At other times treatment(s) will be based on the trainer's compliance and training philosophies. It is not possible to document an SDFT lesion and advise a specific treatment without considering the variables and other factors that enter into the case outcome. I hope to develop the interrelationships of the medical and nonmedical factors that influence treatment selection and case management by illustrating a variety of past experiences. These case examples will provide the reader with the sense of complexity that can surround tendon injury treatment. This is contrary to the literature where simplistic therapeutic approaches are often discussed. It may be that oversimplification of the many considerations may well have resulted in the unfavorable prognosis given for racing after tendon injury.

SDFT INJURY EVALUATION (SEE CHAPTER 21)

In the typical, first-episode SDFT injury, the practitioner is usually summoned to examine the horse for a recent swelling following a race or a workout the day or 2 prior to the clinical signs. Usually, in slight to moderate injuries, horses showing lameness at the trot are in the minority. Palpation reveals slightly painful swelling along the SDFT. I generally advise a sonographic evaluation at this time. I refer to this sonographic evaluation as the *initial* examination. Since the injury is most likely only 24 to 48 hours old, there is some inaccuracy in determining the injury's extent and severity because of the inflammation. I will repeat the sonographic evaluation 2 to 4 weeks later. At that time a more accurate assessment of fiber path compromise is made, and this is referred to as the *baseline* examination to which future repair evaluations will be compared. At 2 to 4 weeks post injury there has been time for hemorrhage resorption, edema resolution, and enzymatic necrotic collagen fiber degradation. I make it a routine procedure to scan both tendons at the initial and baseline evaluations. I make hard copies of at least six, preferably seven levels (see Chapter 21) for CSA data. In the BAPTEN® clinical field trials, over 100 horses were evaluated in this manner, and it was determined to be an accurate, quantitative, morphologic injury assessment to assist the clinician. Basically, the sonographic determinations are used to evaluate the tendon size (cross-sectional area [CSA]), the maximum injury zone (MIZ), the extent and degree of fiber bundle compromise (texture) (HYP), and the fiber alignment in the injured areas (FS). These measurements are made for the (MIZ) and the total of all levels (T) scanned. The MIZ is the level with the largest area of fiber bundle damage regardless of the type. The MIZ is identified because it is thought to represent the "weakest cross-sectional site" in the tendon. However, just as important for SDFT injury severity categorization, the total identifiable fiber bundle compromise is measured. The contralateral limb should be scanned as a comparison and to rule out injury to that structure. If there is no concomitant injury, the six- or seven-level CSA is used for normal values. Therefore, in the initial and/or baseline examination a qualitative sonographic assessment and the following seven quantitative sonographic assessments should be made:

1. MIZ tendon cross-sectional area (MIZ-CSA)
2. MIZ hypoechoic fiber bundle volume (MIZ-HYP)
3. The fiber alignment or fiber score (MIZ-FS)
4. The total CSA (T-CSA)
5. The total compromised levels or hypoechoic fiber bundles CSA (T-HYP)
6. The total abnormal level fiber score (T-FS)
7. The total hypoechoic fiber percentage can be calculated from the above data simply by dividing the T-HYP by the T-CSA and multiplying by 100. This value is called the percent total hypoechoic (% T-HYP).

In the BAPTEN® field trials, it proved useful to use the % T-HYP as a practical means to categorize the tendon injury severity:

Slight injury: This included tendons that had either (a) no identifiable hypoechoic fiber bundles present at any level, but the tendon T-CSA was >20% compared with the contralateral normal tendon or (b) a 1 to 15% T-HYP.

Moderate injury: This included tendons that had a 16 to 25% T-HYP.

Severe injury: This included tendons with a >25% T-HYP.

By categorizing SDFT injuries, treatment success or failure of like injuries can be compared. The results of RTR for tendon injuries, with a variety of treatment regimens, were reported in the First Dubai International Equine Symposium Proceedings (6). In this critical evaluation of return to high-level performance, tendon lesion repair was judged on sonographic evidence of reinjury and RTR, not solely on RTR. Therefore, horses that raced were not considered successful if there was sonographic evidence of reinjury. In that study horses were judged successful only if the repaired tendon injury was sonographically stable while the horse was racing. Tendons that had sonographic evidence of reinjury were considered failures even though they were racing.

From that study it was determined that, regardless of treatment, slightly injured tendons had a better prognosis for RTR than those with moderate injuries, and severely injured tendons had the most unfavorable prognosis for RTR without reinjury. Using % T-HYP determinations will greatly assist clinicians in offering prognostic information and will greatly assist in comparing like injuries when evaluating treatment regimens. In that group of 153 racehorses (Standardbreds and Thoroughbreds) there was a 24% chance of RTR without reinjury when all treatments were considered. The successful group (24%) had treated tendons that had no sonographic evidence of reinjury. As the types of injury management, segregation by severity, and types of treatment are further analyzed the success rate exceeds 24%.

The first step in SDFT injury management is to establish the injury severity. For accuracy and consistency, the % T-HYP is best determined during the baseline sonographic evaluation. There are instances when there is a difference in severity classification between the initial and baseline evaluations.

NOTE: Because the following case discussions make numerous references to the various exercise levels discussed in Chapter 21, they are listed below for convenience (Table 27B.1).

Figure 27B.1 is a recently raced TB presented for SDFT swelling. This initial sonogram reveals a Type 3 SDFT "core" lesion. The MIZ-CSA is 161 mm², and the lesion CSA is 39 mm² (24% of the MIZ-CSA has abnormal texture). There are five zones that have hypoechoic fibers. The T-CSA for seven levels is 769 mm², and the T-HYP is 126 mm². The % T-HYP is 16%. The MIZ-FS is 3 and the T-FS is 12. This would be rated as a moderate SDFT injury (16% T-HYP). This horse was treated with 2 g oral phenylbutazone per day (The Butler Company, Columbus, OH) and a single, intravenous dose of 20 mg of dexamethazone (A&G Pharmaceuticals, Clarksburg, NJ). The tendon was placed in ice 2 hours per day and treated with a mild liniment under cotton leg wrapping. The only exercise permitted was 30 minutes per day of hand walking (EL-1). The limb was treated for 1 month.

Table 27B.1.
Exercise Levels

Exercise Level	Activity
EL 1	ALL walk 30 minutes s.i.d. (in hand/mechanical walker)
EL 2a	1. TB/SH (sport horse)—swim/pony/trot lunge 5–10 min; trot under saddle 5–10 min
	2. STD—swim/pony/trot lunge 5–10 min
EL 2b	1. TB/SH—swim/pony/trot lunge 10–15 min
	2. STD—swim/pony/trot lunge 15 min; *walk* only in bike 30 min
EL 3a	ALL—small paddock equivalent to round pen
EL 3b	ALL—regular paddock exercise
EL 4	TB—DO NOT GO ON TRACK!
	TB/SH—hack in arena w/t/c/ 15–20 min 3 days/week
	STD—job 1 mile *over* 6 min 5 days/week
EL 5	TB—normal galloping 1–2 miles on track
	STD—normal multiple mile jogging on track
	SH—normal arena work, limited low-fence jumping
EL 6	TB—normal gallop plus *slow* breezes
	STD—normal jog miles plus *slow* training miles (over 2:20)
	SH—normal hacking and practice round jumps
EL 7	TB—works/racing
	STD—training miles under 2:20/qualifiers/racing
	SH—regular show ring/events

From BAPTEN® research protocol.

Figure 27B.2 is a sonogram of the same horse as in Figure 27B.1 made 1 month post injury. This baseline examination shows sonographic improvement. The MIZ-CSA reduced to 136 mm², the MIZ-HYP to 33 mm², and there is remarkable Type 3 to Type 1 improvement. There are still five abnormal levels, the T-CSA reduced to 712 mm², and the T-HYP to 96 mm². The % T-HYP reduced to 13%, which is a slight lesion. The MIZ-FS reduced to 1, and the

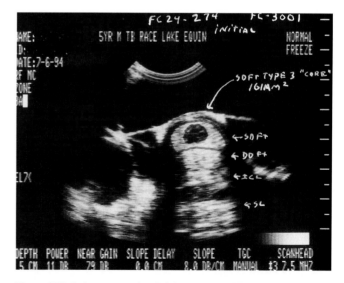

Figure 27B.1. A cross-sectional right metacarpal Zone 3A initial sonogram. Core Lesion Superficial Digital Flexor Tendon. SDFT = superficial digital flexor tendon; DDFT = deep digital flexor tendon; ICL = inferior check ligament (ALDDFT); SL = suspensory ligament (TIOM). (ATL 4600 scanner)

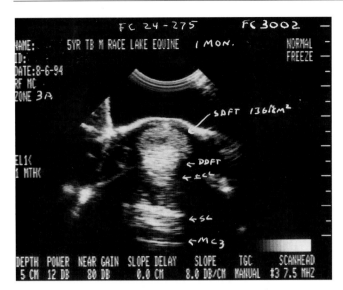

Figure 27B.2. A cross-sectional right metacarpal Zone 3A baseline sonogram of the same horse as in Figure 27B.1 made at 1 month. SDFT = superficial digital flexor tendon; DDFT = deep digital flexor tendon; ICL = inferior check ligament (ALDDFT); SL = suspensory ligament (TIOM); MC3 = third metacarpal bone. (ATL 4600 scanner)

T-FS reduced to 7. Fiber score decrease improves the prognosis. One may conclude from this second examination, that anti-inflammatory medication and hydrotherapy decreased the lesion size and improved the texture by resolving the hematoma and inflammation. At 30 days post injury, obviously, fiber bundle improvement is not due to mature collagen formation. The present 13% T-HYP represents a more accurate evaluation of the tendon fiber compromise.

In contrast to the previous case, Figure 27B.3 is a sonogram of a TB racehorse injured in a recent race. There is a Type 3 SDFT "core" lesion. The MIZ-CSA is 130 mm², and the MIZ-HYP is 21 mm² (16%). The T-CSA is 906 mm², and the T-HYP is 83 mm². At the initial examination the % T-HYP is 9%, which is a slight lesion. The MIZ-FS is 3 and the T-FS is 14. This horse was treated the same as the previous horse. The exercise was limited to 30 minutes daily of hand walking.

Figure 27B.4 is the same horse as in Figure 27B.3 made 3 weeks later. This baseline examination reveals a Type 3 SDFT "core" lesion. The MIZ-CSA increased to 150 mm², and the T-CSA decreased to 787 mm². The MIZ-HYP increased to 42 mm² (28%), and the T-HYP increased to 143 mm². The % T-HYP is presently at 18%, which indicates this to be a more serious injury than originally thought. The MIZ-FS is still 3, and the T-FS is 13. In this case the baseline sonographic examination performed 3 weeks post injury provides a more accurate assessment of fiber path compromise. These data might reflect enzymatic degradation and possibly the influence of pressure necrosis. These findings more accurately assess the injury and may have significant impact on management, prognosis, and treatment. Since my experiences in the BAPTEN® field studies, I routinely inform the trainer during the initial examination, made within 1 to 3 days post injury, that a more accurate injury severity assessment must be made in several weeks for prognosis and for making long-range treatment decisions. This will help determine the time away from training.

Utilizing % T-HYP for SDFT injury classification is a practical tool for determining prognosis and treatment programs. In 1995 a group of 187 superficial digital flexor tendons were examined sonographically during metacarpal swelling evaluation in which SDFT injury was possible or present (6). These horses were segregated into four categories based on sonographic criteria. Category 1 contains horses with suspect tendon injuries or those that had metacarpal swelling not related to tendon injury. Horses with obvious sonographic deep digital flexor tendon, inferior check ligament, or suspensory ligament injury were not included. Category 1 included metacarpal swelling in which the SDFT was suspected to be abnormal (lacked conclusive sonographic

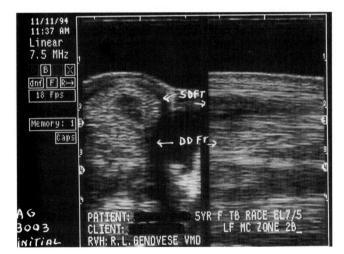

Figure 27B.3. A cross-sectional and sagittal left metacarpal Zone 2B initial sonogram. Core Lesion of the Superficial Digital Flexor Tendon. SDFT = superficial digital flexor tendon; DDFT = deep digital flexor tendon. (Classic 200 scanner)

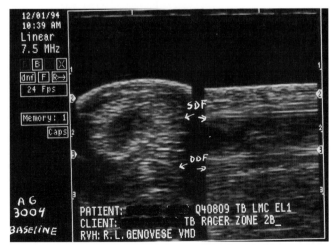

Figure 27B.4. A cross-sectional and sagittal left metacarpal Zone 2B baseline sonogram of the same horse as in Figure 27B.3 made at 3 weeks. SDF = superficial digital flexor tendon; DDF = deep digital flexor tendon. (Classic 200 scanner)

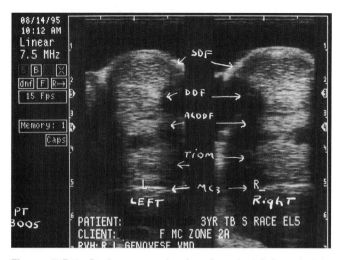

Figure 27B.5. Dual cross-sectional and sagittal left and right metacarpal Zone 2A. Category 1. SDF = superficial digital flexor tendon; DDF = deep digital flexor tendon; ALDDFT = accessory ligament of the deep digital flexor tendon (ICL); TIOM = third interosseous muscle (SL); MC3 = third metacarpal bone. (Classic 200 scanner)

data) or the SDFT was not contributory to the swelling. In the suspect SDFT evaluations for this category, there was <15% T-CSA increase compared with the contralateral limb. In addition, there may or may not be focal hypoechoic fiber bundles identified. However, no SDFT in this category had in excess of 8% T-HYP. In other words, there was not totally conclusive sonographic evidence of SDFT injury in a small percentage of the horses, but certainly there may be some evidence of an early injury. Most Category 1 horses had metacarpal swelling for reasons other than tendon injury. The practical consideration in this category is the decision to cease high-level competition (e.g., racing) or to treat the swelling symptomatically and continue cautiously. I refer to continued use with a favorable response to symptomatic therapy as symptomatic treatment/go on (S/GO) exercise management. This is an exercise management decision reached by the trainer/owner once a diagnosis has been made. The advantage of this exercise management is continued athletic use, and the disadvantage is the possibility of incurring more serious injury. When S/GO is selected, careful clinical and sonographic monitoring are essential. In the 1995 study there were 42 Category 1 horses. Twenty-seven trainers (64%) chose S/GO exercise management. Twenty-three horses (85%) continued their athletic careers and did not sustain a tendon injury. Four horses (15%) did suffer reinjury. Fifteen trainers (36%) decided not to risk injury and removed their horses from training.

Category 2 included 63 horses that had slight SDFT injuries. In this category the T-CSA had a >15% increase compared with the contralateral limb and/or had 1 to 15% T-HYP. Twenty-nine trainers (46%) decided to use S/GO exercise management. Only nine horses (31%) continued their athletic careers and did not suffer reinjury. Twenty horses (69%) suffered further injury and were athletically nonproductive. Thirty-four trainers (54%) decided not to risk further

injury and removed their horses from training. As can be seen, there is a significant difference in the success rate with continued athletic use between Category 1 and Category 2.

Category 3 included 22 horses that had moderate tendon injuries. Tendons in this category had 16 to 25% T-HYP. Only four trainers (18%) selected S/GO exercise management. Twelve trainers (55%) selected long-term rehabilitation. Six trainers (27%) chose retirement to an alternative career. Four horses is a small group on which to base an opinion; however, two horses competed successfully (Standardbreds), and two horses failed (Thoroughbreds).

Category 4 included 29 horses with severe injuries. Tendons in this category had >25% T-HYP. Only four trainers (14%) selected S/GO exercise management. All (100%) failed to continue. Twenty-five trainers (86%) removed their horses from training.

As can be seen from this retrospective study, injury severity categorization, especially in racehorses, by CSA increase from normal and % T-HYP will help determine prognoses for continued athletic use.

Figure 27B.5 is a sonogram of a TB racehorse with slight proximal swelling. The horse was not lame, and there was no painful response to direct digital pressure. There were no textural abnormalities; however, there was a 9% left SDFT T-CSA increase compared with the normal right. This increase was small and equivocal for tendon damage. This Category 1 metacarpal swelling was treated symptomatically with anti-inflammatory medication, the swelling resolved, and the horse was cautiously continued in training and raced without incident. At times it may be difficult to ascertain if the CSA increase is due to a recent SDFT strain or is the result of a previous injury that is presently stable. This situation may occur in a purchase situation or at times when a new groom notices a firm swelling. It is not often possible to sonographically determine a lesion's age based on one sonographic evaluation. Figure 27B.6 is a sonogram of a

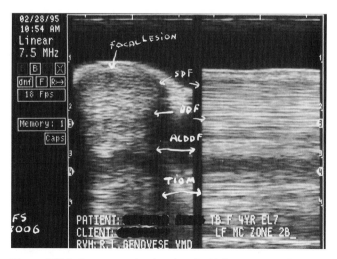

Figure 27B.6. A cross-sectional and sagittal left metacarpal Zone 2B sonogram of a focal superficial digital flexor tendon lesion. SDF = superficial digital flexor tendon; DDF = deep digital flexor tendon; ALDDFT = accessory ligament of the deep digital flexor tendon (ICL); TIOM = third interosseous muscle (SL). (Classic 200 scanner)

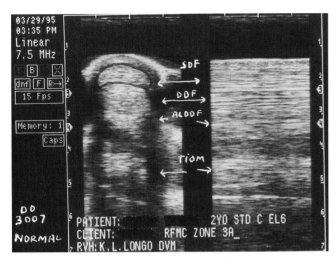

Figure 27B.7. A cross-sectional and sagittal right metacarpal Zone 3A normal sonogram. SDF = superficial digital flexor tendon; DDF = deep digital flexor tendon; ALDDFT = accessory ligament of the deep digital flexor tendon (ICL); TIOM = third interosseous muscle (SL). (Classic 200 scanner)

currently racing TB purchased several months previously. A new attendant noticed a firm left fore SDFT swelling. The trainer could not recall if the swelling was new or present at purchase. There was a Type 1 SDFT lesion and a 15% MIZ-CSA increase compared with the contralateral limb. Fiber alignment was normal. The T-CSA increase was an equivocal 13% (Category 1). It was decided not to chance further injury since there was no conclusive sonographic evidence that this was an older, stable injury. The treatment prescribed was 1 month off at a reduced exercise level and then repeat the sonogram. A repeat examination did not reveal any changes. It was more apparent that this was most likely an older "stable" injury. The horse was returned to training and sonographically monitored without any significant change. The horse competed successfully, and the lesion remained sonographically stable.

One should always proceed with caution when there is even slight sonographic evidence of SDFT abnormality. Even though, based on this study, Category 1 horses have an 85% success rate without reinjury, one must always remember that 15% of them fail. Figure 27B.7 is a normal sonogram of a 2-year-old STD racehorse with low-grade left metacarpal swelling at EL-6. The right limb sonogram has no abnormalities, and the CSA is 82 mm². Figure 27B.8 is a left metacarpal sonogram of the same horse as in Figure 27B.7. There are no significant texture or fiber alignment abnormalities. However, there is a 15% CSA increase, and the tendon was placed in Category 1.

The horse was treated symptomatically, and the training level was slightly reduced; however, serial sonography was not done over the next several weeks. The horse was examined 3 months later with the complaint of persistent left metacarpal swelling at EL-6 (Fig. 27B.9). There is a focal, Type 3 dorsal border SDFT lesion. The MIZ-FS is 3, and the MIZ-CSA is at 157 mm² (65% increase from the previ-

ous scan). The T-CSA increased by 32%. The decision to decrease the EL and continue training was not appropriate for this horse; however, more frequent serial sonography would have forced an EL decrease before the tendon became worse. For the most part, Category 1 metacarpal swelling is not due to SDFT injury, and for that reason there is a reasonably high success rate with symptomatic treatment and continued athletic use. Category 2 horses, however, have slight SDFT injury, and about 30% continue racing with stable lesions. The risk of continued racing is further tendon damage, and most of the time there is a reduced performance level. Economic considerations and the trainer's past experiences interrelate in the decision to continue training. Other factors, including the age of the horse, the racing level, and the lesion location, often affect decision making. In the Dubai International Equine Symposium Proceedings, this author reported on the RTR without reinjury for horses that had slight (Category 2), moderate (Category 3), and severe (Category 4) SDFT injuries treated with various therapeutic regimens and long-term layoff. In that report a group of 18 injured tendons with slight lesions were analyzed. This group had traditional therapy such as pin-firing, external blistering, superior check ligament desmotomy (SCLD), percutaneous tendon splitting (TS), or a combination of several treatments. All of these horses were given >6 months below EL-5. In that group 33% returned to racing and did not have a reinjury. One can appreciate the dilemma facing the trainer when he is told the horse has a slight tendon injury. According to our study groups, there is a 31% chance to continue racing and a 33% chance to return to racing after an expensive and extensive layoff. In the intralesional BAPTEN® clinical field trials with >6 months below EL-5, there was a 67% RTR without reinjury, but only six horses were in this group. If the statistical chance of RTR without reinjury improves, there will be a greater in-

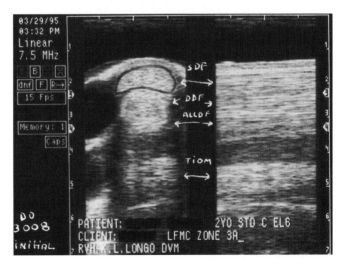

Figure 27B.8. A cross-sectional and sagittal left metacarpal Zone 3A sonogram with normal texture and abnormal CSA. SDF = superficial digital flexor tendon; DDF = deep digital flexor tendon; ALDDFT = accessory ligament of the deep digital flexor tendon (ICL); TIOM = third interosseous muscle (SL). (Classic 200 scanner)

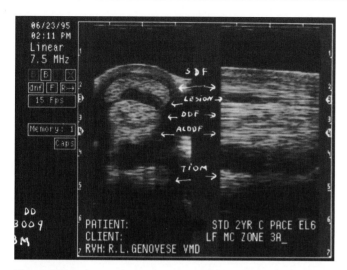

Figure 27B.9. A cross-sectional and sagittal left metacarpal Zone 3A sonogram of the same horse as in Figure 27B.8 made 3 months later. Lesion of the Superficial Digital Flexor Tendon. SDF = superficial digital flexor tendon; DDF = deep digital flexor tendon; ALDDFT = accessory ligament of the deep digital flexor tendon (ICL); TIOM = third interosseous muscle (SL). (Classic 200 scanner)

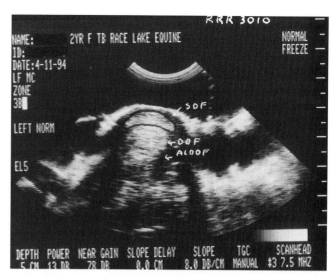

Figure 27B.10. A cross-sectional left metacarpal Zone 3B normal sonogram. SDF = superficial digital flexor tendon; DDF = deep digital flexor tendon; ALDDFT = accessory ligament of the deep digital flexor tendon (ICL). (ATL 4600 scanner)

centive for trainers to allow long-term treatment. Category 2 tendons are important because of the dilemma facing the trainer of continuing or stopping training. However, slight lesions do have better RTR prognoses with long-term treatment.

In traditionally treated, >6-months-off group of 14 Category 3 tendons, only 7% RTR without reinjury. In the BAPTEN®-treated, moderate-injury group of 14 tendons, there was a 50% RTR without reinjury. In the traditionally treated, >6-months-off group of 38 Category 4 tendons, 13% RTR without reinjury. Therefore the more severe the injury, the less chance there is to RTR without reinjury after long-term treatment.

The main concern with slight injury is that the horse will race a few times, most likely suboptimally, and increase the injury severity into a moderate or severe one, decreasing the chance for successful long-range treatment. This possibility should be discussed with the trainer during the early decision-making stages.

Consider the following examples of exercise management and treatment decisions for two TB racehorses: The first horse was an unraced 2-year-old with left metacarpal swelling following a morning breeze. The sonogram did not reveal any abnormal SDFT texture or fiber alignment. However, there was a 23% T-CSA increase. By definition, this is a Category 2 injury (slight). There were no other sonographic abnormalities. It was advised that this colt be given 6 months from training. Since there were no areas of fiber tearing and this was a slight injury, there was no indication for tendon splitting (TS), superior check ligament desmotomy (SCLD), intralesional BAPTEN®, or other treatments. The trainer insisted on external blister application. This horse returned to race as a 3-year-old, and the ten-

don remained asymptomatic through EL increases. The horse had a very successful racing career and never reinjured.

In contrast, the second horse was an expensive, two-year-old, TB filly that developed distal right tendon sheath effusion and slight distal metacarpal swelling. Figure 27B.10 is a normal sonogram, and Figure 27B.11 is a sonogram with thecal fluid increase. There are no tendon texture or fiber alignment abnormalities. There is, however, a slight 15% increased SDFT CSA compared with the left (Category 1). In this instance, in spite of the low-grade abnormalities and the value of this filly, the trainer chose S/GO exercise management with a decreased

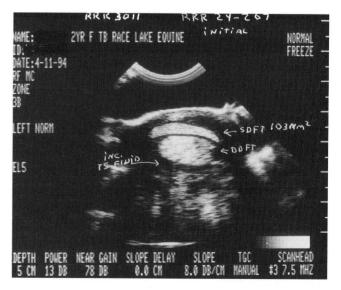

Figure 27B.11. A cross-sectional right metacarpal Zone 3B sonogram. Lesion of the Superficial Digital Flexor Tendon. SDFT = superficial digital flexor tendon; DDFT = deep digital flexor tendon; M.SLB = medial branch of the suspensory ligament; L.SLB = lateral branch of the suspensory ligament. (ATL 4600 scanner)

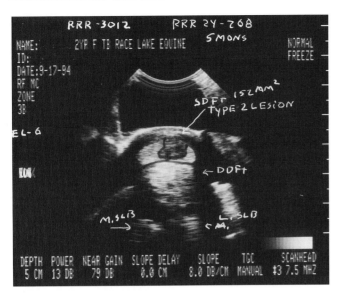

Figure 27B.12. A cross-sectional right metacarpal Zone 3B sonogram. Lesion of the Superficial Digital Flexor Tendon. SDFT = superficial digital flexor tendon; DDFT = deep digital flexor tendon; M.SLB = medial branch of the suspensory ligament; L.SLB = lateral branch of the suspensory ligament. (ATL 4600 scanner)

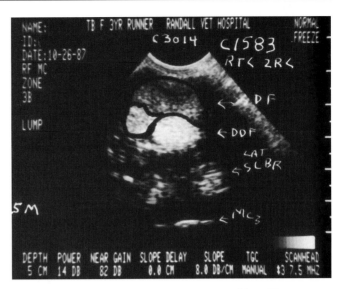

Figure 27B.14. A cross-sectional right metacarpal Zone 3B sonogram. Lesion of the Superficial Digital Flexor Tendon. SDF = superficial digital flexor tendon; DDF = deep digital flexor tendon; M.SLB = medial branch of the suspensory ligament; L.SLB = lateral branch of the suspensory ligament. (ATL 4600 scanner)

exercise level. Figure 27B.12 is a sonogram of the same horse as in Figure 27B.11 made following a light breeze 5 months after the initial examination. The tendon has a Type 2 palmar "trough" lesion. The MIZ-CSA increased to 152 mm², and the MIZ-HYP is 55 mm² (36%). There were six levels with hypoechoic fiber bundles. The T-CSA was 1017 mm², and the T-HYP was 206 mm². There was a 20% T-HYP injury (moderate). It is likely if this filly had been stopped and permitted to mature, her possible career-ending tendon injury could have been avoided. Had this been a seasoned racehorse in the claiming ranks, then S/GO management may have been appropriate. These contrasting cases emphasize the significance of careful exercise management even if the injury is slight.

Exercise level and treatment decisions for slight SDFT injuries are generally the most difficult. These injured horses are seldom lame, there is very little swelling, and it is conceptually difficult for many trainers to accept that this "slight" tendon injury should require a lengthy rest period. Furthermore, in the reality of the racehorse business, it is a situation whereby the owner may shun the long-term treatment program because of minimal physical evidence of injury. Often the situation results in the well-meaning trainer being dismissed. The owner in turn hires a new trainer who may ignore the recommendation and race the horse, which has a 30% chance of success with the S/GO exercise management. The second trainer is applauded. The first trainer lost his job. As trite as this scenario may seem, it is a nonmedical factor such as this that may enter into the equation when a trainer has to make the exercise decision. This in turn influences treatment options and case outcome.

Figure 27B.13 is a TB racehorse examined for slight, mid palmar, metacarpal swelling. There is a small, peripheral, palmar medial focal SDFT lesion. The trainer was informed and advised that an extended rest and treatment program should be set up for this slight injury. The trainer believed that this lesion was not due to work-related tendon strain, but rather to a "rap" and that "he could handle it." The trainer was convinced that if he informed the owner of the veterinarian's advice to give this horse several months off, he would lose his job and a new trainer would be hired. He was further advised that if he chose the S/GO exercise program, sonographic examination should be repeated after each work or race to monitor lesion stability. This was not done.

Figure 27B.14 is a Zone 3B sonogram of the same horse

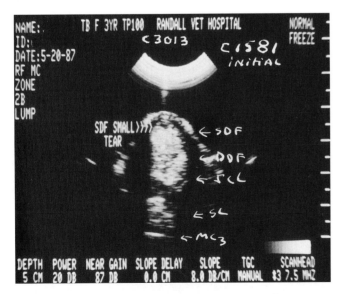

Figure 27B.13. A cross-sectional right metacarpal Zone 2B sonogram. Lesion of the Superficial Digital Flexor Tendon. SDF = superficial digital flexor tendon; DDF = deep digital flexor tendon; ALDDFT = accessory ligament of the deep digital flexor tendon (ICL); TIOM = third interosseous muscle (SL); MC3 = third metatarsal bone. (ATL 4600 scanner)

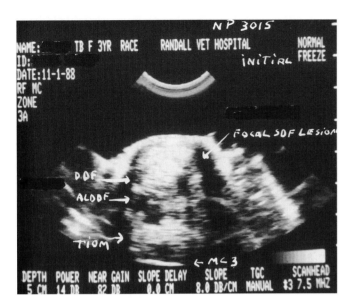

Figure 27B.15. A cross-sectional right metacarpal Zone 3A sonogram. Lesion of the Superficial Digital Flexor Tendon. SDF = superficial digital flexor tendon; DDF = deep digital flexor tendon; ALDDFT = accessory ligament of the deep digital flexor tendon (ICL); TIOM = third interosseous muscle (SL); MC3 = third metacarpal bone. (ATL 4600 scanner)

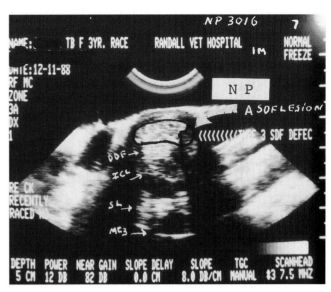

Figure 27B.16. A cross-sectional right metacarpal Zone 3A sonogram. Lesion of the Superficial Digital Flexor Tendon. SDF = superficial digital flexor tendon; DDF = deep digital flexor tendon; ICL = inferior check ligament (ALDDFT); SL = suspensory ligament (TIOM); MC3 = third metacarpal bone. (ATL 4600 scanner)

as in Figure 27B.13. This was the first sonogram since the original injury 5 months prior. The horse had raced several times and performances were substandard. There was an extensive SDFT injury. The injury was now severe and the horse was lame. There was a failed attempt to rehabilitate the horse at this point. The choice to continue was not medically based in this case, and treatment was based on the primary exercise management decision.

Not all S/GO management decisions result in such catastrophic endings. Figure 27B.15 is a TB racehorse that was recently purchased in a sale. There was a slight SDFT lateral border lesion limited to two levels. The horse was sound and the sonogram was done because of the slight tendon enlargement. This scan was performed in the fall of the year, and the trainer stated that the filly was purchased for a broodmare. He realized that there would be some risk of additional injury if this horse raced, but felt that he would be willing to take the risk. He selected S/GO exercise management and informed the owner. A sonogram was performed following each race. The horse was productive and remained clinically asymptomatic. Figure 27B.16 is a sonogram of the same horse as in Figure 27B.15 made 5 weeks and three races after the initial examination. There were slight MIZ-CSA and MIZ-HYP increases. In this instance, with careful sonographic monitoring and a modified training program, this lesion remained relatively stable at EL-7. The symptomatic treatment program and case management resulted in fulfilling the goals of the owner and the trainer. Treatment was based on nonmedical criteria with full understanding of the risks.

Figure 27B.17 is a STD racehorse with swelling and de-

clining performances. There was a focal SDFT lateral border lesion. This was an older horse racing at the claiming level. The trainer stated that if this injury was such that a long-term treatment program was required, the horse would be sold for alternative use. He selected the S/GO exercise program because he felt the horse could perform at its present level if the inflammation could be controlled. A combination of 6 mg triamcinolone (Vetalog, Solvay Animal Health Inc., Mindota Hts, MN) and 20 mg sodium

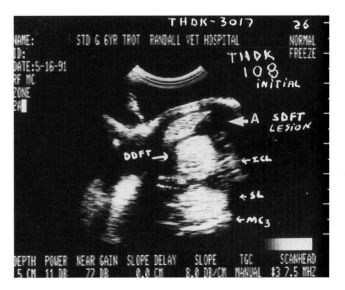

Figure 27B.17. A cross-sectional right metacarpal Zone 2A sonogram. Lesion of the Superficial Digital Flexor Tendon. SDFT = superficial digital flexor tendon; DDFT = deep digital flexor tendon; ICL = inferior check ligament (ALDDFT); SL = suspensory ligament (TIOM); MC3 = third metacarpal bone. (ATL 4600 scanner)

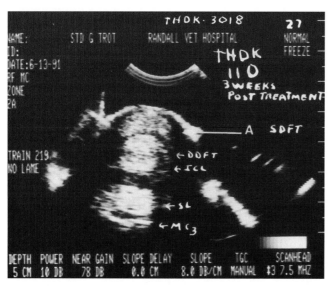

Figure 27B.18. A cross-sectional right metacarpal Zone 2A baseline sonogram of the same horse as in Figure 27B.17 made 3 weeks later. SDFT = superficial digital flexor tendon; DDFT = deep digital flexor tendon; ICL = inferior check ligament (ALDDFT); SL = suspensory ligament (TIOM); MC3 = third metacarpal bone. (ATL 4600 scanner)

hyaluronate (Legend, Miles Shawnee Mission, KS) was injected perilesionally. The exercise level was decreased to EL-5 for 1 month, and sonography was repeated to reassess the injury. The therapeutic concept, in this select case, was to allow time for a baseline evaluation. Even though *intralesional* corticosteroids are contraindicated in tendon or ligament injuries, a low, peritendinous dose was used to resolve the inflammatory response to obtain a more accurate fiber damage assessment. Furthermore, the exercise level was reduced to prevent injury. There is no proven scientific basis for any therapeutic benefit from the hyaluronate.

Figure 27B.18 is a sonogram of the same horse as in Figure 27B.17 made 3 weeks post treatment. There is a marked lesion-texture improvement. This baseline examination indicated the fiber compromise to be significantly less than initially thought, which improved the prognosis of success for S/GO exercise management. This horse raced multiple times at the lower class level and was productive. The lesion remained stable for 1 year and over 20 races. There was a slight relapse the following year, and the same treatment was successfully repeated.

Currently, few TB and STD trainers select S/GO for slight SDFT injuries. Sonography has modified trainer response to tendon injury over the past 10 years. Most trainers prefer not to risk further injury except for those horses where economic decisions intervene. The long-range treatment programs for slight injuries in the author's hands are based on the lesion location, conformation, the maximum EL attained prior to injury, the intended use of the horse, and the projected trainer/owner compliance to a long-range rehabilitation program. If long-range treatment and rehabilitation are selected by the trainer, it is assumed the horse's value and stable economics justify that decision. There are two basic

"time out of training" options available to the trainer: Phase 1 and 2. The length of time from training was derived from the BAPTEN® clinical field trials. In the early stages of BAPTEN® testing, the project design was such that horses, regardless of treatment were elevated to EL-5 prior to completing 6 full months at lower levels. This was called Phase I exercise management. Furthermore, in this author's experience, many traditionally treated horses in the United States were managed with 3 to 6 months out of training. In the Phase I exercise managed BAPTEN® treated horses, the percentage RTR was low. Because of this, a second study was undertaken and horses were given a minimum of 6 months out of training. This was called Phase II exercise management. This use of Phase I or Phase II terminology simplified communication and became firmly entrenched in the overall tendon-injury management. Therefore, for practical purposes, there are three decision-making levels relative to the horse's exercise management and return to athletic use:

1. S/GO (symptomatic treatment with continued competition regardless of training program. Included are horses that are rested for 1 month or less)..
2. Phase I exercise management (includes horses that are kept at exercise levels below EL-5 for 1 to 6 months).
3. Phase II exercise management (includes horses that are kept at exercise levels below EL-5 for 6 or more months).

The practical aspect of this exercise segregation from a therapeutic viewpoint becomes clear as we continue. In the 1996 Dubai International Equine Symposium Proceedings, this author reported a study of 37 tendons of varying injury severity that were provided long-term therapy but were managed as Phase I. The RTR without reinjury was 11%, or, conversely, there was an 89% failure rate regardless of treatment. On the other hand, 26% of a group of 113 horses with a variety of SDFT injuries that were al-

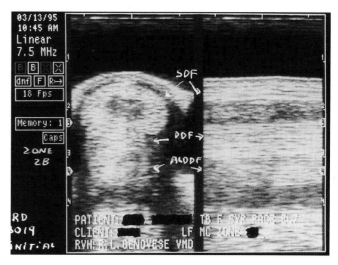

Figure 27B.19. A cross-sectional and sagital left metacarpal Zone 2B sonogram. Core Lesion of the Superficial Digital Flexor Tendon. Initial. SDF = superficial digital flexor tendon; DDF = deep digital flexor tendon; ALDDFT = accessory ligament of the deep digital flexor tendon. (Classic 200 scanner)

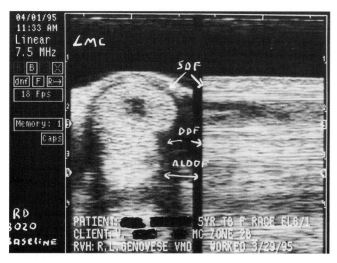

Figure 27B.20. A cross-sectional and sagittal left metacarpal Zone 2B sonogram. Core Lesion of the Superficial Digital Flexor Tendon. Baseline. SDF = superficial digital flexor tendon; DDF = deep digital flexor tendon; ALDDFT = accessory ligament of the deep digital flexor tendon (ICL). (Classic 200 scanner)

lowed long-term therapy, but were managed as Phase II, made a RTR without reinjury. It would appear that there is an improved chance of recovery using Phase II exercise management in long-term treatments. In the BAPTEN®-treated horses, there was a low rate of RTR with Phase I horses and a 45% RTR without reinjury in the Phase II group. Silver et al. (3) have conclusively shown that damaged collagen tissue repair may require a year or more for recollagenization, maturation, remodeling, and injured fiber bundle strengthening. This principle must be kept in mind when interpreting the sonographic repair progress. The BAPTEN® study program supports the principle that treated horses with moderate to severe injuries must be managed in Phase II.

There are many references to treating tendonitis with "controlled exercise," yet few authors specifically defined controlled exercise. Madison (7) and Dyson (8) have outlined controlled exercise programs for SDFT rehabilitation. In the BAPTEN® program there is a defined, Phase II controlled exercise program that has strong sonographic support and end results. For example, the following two horses were enrolled in the intralesional BAPTEN® project: The first horse was a seasoned TB filly that had raced for 2 years until she injured the left fore SDFT. This filly had raced (EL-7) many times prior to injury. Limb conformation was normal, and there were no other apparent musculoskeletal abnormalities. Figure 27B.19 is a sonogram at the initial examination. This recent injury occurred during a race (EL-7). There is a Type 3 "core" SDFT lesion. The MIZ-CSA was 168 mm², and the MIZ-HYP was 34 mm². The MIZ-FS is 3 and the T-FS was 17. The % T-HYP was 12% (slight injury). This injury was treated with daily icing, mild leg liniment application, and limb bandaging. The horse was treated with oral phenylbutazone at the rate of 2 g per day

for 10 days. The horse was permitted 15 minutes daily hand walking. Three weeks later, the baseline sonographic examination was done and the BAPTEN® treatment started.

Figure 27B.20 is the same horse as in Figure 27B.19 made 3 weeks post injury (baseline). There is a Type 3 "core" SDFT lesion. Due to the anti-inflammatory treatment there is a MIZ-CSA to 143 mm² reduction and a T-CSA to 941 mm². The MIZ-HYP is elevated slightly to 36 mm², and the T-HYP has slightly decreased to 110 mm². The MIZ-FS is still 3 and the T-FS is decreased to 11. The % T-HYP remains the same at 12% (slight injury). These are the baseline (0 elapse time) data from which future quantitative evaluations will be made. The tendon lesion was injected intralesionally with BAPTEN® every other day until five treatments were completed. The only other treatment permitted was daily wrapping of the leg using isopropyl alcohol as the liniment. This horse was hand walked (EL-1) 30 minutes daily for 2 months. Figure 27B.21 is a cross-sectional and sagittal left metacarpal Zone 2B sonogram of the same horse as in Figure 27B.20 made two months post baseline. There was no evidence of the "core" lesion; but there are small areas of ill defined, reduced echogenicity. The MIZ-CSA increased to 187 mm² and the MIZ-HYP was 32 mm² (17%). The T-CSA increased to 1271 mm² and the T-HYP decreased to 90 mm². The MIZ-FS was still 3 and the T-FS still 11. The %T-HYP decreased to 7%. There was overall textural improvement, but there was CSA increase. Because of the increased CSA, the client was advised to continue walking and add swimming (non weight bearing exercise EL-2) three days per week for the next 2 months.

Figure 27B.22 is the same horse as in Figure 27B.21 made 4 months post baseline. There was no evidence of the "core" lesion or scattered areas of slightly reduced echogenicity. The MIZ-CSA reduced to 124 mm², and the T-CSA reduced to

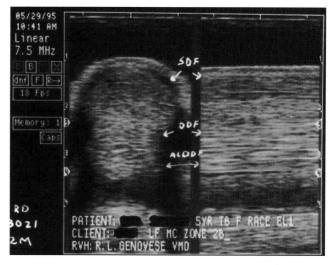

Figure 27B.21. A cross-sectional and sagittal left metacarpal Zone 2B baseline sonogram of the same horse as in Figure 27B.20 made 2 months later. SDF = superficial digital flexor tendon; DDF = deep digital flexor tendon; ALDDFT = accessory ligament of the deep digital flexor tendon (ICL). (Classic 200 scanner)

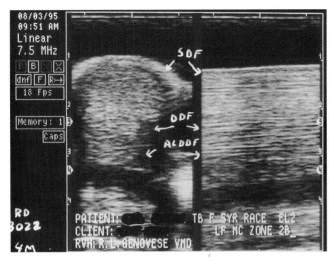

Figure 27B.22. A cross-sectional and sagittal left metacarpal Zone 2B sonogram of the same horse as in Figure 27B.21 made 4 months later. SDF = superficial digital flexor tendon; DDF = deep digital flexor tendon; ALDDFT = accessory ligament of the deep digital flexor tendon (ICL). (Classic 200 scanner)

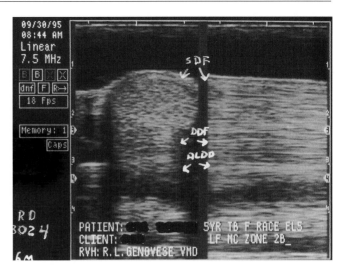

Figure 27B.24. A cross-sectional and sagittal left metacarpal Zone 2B sonogram of the same horse as in Figure 27B.23 made 6 months later. SDF = superficial digital flexor tendon; DDF = deep digital flexor tendon; ALDDFT = accessory ligament of the deep digital flexor tendon (ICL). (Classic 200 scanner)

792 mm². The MIZ-HYP decreased to 17 mm² (15%), and the T-HYP decreased to 94 mm². The MIZ-FS was 2 and the T-FS was still 11. The % T-HYP was still at 12%. As can be seen there has been sonographic evidence of progress. Externally, with the decreased CSA, the leg had an improved appearance. The trainer was advised only to progress to ponying 3 days per week (EL-2) along with the daily walking since the % T-HYP was still elevated. Unfortunately, this trainer made a personal decision to switch from Phase II to Phase I exercise management and started to advance the horse to EL-5. Even though there may be a favorable sonographic appearance at 4 months post baseline examination, the quantitative data and the physiologic principle of necessary time dictates that restraint in EL elevation at this

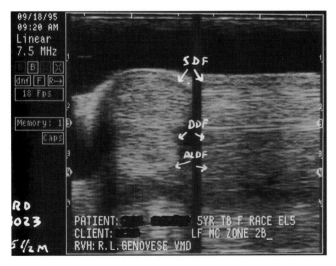

Figure 27B.23. A cross-sectional and sagittal left metacarpal Zone 2B sonogram of the same horse as in Figure 27B.22 made 5½ months later. SDF = superficial digital flexor tendon; DDF = deep digital flexor tendon; ALDDFT = accessory ligament of the deep digital flexor tendon (ICL). (Classic 200 scanner)

time is important. Recollagenization is taking place, but exercise control and more time are required to allow strengthening and fiber alignment remodeling. This was very apparent from the MIZ and T fiber alignment scores.

Figure 27B.23 is a sonogram of the same horse as in Figure 27B.22 made 5½ months post baseline examination. At this time, the advised EL has been exceeded and the horse is now in Phase I exercise management. The horse is at EL-5 3 days per week. There was total hypoechoic fiber bundle resolution and near-normal fiber alignment in spite of the escalated EL. The MIZ-CSA decreased to 89 mm², and the T-CSA further decreased to 736 mm². As a point of reference, the contralateral normal MIZ-CSA was 83 mm² and the T-CSA was 592 mm². The MIZ-HYP was 0 and the T-HYP was 11 mm². The MIZ-FS was 1 and the T-FS was 2. The % T-HYP was 1%. The 4- to 6-month stage of repair is a critical point at which one *must* control exercise. This is the strengthening and remodeling phase. An excessive EL will often cause a reinjury. The take-home lesson of this case exists at this stage of rehabilitation. The sonogram and the quantitative data have shown a favorable treatment response to this point, but the sonographer can be lured into thinking that this justifies "full speed ahead." This is not the case, and restraint of premature EL advances is of the utmost importance. More time at lower exercise levels and a gradual return to EL-5 is indicated once this sonographic appearance is attained. One must respect the time requirement for nonsonographically detectable cross-linking. Furthermore, fiber alignment remodeling will require a minimum of 6 months. If the 4 month post baseline criteria are unfavorable, then even more time below EL-5 would be required. Figure 27B.24 is the same horse as in Figure 27B.23 made 6 months post baseline and at daily EL-5 for 2 weeks. There were no significant textural or fiber alignment abnormalities. The % T-HYP at this time was still a low 2%. But there was an increase of the MIZ-CSA to 157 mm² and the T-CSA to 837

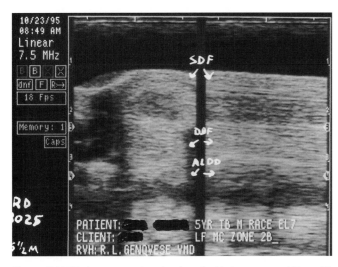

Figure 27B.25. A cross-sectional and sagittal left metacarpal Zone 2B sonogram of the same horse as in Figure 27B.24 made 6¹/₂ months later. SDF = superficial digital flexor tendon; DDF = deep digital flexor tendon; ALDDFT = accessory ligament of the deep digital flexor tendon (ICL). (Classic 200 scanner)

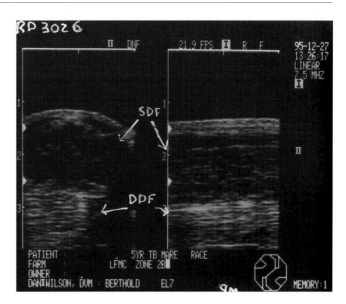

Figure 27B.26. A cross-sectional and sagittal left metacarpal Zone 2B sonogram of the same horse as in Figure 27B.25 made 9 months later. SDF = superficial digital flexor tendon; DDF = deep digital flexor tendon. (Classic 480 scanner)

mm². There was a 79% CSA increase at the MIZ and a 14% CSA increase overall associated. Even though this horse was exercise mismanaged, at this point there was no sonographic evidence of fiber path disruption; however, the CSA increase confirms tendon swelling. The EL should have been reduced to EL-1, but the trainer did not comply.

Figure 27B.25 is a sonogram of the same horse as in Figure 27B.24 made 6½ months post baseline. Prior to this scan the horse had worked twice and raced twice. The first race was credible, and the second race was a poor performance. There was no lameness, but the "core" injury recurred. The MIZ-CSA was 143 mm², and the T-CSA was 844 mm². The MIZ-HYP was 31 mm² (22%), and the T-HYP was 110 mm². The MIZ-FS was 3 and the T-FS was 13. The % T-HYP was 13%. Basically, this horse had a similar injury that it started with almost 7 months prior. The trainer then decided on the S/GO exercise management program, which included only swimming and widely spaced races. Figure 27B.26 is a sonogram of the same horse as in Figure 27B.25. There was a large Type 3 SDFT lesion. The MIZ-CSA was at 267 mm², and the T-CSA increased to 1401 mm². The MIZ-HYP was 198 mm² (74%), and the T-HYP was 738 mm². The MIZ-FS was 3 and the T-FS was 17. The % T-HYP was 53% (severe reinjury).

This case was included to emphasize the importance of exercise management decisions and stricter control over exercise level increases *only* after the necessary time has elapsed. Furthermore, favorable sonographic improvement should not allow reckless exercise increases. One should also heed the sonographic indications that a given exercise level is excessive. In this case, the treatment program was excellent, but the exercise management was not. This was not a treatment failure; in reality, it was an exercise management failure.

Contrasting the previous horse, this TB racehorse sustained a first-episode, right fore SDFT injury after a work

(EL-6). This horse had not attained EL-7 prior to injury as had the previous horse, and this horse had an upright forelimb conformation. Figure 27B.27 is a sonogram with a large, Type 3 SDFT "core" lesion. The MIZ-CSA was 162 mm², and the T-CSA was 1140 mm². The MIZ-HYP was 73 mm², and the T-HYP was 484 mm². The MIZ-FS was 3 and the T-FS was 17. The % T-HYP was 42% (severe injury). Figure 27B.28 is the same horse as in Figure 27B.27 made 2 weeks post injury and serving as the baseline examination. Since the injury the horse was treated with phenylbutazone (2 g per day) and daily icing. A mild liniment was applied, and the leg was wrapped with support bandaging. Due to the degree of lameness there was limited walking allowed. There was a

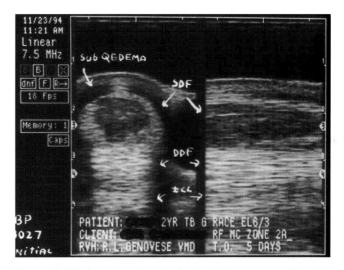

Figure 27B.27. A cross-sectional and sagittal right metacarpal Zone 2A initial sonogram. SDF = superficial digital flexor tendon; DDF = deep digital flexor tendon; ICL = inferior check ligament (ALDDFT). (Classic 200 scanner)

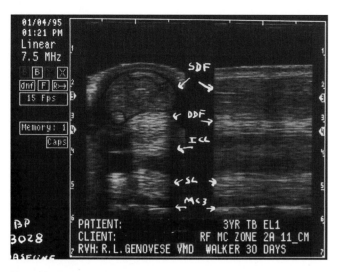

Figure 27B.28. A cross-sectional and sagittal right metacarpal Zone 2A baseline sonogram of the same horse as in Figure 27B.27. SDF = superficial digital flexor tendon; DDF = deep digital flexor tendon; ICL = inferior check ligament (ALDDFT); SL = suspensory ligament (TIOM); MC3 = third metacarpal bone. (Classic 200 scanner)

large, Type 3 SDFT lesion. The MIZ-CSA was 267 mm^2, and the T-CSA was 1556 mm^2. The MIZ-HYP was 216 mm^2 (81%), and the T-HYP was 930 mm^2. The MIZ-FS was 3 and the T-FS was 16. The % T-HYP was 60%. This horse was treated every other day with intralesional BAPTEN® for 5 treatments. No other therapy was permitted. The leg was bandaged daily using isopropyl alcohol as the liniment.

Figure 27B.29 is a sonogram of the same horse as in Figure 27B.28 made 4 months post baseline. The horse was walked 30 minutes daily for the first 2 months, and during the second 2 months the horse was hand walked daily and ponied (EL-2) 1 mile, 2 days per week. This scan shows marked textural improvement. The MIZ-CSA reduced to 209 mm^2, and the T-CSA reduced to 1324 mm^2. The MIZ-HYP reduced to 44 mm^2 (22%), and the T-HYP was 279 mm^2. The MIZ-FS was 3 and the T-FS was decreased to 11. The % T-HYP was 25%.

Figure 27B.30 is the same horse as in Figure 27B.29 made 7 months post baseline. Since the 4-month scan the horse was only permitted hand walking and ponied 1 mile 2 days per week (EL-2). The MIZ-CSA decreased to 173 mm^2, and the T-CSA decreased to 1266 mm^2. The MIZ-HYP decreased to 0, and the T-HYP reduced to 53 mm^2. The MIZ-FS was 0 and the T-FS was 4. The % T-HYP was 4%. This is significant sonographic progress for this severe lesion. The horse gradually increased exercise levels from EL-4 to EL-6 over the next 2 months. This horse was not permitted pasture exercise any time in the recovery period because of hyperactive behavior. During this period sonograms were evaluated prior to increasing exercise levels. There were slight CSA and % T-HYP increases, but they never exceeded acceptable measurement error variation. The % T-HYP always remained below 10%.

Figure 27B.31 is a sonogram of the same horse as in Figure 27B.30 made 9½ months post baseline after the last

work before the first race. The enlarged SDFT had near-normal echogenicity and no evidence of peritendinous fibrosis. The MIZ-CSA was 146 mm^2, and the T-CSA was 970 mm^2. The MIZ-HYP was 0, and the T-HYP was 28 mm^2. The MIZ-FS was 0, and the T-FS was 5. The % T-HYP was 3%. These quantitative sonographic data indicate lesion stability with increasing ELs.

Figure 27B.32 is the same horse as in Figure 27B.31 made 10 months post baseline after three races. The enlarged SDFT had near-normal echogenicity and no evidence of peritendinous fibrosis. The MIZ-CSA is 153 mm^2, and the T-CSA is 1099 mm^2. The MIZ-HYP is 0, and the T-HYP is 26 mm^2. The MIZ-FS is 1, and the T-FS is 4. The % T-HYP is 2%. These data suggest sonographic stability with maximum loading. In contrast to the Phase I–exercise-managed horse, this horse was managed in Phase II and overcame a far more extensive injury. In addition, this tendon attained a higher load post injury than pre injury. It is also worth noting that this horse was never permitted pasture exercise, since its demeanor was such that free choice pasture exercise would have resulted in uncontrolled exercise. Furthermore, this author believes the SQR for less than a year of rehabilitation was significantly better than one would generally expect for an injury of this magnitude.

EXERCISE AND TREATMENT OPTIONS FOR SLIGHT SDFT INJURIES

Slight SDFT injuries can be treated in a variety of ways depending on the exercise management selected by the trainer. In my opinion horses that have tendon swelling without appreciable sonographic evidence of fiber bundle disruption are generally not considered for treatment such as superior check ligament desmotomy (SCLD), intralesional BAPTEN®, or tendon splitting (TS). Phase I– or preferably

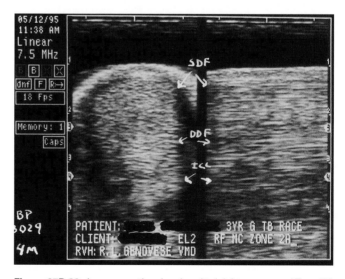

Figure 27B.29. A cross-sectional and sagittal right metacarpal Zone 2A sonogram of the same horse as in Figure 27B.28 made 6 months later. SDF = superficial digital flexor tendon; DDF = deep digital flexor tendon; ICL = inferior check ligament (ALDDFT). (Classic 200 scanner)

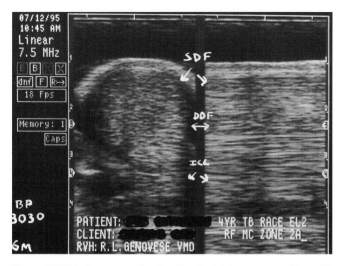

Figure 27B.30. A cross-sectional and sagittal right metacarpal Zone 2A sonogram of the same horse as in Figure 27B.29 made 6 months later. SDF = superficial digital flexor tendon; DDF = deep digital flexor tendon; ICL = inferior check ligament (ALDDFT). (Classic 200 scanner)

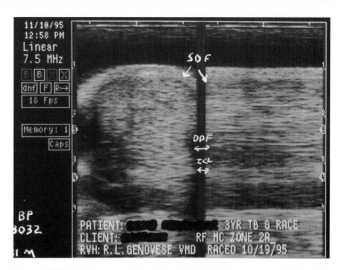

Figure 27B.32. A cross-sectional and sagittal right metacarpal Zone 2A sonogram of the same horse as in Figure 27B.31 made 11 months later. SDF = superficial digital flexor tendon; DDF = deep digital flexor tendon; ICL = inferior check ligament (ALDDFT). (Classic 200 scanner)

Phase II–exercise-managed horses are basically treated with time out of training, and I usually request several lightly irritating external blisters. Admittedly, there is no scientific evidence that external blistering has any therapeutic effect. But from a practical point of view, one must remember that a trainer is controlling the medical care of the horse. Their injury management control is based on established principles they develop over time, and this factor enters into racehorse care. In this situation I have two options as the attending veterinarian advising the trainer: (a) tell my client just to rest the horse for 6 months, and then stand by while the trainer institutes the treatment program of his/her own, or (b) design a sensible program that will be followed, and permit the maintenance of a client/patient/doctor relation-

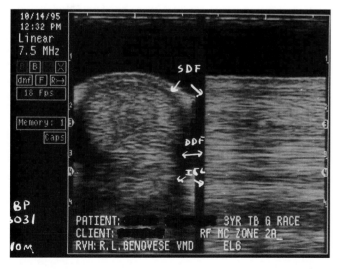

Figure 27B.31. A cross-sectional and sagittal right metacarpal Zone 2A sonogram of the same horse as in Figure 27B.30 made 10 months later. SDF = superficial digital flexor tendon; DDF = deep digital flexor tendon; ICL = inferior check ligament (ALDDFT). (Classic 200 scanner)

ship. I prefer to institute a treatment program that will keep me in contact with my patient and assist in getting the horse the beneficial time off. Furthermore, based on early indications of a possible benefit of PSGAG reported from the UK (5), I would suggest systemic treatment in the first month of rehabilitation. If my client selects S/GO management, I would advise these steps:

1. Downscale the faster training exercises to a minimum (EL-6).
2. Use daily anti-inflammatory treatment systemically and directly to the injured SDFT. I would prefer phenylbutazone at the rate of 2 grams per day.
3. Daily icing or cold-water hydrotherapy .
4. Space races more widely, and select a class level in which the horse can be competitive.
5. Sonographically monitor the horse after each EL-6 or EL-7 event.

I would stress to the trainer that continued high-level exercise can result in further damage and that, as injury severity increases, the prognosis for a successful return from long-term therapy decreases. I also carefully point out that if performances are not productive, S/GO exercise management should be abandoned. If this horse is intended for alternative, less stressful, athletic use, then a Phase I exercise program may well suffice. For high-level competition with Phase II exercise management, horses with this degree of SDFT "strain" have a good prognosis for RTR without reinjury, if the pre injury maximum EL attained was greater than EL-5. If a horse strained the SDFT at EL-5 or less, the prognosis would be guarded for a sustained racing career.

Horses that have a slight SDFT injury (Category 2) and have peripheral, focal hypoechoic lesions are managed in the same manner if S/GO exercise management is selected. If Phase I exercise is selected, I generally advise pin firing, external blistering, and/or physical therapy such as magnetic pads. I have seen successful end results in the STD racehorse with "cryotherapy," but I personally have not used this treatment. Here again, none of these treatment approaches have conclusive scientific evidence of therapeutic value at this time. The only indication of therapeutic benefit is based on favorable anecdotal reports from practitioners. Sonographic examinations should be performed prior to EL-5 and during increase in EL. I do advise sonographic evaluation after each race. I advise systemic PSGAG in the first month post injury. At times, the lesion will resolve and remain stable. The same warnings and disclaimers are always given in S/GO or Phase I–exercise-managed horses. It is difficult to predict the outcome of each case. There are just too many variables that enter into the equation. Some horses with slight lesions are successful and productive, at least for a while, but many fail and the end result is more serious SDFT damage. The TB racehorse fails more often than is successful with S/GO and Phase I management. The STD racehorse seems to be capable of maintaining a stable SDFT lesion and to be more productive than the TB racehorse. Occasionally, in STD racehorses I will administer a perilesional injection of a low-dose (6 mg) triamcinolone coupled with 20 mg sodium hyaluronate, when the trainer is willing to reduce the EL for a month or more post treatment. I do not perform this treatment in the TB racehorse. I am always concerned with inducing a tendon fiber weakness and want to avoid acute breakdown. I have never had acute breakdown secondary to this treatment in STD racehorses with slight peripheral lesions.

The horse in Figure 27B.17 demonstrated an athletically successful outcome of a S/GO-exercise-managed STD racehorse with a peripheral lesion. Obviously, in that instance, the fiber bundle injury was such that at that horse's competitive level there were sufficient intact tendon fibers to sustain racing without further damage. There was no evidence of painful tendinitis, and the horse was productive. However, that situation is unique to that horse, and only by trial and error can the injury's stability be determined. Lesion stability can be determined by serial sonographic evaluations. It is my impression that most competitive horses that have stable focal lesions are those that have a stable MIZ and T-CSA. Peripheral lesions seem more likely to remain stable than "core" lesions. It is also my impression that even though these horses remain clinically asymptomatic, most have decreased quality performance. I believe it is difficult for a horse to race with a peripheral, slightly hypoechoic lesion and be effective at higher competitive levels.

Consider the situation with this 2-year-old STD filly: Figure 27B.33 is Zone 2B sonogram of a recent first-episode SDFT injury. The filly was unraced, but had been at EL-6 several times. The trainer felt the filly had a bright racing future and decided to use Phase II exercise management since she was only a 2-year-old. There was a Type 3 lateral border SDFT lesion. Quantitative data at the initial examination revealed this moderate injury (17% T-HYP) involved five

levels. The trainer did not want any surgical treatment and indicated that he had success with past SDFT injuries with pasture rest and external blistering. Figure 27B.34 is the same horse as in Figure 27B.33 made 6 months post injury at EL-3. There is significant lesion texture improvement, and the MIZ and T-CSA were significantly decreased. There was only 2% T-HYP. The trainer made a slow return to racing fitness and spent several months at EL-5. Figure 27B.35 is the same horse as in Figure 27B.34 made 11 months post injury at EL-6 (2:18-minute training mile). There was reinjury of the same lateral SDFT border area as the original injury. It is worth noting that clinically the horse is not lame and even at high speeds did not have an abnormal gait. The trainer noticed a slight increase in temperature along the lateral SDFT border and requested the sonogram.

At this point the reinjury was slight (12% T-HYP). There has been a great deal of time and money invested in this filly, and there was a Phase II management and treatment failure. One cannot realistically advise a repeat of this treatment for an unproved 3-year-old STD racehorse that has no alternative options other than Amish buggy work. The trainer wanted S/GO management and treatment, realizing that most likely it would not be successful. The lesion was injected perilesionally with 6 mg of triamcinolone and 20 mg of sodium hyaluronate. The horse was raced four times and returned 3 months later for sonographic evaluation. Figure 27B.36 is a sonogram of the same horse as in Figure 27B.35. There was a focal, hypoechoic, lateral border SDFT lesion. The quantitative data indicated there was CSA stability in lieu of four races and the lesion did not progress. The T-HYP was reduced from 12% T-HYP to 9% T-HYP in spite of EL-7. The trainer retired the horse after

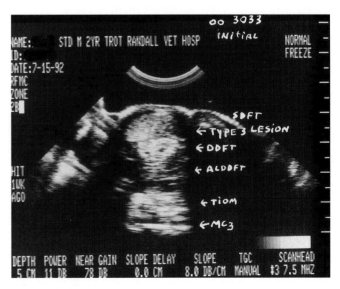

Figure 27B.33. A cross-sectional right metacarpal Zone 2B initial sonogram. SDFT = superficial digital flexor tendon; DDFT = deep digital flexor tendon; ALDDFT = accessory ligament of the deep digital flexor tendon (ICL); TIOM = third interosseous muscle (SL); MC3 = third metacarpal bone. (ATL 4600 scanner)

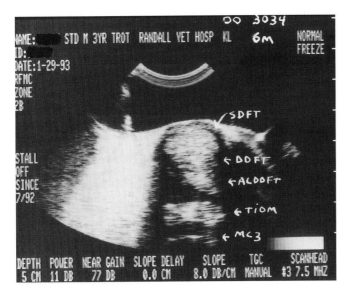

Figure 27B.34. A cross-sectional right metacarpal Zone 2B sonogram of the same horse as in Figure 27B.33 made 6 months later. SDFT = superficial digital flexor tendon; DDFT = deep digital flexor tendon; ALDDFT = accessory ligament of the deep digital flexor tendon (ICL); TIOM = third interosseous muscle (SL); MC3 = third metacarpal bone. (ATL 4600 scanner)

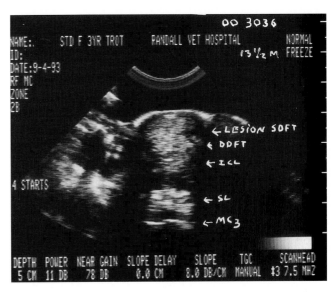

Figure 27B.36. A cross-sectional right metacarpal Zone 2B sonogram of the same horse as in Figure 27B.35 made 13 months later. SDFT = superficial digital flexor tendon; DDFT = deep digital flexor tendon; ICL = inferior check ligament (ALDDFT); SL = suspensory ligament (TIOM); MC3 = third metacarpal bone. (ATL 4600 scanner)

this examination. This horse's retirement was due to lack of racing productivity and not because the horse was clinically lame. The SDFT lesion remained stable at EL-7, but her racing performances were suboptimal.

Even though Phase II exercise management is indicated for slight, peripheral SDFT lesions, on occasion the variables of decision making dictate Phase I exercise management. Like the success rate of S/GO management, it is difficult to predict the outcome of selected cases. Careful case selection of slightly injured tendons may be a significant

part of Phase I management success or failure. Figure 27B.37 is a TB horse racehorse. There is a focal, hypoechoic, lateral border SDFT lesion. The quantitative data indicated only two-level involvement, and the % T-HYP was only 4%. The owner/trainer relationship was such that Phase II exercise management was not an option, but the trainer felt "he could get the horse a couple of months off." One often has to take what one can get. The horse was blistered externally twice (3 weeks apart) and given 6 weeks out of training at EL-1 (mechanical walker 30 minutes a day).

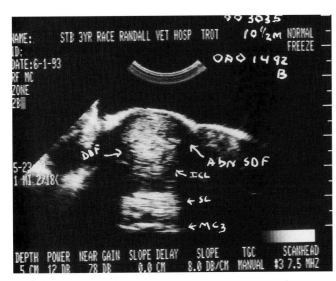

Figure 27B.35. A cross-sectional right metacarpal Zone 2B sonogram of the same horse as in Figure 27B.34 made 11 months later. SDF = superficial digital flexor tendon; DDF = deep digital flexor tendon; ICL = inferior check ligament (ALDDFT); SL = suspensory ligament (TIOM); MC3 = third metacarpal bone. (ATL 4600 scanner)

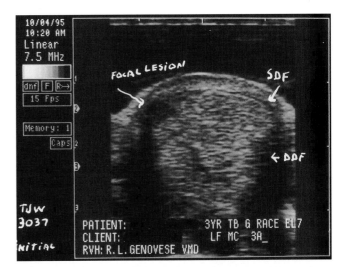

Figure 27B.37. A cross-sectional left metacarpal Zone 3A initial sonogram. SDF = superficial digital flexor tendon; DDF = deep digital flexor tendon. (Classic 200 scanner)

Figure 27B.38 is a sonogram of the same horse as in Figure 27B.37 made 7 weeks post initial examination. There was resolution of the focal hypoechoic lesion. The trainer was aware of the physiologic tendon repair principles and appreciated that sonographic resolution at this time does not necessarily indicate maximum repair. However, the owner insisted the horse return to training-level exercise. The horse progressed gradually up the exercise levels and competed 4 times without recurrence. Unfortunately, for the racing TB this is an unusual end result. However, in this case an early diagnosis may well have been significantly responsible for the favorable outcome. Sonography has greatly improved early detection of SDFT abnormalities. However, with the TB racehorse, even slight peripheral injuries almost always require Phase II exercise management

Figure 27B.39 is an unraced TB filly with slight lateral SDFT swelling following a work (EL-6). There is a focal medial tendon border lesion. There were only two compromised levels, and the lesion was 2% T-HYP (slight injury). This horse was treated with strict Phase I exercise management and was never permitted pasture exercise during rehabilitation. The treatment program was limited to physical therapy (therapeutic ultrasound and magnetic pads). Figure 27B.40 is a sonogram of the same horse as in Figure 27B.39 made 8 months from the initial examination following a morning work (EL-6). There was a large hypoechoic SDFT lesion. The quantitative data indicated a severe reinjury (30% T-HYP), and the filly was retired.

Slight peripheral lesions appear to be more common in STD than TB racehorses, and slight "core" lesions seem more common in TB than STD racehorses. The same principles of S/GO and Phase I management apply for "core" lesions as for peripheral injuries. It is my impression that "core" lesions of the STD and TB are less likely to have successful outcomes with S/GO and Phase I management. I believe this is based in part on basic tendon physiology. First,

the central tendon fibers may be more susceptible to injury and reinjury, and, secondly, the confined inflammatory response may cause more discomfort at maximum tendon loading. Even if these horses remain clinically and sonographically stable, performances seem to be of less quality. Furthermore, I believe that, in addition to focal fiber path compromise, "core" lesions are accompanied by a greater CSA increase, which may indicate more fiber tearing with low-grade tendinitis.

Figure 27B.41 is TB racehorse examined for slight, proximal, palmar metacarpal swelling. The trainer reported that, in spite of a significant drop in class, this filly was not performing well. There was no evidence of lameness. This filly had injured the tendon 2 years previously and had raced in 1994 with optimal performances without clinical signs of tendon discomfort. Presently, physical inspection of the "old" tendon injury indicated stability. However, there was a Type 3 , focal, "core-like" centromedial SDFT lesion. Three levels were involved, and the % T-HYP was 6% (slight reinjury). The trainer indicated that repeat, long-term treatment was not an option. The horse was managed with systemic anti-inflammatory medication and a decreased training program (S/GO exercise management). The filly raced three times at the lowest class level over the next 6 weeks. She finished third twice and next to last in her last race.

Figure 27B.42 is a sonogram of the same horse as in Figure 27B.41 made after the last race. There was a Type 3 SDFT "core" lesion. The injury at this time involved five levels. There was an MIZ-CSA increase from 86 mm^2 to 180 mm^2 and a T-CSA increase from 526 mm^2 to 840 mm^2 since the previous sonographic evaluation in Figure 27B.41. The % T-HYP increased from 6% (slight reinjury) to 24% T-HYP (moderate reinjury). Therefore the S/GO program

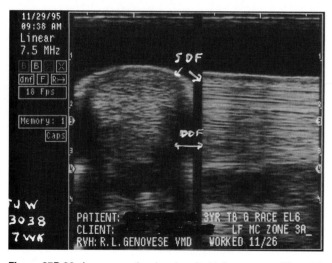

Figure 27B.38. A cross-sectional and sagittal left metacarpal Zone 3A sonogram of the same horse as in Figure 27B.37 made 7 weeks later. SDF = superficial digital flexor tendon; DDF = deep digital flexor tendon. (Classic 200 scanner)

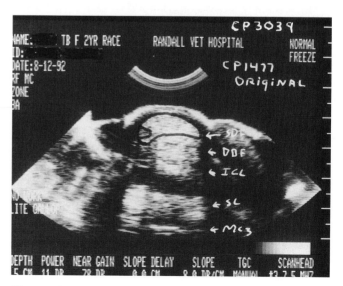

Figure 27B.39. A cross-sectional right metacarpal Zone 3A initial sonogram. SDF = superficial digital flexor tendon; DDF = deep digital flexor tendon; ICL = inferior check ligament (ALDDFT); SL = suspensory ligament (TIOM); MC3 = third metacarpal bone. (ATL 4600 scanner)

was not profitable and if long-range treatment was now selected, there would be a decreased RTR prognosis. The performances also declined more significantly as the degree of tendon compromise increased.

The author's long-term treatment programs for subacute, slight SDFT injury consists of the following:

1. Phase II exercise management
2. Selected treatment program(s)
3. Serial sonographic evaluation for treatment evaluation
4. Exercise management based on quantitative sonographic data
5. In-training sonographic monitoring

At initial injury (acute phase) all injured tendons are treated with anti-inflammatory medication and limited exercise (stall rest and limited hand walking). This period extends 2 to 4 weeks post injury. After the acute phase, a baseline sonographic evaluation is performed and a treatment plan for the subacute phase is started.

Long-term treatment programs for slight SDFT injuries will vary base on several factors. The first consideration is the lesion location. For some peripheral lesions I will advise pin firing. Once again, I realize that research conducted in the United Kingdom established that there was no therapeutic basis for this treatment, but my interpretation of that research is that there was no peritendinous fibrosis increase. This in turn suggested that pin firing did not result in increasing the tendon "strength." My goal with pin firing is to use the firing iron as a form of tendon splitting. It is my personal belief that, properly utilized, the small punctures made are in fact penetrating the peripheral lesion resulting in a pathway to release a hematoma and will result in a temporarily increased peritendinous blood supply. It is not my purpose to cause injury to normal tendon fibers by overly aggressive probe penetration. I limit the firing point penetra-

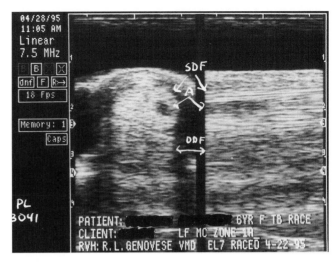

Figure 27B.41. A cross-sectional and sagittal left metacarpal Zone 1A initial sonogram. SDF = superficial digital flexor tendon; A = focal Type 3 lesion of the SDF; DDF = deep digital flexor tendon. (Classic 200 scanner)

tion to the tendon periphery through the paratenon. I prefer the firing iron in this instance to a scalpel blade because I believe I can control the lesion penetration more accurately. Finally, pin firing is a less expensive procedure, and when treatment cost enters the equation, it may be the only affordable treatment. Once commercially available, this author will treat most slight lesions with intralesional BAPTEN®. In the clinical field trials using intralesional BAPTEN®, this author's success rate for RTR was favorable, especially with slightly injured tendons. In either case, I advise hand or mechanical machine walking for 30 minutes daily for the first month and 30 minutes twice a day for the second month. A repeat sonogram is done 60 days post treatment. If the sonographic criteria are favorable for the third and fourth months,

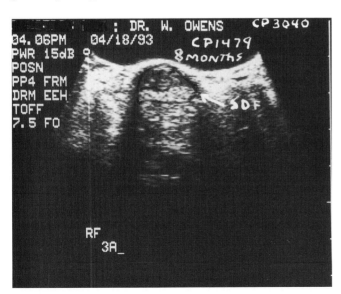

Figure 27B.40. A cross-sectional right metacarpal Zone 3A sonogram of the same horse as in Figure 27B.39 made 8 months later. SDF = superficial digital flexor tendon. (Photo Courtesy of Dr. W. Owen, Oldsmar, FL)

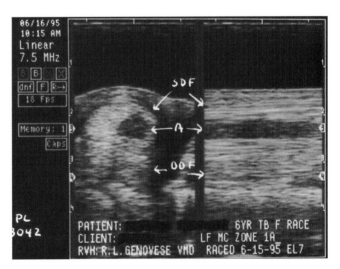

Figure 27B.42. A cross-sectional and sagittal left metacarpal Zone 1A sonogram of the same horse as in Figure 27B.41 made 6 weeks later. SDF = superficial digital flexor tendon; A = focal Type 3 lesion of the SDF; DDF = deep digital flexor tendon. (Classic 200 scanner)

the level can be elevated to the appropriate EL-2 exercise for that breed and trainer. For some trainers and breeds, twice a week ponying is more practical; for others, it may be lunging or swimming. After 4 months a repeat sonogram is done. If the quantitative and qualitative sonographic data are favorable, in some instances the horse will be permitted *small* paddock exercise (EL-3A) for months 5 and 6. Small paddock means a paddock no larger than two round pens. In other instances, with hyperactive horses, I recommend they stay at EL-2 for months 5 and 6. If the sonographic data is not favorable, I recommend decreasing or maintaining the present exercise level depending on the extent of the unfavorable sonographic data. Lately, I have tried to avoid large-pasture, free-choice running at 4 to 6 months post injury, because I believe this can be an excessive EL for many tendon injuries.

After 6 months the tendon is evaluated sonographically. If the qualitative and quantitative criteria are met, then the horse is advanced to EL-4 for 1 month. After 7 months, and if the injury is sonographically acceptable, EL-5 is advised. From that point, the horse is examined sonographically prior to each increase in EL. Increase EL levels are only allowed if sonographic parameters are compatible with lesion stability. Tendons should be scanned after each race, but if this is not feasible, sonographic evaluation after the first 3 or 4 races should be performed for TBs. Obviously, a repeat sonogram is done at any point where there is clinical suspicion of reinjury.

For slight, subacute-stage, "core" injuries the author's treatment program differs. The author's most consistent, current, "core" lesion treatment for the most favorable SQR and RTR is intralesional BAPTEN®. Six horses with slight lesions have been injected with BAPTEN® that have completed the project to the EL-7 stage. In that group, four horses (67%) have competed without reinjury, two (33%) have raced but eventually reinjured, and all reached EL-7. The exercise control and sonographic monitoring is the same as for peripheral injury. If the horse has an upright conformation or SDFT injury at EL-5 or below, I may advise SCLD after the fourth to sixth month of recovery. I would advise this timing for SCLD for two reasons: (a) At this stage the SQR is known. If the repair is poor at 4 to 6 months, I may advise abandoning RTR as a goal and recommend an alternative, less stressful athletic career. In that case, there would be no need for SCLD. (b) At the end of 4 to 6 months, horses are more capable of exercise performance compatible with the SCLD program.

With BAPTEN®-treated tendons I do not use TS. Multiple BAPTEN® injections are made into the tendon lesion at each treatment session with a 25- or 27-gauge needle. For most slight lesions, this usually means 25 to 30 needle punctures on each of 5 treatment days. The multiple needle punctures (125 to 150) effectively are a "tendon lesion needle splitting procedure." If the drug BAPTEN® were not available, my second choice of slight "core" lesion treatment would be a careful TS. I believe that overly aggressive tendon splitting can create additional injury.

TREATMENT OF MODERATE AND SEVERE SDFT INJURIES

Treatment of moderate to severe injuries is also coupled with an extended, Phase II–exercise-management program for the best RTR chance. As a basic rule, assuming that sonographic data are favorable, one can anticipate a return to EL-5 for slight injuries, at the earliest, after 7 months. For moderate injuries, the completion of at least 8 to 9 months below EL-5 and, for severe injuries, at least 10 to 12 months below EL-5 are required. If the sonographic data are unfavorable at any point along the way, this causes a 1- to 3-month delay in return to EL-5. If the sonographic data at 6 to 9 months are consistently poor, I discuss an alternative career for the racehorse. One must always remember that lesser athletic endeavors than racing, including eventing, polo, and steeplechase racing, will tolerate a lesser SQR.

When the goal is returning to high-level exercise such as racing, this author prefers to treat all moderate-to-severe tendon injuries with intralesional BAPTEN®. When that drug is not available, I prefer TS. In selected cases I advise SCLD after 4 to 6 months post injury based on favorable sonographic data; the more serious the injury, the greater the consideration given to SCLD. Exercise levels in all SDFT injuries are based on sonographic data, and I seldom advise large pasture exercise at any point in rehabilitation.

As can be seen, the SDFT treatment can be complex, costly, and time consuming. At the present time this author offers a guarded prognosis for RTR. For these reasons client commitment to necessary time and expense is essential to optimize the chances for RTR. What is even more sobering is to always realize that, in spite of carefully managed rehabilitation programs, no SDFT repair will be the same strength and elasticity of a normal tendon. Finally, one must also remember that the faster the horses must perform, the more functional the repair must be.

SQR ASSESSMENT AND EXERCISE CONTROL BY CASE EXAMPLE

To fully understand my concepts of sonographic management of the injured SDFT by quantitative criteria, I will introduce these principles by case example. The principles and concepts that I share with you were developed from the intralesional, BAPTEN®-treatment field trials. From these experiences, the reader can formulate a program that can be utilized in everyday practice for case management, regardless of the treatment. One will realize that through sonography and quantitative assessment, end results will improve. Furthermore, unfavorable sonographic assessments can result in midstream redirecting of athletic use, which will result in a significant decrease in catastrophic acute breakdowns and eliminate severely damaged tendons.

A Slight SDFT Injury With a Successful RTR

Figure 27B.43 is a TB racehorse that had injured the SDFT the previous year at EL-7. The horse was rested for more

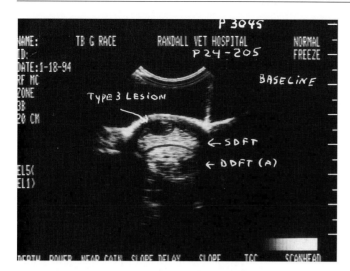

Figure 27B.43. A cross-sectional right metacarpal Zone 3B baseline sonogram. SDFT = superficial digital flexor tendon; DDFT = deep digital flexor tendon. (ATL 4600 scanner)

than 6 months (Phase II exercise management) and treated with external blisters and large pasture exercise (EL-3). The horse was returned to training (EL-5) and reinjured at EL-6. This horse was capable of allowance-class and low-stakes-class performance levels. This scan is the baseline sonogram of the MIZ (Zone 3B), which shows a focal, Type 3 palmar SDFT lesion. There were three levels that had hypoechoic fiber bundles. The quantitative evaluation at baseline was as follows:

MIZ-CSA	159 mm^2
MIZ-HYP	46 mm^2
MIZ-FS	3
T-CSA (6 levels)	690 mm^2
T-HYP	71 mm^2
T-FS	8
%T-HYP	10% (slight reinjury)

There was palpable, sensitive, distal SDFT swelling, but the horse was not lame. In the subacute stage the injured SDFT was injected with intralesional BAPTEN® every other day for five treatments. The horse was hand walked for 30 minutes daily the first month. During the second month the horse was walked by mechanical walker for 30 minutes daily. During the third and fourth months the horse was ridden at the walk 3 days a week and machine walked the other days of the week for 30 minutes. Figure 27B.44 is a sonogram of the same horse as in Figure 27B.43 made 4 months post treatment. There was focal SDFT lesion resolution in the MIZ. At this point only one zone had focal, hypoechoic fiber bundles. The quantitative data at this time at EL-2 after 4 months of rehabilitation were as follows:

T-MIZ	100 mm^2 (37% CSA decrease)
MIZ-HYP	0 (100% improvement)

MIZ-FS	0 (100% improvement)
T-CSA	608 mm^2 (12% T-CSA decrease)
T-HYP	6 mm^2 (92% decrease-improvement)
T-FS 1	(88% improvement)
% T-HYP	2% (improvement)

All quantitative data was favorable. The MIZ and T-CSA decreased greater than 10%. The reduction in CSA is assumed to be due to the following: The fibrous tissue collagen repair fibers are oriented in a proximal-to-distal plane, there is inflammatory process resolution, and there is no recurring injury at the current EL. In my opinion, axially aligned collagen fibers occupy less cross-sectional area than those that are randomly oriented or those with continued inflammation from repetitive, low-level, fiber-bundle injury. The return to isoechogenic fiber density at the lesion sites indicate mature, properly oriented, collagen tissue repair. In the BAPTEN® study a reasonable expectation of hypoechoic tendon-fiber-bundle reduction in the MIZ and T would be 70% quantitative improvement. The MIZ had a normal shape, and no evidence of peritendinous, fibrous-tissue reaction is present. Only Zone 3A has a focal, hypoechoic, fiber-bundle area. The fiber score both of the MIZ and T was greatly improved from 8 to 1, suggesting parallel fiber alignment. The criteria expected at this stage of repair for fiber-alignment score is at least 50% improvement. Fiber realignment is a slow remodeling process, and a 50% reduction at 4 months would be a favorable finding. The conclusion at this stage is that all quantitative assessments have met criteria indicating that a slight increase in the EL is acceptable. It should be noted that the intention is always Phase II management for long-term therapy, even with slight injuries that are making favorable sonographic progress. The fact that this horse has a near-perfect qualitative and quantitative sonographic repair does not

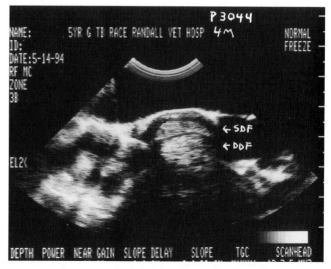

Figure 27B.44. A cross-sectional right metacarpal Zone 3B sonogram of the same horse as in Figure 27B.43 made 4 months later. SDF = superficial digital flexor tendon; DDF = deep digital flexor tendon. (ATL 4600 scanner)

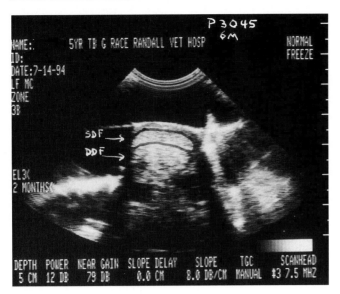

Figure 27B.45. A cross-sectional right metacarpal Zone 3B sonogram of the same horse as in Figure 27B.44 made 6 months later. SDF = superficial digital flexor tendon; DDF = deep digital flexor tendon. (ATL 4600 scanner)

suggest that it should be returned to the training level (EL-5). At least 2 to 3 more months are required for repairing fibrous tissue cross-linking and realignment. Sonographically, cross-linking and collagen maturation cannot be assessed. It is common practice to advise return to EL-5 as soon as the sonogram has reached evidence of maximum sonographic repair. It has been our experience that advancing to EL-5 would most likely result in reinjury in spite of the favorable SQR. Phase I management has a high failure rate; therefore this horse was advanced to only EL-3.

Figure 27B.45 shows the same horse as in Figure 27B.44 made after 6 months of rehabilitation. At the time of this scan, the horse was at large-pasture exercise (EL-3B). There was no evidence of MIZ relapse. There was one level that had a small focal hypoechoic area. The quantitative data were as follows:

MIZ-CSA	100 mm^2 (25% decrease from baseline)
MIZ-HYP	0 (100% improvement from baseline)
MIZ-FS	0 (100% improvement from baseline)
T-CSA	664 mm^2 (4% decrease from baseline) (failed criterion)
T-HYP	10 mm^2 (86% improvement from baseline)
T-FS	2 (75% improvement from baseline)
% T-HYP	2%

At this point the increase to EL-3B resulted in a slight CSA increase. This should serve as a caution that large-pasture exercise at this repair stage can be excessive. Currently, I advise small-pasture exercise if sonographic criteria are met pre EL-3. A small pasture is defined as an area comparable to two round pens. Since most of the sonographic criteria were favorable, this horse was advanced to EL-4,

which included 3 days a week of arena work at the walk, trot, and canter. On the other days, the horse was permitted large-pasture exercise.

Figure 27B.46 is the same horse as in Figure 27B.45 made 7 months post baseline at EL-4. There is a slight, SDFT, palmar-border shape change, but no textural "relapses" were identified. This increased exercise level did result in scattered, focal, hypoechoic fiber bundles at the more proximal levels. The quantitative data were as follows:

MIZ-CSA	110 mm^2
MIZ-HYP	0
MIZ-FS	0
T-CSA	669 mm^2
T-HYP	16 mm^2
T-FS	2
% T-HYP	2%

At this point, the criteria were stable and the horse was advanced to EL-5. After 30 days at EL-5 and pre EL-6, a sonographic evaluation was performed. Figure 27B.47 is a sonogram of the same horse as in Figure 27B.46 There were no sonographic abnormalities. The quantitative data were as follows:

MIZ-CSA	110 mm^2 (31% decrease from baseline)
MIZ-HYP	0 (100% decrease from baseline)
MIZ-FS	1 (66% decrease from baseline)
T-CSA	689 mm^2 (<1% decrease from baseline)
T-HYP	18 mm^2 (75% decrease from baseline)
T-FS	1 (88% decrease from baseline)
% T-HYP	3%

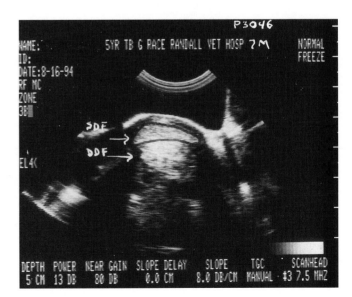

Figure 27B.46. A cross-sectional right metacarpal Zone 3B sonogram of the same horse as in Figure 27B.45 made 7 months later. SDF = superficial digital flexor tendon; DDF = deep digital flexor tendon. (ATL 4600 scanner)

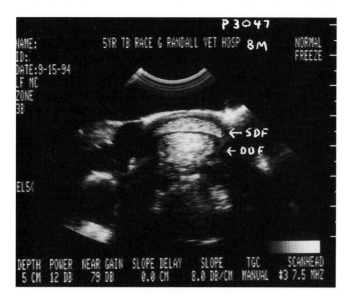

Figure 27B.47. A cross-sectional right metacarpal Zone 3B sonogram of the same horse as in Figure 27B.46 made 8 months later. SDF = superficial digital flexor tendon; DDF = deep digital flexor tendon. (ATL 4600 scanner)

At this stage, the only parameter that was suspect was the T-CSA. Since the MIZ was significantly decreased from the baseline evaluation, the conclusion is that a zone more proximal was slightly strained. In this case it was Zone 2A that increased from 89 mm^2 baseline to 122 mm^2. Overall, this reinjured tendon's texture remained stable, and the T-CSA did not approach a level of concern of 20% increase. The quantitative data remained similarly stable throughout the next racing season. At the completion of eight races, the MIZ decreased to 95 mm^2 and was lesion free. The T-CSA decreased to 640 mm^2, and the % T-HYP maintained at 1 to 3%. The FS ranged from 0 to 2. Figure 27B.48 is a sonogram of the same horse as in Figure 27B.47 made after the eighth race. The SDFT was sonographically stable.

Not all tendons respond in this manner and injured tendons are always susceptible to reinjury at this exercise level. However, this case illustrates favorable quantitative data that can serve as a template for successful case management. This horse remained at the allowance level and only raced once in the lower-stakes race level.

A Slight Injury With an Unsuccessful RTR

A TB racehorse sustained a first episode left fore SDFT injury. The MIZ was Zone 3A, and five levels had identifiable, hypoechoic fiber bundles. The quantitative data were as follows:

MIZ-CSA	142 mm^2
MIZ-HYP	30 mm^2
MIZ-FS	3
T-CSA	730 mm^2
T-HYP	94 mm^2
T-FS	10
% T-HYP	13%

This slight tendon injury was provided Phase II management and the peripheral tendon injury treated with pin firing in the subacute stage. The horse was hand walked for 45 days. This was followed with the first of three monthly external blisters, and the horse was turned out into a large pasture (EL-3B). After the completion of 6 months out of training, the tendon was sonographically evaluated prior to EL-5. Although the textural grade improved from Type 3 to Type 1, there were still five levels that had hypoechoic fiber bundles. The quantitative data were as follows:

MIZ-CSA	155 mm^2 (9% increase from baseline) (failed criterion)
MIZ-HYP	43 mm^2 (43% increase from baseline) (failed criterion)
MIZ-FS	1 (66% improvement from baseline)
T-CSA	696 mm^2 (5% decrease from baseline) (failed criterion)
T-HYP	118 mm^2 (26% increase from baseline) (failed criterion)
T-FS 9	(10% increase from baseline) (failed criterion)
% T-HYP	17% (failed criterion)

In this slightly injured tendon, all of the criteria except the MIZ-FS failed. Based on our research data from the BAPTEN® clinical field trials, these data indicate that this horse is not ready to advance to EL-5. There are six of seven parameters that are not favorable at this time. In spite of this warning, the trainer proceeded with EL-5. The trainer did this because of tradition. The horse had a long layoff, and tendon palpation suggested a stable, "set" tendon injury. One month later and at EL-5, this horse was symptomatic. The tendon was swollen, and there was sensitivity on digital palpation. There was an SDFT reinjury. The quantitative data were as follows:

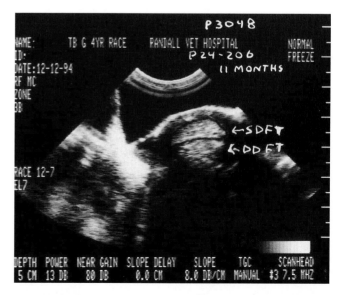

Figure 27B.48. A cross-sectional right metacarpal Zone 3B sonogram of the same horse as in Figure 27B.47 made 11 months later. SDFT = superficial digital flexor tendon; DDFT = deep digital flexor tendon. (ATL 4600 scanner)

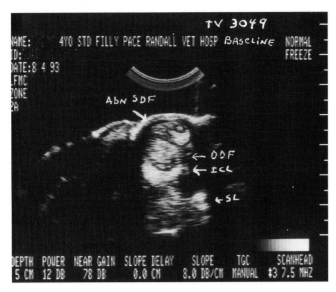

Figure 27B.49. A cross-sectional left metacarpal Zone 2A baseline sonogram. SDF = superficial digital flexor tendon; DDF = deep digital flexor tendon; ICL = inferior check ligament (ALDDFT); SL = suspensory ligament (TIOM). (ATL 4600 scanner)

MIZ-CSA	230 mm^2
MIZ-HYP	101 mm^2
MIZ-FS	3
T-CSA	887 mm^2
T-HYP	310 mm^2
T-FS	13
% T-HYP	35% (severe reinjury)

Using the quantitative data during rehabilitation is useful in guiding exercise levels. Most sonographers are familiar with the appearance of unsatisfactory repair or reinjury, but there are times when the first sign of reinjury or repair instability is a CSA increase. I have found that CSA increase is a sensitive measurement that signals early tendon swelling.

Figure 27B.49 is a STD racehorse presented with a first episode SDFT injury at EL-7. There was a Type 1 lateral SDFT lesion. The quantitative data were as follows:

MIZ-CSA	94 mm^2
MIZ-HYP	41 mm^2
MIZ-FS	1
T-CSA	645 mm^2
T-HYP	136 mm^2
T-FS	6
% T-HYP	21% (moderate injury)

This horse was treated with intralesional BAPTEN® in the subacute stage, and a Phase II management was selected. The horse was hand walked 30 minutes daily for the first post-treatment month and 30 minutes twice a day the second month. Figure 27B.50 is a sonogram of

the same horses as in Figure 27B.49 made 4 months post treatment. At that period in the clinical field trials, we were advising one slow jogging mile (over 6 minutes) 3 days a week for the STD racehorse as a controlled exercise level. However, this level is actually EL-4, which is considered excessive for this stage. There was a marked textural improvement. The quantitative data were as follows:

MIZ-CSA	163 mm^2 (73% increase from baseline) (failed criterion)
MIZ-HYP	0 (100% decrease from baseline)
MIZ-FS	2 (100% score increase from baseline) (failed criterion)
T-CSA	954 mm^2 (48% increase from baseline) (failed criterion)
T-HYP	20 mm^2 (85% decrease from baseline)
T-FS	7 (17% increase from baseline) (failed criterion)
% T-HYP	2%

Only three parameters were favorable at the pre EL-3 stage. Furthermore, there is an alarming CSA increase suggesting ongoing reinjury confirming that the prescan exercise level was excessive. At this time another exercise management mistake was made in suggesting EL-3. This horse should have been reduced to EL-1. However, through misjudgment, large pasture exercise (3B) was advised. Figure 27B.51 is the same horse as in Figure 27B.50 made at 6 months with a definite SDFT "core" lesion. This shows a textural abnormality, in spite of the fact that this horse was only turned out. The quantitative data were as follows:

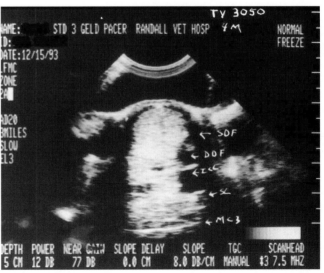

Figure 27B.50. A cross-sectional left metacarpal Zone 2A sonogram of the same horse as in Figure 27B.49 made 4 months later. SDF = superficial digital flexor tendon; DDF = deep digital flexor tendon; ICL = inferior check ligament (ALDDFT); SL = suspensory ligament (TIOM); MC3 = third metacarpal bone. (ATL 4600 scanner)

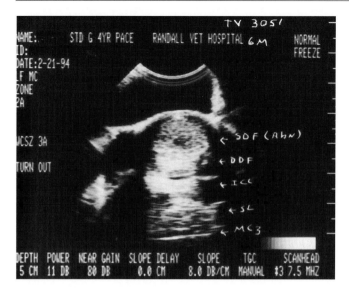

Figure 27B.51. A cross-sectional left metacarpal Zone 2A sonogram of the same horse as in Figure 27B.50 made 6 months later. SDF = superficial digital flexor tendon; DDF = deep digital flexor tendon; ICL = inferior check ligament (ALDDFT); SL = suspensory ligament (TIOM). (ATL 4600 scanner)

MIZ-CSA	230 mm^2 (145% increase from baseline)
MIZ-HYP	21 mm^2 (49% decrease from baseline)
MIZ-FS 1	(0% change from baseline)
T-CSA	1219 mm^2 (89% increase from baseline)
T-HYP	109 mm^2 (20% decrease from baseline)
T-FS	7 (17% increase from baseline)
%T-HYP	9%

At this point, six of the seven criteria were unfavorable to advance to EL-5. However, another misjudgment was made, and a return to EL-5 was advised from simply using a timetable and not appreciating the SQR. Figure 27B.52 is a sonogram of the same horse as in Figure 27B.51 made after the third training mile, 11 months post baseline. This scan reveals a large, Type 3, SDFT "core" lesion. The quantitative data were as follows:

MIZ-CSA	131 mm^2 (39% increased from baseline)
MIZ-HYP	10 mm^2 (76% decreased from baseline)
MIZ-FS	1 (0% change from baseline)
T-CSA	1056 mm^2 (64% increase from baseline)
T-HYP	211 mm^2 (55% increase from baseline)
T-FS	8 (33% increase from baseline)
% T-HYP	20% (moderate reinjury)

This horse's exercise program was mismanaged simply because the emphasis of the SQR was placed on textural evaluation alone along with preconceived concepts of time. The CSA data clearly indicated every EL increase was inappropriate, and the result was a reinjury prior to attaining EL-7. In a retrospective study of 79 Phase II–managed SDFT in-

juries, quantitative data were assessed. These data were reported in the First International Dubai Equine Symposium (6). In that report I used horses with SDFT injuries treated by a variety of methods. All horses had pre–EL-5 data to evaluate the SQR, and all horses had a known athletic outcome. Horses were grouped into those that were successful in RTR without any sonographic indication of reinjury and those that had sonographic evidence of reinjury. There were 15 (19%) injured tendons that were successful and there were 64 (81%) tendons that were reinjured. Of the 15 successful tendons, five had all seven favorable pre–EL-5 sonographic parameters. Ten tendons in the success group had one to three unfavorable sonographic parameters. *None* of the successful group had four to seven abnormal sonographic parameters prior to EL-5. Furthermore, all of the success group started EL-5 with less than 10% T-HYP. There were eight injured tendons in the failure group that had all favorable parameters and 22 tendons in the failure group that had one to three unfavorable sonographic parameters. This would indicate that even the most ideal and near ideal SQR can fail to RTR without reinjury. There were, however, 34 injured tendons that had four to seven unfavorable sonographic parameters that failed. These data indicate that, if injured tendons are managed in Phase II and have four to seven abnormal parameters prior to EL-5, there is a 0% chance for success. Furthermore, if the abnormal parameter is textural, fiber alignment, or % T-HYP, there is greater than an 85% chance of reinjury.

MODERATE AND SEVERE SDFT INJURIES

The acute SDFT injury stage is treated with an anti-inflammatory therapeutic program coupled with hydrotherapy and limited walking. Treatment of the subacute stage (2 to 4 weeks post injury) is similar to slight injuries with the use

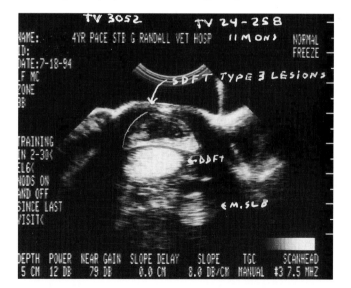

Figure 27B.52. A cross-sectional left metacarpal Zone 3B sonogram of the same horse as in Figure 27B.51 made 11 months later. SDFT = superficial digital flexor tendon; DDFT = deep digital flexor tendon; M.SLB = medial branch of the suspensory ligament. (ATL 4600 scanner)

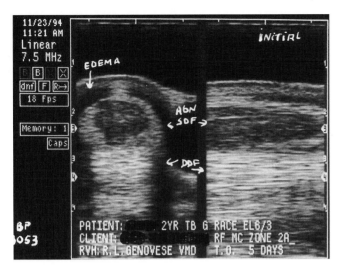

Figure 27B.53. A cross-sectional and sagittal right metacarpal Zone 2A initial sonogram. SDF = superficial digital flexor tendon; DDF = deep digital flexor tendon. (Classic 200 scanner)

of intralesional BAPTEN® when available and, in selected cases, SCLD. If BAPTEN® is not available, I generally advise TS and mild external blistering in TS cases at months 1, 2, and 3 post surgery. I seldom pin fire moderate and severe SDFT injuries, even if the lesion is located peripherally, unless there is persistent trainer/owner request. In addition, EL-5 is prolonged by at least 2 months for moderate and 4 months for severe injuries. In other words, EL-5 with favorable sonographic evaluation is withheld until the completion of 8 months below EL-5 and in severe injuries withheld until completion of 10 months below EL-5.

Figure 27B.53 is an unraced TB made at the initial injury at EL-6. There is a large, Type 2, SDFT "core" lesion. The horse was treated with anti-inflammatory medication (phenylbutazone 2 g per day), daily icing for 2 hours, and topical alcohol and bandaged. Exercise was limited to 5 to 10 minutes of hand walking. At 5 weeks post injury a baseline assessment was made, and the injured tendon was treated with intralesional BAPTEN® as described. The baseline quantitative data were as follows:

MIZ-CSA	267 mm^2
MIZ-HYP	216 mm^2
MIZ-FS	3
T-CSA	1556 mm^2 (seven levels)
T-HYP	930 mm^2
T-FS	16
% T-HYP	60% (severe injury)

For the first 2 months post baseline, the horse was walked 30 minutes daily on a mechanical walker. During months 3 and 4 the horse was ponied for 1 mile 2 days per week and machine walked for 30 minutes 5 days per week. Figure 27B.54 is a sonogram of the same horse as in Figure 27B.53 made 4 months post baseline. There was improved texture and fiber

alignment; however, diffuse hypoechoic fiber bundles can be seen medially. The quantitative data were as follows:

MIZ-CSA	199 mm^2 (25% decrease from baseline)
MIZ-HYP	44 mm^2 (80% decrease from baseline)
MIZ-FS	3 (0% improvement from baseline)
T-CSA	1131 mm^2 (27% decrease from baseline)
T-HYP	279 mm^2 (70% decrease from baseline)
T-FS	11
% T-HYP	25%

The sonographic qualitative evaluation at this time was favorable because the "core" lesion was resolving and there was no significant peritendinous fibrosis. The quantitative measurements improved more than 70%, and CSA decreased more than 10%. The fiber alignment and % T-HYP were still elevated as expected for this period. Fiber realignment is a remodeling process that appears later in the repair stages. Since this was an extremely active horse, it was advised to continue with the EL-2 program. Figure 27B.55 is the same horse as in Figure 27B.54 made 6 months post baseline. There was textural improvement compared with the previous examination and improved fiber alignment. There was no evidence of peritendinous fibrosis. The quantitative data were as follows:

MIZ-CSA	209 mm^2 (22% decrease from baseline)
MIZ-HYP	25 mm^2 (88% decrease from baseline)
MIZ-FS	1 (66% decrease from baseline)
T-CSA	1324 mm^2 (15% decrease from baseline)
T-HYP	158 mm^2 (83% decrease from baseline)
T-FS	6 (63% decrease from baseline)
% T-HYP	12%

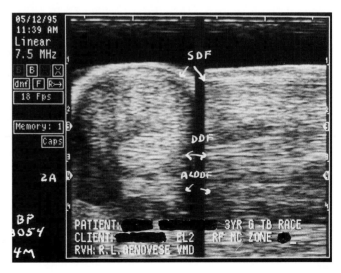

Figure 27B.54. A cross-sectional and sagittal right metacarpal Zone 2A sonogram of the same horse as in Figure 27B.53 made 4 months later. SDF = superficial digital flexor tendon; DDF = deep digital flexor tendon; ALDDFT = accessory ligament of the deep digital flexor tendon (ICL). (Classic 200 scanner)

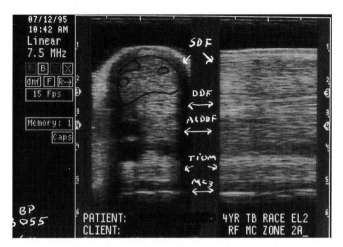

Figure 27B.55. A cross-sectional and sagittal right metacarpal Zone 2A sonogram of the same horse as in Figure 27B.54 made 6 months later. SDF = superficial digital flexor tendon; DDF = deep digital flexor tendon; ALDDFT = accessory ligament of the deep digital flexor tendon (ICL); TIOM = third interosseous muscle (SL); MC3 = third metacarpal bone. (Classic 200 scanner)

At this point, six of the seven evaluations were favorable. The decrease to 12% T-HYP from the baseline of 60% T-HYP was a significant improvement. Reaching the goal of 10% decreased T-HYP pre–EL-5 is slightly ambitious for some severe injuries. The decision was made to start low-level EL-5 and reevaluate sonographically in 30 days to determine if EL-5 should be maintained or if the EL should be reduced for 2 additional months. Generally, for a severe injury the return to EL-5 at the beginning of the 7th month post baseline is premature. There was trainer pressure to proceed to EL-5 because of the time of year (mid July) and the impending winter break. This horse was sonographically guided through training and remained stable through EL-5 and EL-6. Figure 27B.56 is the same horse as in Figure 27B.55 made 9½ months post baseline after the last work and before the first race. There was near-normal echogenicity, parallel fiber alignment, and no significant peritendinous fibrosis. The quantitative data were as follows:

MIZ-CSA	146 mm² (45% decrease from baseline)
MIZ-HYP	0 (100% decrease from baseline)
MIZ-FS	0 (100% decrease from baseline)
T-CSA	970 mm² (38% decrease from baseline)
T-HYP	28 mm² (97% decrease from baseline)
T-FS	5 (69% decrease from baseline)
% T-HYP	3%

These data are consistent with a favorable morphologic repair and remodeling process with lesion stability during increased tendon loading. The horse raced four times before the winter break and remained asymptomatic. It is interesting to note that this horse attained a higher exercise level post injury than pre injury. The tendon remained stable throughout the racing period. There was slight regression with the increased tendon loading but not to a level beyond expected scanning-technique variation.

Figure 27B.57 is the same horse as in Figure 27B.56 made 11 months post baseline, 1 year post injury after four races (EL-7). There was slight textural relapse of the MIZ. The quantitative data were as follows:

MIZ-CSA	183 mm² (31% decrease from baseline)
MIZ-HYP	15 mm² (93% decrease from baseline)
MIZ-FS	0 (100% decrease from baseline)
T-CSA	1059 mm² (32% decrease from baseline)
T-HYP	44 mm² (95% decrease from baseline)
T-FS	8 (50% decrease from baseline)
%T-HYP	4%

Not all tendon injuries will have the same favorable end result as this one. However, this case serves as an example of anticipated favorable qualitative and quantitative assessments, which can serve as guidelines in individual case management. Constant vigilance is necessary for repaired tendons returning to high competitive levels. When quantitative data fail to meet set criteria at critical exercise level increases, the practitioner should advise maintaining or reducing the EL to allow time for more improvement. Not doing so will most likely result in failure. Some tendon injuries never reach the intended goals, and many of these horses should be used for a less stressful athletic career. As the future athletic level is decreased, a less-than-ideal tendon repair may be acceptable.

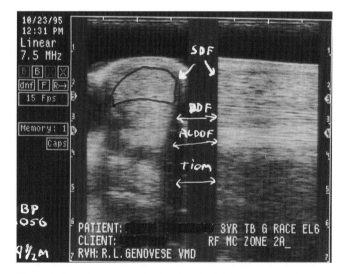

Figure 27B.56. A cross-sectional and sagittal right metacarpal Zone 2A sonogram of the same horse as in Figure 27B.55 made 9¹/₂ months later. SDF = superficial digital flexor tendon; DDF = deep digital flexor tendon; ALDDFT = accessory ligament of the deep digital flexor tendon (ICL); TIOM = third interosseous muscle (SL). (Classic 200 scanner)

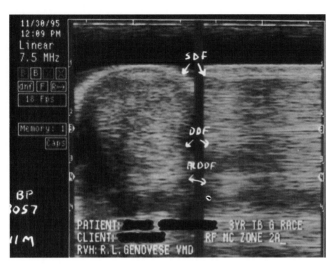

Figure 27B.57. A cross-sectional and sagittal right metacarpal Zone 2A sonogram of the same horse as in Figure 27B.56 made 11 months later. SDF = superficial digital flexor tendon; DDF = deep digital flexor tendon; ALDDFT = accessory ligament of the deep digital flexor tendon (ICL). (Classic 200 scanner)

OVERVIEW

In the author's hands, tendon injury management is developing into a meaningful quantitative science. My methods of quantitative assessment were developed from experience in the BAPTEN® clinical field trials. As a result, I have improved my client information and the sonographic assessment of repair processes. My success rate for return to high competitive levels has improved. There has been a marked reduction in the "banana-shaped" tendons, and catastrophic breakdowns have been significantly reduced. Strict management based on sonographic evaluation and exercise control are essential to the favorable outcome.

I do not believe it is possible to recommend a standard treatment program for SDFT injuries, since each case presents a different set of variables. However, based on past experiences, I have formed some general impressions and principles about SDFT injury treatment and case management.

The exercise management decision by the trainer and/or owner must be the first consideration in the treatment-program development. Trainers often select S/GO exercise management for slight injuries, especially in the STD racehorse. The trainer/owner must be aware of more serious injury risk and the negative effect that may have on any future long-term treatment program. If S/GO exercise management is selected, constant sonographic monitoring is the basis for preventing catastrophic injury. If the horse is not productive and the quantitative assessments indicate an unstable tendon, then the exercise program should be abandoned. Using S/GO management may only apply to select STD racehorses and has a very guarded prognosis for success in the racing TB. Moderate and severe SDFT injuries are generally a failure in both racing breeds with S/GO management, but one can always find a few exceptional successful horses.

Long-term treatment has a greater chance of success with Phase II–exercise management, and this author tries to discourage Phase I management during initial treatment decisions. For slight peripheral lesions I may select pin firing, a series of external blisters, and, for many, intralesional BAPTEN® when available. All treatment programs are coupled with controlled exercise programs. I discourage large-pasture exercise especially within the first 6 months post injury. For the slight SDFT injury that meets favorable sonographic quantitative criteria, I advise EL-1 for the first 2 months, EL-2 for the third through the fourth month, and either the same EL or advancing to small-paddock exercise (EL-3A) for months 5 and 6. The seventh month is an intermediate EL step-up month to evaluate lesion stability (EL-4) consisting of a graded increase in tendon loading. The horse is returned to EL-5 after the 7th month. If the lesion or tendon criteria indicate instability, the EL is maintained or decreased for 1 month and the sonogram is repeated. For moderate injuries, EL-5 is maintained until after the eighth or ninth month and for severe injuries until after the 10th or 12th month. These advances are made with an intermediate EL-4 and sonographic monitoring as well.

For moderate to severe injuries, intralesional BAPTEN® is preferred, and in some cases surgical procedures such as SCLD and/or annular ligament desmotomy (ALD) are performed when indicated in an attempt to improve tendon gliding movement. These procedures are usually performed after the fourth month post baseline. The reason for this is that after 4 months the primary lesion repair can be assessed. If the sonographic data after 4 months is unfavorable, a career change may be suggested, which may obviate the necessity for surgery.

A second treatment option for moderate and severe injuries until BAPTEN® is commercially available would be performing tendon splitting at the time of baseline sonographic injury evaluation. Recently, I have advised systemic PSGAG once a week for 4 weeks immediately post injury combined with anti-inflammatory treatment and limited walking. At 4 weeks post injury, the baseline sonographic evaluation is performed and the primary lesion is split.

Finally, strict sonographic monitoring and exercise-level management is crucial to success. If the CSA has not decreased at follow-up ultrasonographic examinations, the EL should be maintained, or if the CSA has increased, the EL should be decreased. Quantitative assessments of the above-discussed, sonographically measured parameters serve the practitioner in guiding EL management. Ultrasonography can be performed at any time that is necessary, but it is critical at the time of projected EL increases. The following is a recommended schedule of critical ultrasonographic examinations:

1. The initial injury assessment
2. The baseline evaluation (2 to 4 weeks post injury)
3. Pre EL-3A
4. Pre EL-5 (the most critical)
5. Pre EL-6

6. Pre EL-7
7. Serial monitoring during competition (for parameter stability)

CONCLUSION

Physiologic principles of connective-tissue healing dictate that tendon injury repair, especially in the racehorse, results in an inferior tendon when compared with normal. Tendon treatment and case management goals are designed to accomplish the most functional repair possible for a given future athletic career. Veterinary intervention, in my opinion, can affect the outcome. However, the athletic career choice requires careful consideration of variables, sonographic evaluation, proper exercise management, treatment(s), cost, and especially patience. Client and horse compliance is the first major step to fulfill these requirements. There is no argument that the perfect tendon repair can fail, because the repaired tendon was once normal when it failed. It follows that a greater percentage of tendons with poor-quality repair will fail than those with ideal healing. Horses with SDFT injuries must increase tendon loading only after favorable sonographic evaluations. With continued research and the further development of sonographic (or other) criteria to evaluate tendon injury repair, I believe there will be a greater percentage of horses returning to high competitive levels.

Because of this effort to diagnose tendon injuries early and to effectively manage their return to competition, there will be fewer "banana-shaped" tendons and, hopefully, fewer catastrophic breakdowns.

REFERENCES

1. Adams OR. Lameness in horses. 2nd ed. Philadelphia: Lea & Febiger, 1967; pp. 196–200.
2. Asheim A, Knudsen O. Percutaneous tendon splitting. Proc AAEP 1967; pp. 255–262.
3. Silver IA, Brown PN, Goodship AE, Lanyon LE, McCullagh KG, Perry GC, Williams IF. A clinical and experimental study of tendon injury healing and treatment in the horse. Equine Vet J 1983;(Suppl 1):5–22.
4. Bramlage L, Rantanen NW, Genovese RL, Page LE. Long-term effects of superficial digital flexor tendinitis by superior check ligament desmotomy. Proc AAEP 1988;34:655–656.
5. Goodship A. The pathobiology and repair of tendon and ligament injury. Vet Clin North Am 1994;10:322–349.
6. Genovese RL, Reef VB, Longo KL, Byrd JW, Davis WM. Superficial digital flexor tendonditis—long-term sonographic and clinical study of racehorses. First Annual Dubai International Equine Symposium Proceedings 1996; pp. 182–205.
7. Madison J. Acute and chronic tendinitis in horses. The Compendium on Continuing Education 1995; pp. 853–856.
8. Dyson S. Miscellaneous conditions of tendons, tendon sheaths, and ligaments. Vet Clin North Am Equine Pract 1995;2:315–337.

27. Section C

Medical Management of Flexor Tendon Disorders in Horses

EARL M. GAUGHAN, RICHARD M. DeBOWES, AND LISA J. GIFT

Tendon injury is common in horses. The exercise demands and behavioral patterns of horses compounded by their unique musculoskeletal anatomy predisposes them to overload stress and external trauma. Tendon fiber disruption that results from any type of injury can be career limiting and in severe situations, life threatening. Timely and appropriate treatment of horses with tendon injuries can influence outcome and increase the likelihood of a successful return to athleticism.

External traumatic disruption of tendon tissue is often obvious, and a complete physical examination will permit identification of all of the injured tissues. Tendon decompensation that destabilizes the affected limb will result in a classic posture or appearance, typically associated with the loss of tendon integrity, and can be observed on physical examination. For injuries that do not completely disrupt the tendon structure, other diagnostic modalities are often necessary for complete evaluation. Partial tendon laceration and lacerations that involve a tendon within a tendon sheath can be evaluated by physical examination and ultrasound evaluation. Images of the traumatized tendon can assist in treatment selection, can monitor a patient's response to treatment and the progression of tendon healing, and can provide some assistance in determining the appropriate return to an exercise program.

Overload injury to digital flexor tendons is common in horses that perform at high speeds and push the limits of their conditioning. Ultrasonographic evaluation can determine the site and severity of tendon fiber disruption and can provide a means for determining the progression and healing of the injured tendon.

Numerous and widely diverse therapies have been utilized to treat tendon injuries in horses. Some have been successful and many have not. Success may be the result of sufficient amounts of rest from repetitive tendon stress as much as it can be credited to a specific medical or surgical treatment. Many low-grade tendon injuries can be successfully managed with conservative, noninvasive treatment. Horses with more extensive, severe, or repetitive injuries may require more aggressive medical or surgical treatment to achieve an acceptable outcome. Selection of the most appropriate treatment at the most appropriate time is the prevailing challenge to the veterinarian directing the treatment of a horse with an injured flexor tendon.

FIRST AID

Often the immediate care administered to a horse with an injured tendon will dictate the success of a chosen therapy.

Flexor tendinitis is usually the result of overload of tendon fibers composing the tendon body. The physical disruption of these tendon fibers incites a severe inflammatory response. The result is lameness from both the physical loss of intact tendon support and pain originating from, in, and around injured and inflamed tendon and peritendinous tissues.

Immediately after tendon injury, an affected horse should be restrained and prevented from exacerbating the injury and from secondarily traumatizing other structures. A complete physical examination of the horse and assessment of the injury should be performed in all patients when manageable. Occasionally, horses will be too fractious and require chemical restraint for complete physical evaluation and, specifically, evaluation of the injured tendon. Xylazine HCl alone or in combination with butorphanol tartrate can assist restraint and examination. The affected limb should be stabilized and supported immediately at the venue of the injury to prevent additional injury during transportation to a medical or lay-up facility. To the extent possible, the normal load forces on the injured tendon(s) should be neutralized. This can be accomplished with external support using bandage materials, cast materials, and/or splintage. Horses with severe lameness should be transported as would a horse with possible distal limb fracture trauma. Timely, careful management may minimize the secondary disruption and inflammation of associated tendon tissue.

Immediately and for the 24 hours after injury, the application of topical coolants is appropriate to minimize and reduce the initial inflammatory response. Ice packs, chemical coolant packs, and alcohol-ice slurry boots can reduce the vascular, cellular, and chemical responses to the injury. This may be beneficial to the recuperative phase of tendon healing as well by reducing the influx of cellular and chemical mediators of inflammation, which can further retard the naturally deficient healing capabilities of tendons. Application of coolants may also provide some immediate local analgesia for the injured horse. Our recommendation is the application of ice for at least 1 hour as soon after injury as possible. This should be repeated at 4- to 6-hour intervals for the first 24 hours after injury.

The injured limb should be maintained in a neutral position until the horse can bear weight without distress. Bandages with firm pressure and splintage are usually appropriate and can be removed easily for access to the limb.

Administration of anti-inflammatory medication is indicated for horses with tendon injury. Nonsteroidal agents (NSAIDs) should be administered as part of the first aid for affected horses. Phenylbutazone (4 to 8 mg/kg), administered intravenously, serves as a timely and effective option for anti-inflammatory and analgesic therapy. Subsequent administration per os is accomplished adequately (2 to 4 mg/kg). Flunixin meglamine and ketaprofen are related nonsteroidal anti-inflammatory agents that can be substituted for phenylbutazone. While no benefit has been documented for simultaneous administration, the toxic effects resulting from excessive administration of NSAID compounds are well documented. From the authors' clinical perspectives, phenylbutazone appears to have a more clinically desirable result than these other nonsteroidal medications for initial treatment of tendon injury.

The systemic administration of dimethylsulfoxide (DMSO, 1 g/kg, IV or per os) may have beneficial effects for horses with tendon injuries. Affected horses treated with DMSO have been noted to be more comfortable and had less heat, pain, and swelling associated with the affected tendon tissue. The exact mode of action in these cases is unclear. The roles of oxygen (O_2^-) and hydroxyl (HO^-) radicals in tendon injury are not fully appreciated. Systemic administration of DMSO can be accomplished intravenously and per os. The authors have observed more satisfactory clinical results from systemic administration of DMSO solutions than following topical application of DMSO paints or gels. This positive clinical correlation may be due to effective control of the acute inflammatory response by the systemically administered DMSO, which appears to reduce edema and in turn reduce pain and increase regional vascular perfusion.

The systemic administration of polysulfated glycosaminoglycans (PSGAG) and sodium hyaluronate (SH) have been advocated for tendon and joint injury. The local administration of these agents has been investigated in both singular acute and repetitive dosing regimens. These treatments have been associated with equivocal results (1, 2). Hyaluronic acid (HA) is a component of tissue ground substance and has been detected in increased quantities in wounded tissues. It has been postulated that HA has an anti-inflammatory effect that may modify the severity of normal inflammation. Intrathecal sodium hyaluronate has been demonstrated to reduce the number and size of adhesions within the digital flexor tendon sheath of experimental horses, as well as to support improved tendon healing. The administration of sodium hyaluronate solution directly into chemically created core tendon lesions in experimental horses has been associated with reduction in the size of ultrasonographic lesions. However, serial intratendinous injections of sodium hyaluronate did not demonstrate continued improvement (3, 4). Systemic administration of SH and PSGAG has been observed to assist tendon healing and provide an earlier return to exercise (5, 6).

The most important component of immediate and long-term treatment of equine tendon injuries is rest and removal from the type of insult that created the original overload trauma. After transport to the treatment venue, the horse should be confined to a box stall and rested as completely as possible.

TOPICAL THERAPY

An exhaustive list of topical agents has been used to treat horses with injured tendons. Medications and manipulations directed at changing the local tissue temperature, blood flow, and tissue resiliency have been employed for many years. Salves, counter-irritants, coolants, and firing irons have all been used in varying degrees and combinations. With closer scrutiny, the common element in all of these therapies is rest. The difficulty in positively influencing the innately poor healing capabilities of the equine tendon is demonstrated by the months of time necessary to achieve adequate tendon healing. Topical application of therapeutic ultrasound energy has been reported to improve tendon healing in experimental rats. An ultrasound intensity of 1.5 W/cm^2 was employed in this study for this purpose. Ultrasound-treated tendons were observed to have increased collagen synthesis and greater breaking strength when compared with untreated control rat tendons. Therapeutic ultrasound therapy applied to a chemical tendinitis model in racing greyhounds had no obvious beneficial effects (7). Objective assessment of therapeutic ultrasound remains unproven in horses.

Topical hydrotherapy for 15 to 30 minutes two times a day may be beneficial to horses with tendinitis. The massaging action may stimulate local increases in circulation and assist in perfusing the poorly vascularized tendon tissue. Cold water is likely to be best for the first 24 hours after injury. Warm to hot water is likely to be more effective for subsequent applications. Hydrotherapy can be accomplished within a turbulating sleeve or boot, but may be more cleanly performed from a free-running hose. Limbs with open wounds are poor candidates for turbulation systems that encompass the entire limb, as contaminates from the distal limb and hoof can easily be introduced to the wound.

Although long used and accepted, topical agents such as hyperosmotic dressings (sweats), rubrifacients (paints), and counter-irritants (blisters) have not been documented to have a positive effect on tendon healing. Cutaneous alterations in irritation, inflammation, and circulation do not necessarily reflect changes in the tendon environment. Topically applied hyperosmotic dressings such as DMSO, antiphlogestine, and glycerine under vapor barrier bandages, may assist in reducing peritendinous edema. The specific effects of such compounds on tendon tissue remain unknown. More severe chemical irritants have been associated with unnecessary debilitation of treated horses. Red mercury blisters have been associated with renal failure in horses, and its use cannot be recommended.

Thermocautery methods that burn skin and external tissue with a firing iron have also been long accepted in some circles as a traditional therapy for tendinitis. To date there has been no proven positive effect on tendon healing. Recently, thermocautery has been declared an unethical and illegal practice in the United Kingdom. Serious reevaluation of this practice is needed as firing of tendinitis lesions cannot be recommended. Enforced rest of fired horses for prolonged periods is the only reasonable mechanism for any success associated with this painful method of treatment. Locally invasive, nonsurgical therapy of tendinitis has been advocated. Hypodermic needles (16 to 23 gauge) have been introduced into core lesions under ultrasonographic guidance. Serosanguinous fluid contents of hypoechoic core lesions have been aspirated from the lesion site to remove the hematoma and inflammatory mediators that may retard the tendon healing. Results of this practice are equivocal, and no documentation of positive benefit to tendon healing from this practice has been determined.

PARENTERAL THERAPY

The peritendinous administration of sodium hyaluronate (SH) was reported originally to have a positive effect on tendon healing based on a collagenase-induced tendinitis model (1). Subsequent research has failed to verify a distinct advantageous effect on tendon healing as a result of peritendinous SH treatment (2). Other investigations have examined the effect of intralesional injections of SH into collagenase-induced tendinitis lesions. At least one study appears to indicate that injection of SH directly into the tendon core lesion can reduce the acute severity of tendinitis as evidenced by reduction in the ultrasonographic lesion size after SH administration (3). Subsequent work has evaluated repeated administration of SH to the same lesion site and found no additional merit to more than one treatment at the earliest possible time (4). The specific benefit of intralesional administration of SH into tendon core lesions resulting from physical disruption of tendon fibers has not been examined.

Injection of SH into the intrathecal space has been demonstrated to reduce the severity of tendon sheath adhesion formation and to improve tendon healing. This appears to be beneficial for horses with tendinitis and tenosynovitis originating from overload stress or external trauma. Repeated intrathecal administration of SH is suggested at weekly intervals.

Corticosteroid administration to tendinitis lesions has not been associated with favorable improvement in equine tendon healing. Repeated injections of reposital forms of glucocorticoids can predispose tendon tissue to dystrophic mineralization. Repeated injection of glucocorticoid medications may also result in weakening of collagen connective tissues. Prolonged systemic steroid therapy has also been reported to weaken collagen-based connective tissue (8).

Surgical treatment of tendon disease has had widespread acceptance. Adjunctive medical therapy of tendinitis may augment and enhance the results achieved by these surgical procedures. Annular ligament desmotomy can relieve constriction of injured digital flexor tendons and possibly enhance vascular perfusion of tendon parenchyma. This procedure also appears to reduce the pain associated with tendon lesions in the region of the fetlock. Proximal and distal check ligament desmotomies can transfer strain from affected tendons to the associated superficial and deep digital flexor muscles. By distributing stress loads and resultant strain deformation over a greater length of the musculotendinous unit, patients appear to be more comfortable. It is possible but undocumented that such a technique may enhance perfusion by decreasing intratendinous strain deformation and improve the potential for healing the injured tendon. Tendon splitting (Asheim's tenotomy) has been associated with decompression of core lesions and improving peritendinous vascular access to tendon lesions.

EXTERNAL SUPPORT

Tendinitis in horses can cause moderate to severe lameness (Grades 3–5/5). As an important component of first aid, external support is often beneficial to reduce further exacerbation of injury and to reduce stress loads and strain deformation of the injured tendon. The goal of external coaptation is to place the affected limb in a position to neutralize continued strain deformation of the injured tendon. Raising the heel and immobilizing the limb can reduce some of this flexor tendon strain. This can be accomplished with bandage material, splintage (PVC and Kimzy® splints), gelcast, rigid fiberglass casting, or a rigid distal limb boot (Farley boot). Stress loading and strain deformation cannot be reduced completely without fully immobilizing the musculotendinous unit. To approximate such relief for the digital flexor tendons will require a full limb cast for external coaptation. Heel elevation alone can be accomplished with therapeutic shoeing. The amount of elevation should be customized to each horse and can reach 20° of elevation. Extending the heel of the shoe can also provide caudal support of the limb and prevent excessive hyperextension.

ALTERNATIVE THERAPY

Alternative treatment modalities have become more available as lay equestrians and veterinarians alike have searched for nontraditional and potentially more successful methods of managing equine flexor tendinitis. Magnetic field therapy and electrical current treatment have been evaluated as possible treatments for nonspecific limb injury. The application of magnetic field treatments has been associated indirectly with an increase in blood flow to bone in the equine distal limb. Although no work has been performed examining the effect on tendon tissue and vasculature, magnetic field therapy may hold some promise as a treatment of tendon disease in the future. Electrical current therapy has also not been examined in equine tendinitis per se, but this treatment method has not met with acceptance for acceleration of normal osseous healing and was shown to have no effect at all on tendon gap healing in horses. It is likely that electrical current therapy has no place for treating traumatic tendinitis in athletic horses.

Acupuncture and cold laser therapy are commonly encountered treatment choices of modern horse owners and trainers. Acupuncture appears to hold some promise as an adjunctive symptomatic treatment for equine tendinitis, principally as a nonpharmaceutical modality for relief of pain. There appears to be documentable transient analgesic properties associated with the application of these methods. Acupuncture may stimulate the release of the endogenous opiate compounds, endorphines and enkephalines, which in turn provide local transient analgesia. Many other claims have been made for acupuncture and some may have merit. However, at this time very little documented evidence is available that has been substantiated by critical prospective Western scientific evaluation. Similarly, "cold" laser energy is usually applied to acupressure/acupuncture points to achieve the same favorable symptomatic results expected from acupuncture needle application. Critically reviewed scientific data is lacking to substantiate claims of rational treatment success with cold laser therapy.

Chiropractic techniques are being applied with increasing frequency to horses suffering from a variety of musculoskeletal disorders, including flexor tendinitis. Anecdotal evidence abounds that chiropractic provides a useful clinical alternative to conventional medical and surgical treatment. Regrettably, sources of information addressing methodology and application to the equine patient are not available, and evidence of symptomatic or curative relief is scarce. No critically reviewed data are available to substantiate chiropractic as a viable alternative to conventional therapy.

PHYSICAL THERAPY

Physical therapy has been associated with improved tendon healing and return to function in other species. Passive range-of-motion exercise has been associated with stronger and more normal tendon healing in laboratory animals and humans. With the possible exception of swimming, passive exercise is not possible for horses. Early return to range-of-motion exercise by hand may be beneficial to horses, as this is anecdotally reported for horses with tendon lacerations and tenosynovitis. Some controlled walking for horses with tendinitis may be advantageous in assisting vascular perfusion. Repeated hydrotherapy may be helpful in the same situation.

Application of transcutaneous therapeutic ultrasound energy may hold some promise for horses with tendinitis. As stated earlier, experimental laboratory animals experienced stronger tendon healing and increased collagen synthesis after ultrasound treatment. Treatment periods of 10 to 20 minutes with 10 W/cm^2 have been suggested for horses.

The most sound and continuously proven tenant of treatment for tendon disorders in horses is rest of the affected tendon tissue. It is likely that all other treatment modalities can appear successful if enough proper rest is provided. The relative paucity of vascular perfusion of the tendon and the added demands of weight support and exercise of horses make healing very difficult. Complete, neutral, non-weight-bearing rest is virtually impossible for horses. Therefore, adequate rest becomes prolonged and usually involves an ex-

tensive period of box stall confinement. Severe core tendinitis lesions (Grades 3 and 4) can require up to 12 months of rest to allow healing of the disrupted tendon fibers. The time and rest allow revascularization and delivery of peritendinous vascularity to the injured tendon. This in turn delivers the necessary cellular and chemical elements necessary for tendon healing. Lesion severity and individual variation make it difficult to predict accurately the effective duration of rest that will be necessary before appropriate return to exercise is begun. Ultrasonographic examination is the best way to evaluate the affected tendon and the course of healing. Appropriate return to exercise is determined by a return to normal ultrasonographic appearance of the tendon.

A horse with suspected flexor tendinitis should be evaluated by a veterinarian as soon as possible. Although it is unlikely there exists a singly, effective, therapeutic regimen for treatment of acute flexor tendinitis, the typical course of therapy after definitive diagnosis is as follows: Systemic administration of nonsteroidal anti-inflammatory agents (phenylbutazone 4 to 8 mg/kg and DMSO) is performed as soon as possible. The affected limb and tendon tissue should have ice or topical coolants applied to reduce the immediate inflammatory response. The limb should be placed in a heavy bandage, flexed-position splint, or distal-limb support to avoid further trauma to the disrupted tendon.

An ultrasonographic examination of the affected tendons should be performed as soon as possible. This will provide a baseline assessment of location and initial severity of the lesion. We suggest that intralesional administration of sodium hyaluronate (SH) may reduce the progression of tendon fiber inflammation and lesion propagation. Dependent on location and severity of the tendon lesion, check ligament desmotomy and/or a tendon-splitting procedure may be beneficial to the ultimate quality of tendon healing after the initial inflammatory response is controlled or reduced. These procedures appear to be indicated in the acute period after injury and during the early stages of recuperation. After these initial treatment efforts, the affected horse should be confined to a box stall and begin the essential rest period. The tendon lesion should be monitored periodically to assess the ongoing healing process. The affected limb should be supported in a bandage after removal from splintage. Range-of-motion exercise should precede active walking. Manual flexion and extension (10 to 20 repetitions) with the horse standing should be initiated early in the course of rest. Walking should be initiated after clinical pain and lameness are markedly reduced and ultrasonographic evidence of tendon healing is determined. Daily hydrotherapy is performed for 10 to 20 minutes one to three times per day. Return to full exercise is delayed until the horse is sound and tendon ultrasound evaluation is normal. Full healing and return to sound athletic use may require 6 to 12 months.

This course of treatment is successful for most horses with flexor tendinitis. The amount of time out of work is variable and ultrasound examination appears to be the key to proper return to exercise. Medical therapy may support surgical treatment and rest to return athletic horses to competition as early as possible. Yet it must be kept in focus that a horse that has experienced overload tendon fiber disruption is predisposed to repeated occurrence of the injury.

REFERENCES

1. Spurlock GH, Spurlock SL, Parker GA. Evaluation of Hylartin V therapy for induced tendinitis in the horse. Equine Vet Sci 1989; 9(5):242–246.
2. Foland JW, Trotter GW, Powers BE, et al. Sodium hyaluronate in induced equine digital flexor tendinitis. Vet Surg 1991;20(5):336.
3. Gift LJ, Gaughan EM, DeBowes RM, et al. The influence of intra-tendinous sodium hyaluronate on tendon healing in horses. VCOT 1992;5:151–157.
4. Gaughan EM, Gift LJ, Roush J, et al. The influence of sequential intratendinous sodium hyaluronate on tendon healing in horses. VCOT 1995;8:40–45.
5. Gaughan EM, McLaughlin RM, Hoskinson JJ, et al. The influence of intravenous sodium hyaluronate on tendon healing and adhesion formation in horses. In press.
6. Booth LC. Biology of tendon and ligament healing. Proceedings of the 23rd Annual Surgical Forum, ACVS 1995; 77–79.
7. Roush JK, Gaughan EM, Kraft SL. Clinical, histomorphometric and mechanical effects of therapeutic ultrasound on enzyme-induced tendinitis in racing greyhounds. Proceedings of the 29th Annual Scientific Meeting, ACVS 1994.
8. Stashak TS. Methods of therapy. In: Stashak TS, ed. Adams' lameness in horses. Philadelphia: Lea & Febiger, 1987; 840–877.

27. Section D

Tendinitis, the Approach to Treatment

LARRY R. BRAMLAGE

Tendinitis is a frustrating musculoskeletal disease to treat. A rational approach to therapy, however, may make the difference between success and failure. The prognosis for maximal-effort activities such as racing is poorer than for less strenuous activities such as pleasure riding. The prognosis varies for different tendons and limbs. Extensor tendons are able to functionally heal from nearly any injury. The function of an extensor tendon is not dynamic like the flexor tendons. Extensor tendons function like strings that lift or extend joints. Therefore a lost segment of extensor tendon can be readily replaced by fibrous tissue. The treatment of extensor tendon injuries is more appropriately dealt with as a wound-healing topic.

Hind limb flexor tendon injuries carry a more favorable prognosis than forelimb tendon injuries because the hind limb flexor tendons are longer and do not have a well-developed check ligament like the forelimbs. As a result they are more tolerant of healing by fibrosis with the resultant loss of elasticity than are the flexor tendons of the forelimbs. The deep digital flexor tendon is much less frequently injured than the superficial digital flexor tendon. Injury to the superficial digital flexor tendon of the forelimb carries the worst prognosis for return to unimpaired function and therefore, is the most difficult to treat.

CLINICAL SIGNS AND DIAGNOSIS

Inflammation indicates damage, and therefore any heat, swelling, or pain on palpation of the tendons should be noted and followed for progression. Although persistence or recurrence of inflammation are the key indicators of tendon damage, the amount of inflammation is not always a measure of the amount of tendon damage. Injuries near the surface of the tendon show much more heat and swelling than do injuries deep within the tendon. The swelling may subside with therapy, and tendon damage may still be present. If inflammation recurs or persists after the initial episode, diagnostic ultrasound examination is warranted to establish the degree of damage. It is as important to know when there is no injury as it is to know when the tendon is injured. Ultrasound examination aids in the determination of the presence and progression of an injury to a tendon. It may not be necessary for making a diagnosis of tendinitis, but it is important in defining the lesion and therefore in the selection of treatment.

The goals in the initial treatment of tendinitis are to keep the inflammatory response to the minimum necessary to re-

pair the injury, and to prevent the inflammatory response from affecting the normal tendon. The inflammatory response results in edema and, subsequently, fibrous tissue deposition, which is detrimental to the elastic function of the tendon. Fibrous tissue deposition is, however, the only means of repair available in the adult and is therefore necessary for healing. The therapeutic goal is to allow repair to proceed, but to modulate the response and not let it become excessive and inflame the adjacent normal tendon.

THERAPY

Acute Stage (0 to 48 Hours)

The goal in the acutely injured tendon is to control the inflammatory response.

Physical Therapy

Ice is an effective inhibitor of inflammation. It constricts blood vessels, slows hemorrhage, reduces the amount of inflammatory mediators released into the injured tissue, slows the activity of the mediators of inflammation, and reduces the perception of pain. Cold application should be in 30-minute to 1-hour sessions ideally three to four times a day.

Bandaging provides counterpressure against tissue swelling. Constant, firm, uniform pressure will keep tissue planes collapsed and reduce the quantity of tissue fluid that escapes from the vascular system into the tissues. Persistent fluid within the tendon will lead to fibrosis and is detrimental.

Rest is essential during the 48-hour acute inflammatory phase of injury because exercise may worsen the injury. In most instances, shoes should be removed. Since the superficial digital flexor tendon attaches to the pastern area, the heel should be lowered to straighten the fetlock angle and decrease the excursion of the superficial digital flexor tendon. It should not be elevated.

Pharmacologic Therapy

Nonsteroidal anti-inflammatory drugs (NSAIDs) are always indicated as part of the initial treatment of tendon inflammation. Interruption of the prostaglandin cascade, initiated by tissue injury, reduces the inflammatory process. Flunixin meglumine (1.1 mg per kg) should be included in the initial treatment regimen because of its rapid onset of activity. Phenylbutazone (4.4 to 8.8 mg per kg) is preferable for long-term maintenance, due to its longer half-life. Both drugs are often given simultaneously initially to get the fastest and most complete therapy. Other NSAIDs are also available. Their use is a matter of personal preference and appropriate pharmacologic application.

Corticosteroids provide the most powerful anti-inflammatory therapy; however, they also have the undesirable effect of delaying healing and reducing repair strength for up to 1 year after administration if crystalline products are used. Some long-acting corticosteroids may also contribute to soft-tissue calcification. Long-acting corticosteroid therapy is undesirable, but the use of the ultra-short-acting corticosteroid during the acute inflammatory phase can stop the inflammatory process and protect the remaining normal tissue. Anything but short-acting corticosteroids in small doses should be avoided.

Dimethyl sulfoxide (DMSO) is of benefit in the treatment of acute tendon inflammation. It is a free-radical scavenger and will therefore prevent some of the detrimental effects of tissue inflammation. Clinically, however, tendon inflammation is often discovered after free radicals would have been released in the greatest amounts. The generally recommended, systemic, anti-inflammatory dose of DMSO is 2.2 mg per kg given intravenously (IV) and diluted in large volumes of fluid, although as little as 0.5 mg per kg given IV or orally by stomach tube has been described as being useful. There are few instances in which DMSO would be detrimental in the treatment of acute tendinitis.

Hyaluronic acid deposited around the tendon at the site of inflammation has proven beneficial in the treatment of tendon injuries in human hands. The goal is to prevent adhesions and maintain gliding function to preserve fine-motor activity. Although adhesions are of concern in the horse, the main goal is to preserve weight-bearing function. Therefore hyaluronic acid therapy must be weighed as to its cost:benefit ratio in the treatment of flexor tendon injuries in the horse. Injuries to tendons within tendon sheaths may benefit from hyaluronic acid administration into the tendon sheath to preserve the lubrication function of the sheath around the tendon and to prevent the development of adhesions between the sheath and tendon. The recommended dose of hyaluronic acid varies from 20 to 120 mg per treatment. The necessary minimum dose for efficacious coating of a digital tendon sheath probably is near the low end of this range, and the expense of treatment encourages a low dose.

Polysulfated glycosaminoglycans (PSGAGs) may have some use in the early treatment of tendon inflammation. They should be administered into the lesion to be most effective, but can also be given systemically. Though pharmacologically logical as an enzyme inhibitor, the efficacy of PSGAG remains speculative. Scientific documentation and the test of time are necessary. It is probable that they are helpful, but the degree of benefit is not yet established in the clinical situation.

Surgical Therapy

Surgical treatment is not recommended during the 48-hour acute inflammatory phase.

Monitoring

Monitoring the success of treatment in the first 48 hours of tendon injury is by physical examination. The goal is to arrest the progression of the disease.

Subacute Stage (2 to 21 Days)

Acute inflammation should now be arrested. The goals of treatment in the subacute stage of tendon injury are to prevent the spread of inflammation into normal tendon, to reverse the acute inflammation, to minimize permanent damage to the injured tendon, and to initiate the repair process for an orderly and functional reestablishment of the flexor tendon. In the subacute stage, fibrous tissue deposition necessary for repair begins. For the highest quality repair it must be confined to the areas needing repair. Since coagulated tissue fluids and fibrin form the scaffold for fibrosis, edema needs to be controlled. The rapid removal of tissue fluids from the tendon adjacent to the injury minimizes fibrosis in the normal tissue surrounding the injury.

The signs of subacute tendinitis include heat, pain on tendon palpation, swelling, and, depending on the degree of damage, possibly lameness. Three courses of treatment are available: (a) removal from training and rest for an extended period to allow natural repair, (b) disregard the inflammation, provide symptomatic treatment, and allow continuation of exercise, or (c) accurate assessment of the damage with ultrasound examination and initiation of appropriate treatment.

Physical Therapy

Cold therapy should be alternated with warm temperatures for 4 to 6 days after the acute inflammation is controlled to help in removal of tissue fluid. Warm intervals should be three times as long as cold intervals, and the cycle can be repeated as many times as possible each day until the desired result is obtained. Four to 6 days after injury, fibroproliferation begins and fluid removal becomes progressively more difficult. Singular cold therapy can be stopped, and warm temperatures are used to improve circulation and speed repair. Prolonged warm temperatures can be achieved by stimulating circulation through the topical medications, such as rubefacients, and the use of an occlusive bandage (a "sweat bandage"). Pressure bandaging is still useful to counteract swelling.

Hydromassage is a beneficial treatment that entails use of pressurized water from a hose, a "turbolator boot," a water treadmill, or a whirlpool. The water massages the injured tissue, aids in removal of stagnant tissue fluids, and speeds repair by stimulating circulation.

Exercise must be limited until tissue fluid accumulation is halted. At that point, unless complete structural integrity is lost, controlled mild exercise such as walking can begin, but free exercise is not advised. Mild, noninjuring exercise stimulates tissue fluid movement from areas of poor perfusion and stimulates improved perfusion throughout the entire tendon.

Pharmacologic Therapy

Nonsteroidal anti-inflammatory drugs should be continued through this stage. Corticosteroids are contraindicated because their anti-inflammatory properties prevent repair. Topical DMSO can be applied until the tissue fluid has been evacuated. Once the fibroproliferative phase begins, DMSO should be discontinued because it has a detrimental effect on the amount and quality of collagen formation within a scar. Hyaluronic acid therapy is not often used in the subacute-inflammation period. PSGAG therapy needs to be administered early in the acute phase to neutralize the damaging enzymes. Methysulfomethane (MSM) has anti-inflammatory properties and may be a very rich source of available sulfur for tissue repair. The recommended dosage for treatment of injured tendons is 1 to 2 oz of Methysulfomethane-containing feed supplement daily.

Surgical Treatment

Surgeries undertaken during the subacute phase include tendon transplantation, carbon fiber implantation and fragment injection, tendon splitting, and superior check ligament desmotomy. None is universally accepted as the treatment of choice. I prefer superior check ligament desmotomy and tendon splitting in selected cases.

Monitoring

Monitoring the response to treatment is primarily by observation of the clinical signs and repeat ultrasound evaluations. Surgical intervention is aimed at improving the expected course of healing and appearance of the tendon.

Remodeling Stage (21 to 60 Days)

During this stage, treatment guides the repair process and produces a functional tendon or tendon substitute. Repair mechanisms should have started in the vascularized areas of the injured tendon. Medical or surgical steps should have been taken in the subacute period to ensure that the injured area of tendon revascularizes as completely as possible. During the remodeling stage, fibroblasts remodel and replace collagen according to the needs dictated by the local biomechanical forces. The fibroblasts produce as much collagen as is needed and therefore as much scar as is necessary to accommodate the load on the tissues. It is difficult, however, for the fibroblasts to reproduce the elasticity of the stroma necessary for the repairing tendon to function as the original tissue.

Physical Therapy

Temperature-altering methods of therapy lose their efficacy during this healing period. Small recurrences of inflammation can and should accompany proper aggressive rehabilitation programs. Electronic aids such as electromagnetic fields direct electrical stimulation, and many others have been advocated to assist tendon remodeling. Their benefit is questionable, and their use may be detrimental, so it is recommended that they be avoided. Therapeutic laser treatment is losing popularity. Anecdotal success has been derived from treatment with "cold" lasers. The ability of the cold laser to penetrate to the tendon injury is questionable, though evidence does not indicate any detrimental effect of laser treatment.

Irritants were formerly used in this stage of healing in draft horses. These beasts of burden needed strong tendons, and therefore the production of fibrous tissue was encouraged. In the performance horse, however, preservation of a functional tendon is a more desirable end. Firing has been used in varying patterns to reinforce the injured tendon. Though still used in certain locales, firing has lost its popularity. Blistering as a means of stimulating an increased circulation makes sense theoretically and has been used for years. Stimulating remodeling, without the danger of stimulating more fibrosis, is the goal. Mild rubefacients are safer than aggressive counter-irritants. Any topical medication that is injurious to normal tissues is too strong to be useful in minimizing permanent tendon damage. Only mild circulatory stimulants are indicated. Injectable irritants carry the danger of stimulating an increase in unwanted fibrosis.

Bandaging in this phase is not likely to alter the size or character of the healing area. If inflammation reappears, bandaging should be used.

Controlled exercise is indicated during the remodeling stage. If exercise is excessive, fibrous tissue is produced rather than remodeled. If no stress is applied during the remodeling phase, the haphazard end result may resemble a tendon more adapted to pasture exercise than performance. Dosing the exercise regimen is an art and must be done according to the individual patient's needs. It is assumed that, like other tissues, tendon scars reach one-half of their eventual strength in 6 to 8 weeks. Therefore only very light exercise should be allowed for this stage. Paddock exercise is okay once pain to palpation has subsided. At 60 days, gradually increasing loads should be applied. Exercise aids such as underwater treadmills can assist in this process by requiring work against resistance and some weight-bearing while still avoiding strenuous loading. Swimming produces no weight-bearing load on the injured tendon and therefore does not create work-specific remodeling. This disadvantage can be overcome by combining some form of weight-bearing exercise, in addition to or alternating with swimming. In most instances, however, special facilities are not available and are unnecessary. Four weeks of walking followed by 2 to 4 weeks of pasture exercise and then 8 weeks of jogging during or after the pasture exercise is a good start. Jogging keeps the rear-quarter weight on the hind limbs and therefore lightly loads the tendon, stimulating remodeling but staying below the reinjury threshold. I prefer to leave the horse at paddock exercise between 2 and 4 months, but put the horse under saddle or in harness 3 times a week for 10 to 15 minutes for trotting exercise.

There are sources of minor inflammation that must be overcome in the rehabilitation of a tendon. As a tendon is stretched after healing, adhesions must be stretched and in some instances torn to reestablish a full range of motion. Small sites of inflammation within the tendon, which may then spread to other parts of the tendon, appear and can recreate tendinitis. This problem can be overcome with careful retraining. Recognition of the minor inflammation caused by the breakdown of intratendinous and peritendinous adhesions and curtailment of strenuous exercise until the inflammation subsides (generally a matter of days) eliminates the danger created by breaking down the adhesions and prevents the spread of inflammation into the recovering tendon. Adhesion problems are most likely to occur at each major increase in exercise level, for example, from trotting to galloping and from training to racing. The longer the horse has been rested, the more problems one will encounter with adhesions.

SUGGESTED READINGS

Bramlage LR. Superior check ligament desmotomy as a treatment for superficial digital flexor tendinitis: initial report. Proceedings of the 32nd Annual Convention of the American Association of Equine Practitioners 1986; pp. 365-370.

McIlwraith CW. Diseases of joints, tendons, ligaments, and related structures. Adams' lameness in horses. 4th ed. Philadelphia: Lea & Febiger, 1987, p.447.

28. Cardiovascular Sonography

JOHANNA M. REIMER

Equipment selection, examination procedures, and normal anatomy are discussed elsewhere in this volume. The various abnormalities that may be detected in the horse and foal are described in this chapter.

Sonographic evaluation of the heart should not be performed without auscultation of the animal's heart and a thorough knowledge of normal cardiac anatomy. Familiarity with the various disorders that may affect the equine heart and knowledge of the sonographic characteristics of primary lesions and the secondary effects of these disorders on the heart are necessary to interpret the sonographic study properly.

VALVULAR DISEASES

Degenerative Valve Disease

The aortic valve is commonly affected by degenerative changes in older horses. This is in contrast to dogs, in which the mitral valve is typically affected by the degenerative disease of endocardiosis. Auscultation of affected horses typically reveals a decrescendo diastolic murmur that may be accompanied by a musical or "honking" component. This musical or honking tone suggests a fenestration. Valvular lesions range from generalized thickening of one or more valve cusps to nodules, fibrous bands, or full-thickness fenestrations of the cusps (Fig. 28.1). M-mode echocardiography may reveal diastolic vibrations of the aortic valve, mitral valve (Fig. 28.2), or septum, or early mitral valve closure in severe cases. Left atrial and left ventricular chamber dilation may be seen to varying degrees, depending on the severity and duration of aortic regurgitation. Mitral regurgitation may occur as a sequela of aortic regurgitation, because of dilation of the mitral valve annulus (1). Pulsed-wave Doppler studies are useful in determining the extent of the regurgitant jet and estimating the animal's prognosis. Certainly, serial echocardiographic studies enable a more accurate estimation of the course of the disease process. In light of the occurrence of aortic valve disease in predominantly older horses, aortic regurgitation in general is well-tolerated and is infrequently associated with clinical signs in such horses. Often, the horse succumbs for other reasons before the valvular disease leads to congestive heart failure. A worse prognosis may need to be considered for younger horses, depending on the horse's age, workload, and the severity of the regurgitation.

Degenerative changes of the other cardiac valves may also occur. Such valves may appear thicker than normal,

although in some horses with valvular regurgitation due to degenerative disease, gross valvular disease may be difficult to demonstrate echocardiographically. Doppler echocardiography is of benefit in estimating the severity of the regurgitation. Prognosis depends on the the the degree of regurgitation and whether the lesion is right sided or left sided.

Bacterial Endocarditis

Horses with bacterial endocarditis are often febrile and have laboratory evidence of infection. Bacteriologic cure of this disease is possible; however, valvular abnormalities often persist. Horses with bacterial endocarditis may *not* have murmurs, particularly if the infection involves an intact chorda tendinea, or if the lesions are proliferative and large, restricting any regurgitant blood flow.

Lesions caused by bacterial endocarditis are typically large, knobby, or fleshy lesions on the valve leaflets or chordae tendineae (Fig. 28.3). These lesions develop over time; therefore, the sonogram may be negative in the early stages of the disease. Vegetative lesions may be detected on the chordea tendineae, on the leaflets of the tricuspid or mitral valves, or on the cusps of the aortic or pulmonic valves. Rupture of a chorda tendinea may also be detected (Fig 28.4). Valvular regurgitation may or may not be present, although hemodynamically significant valvular regurgitation may ultimately develop, even if not present or minimal at the time of diagnosis. Affected valves often contract with a fibrous scar even with successful antimicrobial treatment, consequently resulting in more severe regurgitation (2). Involvement of the left side of the heart is associated with a grave prognosis, whereas right-sided valvular regurgitation is better tolerated, and the prognosis, at least for life, is more favorable because of the lower pressures in the right side of the heart.

Abnormal valve morphology is often evident in bacteriologically cured vegetative endocarditis; therefore, a diagnosis of active endocarditis should be supported by history, physical findings, and laboratory data. The echogenicity of the lesion may also provide a clue to the stage of the disease. Dense and even calcified lesions can be seen in horses that have "recovered" from the infection (Fig 28.5).

Ruptured Chordae Tendineae

Rupture of chordae tendineae is often suspected when auscultation reveals an unusually loud and honking quality

581

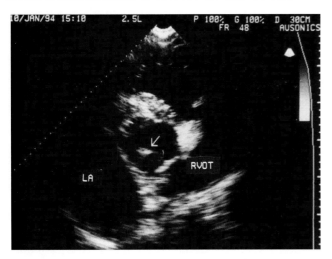

Figure 28.1. Nodular lesion (*arrow*) along the edge of the left coronary cusp of the aortic valve in an aged horse with moderate aortic regurgitation. Right intercostal, short axis view. LA = left atrium; RVOT = right ventricular outflow tract.

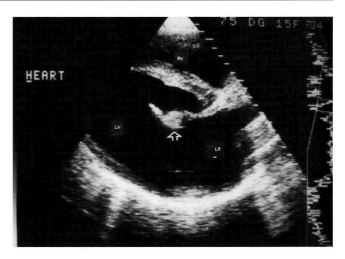

Figure 28.3. Large vegetative lesion on the septal leaflet of the mitral valve (*arrow*) in a foal with bacterial endocarditis. LA = left atrium; LV= left ventricle; RV = right ventricle.

murmur, although the character of the murmur can be of any variety. Chordae tendineae disruption can occur as a result of infection, degenerative processes, or necrosis, or it may be idiopathic. If a major attachment is disrupted in the mitral valve, fulminant pulmonary edema may result. At the other extreme, disruption of a minor attachment may produce a characteristic honking murmur yet only hemodynamically insignificant mitral regurgitation. Tricuspid regurgitation due to ruptured chordae tendineae appears to be less common. Clinical signs are often not as severe; tricuspid regurgitation is better tolerated because of lower pressures in the right heart.

Sonographic diagnosis of a ruptured chorda tendinea is made by the detection of disrupted chordae tendineae or even valve leaflet pointing, prolapsing, or flailing into the atrium during systole (see Fig. 28.4).

Prolapse

Prolapse of the mitral, aortic, or tricuspid valve is not an uncommon two-dimensional echocardiographic diagnosis for murmurs originating from these areas. Mild valvular prolapse, not associated with ruptured chordae tendineae, is a common sonographic finding in the horse; it may be detected sonographically in horses with no associated murmur. In horses with a slight degree of mitral valvular regurgitation, auscultation may reveal a mid-systolic crescendo murmur, which may infrequently be accompanied by a musical component. In the "classic" case, prolapse of the valve is characterized by bulging of the central portion of the involved leaflet into the atrium during systole (or bulging of the aortic valve into the left ventricle during diastole). Regurgitation may or may not be present and may

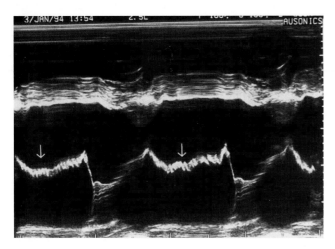

Figure 28.2. M-mode echocardiogram of the mitral valve in an aged horse with aortic valve insufficiency. Notice the fine vibrations of the septal leaflet during diastole (*arrows*).

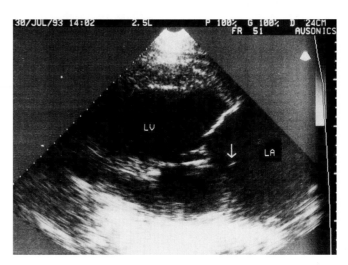

Figure 28.4. Ruptured chorda tendinea (*arrow*) of the mitral valve in an aged horse with acute left-sided heart failure. Left long axis two-chamber view. LA = left atrium; LV = left ventricle.

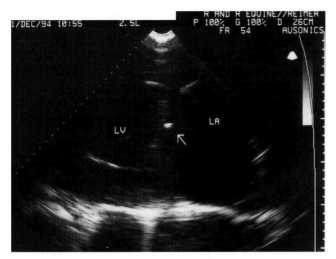

Figure 28.5. Echodense nodule (*arrow*) along the mitral valve of a 2-year-old colt that had bacteriologically cured vegetative endocarditis as a young foal. The horse had severe mitral regurgitation and left atrial and ventricular dilation; he developed congestive heart failure several months later. Left long axis two-chamber view. LA = left atrium; LV = left ventricle.

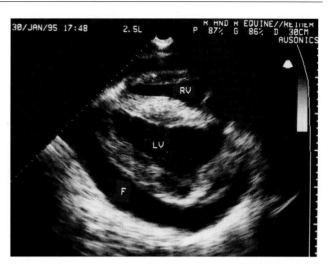

Figure 28.6. Pericardial effusion in a yearling colt with fevers, muffled heart sounds, and jugular pulsations. Right long axis view. F = pericardial fluid; LV = left ventricle; RV = right ventricle.

vary in severity. Prolapse of the mitral valve is suspected to be the most common cause of mid-systolic crescendo murmurs in the horse (3), although valvular abnormalities may be undetectable echocardiographically in horses with such murmurs of mitral regurgitation. Tricuspid valve prolapse may be detected echocardiographically in horses with murmurs of tricuspid regurgitation, which are often band-shaped in quality, regardless of the type of valvular lesion.

Doppler echocardiography is invaluable in assessing the degree of regurgitation. Often, only minimal to moderate regurgitation is found, and the disorder in these horses generally progresses little, if at all, over several years. Again, this type of valvular prolapse should be distinguished from that resulting from loss of valvular support, such as with ruptured chordae tendineae or prolapse of an aortic valve cusp into a ventricular septal defect. These cases may carry a worse prognosis.

MYOCARDIAL DISEASE

Results of auscultation of horses with myocardial disease may be normal if myocardial dysfunction and dilation is mild. Elevated heart rates can be detected in more severe cases. Murmurs of mitral and tricuspid regurgitation may be detected if the heart has dilated to the point where the valve annulus has been stretched apart. Myocardial disease in the horse may result from toxins, such as ionophore antibiotics (monensin and lasolacid), certain plants, viral agents, or immune-mediated phenomena. Myocardial dysfunction may also be seen secondary to chronic valvular disease as the horse develops congestive heart failure.

The diagnosis of myocardial disease is based on reduced myocardial contractility (fractional shortening). Severe noncardiac diseases can also result in myocardial dysfunction, as can persistent ventricular tachycardia and other rhythm dysfunctions. Horses with severe mitral regurgita-

tion have elevated shortening fractions if myocardial function is relatively normal (this is because a substantial amount of blood is ejected into the left atrium rather than into the aorta).

PERICARDIAL DISEASE

Physical findings in horses with pericardial disease include tachycardia, jugular pulsations, muffled heart sounds, and friction rubs (unless pericardial effusion is predominant). Pericardial disease in the horse is often presumed to be infectious (bacterial or viral), although some tumors and hemopericardium may occur. Neonatal foals with fractured ribs occasionally develop hemopericardium.

Pericardial effusion is detected easily in the horse (Fig. 28.6). Fibrin tags can be identified readily, particularly if fluid is present in the pericardial sac. Care must be made not to confuse pleural effusions with pericardial effusions. The lung tip and caudal vena cava are surrounded in pleural effusions, whereas the lung tip overlies the pericardial sac and the caudal vena cava is not visible in pericardial effusion. Certainly, both effusions may be present either as a result of inflammation of both cavities or because the pleural effusion may result from cardiac tamponade.

Cardiac tamponade results when intrapericardial pressure rises above right atrial and right ventriclular pressures. This condition is demonstrated sonographically by collapse of the right atrium or right ventricle during diastole. Clinical signs of right heart failure, including jugular pulsations, peripheral edema, and pleural and peritoneal effusions develop. The degree of cardiac tamponade is based on the rapidity in which effusion accumulates. Severe tamponade may develop with only a small but rapidly accumulating amount of fluid, whereas several liters of slowly accumulating pericardial fluid may be present and may cause few clinical signs. Pericardiocentesis is indicated for the treatment of cardiac tamponade. Digoxin and furosemide are *not* indicated. Myocardial contractility is not affected in

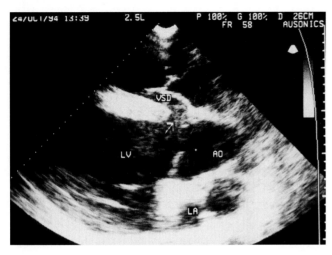

Figure 28.7. Ventricular septal defect (VSD; *arrow*) in a weanling Standardbred colt. Right-sided, long axis left ventricle (LV) outflow view. AO = aorta; LA = left atrium.

patients with pericardial effusion; cardiac output is low because of decreased diastolic ventricular volume caused by increased pericardial pressure. Diuretics further decrease ventricular filling and may well compound the problems of low cardiac output and hypotension.

CONGENITAL CARDIAC DISEASE

Ventricular Septal Defect

Ventricular septal defect (VSD) is the most common congenital cardiac defect in the horse. In the most common type of VSD, the defect is located in the membranous portion of the ventricular septum, it measures up to a few centimeters in size, and the flow of blood through the defect is from left to right. In such cases, auscultation typically reveals systolic murmurs on both the left and right sides of the heart; the right-sided murmur is often the more prominent. Precordial thrills are often present.

VSDs are typically located in the membranous portion of the ventricular septum and are best imaged in the long axis left ventricular outflow plane (Fig 28.7). Defects should be measured in both long axis and short axis planes. Defects measuring less than 2.5 cm in diameter are generally considered to be hemodynamically insignificant in the horse. Although several horses with small VSDs have raced or competed in other athletic disciplines, one may argue that defects of this degree may reduce athletic potential (4). Pulsed-wave Doppler echocardiography can be used to document the presence and relative location of VSDs that may be too small to visualize easily with two-dimensional echocardiography.

Small, hemodynamically insignificant VSDs do not cause cardiac chamber dilation. Large defects typically result in left atrial and left ventricular dilation. Very large defects, some so severe that the ventricles act as a single chamber, or defects lower in the muscular portion of the ventricular septum generally result in right ventricular dilation.

Thorough evaluation of the remainder of the heart is warranted to ensure that no other abnormalities exist; VSDs often accompany other less common congenital defects. Careful auscultation of the heart for the presence of a diastolic murmur of aortic regurgitation and careful echocardiographic evaluation of the aortic valve for prolapse of the right coronary cusp into the septal defect during diastole should be undertaken because this additional problem may adversely affect the long-term prognosis.

Tetralogy of Fallot

Tetralogy of Fallot is the second most common congenital cardiac defect reported in the horse and is characterized by a VSD accompanied by pulmonic stenosis. The severity of the clinical signs and longevity are based on the size of the VSD and the degree of pulmonic stenosis, which determine the degree of right-to-left shunting. The other components of the tetralogy (hypertrophy of the right ventricle and overriding of the aorta) are essentially secondary. Occasionally, a patent ductus arteriosus may also be present (pentalogy of Fallot). Careful study of the pulmonary artery and pulmonic valve assists in the differentiation of this defect from *pseudotruncus arteriosus* (hypoplastic pulmonary artery) and *truncus arteriosus* (in which a single large vessel arises from both the left and right ventricles, which communicate through a VSD; Fig. 28.8).

Tricuspid Atresia

Tricuspid atresia is characterized by the absence of a tricuspid valve, with no communication between right atrium

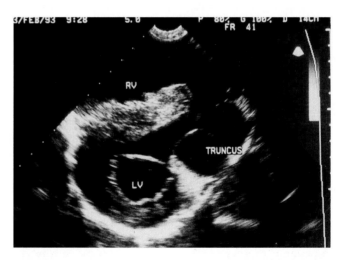

Figure 28.8. Truncus arteriosus (TRUNCUS) in a 2-week-old foal with a load murmur and cyanosis. Right-sided, slightly oblique cross-sectional view at the mitral valve level. LV = left ventricle; RV = right ventricle. Reprinted with permission from Bernard WV, Reimer JM. Examination of the foal. Vet Clin North Am Equine Pract 1994;10: 37–66.

and right ventricle. Two-dimensional echocardiography reveals a thick band of echoes at the level of the tricuspid valve. A large atrial septal defect is also present. A VSD (or patent ductus arteriosus in horses with only a rudimentary right ventricle and pulmonary atresia) must also be present.

Transposition of the Great Arteries

Transposition of the great arteries , a defect in which the aorta arises from the right ventricle and the pulmonary artery from the left ventricle, is characterized sonographically by the image of the great arteries arising in parallel from the ventricles, rather than in the normal spiral fashion. A VSD, atrial septal defect, or patent ductus arteriosus must be present for the animal to be alive.

Many other congenital cardiac diseases have been reported in the foal, including hypoplastic left heart, double-outlet right ventricle, complete atrioventricular canal (endocardial cushion) defect, and single ventricle. When an unusual cardiac defect is encountered, a systematic approach to the echocardiogram is invaluable. Each chamber and valve should be identified, and all the venous and arterial connections should be evaluated as thoroughly as possible.

Patent Ductus Arteriosus

Patent ductus arteriosus as a true isolated congenital defect is extremely rare in the horse. Some neonatal foals have patent ductus arteriosus until they are several days of age. Physical examination reveals a continuous machinery murmur over the heart base, which may be accompanied by a precordial thrill, and bounding arterial pulses. Although the ductus arteriosus normally cannot be imaged with two-dimensional sonography, Doppler echocardiography can be used to demonstrate turbulent flow in the pulmonary artery

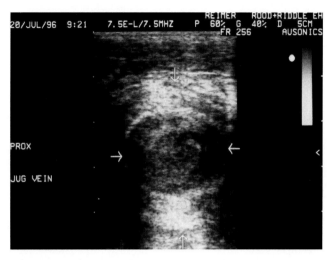

Figure 28.10. Cross-sectional view of jugular vein thrombophlebitis. The wall of the vein is delineated by *vertical arrows,* and the lumen of the vein by *horizontal arrows.* Notice thickening of the wall of the vessel as well as the slightly heterogeneous echogenicity of the thrombus.

in foals with left-to-right shunts. In foals with severe pulmonary hypertension (which may occur in complex congenital heart disease, severe sepsis, or severe pneumonia) and patent ductus arteriosus, pressures between the aorta and pulmonary artery are nearly equal in these cases, a murmur is absent, and Doppler echography is of no aid in documenting right-to-left flow.

Reversion to Fetal Circulation

Reversion to fetal circulation may occur in neonatal foals before fibrosis of the foramen ovale or ductus arteriosus has occurred. If pulmonary hypertension develops before anatomic closure of these structures, these shunts may reopen, and right-to-left shunting, as it occurs in the fetus, may result. Pulmonary hypertension may potentially be a result of severe lung disease (pneumonia, immature lungs) or of septicemia or endotoxemia.

Diagnosis of reversion to fetal circulation can be made easily by bubble study. Agitated saline or the patient's blood is injected rapidly intravenously. If bubbles are identified in the left side of the heart, a right-to-left shunt exists (Fig. 28.9) (5). Documentation of right-to-left patent ductus arteriosus is much more difficult. A similarly performed study with evaluation of the abdominal portion of the aorta for bubbles may be of diagnostic value.

VASCULAR DISEASES

Venous Thrombosis

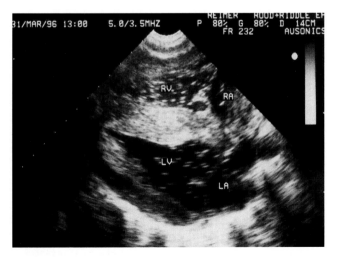

Figure 28.9. Bubble study reveals reversion to fetal circulation in a 3-day-old foal with severe hypoxemia and herpesvirus pneumonia. Bubbles are in all four cardiac chambers. Right-sided long axis four-chamber view. , LA = left atrium; LV = left ventricle; RA = right atrium; RV = right ventricle.

Thrombosis of the jugular vein is not an uncommon problem in the horse. Although thrombosis can be easily determined by clinical examination, sonography enables characterization of the thrombus and surrounding tissues. A sterile thrombus is usually relatively homogenous. Infected or inflamed thrombophlebitis may be characterized by a heterogeneous-appearing thrombus, by cavitation of the thrombus, or by edema of the vessel wall (Fig 28.10) (6). The presence or absence of sepsis should be supported by physical findings and laboratory data. Sonography is of additional value in determining whether swelling is due to enlargement of the vein, edema of the surrounding tissues, or perivascular infection.

Aortoiliac Thrombosis

Affected horses exhibit exercise-induced lameness of the hind limb and poor performance (7). Ejaculatory failure has also been associated with this problem in stallions (8). Results of rectal palpation of the aortic quadrifurcation may be normal in some affected horses. The diagnosis is made by transrectal sonographic evaluation of the terminal aorta and the internal and external iliac arteries using a 7.5- or 5.0-Mhz linear-array transducer. A plaque or thrombus originating from the dorsal or ventral wall may be seen in the terminal aorta. The iliac arteries may be involved to varying degrees, with or without involvement of the terminal aorta (7).

REFERENCES

1. Reef VB, Spencer P. Echocardiographic evaluation of equine aortic insufficiency. Am J Vet Res1987;48:904–909.
2. Dedrick P, Reef VB, Sweeney RW, et al. Treatment of bacterial endocarditis in a horse. J Am Vet Med Assoc 1988;193:339–342.
3. Pipers FS, Hamlin RL, Reef V, et al. Echocardiographic detection of cardiovascular lesions in the horse. J Equine Med Surg 1979; 3:68–77.
4. Reef VB. Echocardiographic findings in horses with congenital cardiac disease. Compend Contin Educ Pract Vet 1991;13:109–117.
5. Cottrill CM, O'Connor WN, Cudd T, et al. Persistence of foetal circulatory pathways in a newborn foal. Equine Vet J 1987;19: 252–255.
6. Gardner SY, Donawick WJ. Jugular vein thrombophlebitis. In: Robinson NE, ed. Current therapy in equine medicine. 3rd ed. Philadelphia: WB Saunders, 1992:406–408.
7. Reef VB, Roby KA, Richarson DW, et al. Use of ultrasonography for the detection of aortic-iliac thrombosis in horses. J Am Vet Med Assoc 1987;190:286–288.
8. McDonnell SM, Love CC, Martin BB, et al. Ejaculatory failure associated with aortic-iliac thrombosis in two stallions. J Am Vet Med Assoc 1992;200:954–957.

29. Evaluation of the Respiratory System

NORMAN W. RANTANEN

INTRODUCTION

The purpose of this paper is to show ultrasonographic examples of thoracic and pulmonary disease. Chapter 7 covered thoracic ultrasound scanning techniques, normal cross-sectional anatomy, ultrasonographic appearance of the highly reflective lung, and limitations of thoracic radiography.

As was seen in Chapter 7, the lung surface (or sound/air interface) is normally flat and smooth. Any irregularity altering the shape of the reverberation artifact is compatible with some disease process. A few, small, pleural irregularities causing gas reverberation artifacts, referred to as "comet tails," are considered to be incidental findings.

ULTRASONOGRAPHIC DIAGNOSIS OF PNEUMONIA

Small Visceral Pleural Surface Irregularities and Consolidations

The small "comet-tail" artifacts described in Chapter 7 should be few in number and confined to the ventral lung borders to be considered incidental findings. An increased number (Fig. 29.1), a mid to dorsal location (Fig. 29.2), or an increased artifact width (Fig. 29.3) is presumptive evidence of lung inflammation (1–3). Horses with exercise-induced pulmonary hemorrhage (EIPH) have these artifacts in the dorsal and caudodorsal regions (3).

If segments of lung are devoid of air, a disease process is likely. When small surface consolidations are present, reverberation artifacts originate deep to the visceral pleural surface (Fig. 29.4). The normal concentric reverberation artifact is divided by the comet tail. This is evidence of lung consolidation from any number of causes. If that portion of the lung contained air, the sound would not penetrate beyond the visceral pleural surface (3).

It is sometimes difficult to decide whether small pleural irregularities are significant in some horses, and ancillary diagnostic tests are always recommended. Clinical examination, including auscultation and percussion, however, is often inconclusive. Complete blood counts and fibrinogen levels are helpful, but may be within normal limits if pneumonia is mild or chronic. It is not possible to determine from sonography alone whether lung surface consolidations are due to, for example, bacterial or viral infection, allergy,

thrombosis, cardiac disease, granuloma, neoplasia, hemorrhage, chronic fibrosis, or fungal pneumonia. Transtracheal wash (TTW) or bronchoalveolar lavage (BAL) is often needed for definitive diagnosis (4). Response to treatment, with resolution of the "comet-tail" artifacts and small consolidations and a return to smooth lung surfaces, can help confirm the diagnosis of lung inflammation.

Medium-Sized Lung Consolidations

Medium-sized lung consolidations are very easily seen during scanning and range from one to several centimeters deep (Fig. 29.5). They are hypoechoic areas usually found along the ventral lung margins, but can be found in any surface location. They can have bizarre shapes, and the severity of the disease process usually correlates with the amount of lung consolidation (5). Clinical signs of respiratory disease and abnormal blood parameters are usually found in horses with moderate consolidation, but not always.

Large Lung Consolidations

These are very obvious, massive segments of lung consolidation, often with no pleural component. They may involve an entire lung lobe segment, allowing visualization of deeper structures not normally seen. Large lung consolidations may contain fluid-filled airways referred to as "fluid bronchograms" (6, 7) (Fig. 29.6). Fluid bronchograms indicate that the lung lobe is completely consolidated and the process has flooded the airway with exudate. If air remains in the airway, it appears as a focal gas echo within the consolidated lung lobe in cross-section and as a bright linear gas echo in long-axis scans (Fig. 29.7, A and B). Pulmonary blood vessels are normally not seen, which may be due to physiologic shunting of blood away from the diseased areas, reducing their size.

Whenever large consolidated lung lesions are found, anaerobic infection should be ruled out. This investigator, however, has examined horses, from which anaerobic organisms were isolated, that had only mild-to-moderate lung consolidation and no visible gas production. Based on this, one should not withhold treatment for anaerobic organisms if only small consolidations and effusions are found.

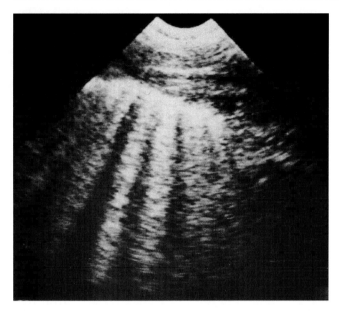

Figure 29.1. An increased number of so-called "comet tail" artifacts consistent with a broad area of pleural irregularity.

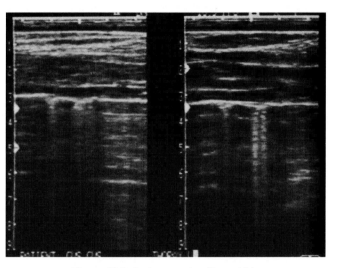

Figure 29.3. An increased artifact width.

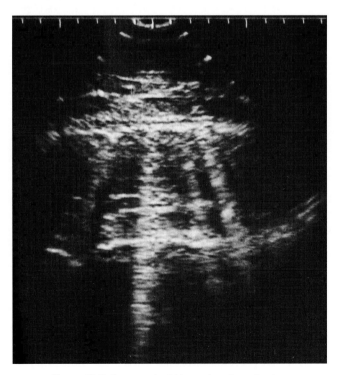

Figure 29.2. An area of mid-lung pleural roughening.

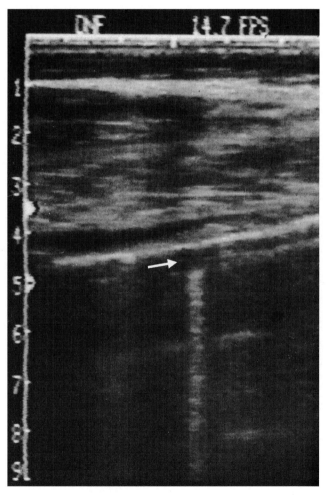

Figure 29.4. This artifact originated from several millimeters below the pleural surface (*arrow*).

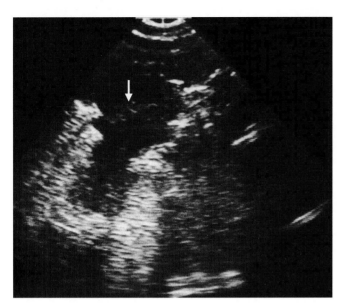

Figure 29.5. A medium-sized lung surface consolidation consistent with significant lung disease (*arrow*).

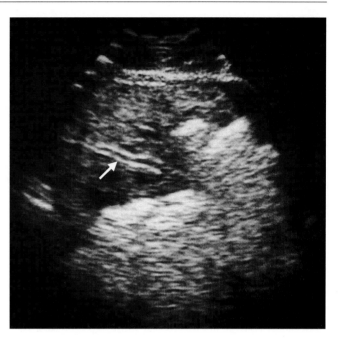

Figure 29.6. A large, consolidated, lung-lobe segment with a fluid-filled airway (*arrow*).

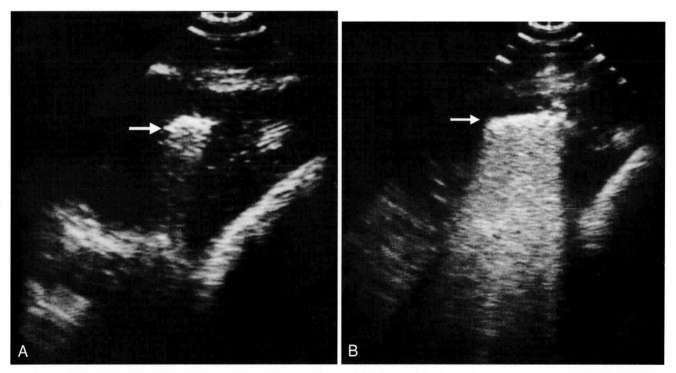

Figure 29.7. A, Cross-section of an airway containing air in a consolidated lung-lobe segment (*arrow*). **B,** The same airway seen in a longitudinal, oblique view (*arrow*).

Follow-up Examination

Whenever significant lung consolidation is found ultrasonographically, a follow-up examination to monitor its resolution is necessary, since extension from the lung into the thoracic space is a common sequel (6). Serial sonography should be performed during the treatment period to monitor drug efficacy. Follow-up examination can be delayed until several weeks posttreatment or earlier if clinical signs recur. This author has followed sites of lung consolidation that persisted longer than 6 months.

Pleuropneumonia

Pleuropneumonia is defined as pneumonia with extension into the thoracic cavity producing pleuritis and pleural effusion. It is a relatively common form of equine respiratory infection. Most, if not all, infectious pleuritis/pleural effusions are extensions of infection from the lung. There is usually some degree of lung consolidation found in most horses with pleuritis, which confirms this supposition (7–12).

Whenever pleural effusion occurs, lung margins are displaced dorsally and a relatively echolucent, fluid-filled space is seen surrounding the lung margins (Fig. 29.8). If the fluid volume is large enough, mediastinal structures are seen. Varying amounts of consolidated lung are usually found. As large fluid volumes compress the ventral lung margins, atelectasis can occur (Fig. 29.9). The lung margins are thin, whereas lung lobes with infiltrative disease may be reduced in size, but are usually not as thin.

Septic pleuritis (empyema) is essentially an abscess with its borders formed by the lungs and thoracic walls. The fluid can have a variable echogenicity and can be homogenous (echolucent) or composite (echogenic) due to inflam-

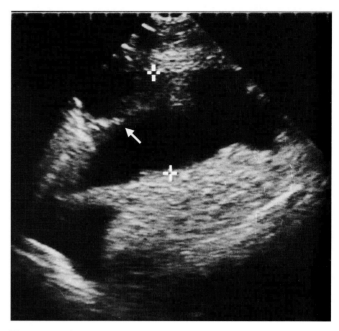

Figure 29.9. Large-volume effusions may cause atelectasis of the lung margin (*arrow*).

matory exudate and fibrin formation. Fluid in the left and right sides of the thorax can vary in amount and character. There is a predilection for the right side to be more severely involved than the left. It is common to find a relatively clear (homogeneous) fluid in the left hemithorax, surrounding the lung and outlining the so-called pericardial diaphragmatic ligament (Fig. 29.10), and composite fluid with copious fibrin formation in the right hemithorax (Fig. 29.11). The reason for this is not entirely clear. Drains are usually placed in the right hemithorax first, and the left is observed to see if it empties, often precluding puncturing both sides.

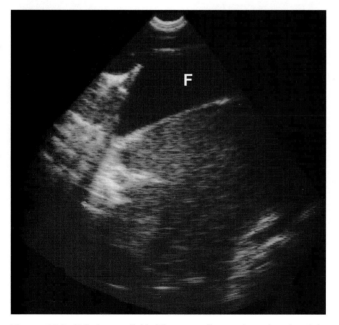

Figure 29.8. Echolucent fluid *(F)* surrounding and moving the right ventral lung margin dorsally and medially from its normal location. Dorsal is to the left.

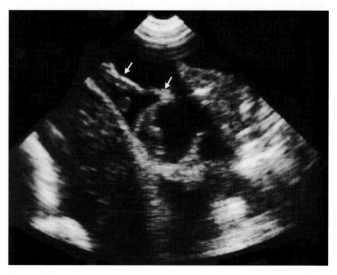

Figure 29.10. Massive, hypoechoic, left hemithorax effusion outlining the so-called "pericardial diaphragmatic ligament" (*arrows*). Dorsal is to the right.

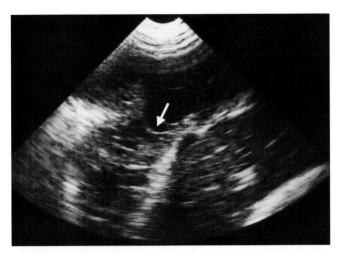

Figure 29.11. The right hemithorax of the same horse shown in Figure 29.10 with a fibrinous inflammatory response. Adhesions are present between the lung and the diaphragm (*arrow*). Dorsal is to the left.

SEQUELAE TO PLEUROPNEUMONIA

Anaerobic Infection

Echogenic air/gas bubbles suggest anaerobic infections (9) (Fig. 29.12). The bubbles are usually of uniform size and appear to be suspended in the fluid. They move with respiratory and cardiac motion. The fluid usually has a foul odor if anaerobic bacteria are present. Gas formation within copious echogenic fibrinous exudate is a serious finding allowing a guarded prognosis.

FIBRINOUS PLEURITIS

Horses with extensive fibrin production in the thorax are special cases with more unfavorable prognoses. Fluid

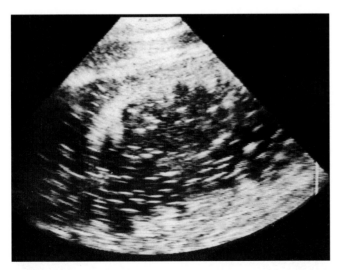

Figure 29.12. Numerous echogenic air bubbles of uniform size present in the inflammatory exudate suggest anaerobic infection. Lateral, beam-width artifact has caused an increased width of the bubbles beyond the transducer's focal zone.

trapped in mature fibrin loculations is difficult or impossible to remove via thoracentesis. Severe fibrinous responses are indications for thoracotomy, usually performed on standing horses, which facilitates drainage and lavage (13). The surgical procedure can be extensive and includes rib resection or may be simplified with a smaller intercostal incision to permit introduction of the fingers or hand. Care must be taken to monitor contralateral pneumothorax development during the procedure. This is easily done ultrasonographically (see below).

Pneumothorax

Radiography is very effective in detecting free air dorsal to the lung; however, pneumothorax is a straightforward ultrasonographic diagnosis. Free air can be easily detected by scanning the dorsal intercostal spaces in a ventral direction. If free air is present, a static gas reverberation artifact will be encountered dorsally that will resemble air-filled lung, but the surface will not glide during respiratory movements. At the ventral margin of the air bubble, where the lung touches the wall, the pleura will be seen moving during respiration. The junction of the moving lung pleura and the static gas echo is the exact ventral extent of the free air. If gliding visceral pleura can be seen extending to the most dorsal reaches of the thorax, significant pneumothorax is ruled out. This is the author's preferred method of continuous monitoring for pneumothorax during unilateral thoracotomy, because it does not interfere with the procedure and is simpler and more accurate than radiography.

Bronchopleural Fistula

In rare cases lung necrosis can be severe enough to create a bronchopleural fistula. The pulmonary parenchyma sloughs, and the airway communicates with the thoracic cavity and the environment (through the upper airway) (9).

Cranial Thoracic Abscess

Because of gravity, fluid is usually present cranial to the heart in most horses with pleural effusion. It should be monitored to ensure that it resolves with medical treatment and/or thoracentesis and does not sequester and form an abscess. Pressure from cranial thoracic abscesses can displace the heart caudally and be life threatening (14). Whenever cardiac structures are found caudal to their normal location during ultrasonography, a cranial thoracic, space occupying process should be ruled out. Figure 29.13 shows pleural effusion cranial to the heart. The mediastinum can be seen with fluid on both sides. It will "float" in the fluid and show undulant motion. Figure 29.14 shows a walled-off cranial abscess that caused caudal cardiac displacement. These need to be monitored, and some may require centesis.

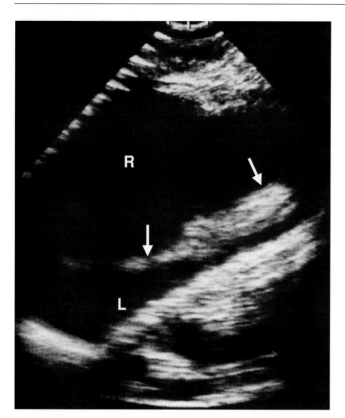

Figure 29.13. Cranial thorax ultrasound scan of fluid outlining the cranial mediastinum (*arrows*). The right side has more fluid than does the left. Dorsal is to the left. The scan head is placed cranial to the heart.

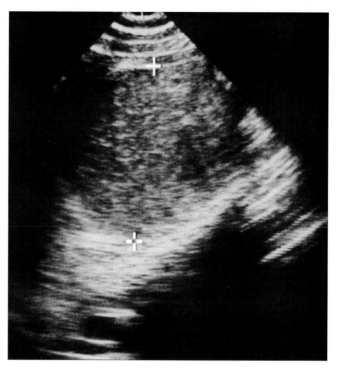

Figure 29.14. Ultrasound scan of an abscess cranial to the heart. The pus is more echogenic than the fluid shown in Figure 29.13.

Pericarditis

Infection within the pericardial sac can occur in some horses. This is an uncommon sequel to pleuropneumonia, but is a significant finding, often causing tamponade leading to cardiac failure. Pericardiocentesis can be performed to obtain exudate for culture and to reduce cardiac tamponade. A possible sequel is restrictive pericarditis caused by extensive fibrosis leading to cardiac failure.

Lung Abscesses

Pulmonary abscesses can be single or multiple and can occur anywhere in the lung (3, 9). They must extend to the lung surface to be diagnosed ultrasonographically because the sound cannot penetrate aerated lung. They are usually characterized by discrete, relatively echolucent, areas of composite fluid within well-defined borders (Fig. 29.15). They vary from less than a centimeter to several centimeters or more. Occasionally, they contain gas produced by anaerobic organisms. The gas is usually at the dorsal limit of the abscess.

It is often difficult to decide if a lung surface lesion is a consolidation due to pneumonia or an abscess. Occasionally, small airways can be seen within a consolidated lung, which may help differentiate lesions. Follow-up examinations should be done to monitor abscess shrinkage.

Horses with clinical signs that suggest an occult or deepseated abscess may require radiography or scintigraphy to confirm the diagnosis (15–17). Radiography is the most commonly used modality to evaluate the pulmonary parenchyma. Radiography does have limitations, however, if abscesses are small or if they are in sites that are superimposed over dense structures like the liver.

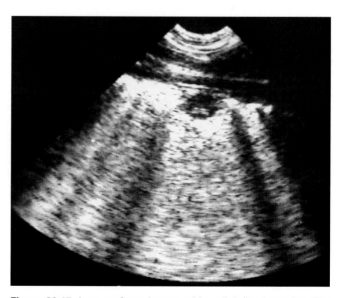

Figure 29.15. Lung surface abscess with well-defined margins. The lack of the normal, concentric, reverberation artifact is noticeable.

CARDIAC ULTRASOUND

Because the heart is in the ultrasonographic field of view and because lung disease can be secondary to cardiac disease, it should be surveyed in all horses with known or suspected lung disease, especially in foals. The reader is referred to Chapter 28 for echocardiography.

Spontaneous Echocardiographic Contrast

Mahony et al. (18) and Kearney and Mahony (19) described ultrasonographically visible, spontaneous, echocardiographic and peripheral venous contrast in horses and in man. This was found in several disease conditions in man and was more prevalent in racehorses with EIPH than in normal horses (Fig. 29.16). In horses, the contrast material consisted primarily of aggregated platelets with some white blood cell aggregation. In human volunteers, aspirin therapy reduced the degree of peripheral spontaneous contrast (19).

This author (in collaboration with Mahony and others) has successfully treated poorly performing racehorses, with a history of EIPH and with spontaneous echocardiographic contrast, with daily, low-level (4 to 8 grams), oral aspirin therapy (unpublished data). Spontaneous contrast was reduced, performance level improved, and, in many horses, the degree of EIPH decreased or stopped. This author suggests that a relationship between echocardiographic spontaneous contrast and EIPH exists. Aggregated blood components (platelets) may exacerbate pulmonary hypertension currently thought to be a major factor in EIPH (20, 21). Further evidence of an embolic phenomenon in racehorses is the occurrence of bone marrow infarcts causing osseus metaplasia in the marrow allowing radiopharmaceutical uptake (22) (Fig. 29.17).

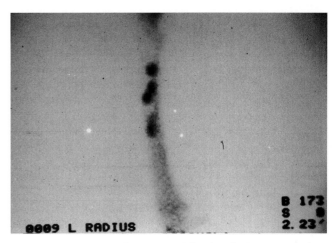

Figure 29.17. A cluster of intense, multifocal, radiopharmaceutical uptake in the central radius of a Thoroughbred racehorse consistent with bone-marrow infarcts.

Miscellaneous Causes of Pleural Effusion

Neoplasia

Thoracic and pulmonary neoplasms are rare in horses (23). Figure 29.18 shows a thoracic ultrasound scan of a thoroughbred mare with an undifferentiated carcinoma causing pleural effusion. While there are no pathognomonic signs of thoracic neoplasia, it should be suspected in horses with refractory pleural effusion. Rapid replacement of thoracic fluid post thoracentesis should arouse suspicion that an unusual diagnosis is imminent, especially if there is minimal evidence of fibrin formation and inflammation. The horse in Figure 29.18 had several apparent tissue growths in various pleural locations. These were similar in appearance on serial examinations, which would be unlikely with septic pleuritis. The importance of cytologic examination of thoracic fluid cannot be stressed enough in these situations.

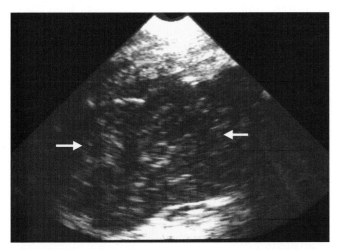

Figure 29.16. Echogenic spontaneous contrast in the right heart of a Thoroughbred racehorse. The left arrow is in the right atrium, and the right arrow is the right ventricle.

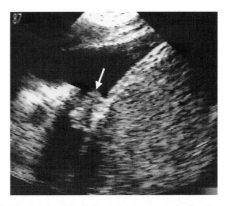

Figure 29.18. A right-sided thoracic ultrasound of a Thoroughbred broodmare with pleural effusion caused by undifferentiated carcinoma. A tumor implant is on the diaphragm surface (*arrow*). Dorsal is to the left.

Granulomatous Infection

Occasionally, horses are encountered with very large, pleural fluid volumes and minimal sonographic evidence of fibrin formation. Figure 29.19 shows a thoracic ultrasonogram of a horse with coccidioidomycosis. There was minimal respiratory distress and massive effusion that would replenish overnight. Careful examination of the lung revealed small surface lesions that proved to be granulomas. Ascites developed after admission, which was another clue that an unusual diagnosis was likely. The horse had positive serology for coccidioidomycosis, and the organism was recovered from the fluid on several occasions.

Trauma

Thoracic trauma with lung contusion and rib fracture may result in lung consolidation and pleural fluid. Rib fractures can often be palpated, radiographed or scanned with high-frequency ultrasound. Usually, there is a history or other evidence of trauma to aid in the diagnosis. Thoracocentesis is performed to confirm the presence of hemorrhage. Caution is indicated if rib fracture fragments are in close proximity to the heart.

Cardiac Failure

Horses in cardiac failure can have significant pleural or pericardial effusion, lung consolidation, or ascites. The fluid is usually hypoechoic, and little or no fibrin is produced. Other signs of cardiac disease are usually present such as auscultable murmur, increased heart rate, exercise intolerance, and respiratory difficulty. Horses with suspected heart disease should have an echocardiogram to help determine the prognosis.

CONCLUSION

Because ultrasound is an easy, efficient modality to obtain important diagnostic and prognostic information in horses with suspected respiratory disease, its use is advocated. In conjunction with conventional radiography, an accurate morphologic assessment of the lungs and thoracic cavity is possible.

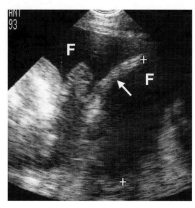

Figure 29.19. A right-sided thoracic ultrasound of a standardbred racehorse with coccidioidomycosis. Fluid effusion *(F)* is present on the pleural and peritoneal sides of the diaphragm *(arrow)*.

REFERENCES

1. Rantanen NW. Ultrasound appearance of normal lung borders and adjacent viscera in the horse. Vet Radiol 1981;22:217–219.
2. Rantanen NW. Ultrasonographic appearance of normal lung surfaces of the horse. J Equine Vet Sci 1993;13(1):621–622.
3. Rantanen NW. Thoracic ultrasound. Proceedings of the 2nd Dubai International Equine Symposium 1997; pp. 125–138.
4. Freeman K. Equine respiratory cytology. Proceedings of the 2nd Dubai International Equine Symposium 1997; pp. 107–124.
5. Rantanen NW. The diagnosis of lung consolidation in horses using linear array diagnostic ultrasound. J Equine Vet Sci 1994; 14(2):79–80.
6. Rantanen NW. Diseases of the thorax. Vet Clin North Am Equine Pract 1986;2:49–66.
7. Byars TD, Becht JL. Pleuropneumonia. Vet Clin North Am Equine Pract 1991;763–778.
8. Rantanen NW, Gage L, Paradis MR. Ultrasonography as a diagnostic aid in pleural effusion in horses. Vet Radiol 1981;22: 211–216.
9. Reef VB. Ultrasonographic evaluation. In: Beech J, ed. Equine respiratory disorders. Philadelphia: Lea & Febiger, 1991; pp. 69–88.
10. Reimer JM, Reef VB, Spencer PA. Ultrasonography as a diagnostic aid in horses with anaerobic bacterial pleuropneumonia and/or pulmonary abscessation: 27 Cases (1984–6). J Am Vet Med Assoc 1989;194:278–282.
11. Reimer JM. Diagnostic ultrasonography of the equine thorax. Compen Contin Educ Pract Vet 1990;12:1321–1327.
12. Rantanen NW. The use of linear array ultrasound in the diagnosis of pleuropneumonia in the horse. J Equine Vet Sci 1994; 14(3):139–140.
13. Grant BD. Thoracotomy. Proceedings of the 2nd Dubai International Equine Symposium 1997; pp. 419–424.
14. Byars TD, Dainis CM, Seltzer KL, Rantanen NW. Cranial thoracic masses in the horse: a sequel to pleuropneumonia. Equine Vet J (North Am Edition) 1991;23:22–24.
15. Farrow CS. Radiographic aspects of inflammatory lung disease in the horse. Vet Radiol 1981;2:7–114.
16. Sande RD, Tucker RL. Radiology of the equine lungs and thorax. Proceedings of the 2nd Dubai International Equine Symposium 1997; pp. 139-158.
17. Votion D, Lekeux P. Equine lung scintigraphy. Proceedings of the 2nd Dubai International Equine Symposium 1997; pp. 159–172.
18. Mahony C, Rantanen NW, DeMichael JA, Kincaid B. Spontaneous echocardiographic contrast in the thoroughbred: high prevalence in racehorses and a characteristic abnormality in bleeders. Equine Vet J 1992;24:129–133.
19. Kearney K, Mahony C. Effect of aspirin on spontaneous contrast in the brachial veins of normal subjects. Am J Cardiol 1995;75: 924–928.
20. West JB, Tyler WS, Birks EK, Mathieu-Costello O. Exercise-induced pulmonary hemorrhage. Proceedings of the 2nd Dubai International Equine Symposium 1997; pp. 353–368.
21. Pascoe JR. Exercise-induced pulmonary hemorrhage: a unifying concept. Proceedings of the 2nd Dubai International Equine Symposium 1997; pp. 369–378.
22. Rantanen NW, Rose J, Grisel GR, Grant BD, Cannon J, Grisel A, Rose E. Apparent bone marrow infarcts in thoroughbred racehorses. J Equine Vet Sci 1994;14:(3):126–127.
23. Robertson JL, Rooney JR. The pathology of the equine respiratory system. Proceedings of the 2nd Dubai International Equine Symposium 1997; pp. 189–240.

30. Gastrointestinal and Peritoneal Evaluation

T. DOUGLAS BYARS AND FAIRFIELD T. BAIN

INTRODUCTION

Equine abdominal ultrasound evaluation provides a noninvasive opportunity to obtain selective information regarding abnormalities without surgical exploration. The horse's abdomen can have pathology, including physical trauma, intraluminal and visceral disease, and extraluminal disorders. Acute and chronic diseases may be diagnosed that have signs ranging from colic to weight loss (1–3). Traditional physical diagnostic procedures include auscultation, rectal palpation, and gastric refluxing, along with the ancillary laboratory evaluation of blood samples and abdominal fluid. Abdominal radiography is rarely performed because of the large capacity equipment required, patient size, and the low diagnostic yield with the exceptions of enteroliths and the subjective evaluation of foal abdomens.

Equine abdominal ultrasound examination is noninvasive, economically practical, and clinically efficient and yields objective and subjective diagnostic information. Negative ultrasonographic findings are valuable in ruling out obvious lesions.

The purpose of this chapter is to encourage ultrasound use as a routine procedure in gastrointestinal diagnostics and to provide explanations of the equipment use and diagnostic interpretations.

NORMAL EQUINE ABDOMINAL ANATOMY

Equine abdominal ultrasound examination requires a basic knowledge of the normal gastrointestinal-tract anatomy relative to the respective positions within the abdominal cavity (4) (see Chapter 4). The normal position of the viscera can be divided into the expected left-sided and right-sided structures and the relationship of the liver, kidneys, and spleen. The reproductive organs, especially the gravid uterus, can cause displacement and preclude the visual ultrasound access to the viscera. The reproductive organs are presented in Chapter 6.

The abdomen may be divided into three zones or areas for ultrasound examination, which have been described as starting from the left and right paralumbar fossae and extending ventrally toward the midline. The ventral abdomen is divided into three areas along the midline from cranial to caudal (5). Visceral structures are considered to be dynamic regardless of whether they are fixed within the abdomen by mesentery. Intraluminal gas can distend and elevate the viscera, while fluid within the lumen causes it to gravitate toward the midline. Viscera that are not restrained by mesentery such as the pelvic flexure are more freely movable within the abdomen and, consequently, can twist or be displaced and may be diagnosed ultrasonographically. A complete anatomic listing of the gastrointestinal attachments and principle vascular structures are available (4).

The stomach lies just caudal to the diaphragm in the left side of the abdomen, and the left ventral and dorsal colon are located just medial and ventral to the spleen. The colon and small intestines can be located in the ventral and left side of the abdomen dorsally to the most distal portion of the paralumbar fossa. The left kidney is medial to the spleen in the nephrosplenic recess, and gas-filled bowel (colon) is not normally located above the nephrosplenic ligament. The liver and spleen can usually be found in the cranial portion of the left abdomen lateral to the midline and just caudal to the diaphragm. The liver is adjacent and usually lateral, but occasionally medial, to the spleen.

The right side of the abdomen contains the right ventral and dorsal portions of the large colon, the cecum, and the duodenum, which traverses along the right side of the greater mesentery. The right kidney is located within the retroperitoneal space cranial to the paralumbar fossa and ventral to the vertebral transverse spinous processes. The right kidney is more cranial within the abdominal cavity than the left kidney and nearer the surface. Figures 30.1 and 30.2 are diagrams of the left and right abdominal viscera and organs with the paralumbar fossas outlined as an area of reference. Figure 30.3 is the dorsal view.

Foal anatomy is undifferentiated from the adult with the exceptions of a relatively greater ease of penetration and viewing area due to the smaller patient size (3). Umbilical abscesses, unique to the foal, may present within the abdomen and do not resemble viscera (see Chapter 35).

Broodmare anatomy is altered by the "space-occupying mass" of the gravid uterus within the abdomen, which varies with the gestational age. The viscera can be displaced cranially and/or dorsally.

ULTRASOUND TECHNIQUE

Clipping the hair is not necessary for abdominal ultrasound examination. The ventral and lateral abdominal surfaces can be moistened with isopropyl alcohol applied liberally with a sponge. Aqueous ultrasound gel can be secondarily applied if desired (5). The examiner should apply the alcohol carefully and not splash it onto the legs or allow it to

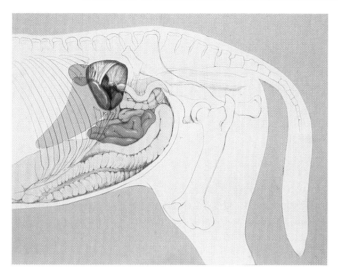

Figure 30.1. A diagram of the left abdomen with the spleen, left kidney, and paralumbar fossa darkened. (Courtesy of D. Biesel, University of Georgia, Athens, GA)

run down the hind limbs. Horses will often be aggravated by the sensation of the alcohol on the limbs and will stamp or move during the examination process. Alcohol with a saturated sponge kept in a closed plastic container is warmer and less noxious to the horse or ultrasonographer. Sector, linear, or convex-array and annular-array scanheads can be used. Depth of penetration dictates the ideal frequency for the examination. The soundbeam will be impeded by the presence of gas-filled bowel or air, which, when peripherally positioned, will prevent imaging deeper abdominal structures.

The stomach is seen as a large, curved, gas-filled structure on the left, caudal to the liver and medial to the diaphragm and spleen. The observation window is best approximately one-third to halfway up on the lateral side of the abdomen.

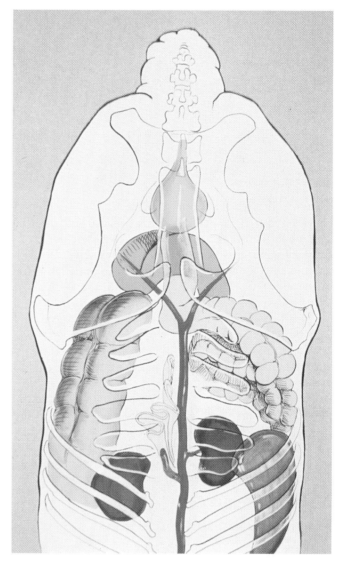

Figure 30.3. A dorsal abdominal view with the relationships of the spleen and right and left kidneys. (Courtesy of D. Biesel, University of Georgia, Athens, GA)

The viscera are dynamic and peristalsis can be observed ultrasonographically. Peristalsis is observed as rhythmic intestinal wall contractions and is more apparent in the small intestines. The small intestinal loops can usually be examined in either cross-section (transverse) or longitudinally by rotating the scanhead 90°. The small intestine most often contains ingesta, which may be observed as propulsive. The only fixed, small intestine segments are the duodenum and duodenal-jejunal flexure on the right side, medial to the right liver lobe and ventral to the right kidney, respectively. The small-intestinal walls vary only slightly in thickness and are smooth without bands or haustra along the serosal surfaces. Care must be taken that tangential planes across bowel walls are not used for measurements. Transverse examination usually reveals the luminal walls to be relatively flaccid

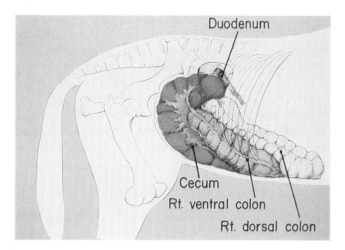

Duodenum

Cecum

Rt. ventral colon

Rt. dorsal colon

Figure 30.2. A diagram of the right abdomen. (Courtesy of D. Biesel, University of Georgia, Athens, GA)

and to partially collapse during peristalsis. The small-intestinal loops usually contact each other or other abdominal viscera and organs. The outer serosal surface is smooth compared with the large colon.

The large colon does not lend itself to either transverse or longitudinal examinations due to the large luminal size and the presence of gas. A thorough evaluation of the near wall, which is slightly thicker and coarser than the smoother, small-intestinal walls, can be made. Haustra appear as depressions or grooves and the taenia are not normally discernible. The large colon less frequently exhibits the peristaltic motion seen with the small intestines, and the most peripheral walls usually occupy the majority of the abdomen, either in contact with the peritoneal surface or apposing the spleen, liver, and diaphragm. The mesenteric attachments are medial and are not seen.

The cecum, a portion of the large intestines, is fixed at its base on the right side in a medial to dorsal direction. The base of the cecum is a thinner-walled, gas-filled structure found along the right paralumbar fossa extending in a ventral direction in conjunction with the large colon.

The small colon is not seen due to its caudal position, medial to the large colon. If transrectal ultrasound is performed, the small colon may be identified by the presence of firm, intraluminal fecal balls. The distal portion is continuous with the rectal antrum and the rectum extending to the retroperitoneal space. The muscles surrounding the pelvis and the pelvic bony surfaces can be identified around the rectum from the pelvic inlet to the anus.

The peritoneum and peritoneal space can be evaluated with ultrasound for the presence of excessive fibrin and fluid. Normal peritoneal fluid should appear as a minimal amount of echolucent (black or homogenous) fluid. The fluid can contain "strands," which are most likely portions of the omentum in the cranioventral abdomen. Excessive fluid displaces loops of bowel from their normal visceral contact and varies in its echogenicity depending on its content. Fluid may range from a homogenous transudate (or uroperitoneum) to a composite (cellular or particulate) exudate, or hemorrhage, which is seen as swirling (ground-glass), cellular waves mixed with echolucent fluid.

ULTRASOUND DIAGNOSIS OF GASTROINTESTINAL TRACT PATHOLOGY

Gastric Lesions

Ultrasound evaluation for gastric lesions is made by determining the thickness and echogenicity of its fundic wall. Gastric emptying (size) is determined by the size, shape, position, and contents (gas or fluid). Mural lesions can be neoplastic or inflammatory. The most common neoplasm is squamous cell carcinoma (Fig. 30.4), and abscesses within the wall can be found. An echogenic, fluid-filled, distended stomach can frequently be observed in septic refluxing neonates and in diseases (proximal enteritis) or colics (6).

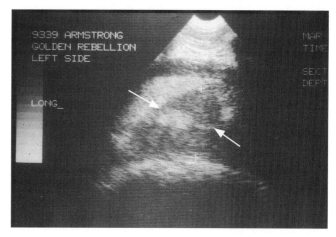

Figure 30.4. Left lateral abdominal ultrasound of a horse with stomach-wall thickening caused by squamous cell carcinoma. Tumor *(arrows)*; spleen *(S)*; stomach gas *(ST)*. (Courtesy of N. W. Rantanen, Fallbrook, CA)

Ventral splenic displacement and increased contact area of the stomach ventral to the lung margin, against the diaphragm, are the significant findings (Fig. 30.5).

Enteritis

Inflammation of the bowel usually results in mural thickening caused by either vascular stasis, edema formation, or cellular infiltrates (1, 6). The small or large intestines often contain excessive fluid. Diarrhea can be observed as ingesta

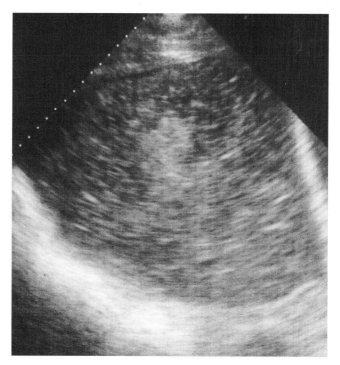

Figure 30.5. A grossly distended stomach of a horse with colic and gastric reflux. The spleen is displaced ventrally out of the field of view allowing greater stomach contact with the diaphragm.

with echodense particulate fluid, which may "layer" with the more echolucent fluid dorsal to the more particulate solid sediment (Fig. 30.6). In disorders causing gastric reflux (proximal duodenojejunitis) or severe ileus, the stomach can be profoundly enlarged in the left side in adults and more ventrally in neonates (Fig. 30.5). The bowel loops may have fluid-filled and gas-filled segments and, commonly, are hypomotile. Loops of bowel may be moderately distended, but are rarely turgid unless either a surgical lesion or absolute ileus is present. The small-intestinal walls can be flaccid and assume a triangular lumen during peristalsis as opposed to tight, rounded segments of intestine consistent with strangulation and/or obstruction (Fig. 30.7). The intestines are usually in contact with each other unless displaced by excessive peritoneal fluid.

Strangulation/Obstruction

Strangulation/obstruction lesions of the small and large intestines are seen with volvulus, torsion, entrapment (e.g., through the epiploic foramen), hernia, mesenteric rent, or incarcerating lesions such as adhesions or lipomas. The intestinal walls may be thickened, and, especially with the small intestine, distention can appear as excessively turgid and static, suggesting "trapped" bowel (2, 6) (Fig. 30.8). Turgid, gas-filled, small-intestinal loops may be in the dorsal abdomen and may not be seen due to the midline position and impedance from the large colon. The above findings correlated with the clinical signs are important when deciding to surgically intervene and are more relevant in young horses too small for rectal examination.

Large Colon Ultrasound

Ultrasound evaluation of the large colon does not uniformly aid in the diagnosis of lesions of the large colon responsible for colic. The size of the large colon with the extensive gas echo does not lend to a specific ultrasound diagnosis with

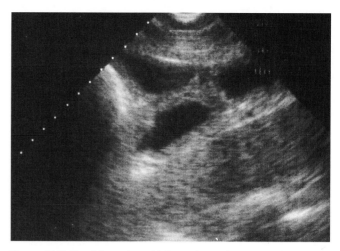

Figure 30.7. Small intestine with loss of tone forming roughly "triangular" shapes.

the exception of the more obvious displacements of nephrosplenic entrapments (7) and potentially diaphragmatic hernias. Edematous bowel or intraluminal fluid with ingesta may be interpreted as either an enteritis or potential strangulating obstruction (Fig. 30.9). Solid, nonmovable ingesta within the large colon can be consistent with an impaction when combined with the clinical signs, rectal examination, laboratory evaluation, and ancillary ultrasound evaluation.

Intussusceptions

The ultrasound diagnosis of intussusceptions has been described and is more common in foals (8, 9). The intussusceptum may be thicker and more edematous than the walls

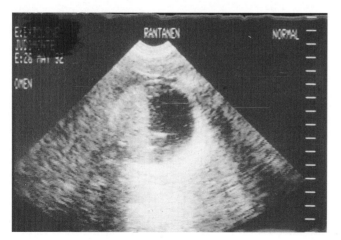

Figure 30.6. Cross-section of a small intestine with "layering" of contents. Ventral is to the left. (Courtesy of N. W. Rantanen, Fallbrook, CA)

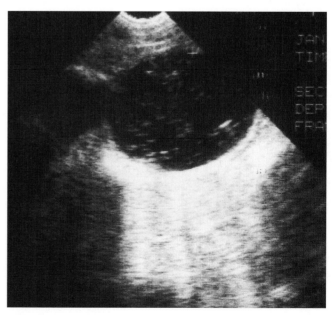

Figure 30.8. A dilated, 7.5-cm segment of small intestine caused by obstruction.

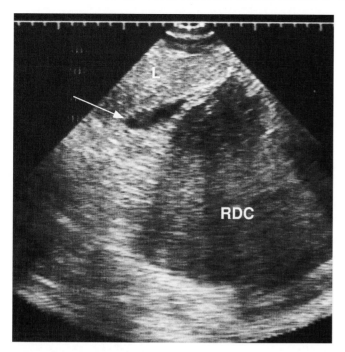

Figure 30.9. Fluid-filled large colon in a horse post colic surgery. The colon is usually gas-filled, and the luminal surface is normally not imaged. *RDC* = right dorsal colon; *L* = liver; *arrow* = duodenum. (Courtesy of N. W. Rantanen, Fallbrook, CA)

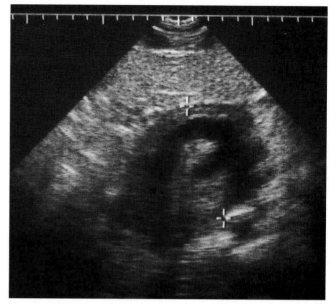

Figure 30.10. Adult horse with ileocecal intussusception. A portion of the lesion was able to be imaged and was confirmed at surgery. The presence of a gas reverberation echo is consistent with a gut lumen in this case. (Courtesy of N. W. Rantanen, Fallbrook, CA)

of the outer intussuscipiens. Fluid and ingesta can occupy the intraluminal portions of both segments of the bowel involved with the intussusception and provide for an ultrasound contrast and space to aid in the visual diagnosis. Intussusceptions should be viewed by both longitudinal and transverse ultrasound examination with the transverse view being capable of providing the characteristic "target lesion" (Chapter 35). Intussusceptions may be multiple, most frequently involving the small intestines; may include ileocecal or cecocolic lesions; and, more rarely, may involve the small colon (Fig. 30.10). Small-colon lesions would most likely require ultrasound examination per rectum rather than transabdominal.

Nephrosplenic Entrapment

Nephrosplenic entrapment is also referred to as left dorsal displacement of the large colon (LDDLC) and is seen ultrasonographically as a gas echo dorsal to the spleen, which covers a variable amount of the dorsal splenic border, or when the gas-filled colon is observed lateral to the spleen (Fig. 30.11**A**). Nonvisualization of the left kidney is commonly seen with entrapment. Transabdominal ultrasound is further utilized to monitor nonsurgical correction of the displacement by a rolling procedure (7) (Fig. 30.11**B**).

Abdominal Abscessation

Contained infections within the abdomen can arise as acquired mesenteric lymph node abscesses, walled-off extralu-

minal abscesses, and mural abscessation of the visceral walls. The ultrasonic appearance of abscessation will present as space-occupying masses that may be densely organized and contain echogenic cellular particulate material and rarely have independent motion. Gas echoes and a fluid line may be contained within the abscess. The abscess can vary from a few centimeters to very large intra-abdominal masses that may compress bowel and interfere with fecal transport (Fig. 30.12). If bowel is contained within an abscess, the motion of ingesta and the outline of the visceral luminal walls will usually be apparent within a larger, nonmovable mass of adhered or pendulous tissue. Ultrasound can be further utilized to direct needle aspiration of peripheral abdominal abscesses (Chapter 38).

Extraluminal Abdominal Fluid

Peritonitis

Cellular echogenic particles in excessive fluid can be observed with ultrasound. The fluid will displace the viscera that are no longer in contact with each other or the abdominal organs. The fluid may contain fibrin strands and fibrin can frequently be seen attached to the serosal surfaces of the viscera (Fig. 30.13). Occasionally, the serosa can appear to be thickened with an echolucent line of fluid between the serosa and mucosa, or dense fibrin can be found in chronic cases (Fig 30.14). Gas echoes within the free abdominal fluid usually indicate peritonitis secondary to bowel perforation or gastric rupture.

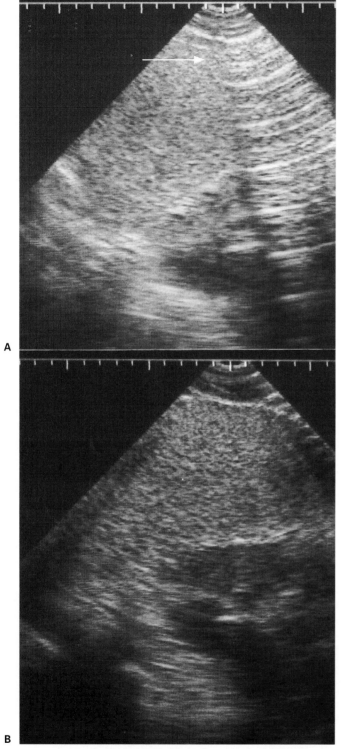

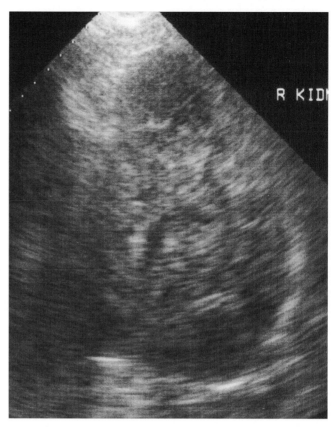

Figure 30.12. A large, 17-cm, mesenteric abscess. Note the composite appearance of the contents and partial wall visualization.

Figure 30.11. A, Gas-distended bowel *(arrow)* blocking sound to the dorsal spleen *(S)* and left kidney *(LK)* in a horse with nephrosplenic entrapment. **B,** Ultrasound of the same anatomic plane of the horse in Figure 30.11A after manipulation to reduce the nephrosplenic entrapment. The gas echoes are no longer visible. (Courtesy of N. W. Rantanen, Fallbrook, CA)

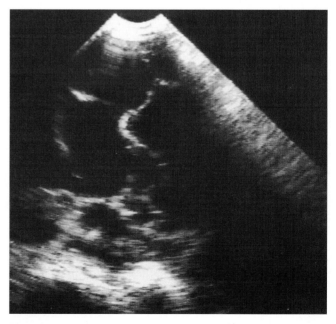

Figure 30.13. Acute peritonitis secondary to intestinal rupture with fibrin strands and composite fluid.

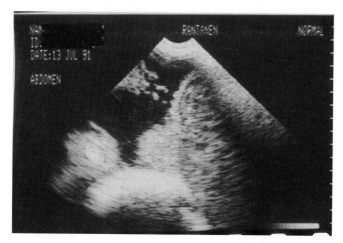

Figure 30.14. Thoroughbred broodmare with chronic peritonitis. There is composite fluid and dense fibrin formation on the serosal surfaces *(arrows)*. One colon segment was fluid-filled because of the functional ileus allowing the lumen to be imaged.

Hemoperitoneum

Acute abdominal hemorrhage usually appears as a uniformly cellular fluid with a swirling motion due to diaphragm movement. Intimate bowel contact with adjacent visceral loops of intestine and abdominal organs will be displaced by the hemorrhage depending on the volume. The cellular component is relatively homogenous with a ground-glass appearance. As the hemorrhage organizes, its appearance changes to a more coarsely echogenic pattern. Organized clots may more firmly displace the intestines, but have no independent motion and may contain channels or compartments of echolucent fluid consistent with serum (Fig. 30.15).

Uroperitoneum

Uroperitoneum can occur in foals secondary to congenital defects, tears, or septic and necrotic urogenital tract lesions. In older foals and adults the urogenital tract can be compromised by external trauma such as kicks or collisions, internal trauma such as foaling, or necrosis secondary to urolithiasis and hydronephrosis. Uroperitoneum appears as echolucent fluid displacing bowel and may have sparse particulate echoes. The omentum will often be observed as free-floating in foals and can be confused or mistaken for fibrin strands (Chapter 35).

Transudates

Transudates appear as echolucent fluid without obvious cellular content. Excessive abdominal transudate can form secondary to neoplasia, hypoproteinemia, or congestive heart failure. Whenever neoplasia is suspected, ultrasound examination should include a search for abdominal masses, abdominal organ infiltrates, and nodularity of the capsular surface of abdominal organs, the parietal peritoneum, or the diaphragm (Fig. 30.16).

Diaphragmatic Hernias

Colic can occur secondary to diaphragmatic hernias and ultrasound may provide for a definitive diagnosis. Ultrasound of the thorax can reveal viscera beyond the diaphragm and in direct contact with the lungs and heart (Fig. 30.17). Fluid or hemorrhage may also be present within either the abdominal or thoracic cavities and further provide a background contrast for identification of the misplaced abdominal organs.

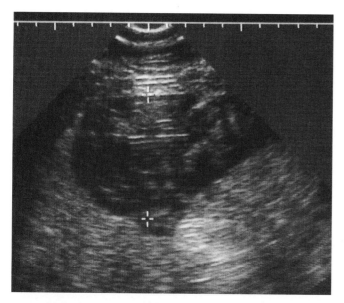

Figure 30.15. Echogenic blood in the peritoneal cavity, which may be seen to "swirl" with diaphragm motion. There are transverse reverberation artifacts arising from the abdominal wall in the center of the hemorrhage. (Courtesy of N. W. Rantanen, Fallbrook, CA)

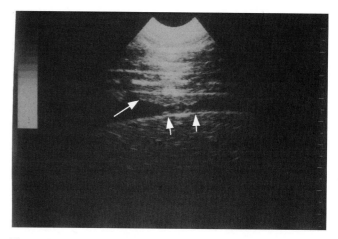

Figure 30.16. Horse with carcinomatosis secondary to gastric squamous cell carcinoma. Large arrow is pointing to tumor growth on the peritoneal surface of the diaphragm *(D)*. Small arrows are pointing at small tumor implants on the liver surface. The tumors are made more obvious because of the surrounding echolucent ascites, which is usually found with carcinomatosis. (Courtesy of N.W. Rantanen, Fallbrook, CA)

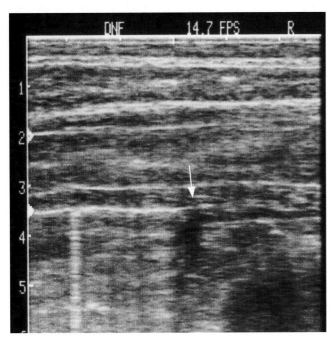

Figure 30.17. Lung *(L)* adjacent to an intestinal wall *(I)* of an adult horse with diaphragmatic hernia. The normal diaphragm image is missing from its location *(arrow)*. (Courtesy of N. W. Rantanen, Fallbrook, CA)

CONCLUSION

Ultrasound diagnostics have been described as superior to conventional diagnostics in specific lesions of the equine abdominal cavity (5) and provide real-time visual assessment of abdominal lesions and diseases in all species (10). In most cases the diagnosis is not definitive, but can explain other clinical and laboratory findings. In the age-old dilemma of seeking answers to abdominal disorders in the horse, short of invasive surgical procedures, diagnostic ultrasound provides an enormous advance in the veterinarian's approach to diagnosis and appropriate treatments.

REFERENCES

1. Rantanen NW. Diseases of the abdomen. Vet Clin North Am 1986;2(1):67–88.
2. McGladdery AJ. Ultrasonography as an aid to the diagnosis of equine colic. Equine Vet Educ 1992;4:248–251.
3. Reef VB. Diagnostic ultrasonography of the foal's abdomen. In: McKinnon AO, Voss JL, eds. Equine reproduction. Philadelphia: Lea & Febiger, 1993; pp. 1088–1094.
4. Pfeiffer CJ, MacPherson BR. Anatomy of the gastrointestinal tract and peritoneal cavity. In: White N, ed. The equine acute abdomen. Philadelphia: Lea & Febiger, 1990; pp. 2–7.
5. Klohnen A, Vachon AM, Fischer AT. Use of diagnostic ultrasonography in horses with signs of acute abdominal pain. J Am Vet Med Assoc 1996;209:1597–1601.
6. Reimer JM. Practical field uses of the ultrasound machine for evaluation of problems in the foal. AAEP 42nd Proceedings 1996; pp. 236–238.
7. Santschi EM, Slone DE, Frank WM. Use of ultrasound diagnosis of left dorsal displacement of the large colon and monitoring its non-surgical correction. Vet Surg 1993;22:281–284.
8. Bernard WV, Reef VB, Reimer JM, et al. Ultrasonographic diagnosis of small-intestinal intussusception in three foals. J Am Vet Med Assoc 1989;194:395–397.
9. McGladdery AJ. Ultrasonographic diagnosis of intussusception in foals and yearlings. AAEP 42nd Proceedings 1996; pp. 239–240.
10. Dominique G, Nyland TG, Fisher PE, Kerr LV. Ultrasonographic evaluation of gastrointestinal diseases in small animals. Vet Radiol 1990;31:3, 134–141.

31. HEPATIC EVALUATION

NORMAN W. RANTANEN AND T. DOUGLAS BYARS

INTRODUCTION

Detailed topographical and cross-sectional abdominal anatomy is presented in Chapter 4. The liver should be examined from both the right and left sides. It extends from the diaphragm to the mid to caudal abdomen. Although it can be found bilaterally, more liver mass is usually on the right where it extends ventral to the right lung angling obliquely to the right kidney. The more compact left lobe is adjacent to the spleen in the left cranial abdomen. In adult horses, transducers with 3.0-MHz (or lower) crystals should be used to scan the liver. In foals, 5.0 and, in some cases, 7.5 MHz can be used.

Liver diseases in horses can be acute or chronic and are not rare entities encountered in equine practice. The approach to each patient varies depending on the history and clinical signs. Often, liver failure can be diagnosed, but a definitive diagnosis is elusive. Antemortem diagnosis is aided by the veterinarian's ability to biopsy and culture the liver and receive microbiologic and histopathologic diagnostic support (1, 2). The results of these diagnostic procedures, however, can require 48 to 72 hours or longer. As in human medicine, ultrasonographic evaluation of the liver provides an immediate visual, although sometimes subjective, liver assessment (2, 3). The knowledge of liver size, shape, position, texture, and relationship with adjacent structures can greatly influence differential diagnoses and case management. For example, the liver may be incarcerated within the thoracic cavity secondary to a diaphragmatic hernia, or there may be characteristic changes in size and architecture compatible with a particular disease entity.

HISTORICAL INFORMATION

Many liver disease diagnoses are suspected from the patient's history and the presence of the disease in other horses. The vaccination history is important in determining whether an equine origin biologic has been used in recent months or if the patient has received or given blood or serum products (4). Diet is important in determining access to toxic plants such as those containing pyrrolizidine alkaloids, either by grazing in pastures or through feed contamination (i.e., Amsinckia, Alsike clover, Crotalaria, and Senecio plants) (5, 6). The number of affected horses, their body condition, and the rapidity of onset of clinical signs are important liver disease features. In less obvious cases, access to toxic products such as drugs, chemicals, or heavy metal (i.e., copper, iron, selenium) or parasites should be considered. Acute deaths suggest diseases such as Theiler's disease in adults and Tyzzer's disease in foals.

Individual horses that do not share common histories with other horses may have congenital defects (i.e., portal-caval shunts), neoplasms, cholelithiasis, recent external trauma (i.e., accident) or internal trauma (i.e., parturition), or idiopathic liver failure. Recurrent colics, anorexia, and weight loss are important clinical signs. Findings of portal congestion, hepatic nodularity, echogenic parenchymal densities that cast "acoustic shadows," and abdominal or thoracic cavity hemorrhage are examples of important and immediate findings that are possible with diagnostic ultrasound examination.

CLINICAL SIGNS OF LIVER DISEASE

The immediate complaints of liver failure may include weight loss, partial or complete anorexia, behavioral changes, neurologic signs ranging from dysphagia to coma, or merely decreased performance. Physical findings may be limited to elevations in vital signs and the presence or absence of icterus. Mucous membranes can also be toxic to hyperemic (magenta colored), secondary to polycythemia. More frequent observations made in horses with liver disease include head pressing, persistent yawning, belligerence, depression, or dementia and polydipsia-polyuria to anuria in the fatty-liver syndrome. Some horses have a vasculitis, including coronary band edema, without laminitis. Photosensitization (sunburn) of the nonpigmented body surface is a frequent but inconsistent feature of liver disease, as are corneal ulcers secondary to keratitis. Liver disease can often be confused with primary neurologic insults such as dysphagia, upper respiratory stertor (6), blindness (amaurosis), circling, seizures, and coma.

DIAGNOSIS

Liver disease can be diagnosed clinically, but often requires laboratory conformation to rule out other differentials such as hemolytic diseases and icterus secondary to internal hemorrhage resorption (7). Distinct liver disease features include elevations of parenchymal liver enzymes (SGOT, sorbitol dehydrogenase [SDH], gamma GT) or the combined elevations of liver clearance enzymes (Gamma GT and alkaline phosphatase) found in biliary obstruction. The BUN can be decreased (less than 10 mg/dL) and the bilirubin increased (>2.2 mg/dL). Bilirubin increases should not be confused with anorectic icterus, which can cause transient bilirubin elevations upward to 6.0 mg/dL. Fractionation of indirect to direct bilirubin concentrations can aid in differentiating prehepatic and posthepatic disease (normal is 4:1). Glucose concentrations may be low, and hematocrits may be high.

Protein levels may be elevated with a relative decrease in albumin concentrations and increased beta globulins. Blood ammonia levels may be increased, especially in hepatic coma. Lipemia may be present, especially with fatty liver disease (8). Alpha-fetoprotein levels can indirectly support hepatic carcinoma diagnosis if significantly elevated above controls. Profound leukopenia and hypoglycemia are usually found in foals with Tyzzer's disease.

Liver function tests include dye injections (bromosulfophthalein [BSP], indocyanine green) and determinations of clearance times. The BSP dye test remains the most commonly used in clinical practice, but it has become difficult to obtain the dye or locate a laboratory to conduct the test.

Ultrasound has become an important diagnostic modality in the evaluation of suspected liver disease, but often does not allow a definitive diagnosis to be made. Transcutaneous biopsy is a more direct antemortem test to determine liver failure causes (see Chapter 38). At least 75% of the liver must be failing to function to produce clinical signs. Biopsies formerly were blindly conducted through the right T 11th to 12th intercostal space. Ultrasonographic examination, however, provides specific guidance for liver biopsy, and it is possible to target specific suspected abnormal areas within the liver lobes or to safely harvest tissue from several representative sites. Tissue samples can be cultured, as well as examined, histopathologically. Complications from liver biopsy are infrequent and include hemorrhage and peritonitis. Coagulation tests may be performed prior to biopsy, but are rarely abnormal, and normal values do not exclude the potential for hemorrhage.

TREATMENTS

Treatment of liver disease is beyond the scope of this text, but certain principles are worth mentioning. Treatment is mostly empirical except in cases with definitive diagnoses. Dietary adjustment to low protein and high energy carbohydrates are basic if the patient is eating. Vitamin B-complex supplements are indicated; however, the fat soluble vitamins, A and D, may be contraindicated since liver metabolism is disrupted and toxic levels are possible. Fluid therapy is beneficial and antibiotics are indicated in horses with suspected or known sepsis. Oral neomycin (100 mg/kg sid) is recommended in horses with liver disease to decrease gastrointestinal bacterial nitrogen contributions to ammonia production, which is associated with hepatic coma. Other treatments that may lessen hepatic coma are lactulose (150 to 200 mL tid to qid to an adult horse) and increasing the branched-chain amino acids while decreasing the aromatic amino acids.

Surgery is rarely indicated in cases of liver disease unless persistent cholelithiasis or bile duct cysts are present, or liver incarceration (i.e., diaphragmatic hernia or liver torsion) is known to exist.

PROGNOSIS

The prognosis for liver disease is guarded to unfavorable until a favorable clinical response to treatments is found and horses consistently improve. The liver is an organ with effective regenerative capabilities, and if the original insult has been relieved, the prognosis may be changed to more favorable if clinical and laboratory evaluations are consistent with functional healing.

ULTRASONOGRAPHIC APPEARANCE OF SPECIFIC DISEASES

Liver diseases may be roughly grouped into those that cause a reduction or an increase in size of the organ. Obviously, there will be some variation and overlap depending on the stage of any particular disease. Age must also be taken into account in older horses since right liver lobe atrophy causes a normal decrease in organ size and the liver may not be visible on the right. It is impossible to determine if a slight or mild increase or decrease in organ size is present unless serial examinations are done on the same patient. Moderate-to-extreme size changes are more obvious. Since there are no reported normal parameters for liver size and it is possible for the liver architecture to be sonographically normal in diseased horses, a definitive ultrasonographic diagnosis usually cannot be made without correlation with laboratory and biopsy data. Definitive diagnosis of some conditions like cholelithiasis, however, can be made.

NORMAL TO SMALL LIVER

Theiler's Disease (Serum Sickness)

Theiler's disease usually results in an acute hepatic failure in mature horses within 30 to 60 days of receiving an equine origin biologic product (e.g., tetanus antitoxin). The incidence of this problem was more frequent in years past when equine herpes type I and other equine blood origin products were more frequently used in practice. Currently, use of these products is rare, yet serum sickness is a clinical entity still encountered in practice. Recent epidemiologic surveys have suggested that 50% or less of confirmed serum sickness cases have historical documentation of receiving an equine origin biologic product suggesting that unknown causes exist for the syndrome (TJ Divers, personal communication).

The clinical signs of this liver disease are usually acute with laboratory evidence of liver failure associated with acute hepatic necrosis. Hepatic enzymes can be markedly elevated. Horses are jaundiced and often have vascular hyperemia of the mucous membranes with prominent scleral injection. Since the onset is acute, body condition is usually good.

Ultrasonography is generally associated with difficulty in finding the liver. If located, the reduced size and a relatively normal texture are the usual sonographic findings. As mentioned above, treatment is empirical. The use of corticosteroids is controversial (GP Carlson, personal communication). A favorable response to supportive treatment usually allows a favorable prognosis to be given.

Hepatic Fibrosis

Chronic liver disease can eventually progress to fibrosis of the hepatic subendothelial space and cause a reduction in liver size, although hepatomegaly may be seen. The alteration of fibrinogenesis is a change to a high-density matrix secondary to the prolonged insult (9). In horses, idiopathic fibrosis occurs, but, more commonly, chronic toxicities such as dietary sources of pyrrolizidine alkaloid plants (Amsinckia, Crotalaria, and Senecio species) occur in horses located in geographic regions where either these plants exist or contaminated hay is fed. Chronic active hepatitis, hepatosis, and cholangitis are further potential causes of liver fibrosis. In these cases, rarely is the primary cause determined since horses are usually not seen clinically until liver fibrosis is advanced.

Ultrasonographic findings can include an increased echogenicity of the liver parenchyma and a reduced liver size with rounded peripheral borders or a dense, enlarged liver (Fig. 31.1). Biopsy is used to diagnose advanced liver fibrosis. An unfavorable prognosis is usually offered with advanced fibrosis, although medicating with colchicine has been utilized to inhibit fibrosis, possibly by reducing inflammation.

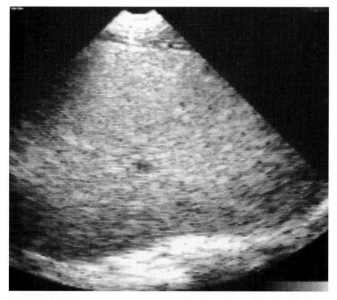

Figure 31.1. Ultrasound scan of the right liver lobe of a thoroughbred with severe hepatic fibrosis and necrosis. The liver is enlarged and more dense than normal and has a nodular appearance. (From Rantanen NW. Diseases of the liver. Vet Clin North Am Equine Pract 1986; 2:105–114. Reprinted with permission of WB Saunders.)

NORMAL TO ENLARGED LIVER

Neoplastic Diseases

Any metastatic neoplasia can potentially involve the liver and increase its size. The more commonly encountered metastatic cancers in horses include lymphosarcoma in any age group and melanomas usually seen in older gray horses. Infiltration into the hepatic parenchyma may produce solitary or multiple lesions. The tumors are rarely responsible for liver disease causing the horse's demise. Ultrasonographic characteristics have been described (10). Figure 31.2, **A** and **B**, are ultrasound scans made in two areas of the liver of a 3-year-old thoroughbred with lymphosarcoma. The tumor had developed in multiple sites in the thorax, abdomen, and diaphragm (lymphosarcomatosis). The tumor has a markedly different texture than normal liver. There was a sharp demarcation of the tumor surface. Figure 31.3 is a grossly enlarged liver in a thoroughbred broodmare with a biopsy diagnosis of malignant lymphoma. The spleen can be seen displaced medially by the massively enlarged liver.

Hepatic carcinoma is a primary liver neoplasia that causes signs of liver failure. They usually occur as multiple, diffuse, small, liver nodules. A specialized blood test for elevated alpha-fetoproteins can support the diagnosis of a primary carcinoma, but has not been shown to increase with metastatic liver tumors. The range of ages affected by hepatic carcinoma is broad, and it has been diagnosed in yearlings. The liver usually has diffusely distributed, multiple, small, echogenic nodules within the parenchyma and as subcapsular surface elevations (Fig. 31.4, **A** and **B**).

Cholangitis, Cholestasis, and Cholelithiasis

These diseases of biliary obstruction are caused by inflammation of the biliary tree (cholangitis) (11) or blockage by either singular or multiple choleliths. Cholangitis is characterized by visualization of the bile ducts normally not seen during ultrasonography (Fig. 31.5). They are seen as small, "tubular" structures uniformly distributed throughout the liver. Supportive care and antibiotics known to function in the enterohepatic cycle are the basis of therapy.

Variable-sized choleliths can be found diffusely throughout the bile ducts, or they may be few in number and large. Ultrasonographic findings include a mottled, echogenic liver parenchyma and echogenic intrabiliary densities that may or may not produce acoustic shadows (12). Some degree of hepatomegaly is usually present; however, mild-to-moderate enlargement is difficult to assess. Figure 31.6, **A** and **B,** are ultrasound scans of a thoroughbred broodmare with a massive hepatomegaly secondary to cholelithiasis producing bile duct obstruction. Mineralized and nonmineralized choleliths were found throughout the liver.

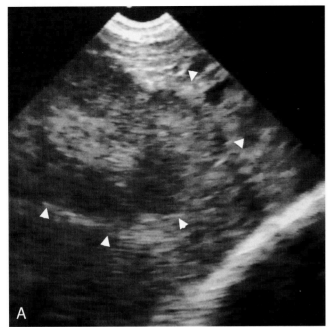

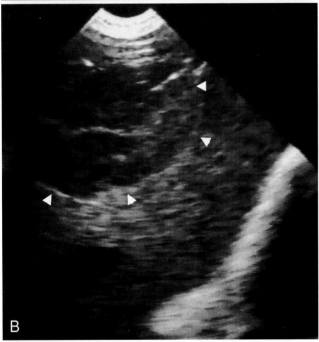

Figure 31.2. A and **B,** Ultrasound scans of the right liver lobe made at two different sites of a 3-year-old thoroughbred with lymphosarcoma *(arrows)*. There was a marked alteration in the normal liver texture. This tumor was widespread and had invaded the thorax, as well as the diaphragm and liver.

Choleliths are treated surgically if singular and near the major papilla; however, multiple choleliths causing marked hepatomegaly allow an unfavorable prognosis to be given. Cholangiocellular carcinomas of the biliary system have been described (13). Laboratory tests supporting a diagnosis of cholestasis include increased alkaline phosphatase and gamma glutamyl transferase (gamma GT) levels.

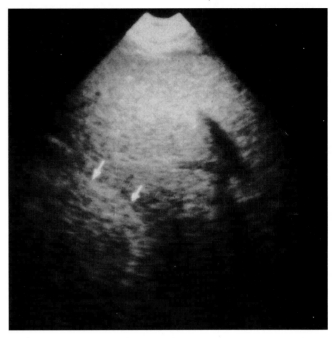

Figure 31.3. Ultrasound scan of a grossly enlarged, left liver lobe of a thoroughbred mare with malignant lymphoma. The arrows are pointing out the liver/spleen interface. (From Rantanen NW. Diseases of the liver. Vet Clin North Am Equine Pract 1986;2:105–114. Reprinted with permission of WB Saunders.)

Fatty-Liver Syndrome

The fatty-liver syndrome is most commonly observed in ponies. The disease can also occur in horses and is usually associated with a profound change in diet and metabolism. It most commonly occurs in pregnant mares and presents shortly after parturition. The clinical signs are consistent with hepatic failure. Laboratory samples reveal marked hyperlipidemia (lipemia) along with increased liver indices. If coexisting renal disease is present, this is usually seen clinically as an anuric renal crisis. The prognosis is such cases is unfavorable.

Ultrasound can be used to confirm hepatomegaly and an abnormal texture. A biopsy can be performed for definitive diagnosis; however, the predominant history and lipemia are usually sufficient for diagnosis.

Treatment is supportive, but with the addition of heparin sulfate, 40 to 80 IU/kg tid or qid, intravenous or subcutaneous, in hopes of stimulating sufficient lipase activity for lipid mobilization. The response to treatment is usually poor.

Nonneoplastic Intrahepatic Masses

Masses such as intrahepatic abscesses, hematoma/seromas, and cystic lesions of the biliary system can be found. Figure 31.7 is an ultrasound scan of a thoroughbred stallion's liver made during a search for a cause for hypertrophic osteopathy and sporadic mild colic. A 3-cm apparent bile duct en-

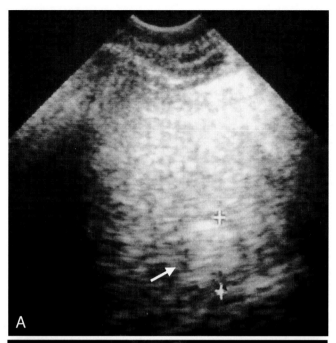

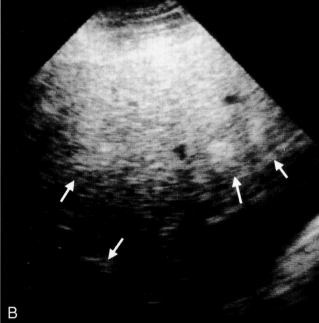

Figure 31.4. A and **B,** Two ultrasound scans of the right liver lobe showing diffuse echogenic nodules in a thoroughbred yearling with hepatic carcinoma.

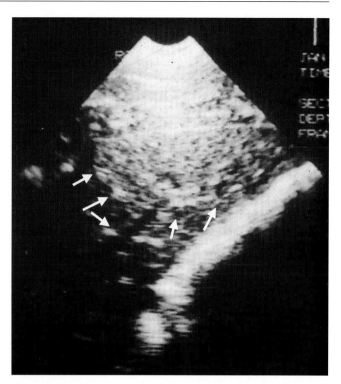

Figure 31.5. Ultrasound scan of the right liver lobe of a 3-year-old thoroughbred racehorse with cholangitis that was confirmed by biopsy. There are more "tubular" structures in the liver than normal *(arrows)*.

largement (cyst?) was found. At exploratory surgery, a large hematocyst was found in the stomach that protruded through the pylorus, periodically blocking the bile-duct orifice. This may have created the cyst. The stomach mass was removed and was thought to be the cause of the osteopathy.

Diagnostic ultrasound can be utilized to locate focal lesions and guide needles for percutaneous sampling or complete drainage. Culture and cytologic examination are rec-

ommended for aspirated samples. If lesions are large, treatment may require a celiotomy. Cystic lesions may be the result of choleliths or bile-duct blockage not visible by ultrasound examination as in the horse in Figure 31.7.

Hepatic Displacements or Entrapments

These entities are trauma associated and include intrathoracic hepatic displacement due to diaphragmatic hernia or intra-abdominal compression of the liver secondary to displacement. Liver torsion has been described (14). Figure 31.8 is a photograph of a mixed-breed mare's liver that was inadequately visualized ultrasonographically. Only a small window to the liver was found, and scans were not definitive. It is an example of severe liver compromise due to blood supply interruption. A complete necropsy was not allowed, but the liver was removed for examination through a small incision.

Tyzzer's disease

Tyzzer's disease is caused by a bacillus piliformis hepatic infection affecting foals from 9 to 22 days of age. The disease is usually peracute with some foals being found dead without known preexisting clinical signs. Foals may be stuporous, comatose, and in shock. Icterus is usually present, but may not be profound. The diagnosis is supported by confirmed cases that have occurred within an area and labo-

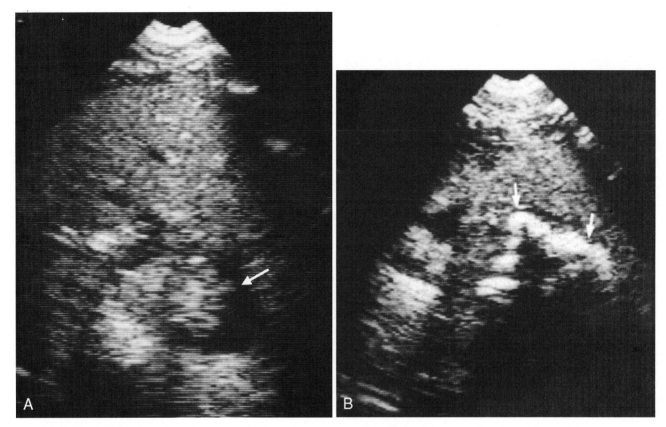

Figure 31.6. A and **B,** Ultrasound scans of a thoroughbred broodmare with clinical signs of liver failure. There are numerous dilated bile ducts with nonmineralized **(A)** *(arrow)* and mineralized choleliths producing acoustic shadowing **(B)** *(arrows).* (From Rantanen NW. Diseases of the liver. Vet Clin North Am Equine Pract 1986;2:105–114. Reprinted with permission of WB Saunders.)

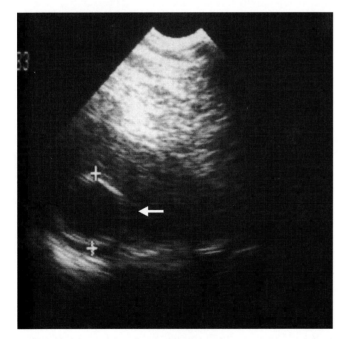

Figure 31.7. Ultrasound scan of the right liver lobe of a thoroughbred stallion showing a well-defined, 3-cm cyst. This was found during a search for a space-occupying mass causing hypertrophic osteopathy. A gastric hematocyst that was periodically occluding the bile duct orifice was eventually determined, during exploratory surgery, to be the cause of the osteopathy. The cyst was most likely secondary to the bile duct occlusion.

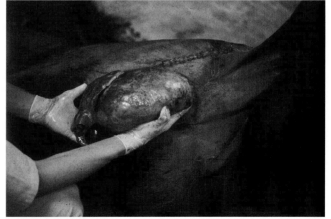

Figure 31.8. This mixed-breed mare had signs of liver failure, and only a small portion of the liver could be seen on ultrasonographic examination. The liver was very small and had rounded borders. Vascular impairment was diagnosed.

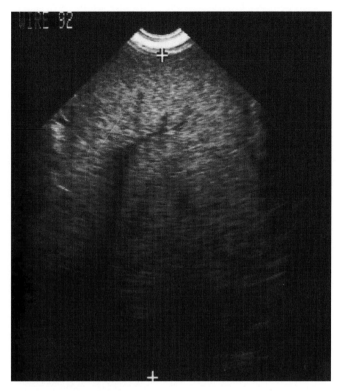

Figure 31.9. Grossly enlarged liver in a foal with Tyzzer's Disease. The liver extended caudally to the umbilical level.

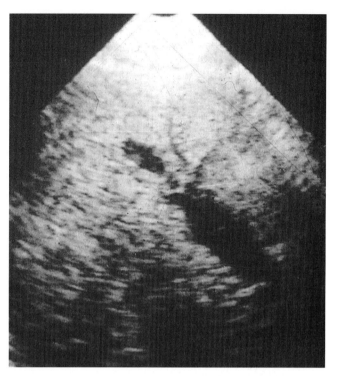

Figure 31.10. Ultrasound scan of a grossly enlarged, right liver lobe of a 2-year-old thoroughbred racehorse with a history of poor performance. The liver is grossly congested secondary to cardiac failure caused by a 3.0-cm, interventricular, septal defect. The hepatic vein is enlarged to 2.5 cm in diameter, and the smaller veins are visible, which is abnormal.

ratory evidence of severe hypoglycemia and leukopenia in the presence of hyperbilirubinemia and elevated liver enzymes.

Ultrasound can aid in the diagnosis by the presence of profound hepatomegaly. The liver will usually encompass a greater majority of the abdominal cavity (Fig. 31.9). A definitive diagnosis can be made postmortem or would require recovery of the causative organism from an antemortem liver biopsy. Biopsy may be contraindicated due to internal hemorrhage risk and the low probability of isolating the bacillus piliformis organism from cultures. Microbiologic observation of the organism within tissues requires special staining procedures.

Treatment of Tyzzer's disease should not be considered futile and requires rapid intravenous replacement of glucose, fluid therapy, and antibiotics and the prolonged use of total parenteral nutrition (TPN) made from 50% dextrose plus amino acids. Recovery can require 2 to 3 days of intensive care, but can be complete without permanent liver damage.

Hydatidosis

Hydatidosis has been considered a foreign disease entity caused by liver fluke infestation; however, it has recently been described from a horse indigenous to the United States (15). Other recent reports have been from horses with European origins (16, 17). Ultrasound examinations have not been described, although singular or multiple fluid-filled lesions would be expected to be visualized within the liver

parenchyma. Black's disease *(Clostridium novyi)* can occur in horses and may be associated with liver flukes.

Indirect Liver Disease: Congestive Heart Failure

Congestive heart failure can result in liver edema and a low-to-moderate grade of peritoneal effusion caused by hepatic capsular leakage of lymphatic fluid. In some cases the leakage may produce ascites. Ultrasonography usually reveals an enlarged liver with rounded margins and excessive peritoneal fluid. Hepatic vessels are dilated, and a hyperechoic turbulent blood flow is seen, which at times is bidirectional in some horses. Figure 31.10 is an ultrasound scan of a 2-year-old thoroughbred racehorse with a congested liver secondary to a large interventricular septal defect and cardiac failure. The liver was massive and the vessels were markedly dilated causing the smaller, more peripheral veins to be visible.

HEPATIC CALCIFICATION

Calcifications within the liver can be incidental findings. Single or multiple foci of calcification about 1 cm in diameter producing acoustic shadows are occasionally found scattered throughout the hepatic parenchyma (Fig. 31.11). Care must be taken to determine if they are small choleliths within bile ducts. If the calcifications are intraluminal, some

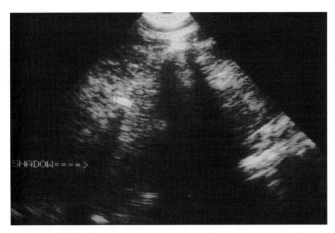

Figure 31.11. Incidental, 1-cm calcification found during routine hepatic ultrasonography. The calcification produced an acoustic shadow. A similar, but larger shadow from the rib is to the right.

evidence of hypoechoic fluid on their borders should be seen if bile stasis is present. Occasionally, echogenic foci are found that do not cast acoustic shadows and are apparently within dilated bile ducts. These are most likely inspissated bile or nonmineralized choleliths (Fig. 31.12).

Rarely, bile-duct calcification producing acoustic shadows is found (Fig. 31.13, **A** and **B**). The pattern has a similar distribution as the visible bile ducts in horses with cholangitis (see Fig. 31.5). The difference is the presence of calcification producing the shadows. This may be a result of

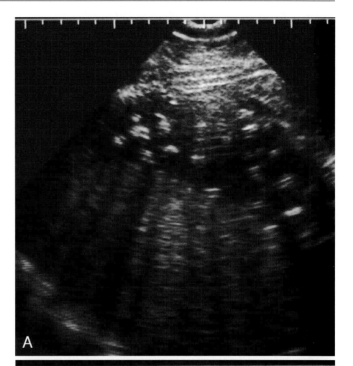

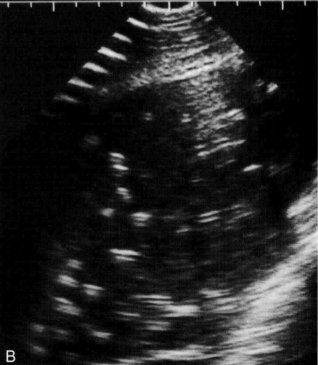

Figure 31.13. A and **B,** Ultrasound scans of the left **A,** and right **B,** liver lobes of an aged mare with echogenic bile duct walls, some of which produced acoustic shadowing through the spleen image **A.** This proved to be an incidental finding during routine examination for an infectious lesion.

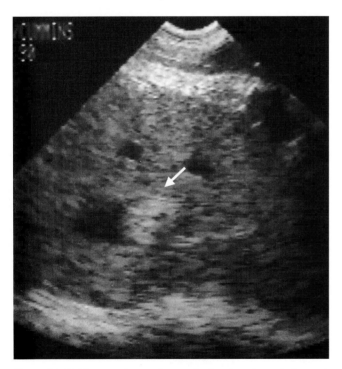

Figure 31.12. Ultrasound scan of a standardbred racehorse being evaluated for pneumonia showing an incidentally found, nonmineralized bile concretion with a dilated bile duct. It was the only one found, and no signs of liver disease were present.

chronic inflammation of the ducts. So-called "pipestem" liver in cattle is caused by liver flukes. If no clinical evidence of liver disease is present, the calcified ducts are most likely incidental findings.

CONCLUSION

Valuable diagnostic information regarding liver disease can be obtained relatively easily with standard ultrasound equipment in adult and neonatal horses. Determining the size, shape, texture, and position of the liver provides data that cannot be obtained by other noninvasive methods. The ability to safely and accurately biopsy the liver with ultrasound guidance has allowed clinicians to be more invasive in the diagnostic approach. While certain diseases have characteristic ultrasonographic appearances, many do not, and biopsies are necessary for definitive diagnoses.

REFERENCES

1. Modransky PD. Ultrasound-guided renal and hepatic biopsy techniques. Vet Clin North Am Equine Pract 1986;2:115–126.
2. Rantanen NW. Diseases of the liver. Vet Clin North Am Equine Pract 1986;2:105–114.
3. Longmaid HE, et al. Noninvasive liver imaging. New techniques and practical strategies. Seminars in ultrasound, CT-MR. 1992;13:377–398.
4. Abdelkader SV, Gudding R, Nordstoga K. Clinical chemical constituents in relation to liver amyloidosis in serum producing horses. J Comp Path 1991;105:203–211.
5. Cornick JC, Carter GK, Bridges GH. Kleingrass-associated hepatotoxicosis in horses. J Am Vet Med Assoc 1988;193:932–935.
6. Pearson EG. Liver failure attributable to pyrrolizidine alkaloid toxicosis and associated inspiratory dyspnea in ponies: three cases (1982–1988). J Am Vet Med Assoc 1991;193:1651–1654.
7. Divers TJ. Biochemical diagnosis of hepatic disease and dysfunction in the horse. Equine Pract 1993;15:15–17.
8. Watson TD, Murphy D, Love S. Equine hyperlipaemia in the United Kingdom: clinical features and blood biochemistry of 18 cases. Vet Rec 1992;131:48–51.
9. Friedman SL. The cellular basis of hepatic fibrosis. N Engl J Med 1993;328:1828–1835.
10. Chaffin MK, Schmitz DG, Brumbaugh GW, Hall DG. Ultrasonographic characteristics of splenic and hepatic lymphosarcoma in three horses. J Am Vet Med Assoc 1992;201:743–747.
11. Clabough DL, Duckett W. Septic cholangitis and peritonitis in a gelding. J Am Vet Med Assoc 1992;200:1521–1524.
12. Reef VB, Johnston JK, Divers TJ, Acland H. Ultrasonographic findings in horses with cholelithiasis: eight cases. J Am Vet Med Assoc 1990;196:1836–1840.
13. Mueller PO, et al. Antemortem diagnosis of cholangiocellular carcinoma in a horse. J Am Vet Med Assoc 1992;201:899–901.
14. Turner TA, et al. Hepatic lobe torsion as a cause of colic in a horse. Vet Surg 1993;22:301–304.
15. Miller S, Hoberg EP, Brown MA. Autochthonous echinococcosis in a horse. (In Letters to the Editor.) J Am Vet Med Assoc 1993;203:1117.
16. Binhazin AA, Harmon BG, Roberson EC, Boerner M. Hydatid disease in a horse. J Am Vet Med Assoc 1992;200:958–960.
17. Razabek GB, Giles RC, Lyon ST. Echinococcus granulosis hydatid cysts in the livers of two horses. J Vet Diagn Invest 1993;5:122–125.

32. Ultrasonographic Evaluation of the Urinary Tract

JOSIE L. TRAUB-DARGATZ AND ROBERT H. WRIGLEY

INDICATIONS

Many diagnostic techniques can be used in the evaluation of the urinary tract of the horse, including urinalysis, urine specific gravity, urine culture, sodium sulfanilate clearance, evaluation of enzymuria, calculation of fractional clearance of electrolytes, rectal palpation of the urinary bladder and left kidney, endoscopy of the urethra and urinary bladder, excretory urography, retrograde contrast study of the urethra and urinary bladder, and diagnostic ultrasonography of the urinary bladder and kidneys. In-depth discussion of the indication and interpretation of all these diagnostic tests is beyond the scope of this chapter; however, excellent reviews of this material exist (1–3). Ultrasonography has the advantage of being relatively noninvasive and allowing the imaging of both kidneys and the urinary bladder.

Kidneys

Diagnostic ultrasonography of the kidneys is recommended whenever other diagnostic tests indicate abnormal renal function, pyelonephritis, hematuria of renal origin, or abnormal size or texture of the kidneys (1). Kidney size, shape, location, and ratio of thickness of medulla to cortex can be determined with ultrasonography. For example, horses with chronic renal failure often have a history of weight loss, physical findings that rule out more common causes of weight loss, and a biochemistry panel and urinalysis consistent with azotemia with isosthenuria. The next step at our hospital is to perform renal ultrasonography. We have found ultrasonography of the kidneys to be a reliable, noninvasive method of differentiating acute from advanced chronic renal failure in the horse. Thus, diagnostic ultrasonography is an aid in developing a therapeutic plan and in determining a prognosis. Diagnostic ultrasonography can be used to guide a needle biopsy of either kidney (see Chap. 38).

Ureters

Imaging of the ureters is indicated when obstruction or enlargement of the ureters is suspected based on rectal palpation.

Urinary Bladder

Diagnostic ultrasonography of the urinary bladder is indicated when a mass is palpated in or associated with the bladder per rectum, in suspect bladder atony, or when the integrity of the bladder is in question, such as in horses with a ruptured bladder, hematuria, and stranguria.

PREPARATION OF THE PATIENT AND REQUIRED EQUIPMENT

During the examination, the horse should be restrained in stocks, preferably in a room where the light can be dimmed. The left kidney of the horse can be imaged transrectally, whereas both kidneys can be imaged percutaneously. To allow for optimal imaging, the hair in the region to be scanned should be clipped and shaved, and a coupling gel should be applied to the patient's skin and to the transducer. This gel should be cleaned from the skin at the termination of the procedure to minimize skin irritation. It may not be necessary to clip and shave most horses to evaluate the size, shape, and position of the kidneys. Although clipping and shaving the hair allow for the best image, this procedure may be impractical.

Racehorses and show horses with fine hair coats that are well groomed can often be examined without clipping and shaving the hair, thus improving acceptance of the procedure by the horse's owner. The use of isopropyl alcohol on the hair causes the coat to lie flat and thus eliminates air. (Be sure isopropyl alcohol is safe for your transducer head.) Aqueous gel can be used over the alcohol if desired; however, most abdominal scans can be performed with excellent image quality with just alcohol (NW Rantanen, personal communication). With the improvement in transducer materials, most well-groomed horses can be scanned with just aqueous gel smoothed on the hair (NW Rantanen, personal communication).

The right kidney is located under the last few ribs (fourteenth to sixteenth) ventral to the lumbar processes, generally at a level between the upper and lower margins of the tuber coxae (4). The left kidney is located in the seventeenth intercostal space or the paralumbar fossa ventral to the lumbar processes and at a level between the tuber coxae and the tuber ischii (4). Scanning of the kidneys percutaneously is best done with a real-time sector scanner with a 5-Mhz transducer for the right kidney and a lower-frequency transducer (2.5 to 3.5 Mhz) for the left kidney. In smaller horses or foals, a 5-Mhz or higher-frequency transducer (7 to 7.5 Mhz) may be used.

The left kidney and urinary bladder can be imaged through the horse's rectum. If the right kidney or ureters are enlarged, they may be imaged through the rectum in some cases. When imaging these structures through the rectum, a 5-Mhz linear-array transducer is optimal. All feces should be removed from the rectum. A water-soluble gel used as a lubricant for rectal palpation is applied to the transducer to improve contact with the rectal mucosa. The transducer is then manually positioned on the structure of interest. Any lubricant that contacts the perineum should be cleaned from the skin at the termination of the procedure to minimize irritation.

NORMAL ULTRASONOGRAPHIC APPEARANCE

Kidneys

The normal ultrasonographic appearance of the kidneys of the horse has been described by several authors (4–7). The kidney parenchyma is normally the least echogenic organ tissue in the abdomen, although older horses may have kidneys with echogenicity similar to that of the liver (4). The right kidney is located deep to the most caudal few ribs (Fig. 32.1). The left kidney is located in the seventeenth intercostal space or paralumbar fossa. The spleen often provides an acoustic window to the left kidney (Fig. 32.2). Occasionally, the kidney cannot be imaged because bowel containing gas interposes between the kidney and the body wall. When bowel interferes with the examination, repeating the examination later generally allows imaging of the kidney (6).

The renal structures that can be identified in normal horses include the renal cortex, medulla, pelvis, and interlobar vessels (5), although not all structures are simultaneously visible on all scans (6). The cortex appears as a homogeneous area of fine echoes; it is less echogenic than the adjacent retroperineal and splenic tissue and is approxi-

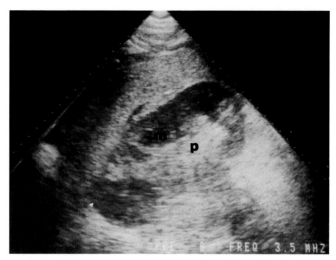

Figure 32.2. Dorsal sonogram of the left kidney made with a 3.5-Mhz sector transducer placed in the left flank just caudal to the eighteenth rib. The more superficial spleen forms an acoustic window to the deeper left kidney. The renal cortex was relatively hypoechoic to the overlying spleen. The hypoechoic medulla (m) was visualized adjacent to the hyperechoic centrally located renal pelvis (p) and sinus.

mately 2 cm thick (5) (see Fig. 32.2). The medulla is a hypoechoic or anechoic region deeper to the superficial cortex. Normally, a distinct demarcation can be detected between the cortex and the medulla. The renal pelvis can be visualized as a bright echogenic line or band in the center of the kidney (5). Interlobar vessels are apparent as small circular or linear structures evenly spaced within the medulla. The vessels have anechoic centers with echogenic walls.

Sonograms of the left kidney obtained through the rectum using a 5-Mhz or higher-frequency linear-array transducer are superior to those obtained by percutaneous scanning, although the kidney is often larger than the transducer field can encompass, and multiple scans are needed to evaluate the entire kidney. The technique is described earlier in this chapter.

Urinary Bladder

Ultrasonography of the adult horse urinary bladder is performed through the rectum as described previously. The bladder appears as a circumscribed, hyperechoic-filled structure in the pelvic area. The bladder normally contains multiple echogenic areas that represent calcium carbonate crystals and proteinaceous material (1). Horses eating alfalfa hay have more calcium carbonate crystals in the urine and thus more of this echogenic material in the bladder than those eating grass hay or pasture. The calcium carbonate crystals can be seen swirling in the bladder if mild pressure is applied to the bladder with the transducer. Normal ureters generally cannot be imaged ultrasonographically. The urinary bladder of the neonate can be imaged percutaneously as described in Chapter 5.

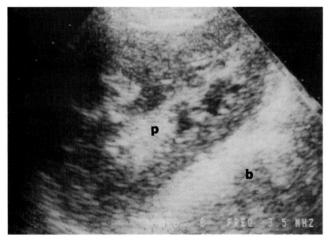

Figure 32.1. Dorsal ultrasonogram, right kidney of a normal horse. This image was obtained by placing a 3.5-Mhz sector transducer in the dorsal right seventeenth intercostal space. The centrally located hyperechoic renal pelvis (p) and sinus were visualized. Several hypoechoic medullary pyramids were surrounded by the uniform echogenicity of the cortex. Hyperechoic content of the adjacent bowel (b) is seen medial to the kidney.

ULTRASONOGRAPHICALLY IMAGED ABNORMALITIES

Kidneys

In acute renal disease, renal anatomy generally remains normal ultrasonographically, except the kidneys may appear larger than normal and less echogenic (1, 4). Perirenal edema may also be visualized ultrasonographically in some horses with acute renal failure.

Most causes or types of chronic renal failure in the horse cannot be differentiated from each other with sonography. The major ultrasonographic changes associated with most types of chronic renal failure are similar and include fibrosis or calcification in the renal parenchyma, calculi in the renal pelvis, loss of renal parenchyma resulting in kidneys that are smaller than normal, and loss of distinction between the cortex and the medulla. Thus, to define the specific type of renal disease requires a renal biopsy, and even with the benefit of histopathologic study, end-stage renal disease often appears similar despite the original cause. In many cases, renal biopsy may be academic because, if both kidneys have ultrasonographic evidence of chronic disease, the prognosis is grave and the benefit of therapy limited. Thus, the primary role of diagnostic ultrasonography of the kidneys in the horse, in our experience, is to differentiate acute from chronic renal disease, thus allowing prognostication and assistance in obtaining a renal biopsy when indicated.

Increased echogenicity to the renal parenchyma, small or irregularly shaped kidneys with poor cortical medullary differentiation, and cystic or calcific areas in the parenchyma are the ultrasonographic changes associated with chronic renal disease (1, 4, 5). Kidneys that are smaller than normal with poor cortical medullary differentiation and increased

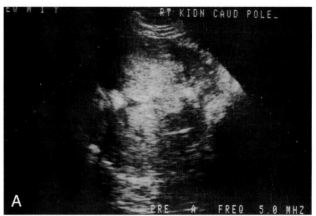

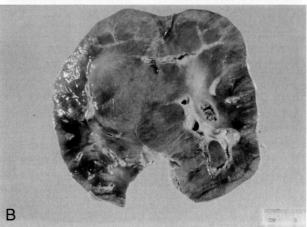

Figure 32.4. A, A 19-month-old American Saddlebred presented with a history of anorexia and lethargy. The owner had noted that the horse seemed to drink excessively. Serum biochemistry revealed markedly elevated blood urea nitrogen and creatinine levels. Ultrasonography of the right kidney showed irregular hyperechoic tissue in the area of the medulla and irregular distortion to the border of the renal cortex. A similar, although less severe, change was present in the left kidney. **B,** Cross section of right kidney at necropsy. Histology of the right kidney revealed interstitial fibrosis between dilated renal tubules and sclerotic glomeruli associated with juvenile renal dysplasia.

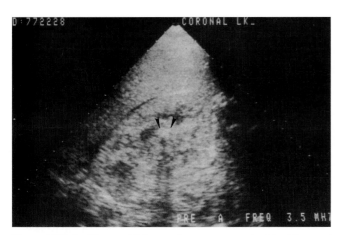

Figure 32.3. An 11-year-old Quarter horse presented with a history of weight loss. Serum biochemistry revealed elevated blood urea nitrogen and creatinine levels. Ultrasonography of the left kidney revealed the cortex to be abnormally echogenic. Differentiation of the normally hyperechoic regions of the renal sinus and pelvis also seemed to be lost. Hyperechoic foci (*arrowheads*) with incomplete far-field shadowing were also present. Histology of the kidney revealed severe chronic membranoproliferative glomerulonephritis.

parenchymal echogenicity are consistent with renal fibrosis (Fig. 32.3) (4). A kidney can be smaller than normal in horses with renal hypoplasia and dysplasia. Irregular distortion of the border of the renal cortex and irregular hyperechoic tissue in the area of the medulla were imaged in a young horse with juvenile renal dysplasia (Fig. 32.4). Bright echogenic areas with acoustic shadowing deep to these areas is consistent with renal calculi or calcification (Fig. 32.5) (5). Multiple large, circumscribed anechoic areas in the renal parenchyma represent polycystic kidney disease, which is associated with chronic renal failure in the horse (Fig. 32.6) (8). Hydronephrosis can be recognized by the presence of an enlarged hypoechoic to anechoic center of the kidney with a dilated adjacent ureter (Fig. 32.7). Renal neoplasia is uncommon in the horse, but it has been imaged ultrasonographically (5). Renal neoplasms can appear as uniform hypoechoic or hyperechoic masses, or they may

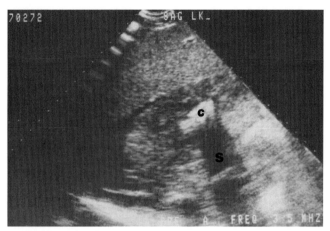

Figure 32.5. A 1-year-old Thoroughbred colt presented in a depressed and disoriented state. The colt was small for its age and thin. Serum biochemistry revealed elevated blood urea nitrogen and creatinine levels. Ultrasonogram of the left kidney revealed a small amount of surrounding free fluid. The adjacent renal cortex had a patchy hyperechoic echo pattern. In the center of the kidney, an intensely hyperechoic focus with far-field acoustic shadowing (S) was present. No sign of hydronephrosis was present. The colt continued to deteriorate and eventually became recumbent. At necropsy, the renal pelvis was filled with calculi (C) bilaterally. Histology of the kidneys revealed interstitial fibrosis, diffuse tubular dilatation, and atrophy consistent with a diagnosis of renal dysplasia.

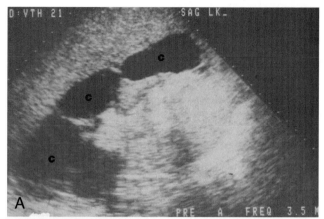

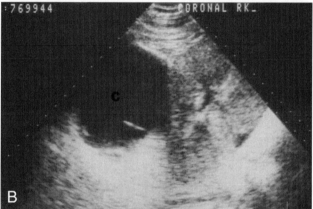

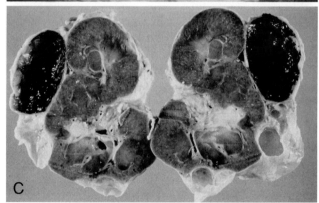

have a complex pattern secondary to areas of tumor necrosis (Fig. 32. 8) (5). Renal abscesses and hematomas tend to have irregular margins and centers that are homogeneous and hypoechoic compared with the renal parenchyma (5). Ultrasonographically guided biopsy of the kidney and associated masses is described in Chapter 38.

Urinary Bladder

Abnormalities of the urinary bladder that can be imaged ultrasonographically include cystic calculi, sludging of calcium carbonate in the ventral bladder in horses with bladder atony, and masses associated with or present in the bladder (1). Cystic calculi can generally be diagnosed by rectal palpation alone, but ultrasonography enables accurate measurement of the calculus and determination of the number of calculi. The calculus appears as a highly echogenic area in the bladder giving rise to acoustic shadowing (Fig. 32.9) (1, 9). Sludging of calcium carbonate crystals in the bladder appears as an abrupt level of amorphous echogenicity in the ventral portion of the bladder. Manipulation of the bladder generally causes the crystals to disperse into the urine. Masses within the bladder can be imaged ultrasonographically. A large hematoma was imaged in the bladder of a young foal with hematuria (Fig. 32.10). Uroperitoneum of the neonate with or without rupture of the urinary bladder can be diagnosed with the aid of ultrasonography (Fig. 32.11).

Figure 32.6. A, A 10-year-old paint horse presented with a history of weight loss. On clinical examination, the horse appeared to be normal. However, serum biochemistry revealed mildly elevated blood urea nitrogen and creatinine levels. Ultrasonography of the left kidney revealed several circumscribed anechoic cysts (c) replacing the renal cortex. The underlying medulla could not be differentiated from the hyperechoic renal sinus. **B,** Dorsal ultrasonogram of the right kidney revealed a large anechoic cyst (C) compressing the adjacent cranial renal cortex. An ultrasound-guided aspirate of the largest cyst yielded more than 400 mL of fluid. The fluid was clear and had a specific gravity of 1.006 with the occasional neutrophil, monocyte, and mast cell. The blood urea nitrogen and creatinine levels gradually increased over several months; also, the horse deteriorated clinically and was euthanized. **C,** A cross-section of the right kidney at necropsy confirmed cortical cysts and a hematoma distorting the architecture of the kidney.

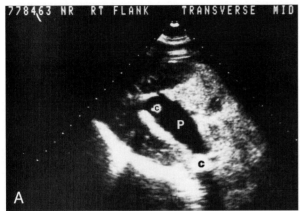

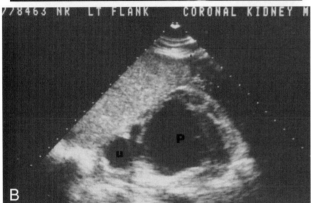

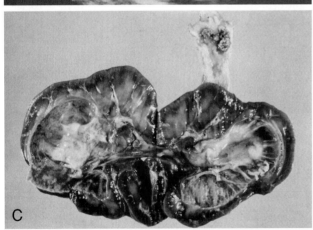

Figure 32.7. A 5-year-old quarter horse presented with a history of weight loss over the previous month. The horse was observed by the owner to be polydipsic and polyuric. Serum biochemistry revealed elevated blood urea nitrogen and creatinine levels. **A**, The ultrasonogram of the right kidney revealed a distended renal pelvis (P). A hyperechoic focus with far-field acoustic shadowing was present in the most medial aspect of the pelvis (c). A second smaller, hyperechoic focus (c) with incomplete far-field shadowing was present in the more superficial portion of the dilated renal pelvis. The ultrasonographic diagnosis was hydronephrosis resulting from multiple calculi. **B**, The ultrasonogram of the left flank revealed a normal spleen. The underlying kidney had been mostly replaced by severe dilation of the renal pelvis (P), and only a thin rim of remnant renal tissue remained. A second anechoic structure medial to the kidney was caused by a dilated ureter (u). **C**, Cross-section of the left kidney obtained after euthanasia some weeks later revealed hydronephrosis caused by a calculus lodged in the proximal ureter.

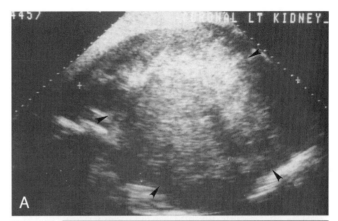

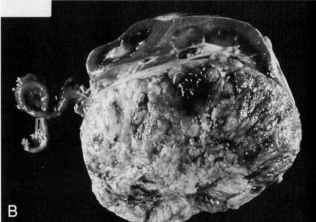

Figure 32.8. A, During a rectal examination of an 11-year-old quarter horse, a large mass was palpated in the region of the left kidney. Ultrasonography showed that a large, complex echo-patterned mass (*arrowheads*) had replaced the left kidney. **B**, The mass was too large to be removed surgically. At subsequent necropsy, the large mass was found to have replaced most of the left kidney. Histology revealed a renal adenocarcinoma.

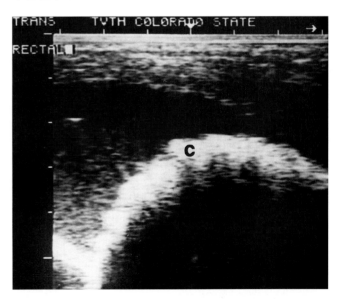

Figure 32.9. A 16-year-old castrated male quarter horse presented with a history of chronic hematuria and constant dribbling of urine. On rectal examination, a hard mass was palpable in the region of the urinary bladder. A transrectal ultrasonogram revealed a large hyperechoic calculus (C) in the urinary bladder. The calculus was removed by cystotomy.

Ureters

Transrectal and percutaneous imaging techniques have been used to confirm bilateral ureteral and renal recess dilation. In one report, a calculus was imaged in both ureters (10). All palpable calculi in the left ureter were surgically removed by ventral laparotomy to allow exteriorization of bowel with a paralumbar incision to permit access to the left ureter (10). Postoperatively, the horse failed to have improved renal function even with patency reestablished to the left ureter. Percutaneous, ultrasonographically guided nephrostomy of the right kidney was used as a diagnostic technique to assess right renal function and a possible therapeutic method for decreasing azotemia (10). Temporary percutaneous nephrostomy was reported to be an effective and practical therapeutic and diagnostic tool (10). The technique requires surgical and ultrasonographic skill and is more feasibly done on the right kidney, but it is possible on the left kidney. The horse in this report had an improvement in azotemia because of the percuta-

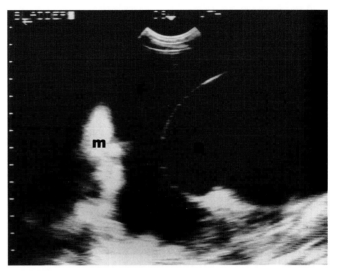

Figure 32.11. A 14-day-old foal suffered from depression and a gradually enlarging abdomen. Transabdominal ultrasonography identified anechoic free fluid in the abdomen (F) as well as outlining the mesentery (m). The urinary bladder appeared intact (B) and was easily identified because of the anechoic fluid within it and surrounding the wall. Subsequent explorative surgery revealed that the uroabdomen was caused by a rupture of the left ureter.

neous nephrostomy, but the animal died of a cecal rupture from a cecal impaction 6 days after the percutaneous nephrostomy tube was placed (10). Ultrasonography accurately detected the extent of calculi, but failed to assess renal parenchymal changes sufficiently to predict renal function in this horse (10).

REFERENCES

1. Traub-Dargatz JL, McKinnon AO. Adjunctive methods of examination of the urogenital tract. Vet Clin North Am Equine Pract 1988;4:339–358.
2. Kohn CW, Chew DJ. Laboratory diagnosis and characterization of renal disease in horses. Vet Clin North Am Equine Pract 1987;3:585–617.
3. Divers TJ. Diseases of the renal system. In: Smith BP, ed. Large animal internal medicine. St. Louis: CV Mosby, 1990:872–887.
4. Reef VB. The use of diagnostic ultrasound in the horse. Ultrasound Q 1991;9:1–35.
5. Kiper ML, Traub-Dargatz JL, Wrigley RH. Renal ultrasonography in horses. Compend Contin Educ Pract Vet 1990;12:993–999.
6. Pennick DG, Eisenberg HM, Teuscher EE, et al. Equine renal ultrasonography: normal and abnormal. Vet Radiol 1986;27:81–84.
7. Rantanen NW. Disease of the kidney. Vet Clin North Am:Eq Pract Diagnostic Ultrasound 1986;2:89–105.
8. Bertone JJ Traub-Dargatz JL Fettman, MJ. Monitoring the progression of renal failure in a horse with polycystic kidney disease: use of the reciprocal of serum creatinine concentration and sodium sulfanilate clearance half-time. J Am Vet Med Assoc 1987;191:565–568.
9. Kaneps AJ, Shires GMH, Watrous BJ. Cystic calculi in two horses. J Am Vet Med Assoc 1985;187:737–739.
10. Byars TD, Simpson JS, Divers TJ, et al. Percutaneous nephrostomy in short-term management of ureterolithiasis and renal dysfunction in a filly. J Am Vet Med Assoc 1989;195:499–501.

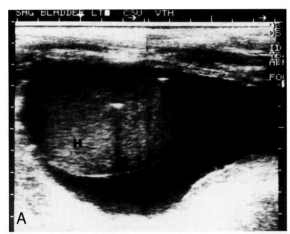

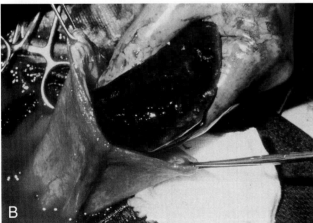

Figure 32.10. A, A 30-day-old Shire colt presented for severe hematuria. Urinalysis revealed gross hematuria and large numbers of gram-positive rod-shaped bacteria. Urine culture identified *Clostridium perfringens* and *C. sporogenes*. Transabdominal ultrasonography revealed an encapsulated hypoechoic mass (H) within the urinary bladder. The hyperechoic reverberating foci present within the mass were probably gas bubbles. **B,** Cystotomy revealed a large organized hematoma in the lumen of the urinary bladder.

33. Ultrasonic Evaluation of the Spleen

JOSIE L. TRAUB-DARGATZ AND ROBERT H. WRIGLEY

INDICATIONS

The spleen of the horse is one of the more easily imaged organs in the abdomen; however, the spleen seldom becomes diseased. Indications for ultrasonographic evaluation of the spleen include a rectally palpable mass in the spleen, abnormal contour or texture of the spleen as palpated through the rectum, suspicion of lymphosarcoma based on abdominal fluid cytologic or hematologic findings, weight loss of undetermined origin, suspected hemoperitoneum due to splenic rupture, and identification of the location of the spleen when performing an abdominocentesis.

PREPARATION OF THE PATIENT AND REQUIRED EQUIPMENT

The spleen can be imaged ultrasonographically either percutaneously or through the horse's rectum. The choice of approach for ultrasonography depends on the site of suspected disease. The multiple wide ribs of the left body wall block transmission of the ultrasound beam, so percutaneous imaging can only be performed when the transducer is located in the intercos tal spaces. Real-time sector scanners are optimal for percutaneous imaging. The transducer is moved along the intercostal space to obtain transverse images and is then turned 90° to obtain dorsal images. Linear-array transducers may also be used, but only transverse images are helpful because much of the spleen is hidden behind rib shadows if the transducer is turned from an axial orientation. However, by maintaining an intercostal location and by rocking the linear-array transducer cranially and caudally, the remaining splenic tissue deep to the ribs can be evaluated. The highest-frequency transducer with sufficient penetration to display the mesenteric surface of the spleen should be used to obtain optimum image quality (10). A 5-Mhz transducer is ideal to scan the spleen in most adult horses. A 3.5-Mhz transducer may be required to penetrate thicker spleens and may also yield excellent-quality images with percutaneous imaging. To obtain optimal percutaneous ultrasonographic images of the spleen, the hair on the left side of the horse is clipped from the left paralumbar fossa to the left seventh intercostal space, extending dorsally to the lower border of the lung and the ventral body wall (1–5). Acoustic coupling gel is applied to the patient's skin and to the transducer. This gel should be cleaned from the patient's skin at the conclusion of the procedure to avoid skin irritation. It may not be necessary to clip and shave most horses to evaluate the size, shape, and position of the spleen. Although clipping and shaving the hair allow for the best image, the procedure may be impractical.

Racehorses and show horses with fine hair coats that are well groomed can often be examined without clipping and shaving the hair, thus improving acceptance of the procedure by the horse's owner. The use of isopropyl alcohol on the hair causes the coat to lie flat and thereby eliminates air. (Be sure isopropyl alcohol is safe for your transducer head.) Aqueous gel can be used over the alcohol if desired; however, most abdominal scans can be performed with excellent image quality with just alcohol (NW Rantanen, personal communication). With the improvement in transducer materials, most well-groomed horses can be scanned with just aqueous gel smoothed on the hair (NW Rantanen, personal communication). The scan is performed by moving the transducer up and down in the intercostal spaces, beginning with the cranial spleen at the seventh intercostal space and ending in the paralumbar fossa.

The caudodorsal portion of the spleen, essentially that portion that can be palpated rectally, can be imaged through the horse's rectum. If a mass or abnormal texture or contour of the spleen can be palpated rectally, an attempt should be made to image the lesion ultrasonographically. All feces are removed from the rectum, and the horse is restrained as it would be for rectal palpation. A water-soluble lubricant used for rectal palpation is placed on the transducer to improve contact with the rectal wall. A 5-Mhz linear-array transducer provides excellent images of the spleen when used through the horse's rectum.

NORMAL ULTRASONOGRAPHIC APPEARANCE

The splenic parenchyma is the most echogenic organ tissue in the abdomen (1). The spleen has a fine, speckled echo pattern similar to that of the spleen of other domestic animals and humans (4) (Fig. 33.1). The spleen acts as an acoustic window for imaging the left kidney in the horse, and the echo intensity of the two organs can be compared (Fig. 33.2). The splenic parenchyma should normally generate more echoes than the renal cortex. Multiple splenic veins are detected in the parenchyma. The cranial edge of the spleen can be visualized just caudal to the liver in the left seventh to eighth intercostal space just above the costochondral junction (Fig. 33.3). The spleen is normally more echogenic than the liver; thus, the two parenchymal organs are distinguished by their echo pattern and by the finding that the spleen continues as a contiguous echo pattern back to the paralumbar fossa. The spleen can course from the left side of the horse across the ventral midline (4). Thus, if resistance is felt when performing an abdominocentesis and

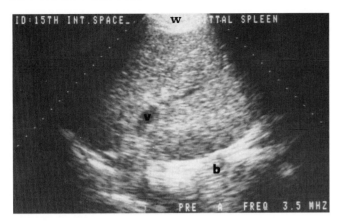

Figure 33.1. Ultrasonogram of a normal equine spleen. This scan was obtained by placing a 3.5-Mhz sector transducer at the left fifteenth intercostal space with the transducer oriented in a dorsal plane parallel to the ground. This dorsal plane was oriented cranial to the left and caudal to the right of the image. The edges of the adjacent ribs create shadowing artifacts that limit visualization of the spleen in this horse. The splenic parenchyma consisted of hypoechoic echoes compared with the brighter echoes of the overlying abdominal wall (w) and deep bowel (b). A splenic vein (v) was visualized coursing through the parenchyma toward the mesenteric border of the spleen.

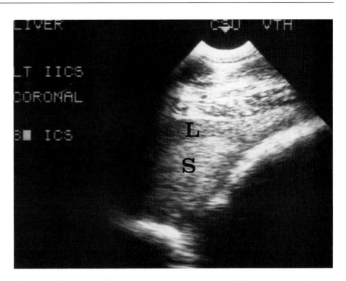

Figure 33.3. Cranial edge of the normal spleen (S) visualized adjacent to the liver (L) in the eighth intercostal space. The spleen is more echogenic than the liver.

the reason is not evident, ultrasonography of the site may reveal that the splenic capsule is the reason for the resistance, and another site should be chosen.

The size of the spleen in the horse varies, depending on the degree of splenic contraction that can be affected by multiple factors including exercise, excitement, and certain drugs. To our knowledge, the effect of such factors on the ultrasonographic appearance of the spleen in the horse has not been reported. Thus, it is difficult to make a diagnosis of splenomegaly in the horse based on ultrasonography.

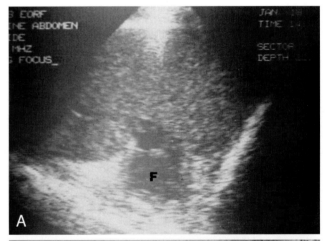

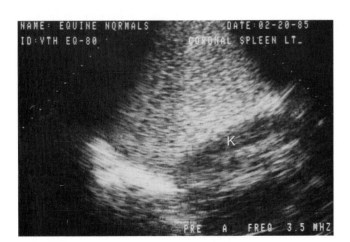

Figure 33.2. Ultrasonogram of a normal horse made in the left flank with a 3.5-Mhz transducer oriented in a dorsal plane. Normal splenic parenchyma is relatively more echogenic than the adjacent cortex of the left kidney (K).

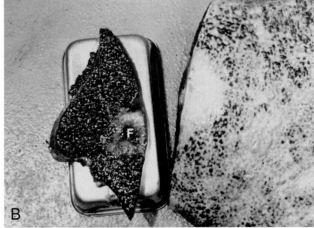

Figure 33.4. A, An 8-year-old Percheron mare presented with a history of weight loss. Splenic ultrasonography revealed hypoechoic foci throughout the spleen. On this ultrasonogram, a hypoechoic focus (F) was present in the medial aspect of the spleen. **B,** The lesions in the horse in **A** were confirmed on gross examination of the spleen at necropsy. Histology revealed focal areas of lymphosarcoma.

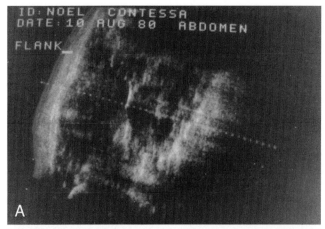

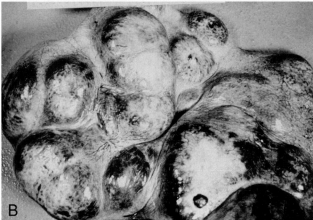

Figure 33.5. A, A 15-year-old Arabian mare was examined because of mild recurrent colic. Rectal palpation detected a large firm mass in the area of the left kidney and spleen. Ultrasonography revealed that much of the spleen had been replaced by hypoechoic to anechoic circumscribed foci. **B**, During laparotomy, in the spleen and in the mesentery mottled masses were found that had melanocytes on cytologic examination. At necropsy, focal areas of melanoma were seen protruding from the surface of the spleen.

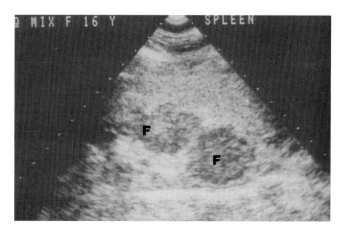

Figure 33.6. A 16-year-old mare presented with a chronic history of weight loss and distended abdomen. Abdominal sonography revealed free fluid in the abdomen and multiple hypoechoic foci (F) in the spleen. Subsequent necropsy revealed a gastric squamous cell carcinoma with widespread metastasis throughout the abdomen, including metastatic neoplasia in the spleen.

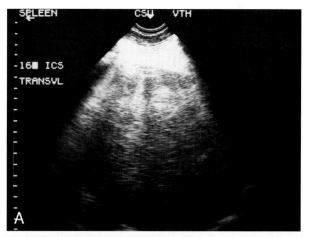

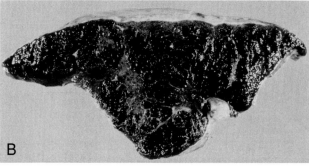

Figure 33.7. A, A 24-year-old Arabian horse presented with a history of ventral abdominal edema and mild colic. An enlarged spleen was found on rectal examination. Hematology revealed anemia, and abdominal paracentesis yielded a free flow of blood. The ultrasonogram at the sixteenth intercostal space showed that the spleen contained a heterogeneous echo pattern with hyperechoic and hypoechoic foci having ill-defined borders. **B**, At exploratory laparotomy of the horse in **A**, blood was present in the peritoneal cavity. The spleen was enlarged and distorted. At subsequent necropsy, the splenic arteries were found to be thrombosed and the cut section of the spleen showed patchy areas of intrasplenic hemorrhage and necrosis.

ABNORMAL ULTRASONOGRAPHIC APPEARANCES

The most common abnormality of the equine spleen that can be detected ultrasonographically is neoplasia. Several reports exist of ultrasonographic detection of neoplasia involving the spleen (1, 6–9). Types of neoplasia that can cause ultrasonographic alterations in the spleen include lymphosarcoma and melanoma (6–9). Lymphosarcoma of the spleen can appear as a large, poorly defined region with a complex echo pattern. Much of the mass is hypoechoic, with linear and curvilinear echogenic lines and hyperechoic reflections throughout (7), or as hypoechoic, well-marginated circular masses (7, 8) (Fig. 33.4). Metastatic neoplasia involving the spleen can appear poorly defined hypoechoic masses scattered throughout the spleen (7) (Figs. 33.5 and 33.6). In one horse presented for mild colic and thought to have an enlarged spleen based on rectal palpation, thrombosis of the splenic vessels with subsequent splenic congestion and necrosis appeared ultrasonographically as hyperechoic and hypoechoic foci throughout the spleen (Fig. 33.7). Granulomatous masses and abscesses in the spleen may be identified with ultrasonography (1). The differentiation of "mass"-like structures, such as neoplasia, granuloma, and abscess, on occasion, may be difficult with ultrasonography alone. Thus, further diagnostic procedures, including a hemogram and biochemistry profile as well as a biopsy or aspiration of the mass guided by ultrasonography or exploratory laparotomy, are indicated to confirm the disease.

Most horses with nephrosplenic entrapment can be diagnosed on transrectal palpation. However, in the few horses that cannot be adequately palpated (small horses or uncooperative horses), the absence of intestine in the nephrosplenic area ultrasonographically tends to rule out nephrosplenic entrapment (NW Rantanen, personal communication). Some examiners have found ultrasonographic examination of the nephrosplenic space a reliable means of confirming and monitoring the success or failure of rolling the horse to alleviate the entrapment nonsurgically (10). The presence or absence of gas-filled intestine is not a definitive finding, but rather, nonvisualization of the left kidney and the characteristic cutoff of most of the dorsal aspect of the spleen by the gas-filled bowel are the most reliable findings (10).

REFERENCES

1. Reef VB. The use of diagnostic ultrasound in the horse. Ultrasound Q 1991;9:1–35.
2. Rantanen NW. Diseases of the abdomen. Vet Clin North Am Equine Pract 1986;2:67–89.
3. Yamaga Y, Too K. Diagnostic ultrasound imaging in domestic animals: fundamental studies on abdominal organs and fetuses. Jpn J Vet Sci 1984;46:203–212.
4. Rantanen NW. Ultrasound appearance of normal lung borders and adjacent viscera in the horse. Vet Radiol 1981;22:217–219.
5. Byars JD, Halley J. Uses of ultrasound in equine internal medicine. Vet Clin North Am Equine Pract 1986;2:256.
6. Marr CM, Love S, Pirie HM. Clinical, ultrasonographic and pathological findings in a horse with splenic lymphosarcoma and pseudohyperparathyroidism. Equine Vet J 1989;21:221–226.
7. Chaffin MK, Schmitz DG, Brumbaugh GW, et al. Ultrasonographic characteristics of splenic and hepatic lymphosarcoma in three horses. J Am Vet Med Assoc 1992;201:743–747.
8. Traub JL, Bayly WM, Reed SM, et al. Intra-abdominal neoplasia as a cause of chronic weight loss in the horse. Compend Contin Educ Pract Vet 1983;5:S526–S536.
9. Rantanen NW. Ultrasonographic examination of the abdomen of the horse. Proc Am Assoc Equine Pract 1993;39:7–8.
10. Santschi EM, Slone DE, Frank WM II. Left dorsal displacement of large colon (LDDLC) in the Thoroughbred: diagnosis and monitoring of nonsurgical correction via ultrasound. In: Proceedings of the Fourth Equine Colic Research Symposium. Athens, GA,1991:57.

34. THORACIC EXAMINATION of the NEONATE

NORMAN W. RANTANEN

Ultrasonographic anatomy and scanning techniques peculiar to neonates were presented in Chapter 5. It is important to stress that thoracic ultrasonography can be accomplished with a minimum of effort in foals and provides important diagnostic information concerning the status of the lungs, thoracic space, and heart. Cardiology was covered in Chapters 2 and 28; however, potential cardiac disease always needs to be considered in sick foals. The purpose of this chapter is to stress the importance of diagnostic ultrasound in the diagnosis, prognosis, and management of thoracic disease in foals. All of the principles of thoracic ultrasound discussed in Chapters 3 and 29 apply to foals. The echogenic lung appears similar to the adult lung, as do the lesions that affect the lung surface and thoracic space. A major difference in the cranial thorax is the presence of the thymus, which is not normally seen in adults.

The incidence of foal pneumonia is high. In one report pneumonia was found in 39 (53%) of 74 septicemic or post-septicemic neonatal foals that died or were euthanized (1). Bones and joints and the gastrointestinal tract had the next highest lesion incidences. Therefore it is important to consider sick foals as potentially having multiple sites of infection. The lungs, heart, and umbilicus should always be ruled out as sites of infection. Any foal (or weanling) with a lameness, peripheral swelling, or fever should be suspect as having infection in one or more of those areas. The two common clinical findings in foals with bacterial endocarditis, for instance, are lameness and fever spikes (Byars TD, personal communication).

LUNG CONSOLIDATION

The normal, aerated lung in foals has a similar appearance as the adult lung (Fig. 34.1). Small comet tails and small surface consolidations are similar to those described in Chapter 29 (Fig. 34.2, **A** and **B**). As in adults, any condition that alters the lung surface or replaces air in the subpleural lung will produce a different reverberation artifact than that normally seen. Ultrasonographic findings of an altered sound/air interface of the lung are nonspecific and usually do not indicate a specific lung disease with few exceptions (e.g., Rhodococcus equi abscesses).

PLEUROPNEUMONIA

Extension of pneumonia into the thoracic space is thought to be uncommon in foals; however, in one report the age range of 153 horses with pleuropneumonia was given as 4 days to 24 years (2). It is not unusual to encounter pleural effusions in neonates that require placement of indwelling catheters (Byars TD, personal communication). Therefore ultrasonography of the thorax to rule out effusion is indicated in foals with respiratory disease. Overlooking a significant septic effusion or a sequestered cranial thoracic abscess (3), both of which can be sequelae to pleuropneumonia, might have grave consequences. Ultrasonographic findings are similar to those in older horses.

Pneumonia in Conjunction with Umbilical Infection and/or Vegetative Endocarditis

Foal pneumonia can be found in conjunction with other sites of infection. Umbilical infection, which can be occult with a normal-appearing external umbilicus, is a potential bacteremic source for other parts of the body (Chapter 35). It is commonly associated with secondary joint infection, and pneumonia will often be present.

Vegetative valvular endocarditis can affect any heart valve, but has been most commonly found on the mitral valve by this author. It is not uncommon to find some degree of concomitant pneumonia with mitral vegetation. Tricuspid vegetations almost always have "seeded" the lungs with bacterial emboli.

PULMONARY ABSCESSES

Lung abscesses can be due to a variety of organisms; however, in foals ranging from about 1 to 6 months old, *Rhodococcus equi* is a common cause. The disease can cause acute deaths or more chronic signs. Well-defined, variable-sized abscesses distributed over the lung surfaces are highly suggestive of *R. equi* infection in this age group (Fig. 34.3, **A** and **B**). Ultrasonographic examination is a valuable screening method in nurseries where Rhodococcus infection is suspected. Usually, a minimum of restraint is needed to examine foal lungs. Alcohol can be used to cause the hair to

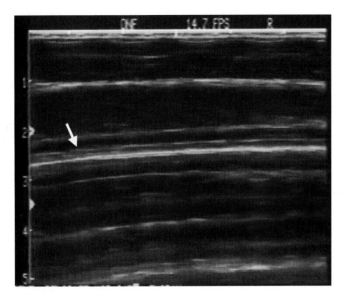

Figure 34.1. Normal 7.5-MHz ultrasonographic appearance of foal lung surface *(arrow)*. It is highly reflective as in adults, and the reverberation artifact is similar.

lie flat and clipping is not required. Both lungs, including the cranial lobes, should be carefully searched for abscesses, pleural roughening and surface consolidation. Pleural effusion is seldom seen in foals with Rhodococcus infection.

TRAUMA

Hemothorax/Pneumothorax

Foals are more susceptible to thoracic trauma than adults because of their small size. Trauma during parturition can also occur. In neonates, free thoracic fluid or air in an otherwise healthy-appearing foal, should cause suspicion of lung trauma and hemorrhage. Fractured ribs should be carefully searched for by palpation and radiographic and ultrasonographic examinations (4) (Fig. 34.4). Foals with rib fractures should be confined to reduce the possibility of lung or heart puncture. Pneumothorax can also occur as a result of mechanical ventilation and can spontaneously occur in some foals.

DIAPHRAGMATIC HERNIA

Presence of abdominal viscera in the thorax can be seen ultrasonographically as intimate contact between thoracic and abdominal viscera with no evidence of the diaphragm between them. Liver or gas-filled small or large intestine may be present in the thorax. Gas-filled viscera may cause confusing shadows initially; however, observation of peristalsis can confirm intestine in most cases. Each presentation will be peculiar to the size of the diaphragm defect and the particular viscera herniated in the thorax (Fig. 34.5). Small hernias deep to aerated lung may not be seen. In foals, especially, the ease of radiographic examination dictates that it

should be used not only for suspected diaphragmatic hernia but for any suspected thoracic or pulmonary disease. Ultrasound can provide a screening examination for diaphragmatic hernia in the field or nursery for foals and may be the only diagnostic method for adults if large-capacity radiographic equipment is not available.

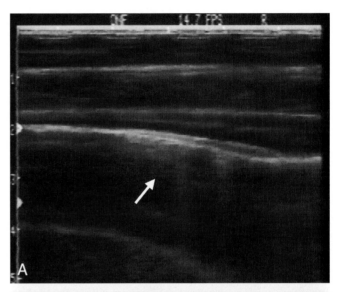

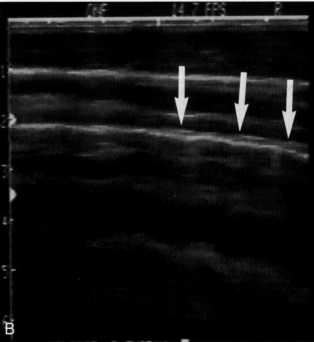

Figure 34.2 A. An area of lung inflammation producing an abnormal sound beam/air interface *(arrow)* in a quarterhorse foal with pneumonia. Vertical streaks are arising from the abnormal area. There is a slight depression in the lung surface. **B.** A subtle area of pleural roughening in a foal with a confirmed pneumonia. The change is subtle, and 7.5 MHz is required to detect this degree of change *(arrows)*.

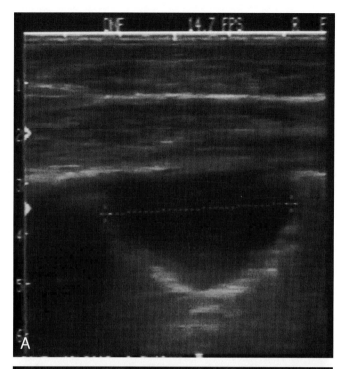

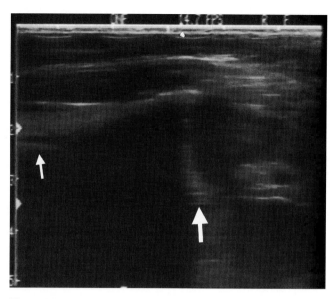

Figure 34.4. Longitudinal ultrasound scan of a foal's rib with a break in the profile of the bone *(small arrow)*. The costochondral junction can be seen *(large arrow)*.

Since ultrasonography provides different diagnostic information than radiography, it should also be routinely used in evaluation of the foal thorax. Thoracic ultrasonography can be accomplished with a minimum of patient preparation and restraint. It can provide important diagnostic information when radiography is not available and can influence treatment decisions in the field or nursery. The two modalities used together provide a thorough examination of the lungs, heart, and thoracic space. Since foals often have more than one site of infection, concomitant umbilical and cardiac ultrasound examination can add important diagnoses relative to the patient's status.

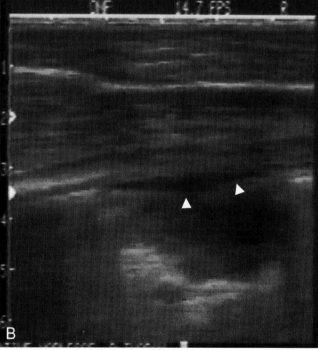

Figure 34.3 A. Ultrasonographic, 7.5-MHz image of a 3.3-cm, *Rhodococcus equi* abscess on the lung surface. **B.** Image made near the margin of the same abscess as in **A** showing a depression in the lung surface *(arrowheads)*.

CONCLUSION

Because of their small size, thoracic radiography of the foal can be performed as a routine procedure, often with portable equipment and rare-earth radiographic screens.

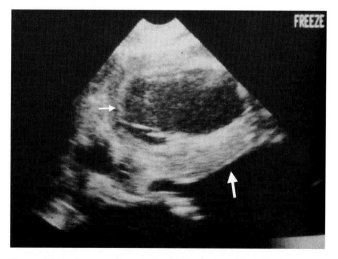

Figure 34.5. Ultrasound scan of a foal's thorax with a diaphragmatic hernia. There is a loop of small intestine *(small arrow)* adjacent to the right ventricular wall *(large arrow)*. (Image courtesy of T. D. Byars)

REFERENCES

1. Brewer BD. Neonatal infection. In: Koterba AM, Drummond WH, Kosch PC, eds. Equine clinical neonatology. Philadelphia: Lea & Febiger, 1990; pp. 295–316.
2. Byars TD, Becht JL. Pleuropneumonia. Vet Clin North Am Equine Pract 1991;7:63–78.
3. Byars TD, Dainis CM, Seltzer KL, et al. Cranial thoracic masses in the horse: a sequelae to pleuropneumonia. Equine Vet J (North Am Edition) 1991;23:22–24.
4. Bernard WV, Reimer JM. Examination of the foal. Vet Clin North Am Equine Pract 1994;10:37–66.

35. Abdominal Sonography of the Foal

JOHANNA M. REIMER AND WILLIAM V. BERNARD

The small size of the foal, combined with the preponderance and variety of abdominal diseases in the foal, makes sonography of the abdomen an invaluable diagnostic technique in these patients. Umbilical remnant infections, bladder ruptures, small intestinal diseases, and abdominal abscesses are some of the common problems encountered in the foal, and all are readily evaluated with sonography. This chapter reviews the sonographic appearances of several such abdominal disorders of the foal. Transducer selection and the appearance of normal abdominal structures are discussed and illustrated in Chapter 5.

UMBILICAL REMNANTS

Abnormalities of the umbilical remnants are readily diagnosed with ultrasonography. The most important indication for umbilical ultrasound is to determine whether infection of any of the internal umbilical structures is present. Trauma can also occur to these structures at birth. Differentiation of traumatic injuries from sonographic changes due to infection must be made as carefully as possible to avoid overtreatment or undertreatment.

Umbilical Remnant Infections

The potentially disastrous consequences of internal umbilical remnant infections make sonography of these structures an economically justifiable procedure. Internal umbilical infection may be a source of septicemia in the neonate and a potential source of septic arthritis, physitis, or osteomyelitis. Dissemination of umbilical infections can potentially occur at other sites, such as the meninges, eye, and heart valves. Abscesses can leak and even rupture, leading to peritonitis and adhesions. Uroperitoneum is an additional complication if the bladder apex is involved. Many foals may well have unrecognized umbilical infections that resolve without treatment and without untoward effects on the foal. However, in the provision of optimal patient care, the importance of umbilical ultrasonography should be realized.

Many internal umbilical infections can be treated successfully medically. Sonography provides a means to select medical versus surgical management of these cases and to monitor the response to therapy in those managed medically (1). Foals with sizable umbilical abscesses that require long-term antimicrobial agents for coincident infections may respond well to treatment, and the owner is spared the expense of surgery. Conversely, surgical excision of similar umbilical abscesses may be the more economical choice in foals that are otherwise healthy.

The most common problems prompting umbilical sonography include septicemia, septic arthritis, physitis, or osteomyelitis, other bacterial infections remote from the umbilicus, abnormal leukograms, elevated fibrinogen levels, dysuria, patent urachus, elevated temperature, thickened umbilical stump, drainage of pus from the umbilical stump, and perinavel edema (1).

Internal umbilical infections are most commonly recognized in foals under 2 months of age (2), although an internal umbilical remnant infection was not discovered in one case until the foal was 16 months of age (3). Review of internal umbilical infections diagnosed by our ultrasound service over a 2-year period revealed palpable abnormalities of the stump at the time of the sonogram in only 30% of those foals with internal umbilical abscesses (1), a finding similar to that reported by others (4). Any history of drainage from the umbilical stump is highly indicative of internal umbilical abscessation, even if the external umbilicus is normal at the time of sonographic evaluation. Of foals with internal umbilical infections diagnosed by our service, only 25% had a history of pyrexia, and only 30% had abnormal leukograms or elevated fibrinogen levels. However, the majority of these foals with fevers, leukocytosis, or hyperfibrinogenemia also had a concurrent infection remote from the umbilicus. Therefore, the percentage of foals with either pyrexia or abnormal hemograms primarily attributable to umbilical infection may actually be lower.

Diagnosis of internal umbilical infections is easy, but in some cases differentiation of infection from fibrosis (presumably due to trauma at birth) can be difficult. Moreover, the sonographer must realize that infection may be present within an umbilical structure in the absence of abnormal enlargement of the structure.

Abnormalities of the Urachus

A lumen or centrally located pocket within the urachus most often indicates purulent fluid (Fig. 35.1). The sonographer should note not only the dimensions of the urachal remnant, but also the dimensions of the fluid pocket (1). Longitudinal views should also be obtained, because abscessation may be present over most of the length of the urachal sheath, or it may be located only within a small segment. Urachal abscesses can be deformed to varying degrees, depending on the amount of bladder distention, so it is important to obtain longitudinal views, particularly if serial sonograms are to be compared (Fig. 35.2).

The contents of the fluid pocket should be examined for gas, which may indicate anaerobic infection (4). Gas echoes

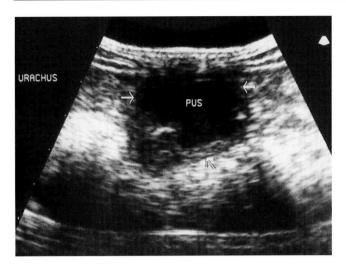

Figure 35.1. Cross-sectional view of a urachal abscess. *Arrows* delineate the borders of the urachus.

may be dispersed within the fluid, or a dorsal gas cap may be present (Fig. 35.3). However, gas echoes may also be seen within the urachal lumen if the abscess is draining to the outside.

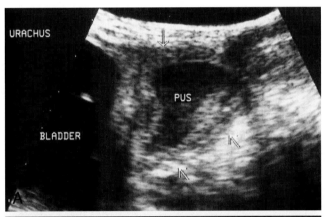

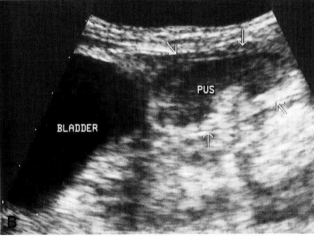

Figure 35.2. A and **B**, Longitudinal views of a urachal abscess in a 21-day-old Thoroughbred colt (same foal shown in Figure 35.1) obtained 3 days apart (arrows). The abscess is distorted by the degree of bladder distention.

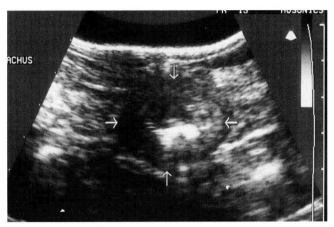

Figure 35.3. Closed urachal abscess with a dorsal gas cap in an 8-day-old Thoroughbred foal. The borders of the urachal sheath are delineated by *arrows*. *Bacteroides fragilis* was cultured at surgery.

Abscesses should not be confused with serouslike cysts or seromas, which are typically seen near the periphery of the urachal sheath (Fig. 35.4). Generalized enlargement of the urachus can be a result of infection or fibrous tissue. Seromas are characterized by loculated anechoic tissue and should not be confused with infection. A homogenous appearance to the remnant is more typical of fibrous tissue, whereas infection may be more heterogenous. However, differentiation of trauma from infection can still be difficult. Follow-up sonograms of urachal remnants in which the diagnosis is unclear are often of benefit. Further enlargement of the structure should make one suspicious of infection, whereas no change or reduction in the size of the remnant (without treatment) is compatible with fibrosis. In foals with urachal infections in which the urachus is enlarged and heterogenous, a response to medical treatment can be manifested sonographically as a reduction in overall size of the structure and organization of the infected material into a discrete fluid pocket or complete resolution of the abnormality (Fig. 35.5) (1).

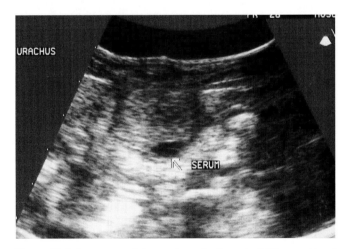

Figure 35.4. Sonogram of the urachus of a 2-week-old Thoroughbred foal depicts a small seroma-like structure at the periphery of the urachal sheath.

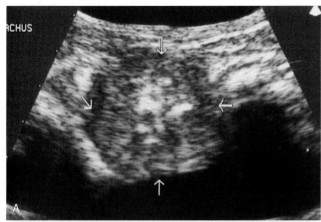

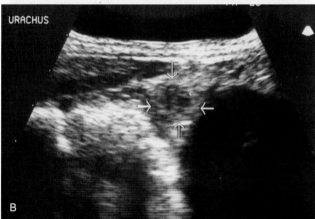

Figure 35.5. A, Enlarged urachal remnant (arrows) in a 19-day-old Thoroughbred foal with purulent material draining from the umbilical stump. The heterogenous appearance of the urachal sheath is consistent with infection or inflammation. **B,** Sonogram of the urachus of the same foal obtained after approximately 2 weeks of oral antimicrobial therapy (arrows).

Urachal diverticula may also be easily identified sonographically. The longitudinal view reveals an outpouching of the bladder apex ranging in size from a small projection (Fig. 35.6) to a large, fingerlike protuberance into the urachus. The cross-sectional view reveals a fluid pocket that communicates, without narrowing, with the bladder apex. Urachal diverticula can therefore be easily mistaken for urachal abscesses if the urachus is not followed in its entirety to the bladder apex, or if a longitudinal view is not obtained.

Abnormalities of the Umbilical Arteries

As stated in Chapter 5, normal variations exist in umbilical artery wall thickness, dimensions, and echogenicity of the contents of the lumen. Because both blood clots and purulent material can range in echogenicity from anechoic to echogenic, differentiation of arterial abscessation from clot can be difficult unless the structure is overtly enlarged. Marked thickening of the umbilical artery wall can occur in concert with urachal infection, but it should not be interpreted as absolute infection of the artery itself (Fig. 35.7).

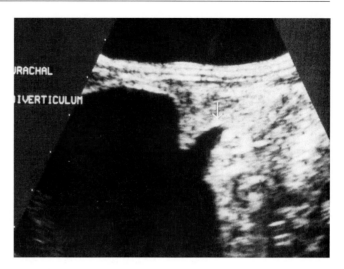

Figure 35.6. Longitudinal view of a urachal diverticulum (arrow) in a 2-day-old Thoroughbred colt with strangury.

Of the umbilical remnants excised at our clinic because of urachal abscessation, most arteries with such an appearance contain only a sterile clot. Foals with similar sonographic findings treated medically for urachal infections often have a rapid (within a few days) reduction in the perivascular thickening. Additionally, a widely dilated arterial lumen, without perivascular thickening, may only be a sterile clot (Fig. 35.8). However, a widely dilated arterial lumen and marked perivascular thickening are highly suggestive of arterial abscessation, particularly if other remnants are involved (Fig. 35.9).

A decision to excise the umbilical remnants surgically based on involvement of an umbilical artery should therefore be made with caution and only after careful sonographic evaluation. It is also unusual for an umbilical artery

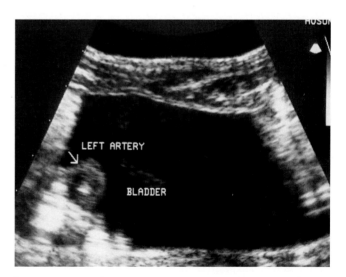

Figure 35.7. Left umbilical artery (*arrow*) of a 12-day-old Thoroughbred colt with urachal and umbilical vein abscessation. Notice the echodense arterial lumen and the perivascular thickening or edema.

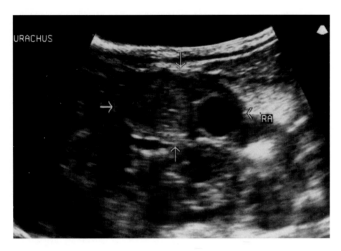

Figure 35.8. Blood clot in the right umbilical artery (RA) of an 8-day-old Thoroughbred foal with a urachal abscess (arrows). The blood clot was confirmed to be sterile at surgery.

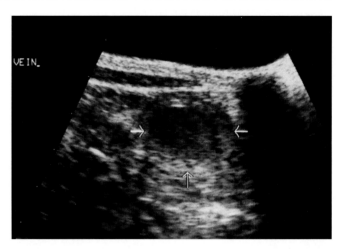

Figure 35.10. Umbilical vein abscess in an 8-day-old Thoroughbred colt. The vein is markedly enlarged (arrows) and echogenic fluid is within the lumen.

infection to be present without concurrent urachal infection.

Abnormalities of the Umbilical Veins

Perivascular thickening of the umbilical vein can also be seen as a response to adjacent urachal infection, and it should not be immediately interpreted as indicative of infection of the vein itself. As with the umbilical arteries, this perivascular response resolves quickly with appropriate medical therapy of the infection. Gross distention of the lumen with fluid most commonly indicates infection of the vein (Fig. 35.10). The umbilical vein should be followed from the stump to the liver, to avoid missing any segments of the vein that may be more severely affected. Homogenous enlargement of the vein can also occur as a

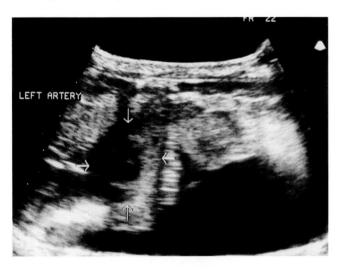

Figure 35.9. Left umbilical artery abscess in a Thoroughbred colt with a urachal abscess. Notice the widely dilated arterial lumen with somewhat echogenic fluid and the perivascular thickening (arrows). Purulent material was present in both the artery and the urachus at surgery.

result of trauma, but the lumen of the vein should not be overtly enlarged.

Management of Umbilical Infections

Most internal umbilical infections diagnosed in our practice over a 2-year period were successfully managed medically (1). Although many of these were small abscesses, even foals with large internal umbilical abscesses responded to medical treatment (see Fig. 35.1). Surgical excision should probably still be considered most strongly in foals with extensive umbilical vein abscessation that extends to the liver. However, a 24- to 72-hour course of preoperative antimicrobials may reduce bacterial contamination at surgery and may improve outcome (1).

Umbilical infections often contain both Gram-positive and Gram-negative bacteria; therefore, broad-spectrum antimicrobials should be administered (3). Antimicrobials effective against B streptococci and Gram-negative enteric organisms should be strongly considered because these pathogens are common isolates. Staphylococcal organisms are also occasionally identified (3). The presence of gas echoes within a closed abscess should prompt therapy with antimicrobials efficacious against anaerobic organisms (1, 3, 4). Ideally, culture of any purulent material should be performed, so appropriate antimicrobial selection is ensured. Ultrasound-guided aspiration of closed urachal abscesses may be feasible, although we are unaware of any attempts to perform this procedure. The sonographer should ensure that the remnant is in full contact with and fibrosed to the body wall, to avoid peritoneal contamination.

Drainage should be encouraged, as with any abscess. Duration of antimicrobial therapy required depends on the size of the abscess and on the sensitivity of the organisms to the therapy selected. Most foals treated medically at our clinic were treated for 2 to 3 weeks (1). The antimicrobials used in the management of these cases included the following:

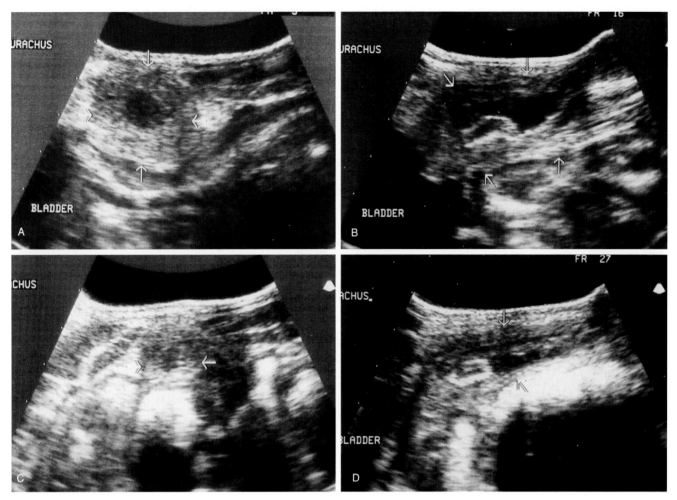

Figure 35.11. Cross-sectional (**A**) and longitudinal (**B**) sonograms of a 14-day-old Thoroughbred colt with a urachal abscess. Notice the central fluid pocket and the thickened tissue of the urachal sheath surrounding the fluid pocket (arrows). The tubular structure within the fluid is an umbilical artery. Cross-sectional (**C**) and longitudinal (**D**) views of the same foal after 6 days of antimicrobial therapy. Notice the marked reduction in size of both the entire urachus and of the fluid pocket.

intravenous penicillin combined with either an aminoglycoside or trimethoprim–sulfamethoxazole (TMS); TMS alone; or TMS in combination with intramuscular penicillin or an oral cephalosporin (cefuroxime) (1). Rifampin was added to the treatment regimen in some cases. Metronidazole was used when gas echoes were identified sonographically in closed abscesses, or when a foul odor was noted from any discharge from the umbilical stump. Shorter duration of therapy may well result in sterilization of the infected tissue, before complete sonographic resolution (1).

Sonographic changes consistent with resolution of the infection include reduction in perivascular or urachal sheath thickening and reduction in the size of the fluid pocket (Fig. 35.11). Additional sonographic changes consistent with resolution of the infection include organization of a diffusely enlarged urachus into a smaller diameter urachus with development of a central fluid pocket, increased echogenicity (inspissation) of the fluid, and mineralization (1). In some cases, the abscess may rupture (without incident) into the bladder.

Sonographic evidence of therapeutic response may not be noted for 3 to 7 days (1). Failure of medical therapy is indicated by enlargement of the affected remnant (entire diameter or size of the abscess). Clinically, persistence of fever or lack of improvement of the hemogram should prompt a change in antimicrobial therapy or surgical resection. However, most foals with umbilical infections seen by our service had neither fevers nor hemogram abnormalities. Therefore, sonographic monitoring is imperative.

In foals undergoing long-term antimicrobial therapy for another septic process, surgical resection may *not* be necessary because dissemination of bacteria from the umbilical abscess may no longer be a threat (1). Surgical resection may be considered more appropriate and economical in neonatal foals with extensive umbilical remnant infections that are otherwise healthy. The presence of gas echoes indicative of anaerobic infection may also prompt one to consider surgical resection.

In summary, considerations for the management of umbilical remnant infections include the age of the foal, size of the abscess, involvement of other structures (aside from perivascular thickening), fevers or abnormal hemograms attributable to the umbilical infection (rule out other sources for these findings), anaerobic infections, clinical and economic situations, and culture and sensitivity results. If medical therapy is selected, follow-up sonograms must be performed to ensure that therapy is appropriate, because even very small abscesses can become large, extensive infections with potentially deleterious consequences. Continuation of treatment until one sees complete sonographic resolution of the abscess may not be necessary, because sterilization of the infected material may occur well before sonographic resolution (1).

UMBILICAL SWELLINGS

External umbilical swellings are best investigated with diagnostic ultrasound, to confirm or rule out infection or inflammation of the internal remnants or the umbilical stump. Other causes of umbilical swellings or perinavel edema can be elucidated with ultrasound. Sonographically derived measurements of the umbilical defect can be obtained, if not apparent on palpation. Additionally, the contents of the hernial sac and the viability of any intestine within the sac can be determined. A common cause of diffuse edema originating in the umbilical area, which can become extensive, is tearing of the peritoneum at the umbilical stump with leakage and dissection of peritoneal fluid into the subcutaneous tissues (Fig. 35.12). Warmth is often detected in the umbilical region; however, this is likely caused by the oozing of the warm peritoneal fluid into the subcutaneous tissues, rather than by cellulitis. Of six cases identified sonographically by our service thus far, the

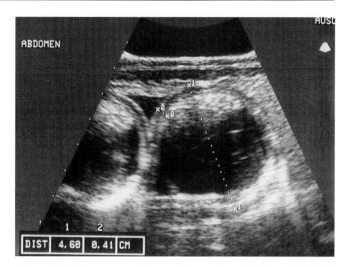

Figure 35.13. Sonogram of the small intestine of a Thoroughbred foal with a small intestinal volvulus. Notice the taut appearance of the intestinal wall and the sedimentation of echodense material to the dependent side of the loop of intestine (top of the image).

defect in the body wall was small (less than 1.5 cm), and all patients responded to bandaging and restricted exercise for 7 to 10 days, without antimicrobial therapy.

GASTROINTESTINAL TRACT

Small Intestinal Disorders

Sonography enables visualization of intestinal distention, lumen contents, wall thickness, and motility (5). Although only a portion of the small intestine can be visualized with ultrasound, diseased intestine often lies against the dependent portion of the abdomen (6). The actual intestinal lesion, such as a volvulus, cannot be directly visualized; however, the clinician can observe the response of the adjacent intestine and can better surmise the nature of the disorder. Taut, amotile, fluid-filled small intestine (Fig. 35.13), occasionally accompanied by a slight peritoneal effusion, is an anticipated result of a strangulating small intestinal disorder. As a strangulating lesion persists, peritoneal effusion, and a more flaccid and edematous appearance to the intestinal wall, with no evidence of motility, is anticipated (Fig. 35.14).

Differentiation of diseases requiring surgery from enteritis with functional ileus can be difficult. Gas echoes along or even within the intestinal wall, sometimes accompanied by substantial peritoneal effusions if there is transmural necrosis, can be identified in foals with severe necrotizing enteritis. The wall of the intestine may even appear thin and friable in such cases (7). These cases can be difficult to differentiate from strangulating obstruction in the final stages.

The wall thickness and degree of distention of the affected loops of bowel are generally uniform among the involved segments of intestine in foals with mechanical obstructions. Normal-appearing intestine (which would be distal to the involved intestine) may also be identifiable. In foals with

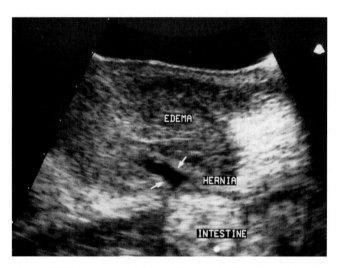

Figure 35.12. Sonogram of the umbilical region (longitudinal view) of a 3-month-old foal with sudden onset of progressive warm, non-painful ventral edema. Notice the small (less than 1 cm) gap in the body wall at the umbilical region, the fluid-filled outpouching into the subcutaneous tissues (arrows), and the edematous hypoechoic tissue (presumably extravasated peritoneal fluid) in the umbilical region. A diagnosis of a peritoneal tear at the umbilical region was made. A belly bandage was applied, and the foal recovered uneventfully.

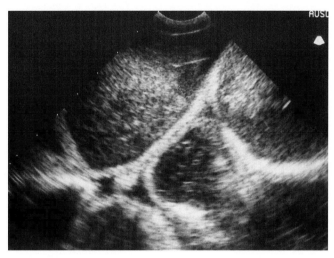

Figure 35.14. Sonogram of the small intestine of a foal with a history of severe abdominal pain. At the time of the examination, the foal was no longer experiencing pain but was in shock. The distended loops of intestine appear flaccid. Peristaltic activity was not observed. Based on the history, physical examination, and sonogram, a diagnosis of strangulated small intestinal obstruction was made. A small intestinal volvulus with necrosis of the involved segment was confirmed at surgery. Reprinted with permission from Bernard WV, Reimer JM. Examination of the foal. Vet Clin North Am Equine Pract 1994;10:53.

enteritis, the affected loops of intestine may be distended to varying degrees, and it is unusual to identify normal segments of small intestine. Fortunately, most foals with enteritis have visibly hypermotile intestine and are not difficult to differentiate from foals with intestinal lesions requiring surgery. Intestine proximal to an obstruction in the acute stages may also appear fluid filled and hypermotile. Incomplete mechanical obstructions, such as adhesions involving a short segment of intestine, may appear as

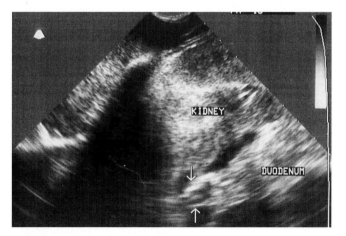

Figure 35.15. Sonogram of the right kidney and duodenum of a 4-month-old foal with a duodenal stricture. The duodenum is easily visualized in this individual because it is surrounded by peritoneal fluid and the lumen is collapsed and contains no gas. The stricture is delineated by *arrows*.

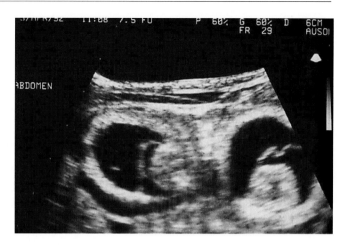

Figure 35.16. Cross-sectional sonogram of a loop of a small intestinal intussusception. Notice the central intussusceptum within the lumen of the intussuscepiens. The cross-sectional segment on the left also demonstrates an intussusception of the intussusception. Reprinted with permission from Bernard WV, Reimer JM. Examination of the foal. Vet Clin North Am Equine Pract 1994;10:53.

one or two loops of distended hypomotile intestine, adjacent to normal intestine.

A segment of the duodenum is visible immediately caudal and ventral to the right kidney. Although duodenal strictures may occur in other segments of the duodenum, the sonographer may be able to identify a stricture in this region (Fig. 35.15).

Small intestinal intussusception is clearly visible sonographically in the foal (Fig. 35.16) and obviates radiography and abdominocentesis. The sonogram reveals a distended segment of intestine with an echogenic center surrounded by fluid when imaged in cross-section. The involved intestine has a "bull's-eye" or target appearance (8).

Grossly thickened small intestinal walls can be visualized sonographically and may result from various disorders. Bowel wall edema may be identified postoperatively in foals with surgically corrected mechanical obstructions or in foals with enteritis or mild abdominal pain of unknown cause (Fig. 35.17). Thickening of the intestinal wall as a result of fibrosis or cellular infiltrate appears more echogenic than thickening due to edema. The significance of intestinal wall thickening should also take into consideration the peristaltic activity of the segment, the patient's history, and the physical findings.

With the exception of small intestinal intussusception, a diagnosis can only be *inferred* from the sonogram. The sonographic findings must be assimilated with the history, physical examination, and laboratory data. Serial sonographic evaluations are often of tremendous benefit if the diagnosis is unclear (5).

Colon Disorders

Meconium impactions can occasionally be identified sonographically, and they have a soft tissue echogenicity (Fig.

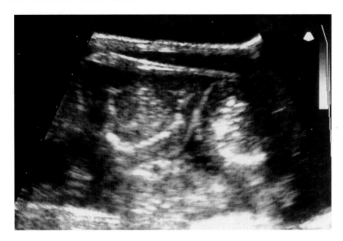

Figure 35.17. Sonogram of a Thoroughbred weanling with mild to moderate abdominal pain. Notice the thick edematous intestinal wall and the numerous gas echoes within the lumen. The abdominal pain resolved, and the segment of intestine was more normal in appearance by the following day.

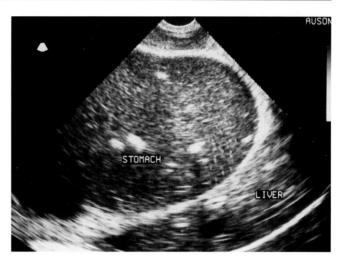

Figure 35.19. Sonogram (longitudinal view) of the abdomen of a foal with abdominal pain shows fluid and milk curd within a distended stomach.

35.18). The bladder can be used as an acoustic window to try to visualize the obstruction if it is located in the proximal rectum or distal small colon. Any gas-filled intestine surrounding the impaction obscures it from view. Occasionally, meconium impactions can be visualized in the large colon. The sonographer must be careful to ensure that this is solid obstructing material, because meconium can appear similar to normal large intestinal contents. Large and small colon disorders are otherwise infrequent in the neonate.

Gastric Disorders

The stomach is often difficult to image because of the foal's deep-chested conformation. Occasionally, the stomach may be distended with fluid or gas and may be readily identified

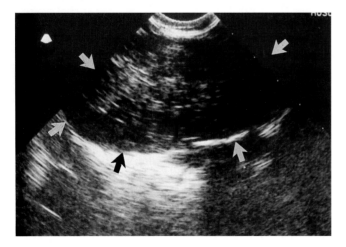

Figure 35.18. Sonogram of the abdomen of a 24-hour-old Thoroughbred colt with meconium impaction in the large colon. Notice the almost soft-tissue echogenicity of the meconium (*arrows*).

(Fig. 35.19). If the foal has gross gastric distention, gastric decompression by nasogastric tube should be performed (4). Although sonography has been used to demonstrate gastric ulceration in the dog, the view of the stomach is too limited and the image quality is inadequate to use the technique in the foal with any reliability.

PERITONEUM

Peritoneal effusions can be readily characterized sonographically. The foal should be standing, if possible, so peritoneal fluid is easily identified. Although peritoneal fluid may not be grossly visible, this should not preclude abdominocentesis if such information is desired and if no gross intestinal distention is noted.

Peritoneal fluid echogenicity can reflect the cellularity of the fluid. Echogenic fluid may indicate peritonitis (4) or hemoperitoneum, whereas anechoic fluid is compatible with a low cell count. However, sonography alone is not a reliable way to make a diagnosis of the type of fluid within the peritoneal cavity. For example, a large amount of anechoic peritoneal fluid may be seen in foals with a ruptured bladder (Fig. 35.20) (4, 7) or acute gastrointestinal rupture (1). Occasionally, gas echoes may be seen within the peritoneal fluid if the foal has gross intestinal contamination of the abdomen. Foals with ruptured bladder may have echogenic peritoneal fluid, either from peritonitis or from urinary sediment, and it may be difficult to differentiate foals with these disorders from those with intestinal perforation. Anechoic peritoneal effusions can also occur secondary to intestinal disorders or for unknown reasons. The history, physical findings, and applicable blood studies should be assimilated with the sonogram before making a diagnosis. Abdominocentesis should be performed in appropriate cases for visual examination and analysis, if necessary.

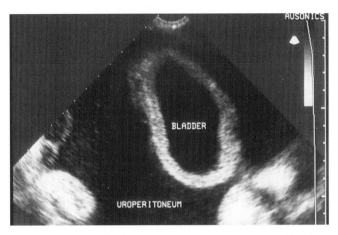

Figure 35.20. Sonogram of a foal with uroperitoneum resulting from a ruptured bladder. Notice the somewhat flaccid appearance to the bladder and copious amounts of anechoic peritoneal fluid. Reprintd with permission from Bernard WV, Reimer JM. Examination of the foal. Vet Clin North Am Equine Pract 1994;10:53.

URINARY TRACT

Abnormalities of the Bladder

Ruptured bladder is the most common disorder affecting the urinary tract in the foal. In acute cases, little urine may be present within the abdominal cavity; therefore, views from the most dependent portion of the abdomen are critical. As described in the section of this chapter on the peritoneum, the echogenicity of the fluid can vary, although anechoic fluid is most typical of uroperitoneum.

Because most tears occur at the dorsal aspect of the bladder, direct visualization of the tear is often not possible. The bladder may also contract enough so even a large tear is not visible sonographically. Bladders may be moderately filled but appear "flaccid." Ruptured bladders may also appear normal, and they can become full and turgid without any evidence of a tear (such an appearance is expected with small defects or urachal tears). The urachus should also be evaluated closely for any evidence of a urachal tear. The clinician should interpret the sonogram in light of laboratory data, including serum electrolytes and creatinine, and results of abdominocentesis.

The urine within the bladder of the foal is typically anechoic; however, mucus and white blood cells may accumulate within the bladder in foals that have undergone repeated catheterizations or in foals with a urachal abscess that has ruptured into the bladder. Large blood clots, presumably associated with trauma to the umbilical cord or the bladder at birth, may also be identified within the bladder.

Abnormalities of the Kidneys and Ureters

Congenital renal defects are uncommon in the foal, but they are amenable to sonographic evaluation. Kidneys may appear very small, with large cystic cavities. Acute renal failure may produce no appreciable changes in the kidney, but some foals may have gross renomegaly or perirenal edema.

The kidneys may also be less echogenic than normal. Sonographic changes consistent with chronic renal disease, such as small kidneys with an irregular contour, require time to develop and may not be expected in a young foal.

The ureters are normally not visible sonographically. Ureteral defects can therefore be difficult to image. A large amount of anechoic fluid in the retroperitoneal space is consistent with a ureteral defect. Gross enlargement of the ureter, to the point where it is visible sonographically, may occur with obstruction; however, this disorder is also uncommon in the foal.

ABDOMINAL ABSCESSATION

Foals with suspected abdominal abscessation are candidates for sonographic evaluation. Because abdominal abscesses are more common in the older foal, small abscesses may be difficult to detect because of the larger size of the patients and the more developed and gas-filled large colon. Large abdominal abscesses may be identified sonographically transcutaneously, thus confirming the diagnosis noninvasively. The approximate size of the abscess and the characteristics of the contents of the abscess cavity (liquid pus, versus thick whorls of fibrin and pus) can be gleaned from the ultrasound examination. Sonography is also a means by which to monitor therapeutic response in foals that are treated medically or to monitor the success of marsupialization.

The abdomen should be thoroughly clipped, as for exploratory celiotomy. Although large abscesses may be identified readily, detection of smaller abscesses may require extensive, careful scanning. Gas-filled intestine may obscure visualization of an abscess, but eventually the abscess may become evident once the gas moves out of the plane of view. In some older foals with good appetites, it may be worth performing the ultrasound examination after fasting the foal for 12 to 24 hours.

The typical sonographic appearance of an abdominal abscess is similar to that of parenchyma, it is slightly heterogenous, and it can resemble the contents of the large colon if there is little gas mixed in with the ingesta (Fig. 35.21). Normal structures, such as the liver, spleen, and colon, should not be mistaken for an abscess. Liver and spleen can be easily distinguished by their anatomic location. Ingesta within the colon appear mobile, as a result of peristaltic activity.

Additional sonographic findings that may be noted with abdominal abscessation include echogenic peritoneal fluid, distended mesenteric vessels, and sometimes smaller abscesses within the mesentery adjacent to the body wall.

Sonographic monitoring of the size of the abscess can be of value in monitoring the response to therapy. One month of antimicrobial therapy may be required before any obvious change in abscess size is noted; antimicrobial therapy is required for even longer for successful treatment of most cases.

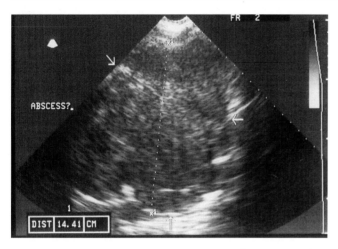

Figure 35.21. Abdominal abscess in a weanling Thoroughbred foal. The abscess is delineated by *arrows*, and a cursor is positioned through it. Notice the heterogenous appearance to the abscess contents, which might be confused with gastrointestinal contents.

LIVER AND SPLEEN

Liver and splenic disorders are uncommon in the foal. Acute hepatitis, as might be seen in foals with Tyzzer's disease, may result in hepatomegaly and a swollen or slightly rounded appearance to the liver edges. Hepatomegaly is a subjective assessment, and the sonographer must be familiar with the normal borders of the liver to make this judgment. Hepatomegaly may also be a result of hepatic congestion. The liver may also appear less echogenic than normal in such cases. Because the echogenicity of the liver may be artifactually altered by gain settings, a comparison of liver echogenicity with that of the right kidney and the spleen should be made as part of the sonographic evaluation. The results of sonographic evaluation rarely provide a specific diagnosis, although the nature (acute, chronic, diffuse, focal, biliary) of the disorder may be revealed. Even in severe acute liver diseases, gross sonographic changes may not be evident. Biopsy should be performed in appropriate cases to accurately diagnose liver disorders. The clinician should also be aware that the liver may become displaced caudally in foals with diaphragmatic hernias in which the intestine (not liver) is entrapped in the thoracic cavity.

REFERENCES

1. Reimer JM. Ultrasonography of umbilical remnant infections in foals. Proc Am Assoc Equine Pract 1993;39:247–248.
2. Reef VB, Collatos C, Spencer PA, et al. Clinical, ultrasonographic, and surgical findings in foals with umbilical remnant infections. J Am Vet Med Assoc 1989;195:69–72.
3. Collatos CC, Reef VB, Richardson DW. Umbilical cord remnant abscess in a yearling colt. J Am Vet Med Assoc 1989;195: 1252–1254.
4. Reef VB. Equine pediatric ultrasonography. Compend Contin Educ Pract Vet 1991;3:1277–1285.
5. Reimer JM. Ultrasonography of the gastrointestinal tract of the foal. In: Proc 2nd Internatl Sci Vet Echoc 1993:91–92.
6. Reef VB. Diagnostic ultrasonography of the foal's abdomen: In McKinnon AO, Voss, JL, eds. Equine reproduction. Philadelphia: Lea & Febiger,1993;1088–1094.
7. Reimer JM. Sonographic evaluation of gastrointestinal diseases in foals. Proc Am Assoc Equine Pract 1993;39:245–246.
8. Bernard WV, Reef VB, Neimer JM, et al. Ultrasonographic diagnosis of small-intestinal intussusception in three foals. J Am Vet Med Assoc. 194:395-397, 1989.

36. Equine Diagnostic Ocular Ultrasonography

DAVID A. WILKIE AND BRIAN C. GILGER

EQUIPMENT

Ocular ultrasonography as a diagnostic tool includes both amplitude-mode (A-scan) and brightness-mode (B-scan) ultrasound. In veterinary ophthalmology, B-scan ultrasound provides a two-dimensional real-time image and is the most common mode of ultrasound in a clinical setting. Ultrasonography is a safe and painless method of examining intraocular and retrobulbar structures in an awake animal.

When ocular ultrasonography is performed, high resolution is desirable, but great tissue penetration is not essential. In the selection of a transducer probe for ocular ultrasonography, several variables should be considered. It is best to use a sector scanner with a small scan head diameter (footprint) to facilitate optimal placement on the cornea. Transducer probes are available in a range of frequencies. The frequency of the transducer is inversely proportional to the wavelength of the sound beam. Depth of sound beam penetration is proportional to wavelength. Therefore, a low-frequency transducer (5 Mhz) gives greater tissue penetration but poor near-field axial resolution, and a high-frequency transducer (10 Mhz) gives lower tissue penetration but high near-field axial resolution (Figs. 36.1 to 36.3). In simple terms, the higher the transducer frequency, the better the visualization of superficial structures such as those found within the eye. The optimal ophthalmic transducer is a 10-Mhz instrument with a focal range of 3 to 4 cm (see Fig. 36.3). This probe provides adequate depth of penetration to visualize the retrobulbar structures, enhanced resolution, and ability to visualize the anterior intraocular structures such as the iris, ciliary body, anterior and posterior chambers, and cornea. Alternately, a 7.5-Mhz transducer provides clear ophthalmic images (see Fig. 36.2). It has a focal range of 2 to 5 cm and a better depth of penetration for visualization of retrobulbar structures. However, the anterior segment of the globe is lost in the near-field reverberation artifact. To overcome the near-field loss, use of a stand-off device, increased application of sterile coupling gel, or examination through the horse's closed eyelids may help when using a 7.5-Mhz transducer (Figs. 36.4 and 36.5).

In addition to the transducer and ultrasound machine, some form of documentation is required to allow freeze-frame evaluation, to obtain measurements, to create records for current and future reference, and to permit consultation with colleagues.

NORMAL OCULAR ANATOMY

In general, ultrasonographic images are described as hyperechoic, hypoechoic, and anechoic. Four major ocular acoustic echoes are noted within a normal eye: anterior cornea, anterior lens capsule, posterior lens capsule, and retina–choroid–sclera (see Fig. 36.5). When ultrasound energy traveling along an axial beam travels across these interfaces, energy is reflected back to the transducer in the form of an echo and is seen as an echodensity. Additional echodensities may be generated by the iris, corpora nigra, ciliary body, optic nerve, orbital fat, muscles, and other orbital structures. The optic nerve head–lamina cribrosa appears as a hyperechoic structure, with the optic nerve itself seen as a hypoechoic structure extending posteriorly from the optic nerve head. The orbital muscle cone appears as an echodensity extending posteriorly from the equatorial region of the globe and converging toward the orbital apex. The anterior and posterior chambers, lens cortex and nucleus, and vitreous chamber are normally anechoic. The measurements of the globe and intraocular structures of the extirpated normal equine eye as determined by use of a 7.5-Mhz B-mode sector transducer has been reported (Table 36.1 and Fig. 36.6) (1). These measurements differ slightly from the reported normal values obtained by other methods because they were obtained on extirpated globes, which may be subject to some variability.

INDICATIONS

Ocular ultrasonography is indicated whenever an opacity of the transmitting media of the eye (cornea, aqueous humor, lens, vitreous humor) prevents a complete ophthalmic examination. In addition, evaluation of intraocular mass lesions, differentiation between solid and cystic structures, examination for a foreign body, axial length determination, and examination of retrobulbar orbital structures are all indications for performing ocular ultrasound.

The most common clinical indications for ocular ultrasound are to evaluate for the presence of a retinal detachment in eyes with a cataract, to assess posterior segment damage and examine for the presence of a foreign body after trauma, and to evaluate intraocular structures in eyes with severe corneal opacification. In addition, orbital evaluation can be performed in instances of exophthalmos or orbital trauma.

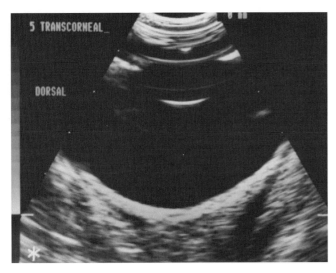

Figure 36.1. Normal ocular ultrasound performed transcorneally using a 5-Mhz transducer. The near artifact extends into the anterior lens, and no useful anterior segment detail is visible.

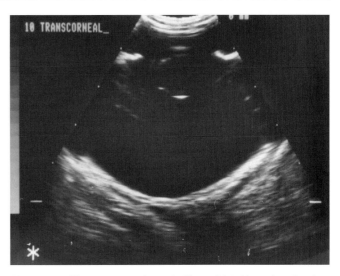

Figure 36.3. The same eye shown in Figure 36.1. Normal ocular ultrasound performed transcorneally using a 10-Mhz transducer. The entire anterior and posterior lens is visible as is the iris and a portion of the anterior chamber.

Ocular ultrasound is an addition to, not a replacement for, routine ophthalmic examination including assessment of menace, blink and pupillary light response, fluorescein staining, nasolacrimal evaluation, determination of intraocular pressure, and examination of anterior and posterior segments using a bright focal light source and direct and indirect ophthalmoscopy, respectively.

TECHNIQUE

To perform a complete ultrasound examination of the globe and orbit in the horse some form of tranquiliza-

tion and regional nerve blocks may be required. Topical anesthesia of the cornea (proparacaine 0.5%, Alcaine, Alcon Laboratories) is always used. Xylazine (Rompun, Haver-Lockhart) 0.5 to 1.0 mg/kg intravenously, in combination with butorphanol tartrate (Torbugesic, Bristol Laboratories) 0.01 mg/kg intravenously, will facilitate examination.

Sensory innervation of the globe and adnexa is provided by the trigeminal nerve (CN V), and motor innervation is supplied by the facial nerve (CN VII). The auriculopalpebral branch of CN VII and the supraorbital (frontal) branch

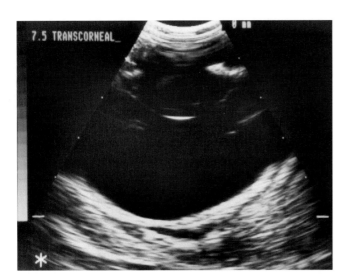

Figure 36.2. The same eye shown in Figure 36.1. Normal ocular ultrasound performed transcorneally using a 7.5-Mhz transducer. The near artifact extends into the anterior chamber and visualization of lens detail is improved.

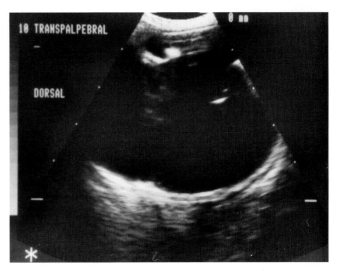

Figure 36.4. The same eye shown in Figure 36.1. Normal ocular ultrasound performed transpalpebrally using a 10-Mhz transducer. Significant artifact occurred with this technique as the result of poor probe contact, palpebral hair, and air in the conjunctival cul-de-sac. The corpora nigra is visible as an echodensity at the pupillary margin of the iris.

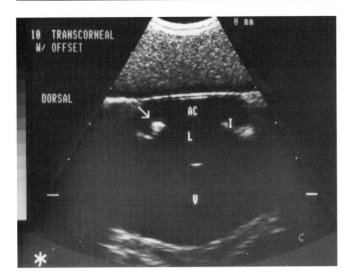

Figure 36.5. The same eye shown in Figure 36.1. Normal ocular ultrasound performed transcorneally using a tissue-equivalent offset device and a 10-Mhz transducer. The anterior segment, including the axial cornea, is clearly visible. With use of an offset device the orbital tissues are not visible with a 10-Mhz transducer. AC = anterior chamber; I = iris; L = lens; V = vitreous; *arrow* = corpora nigra.

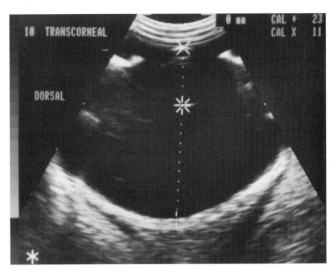

Figure 36.6. Normal eye examined transcorneally using a 10-Mhz transducer. The anterior-posterior dimension of the lens (11 mm) and the lens-vitreous dimension (23 mm) are shown.

of CN V are the regional nerves blocked most commonly to facilitate examination. These nerve blocks provide akinesia and anesthesia, respectively, of the superior eyelid. The auriculopalpebral nerve can be palpated as it courses over the zygomatic arch in the area of the temporofrontal suture. Using a 25-g 5/8-inch needle, the nerve is blocked by injection of 3 to 5 mL of mepivacaine HCl (Carbocaine, Winthrop Laboratories) over the zygomatic arch in this area. The supraorbital nerve is blocked as it emerges from the supraorbital foramen of the frontal bone. This foramen is palpated, a 25-g 5/8-inch needle is inserted into the foramen, and 2 mL of mepivacaine HCl is injected. Another 2 to 3 mL is infiltrated subcutaneously as the needle is removed (2). Additional sensory nerves, the infratrochlear, lacrimal, and zygomatic branches of CN V are not routinely blocked.

Sterile ultrasound coupling gel or K-Y jelly is placed on the transducer tip or on the corneal surface. Cellulose-based coupling gels should be avoided because they may cause corneal irritation. The transducer is then placed directly on

Table 36.1.
Measurements of the Extirpated Equine Globe Obtained by B-Mode Ultrasonography

Structure	Measurement (mm) ± SD
Anterior chamber depth	4.22 ± 1.29
Lens anterior–posterior dimension	11.93 ± 1.10
Vitreous	17.37 ± 1.98
Globe anterior–posterior dimension	39.4 ± 2.30

(Reprints with permission from Rogers M, Cartee RE, Miller W, et al. Evaluation of the extirpated equine eye using mode ultrasonography. Vet Radiol 1986;27:24–29.)

the cornea (see Fig. 36.3), or the scan may be performed through the horse's closed eyelids (see Fig. 36.4) or an offset device (see Fig. 36.5). Performing the examination through the eyelids or an offset device facilitates examination of the anterior portions of the globe, whereas direct corneal contact provides a superior image of the posterior segment and orbit. A suitable tissue-equivalent offset device is available with most transducers, or alternately, a water-filled balloon or excess coupling gel can be used. Care is taken to eliminate all air bubbles from the water-filled balloon or significant reverberation artifact will occur. When imaging through horse's eyelids or an offset device, it may be necessary to increase the gain setting. The globe is imaged in both horizontal and vertical planes through the visual axis. Oblique positioning of the probe should also be used for a complete examination. At the completion of the study, the coupling gel should be irrigated from the eye and conjunctiva using sterile Collyrium (eyewash).

ARTIFACTS

The normal lens refracts the sound waves from the transducer resulting in a faster passage of sound through the peripheral as compared with the central lens (3, 4). This feature may cause the posterior eye wall to appear to be closer to the probe and to be seen as two discrete retinal elevations at the retinal surface the size of which varies with the scan angle. This artifact has been termed "Baum's bumps" (3, 4).

Reduplication echoes result from the echo passing from an intraocular structure to the transducer and back again. Because it takes longer for this echo to reach the probe and to return into the eye to be imaged, the artifact always appears deeper in the globe than the tissue of origin. The typical reduplication echo occurs from the lens capsule to the transducer and back again and appears as linear hyperechodensities in the middle to posterior axial vitreous and can be confused with vitreous hemorrhage, inflammatory debris, or degeneration (3, 4).

Absorption artifact occurs when a dense structure such as a cataract or intraocular foreign body results in an acoustic shadow. This phenomenon occurs because of the almost complete reflection of sound from the dense structure, with little or no sound passing beyond to image the deeper tissues. This artifact appears as an anechoic area posterior to the hyperechoic structure and can be confused with a mass lesion (3, 4).

Additional artifacts occur when failure to use adequate coupling gel results in a gap between the transducer and the eyelid or cornea.

ABNORMALITIES

Ocular Trauma

Of all the indications for ocular ultrasonography in the equine patient, evaluating ocular trauma is perhaps ultrasound's greatest value. Ultrasonography helps to determine the extent and severity of the injury, assists in treatment selection, and allows the clinician to give a more accurate prognosis. In many instances, ultrasonography is the only examination method of value in an eye that is otherwise severely painful and opaque. In instances of severe eyelid swelling, the examination can be performed directly through the horse's eyelids. Care should be taken to avoid further traumatizing the globe by exerting excessive pressure on it with the ultrasound probe. In addition, the clinician should avoid exposing the horse's intraocular contents to the coupling gel in instances of corneal laceration or uveal prolapse. In addition to ultrasound, a routine, complete ophthalmic examination should be performed on globes that have sustained a traumatic injury. This includes, but is not limited to, assessment of menace, blink and pupillary light response, fluorescein staining, nasolacrimal evaluation, and determination of intraocular pressure and examination of anterior and posterior segments using a bright focal light source and direct and indirect ophthalmoscopy, respectively.

Trauma to the globe can be categorized as blunt (concussive) and sharp (penetrating or perforating). Of these categories, sharp trauma tends to have a better prognosis resulting often in severe, but focal damage to the globe. Sequelae of penetrating trauma include shallow anterior chamber, fibrin in the anterior chamber, lens capsule rupture, hyphema, retinal detachment, vitreous hemorrhage, and possibly rupture of the posterior eye wall. Blunt or concussive trauma causes a rapid increase in the intraocular pressure and often results in an expulsive rupture of the weak areas of the globe such as the limbus or posterior pole. Such an expulsive rupture expels intraocular contents (lens, uvea, vitreous, and retina) out of the eye and onto the face or into the surrounding environment. In addition, hyphema, vitreous hemorrhage, retinal detachment, cataract, lens (sub)luxation and rupture, and choroidal detachment can all occur with blunt trauma.

If the entire lens is visible 360° around its periphery, a cortical cataract may be present, or hemorrhage or a cyclitic membrane may be surrounding the lens capsule. The presence of hemorrhage or inflammatory membranes around the lens often results in posterior synechia, capsular cataract, and possibly secondary glaucoma in the weeks and months following an injury.

Retinal detachment may occur at the time of injury associated with vitreous loss and/or subretinal hemorrhage or can develop subsequent to injury as the result of traction from organizing vitreous hemorrhage or fibrosis.

In instances of severe trauma, it may be of benefit to obtain measurements of identifiable structures to assess the damage. For example, a reduction in the lens–posterior eye wall axial length may indicate a posterior lens luxation, whereas an increase may indicate an anterior lens luxation or a posterior eye wall rupture. In most instances of rupture of the posterior eye wall, the globe exhibits hypotony and hyphema. On ultrasound, vitreous and orbital hemorrhages are usually present and appear uniform in echodensity, blending together because a fibrous tunic no longer separates these two spaces. In addition, the normally hyperechoic posterior eye wall is not identifiable (Fig. 36.7).

Using ultrasound to evaluate the eye for intraocular foreign bodies is often unrewarding. For a foreign body to be visual on ultrasonography, it must be of sufficient size (larger than 1.0 mm) (3) and must have a surface that will reflect enough energy to be visualized as compared with the surrounding tissue. In general, metal is highly reflective and results in echodensity with shadowing behind as a result of absorption of sound by the object. Glass and organic material tend to be less echodense and more difficult to diagnose on ultrasound.

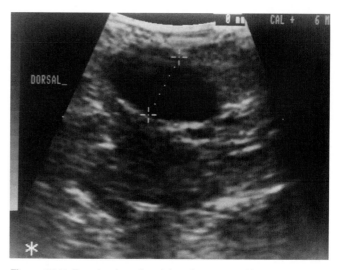

Figure 36.7. Examination of a globe after severe blunt trauma. The lens is visible as an anechoic structure. This is an axial scan and the anteroposterior lens is marked, showing that the lens is tipped on the anteroposterior axis indicating subluxation. The echodensity seen anterior and posterior to the lens (vitreous cavity) is hemorrhage. The posterior eye wall is not well defined because it has been ruptured.

Intraocular Mass Lesions

Intraocular mass lesions consist of inflammatory, neoplastic, and cystic structures and most commonly arise from the anterior uvea (iris, ciliary body). In addition, choroidal mass lesions can occur, although rarely.

Inflammatory material such as fibrin and hypopyon may accumulate in the anterior chamber as a result of anterior uveitis. Clinically, this material is usually evident on penlight examination of the anterior segment, but in severe cases of anterior uveitis, diffuse corneal edema may be present and an ultrasound examination may be indicated. Fibrin appears as a series of disconnected echodensities throughout the anterior chamber, whereas hypopyon is most often seen ventrally and is more uniform in its echodensity. In addition, the ciliary body and vitreous should be examined for involvement in the inflammatory process, and the lens should be examined for secondary cataract formation. Intraocular pressure (IOP) determination is also indicated in these eyes; the pressure is expected to be low in instances of anterior uveitis. Elevation in IOP suggests glaucoma secondary to the inflammatory process and obstruction of the outflow pathway for aqueous humor.

Uveal cysts are brown-black in appearance and arise from the pigmented epithelium of the iris and ciliary body. They may remain attached to the tissue of origin, or they may break free and float in the anterior chamber. The differential diagnosis of a pigmented lesion of the anterior uvea includes intraocular melanoma. A free-floating pigmented mass or one that transilluminates is considered a cyst because these are not characteristics of neoplasia. Mass lesions that remain attached or are densely pigmented and fail to transilluminate are either cysts or melanomas. To distinguish between these lesions requires ocular ultrasonography or histopathologic examination. On ultrasound, a cyst has an echogenic wall, but an anechoic, fluid-filled center, whereas a melanoma appears homogeneous in its acoustic density (Fig. 36.8). Because many of these mass lesions arise from the anterior uvea, an offset device, extra coupling gel, or scanning through the horse's closed eyelids is required to visualize the lesion adequately. Uveal cysts are benign and do not require treatment.

Neoplasms of the anterior uvea include primary (melanoma, adenoma, adenocarcinoma) and secondary lesions, of which lymphosarcoma is the most common. Choroidal neoplasms include melanoma and metastatic tumors. Reports of intraocular neoplasia in the horse are rare. Focal neoplasms of the anterior uvea can undergo surgical biopsy, and in some instances, the biopsy may be excisional and curative. This type of intraocular surgery requires specialized equipment and is considered a referral procedure. For a complete discussion of equine intraocular neoplasia, the reader is directed to consult additional sources (5).

Cataract and Lens Luxation

In a normal eye, the lens appears as two distinct echodensities seen at the anterior and posterior axial lens capsules (see Fig. 36.3). The anterior echo is slightly convex, whereas the posterior echo is concave in relation to the probe. Internally, the lens is anechoic, and peripherally, echo is reflected away from the probe. Abnormalities of the lens that can be detected on ultrasonography include abnormalities of lens size, cataract, (sub)luxation, and lens rupture.

Cataract appears as increased internal echoes within the lens or as increased visualization of the lens periphery other than the anterior and posterior axial portions (Fig. 36.9). The size and intensity of the echoes depend on the extent and severity of the cataract. Ultrasound may be used to diagnose a cataract in a posttraumatic globe or in an eye with opacity of the cornea or anterior chamber. Additionally, ultrasound is used to evaluate the posterior

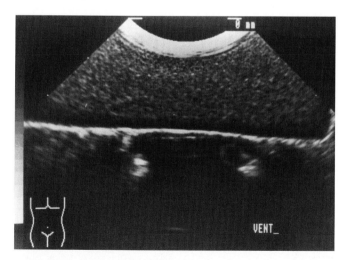

Figure 36.8. Transcorneal ultrasound using a tissue-equivalent offset device. Clinically, a pigmented mass lesion was noted to be attached to the ventral iris margin. On ultrasound, this mass has an echodense periphery but an anechoic center, indicating that it is hollow. The diagnosis is an iris cyst.

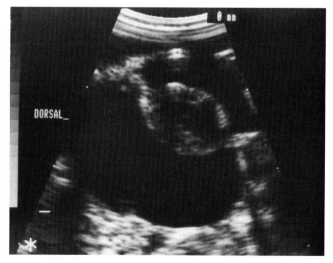

Figure 36.9. An intumescent cataract is present. The lens is visible 360° and has internal echodensities indicating a cataract. The antero-posterior lens measurement is increased indicating that the cataract is intumescent. The posterior segment is normal.

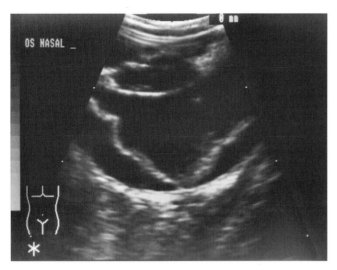

Figure 36.10. Transcorneal ultrasound using a 10-Mhz transducer. A cataract and retinal detachment are present. The retina remains attached at the optic nerve and ora ciliaris retina. The cataract is hypermature.

segment for abnormalities of the vitreous or retina in an eye with a cataract (Fig. 36.10) (6). To ensure that the posterior segment is normal anatomically, an ultrasound evaluation in an eye with a cataract is essential if cataract surgery is planned.

Abnormalities of lens size, measured from anterior to posterior at the axial position, include both increased and decreased lens dimensions. Enlargement of the lens is typically seen in association with a cataract and is the result of imbibition of fluid by the cataract resulting in swelling of the lens. Such a lens is said to be intumescent (see Fig. 36.9). An acquired decrease in lens size occurs as a result of resorption of liquefied cortical material, as is seen with a hypermature cataract (Figs. 36.10 and 36.11). Microphakia, a congenitally small lens, may be seen alone or in association with other congenital intraocular abnormalities.

Lens (sub)luxation may occur as a primary disease, or it may be secondary to trauma, inflammation, or glaucoma. With trauma or inflammation, the anterior segment may be opaque as a result of edema or hemorrhage, thereby complicating the diagnosis of lens luxation. In such instances, ocular ultrasound allows examination of the lens and its position. When performing an examination of these eyes, it is of benefit to freeze the image and to obtain measurements of the intraocular structures and their relationships with each other. Difficulty in obtaining a simultaneous echo of both the anterior and posterior lens capsule or changes in the anterior–posterior axial measurements of the lens or lens and posterior eye wall may indicate a (sub)luxation of the lens. In addition, the lens should be evaluated for internal echoes, which indicate cataract.

Vitreous Abnormalities

The vitreous cavity is normally anechoic, appearing dark or black on ultrasonography. Abnormalities of the vitreous appear as echodensities and include hemorrhage, inflammation, degeneration (syneresis), asteroid hyalosis, and detachment.

Vitreous is composed primarily of water, collagen, and glycosaminoglycans (principally hyaluronic acid). It has been described as a coiled spring with water bound between the coils. This property gives the vitreous elasticity. Degeneration or liquefaction of the vitreous decreases the vitreous gel and increases the free water content. Vitreous degeneration increases with age, can result from intraocular inflammation, and is associated with hypermature cataract formation (6). As the vitreous gel and water separate, interfaces are created that result in echodensities ultrasonographically. These appear as multiple, variable echogenic lines within the vitreous cavity and are best visualized by increasing the far-field gain setting on the ultrasound unit (6). Clinically, vitreous degeneration may appear normal or as fine strands of gray-white material swirling in the vitreous cavity as the globe moves. The significance of vitreous degeneration in animals is not well defined, but it may possibly predispose animals to retinal detachment.

Vitreous hemorrhage, in the equine eye, typically occurs as a result of ocular trauma and is usually associated with anterior segment hemorrhage (hyphema). Vitreous hemorrhage appears as discrete to diffuse moderate amplitude echoes that may demonstrate motion when evaluated during a real-time kinetic study. The presence of vitreous hemorrhage is a poor prognostic indicator and represents damage to the ciliary body, retina, or choroid. In many instances, eyes with severe vitreous hemorrhage develop cataract and retinal detachment or degeneration, and they often become phthisical.

Inflammation of the vitreous (hyalitis) is seen in association with inflammation of the anterior or posterior uvea; the most frequent syndrome in which this occurs is equine recurrent uveitis. Vitreous inflammation appears as multifocal, disconnected variable echodensities within the vitre-

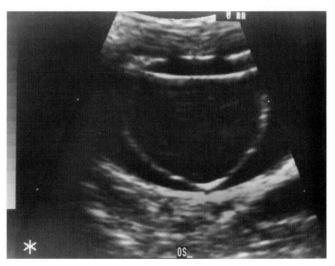

Figure 36.11. Severe resorption of lens, indicated by small anteroposterior dimension, associated with a hypermature cataract. In addition, a retinal detachment is present.

ous cavity. In addition, fibrin, hypopyon, and retinal detachment may be present if the inflammation extends to other structures. Vitreous degeneration is a sequela of inflammation of the vitreous.

The presence of calcium phosphate crystals, suspended in the vitreous humor, is termed asteroid hyalosis. Clinically, these crystals appear as white particulate material suspended within the vitreous. On ultrasound, they appear as highly reflective, discrete, freely moving echoes. These echoes persist even as the gain setting is decreased. Asteroid is common in older dogs, but rare in the horse. It is not clinically significant, and no treatment is indicated.

Retinal Detachment

In a normal eye, the retinal echo is indistinguishable from the underlying choroidal and scleral echo. The retina becomes apparent as a distinct echodensity with a separation of 0.5 to 1.0 mm (3). Retinal separation or detachment can be congenital or secondary to trauma, inflammation, neoplasia, hypertension, or idiopathic causes. Retinal detachments can be partial or complete and may or may not be associated with a tear in the retina. When detached, the retina appears as an echodense linear structure, most often attached at the optic disc posteriorly and the ora ciliaris retinae anteriorly, resulting in the classic funnel or gull-wing appearance (see Figs. 36.10 and 36.11). Retinal detachment can be complete or partial, and in some instances, the retina can become disinserted from the ora (usually dorsally) and collapses onto itself. Initially, retinal detachments undulate when viewed in real-time imaging, but eventually, the retina becomes fixed and less mobile. When evaluating a retinal detachment, it is important to examine the subretinal space and to evaluate the echo from this space. An anechoic subretinal space indicates fluid such as a transudate that may resorb, whereas the presence of echodense material in the subretinal space may indicate hemorrhage or infiltration of neoplastic or inflammatory cells and carries a less favorable prognosis. The differential diagnosis of a hyperechoic linear structure in the vitreous includes choroidal detachment, vitreous hemorrhage, vitreous detachment, vitreous degeneration, traction bands, and artifacts such as reverberation from the lens.

Abnormalities of Globe Dimensions

Ultrasound can be used to quantitate the axial dimensions of the globe and intraocular structures. The ultrasound dimensions of the extirpated equine globe noted in Table 36.1 are shorter in length than the ocular dimensions previously reported for the equine eye. Abnormalities of globe dimensions include enlargement of the globe (buphthalmos), decrease in globe size (microophthalmos, phthisis bulbi), increased or decreased lens dimensions, and changes in the relationships of intraocular structures with each other.

Orbital Abnormalities

Orbital contents include the extraocular muscles, fat, vascular tissues, glands, and the optic nerve. Ultrasound examination of the equine orbit is best performed using a 7.5-Mhz probe, which allows deeper tissue penetration than is obtainable with a 10-Mhz probe. Typically, orbital ultrasonography is performed in instances of exophthalmos to examine for retrobulbar space-occupying lesions or after orbital trauma to assess type and extent of damage.

Although exophthalmos is rare, the differential diagnosis of exophthalmos should include trauma, hemorrhage, extension of nasal or sinus disease, cellulitis or abscess, cyst, and neoplasia. Clinical signs and signalment, in addition to ultrasound, skull radiographs, and cytologic and histopathologic findings, may be required to confirm a diagnosis. In general, cellulitis or abscess is painful and rapid in onset, whereas neoplasia is more gradual in progression and less painful. Neoplasms of the equine orbit may include sarcoid, squamous cell carcinoma, melanoma, mast cell tumor, lymphosarcoma, lipoma, and undifferentiated carcinoma (5). If an orbital mass lesion is present on ultrasonography, an attempt is made to characterize it as cystic or solid and with regard to location within the orbit. If a mass lesion is detected, one can then obtain an ultrasound-guided fine-needle aspirate or biopsy to assist in the diagnosis.

After trauma to the orbit and associated structures, ultrasound may be used to evaluate the retrobulbar space. The orbit is examined for evidence of fractures, hemorrhage, and swelling or compression of the optic nerve, and the posterior wall of the globe is evaluated for explosive-type injury with expulsion of the intraocular contents into the orbit. In addition, the intraocular contents should be examined in such cases both by ophthalmoscopy and ultrasonography, the orbit and associated facial structures should be palpated, and the horse's skull should be radiographed to ascertain the extent of injury.

In summary, ocular ultrasonography is a safe, rapid, and essential tool to help evaluate, give an accurate prognosis, and plan treatment in eyes with opacity of the transmitting media.

REFERENCES

1. Rogers M, Cartee RE, Miller W, et al. Evaluation of the extirpated equine eye using B-mode ultrasonography. Vet Radiol 1986;27: 24–29, 1986.
2. Wilkie DA. Ophthalmic procedures and surgery in the standing horse. Vet Clin North Am Equine Pract 1991;7:535–547.
3. Koplin RS, Gersten M, Hodes B. Real time ophthalmic ultrasonography and biometry: a handbook of clinical diagnosis. Thorofare, NJ: Slack, 1985.
4. Byrne SF, Green RL. Ultrasound of the eye and orbit. St Louis: CV Mosby, 1992.
5. Lavach JD. Large animal ophthalmology. St Louis, CV Mosby, 1990.
6. van der Woerdt A, Wilkie DA, Myers W. Ultrasonographic abnormalities in the eyes of dogs with cataracts: 147 cases (1986–1992). J Am Vet Med Assoc 1993;203:838–841.

37. Ultrasound of the Endocrine System

NORMAN W. RANTANEN

INTRODUCTION

Ultrasound's role in the diagnosis of equine endocrine diseases is almost entirely limited to the thyroid gland. Diseases of the hypothalamus, the pituitary gland, the pancreas, and the adrenal glands are relatively rare in horses (1) and are most likely not readily diagnosable with current ultrasound techniques. The hypothalamus and pituitary are encased in the cranial vault, and the pancreas and adrenal glands are located near the dorsal midline of the body and are not routinely scanned in horses. Transrectal imaging at high frequencies would have to be performed because of their small size since transcutaneous scanning would require low frequencies with poor lateral resolution in the far field.

The thyroid gland, however, is a superficial structure found at the level of the larynx and can be imaged if necessary. It is comprised of two lobes that may be connected by a thin layer of connective tissue in the adult. The average gland weighs about 15 g/lobe and is 5 cm × 2.5 cm × 2 cm (1).

The purpose of this chapter is to present the scanning technique for thyroid glands and to show normal and abnormal scans. Even though the reported incidence of carcinoma is rare, veterinarians may be called on to evaluate cervical masses, and thyroid disease should be in the differential diagnosis. There are several reports of malignant thyroid tumors cited in the literature indicating that thyroid malignancies can produce clinical signs and can metastasize (2–6). Because of the location, tumors of the parotid salivary gland or lymph nodes need to be ruled out.

Hypothyroidism (goiter) in neonates will not be covered in this chapter. The thyroid may be enlarged in this condition and is pathognomonic if present, but this disease is usually investigated by determining blood values and response to treatment. Functional hypothyroidism in adult horses is a controversial issue with no imaging considerations, and hyperthyroidism, not documented in horses, will not be discussed.

SCANNING TECHNIQUE

The normal thyroid gland is readily palpable as two relatively firm enlargements lateral to the larynx. Ultrasound scans must be performed with high frequency (e.g., 7.5 MHz) for maximum resolution. Alcohol is effective to eliminate trapped air from the hair, and high quality scans are usually possible. It helps to keep the head straight or turned slightly away from the side being scanned to allow contact with the gland beneath the skin. The transducer is held directly over the gland. Standoff pads or devices are usually not needed, especially if the gland is enlarged. Occasionally,

large masses require 5.0-MHz transducers, especially if the hair is very thick. The transducer should be slowly passed over the gland in opposing planes to ensure covering the entire structure. Measurements of the gland and any internal structures should be made and photographs taken for future comparison. The normal thyroid has a homogeneous, fine, "stippled" texture (Fig. 37.1, **A** and **B**). In cross-section, the carotid artery and the laryngeal wall can be seen contacting the gland.

THYROID ENLARGEMENT

Benign

The most commonly found thyroid gland enlargement is benign adenoma (Fig. 37.2). The gland is uniformly enlarged and may have small cystic structures within it. There are usually no recognizable blood vessels.

Malignant

Whenever the normal or adenomatous thyroid gland cannot be found and there is a large mass present in the cranial cervical region, thyroid carcinoma should be considered. Figure 37.3 is an ultrasound scan of a mare with a large, cranial cervical swelling. The swelling extended to both sides of the neck. It was composite with a large fluid component and wispy strands of tissue extending across the fluid space. Biopsy confirmed neoplasia, and it was removed surgically. Histopathologic examination confirmed a follicular thyroid adenocarcinoma. The mare made an uneventful recovery. Whether the composite appearance found in this tumor is a consistent finding in thyroid malignancies is not known. Aspiration and biopsy should be performed to confirm the diagnosis. Recommending surgical excision seems to be logical based on the success in this horse.

CYSTS

As stated above, small cysts are occasionally found in enlarged thyroid glands thought to be adenomas. Whenever multiple cysts of variable size are found, biopsy may be indicated. Figure 37.4, **A** and **B**, are ultrasound scans of a mare with a prominent thyroid gland. There were multiple cystic structures up to 1 cm in diameter scattered throughout the gland. This case has not been resolved, but this gland enlarged to softball size on one occasion, but then regressed within 3 days after administration of a nutritional supplement containing sulfur that is designed to reduce inflammation. Biopsy may be indicated in glands of this type that exhibit strange behavior.

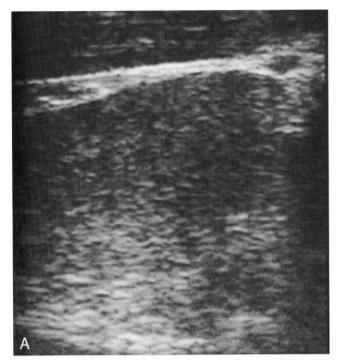

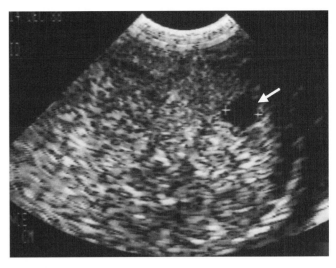

Figure 37.2. Ultrasound scan of an enlarged thyroid (benign adenoma) in a normal American Saddlebred stallion. There was a small cyst *(arrow)* in the gland. This sector scan was made at 5.0 MHz because of the hair thickness and cold winter temperature, both of which impede sound transmission. This accounts for the more coarse texture compared with Figure 37.1.

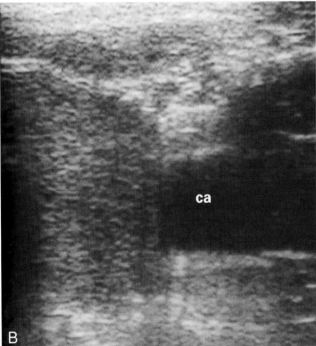

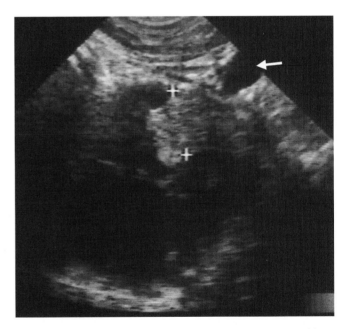

Figure 37.1. A. Ultrasonogram of one normal thyroid lobe of a part Arab mare made in long axis. The scan was made with a 7.5-MHz linear-array transducer by direct contact with an alcohol skin preparation. **B.** Cross-section of the same thyroid lobe as in **A**. The carotid artery *(ca)* is adjacent to the gland.

Figure 37.3. Ultrasound scan of an 8-cm (in cross-section) thyroid carcinoma. It extended to both sides of the neck. Note the solid tissue outlined by the cursors and the large fluid component. The carotid artery is in the upper right *(arrow)*.

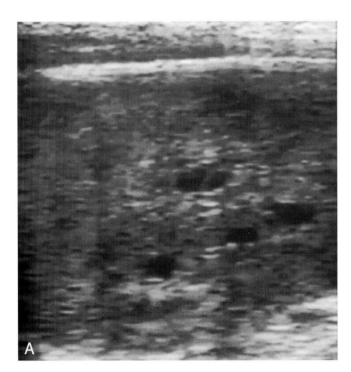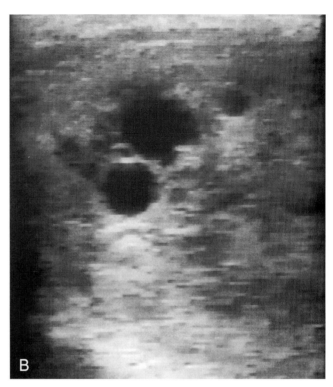

Figure 37.4. A and **B.** Two 7.5-MHZ linear-array ultrasound scans of a thyroid gland with multiple cystic structures throughout.

CONCLUSION

Thyroid tumor must be considered when examining horses with cranial cervical masses. Differentiating tumors of thyroid origin from salivary gland or lymph node may be possible. The incidence of malignant thyroid disease in horses is low and has a guarded prognosis with surgical removal.

REFERENCES

1. Dybdal NO. Endocrine and metabolic diseases. In: Smith BP, ed. Large animal internal medicine. 2nd ed. St. Louis: CV Mosby, 1996; pp. 1444–1455.

2. Held JP, Patton CS, Toal RL, et al. Work intolerance in a horse with thyroid carcinoma. J Am Vet Med Assoc 1985;187:1044–1045.

3. Haeni H, Von Tscharner C, Streub R. Thyreoideacarcinoma mit knocken metastasen beim pferd. Schweizare Tierheilkd 1979;121: 413–420.

4. Hillidge CJ, Sanecki RK, Theodorakis MC. Thyroid carcinoma in a horse. J Am Vet Med Assoc 1982;181:711–714.

5. Lehr L. Struma adenocarcinom mit metastasen bei einem pferd. Wien Tieaerztl Monatasschr 1934;21:111–112.

6. van der Velden MA, Meulenaar H. Medullary thyroid carcinoma in a horse. Vet Pathol 1986;23:622–624.

38. ULTRASOUND-GUIDED BIOPSY

RUSSELL L. TUCKER

One of the most valuable ultrasound applications in veterinary medicine is ultrasound-guided fine-needle aspiration and core biopsy of tissues. The ability to visualize the pathway and position of the biopsy needle greatly improves the diagnostic success and reduces complications associated with blind percutaneous biopsy. Ultrasound-guided biopsy is also quicker and less invasive than most surgical biopsy techniques. Ultrasound-guided biopsy procedures have been described for many small-animal applications (1–11). The fundamentals of ultrasound-guided biopsy are similar in all species, and applications in horses parallel the uses in small animals. A recent publication of ultrasound-guided biopsy techniques in small animals provides an in-depth review (12). The first reprinted use of ultrasound-guided biopsy in horses appeared in 1986 (13).

Portable ultrasound systems are ideal for most equine, ultrasound-guided, biopsy procedures. The need for additional equipment is minimal. Ultrasound-guided biopsy is performed using real-time B-mode imaging with conventional transducers. The depth of the target tissue will determine which transducer will be selected. The higher-frequency transducers (7.5 to 10 MHz) are optimal for biopsy of superficial structures. The increased resolution of the higher-frequency transducers facilitates visualization of the superficial tissues and biopsy needles. Deeper tissues will require the use of lower-frequency transducers (3.5 to 5.0 MHz). In general, the highest-frequency transducer, which will penetrate to the desired depth of tissue collection, should be used to perform biopsies.

Linear-array or sector-array transducer designs can be used for ultrasound-guided biopsy. Many transducers are manufactured with a needle slot or will accept a needle-guide attachment to direct the biopsy needle into the tissues within a predetermined pathway (Fig. 38.1). The attachable needle guides accept a variety of needle sizes and can be sterilized for reuse. Ultrasound systems with this type of needle guide allow the sonographer to display an on-screen outline showing the course the needle will travel (Fig. 38.2). The transducer must be positioned such that the target tissue is within the outlined path. This method of biopsy has the distinct advantage of displaying the entire path of the needle through the overlying tissues and aids in avoiding critical structures. The disadvantage of this method is the restricted insertion angle of the needle into tissues, which may limit the biopsy path. Some equipment manufacturers offer a selection of needle guides with varying needle insertion angles. Alternatively, many experienced sonographers prefer to use a "freehand" biopsy technique. In this technique, the biopsy needle is directed into the tissue with one hand, while the other hand maintains the transducer position (Fig. 38.3).

This technique permits greater freedom in the site of needle insertion relative to the transducer position. The sonographer determines the optimal entrance site for and angle of the biopsy needle relative to the target tissue. Sonographers must become familiar with the ultrasound beam characteristics of each transducer when using the freehand technique. Ideally, the course of the needle is maintained within the narrow beam to allow visualization of the needle as it is directed toward the target tissue (Fig. 38.4). The optimal visualization of the biopsy needle occurs when the needle is perpendicular to the emitted ultrasound beam. In many applications, the anatomic restrictions and the ability to redirect the needle makes the freehand technique the safest and easiest method to obtain diagnostic tissue samples.

Ultrasound-guided fine-needle aspirates are performed when small tissue samples are desired for cytologic analysis or culture. Many different types of biopsy needles are available for fine-needle aspirates. The size and length of the biopsy needle is determined by each situation. For fine-needle aspirates, disposable spinal needles are commonly used. These needles are inexpensive and are available in a wide variety of gauges and lengths. The spinal needle can be inserted with the central stylet in place to avoid plugging the needle with unwanted tissue. The best visualization of the needle is accomplished when the needle bevel is facing the transducer. The echogenicity of the needle can be enhanced by roughing the needle surface with a metal file to increase the specular reflections from the needle surface. Highly reflective, Teflon-coated biopsy needles are commercially available, but are considered unnecessary by most sonographers.

Once the needle is positioned within the target tissue, the stylet can be removed and the tissue sample collected. A syringe can be attached directly to the needle hub to apply repetitive suction to aspirate tissues. Excessive suction may yield a sample contaminated with blood degrading the diagnostic quality of the collected tissue. Suction should be discontinued before the needle is withdrawn from the tissues to avoid blood contamination. Many sonographers prefer to use an intravenous extension tube connected between the needle hub and the syringe. This method makes the aspiration procedure easier and allows an assistant to perform the syringe suction while the sonographer maintains the transducer position and redirects the needle if so desired. Other sonographers advocate a rapid oscillation of the needle within the target tissue without the use of suction to harvest the tissue sample. This technique minimizes the cellular destruction resulting from overzealous suction. When properly performed, the oscillation method will yield a superior cellular sample compared with the syringe suction technique

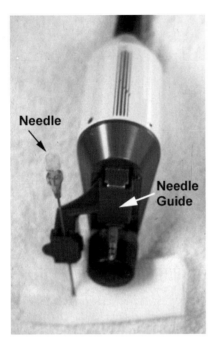

Figure 38.1. Biopsy needle guide attached onto a mechanical sector transducer. The plastic guide accepts various sizes of biopsy needles, which are directed into the tissue at a fixed angle relative to the transducer.

in solid tissues. Fluid aspirates usually require negative pressure to remove diagnostic or therapeutic volumes of fluid. A three-way stopcock can be used to facilitate removal of large amounts of fluid. Experience and personal preference will help to determine which aspiration technique is indicated in each case.

Ultrasound-guided core samples can be obtained using a variety of biopsy instruments. The larger, tissue-core, biopsy needles are easier to visualize in the ultrasound beam than are the smaller needles used in fine-needle aspirates; how-

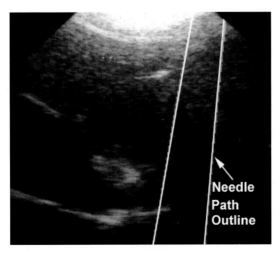

Figure 38.2. Display of needle path on the ultrasound monitor showing the course the needle will travel when using the attachable needle guide. The needle guide confines the needle within the outlined tract as it is inserted into the target tissue.

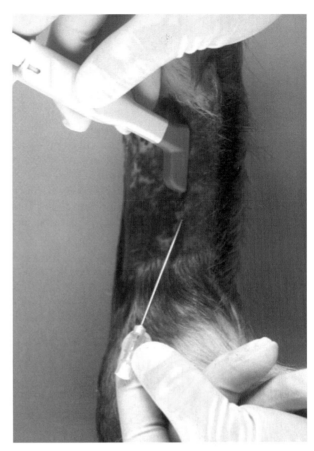

Figure 38.3. Ultrasound-guided biopsy using the freehand technique. The transducer is held in one hand, while the needle is inserted with the other hand. The operator selects the biopsy needle entrance site and angle relative to the transducer position.

ever, increased complications have been reported with the use of core biopsy needles. Conventional, tissue-core, biopsy needles can be used, but often yield poor tissue samples. It is difficult to insert the hand-driven biopsy needles in a manner that will collect adequate tissue-core samples. Operation of these needles requires the coordinated use of both hands, and an assistant is necessary if the sonographer wishes to visualize the needle position during the biopsy procedure. Therefore most experienced sonographers use some type of an automatic, spring-activated, core biopsy instrument when tissue-core samples are desired. Nondisposable, autoclavable biopsy systems that accept a variety of needle sizes are available. These instruments employ a spring-activated mechanism to thrust the biopsy needle into the target tissue (Fig. 38.5). With proper handling, the biopsy needles for these devices can be resterilized and reused several times. Such devices yield the best tissue-core samples, but are relatively expensive. Alternatively, inexpensive, plastic, core biopsy instruments are now available in many sizes. These devices, although marketed for single use, can often be reused following resterilization. The spring-activated mechanism of these devices is similar to the nondisposable types. With proper care, the disposable core biopsy devices will

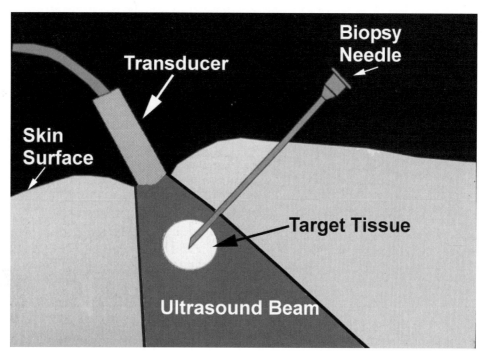

Figure 38.4. Schematic of the freehand biopsy technique. The needle is maintained within the ultrasound beam as it is inserted into the target tissue. The needle is best visualized when perpendicular to the ultrasound beam.

yield multiple diagnostic tissue samples and are popular for veterinary applications (Fig. 38.6).

Patient preparation for the biopsy procedure depends on the intended biopsy site. In most circumstances, it is optimal to place the horse in some type of restraint stocks that will allow safe access to the biopsy region. For biopsy of the legs, neck, and head areas, mild sedation may be all that is required. A local anesthetic can also be infiltrated into the entrance site prior to biopsy-needle introduction. The area should be first scanned to clearly visualize the target tissue

and to determine the most appropriate biopsy pathway. Overlying tissues should be carefully examined to discover any critical structures that may interfere with the path of the needle. Once the needle path has been selected, the entrance site should be prepared in an aseptic manner. Iodinated surgical preparation solutions may stain transducers, and non-iodinated preparation solutions such as Nolvsan are preferred. If iodinated solutions are used to prepare the skin surface, a final wipe with diluted alcohol can be used to remove the solutions. Some transducers are damaged by full-

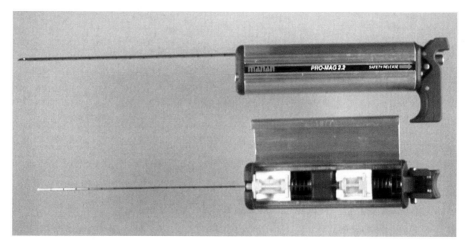

Figure 38.5. Example of automated biopsy instrument: Pro-Mag™ Automatic Biopsy System (Manan Medical Products, Northbrook, IL 60062). The spring-activated biopsy gun accepts various sizes of needles to obtain tissue-core samples. Two sizes are available, which collect 17-mm or 8-mm tissue samples. The system features a safety release to prevent accidental triggering.

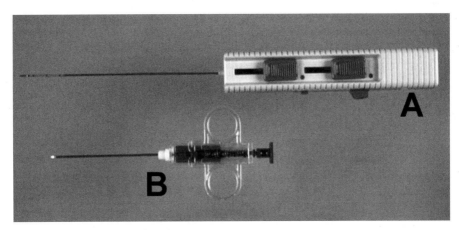

Figure 38.6. Examples of disposable automated biopsy instruments: **(A)** ASAP™ Biopsy System (Medi-tech, Boston Scientific Corp, Watertown, MA 02172) and **(B)** Temno™ Biopsy Device (Bauer Medical Inc, Clearwater, Fl 34620). These spring-activated devices are operated with one hand.

strength alcohol, and equipment manufactures should be consulted before using preparation solutions. Sterile acoustic coupling gel is applied to the prepared surface to facilitate transducer contact. A scalpel blade can be used to puncture the skin to simplify introduction of the biopsy needle. This is common practice when using the longer needle lengths, which are flexible and may bend when entering thick skin if no puncture was initially performed.

If the transducer will be positioned close to the needle entrance site, or if a needle-guide attachment will be used, the transducer should be placed in some type of sterile cover or wrap to maintain sterility. Sterile transducer covers are available from several commercial sources. Other methods have included placing the transducer into a sterile glove or condom, or by wrapping the transducer in sterilized plastic materials (Fig. 38.7). A small amount of sterile coupling gel is placed inside the sterile cover to maintain transducer acoustic contact. If the freehand biopsy technique is used, the transducer may be positioned a safe distance from the needle entrance site and will eliminate the need for a sterile transducer cover.

The collected tissue samples should be immediately fixed or processed for evaluation. For fine-needle aspirates, several clean glass slides should be prepared and ready to receive collected tissues. The diagnostic quality of the sample will be improved if the collected tissue is quickly spread over the slide surface. Aspiration samples are best expelled as small volumes that are promptly spread over the slide mounts. It is better to generate several slides with thin, cellular smears rather than thick, poorly spread biopsy samples. Culture media and swabs should also be prepared and ready to accept collected material. Tissue-core samples are frequently placed in 10% buffered formalin solutions or used to make impression smears on slide mounts. If multiple core samples are desired, the collected tissue can be removed from the biopsy needle with a sterile needle or rinsed off the biopsy needle with sterile saline solution. Inadequate sample volume is a common problem reported by sonographers inex-

perienced in performing biopsy procedures. Multiple samples can usually be safely obtained when the proper techniques of ultrasound-guided biopsy are practiced. Biopsy experience and consultation with persons evaluating the

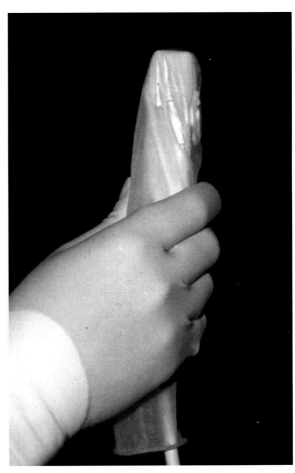

Figure 38.7. Sector-array transducer covered with a sterilized condom. Sterile coupling gel is placed inside of the condom to maintain acoustic transmission.

samples will help sonographers determine when an adequate sample has been obtained.

Following the biopsy procedure, the biopsy site should be carefully re-imaged to check for complications. Hemorrhage is the most common complication associated with ultrasound-guided biopsy. Bleeding may occur within or around the sampled tissue or may result from puncture of adjacent vessels. Hemorrhage will appear as hypoechoic regions within the sampled tissues or may collect in dependent areas at some distance from the biopsy site. Potential areas of hemorrhage accumulation should be imaged before completing the final examination. Most bleeding created from biopsy procedures is self-limiting and insignificant. If hemorrhage is detected, re-examination in 5 to 10 minutes should determine if the bleeding has stopped or if further intervention is warranted. In patients suspected of having coagulation abnormalities, or if the biopsy path is likely to induce unavoidable hemorrhage, the coagulation status of the horse should be evaluated prior to the biopsy procedure.

In addition to biopsy guidance, ultrasound imaging can be helpful with other interventional procedures. Transcutaneous placement of drainage catheters can be facilitated with ultrasound imaging. Ultrasound-guided thoracentesis has been very beneficial for the removal of pleural effusions. The ability to visualize the drainage catheter aids in the optimal placement for fluid removal. Transcutaneous drainage of thoracic and abdominal abscesses has also been accomplished with ultrasound guidance (Fig. 38.8).

The principles and limitations of ultrasound imaging must be considered when attempting any guided biopsy procedures. Air and bone are strong reflectors of ultrasound, which limit biopsy applications. Thoracic or abdominal lesions that are deep to aerated lung or gas-filled bowel loops are obscured from transcutaneous ultrasound imaging. Intracavitary lesions that are close to the skin surface or surrounded by fluid may be adequately imaged with ultrasound allowing for guided biopsy. Initial scanning should determine which lesions are well suited for ultrasound-guided biopsy techniques.

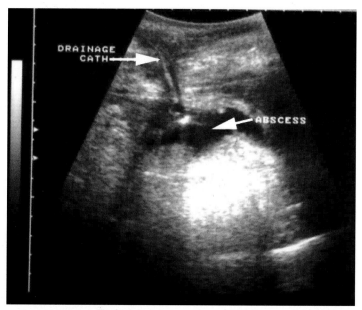

Figure 38.8. Transcutaneous, ultrasound-guided, catheter placement to drain a large, periuterine abscess in a mare. In this parasagittal view from the ventral abdomen, the catheter can be seen as the hyperechoic structure entering the abscess containing fluid and gas.

REFERENCES

1. Hagar DA, Nyland TO, Fisher P. Ultrasound-guided biopsy of the canine liver, kidney, and prostate. Vet Radio 1986;26(3):82–88.
2. Smith S. Ultrasound-guided biopsy. Vet Clin North Am Small Anim Pract 1985;15(6):1249–1262.
3. Hoppe FE, Hagar DA, Poulos PW, et al. A comparison of manual and automatic ultrasound-guided biopsy techniques. Vet Radio 1986;27(4):99–101.
4. Kerr LY. Ultrasound-guided biopsy. Calif Vet 1988;42(3):9–10.
5. Papageorges M, Gavin PR, Sande RD, et al. Ultrasound-guided fine-needle aspiration: an inexpensive modification of the technique. Vet Radio 1988;29(6):269–271.
6. Smith S. Ultrasound-guided biopsy. Semin Vet Med Surg (Small Anim) 1989;4(1):95–104.
7. Selcer B, Cornelius LM. Percutaneous liver biopsy. Using the ultrasound-guided biopsy instrument. Vet Med Rep 1989; 1(3):412–416.
8. Lamb CR. Abdominal ultrasonography in small animals: examination of the liver, spleen and pancreas. J Small Anim Pract 1990; 31(1):5–14.
9. Leveille R, Partington BP, Biller DS, et al. Complications after ultrasound-guided biopsy of abdominal structures in dogs and cats: 246 cases (1984–1991). J Am Vet Med Assoc 1993;203(3): 413–415.
10. Finn-Bodner ST, Hatchcock JT. Image-guided percutaneous needle biopsy: ultrasound, computed tomography, and magnetic resonance imaging. Semin Vet Med Surg (Small Anim) 1993; 8(4):258–278.
11. Thomas WB, Sorjonen DC, Hudson JA, et al. Ultrasound-guided brain biopsy in dogs. Am J Vet Res 1993;54(11):1942–1947.
12. Nyland TO, Mattoon JS, Wisner ER. Ultrasound-guided biopsy. In: Nyland TO, Mattoon JS, eds. Veterinary diagnostic ultrasound. Philadelphia: WB Saunders, 1995; pp. 30–42.
13. Modransky PD. Ultrasound-guided renal and hepatic biopsy techniques. Vet Clin North Am Equine Pract 1986;2:115–126.

APPENDIX OF ULTRASOUND EQUIPMENT AND MANUFACTURERS

ULTRASOUND EQUIPMENT FOR EQUINE VETERINARIANS

The following ultrasound equipment information was supplied by manufacturers or distributors. This information is provided to give the reader an overview of available ultrasound equipment for the equine veterinarian and is not meant as an endorsement of any particular product.

Advanced Technology Laboratories (ATL)
22100 Bothell Everett Highway
Post Office Box 3003
Bothell, WA 98041-3003
USA
Phones: 206-487-7000, toll-free 800-982-2011; Fax: 206-485-6080

Apogee 8OOPLUS Ultrasound System

The Apogee 8OO PLUS system provides complete diagnostic capabilities, with excellent image quality, sensitive color Doppler, and many advanced features. This mobile, in-clinic system has 256 gray shades and 128 color hues, with multifrequency capability and broadband scanhead compatibility. Complete calculations and analysis packages, Cineloop image review, Color Power Angio™ imaging, and complete cardiac capabilities, including multiplane transesophageal echocardiography, are part of the standard configuration.

The advanced, multifrequency, beam-forming capability provides a frequency range of 2 to 12 MHz, optimizing resolution and penetration and requiring fewer scanheads. The complete range of scanheads includes broadband linear arrays, broadband convex phased arrays, broadband curved arrays, multiplane transesophageal, intracavitary, TCD, and CW Doppler.

HDI 3000

The HDI 3000 is a mobile, in-clinic system with a large, high-resolution monitor. The system uses ATL's tissue-specific imaging for total system optimization. The HDI 3000 was designed to be easy to learn and use. It provides a high level of diagnostic performance across all imaging modes and applications.

The HDI 3000 has 3D Color Power Angio™ (3D CPA) imaging, providing fuller appreciation of the architecture of vascular anomalies and pathology. Access™ Disk Link provides storage and retrieval of ultrasound images in original digital quality.

Aloka Company Limited
10 Fairfield Boulevard
Wallingford, CT 06492

USA
Phones: 203-269-5088, toll-free 800-442-5652;
Fax: 203-269-6075

Aloka SSD-500V Micrus

The Aloka 500V Micrus is a portable ultrasound system weighing 22 pounds, with a 7-inch black-and-white monitor, 64 gray shades, and a fold-up keyboard. It provides clinical versatility through user-selectable display modes. The standard B-mode can be displayed as a single image or dual image by utilizing the split-screen capability.

In addition, the Micrus provides M-mode (motion mode) for the display and assessment of cardiac motion. This M-mode can be displayed either separately or combined with a simultaneous real-time B-mode image.

The Micrus includes comprehensive measurement and analysis capability, cardiac calculations, and built-in gestational-age tables. The Micrus provides versatility through a wide range of optional convex and linear-array transducers from 3.5 MHz to 7.5 MHz.

Aloka Flexus SSD-1100

The Aloka Flexus is an in-clinic system, approximately 100 pounds, with a 12-inch swivel monitor, and 256 gray shades. It supports a wide range of transducers, including all of the 500V transducers and convex, linear, and mechanical-sector transducers from 2 to 10 MHz.

The system has comprehensive measurement and analysis software for cardiac calculations, distance, area by ellipse, area by trace, ratio, and histogram. It is B-Mode, M-Mode, and Doppler capable, and an optional ECO display unit is available. The Cine Memory option stores eight screens in still memory, 24 frames of B-Mode, and 24 screens of M-Mode.

Diasonics Ultrasound, Inc.
2860 De La Cruz Blvd.
Santa Clara, CA 95050
USA
Phones: 408-496-4700, toll-free 800-937-9373;
Fax: 408-496-3556

Gateway Series

The Gateway Series is a high-performance, digital-array–based, triplex ultrasound system that features 2D Array Imaging, spectral and color Doppler, Ultrasound Angio™, Vascular Topography™, and automated calculations. The Gateway features a family of Matched-Impedance probes (2.25 to 12 MHz) optimized for all clinical applications. The digital-image management system stores hundreds of images for immediate review or recall at a later time. DICOM compatibility provides networking for LAN, WAN, or worldwide connectivity.

Vingmed CFM Series

The Vingmed CFM Series is an industry-leading family of imaging/Doppler ultrasound systems optimized for diagnostic echocardiography. Vingmed Doppler, the worldwide gold standard, allows accurate detection of a wide range of hemodynamic conditions. The CFM integrates a complete family of multifrequency transthoracic probes (2.25 to 7.5 MHz) and adult/pediatric multiplane transesophageal probes (5.0 to 7.5 MHz). The CFM features high-speed digital processing, extensive patient image archiving, on-line digital stress echo capability, and custom patient reports. The EchoPAC™ and Mobile Access™ workstations allow either on-line or off-line echo analysis from any location via a DICOM-compatible networking capability.

Synergy Series

The Synergy Series is a state-of-the-art, Pentium-based triplex system for the radiology and shared-service environments. The flexible architecture provides superior imaging and Doppler (spectral, color, and power) to ensure diagnostic accuracy and efficient patient throughput. The system features a family of probes (3.5 to 10 MHz) for all diagnostic applications. The digital archiving features patient folders that hold diagnostic images and clinical reports for on-line and off-line review and analysis. The midrange Synergy system is compact and lightweight for use in a hospital, clinic, office, or mobile location.

Compact

The Compact is a versatile, cost-effective, portable, duplex ultrasound system that provides superior gray-scale imaging and quantitative spectral Doppler using a family of linear and mechanical-sector probes (2.5 to 10 MHz). The system incorporates easy-to-use, programmable protocols for all applications. The flexible architecture allows the system to expand with new clinical requirements and ensures convenient upgradeability.

Dynamic Imaging Limited

9 Cochrane Square
Brucefield Industrial Park
Livingston, EH54 9DR
Scotland, UK
Phone: +44 (0) 1506 415282; Fax: +44 (0) 1506 410603

Concept Veterinary Ultrasound

Concept\MLV combined with a 7.5-MHz, linear-array rectal probe is ideal for equine applications, including reproduction studies and musculoskeletal work. Concept\MLV is

a dedicated linear scanner with a dual-frequency facility. It comes complete with a comprehensive software and measurement package. This is a portable system and weighs approximately 11 kg.

Concept\MCV provides the same image quality and functions of Concept\MLV in terms of equine scanning, but where the veterinarian's applications extend beyond equine work, the addition of microconvex probes can be used for small-animal studies.

Concept\GV provides additional diagnostic capabilities to those of Concept\MLV and Concept\MCV. The selection of a 2.25-MHz mechanical-sector probe allows equine cardiology and abdominal work. Concept\GV is capable of accepting linear, convex, microconvex, and mechanical-sector probes.

Hitachi Medical Corporation of America

Hitachi Medical Systems
660 White Plains Road
Tarrytown, NY 10591
USA
Phone: 914-524-9711; Fax: 914-524-9716

Hitachi EUB-405 PLUS

The *Hitachi EUB-405 PLUS* is a portable, digital, ultrasound system incorporating the latest in microelectronic technology, allowing the user to make comprehensive measurements with direct key access and a trackball. There are autocalculation worksheets for obstetric and urologic data and biopsy software providing accurate guidelines on-screen to plot the path of the needle.

The system is capable of utilizing all of the high-density (maximum 192 channels) probes and is configured to support Hitachi's dual-frequency probes and the 200°, steerable, endocavitary probe.

The display modes are M mode, 2D (B mode), 2D/M mode, and split-screen 2D mode. Both convex and linear-array scanning methods can be utilized.

The *Hitachi EUB 525* is a mobile, in-clinic, ultrasound system with a 12-inch, high-resolution color monitor on a compact wheeled chassis. It can be coupled with the full line of multipurpose and specialty probes. The continuous, variable, sliding receive filter utilizes the entire frequency spectrum and optimizes both near-field and far-field resolution. The system is capable of performing all Doppler and color flow studies.

The crystal technology of the Hitachi probes allows for maximum use of the available frequency spectrum, which allows shifting frequencies from 2.5 MHz to 10 MHz. Both convex and linear-array scanning methods can be utilized. The system has the ability to display a full 200° field of view with the V33W endocavity probe.

The display modes are M mode, 2D (B mode), 2D/M mode, 2D/Spectral Doppler mode, 2D/Spectral Doppler/M mode, 2D/Color Flow mode, 2D Spectral Doppler/Color Flow mode, and CW Doppler mode.

Medison America, Inc.

5880 W. Las Positas Blvd. #52
Pleasanton, CA 94588
USA
Phone: 510-463-1330; Fax: 510-463-2646

Medison Veterinary Ultrasound

Medison ultrasound systems are compact, portable, and easy to use. The latest technology and features are offered such as 256 shades of gray, reliable solid-state veterinary probes for tendon and transrectal scanning, and a special transvaginal probe with a biopsy guide for follicular cyst aspiration and embryo transfers. The SonoVet 600 has a fold-up keyboard and weighs 22 pounds for veterinarians who require hand-held portability.

Pie Medical Equipment

Philipsweg 1
6227 A J Maastricht
The Netherlands
Phone: (+31) 433824600; Fax: (+31) 43 3824601

Scanner 480 Vet

The Scanner 480 Vet is a multipurpose ultrasound scanner for the veterinarian. The 5/7.5 MHz DF endorectal probe is known for its high image quality and is used for pregnancy detection and evaluation of the ovary in horses and cows and for pregnancy detection in small animals. The 7.5-MHz LA small-size, linear-array probe is ideal for examination of tendons.

Scanner 100 Vet

The Scanner 100 VET uses the very latest in ASIC (Application Specific Integrated Circuit) technology, which enables high image quality to be built into a compact, portable system, with a 9-inch monitor and a built-in battery. The Scanner 100 VET also includes an extensive software package of animal-specific software for cardiology, fetal age, and equine tendon and a built-in floppy disk drive on which digital images and data can be stored. The scanner can be used for pregnancy detection in horses, cows, and smaller animals such as swine, sheep, goats, dogs, and cats.

The Scanner IOOLC supports the high-resolution linear and convex probes, and the 100S supports the versatile, multiangle, sector and annular-array probes.

Scanner 200 Vet

The Scanner 200 Vet is suited for imaging in a variety of reproductive, abdominal, cardiac, and small-parts examinations. The Scanner 200 VET is also a diagnostic tool for the highly specialized and exotic, mixed-species practice. In addition, the Scanner 200 VET can perform quality cardiology examinations.

The built-in Cineloop and the feline-specific cardiac calculations, the weight-based canine cardiac calculation tables, and the equine-specific cardiac calculation table make the clinical data produced more pertinent to the patient being examined.

With the Animal Science probe, images of backfat and rib eye of beef cattle, hogs, and sheep can be performed. An extensive calculation package for backfat measurements and determination of intermuscular fat is included.

Scanner 250 Vet

The Scanner 250 is a multifunctional scanner suitable for the larger, small-animal clinics or veterinary hospitals. The scanner has a large screen in comparison with the portable products. Three probes can be connected simultaneously, and an ECG and Cineloop can be built in to facilitate cardiac examinations of small animals. The built-in feline-specific cardiac calculations, the weight-based canine cardiac calculation tables, and the equine-specific cardiac calculation table make the clinical data produced more pertinent to the patient being examined.

Index

Note: Numbers in *italics* refer to illustrations; numbers followed by *t* indicate tables

Renosplenic entrapment, 66

Reports, standardized, 105–106

Reproductive senescence, sequence of progression into, 209, 210

Reproductive tract, examination procedures and normal anatomy
mare, 79–95
stallion, 96–100

Resistance index, 177

Resolution, 79

Resolution and penetration, balancing, 17

Respiratory distress syndrome, neonatal, 178

Respiratory system evaluation
anaerobic infection, 591, 591
bronchopleural fistula, 591
conclusion, 594
cranial thoracic abscess, 591, 592
fibrinous pleuritis, 591
lung abscesses, 592, 592
pericarditis, 592
pleural effusion, causes of
cardiac failure, 594
granulomatous infection, 594, 594
neoplasia, 593, 593
trauma, 594
pneumonia, ultrasonographic diagnosis of
follow-up examination, 590
large lung consolidations, 587, 589
medium-sized lung consolidations, 587, 589
pleuropneumonia, 590, 590, 591
small visceral pleural surface irregularities and consolidations, 587, 588
pneumothorax, 591
spontaneous echocardiographic contrast, 593, 593

Rest, treatment for tendon disorders, 575, 577

Retinaculum flexorum (RF), distention of, 490, 490

Retinal detachment, 640, 643

Reverberation artifacts, 94, 95, 121, 121–122, 122

Reversion to fetal circulation, 585, 585

Rhodococcus equi infection in neonate, 623–624, 625

Rubefacients, 573, 579

S. zooepidemicus, in semen, 184

Sagittal proximal sesamoid fracture, 468

Salmonella abortus equi, 99

Scaling factors, 3

Scanhead(s), 5–6
connectors, 9

Scanning errors, minimizing, 80

Scar remodeling, 318

Scattering, 2, 3, 4, 4

SCLD. *See* Superior check ligament desmotomy (SCLD)

Scrotal contents, 97–100, 253–269
arcuate arteries, 254, 256, 257, 257
body of the epididymis, 253–254, 255
cauda epididymis, 254, 254, 256
central vein, 253, 254
enlarged scrotum, diagnosis of, 257–261
cauda epididymis enlargement, 258, 259
common sites involved, 258
fluid accumulation, 258, 258

generalized edema *vs.* hydrocele, 258, 259
inguinal hernia, 258, 258
spermatic cord enlargement, 258, 259
spermatic cord torsion, 258–260, 259, 260
epididymides, examination of, 262, 264, 265, 265
manual examination of, 253
measurement of the testes, relationship of DSO and, 267–268, 268
parenchyma, 254, 255
penis, examination of, 265, 265–266, 267
sedation of the animal, 253
spermatic cord, 253, 254, 255, 257, 257
structures, 254
"Swiss cheese" appearance, 254, 256
testes, examination of, 262, 262–263
ultrasound as diagnostic aid, 253

Scrotal skin and investments, 98

Seasonal influence on ovulations, 209, 210

Section thickness artifacts, 121

Sector scanners
for abdominal ultrasonography, 48–49
linear phased arrays *vs.,* 103
reproductive ultrasonography, 79, 81
types of, advantages/disadvantages of, 103

Sedation, to facilitate examination, 32

Semen
bacteria and fungi in, 184
frozen, breeding with, 82–83

Seminal colliculus, 272, 273, 274, 277

Seminal extenders, antibiotic, use of, 184–185

Seminal vesicles. *See* Vesicular gland

Sepsis
chronic CS swelling with sepsis, 427, 427
subcutaneous fluid accumulation due to, 329, 329

Septic physitis, 77

Septicemia, in the neonate, 627

Seromas, urachal, 627–628, 628

Sertoli-cell tumors, testicular, 99

Serum sickness, 604–605

Sex determination. *See* Gender determination

S/GO management
SDFT treatment, 552–553
steps in S/GO management, 557
Thoroughbreds *vs.* Standardbreds and, 377

Shadowing, 94, 95, 96
acoustic, 62, 122, 122–123

Shape change, SDFT, 305–307, 306–309

Shoe boil, 536

Shoeing, therapeutic, 574

Short digital extensor muscle, 525

Shoulder
bicipital (intertubercular) bursitis, 492
fracture of the supraglenoidal tubercle, 492, 493
normal ultrasonography, 492, 492
traumatic tendinopathy of the brachial biceps, 492, 492, 493

Shunts or jets
Doppler echocardiography examination, 39
portosystemic, diagnosis of, 76

Size and shape, modifications of, in diagnostic approaches to tendons and ligaments, 475

Skeletal musculature, direction-dependent echogenicity in, 119

Slides (35mm), reproducing, 79–80

Sodium hyaluronate (SH), 453, 558
first aid for tendinitis, 573
peritendinous administration *vs.* intrathecal, 574

Sonographic quality of repair (SQR), 544

Sound reflection artifacts, 119, 120

Sound velocity artifacts, 119–120

Speckle, 5

Spectral display, 14, 14

Specular reflection, 4, 4, 94, 95

Sperm granuloma, 253

Spermatic cord, 253, 254, 255, 257, 257

Spermatic cord enlargement, 258, 259

Spermatic cord torsion, 98–99, 253, 258–260, 259, 260
permanent, 259–260, 261
transient, 259, 260

Spermatocele, 253

Spermatozoa
antigenic properties of, 99–100
life span of, after insemination, 86

Spleen
abnormalities, 620–621, 621–622
as acoustic window to the left kidney, 614, 614
equipment, 619
indications for sonogram evaluation, 619
preparation of the horse, 619
size of, 620
ultrasonography, 41, 41, 54, 56–58, 57, 58, 63, 64
of the foal, 636
indications for scanning, 57–58
liver-spleen interface, 52, 53
neonatal, 76–77
normal anatomy, 57, 57
normal ultrasonographic appearance, 619–620, 620
sonographic appearance, 57, 58
splenic enlargement due to chemical constraint, 57
technique, 57

Stallion, examination procedures and normal anatomy, 96–100
ampullae, 96
epididymis, 100
inguinal rings, 97, 97
pelvic urethra, 97
penis, 100
prepuce, 100
reproductive tract
external, 97
internal, 96
scrotal contents, 97–100
scrotal skin and investments, 98
spermatic cord, 98–99
testicle, 99–100, 100
vaginal cavity, 97–98, 98
vesicular gland, 96–97

Standardbreds
incidence of multiple ovulation in, 233
incidence of twins in, 141, 149
Thoroughbreds *vs.* Standardbreds and S/GO management, 377

Stand-off pad, 110
handheld, 74
materials for, 103–104